ADVANCED PRACTICE PSYCHIATRIC NURSING

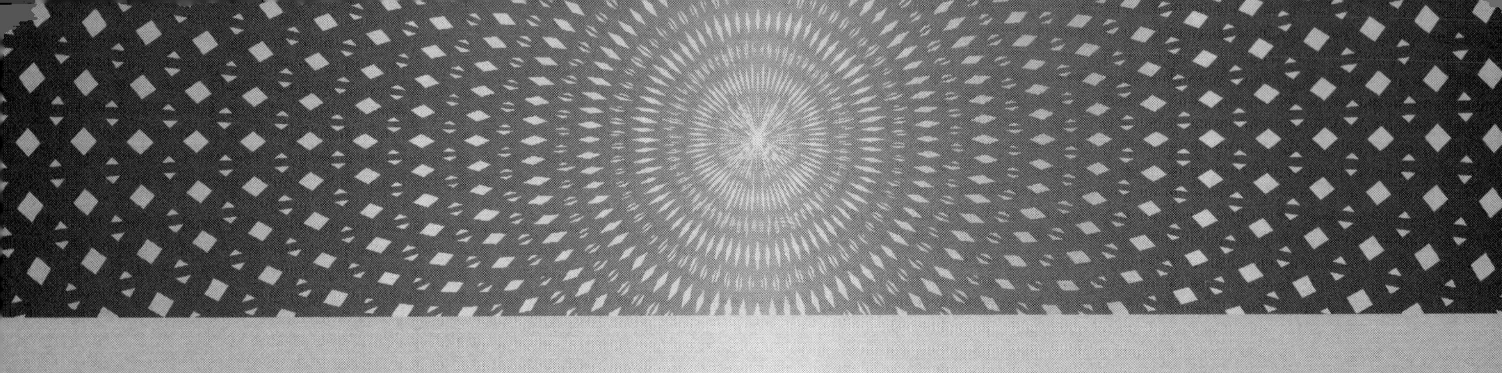

Kathleen R. Tusaie, PhD, APRN-BC, is associate professor and lead faculty for the Family Psychiatric-Mental Health Nurse Practitioner program at the University of Akron and maintains a private practice. Dr. Tusaie is certified as a psychiatric mental health clinical nurse specialist (CNS) by American Association of Colleges of Nursing (AACN). She also holds certificates in Advanced Pharmacology, Multicultural Nursing, Eye Movement Desensitization and Reprocessing (EMDR), Psychoneuroimumunology, Brief Psychotherapy, CBT, Clinical Hypnosis, and Bowan Family Therapy. In addition to the University of Akron, she has taught at the University of Pittsburgh and Pennsylvania State University School of Nursing. Dr. Tusaie's research focuses on resilience and positive psychology. She has published on various psychiatric nursing topics and has presented at national and international conferences.

Joyce J. Fitzpatrick, PhD, MBA, RN, FAAN, is the Elizabeth Brooks Ford Professor of Nursing, Frances Payne Bolton School of Nursing at Case Western Reserve University in Cleveland, Ohio, where she was Dean from 1982 through 1997. She has received numerous honors and awards, including the *American Journal of Nursing* Book of the Year Award 18 times. The works of Dr. Fitzpatrick are widely published in nursing and health care literature. Her most recent Springer books are *The Doctor of Nursing Practice and Clinical Nurse Leader: Essentials of Program Development and Implementation for Clinical Practice; 201 Careers in Nursing; Encyclopedia of Nursing Research: Third Edition;* and *Psychiatric Mental Health Nursing: An Interpersonal Approach* (with Jones & Rogers).

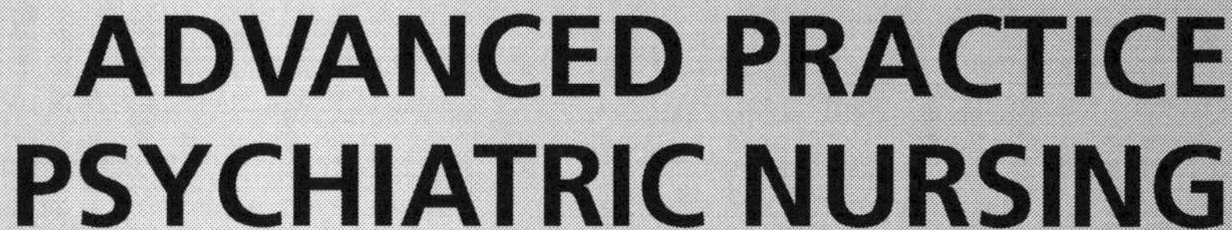

ADVANCED PRACTICE PSYCHIATRIC NURSING

Integrating Psychotherapy, Psychopharmacology, and Complementary and Alternative Approaches

Kathleen R. Tusaie, PhD, APRN-BC
Joyce J. Fitzpatrick, PhD, MBA, RN, FAAN
EDITORS

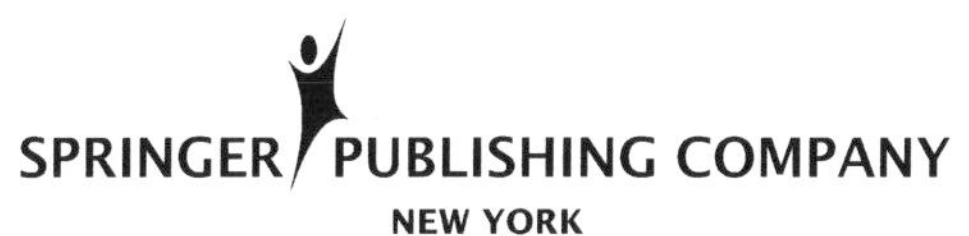

SPRINGER PUBLISHING COMPANY
NEW YORK

Springer Publishing Company, LLC
11 West 42nd Street
New York, NY 10036
www.springerpub.com

Acquisitions Editor: Margaret Zuccarini
Composition: Newgen Imaging

ISBN: 978-0-8261-0870-8
E-book ISBN: 978-0-8261-0871-5

13 14 15/ 5 4 3 2

Library of Congress Cataloging-in-Publication Data:
Advanced practice psychiatric nursing : integrating psychotherapy, psychopharmacology, and complementary and alternative approaches / [edited by] Kathleen R. Tusaie, Joyce J. Fitzpatrick.
p. ; cm.
Includes bibliographical references and index.
ISBN 978-0-8261-0870-8 — ISBN 978-0-8261-0871-5 (e-book)
I. Tusaie, Kathleen R. II. Fitzpatrick, Joyce J., 1944-
[DNLM: 1. Advanced Practice Nursing—methods. 2. Psychiatric Nursing—methods. 3. Mental Disorders—nursing. WY 160]
LC classification not assigned
616.89'0231—dc23 2012021971

Printed in the United States of America by Gasch Printing

For
our families, mentors, and colleagues
What is good is given back…

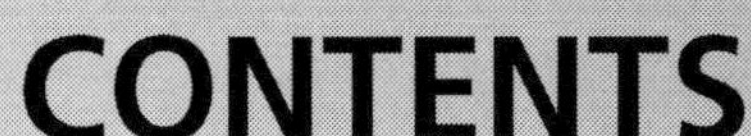

CONTENTS

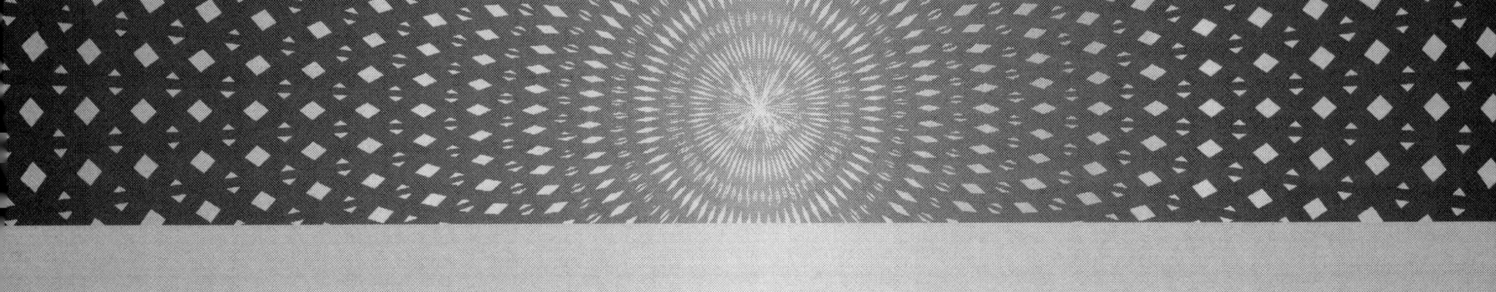

Lisa Barry, MSW, PMH-NP, BC
Advanced Practice Psychiatric Nurse
Casco Bay Medical
Portland, Maine

Ricardo Broach, RN, MDiv, MS, LPC-NCC
Private Practice
Milwaukee, Wisconsin

Carrie Cichocki, MSN, CNS, NP
Psychiatric Consultation-Liaison
Fairview Hospital, Cleveland Clinic
Cleveland, Ohio

Kathleen R. Delaney, PhD, PMH-NP, FAAN
Professor
Rush College of Nursing
Chicago, Illinois

Carol Enderlin, PhD, RN
Clinical Assistant Professor
College of Nursing
University of Arkansas for Medical Sciences
Little Rock, Arkansas

Deborah B. Fahs, DNP, APRN
Professor and Lecturer
Yale University School of Nursing
New Haven, Connecticut

Joyce J. Fitzpatrick, PhD, MBA, RN, FAAN
Elizabeth Brooks Ford Professor of Nursing
Frances Payne Bolton School of Nursing
Case Western Reserve University
Cleveland, Ohio

Matthew Hadley, RN, DNP, PNP-BC, FNP-BC, APN
Pediatric Nurse Practitioner and CNS Specialty Coordinator
Clinical Assistant Professor
College of Nursing, University of Arkansas for Medical Sciences
Little Rock, Arkansas

Rita Hanuschock, MSN, CNS, CNP
Nurse Practitioner
Alcohol and Drug Recovery Center, Cleveland Clinic
Cleveland, Ohio

Melodee Harris, PhD, APN, GNP-BC
Associate Professor, Carr College of Nursing
Harding University
Searcy, Arkansas

Anita Thompson Heisterman, MSN, RN, FNP, PMHNP-BC
Assistant Professor
University of Virginia School of Nursing
Charlottesville, Virginia

Bona Hong, BSN
Student
University of Pittsburgh School of Nursing
Pittsburgh, Pennsylvania

Linda Jacobson, MAED, MSN, APRN-BC
Outpatient Psychiatric Nurse Coordinator
Maine Medical Center
Department of Psychiatry
Portland, Maine

Kathyrn Johnson, MSN, APNP
Associate Clinical Professor
Department of Community Health Systems
University of California
San Francisco, California

Jeffrey S. Jones, DNP, PMHCNS-BC, LNC
Private Practice and Visiting Faculty
University of Akron
Akron, Ohio

Kirstyn M. Kameg, DNP, RN, PMHNP-BC
Associate Professor
Robert Morris University School of Nursing and Health Sciences
Moon Township, Pennsylvania

CONTRIBUTORS

Irene Kane, PhD, RN, HFS, CNAA
Assistant Professor
University of Pittsburgh School of Nursing
Pittsburgh, Pennsylvania

Norman L. Keltner, EdD, APRN
Professor
University of Alabama
Birmingham, Alabama

Robert Krause, MSN, APRN-BC
Assistant Clinical Professor
Yale School of Nursing
New Haven, Connecticut

Martha E. Kuhlmann, MSN, FNP, PMHCNS
Family Psychiatric Mental Health Nurse Practitioner Specialty Coordinator
Clinical Assistant Professor
College of Nursing
University of Arkansas for Medical Sciences
Little Rock, Arkansas

Marla McCall, MSN, PMHNP-BC
PhD student
North Valley Behavioral Health, University of Arizona
Tucson, Arizona

Anita Mitchell, PhD, RN, FNP-BC, APN
Clinical Associate Professor
College of Nursing, University of Arkansas for Medical Sciences
Little Rock, Arkansas

Ann M. Mitchell, PhD, RN, FAAN
Associate Professor
University of Pittsburgh School of Nursing

Beth Phoenix, PhD, RN, CNS
Clinical Professor
Department of Community Health Systems
University of California
San Francisco, California

Karen M. Rose, PhD, RN
Assistant Professor of Nursing
University of Virginia
Charlottesville, Virginia

Austyn Snowden, PhD
Reader in Mental Health, Nursing, and Midwifery
University of West Scotland, Paisley Campus

Ereka R. Spino, BSN, RN
DNP student
Robert Morris University School of Nursing and Health Sciences
Moon Township, Pennsylvania

Debbie Steele, PhD
Assistant Professor
Psychiatric Mental Health Nurse Practitioner Program Coordinator
California State University
Fresno, California

Arlene Sullivan, MNSc, APN
Baptist Health Sleep Center Nurse Practitioner
Little Rock, Arkansas

Marianne Tarraza, MSN, PMHNP-BC
Administrative and Clinical Director
Integrated Behavioral Healthcare
Scarborough, Maine

Kathleen R. Tusaie, PhD, APRN-BC
Associate Professor and Lead Faculty
Family Psychiatric-Mental Health
Nurse Practitioner Program
University of Akron College of Nursing
Akron, Ohio

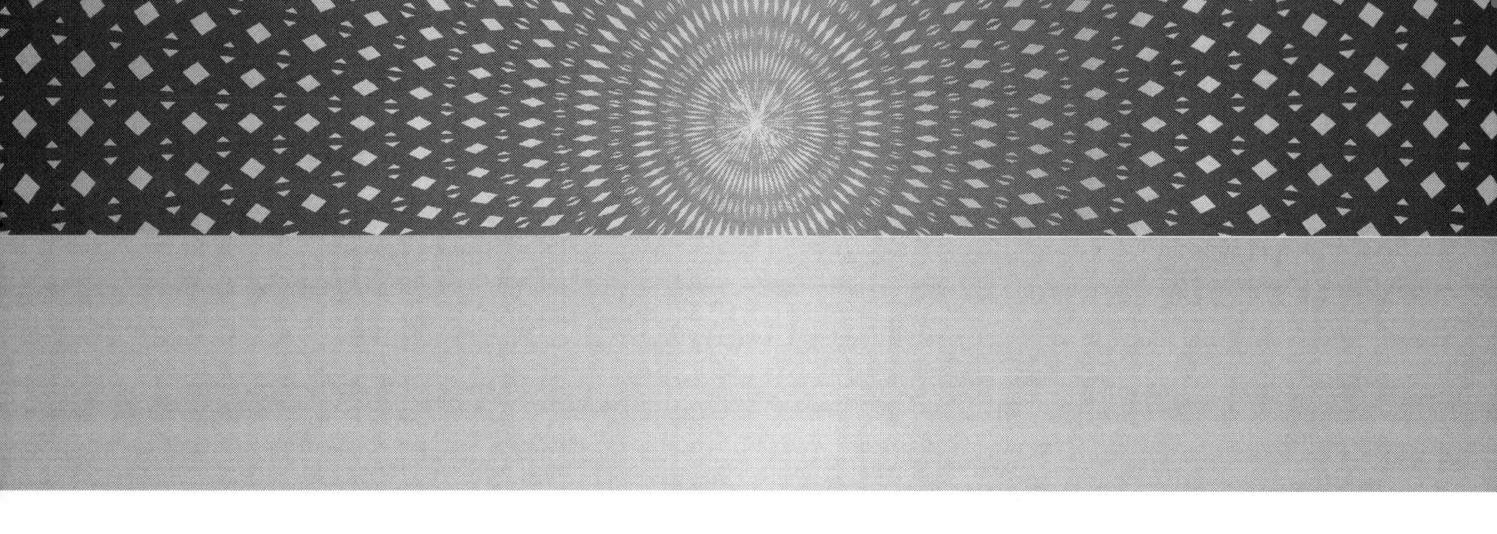

When I finished reviewing the copious materials for this text I was reflecting on my own history. More than 60 years ago I finished my required 1095 days and learned everything there was to know about nursing in that length of time. But what was clear from my reminiscence was how much our field of practice has changed in the last six decades. A certain amount of change has to be expected, but the rate of change has exponentially increased in the last decade. And it is these changes that have led to the production of this compendium of information about the field of advanced practice psychiatric mental health nursing.

This impressive text leans on the scope and standards documents developed by the specialty psychiatric mental health nursing associations (the American Psychiatric Nurses Association and the International Society of Psychiatric-Mental Health Nurses) in collaboration with the American Nurses Association. In the 1960s, Peplau introduced the advanced practice role and emphasized psycho-therapeutic relationships. Prior to that, the roles in psychiatric mental health nursing were largely concerned with developing administrative and teaching skills. However, it is important to acknowledge that the psycho-therapeutic emphasis in the advanced practice role seems to have been shrinking in its influence since those in the role took on the additional responsibility of prescriptive privileges and practices.

This text, however, moves us toward the paradigm that I believe will dominate the next few decades. We are now making good on the long asserted belief that the nursing phenomenon always included a holistic perspective, what some of our theorists have called a unitary vision of persons. Thus, at the moment, the leaders in the field are giving much energy and thought to how we put body and mind together. This text attempts to do that as it reflects the expanding scope and complexity that now

FOREWORD

encompasses the advanced practice role. The book should serve as a review for nurses who are studying for certification exams. It also should be very useful for coursework in Doctor of Nursing Practice programs as well as the masters programs in psychiatric mental health nursing.

It's important to note that each of the chapters in this text represents a sub-field of practice. I would predict that each of these will become full-fledged specialties with their own scope and standard statements in the near future. It would seem to be inevitable if not inescapable that one cannot become a master of all of the areas listed in the text. Thus to some extent the book serves as an introduction to areas of sub-specialization. The authors have carefully included references and citations to all the various sources for the rules and regulations that govern advanced practice. The references alone in this text provided rich source for further exploration in any one of the sub-fields.

As we move forward in this new era of health care that is conceptualized as being more integrative than anything we have seen before, this text provides a road map for the path ahead. What is remarkable here is that it is patently clear that advanced practice psychiatric nursing is useful, and indeed needed, in every field of health care. To the end that the collective mission in nursing is to keep and honor the social contract with the public, it is imperative for each of the sub-specialties delineated in this text to become well-populated with highly competent, very skilled advanced practice nurses.

Grayce M. Sills, PhD, RN, FAAN
Professor Emerita
The Ohio State University

This is a book that has been waiting to be written. It is both *by and for* Advanced Practice Psychiatric Mental Health Nurses (PMH-APRN) in direct care. When, in the early 1990s, the National Institutes of Health (NIH) created the Office of Alternative Medicine, much research had already begun on a variety of therapies considered at the time to be outside the scope of our medical practice model. Among these were relaxation training, therapeutic massage, hypnosis, biofeedback, herbs, and a host of others too numerous to mention. The intervening two decades have seen a general acceptance of many of these approaches, both within the traditional health care community and in the general public. At the same time, traditional psychotherapy models were pressured to become more efficient and cost-effective. And, of course, the ability to prescribe, as well as the range of pharmaceutical agents available to practitioners, has dramatically expanded. The result of these positive trends has compelled PMH-APRNs to expand their knowledge base to a bewildering range not seen before. Most individual practitioners as well as graduate schools have made a profound effort to acknowledge this emerging knowledge base. It is to and for these practitioners, teachers, and students that this book was written. It is indeed an attempt to help organize the thinking and broaden the perspective of the readers.

Each chapter reflects not only state-of-the-art knowledge but also decades of clinical wisdom. The book does not ignore the *Diagnostic and Statistical Manual of Mental Disorders* (*DSM-IV-TR*); we all are grateful for its value in organizing our thinking. Rather, this text draws its focus from commonly seen clinical constellations of symptoms. By that we mean to say that symptom clusters indeed determine both the initiation of treatment and the strategic choices we all face in clinical practice. Further, the book well serves the concept of *integrative care*. It blends traditional psychotherapy with medications and alternative complementary approaches to both familiarize and empower the clinical effectiveness of interventions.

Most advanced practice nurses inevitably will find themselves in a systemic culture of orthodoxy. While few systems willfully exclude any effective intervention, all systems seek to gain efficiency and cohesion. This principle discourages the exercise of broad thinking. It is therefore *the purpose of this book to validate and encourage PMH-APRNs to draw from as wide an information base as possible during clinical practice.*

Building on the interpersonal, psychodynamic roots of our specialty, this text provides a virtual buffet of valuable interventions from which clinicians and clients can co-create the most effective, individualized interventions.

An important focus of this innovative text is that it meets the practice standards included in the APNA and ISPN position statement that requires all PMH-APRN nurses *have skills in psychotherapy,* as well as assessment and psychopharmacology, and *that graduate courses address issues across the life span, not just issues pertaining to the adult patient.*

PREFACE

The book is divided into four sections:

- *Section I: The Dynamic Nature of Advanced Practice Psychiatric Mental Health Nursing* provides an overview of the theoretical and evidence base for practice and an exploration of the concept of *shared decision making or reaching concordance* between clinician and client.
- *Section II: Foundations for Integrated Practice* explores the foundations necessary for the practitioner to implement integrated practice. In this section, the synergistic effects of integrating practice concepts are discussed. Following chapters present the overviews of psychotherapy, psychopharmacology, and complementary and alternative approaches in the context of the stages of treatment.
- *Section III: Integrative Management of Specific Syndromes* applies the information from previous chapters and focuses on integrative management of specific syndromes. This includes chapters that discuss mood disorders, anxiety, psychotic symptoms, sleep disturbances, disordered eating, cognitive impairment, disordered attention, self-directed injury, and other directed violence. Each of these chapters follows a template so information is easily accessed, both for the APRN student and for the PMH-APRN practitioner. Furthermore, each chapter contains at least one decision tree regarding initiation of treatment. This format is expected to assist examination of available, effective options while considering variables that influence decision making. An important component of the text is the across the spectrum of age considerations, highlighted consistently throughout these chapters by the headings Aging Alerts and Pediatric Pointers.
- *Section IV: Special Considerations* covers aspects of managing substance misuse, medical problems, pregnancy, and forensic issues that often co-occur with psychiatric syndromes. The final chapter explores global perspectives, connections, and mentoring.

Within the pages of *Advanced Practice Psychiatric Nursing: Integrating Psychotherapy, Psychopharmacology, and Complementary and Alternative Approache*s, it is our sincere hope that readers will find information needed to assist in the complex decisions necessary in today's psychiatric-mental health clinical practices.

We are indebted to the chapter authors, all expert clinicians and scholars in their field. We wish to thank them for their participation and hope that this exercise of translating their clinical knowledge to a publication will be as beneficial to them as it will be to future generations of clinicians and advanced practice psychiatric nursing students.

We also wish to acknowledge and thank Margaret Zuccarini, Springer Editor, for her encouragement and involvement in all aspects of this book. We would not have had such an easy journey without Margaret's assistance.

Kathleen R. Tusaie
Joyce J. Fitzpatrick

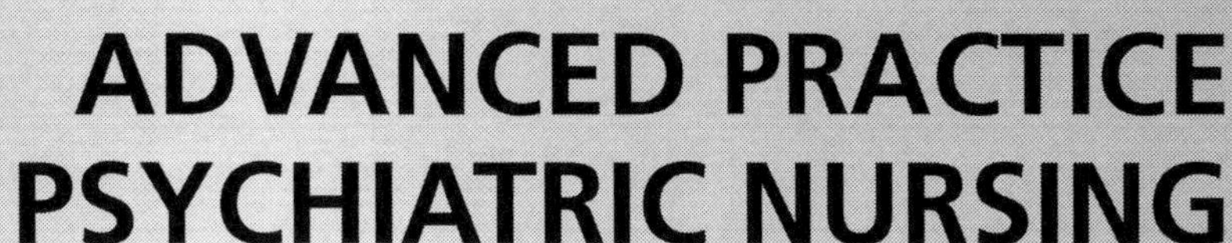

ADVANCED PRACTICE PSYCHIATRIC NURSING

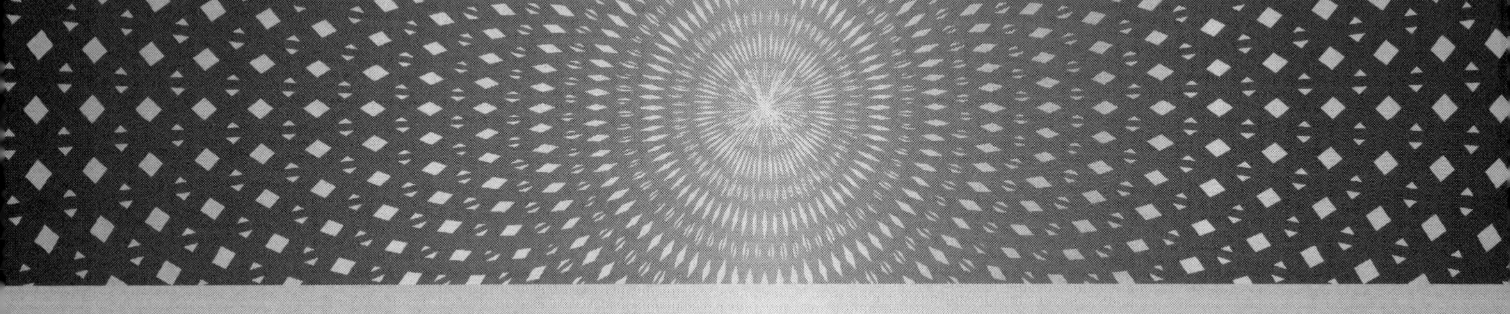

SECTION I

The Dynamic Nature of Advanced Practice Psychiatric Mental Health Nursing

CHAPTER CONTENTS

Theories provide a way of understanding the world and serve to describe, explain, predict, or control phenomena. A widely accepted definition of theory is that it is an organized set of concepts that explains a phenomenon or set of phenomena (American Psychological Association, 2009). Theories can be categorized based on their level of abstraction as grand theories, middle range theories, and micro level theories (Smith & Liehr, 2008). There are many theoretical understandings that advanced practice psychiatric mental health nurses (APRNs) use to guide their practice. These theories include some derived from the nursing meta-paradigm of understandings of the concepts of persons, environment, health, and nursing (Fawcett, 1984), as well as theories borrowed from other disciplines and applied in professional nursing practice. A number of nurse scientists currently are in the process of extending theory development for the discipline. Middle range theories developed by psychiatric nurses that have wide applicability in practice include the theory of uncertainty in illness developed by Mishel (1988) and expanded by Mishel and Clayton (2003), the theory of meaning developed by Stark (2003), and the theory of self-transcendence developed by Reed (2003). Thus we can anticipate a growth in theoretical knowledge development in the future. Knowledge derived from the expert practice

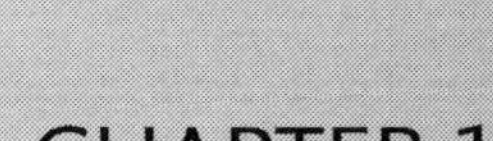

CHAPTER 1

Theoretical Understandings and Evidence Base for Practice

Joyce J. Fitzpatrick

of APRNs, coupled with the knowledge derived from research, contributes to the advancement of clinical practice.

COMMONLY USED THEORIES IN PSYCHIATRIC MENTAL HEALTH PRACTICE

The literature is replete with discussions of theories that inform therapeutic interventions in psychiatric mental health disciplinary practices. These include psychodynamic, biological, social psychological, behavioral, cognitive, humanistic, and change theories. These theories have influenced nursing knowledge development and professional practice in psychiatric mental health nursing.

APRN professional practice should be theoretically based and the practitioner should be cognizant of the influence of theory on the choice of interventions. Building the theoretical knowledge derived from within the nursing discipline and across disciplinary boundaries is an important component of advancing the science and improving practice. Several prominent theoretical perspectives are presented as foundational to developing understandings of practice in specific targeted areas.

PSYCHODYNAMIC THEORIES

The most well known psychodynamic theory is that of psychoanalysis proposed by Sigmund Freud. Many of the assumptions of this theoretical perspective serve as the foundation for psychodynamic theories. Freud's students, Carl Jung and Alfred Adler, developed their psychodynamic theories based on their work with Freud. Others who developed psychodynamic theories included Karen Horney and Erich Fromm. The basic psychodynamic understanding is that there are conscious and unconscious mental processes that influence thoughts and behavior. The goal in therapy is to develop understandings of the unconscious mental processes and use this understanding to address mental health issues. Many of the concepts in psychodynamic theories are used in psychiatric mental health nursing practice. These include the concepts of defense mechanisms, transference, and counter transference.

COGNITIVE THEORIES

Several cognitive theories have influenced the development of psychiatric mental health nursing; many of these are used to guide professional practice and research. Examples include the theories of Bandura

(1963, 1977), who is well known for his work on self efficacy, a theory that also permeates the work of other social scientists; and Beck (1997), best known within nursing for his theoretical and empirical work on depression and the development of measures of depression and hopelessness. Cognitive theories as a group are focused on understanding that human behavior is guided primarily by thought processes. Thus, cognitive therapy is focused on helping individuals understand and change their thought processes in order to change their behavior. Cognitive therapy is often combined with a behavioral approach. One of the therapies commonly used by psychiatric mental health advanced practice nurses (PMH-APRNs) is Cognitive Behavioral Therapy (CBT).

BEHAVIORAL THEORIES

Behavioral theories stem from the early work of Pavlov (1927), who studied the stimulus-response cycle and explained human behavior from this perspective. In particular, Pavlov focused on classical conditioning, in which he demonstrated a direct connection between thought processes and physiological responses. Other early behavioral theorists include Thorndike (1916), who developed a learning theory focused primarily on a problem-solving approach, and Skinner (1935), who described the stimulus-response model of learning. Both of these behavioral theories have influenced the science and professional practice of nursing. The problem-solving approach is foundational to the nursing process as well as to much of the CBT models that are used in psychiatric nursing practice. The stimulus-response model developed by Skinner influenced the work of contemporary nursing theorist, Callista Roy (1980), who developed an adaptation model of nursing.

PSYCHOSOCIAL THEORIES

There are a number of theories in the literature that are based on the psychosocial perspective. Theoretical perspectives that have influenced the development of the psychiatric mental health field across disciplines and professions can be categorized in a variety of ways, depending on the understandings of the core concepts and the guiding principles of the theories. Most of these theories can be understood to have psychosocial dimensions, including theories that can be classified as development, interpersonal, and humanistic. Some of the most influential theoretical perspectives on the development of PMH-APRN practice are presented.

DEVELOPMENTAL THEORIES

Development theories are focused on stages of human development over time, often sequentially. The theory of Erik Erikson (1963, 1968) is most widely used in nursing and adds the cultural dimension to an understanding of the psychosocial aspects of development. Erikson delineated stages of development that were age-based, each characterized by conflicts. He framed these as trust versus mistrust, autonomy versus shame and doubt, initiative versus guilt, industry versus inferiority, identity versus role diffusion, intimacy versus isolation, generativity versus stagnation, and ego integrity versus despair. Much of the work of crisis theory is framed from Erikson's theoretical perspectives along with their psychodynamic roots. According to Erikson, successful resolution of a crisis within the stages of development leads one to develop more resources for future crisis resolution.

INTERPERSONAL THEORIES

The interpersonal theory and work of Harry Stack Sullivan (1953) has influenced nursing theory and professional practice, as has work of Peplau (1952) and colleagues. Sullivan's theory is based on the understanding of personality as energy, which can be manifest as tensions or transformations. Sullivan also referred to behavior as dynamic. He was particularly interested in interpersonal relations, not just between the therapist and the patient, but also as a basis for understanding all of human behavior. He attributed health and illness to the ways in which one interacted with others. Sullivan also attributed one's image of self, that is, self-esteem, to the relationships with others, particularly in the formative years. Seven stages of development were described by Sullivan, thus his theory has much in common with developmental theories that see this component as core to understanding human behavior. The stages of development were described as infancy, childhood, the juvenile era, preadolescence, early adolescence, late adolescence, and adulthood. Further, Sullivan pioneered the notion of the participant observer in therapy, a concept and technique that permeates much of the PMH-APRN therapy work.

HUMANISTIC THEORIES

Humanistic theories and therapies are rooted in an understanding of human potential for goodness and a focus on the positive. Two humanistic theories that are predominant in PMH-APRN understandings and practices are those of Abraham Maslow (1970) and Carl Rogers (1980). Maslow's theory also has been labeled as a developmental theory for its emphasis on stages of human development. Maslow presented an understanding of the hierarchy of needs of individuals that often parallels the chronological developmental process. These needs include physiological and survival needs, safety and security needs, love and belonging needs, esteem needs, and self-actualization needs. According to Maslow the lower level needs must first be met in order for individuals to progress through other developmental stages. Beginning nursing students are often introduced to this model as a way of understanding human behavior as it presents a holistic perspective, particularly as holism is defined from a biopsychosocial perspective.

Carl Rogers's (1980) theory and therapy also have resonated with PMH-APRNs in their practice. Rogers focused on the concept of empathy, a concept that guided the development of client-centered therapy. Rogers proposed that a key dimension of the success of therapy is the therapist's unconditional positive regard for the person receiving therapy. This principle is an important foundation for an integrative approach that has been embraced by PMH-APRNs who build on the individual's strengths to determine treatment goals. Nursing work is empathetic and the relationship between nurse and patient reflects this empathy. This interpersonal approach of Rogers, along with the interpersonal approach of Sullivan (1953), influenced the theoretical understandings of Peplau (1952) and the therapeutic relationship emphasis she proposed.

BIOLOGICAL THEORIES

Selye's (1956) theory and research on the physiological responses to stress, and the description of the adaptation responses of the individual, including at the cellular level as well as at the system level, has received much attention in the nursing literature. Selye described the fight-or-flight mechanism within the general adaptation syndrome. He described three stages within adaptation: the alarm reaction, resistance, and exhaustion. The adaptation model developed for nursing by Roy (1980) and the Stuart Stress Adaptation Model (Stuart, 2008) specific to psychiatric nursing are examples of nursing theories that have a strong biological emphasis, as they are built on the core concept of stress found in Selye's work. However, both of these nursing models also have incorporated other dimensions, reflecting the holistic meta-theoretical perspective of nursing.

GENERAL SYSTEMS THEORY

General systems theory, sometimes referred to as GST or more broadly, systems theory, was proposed by Ludwig von Bertalanffy (1968) as a method of theoretical thinking that would be more holistic and include understandings of several dimensions of human functioning. Von Bertalanffy described two types of systems, open and closed; human systems are understood as open systems, in continuous interaction with the environment, and thus, constantly changing through this interaction. Importantly, von Bertalanffy asserted that the system could not be understood by viewing the parts. Rather, the whole system is greater than the sum of the parts. Further, there is continuous interaction between and among the parts of the system; this interaction affects the functioning of the entire system (von Bertalanffy, 1968).

GST has been used in a wide range of applications, both in relation to understandings of humans and innate systems such as organizations and institutions. Several other theorists have used GST as a foundation for their own theoretical work. The most well known examples of the conceptual and theoretical application of GST in nursing science are the theories of Martha Rogers (1970) and Betty Neuman (2002). Additional nursing theories related to Rogers's

Science of Unitary Human Beings include those of Fitzpatrick (1983) and Margaret Newman (1986). The middle range theory of self-transcendence developed by Pamela Reed (2003) also can be traced to Rogers's theory of unitary human beings. Fitzpatrick and Reed have engaged in a number of research projects from the 1980s to the present to test the propositions in these theories (Fitzpatrick & Reed, 1980; Hunnibell, Reed, Quinn-Griffin, & Fitzpatrick, 2008; Palmer, Quinn-Griffin, Reed, & Fitzpatrick, 2010; Sharpnack, Quinn-Griffin, Bender, & Fitzpatrick, 2011; Thomas, Burton, Quinn-Griffin, & Fitzpatrick, 2010; You et al., 2009). Originally, this collaborative research was based on the Crisis Theory Model, integrated with the Rogerian nursing science perspective. More recently, the focus of their research has been on the concept of self-transcendence, which is at the core of Reed's middle range theory.

Martha Rogers (1970) was one of the first nurse theorists who presented a model of holism within nursing; she viewed persons as open systems, in continuous interaction with, and continuously exchanging energy with the environment. For Rogers, the whole is greater than the sum of the parts; thus this conceptualization is particularly suited to an integrative approach to psychiatric mental health nursing practice. According to Rogers, persons move through the life process in a pattern that is constantly evolving. Rogers delineated three principles that postulate the direction of unitary human development: resonancy, helicy, and integrality. There is considerable research based on Rogers's model, and a number of new theoretical perspectives were derived from the Rogerian conceptualization. Further, several authors have described the applications to professional practice (Hemphill & Quillin, 2005).

Betty Neuman's Systems Model also is consistent with an integrative approach within psychiatric mental health nursing. Within the Neuman Systems theory, persons are viewed as clients and a wellness perspective is emphasized (Neuman, 1989). Neuman proposed that the client or client system is a dynamic composite of the interrelationships among physiological, psychological, sociocultural, developmental, spiritual, and basic structure variables. Thus, this is a holistic view of persons, but differs from Rogers (1970) who proposed that the whole cannot be understood by considering the parts. There is considerable research and professional practice derived from the Neuman Systems Model and several nursing education programs use this model to guide their curricula (Walker, 2005).

CHANGE THEORIES

There are several change theories that have been applied to explain health and illness behaviors in general, and mental health in particular. Two of the most prominent change theories are the theory of reasoned action and planned behavior (Azjen, 1991), and the Stages of Change Model (Prochaska & Velicer, 1997).

THE THEORY OF REASONED ACTION AND PLANNED BEHAVIOR

This theory has guided considerable research in nursing, particularly as related to attitude and behavior change. Azjen's (1991) theoretical premise is that the intention to change determines behavior change. In order for an individual to change behavior there must be a positive attitude toward the behavior. Further, the influence of the individual's social environment is important, that is, the normative factors in one's environment. Thus, the beliefs of one's peers are particularly important in shaping one's own beliefs and attitudes. According to this theory, it also is important that the individual perceive that he or she has control over the desired behavior, and the resources and skills to perform the behavior. This theoretical understanding is similar to the concept of self efficacy that is central to the social learning theory developed by Bandura (1963). Bandura's theory has been used extensively to guide nursing research.

TRANSTHEORETICAL MODEL

This Transtheoretical Model of Behavior Change is sometimes referred to as the Stages of Change Model or simply by the acronym TTM. This model incorporates understandings from several theories of psychotherapy, thus the name. TTM is the predominant model used in health behavior change research and practice. The core concepts in TTM are stages of change, processes of change, decisional balance, and self-efficacy. The basic understanding is that an individual moves through a series of stages in making any personal changes. These include the following six stages:

1. **Pre-contemplation**—at this stage the individual is not aware that their actions are problematic and thus are not likely to take action.
2. **Contemplation**—the individual has beginning awareness that the behavior is causing a problem, and starts to consider the pros and cons of the problematic behavior.
3. **Preparation**—the individual intends to take action in the immediate future, and may take small steps toward change in this stage.
4. **Action**—the individual takes explicit action to change the problematic behavior, and positive changes occur as a result.
5. **Maintenance**—the individual actively works to prevent relapse; this stage lasts as long as the problematic behavior no longer occurs.
6. **Termination**—the individual has no temptation to return to the problematic behavior and is confident that he or she will not return to the problematic behavior (Prochaska & Velicer, 1997).

Not all of the above six stages are included in all of the versions of TTM or in the research that is based on the model; the stages of pre-contemplation, contemplation, action, and maintenance are the most frequently addressed. Also, some of the delineations of TTM include discussion of a relapse stage, in which the individual reverts to previous problematic behavior (Prochaska & Velicer, 1997).

There are several processes of change embedded in the TTM. These include cognitive, affective, and evaluative processes. According to Prochaska and colleagues, it is important to match the process to the stage of change (Prochaska & Norcross, 2007). For example, in the contemplation stage individuals must develop some cognitive awareness of the problematic behavior, and understand the pros and cons of continuing or changing the behavior. They must be able to express their feelings regarding the effects of the problematic behavior on their lives.

Several components of the TTM can be used in therapy to assist the individual in gaining self-awareness and focusing on one aspect of his or her life, albeit an aspect that may be having widespread ramifications. In the contemplation phase, the individual is assisted in understanding the decisional balance that exists, that is, weighing the pros and cons of the current behavior and the contemplated behavior change. There are several therapeutic techniques that have been described to assist individuals in behavior change. Examples include consciousness raising (through cognitive processes), realizing that the new behavior reflects who they want to be (self evaluation or reevaluation), recognition of how the unhealthy behavior affects others (environmental evaluation), awareness that society is more supportive of the new behavior (social liberation), and substituting healthier behaviors for the problematic behavior (counter conditioning). The overall goal of the therapeutic process is to reach a stage of self-efficacy in which the individual has confidence that he or she will not relapse to the problematic behavior (Prochaska & Velicer, 1997).

The TTM has been used to address many unhealthy behaviors, such as smoking. The smoking behavior may not only be causing deleterious health effects for the individual, but also may be affecting his or her interpersonal relationships with family and friends who may opposed to the negative behavior. As the smoking behavior changes through therapy with the TTM, so also will the interpersonal relationships. The individual's awareness of the holistic change in his or her life is an important component of the therapy. Also, as the individual makes a commitment to the new behavior, individuals close to him or her may assist in the maintenance phase through participating in a helping relationship. These helping people, including the therapist, work to keep the individual accountable to his or her commitments through support, encouragement, and understanding.

NURSING THEORIES SPECIFIC TO PSYCHIATRIC NURSING

Hildegard Peplau is considered the founder of psychiatric nursing. She developed her theory of interpersonal relationships in the early 1950s, and published her classic book, *Interpersonal Relations in Nursing*, in 1952. According to Peplau, the person is a developing self-system composed of biochemical, physiological, and interpersonal characteristics and needs (Peplau, 1992). Anxiety was an important concept within Peplau's understanding of persons. She proposed that anxiety is produced when the individual is threatened in some way, and the nursing role is to assist persons to understand that anxiety and learn new behaviors to use the anxiety to effect a positive outcome (Peplau, 1963). The nurse develops a therapeutic interpersonal relationship with patients in order to help them to learn and change. Peplau's work has been traced to the influence of Harry Stack Sullivan and other theorists who emphasized the interpersonal process as the core concept. In addition to her theoretical contributions, Peplau also developed the first graduate level psychiatric nursing program, and prepared the early specialists in psychiatric mental health nursing. Peplau described six roles for the nurse: stranger, resource person, teacher, leader, surrogate, and counselor. She also delineated the sequence of the interpersonal nursing process as including four phases of development: orientation, identification, exploitation, and resolution. For Peplau, communication, both verbal and nonverbal, was a cornerstone of therapeutic work. Overall, Peplau's influence on the field of psychiatric mental health nursing specifically, and of nursing more generally, is legendary.

Gail Stuart has proposed the Stuart Stress Adaptation Model to guide psychiatric mental health nursing practice (Stuart, 2008). In this model she integrates knowledge from the biological, psychological, socio-cultural, environmental, and legal-ethical theoretical perspectives. Underlying this model are five basic assumptions, including: (1) nature is ordered in a social hierarchy that goes from the simplest unit to the most complex; (2) nursing care is provided within a biological, psychological, sociocultural, environmental, and legal-ethical context; (3) health/illness and adaptation/maladaptation are two distinct continuums, and health/illness has its roots in the medical model whereas adaptation/maladaptation comes from a nursing world view; (4) primary, secondary, and tertiary levels of prevention are included by describing four distinct levels of treatment: crisis, acute, maintenance, and health promotion; and (5) the model is based on the nursing process and the standards of care and professional performance for psychiatric nurses (pp. 44–45).

INTERRELATIONSHIP BETWEEN THEORY AND RESEARCH

Theory and research are the two core components of science. Theory may be used to guide research through a deductive process or research may be used to generate theory, through an inductive process. Many examples of the relationship between theory and research can be found in the psychiatric mental health nursing advanced practice literature. These studies have been related to the theories in other disciplines from which some of the nursing theories have been derived, and also specifically to the nursing theories, including those particular to psychiatric mental health nursing such as the theory of Peplau.

Beeber (1996, 1998), for example, has described the treatment of depression through the use of the therapeutic nurse-patient relationship model described by Peplau. Peden (1993) also used Peplau's model to guide her research on women with depression. And Forchuk and colleagues have conducted a number of studies of the therapeutic process according to the stages outlined by Peplau (Forchuk, 1992, 1994; Forchuk et al., 1998). Fawcett and Giangrande (2001) detailed the substantial research undertaken based on the Neuman Systems Model. Malinski (1986) has described the research related to Rogers's model of unitary human beings.

Another area of research that demonstrates the integration of theory and professional practice, and builds on the integrative perspective in psychiatric mental health nursing is that of resilience. There are several nurse researchers exploring this concept. The early theoretical work of Polk (1997) to develop a middle range theory of resilience in nursing, the historical review of the concept presented by Tusaie and Dyer (2004), and the further theoretical and methodological work of Zauszniewski and Bekhet (2010) set the stage for future scientific work for a perspective that builds holistic understandings and provides a foundation for integrated interventions.

DISTINCTIONS BETWEEN RESEARCH AND EVIDENCE-BASED PRACTICE

Research is one form of evidence that can be used to guide clinical practice. The discovery processes that guide research and evidence-based practice are similar, and thus, at times, there is a lack of clarity about which process is being applied. Both processes, for example, require a sourcing of the literature, and a synthesis of what is known about a phenomena and what needs to be discovered. While research is based on the review of the scientific literature, evidence-based practice takes into account other sources of knowledge, including expert clinical knowledge.

The steps in the research process include: identification and explication of the problem for study, identification of the purpose of the study, review of the scientific literature (including theoretical and research literature), delineation of the research method to be used to address the problem, implementation of the research methodology, presentation and discussion of findings, and interpretations based on the previous literature.

The four basic steps in the evidence-based practice process include: (a) converting the information needed into an answerable question; (b) finding the best evidence; (c) appraising the search results for validity and usefulness; and (d) applying the findings to clinical practice. The basic goals of evidence-based practice are to reduce variations in care that is provided, increase the cost-effectiveness of care, lead to efficient and effective decision making, and improve interventions and patient outcomes.

The PICO Model is often used in evidence-based practice, particularly when teaching evidence-based practice to professionals new in practice. The PICO model includes the following components to guide the clinician:

P = Who is the **Patient Population**?
I = What is the potential **Intervention** or area of **Interest**?
C = Is there a **Comparison** intervention or **Control** group?
O = What is the desired **Outcome**?

These questions guide professionals in designing evidence-based practice projects that are directly relevant to the persons being cared for at that point in time. Further, several levels of evidence are accessed in using any evidence-based practice model and the clinician must evaluate the evidence before application to practice. Cochrane reviews (which are primarily focused on research that includes randomized clinical trials) are considered the highest level of evidence. Other systematic reviews are the next level of evidence, followed by other research evidence, such as that from single site studies in which the methodology might be questioned. Evidence garnered from expert clinical practice should also weigh into the evidence-based practice applications.

While it is important to emphasize the empirical research according to the methods described, it also is important to consider other sources of evidence, particularly within a professional discipline such as nursing. Fawcett, Watson, Neuman, Walker, and Fitzpatrick (2001) argue for using a model that includes all of the evidence gathered from the ways of knowing delineated by Carper (1978), in her seminal work on ways of knowing in nursing. Carper described the personal, ethical, and aesthetic ways of knowing in addition to the empiric way of knowing. Too often in evidence-based practice, these other ways of knowing are not fully addressed or are dismissed in preference for empirical knowing. Within an integrative practice model multiple ways of knowing and interacting are encouraged. Thus, the psychiatric mental health nurse practicing from a holistic perspective would have an inclusive approach in evaluating the evidence.

SUMMARY

While there are a number of theoretical perspectives that have influenced the development of nursing theory and professional practice, the emphasis on nursing science, including theory development and research, holds the most promise for the further development of PMH-APRN practice. The integration of a range of therapeutic interventions is particularly relevant to the holistic perspective of nursing science.

A wide range of opportunities exist for psychiatric nurses, especially in advanced practice and particularly in demonstrating the positive results of the integrative approach to mental health care that is so essential to individuals, families, groups, and communities. The expectation is that both the science and the professional practice will expand, and that the leaders and practitioners in psychiatric mental health nursing will chart the course for holistic interventions for generations to come.

REFERENCES

American Psychological Association. (2009). *APA online.* Retrieved from http://www.psychologymatters.org/glossary.html

Azjen, I. (1991). The theory of planned behavior. *Organizational Behavior and Human Decision Processing, 50*, 179–211.

Bandura, A. (1963). *Social learning and personality development*. New York, NY: Holt, Rinehart, and Winston.

Bandura, A. (1977). *Social learning theory*. Englewood Cliffs, NJ: Prentice Hall.

Beck, A. T. (1997). The past and the future of cognitive therapy. *Journal of Psychotherapy Practice and Research, 6*(4), 276–284.

Beeber, L. S. (1996). Pattern integration in young depressed women: Parts I and II. *Archives of Psychiatric Nursing, 10*(3), 151–164.

Beeber, L. S. (1998). Treating depression through the therapeutic nurse-client relationship. *Nursing Clinics of North America, 33*(1), 153–157.

Carper, B. A. (1978). Fundamental patterns of knowing in nursing. *Advances in Nursing Science, 1*(1), 13–24.

Erikson, E. (1963). *Childhood and society* (2nd ed.). New York, NY: Norton.

Erikson, E. (1968). *Identity: Youth and crisis*. New York, NY: Norton.

Fawcett, J. (1984). The metaparadigm of nursing: Present status and future refinements. *Image, 16*(3), 84.

Fawcett, J., & Giangrande, S. K. (2001). The Neuman Systems Model and research. In B. Neuman & J. Fawcett, (Eds.), *The Neuman systems model* (4th ed., pp. 351–354). Upper Saddle River, NJ: Prentice Hall.

Fawcett, J., Watson, J., Neuman, B., Walker, P., & Fitzpatrick, J. (2001). On nursing theories and evidence. *Journal of Nursing Scholarship, 33*(2), 115–120.

Fitzpatrick, J. J. (1983). A life perspective rhythm model. In J. J. Fitzpatrick & A. L. Whall, (Eds.), *Conceptual models of nursing: Analysis and application* (pp. 295–302). Bowie, MD: Brady.

Fitzpatrick, J. J., & Reed, P. G. (1980). Stress in the crisis experience: Nursing interventions. *Occupational Health Nursing, 28*, 19–21.

Forchuk, C. (1992). The orientation phase of the nurse-patient relationship. *Perspectives in Psychiatric Care, 28*(4), 7–10.

Forchuk, C. (1994). Peplau's theory based practice and research. *Nursing Science Quarterly, 7*(3), 110–112.

Forchuk, C., Westwell, J., Martin, M., Azzapardi, W. B., Kosterewa-Tolman, D., & Hux, M. (1998). Factors influencing movement of chronic psychiatric patients from the orientation to the working phase of the nurse patient relationship. *Perspectives in Psychiatric Care, 34*(1), 36–44.

Hemphill, J. C., & Quillin, S. I. (2005). Martha Rogers' model: Science of unitary beings. In J. J. Fitzpatrick & A. L. Whall (Eds.), *Conceptual models of nursing: Analysis and application* (4th ed., pp. 247–272). Saddle River, NJ: Pearson.

Hunnibell, L., Reed, P., Quinn-Griffin, M. T., & Fitzpatrick, J. J. (2008). Self transcendence and burnout in hospice and oncology nurses. *Journal of Hospice and Palliative Care Nursing, 10*(3), 172–179.

Malinski, V. (Ed.). (1986). *Explorations of Martha Rogers' Science of Unitary Human Beings*. Norwalk, CT: Appleton Lange.

Maslow, A. (1970). *Motivation and personality*. New York: Harper and Brothers.

Mishel, M. M. (1988). Uncertainty in illness. *Image: Journal of Nursing Scholarship, 20*, 225–231.

Mishel, M. M., & Clayton, M. F. (2003). The theory of uncertainty in illness. In M. J. Smith & P. R. Liehr (Eds.), *Middle range theory for nursing* (pp. 25–48). New York, NY: Springer Publishing.

Neuman, B. (1989). *The Neuman systems model* (2nd ed.). Norwalk, CT: Appleton & Lange.

Neuman, B. (2002). The Neuman systems model. In B. Neuman & J. Fawcett. (Eds.), *The Neuman systems model* (4th ed., pp. 347–359). Upper Saddle River, NJ: Prentice Hall.

Newman, M. A. (1986). *Health as expanding consciousness*. St. Louis, MO: Mosby.

Palmer, B., Quinn-Griffin, M. T., Reed, P., & Fitzpatrick, J. J. (2010). Self transcendence and work engagement in acute care staff registered nurses. *Critical Care Nurse Quarterly, 33*(2), 139–148.

Pavlov, I. P. (1927). *Conditioned reflexes: An investigation of the physiological activity of the cerebral cortex. Translated and Edited by G.V. Anrep*. London, UK: Oxford University Press. http://en.wikipedia.org/wiki/Oxford_University_Press\ Oxford University Press

Peden, A. R. (1993). Recovering in depressed women: Research with Peplau's theory. *Nursing Science Quarterly, 6*(3), 140–146.

Peplau, H. E. (1952). *Interpersonal relations in nursing*. New York, NY: Putnam.

Peplau, H. E. (1963). Interpersonal relations and the process of adaptation. *Nursing Science, 1*, 272–279.

Peplau, H. E. (1992). Notes on Nightingale. In F. Nightingale. *Notes on nursing: What it is and what it is not* (Commemorative ed., pp. 48–57). Philadelphia, PA: Lippincott.

Polk, L. (1997). Toward a middle range theory of resilience. *Advances in Nursing Science, 19*(3), 1–13.

Prochaska, J. O., & Norcross, J. C. (2010). *Systems of psychotherapy: A transtheoretical analysis* (7th ed.). San Francisco, CA: Brooks & Cole.

Prochaska, J. O., & Velicer, W. F. (1997). The transtheoretical model of behavior change. *American Journal of Health Promotion, 12*(1), 38–48.

Reed, P. G. (2003). The theory of self-transcendence. In M. J. Smith & P. R. Liehr (Eds.), *Middle range theory for nursing* (pp. 145–166). New York, NY: Springer Publishing.

Rogers, C. (1980). *A way of being*. Boston, MA: Houghton Mifflin.

Rogers, M. E. (1970). *Introduction to the theoretical basis of nursing*. Philadelphia, PA: F. A. Davis.

Roy, C. (1980). The Roy adaptation model. In J. P. Riehl, & C. Roy. (Eds.), *Conceptual models for nursing practice* (2nd ed., pp. 179–188). Norwalk, CT: Appleton, Century Crofts.

Selye, H. (1956). *The stress of life*. New York, NY: McGraw-Hill.

Sharpnack, P. A., Quinn-Griffin, M. T., Bender, A., & Fitzpatrick, J. J. (2011). Self transcendence and spiritual well being in the Amish. *Journal of Holistic Nursing, 29*(2), 91–97.

Skinner, B. F. (1935). The generic nature of the concepts of stimulus and response. *Journal of General Psychology: 12*(1), 40–65.

Smith, M. J., & Liehr, P. R. (2008). *Middle range theory for nursing* (2nd ed.). New York, NY: Springer Publishing.

Stark, P. L. (2003). The theory of meaning. In M. J. Smith & P. R. Liehr (Eds.). *Middle range theory for nursing* (pp. 125–144). New York, NY: Springer Publishing.

Stuart, G. W. (2008). The Stuart Stress Adaptation Model of psychiatric nursing care. In G. W. Stuart, *Principles and practice of psychiatric nursing* (9th ed., pp. 44–56). Philadelphia, PA: Elsevier.

Sullivan, H. S. (1953). *The interpersonal theory of psychiatry*. New York, NY: Norton.

Thomas, J., Burton, M., Quinn-Griffin, M. T., & Fitzpatrick, J. J. (2010). Self transcendence and spiritual well being among women with breast cancer. *Journal of Holistic Nursing, 28*(2), 115–122.

Thorndike, E. L. (1916). *The elements of psychology* (2nd ed.). New York, NY: A. G. Seiler.

Tusaie, K., & Dyer, J. (2004). Resilience: A historical review of the construct. *Journal of Holistic Nursing, 18*(1), 3–10.

von Bertalanffy, L. (1968). *General systems theory: Foundations, developments, applications.* New York, NY: Braziller.

Walker, P. H. (2005). Neuman's systems model. In J. J. Fitzpatrick & A. L. Whall (Eds.), *Conceptual models of nursing: Analysis and application* (4th ed., pp. 347–359). Saddle River, NJ: Pearson.

You, K. S., Lee, H., Fitzpatrick, J. J., Kim, S., Marui, E., Lee, J. S., & Cook, P. (2009). Religiosity, spirituality, depression, and perceived health among Korean elders in the community. *Archives of Psychiatric Nursing, 23*(4), 309–322.

Zauszniewski, J., & Bekhet, A. (2010). Resilience in family members of persons with serious mental illness. *Nursing Clinics of North America, 45*(4), 613–626.

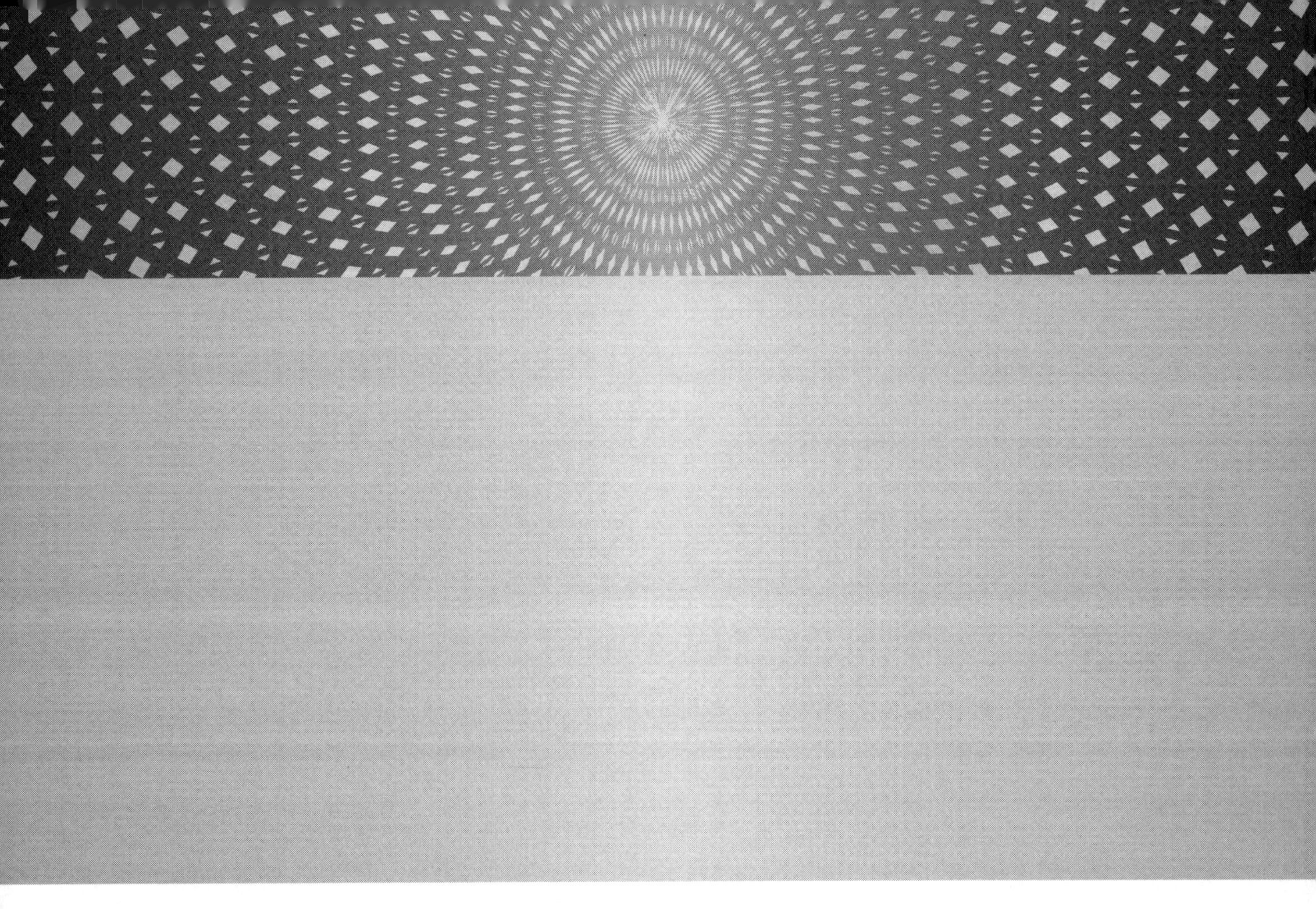

CHAPTER CONTENTS

The relationship between the Psychiatric Mental Health Advanced Practice Nurse (PMH-APRN) and the client is the foundation for any assessment or intervention. The components of building a therapeutic relationship have been described by several nurse authors, beginning with Peplau (1952). However, recent studies have moved on to explore the process of decision making within that therapeutic relationship. The focus is a shift from a paternalistic pattern to one of collaboration, negotiation, and the process of reaching concordance as partners. With this perspective, both the PMH-APRN and the client are viewed as experts. The client is an expert in terms of the lived experience as well as personal values and the PMH-APRN in terms of available evidence, diagnosis, and treatment options in addition to personal values and experiences.

In an ideal world, everyone would be in possession of all necessary evidence to support any decision they were making. The meaning of this evidence would be discussed openly in order to facilitate further understanding where necessary. Different views of the world would be understood and valued in order to ascertain how these perspectives may impact on the person concerned. This is a definition of concordance.

In reality, there are limits to the evidence available. Sometimes there is little time or willingness to discuss

CHAPTER 2

Shared Decision Making: Concordance Between Psychiatric Mental Health Advanced Practice Nurse and Client

Austyn Snowden and Kathleen R. Tusaie

relevant issues in depth. Some views of the world are often considered more worthy than others. In this chapter we will briefly review the ethics underpinning these issues to use the principles of concordance as a framework to examine common aspects of clinical practice. We use medication management to contextualize this discussion where appropriate, but the principles underpinning concordance apply to all aspects of practice.

We show that concordance should be viewed as the ethical goal of partnership, and that partnership can be broken down into achievable goals. We consider the place of knowledge, health beliefs, and collaboration as aspects of successful practice. We demonstrate that telling people what to do, no matter how good that advice may be, is only partially successful. Instead we examine some strategies available to approach concordance. Key terms discussed include *concordance, compliance, adherence, medicine management, partnership, collaboration, health beliefs*, and *knowledge*.

The purpose of this chapter is to provide a theoretical background to many of the specific issues discussed later in this textbook. The perspectives of the authors will be grounded in mental health nursing in the United States and the United Kingdom. The overall thesis is that these themes are requisite to a positive outcome. First, we define some terms.

ADVANCED PSYCHIATRIC MENTAL HEALTH NURSING PRACTICE

In the United States, the American Nurses Association and the National Organization of Nurse Practitioner Faculties (NONPF) have stated that the profession values the promotion of active patient participation in treatment decisions (NONPF, 2003). The scope of practice of the PMH-APRN is regulated by state law; consequently there are some differences across states, both in terms of basic scope of practice and prescriptive authority. Although the United States and the United Kingdom have different structures for the education and licensing of nurses specializing in mental health treatment, the core values are similar.

In the United Kingdom, there is no universal advanced nursing role equivalent to the United States. There are many nurses employed as advanced practitioners but their roles can differ widely. Nursing in the United Kingdom is regulated by the Nursing and Midwifery Council (NMC) and it is their responsibility to set standards for practice. The NMC protects the public by registering all suitably qualified nurses as fit for practice in one of four branches: adult, mental health, children, and learning difficulty. Despite the content and skills differences of these four branches, all registered nurses abide by the same NMC Code of Conduct (Nursing and Midwifery Council, 2010), which informs the public what level of skill and expertise they may expect from a qualified nurse. The NMC further recognizes three recordable qualifications: teaching, specialist practice, and prescribing. However, despite protracted discussion aimed in a general sense at integrating these recordable skills into a registration for advanced nursing practice, agreement has yet to be achieved. As one of the consequences, the definition of advanced nursing differs across the United Kingdom.

EXHIBIT 2-1: DEFINITION OF TERMS

TERM	DEFINITION
Concordance	Process of developing a mutually agreed treatment plan
Compliance	Act of following an instruction
Adherence	Process of sticking with a course of treatment

CONCORDANCE

Concordance is not a synonym of compliance or adherence. Concordance is a way of working together with people. For example, in relation to medicine taking, concordance entails a collaborative process incorporating aspects of choice, self-determination, and empowerment. The aim of a concordant alliance is to maintain an optimal therapeutic effect from medicine taking, *not to inculcate compliance or adherence*, although these may be the *outcomes* of concordance. Compliance and adherence are acceptable within a concordant framework. Yet, they are distinct concepts.

Confusion arises because concordance, compliance, and adherence are often used interchangeably in the literature. This is more than a semantic issue. For example, Latter, Maben, Myall, and Young (2007) conducted a study designed to ascertain the degree to which nurses were practicing the principles of concordance. This is an important study because the nurses thought that they were practicing the principles of concordance, whereas the study found they were not. Latter et al. (2007) found that the *language* of medicine management had changed. Instead of talking about compliance nurses talked about patients' concording with their medicine regimes. In their practice, medicine management activity remained focused on the goal of compliance. Conceptual clarity is therefore a fundamental starting point in any discussion of concordance. Within this chapter the terms concordance, adherence, and compliance are defined as presented in Exhibit 2-1. They are all very important concepts, and all have a place in quality clinical practice, but they are not the same.

BACKGROUND

The principles of autonomy, justice, beneficence, and nonmaleficience are embedded in Western law. They underpin human rights legislation and form the basis of the code of conduct for nurses. In regard to mental health care the principles are explicitly linked to mental health legislation. These principles provide for a set of values taught to all mental health nurses in order to translate these ideals into practice, where reciprocity and person-centered care drive all therapeutic relationships, and partnership is valued as central. Medical and scientific information is combined with personal values to form preferences, which in turn shape decisions, behavior, and outcomes (Wills & Holmes-Rovner, 2006).

However, in practice it is not always easy to work in partnership. For example, how do you build partnerships with people who are compulsorily detained, or have severe cognitive impairments? These are enduring debates (Barker, 2011; Coffey & Byrt, 2011; Lavelle & Tusaie, 2011) and the solutions are complex. However, the decisions and actions can all be explained in relation to the ethical principles discussed above. Trying to achieve the best outcome and actively avoid harm by balancing the principles of autonomy with the agreed needs of wider society provides a framework to discuss all clinical actions.

One of the more difficult issues is that partnership in health care generally involves a relationship of unequal partners, in that the health professional is usually in possession of specialist knowledge and expertise the other partner does not have. Of course this is not always the case, but it is a good place to start.

KNOWLEDGE

Consider the role of knowledge in this triad of themes. Knowledge is in many ways the most straightforward aspect of any clinical session. It is not a sufficient condition, as we will see. However, it is a necessary condition, in that without it no amount of collaborative discussion around health beliefs would be complete. To use medicine management as an example, without in depth knowledge of pharmacodynamics and pharmacokinetics, even the best relationship will not be able to address the most fundamental questions: for example, why am I taking this drug? In order to answer this question you need to know what the drug is for, what it is supposed to do, and how it is supposed to do it.

This may seem absolutely obvious, and of course it is. However, a lot of important agendas fight for their place in nursing curricula, and apparently obvious knowledge can get overlooked in the evolution of nursing. For example, in relation to medicine management in the United Kingdom, there is evidence that pharmacology knowledge is not as good as it should be (Department of Health, 2006; Hemingway, Stephenson, & Allmark, 2011; Jones, Robson, Whitfield, & Gray, 2010). It is therefore briefly worth considering why this is the case in order to consider how certain aspects of knowledge can slip off the agenda. There may be comparative issues with whatever your speciality is, given that the focus of your specialist intervention may also have changed as a function of the partnership agenda. For example, cancer care is changing as a function of the increasing recognition that individually tailored interventions targeted at reducing distress generate better outcomes for people with cancer (Snowden et al., 2011a, 2011b).

Against this background it might become tempting to think that ascertaining individual knowledge was more relevant than traditional methods of treatment. This is of course nonsense. Both complement each other. However, a comparable argument can be made that the diminution of pharmacology knowledge among mental health nurses can be viewed as a paradoxical artifact of person-centered care. In other words, in quite rightly focusing on the creation of partnerships grounded in respect and dignity, unfashionable knowledge with its roots in a supposedly less enlightened era often has been considered less important, despite its enduring central importance.

The education of PMH-APRNs in the United States has drifted away from the relationship focus and more onto a medical model approach. However, recent evaluations of this educational pattern have resulted in the Licensure, Accreditation, Certification, Education (LACE) initiative, which requires more consistency in curriculum and inclusion of the four Ps—Pathophysiology, Pharmacology, Physical Assessment, and Psychotherapy (American Psychiatric Nurses Association, 2011).

This situation can be understood as a function of recent analyses of the place and function of mental health care within postmodern society. For example, the credibility of medication in mental health care has been challenged by eloquent deconstructions of the medical model (Bentall, 2003; Moncrieff, 2007) and sophisticated criticism of classification of mental illness (Fleming & Martin, 2009; Kutchins & Kirk, 1997). These critiques and others have reinforced a mistrust of "treatment" within mental health services, particularly in relation to medication. At the same time, the increasing recognition of the limits of reductionist biology and hence pharmacology (Noble, 2002; 2006) has been paralleled with the rise of evidence-based alternatives to medicines such as cognitive behavior therapy (Hall & Iqbal, 2010). All of these developments appear to be grounded in the ethics of human rights (Barker, 2011), which offers further moral credibility to non-medical perspectives of mental health and the importance of a range of treatment modalities.

In other words, what is important to know is culturally constructed. However, this construction needs to encompass all impact factors. An essential component of this is that psychotropic prescribing has continued to rise year after year (Information and Statistics Division, 2011). This makes medication the most widely utilized intervention in mental health by some considerable margin. Uncritical rejection of medicines is therefore wholly inappropriate at the present time. PMH-APRNs need in-depth knowledge of medicines. Partnership and person-centered care are also needed. Knowledge about the intervention you are applying remains absolutely fundamental. So, in relation to medication administration, knowledge of psychopharmacology is an absolutely essential component of concordance. The same is true of whatever intervention you are discussing.

HEALTH BELIEFS

The starting point for this section is that people have different health beliefs and that these beliefs have a significant impact on subsequent behavior, including actual outcome of treatment. We do not have to go very far to find convincing evidence for this. Consider the placebo effect. In brief, the placebo effect describes the effect by which an inert substance exerts a therapeutic effect. Benedetti has spent an entire research career trying to understand the neurobiological underpinnings of this mechanism and produced some fascinating evidence. For example, he has shown that if people take diazepam without knowing, then it has no anxiolytic effect. He has also shown that pain can be reduced in people who believe they are receiving pain-relieving medication, even when they are receiving opioid-blocking medication, as long as the *administer* of the medicine also believes it will relieve the pain (Benedetti et al., 2005). Further reading of Benedetti's work is recommended at the end of this chapter. However, even this brief explication suggests that the beliefs of everyone involved in medicine management have an impact on the efficacy of that medicine. To a certain degree, expectations dictate outcome.

Of further significance is how these expectations translate into action. Nichol, Thompson, and Shaw (2011) explored the dynamics of beliefs about complementary and alternative medicines (CAM) within families. They found that mothers tended to "champion" CAM, whereas fathers and children remained more skeptical. This would suggest, if generalizable, that these mothers would be more likely to try CAM and get a benefit from it. Understanding this and comparable evidence would arguably lead to a better understanding of subsequent behavior and the likelihood of a particular course of action being coherent and therefore beneficial. We acknowledge this is a big leap, but there have been attempts to connect these hypotheses in practice. Marland and Cash (2005) attempted to understand medicine-taking behavior in mainstream psychiatry by analyzing how people interacted with it. They identified three broad types of medicine-taking behavior. The clinical utility of this for the pertinent professional is to recognize which type of behavior people exhibit in order to tailor further intervention accordingly. The types were:

1. ***Deferential compliant type***. This type defines the person who leaves all medicine-taking decisions to the prescriber and complies even in the absence of insight.
2. ***Direct reactive type***. The person denies the need for medicines and ceases to take medicine when well to assert wellness, or in reaction to side effects or stigma.
3. ***Active discernment and optimising type.*** This includes people with the ability and will to reflect on past experiences. This type is further divided into two stages:
   - *Experimental-reflective stage*. The person insightfully and actively experiments to achieve the optimum medicine regime. This can be carried out unilaterally or in concordance with the prescriber. It may involve reducing the medicine taken to see if beneficial effects can be maintained and side effects reduced, and "recovery testing," which is ceasing to take medicines to prove or disprove their need.
   - *Consolidation stage*. In this stage, the service user has found an effective way of using medicines and is reluctant to consider any changes.

The typology presents one view of how different people have different beliefs and behavior when it comes to engaging with medicine. This is likely to be true of all interventions. Using this typology as an example, it can be seen that if *concordance* is prioritized as an outcome instead of adherence or compliance then this can be achieved with *any of these types of people*. It does not matter what their beliefs or actions are; only that everyone understands them. This equation of course also includes the nurse, and would require the nurse to reflect on his/her own beliefs about the treatment they are suggesting and to clarify the impact of these beliefs of the recipient. By testing these assumptions in practice both parties have an opportunity to align their interactions to the optimal outcome, which needs to be *mutually defined* (see Figure 2-1).

We need to recognize that people's beliefs about health are a fundamental aspect of concordance. Treatment will be less successful if it is discordant with how people view their world. Figure 2-1 illustrates that, regardless of health beliefs, concordance can always be achieved as long as the specific needs of the particular *relationship* are met. We would argue this is a transferable aspect of any clinical intervention. This is discussed in more detail next.

COLLABORATION

We have ascertained the importance of context specific knowledge and the role of people's health beliefs in approaching concordance. The missing element relates to the process of integrating these aspects. This is best done through collaboration, highlighted as the dynamic connection between the two parties in Figure 2-1. In theory, collaboration is broadly seen as a universal good. However, in practice it becomes problematic very quickly.

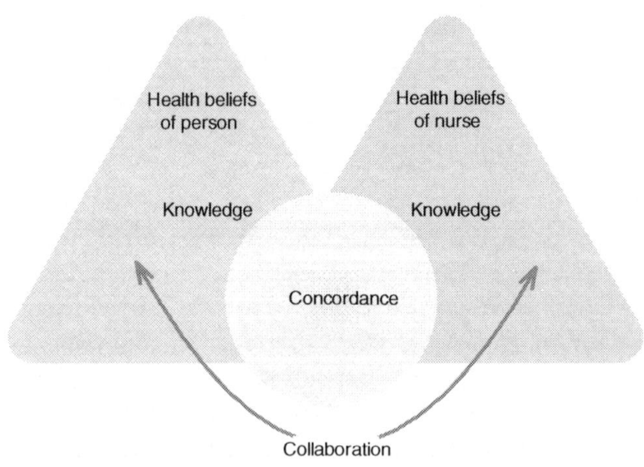

Figure 2-1 The Construction of Concordance

We have already touched on issues of unequal knowledge, and the literature on power relations in health care is voluminous and equivocal. However, even without attention to the power relation issue, collaboration is very complex. From a purely practical perspective collaborating does not necessarily save time, and therefore may not be seen as an option for busy clinicians. There is also evidence that some nurses feel they do not have the skills to operate in a truly collaborative manner (Snowden et al., 2011a, 2011b). Clinicians consistently express fear of opening "cans of worms" they feel unable to manage (Latter et al., 2010). This is a cliché we have heard many times as clinicians.

However, as with many anxieties they are rarely borne out as feared. For example, Snowden et al. (2011a, 2011b) found that collaborating did not take any longer than treatment as usual in a randomized controlled trial of distress management. They measured the time taken in a clinical session and it was equivalent for the experimental and treatment as usual group. Interestingly, the belief that it would take more time persisted in these clinicians, even when presented with this evidence. Applying evidence into practice is a further issue, as it meets much resistance on the way. Latter et al. (2010) also showed that if a collaborative consultation opens up a "can of worms" this is neither unwelcome nor unmanageable. Rather, there is evidence it is a worthy pursuit, and it can only be achieved by asking people what they actually do:

> I've opened a can of worms with some patients. I had been laboring under the misapprehension that they were actually managing quite well, that they understood what they were doing, that they were taking their medications...I've found that's not the case. I've had to start working harder with them and getting to grips with what exactly is going on...I'm hoping that in the end, in the long term, it will actually reduce work, I mean its short-term misery for long-term gain so it's fine.
>
> (Community matron 1, cohort 2, 1 month interview; Latter et al., 2010, p. 1135)

Of course some people may want to keep their cans of worms firmly closed and we would argue it is their right to do so. As with Marland and Cash's typology, some people may not expect or want anything to do with medicine-taking decisions (Manias, 2008). Stenner, Courtenay, and Carey (2011) found that regardless of the level of information patients wanted, when it came to making decisions about treatment, most preferred the prescriber to use their professional judgment to offer the best treatment option for them.

However, this can still be a *collaborative* process. It just makes knowledge of medicines' actions and interactions even more important, as in these cases the recipient is relying on the health professional to tell them everything they need to know. These "deferential compliant" people still need to understand and be understood, and this can only be achieved through collaboration. However, although this is increasingly recognized as a worthy aim there is evidence that clinicians may not be giving people the information they actually need (Ekman, Schaufelberger, Kjellgren, Swedberg, & Granger, 2007). In Latter and colleagues' (2007) words, the "paradigm shift to a concordance model that emphasizes partnership through explanation of the risks and benefits of treatment options and fully informed patients able to make decisions about treatment options, was not yet integrated into practice."

There have been an increasing number of efforts to address integration of the concordance/shared decision making model into practice. Latter et al. (2010) found nurse prescribers could be taught skills to further improve their communication skills. They focused on teaching nurses how to elicit patients' *beliefs* about their medicines in order to better support their medicine taking. The results were significant, and showed that there is considerable space for better collaboration here. A second example is the work of the United States Substance Abuse and Mental Health Services Administration (SAMSHSA). They have held a national conference as well as several web-based conferences on shared decision making and have multiple resources available for clinicians as well as clients. There are tip sheets to assist clinicians in eliciting active participation as well as tip sheets for clients to guide them in more active participation. These can be viewed and downloaded at http://mentalhealth.samhsa.gov/consumersurvivor/shared.asp

Another example of encouraging the practice of shared decision making is the pilot work of Mahone and associates (2011) with seriously mentally ill individuals and their prescribers. They have identified system and client-based barriers as well as new skills needed by both prescribers and clients. This is work in progress, but includes important issues relevant to concordance.

In summary, while we do not understand why, it seems that if people believe their medicine can do what they think it should do then it has a better chance of achieving that outcome. It is therefore important to understand what people think the medicine should do. This "coherence thesis" may go some way to explain the efficacy of homeopathy for example, which has consistently been shown to be a function of the consultation process. For example, in a rheumatology trial, homeopathic consultation was shown to be beneficial (Brien, Lachance, Prescott, Mc Dermott, & George, 2010), whereas the homeopathic remedy alone was not. This is a consistent finding within this literature, illustrating the power of *collaboration,* a fundamental tenet of homeopathic consultations.

Skilled clinicians therefore need to understand the importance of their own beliefs within this collaboration. Unlike Goldacre (2009), who dismisses homeopathy as nonsense, we would suggest that finding out that someone believes in homeopathy tells you a great deal about the person you are collaborating with. There is no need to make a value judgment about this. We would instead argue that if you believe strongly that homeopathy is nonsense then forcing this view on others may not always be therapeutically justified. Perhaps all you will succeed in doing is removing a vestige of hope.

We acknowledge that this is a moral minefield, and that colluding with beliefs you do not share is damaging. However, tolerance of different beliefs is not collusion, and we do not believe there is any disingenuous function of attempting to establish middle ground towards the end of clinical improvement. Instead, we follow Latter et al. (2007) who suggest we need to develop further educational approaches that would help facilitate exploration of facilitating *genuine* concordance. This is about stepping outside any semblance of paternalism or imposition of strongly held beliefs and maintaining an open mind. Collaboration is always possible between people with open minds.

IMPROVING CONCORDANCE

This last section considers actions the clinician can take in relation to the issues discussed above. So, how can they improve their knowledge? How can health beliefs be ascertained? How is genuine collaboration best facilitated? These questions are answered in turn, and further reading is suggested at the end of the chapter.

KNOWLEDGE

Knowledge can be attained if you know where to look and what to look for. The process requires insight into the type of knowledge required and the quality of the knowledge considered. There are two important meta-processes that can be summarized as questions: What do I need to know? What is the quality of the information I have?

We will discuss these in turn.

What Do I Need to Know?

This question is context specific. For example, the knowledge required to practice as a nurse in the United States is taught in educational programs preparing registered nurses, and tested through a national examination (NCLEX) developed by the National Council of State Boards of Nursing. In the United Kingdom the knowledge required to practice is specified by the NMC (Nursing and Midwifery Council, 2010). Students need to provide evidence that they have achieved competence in all the requisite domains. Considering medicine management as an example there is an expectation of a progressive increase in knowledge throughout the educational programs. So every nurse is expected to understand pharmacodynamics and pharmacokinetics, their scope, and the underpinning governance arrangements ensuring safety within the system. This knowledge is largely accessible and straightforward to learn in that anatomy and physiology are broadly generalizable, as are drug pathways and biological actions of drugs.

In the United States, for PMH-APRNs, a master's program in nursing must be completed that addresses the Essentials of Master's Education in Nursing (American Association of Colleges of Nursing, 2011) in the curriculum as well as the psychiatric nurse practitioner competencies (NONPF, 2003). See Exhibits 2-2 and 2-3 for details. This concludes with the successful completion of a national certification exam, such as those offered by American Nurses Credentialing Center (ANCC, 2011; www.nursescredentialing.org).

To apply this to the therapeutic level, if you are prescribing or administering a drug, you would need to know

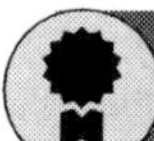

EXHIBIT 2-2: SUMMARY OF THE ESSENTIALS FOR MASTER'S EDUCATION IN NURSING

1. Background for Practice From Sciences and Humanities
2. Organizational and Systems Leadership
3. Quality Improvement and Safety
4. Translating and Integrating Scholarship Into Practice
5. Informatics and Health Care Technologies
6. Health Policy and Advocacy
7. Interprofessional Collaboration
8. Clinical Prevention and Population Health
9. Master's Level Nursing Practice

Source: American Association of Colleges of Nursing, 2011.

exactly what that drug was supposed to do, how it does it, and most importantly, what can go wrong. You also need to know whether this is the right course of treatment. This requires aligning the presenting problems with the purpose of the proposed treatment, and depends on structured and accurate assessment. There are many validated tools available to support this assessment process, and many of them are discussed throughout this book.

Although this knowledge is broadly generalizable as suggested, it can of course vary in every case. The same drug or therapy can be therapeutic in one individual and toxic or ineffective in another. Technology is increasingly helpful in this regard, but its utility and application remain dependent on being able to answer the next question.

What Is the Quality of the Information I Have?

In order to apply any knowledge in practice we have to be able to critically appraise it. This is an essential but difficult aspect of practice. Some clinicians lack the confidence to apply new evidence in everyday practice (Graue, Bjarkøy, Iversen, Haugstvedt, & Harris, 2010). For others it may be a practical matter, with lack of time being cited most frequently as the reason for not engaging with new research (Graue et al., 2010).

The amount of new research can indeed appear overwhelming. However, more concerning than this is Kruger and Dunning's enduring finding (Ehrlinger, Johnson, Banner, Dunning, & Kruger, 2008) that those with the least skill are the most unaware of their own deficits. These people are therefore the least likely to engage with critical appraisal while probably being in most need of it. The interested reader is encouraged to engage with the primary evidence for this claim, as its impact on nurse education needs to be formally assessed. For those few who do recognize the value of the best quality evidence, having found, understood, and appraised the issue under investigation, getting it into practice is extraordinarily difficult as we mentioned earlier. Glasziou and Haynes (2005) articulated the numerous pitfalls between even the best quality evidence and clinical practice.

EXHIBIT 2-3: CORE COMPETENCIES FOR PSYCHIATRIC NURSE PRACTITIONERS

1. Health promotion, health protection, disease prevention and treatment
   a. Assessment
   b. Diagnosis
   c. Plan of care and implementation
2. Nurse-patient relationship
3. Teaching-coaching
4. Professional role
5. Managing and negotiating health care delivery practice
6. Monitors and ensures quality of health care practice
7. Cultural competence

Source: National Panel for psychiatric nurse practitioner Competencies (2003).

In summary, the model shows that all sorts of different quality evidence clamors for our attention through reviews, guidelines, and single studies of varying rigor. Myth, opinion, and poor research enter the practice pipeline along with the high quality information. Glasziou and Haynes suggest that all this information then goes through numerous phases, from initially appearing on people's radars to becoming routine practice with numerous places to drop out on the way. For example, if people do not have the skills to adopt the new technique, or if the new technique does not quite apply in your area, then it will not make it into routine practice.

We acknowledge that applying knowledge in practice is complex and extremely difficult for a number of reasons. A persistent theme is that many people find critical appraisal difficult to do, and subsequently utilize all sorts of conscious and unconscious techniques to avoid it. This is a mistake. We cannot rely on others to tell the difference. Understanding the difference between good and poor research is an essential skill for every clinician. It is a crucial aspect of concordance. Knowledge cannot be shared in a contextually relevant manner without a deep understanding of the quality and scope of that knowledge.

The art of critical appraisal is beyond the scope of this chapter. This is because, akin to the "what do I need to know" question, critical appraisal skills vary with every question, method, and analytic technique. The essential aspect is to ask coherent questions of the topic under review. As a way in, we direct the reader to Trisha Greenhalgh's *How to Read a Paper* (Greenhalgh, 2010). This is an excellent resource and offers practical guidance focused on coherence of questioning.

HEALTH BELIEFS

Health belief models have been recognized as important since at least the 1950s. Although the links between these models and subsequent behavior is not clear (Carpenter, 2010), there is little doubt that understanding someone's health beliefs enables more collaborative discussion and improves insight into the reasons people may or may not follow an agreed treatment plan. One of the original health belief models (Rosenstock, 1966) structured questions around:

- Perceived susceptibility (an individual's assessment of his or her risk of getting the condition)
- Perceived severity (an individual's assessment of the seriousness of the condition, and its potential consequences)
- Perceived barriers (an individual's assessment of the influences that facilitate or discourage adoption of the promoted behavior)
- Perceived benefits (an individual's assessment of the positive consequences of adopting the behavior)

Other factors have subsequently been added to various iterations such as cost, demographics, and locus of control issues. For example McCann, Clark, and Lu (2008) synthesised the literature on explanatory models of medication adherence in individuals with chronic mental illness in order to construct a pertinent health belief model. The outcome of this synthesis was the "self-efficacy model of medication adherence." This model extends existing health belief models such as Rosenstock's to also explicitly incorporate social and contextual issues, relevant to this particular topic. Although the model refers to aspects of adherence as opposed to concordance it is very useful in that, like Marland's model, it identifies relevant factors of medicine-taking behavior, and as such raises awareness of the necessity for nurses to consider these factors in any discussion on health beliefs regarding medicine.

In a practical sense then, eliciting someone's health beliefs is straightforward. In order to use McCann and colleagues' model you would need to discuss what people thought their medication would do for them. You would need to ascertain their support structures and the relationships they had with various health professionals. Personal issues, stigma, and complexity are all better understood through collaborative application of expert knowledge. As far as perceived medicine efficacy goes, if you know the prescribed medicine can cause embarrassing movement disorders and akathisia, then the impact of these effects needs to be discussed and mutually understood. This will allow everyone to discuss openly the likely impact of these effects.

In a more general sense, regardless of specific content the purpose of health belief models is to construct some sort of risk-benefit analysis. From a concordance perspective the health belief models facilitate the provision of relevant individualised information to help answer the following question: What is the risk to me of taking this course of action? Is that risk worth the benefit?

In essence then, ascertaining someone's health beliefs is simply a matter of asking. Latter et al. show how important this simple action is:

> I asked a gentleman, "what are your beliefs around diabetes? What does it mean to you?" And he just turned round and said, "I'm going to lose my legs." He's a gardener I'd been seeing for a year up until that point and I thought, "how do I not know this about you?"
>
> (Community matron 2, cohort 3, 1 month interview; Latter et al., 2010, p. 1133)

COLLABORATION

In the previous section on collaboration we clarified its importance in relation to clinical outcome. Here we will briefly give examples of how to do this. We will discuss two evidence-based interventions that have been shown to improve collaboration; the distress thermometer (DT) and timelines. Both were initially conceived as assessment tools but some clinicians have found that utilising them in practice facilitated collaborative work. In other words, the act of assessing using these particular tools has functioned in two interlinked and essential ways. The tools provide pertinent information, and when utilized as part of a therapeutic encounter they also give the signal that the person collating this information is actually interested in this information. This of course depends on the quality of the therapeutic encounter, but there is increasing evidence that collaboration can be facilitated through good and genuinely pertinent assessment, and that this is very highly valued by people (Snowden et al., 2011a, 2011b).

For example, the DT is a well validated tool for measuring distress in people with cancer (Mitchell, 2007). The DT is a screening tool (Richardson, Tebbit, Brown, & Sitzia, 2006). It has been validated in a wide range of studies and is reliable. This is extremely important as, akin to our discussion on the importance of knowledge, the quality of the assessment method dictates the quality of the information returned. From this validation process we know that the DT produces clinically meaningful data (Mitchell, 2010). The DT entails an analogue scale with 0 indicating no distress and 10 extreme distress. It is accompanied by a problem list (PL): a check-box list of specific issues categorized into five domains: physical, practical, family, emotional, and spiritual problems or concerns. Participants rate their distress, check any problems they have, and finally indicate and rank their three most pressing problems in priority order.

The initial purpose of the tool was to screen people in order to know which ones to refer on for further support. However, pragmatic clinicians have recognized the potential to move beyond this screening utility and enhance the consultation process as well. For example, Lynch and colleagues found that the DT:

> ... brought up issues during consultations which might not normally have been discussed, enabling [nurses] to use consultation time more effectively by focusing on patient concerns. It also demonstrated to patients and their carers that the health care team were interested in all aspects of patient well-being.
>
> (Lynch, Goodhart, Saunders, & O'Connor, 2010)

In other words, the act of gathering information fulfilled the dual role discussed. Completing the DT not only indicated clinical levels of distress and its cause, but also gives a signal that the clinicians *wanted to know*. The impact of this is both simple and effective, and further studies have shown that this interest is reciprocated. Patients who feel that their clinicians are genuinely interested in them are more likely to try to follow the agreed treatment plan (Swanson & Koch, 2010).

This is not new to PMH-APRNs, who have implicitly utilized the therapeutic relationship as their major tool throughout their history (Porter, 2002). What is added by the DT evidence is that this collaboration can be better structured through the use of appropriate techniques. For example, collaboration has been shown to be better facilitated through the use of timelines (Marland, McNay, Fleming, & Mccaig, 2011a). History offers a lens to explain why people behave the way they do. Timelines construct this history for the individual and so offer insight into themes or stressors that may be pertinent for the future (Marland, McKay, McCaig, & Snowden, 2011b). Timelines work best when constructed in collaboration with the nurse in order to clarify and discuss previous events and reactions to events. This activity means that relapse can facilitate learning instead of being seen as failure (Ford, 2000). Thus, difficult to understand symptoms (Snowden, 2009) become more understandable through construction of a timeline. The challenges and approaches to achieving concordance with clients experiencing specific psychiatric symptoms are discussed throughout this book. By sharing someone's journey you are showing that you *want* to understand. Again, this act of collaboration is functional in itself. It engenders hope.

Timelines therefore fulfill a dual function similar to the DT in a clinical sense. They provide practical information related to external stressors and relate these to the impact on the individual. Discussing these in a systematic manner ensures both parties are talking about the same thing and working toward the same ends. This is an essential aspect of collaboration.

SUMMARY AND CONCLUSION

We started this chapter by describing the ethical principles underpinning psychiatric-mental health nursing. We showed that any intervention can be described by pointing out the various tensions inherent within these principles. We then focused on the construction of concordance as an end in itself, to show how this is a more ethical aim than blind compliance or adherence. By breaking this aim down into the manageable and measurable constructs of knowledge, health beliefs, and collaboration, we hope that you now agree that concordance is not only ethical, but also practically achievable.

I (Snowden) have been interested in the way people construct their worlds for as long as I can remember, and I have never seen the value of trying to force my views onto others. This has never been a moral stance, it's just that as a rule it does not tend to work. Consequently, I have been more interested in processes that do appear to work. This is difficult to generalize from, and I suppose that is one of the main problems with trying to convey this type of approach, but let me give you an example to finish. My last clinical role was as a community psychiatric nurse with an older adult team in Greenock, Scotland. Much of this job involved ensuring people were managing well at home, often in relation to their medicine. People with cognitive problems in particular sometimes had additional challenges trying to remember their particular routines. One of the most widely used interventions for this was the dosette box, a weekly delivered compartmentalized supply of that individual's prescription for the week. One of my roles was to ensure this process went smoothly and that people were managing safely.

One of the women on my caseload was clearly struggling with her medicine regime so I suggested a dosette box for her and she agreed to give it a go, because I explained it would help her organize her routine and remember when she had already taken her medicines. I arranged her dosette box with the local pharmacist and then ensured safe delivery and receipt. When I popped in to check how she was getting on a couple of days later, I found she had taken all the medicines out of their individual compartments and placed them in individual egg cups in her kitchen. She said she preferred it that way. I personally could not understand the rationality behind this, but instead of challenging her, asked if I could visit her again shortly. I counted all the medicines in the egg cups and calculated the number that should be there for my next visit. When I next visited, the correct number was in each egg cup. I repeated this for several visits, mostly random ones as I wanted to rule out any "visiting bias," or extra preparation she may have made for my impending visit. Each time the number in the egg cups was correct and she was very happy with her new system. I still have no idea why she chose to do something so apparently complicated (to me) with a system designed to simplify the situation, but it worked for her. She was on top of her medicine regime. The dosette box had worked, but not in any way I could have predicted.

It was therefore no surprise to me when I undertook a review of medicine aids designed to support compliance/adherence and found that none was superior to the other (Snowden, 2008a). I found lots of randomized controlled trials and systematic reviews of educational interventions, dosette box utility, and various warning systems targeted toward enhancing compliance/adherence in medicine taking. All were only partially successful. The only interventions that were consistently successful were those described as "individually tailored" interventions. In light of this chapter it is not hard to understand why. None of the interventions targeted toward compliance or adherence were successful because they omitted the most important aspect of medicine management in this group: concordance. The only intervention that accounted for this worked. For example, it is hard to imagine how egg cups could be incorporated into any systematic intervention. I honestly couldn't recommend it. But the egg cups worked in this individual case.

Hopefully you will agree that concordance is not only ethically superior to any other type of intervention, it is also more efficient. Any treatment plan grounded in shared understanding of the likely impact of that plan is more likely to succeed than any other prescriptive intervention. Yet despite the intuitive simplicity of this point we have shown that practicing the principles of concordance is difficult. Elucidating someone's health beliefs is easier said than done, and collaboration is rarely as good as clinicians think it is (Latter et al., 2007).

Yet, concordance is also extraordinarily simple. It aligns with the principles of person-centered care at the forefront of modern mental health treatment (Scottish Government, 2010). Nurses specializing in mental health are demonstrably good at collaborating with people with severe mental health problems (Shattell, McAllister, Hogan, & Thomas, 2006). Elucidating someone's health beliefs can simply be the product of a single question, and recognizing that asking it is important (Latter et al., 2010). The need for evidence-based knowledge to back these skills up is increasingly recognized (Hemingway et al., 2011). If these findings are indicative of a larger trend then they are all moving in the right direction.

ANNOTATED BIBLIOGRAPHY RELATED TO CONCORDANCE

Promoting Concordance in Mental Health (2011c) Edited by Glenn Marland, Lisa Mcnay, and Austyn Snowden
This book uses unfolding narratives to present three different cases of concordance in practice. It presents a practical, skills-based approach to the promotion of concordance. It provides clear methods for mental health practitioners working in a variety of settings. This includes case studies, examples, and practical guidance for concordance. Many of the ideas discussed in this chapter are expanded within this text. The focus is again on medicine management and so the knowledge required to underpin safe practice is detailed in a dedicated chapter. The final chapter analyzes the construct of concordance in detail. However, the majority of the text is devoted to the practical application of concordance, showing techniques to facilitate it, including examples both well meaning and not, of how concordance can go wrong.

Evaluating Research for Evidence-Based Nursing Practice (2009) by Jacqueline Fawcett and Joan Garity
This book provides excellent guidelines for thoughtful evaluation of research studies as well as strategies for integrating research findings into practice. A CD with learning examples is also provided.

Prescribing and Mental Health Nursing (2008b) by Austyn Snowden
This book is separated into two parts. The first focuses on the history and development of mental health nursing and prescribing rights more generally. Of particular relevance is the discussion on the historical development of psychiatric drugs. The book shows the largely fortuitous nature of these developments. It illustrates how drug treatment of certain patterns of distress led to the clustering of these symptoms for the purpose of psychiatric classification, rather than the other way round. For example, panic disorder didn't exist as a distinct concept until a drug was

found to have subdued a cluster of symptoms previously thought to be aspects of anxiety. Unsurprisingly, this drug remains the mainstay of treatment for panic disorder.

The second part of the book looks at the evidence for drug treatment of certain classifications of disorder. It focuses on the avoidance of "side effects" in that each chapter has a section entitled "what's the worst that can happen?" These issues are essential knowledge within any concordant discussion on medicine taking. They establish the parameters of risk that may need to be discussed.

The Music of Life (2006) by Denis Noble
This book articulates with great clarity the limits of any reductionist view of biology. Professor emeritus Noble is a geneticist at the forefront of studies of the human genome and is therefore perfectly placed to explain exactly what we can and can't conclude from this work. There are many of these types of books out there attempting to explain how everything fits together, and nearly all end up tying themselves in knots with the circularity of the puzzles they create for themselves. Noble's position is refreshingly scientific yet simultaneously humble and articulate. His rejection of top-down and bottom-up explanations of behavior in favor of "middle out" multilevel processes leaves considerable room for an evidence-based explanation of the importance of concordance within a purely biological narrative.

The Myth of the Chemical Cure (2009) by Joanna Moncrieff
Moncrieff presents a lucid and compelling deconstruction of the classification of mental illness. She does this by focusing on the actions of psychiatric drugs in isolation from their contextualized purpose. She argues strongly against any disease based representation of "mental illness" and presents evidence to support her position. There are limits to her position, and like any radical perspective she can be criticized for minimizing the potential benefit of the treatments she criticizes. Nevertheless her account provides a coherent challenge to modern psychiatry, and should be critically appraised by anyone working within the system. Anyone who wants a "value free" account of psychotropic drugs should include this in their reading.

Placebo Effects (2009) by Fabrizio Benedetti
The notion of value judgements is further examined here in great detail through the construct of the placebo effect. The idea that a placebo effect is a worthless effect, that it is "all in the mind" and therefore somehow less worthy than a real, physical effect is beautifully challenged within this body of work. Not only does Professor Benedetti show that this thinking is wrong, but that the biological assumptions are more complex than these simplistic ideas would suggest. Placebo effects are "real" effects. Linking this to the ideas expressed in Noble's book, it seems there is a further role for concordance based around Benedetti's findings. If beliefs play such a demonstrable role in biological outcomes, as demonstrated here, then aligning treatment with expectations is essential. This is concordance.

REFERENCES

American Association of Colleges of Nursing (2011). *The essentials of master's education in nursing.* Retrived June 15, 2012 from www.aacn.nche.edu/education-resources/MastersEssentials11.pdf

American Psychiatric Nurses Association. (2011). American Psychiatric Nurses Association/International Society for Psychiatric Nursing Joint Task Force Recommendations on Implementation of the Consensus Model for APRN Regulation: Licensing, Accreditation, Credentialing, and Education (LACE). Retrieved from http://www.apna.org

Barker, P. (2011). *Mental health ethics.* New York, NY: Routledge.

Benedetti, F. (2009). *Placebo effects.* Oxford, UK: Oxford University Press.

Benedetti, F., Mayberg, H. S., Wager, T. D., Stohler, C. S., & Zubieta, J.-K. (2005). Neurobiological mechanisms of the placebo effect. *Journal of Neuroscience, 25,* 10390–10402. doi: 10.1523/JNEUROSCI.3458–05.2005.

Bentall, R. P. (2003). *Madness explained: Psychosis and human nature.* London, UK: Penguin.

Brien, S., Lachance, L., Prescott, P., McDermott, C., & George, L. (2010). Homeopathy has clinical benefits in rheumatoid arthritis patients that are attributable to the consultation process but not the homeopathic remedy: A randomized controlled clinical trial. *Rheumatology, 50,* 1070–1082. doi: 10.1093/rheumatology/keq234

Carpenter, C. J. (2010). A meta-analysis of the effectiveness of health belief model variables in predicting behavior. *Health Communication, 25,* 661–669.

Coffey, M., & Byrt, R. (2011). *Forensic mental health nursing ethics, debates, dilemmas.* London, UK: Quay Books.

Department of Health. (2006). *Improving patients' access to medicines: A guide to implementing nurse and pharmacist independent prescribing within the NHS in England.* London, UK: Author.

Ehrlinger, J., Johnson, K., Banner, M., Dunning, D., & Kruger, J. (2008). Why the unskilled are unaware: Further explorations of (absent) self-insight among the incompetent. *Organizational Behavior and Human Decision Processes, 105,* 98–121. doi: 10.1016/j.obhdp.2007.05.002

Ekman, I., Schaufelberger, M., Kjellgren, K. I., Swedberg, K., & Granger, B. B. (2007). Standard medication information is not enough: Poor concordance of patient and nurse perceptions. *Journal of Advanced Nursing, 60,* 181–186. doi: 10.1111/j.1365–2648.2007.04397.x

Fawcett, J. & Garity, J. (2009). *Evaluating research for evidence-based practice.* Philadelphia, PA: FA Davis.

Fleming, M. P., & Martin, C. R. (2009). A preliminary investigation into the experience of symptoms of psychosis in mental health professionals: Implications for the psychiatric classification model of schizophrenia. *Journal of Psychiatric and Mental Health Nursing, 16*, 473–480. doi: 10.1111/j.1365–2850.2009.01404.x

Ford, B. (2000). *Coping with setbacks and staying well: Training manual.* York, UK: York Health Services NHS Trust.

Glasziou, P., & Haynes, B. (2005). The paths from research to improved health outcomes. *Evidence-Based Medicine, 9*, 100. doi: 10.1136/ebm.9.4.100

Goldacre, B. (2009). *Bad Science.* London, UK: Harper Perennial.

Graue, M., Bjarkøy, R., Iversen, M., Haugstvedt, A., & Harris, J. (2010). Integrating evidence-based practice into the diabetes nurse curriculum in Bergen. *European Diabetes Nursing, 7*, 10–15. doi: 10.1002/edn.148

Greenhalgh, T. (2010). *How to read a paper: The basics of evidence-based medicine* (4th ed.). Hoboken, NJ: Wiley-Blackwell.

Hall, K., & Iqbal, F. (2010). *The problem with cognitive behavioural therapy* (p. 83). London, UK: Karnac Books. Retrieved from http://books.google.com/books?id=lohLde3–3HkC&pgis=1

Hemingway, S., Stephenson, J., & Allmark, H. (2011). Student experiences of medicines management training and education. *British Journal of Nursing, 20*, 291–298. Retrieved from http://www.informaworld.com/index/739426355.pdf

Information and Statistics Division. (2011). *Antidepressant prescribing statistics.* Retrieved from www.isdscotland.org/isd/information-and-statistics.jsp?pContentID=3671&p_applic=CCC&p_service=Content.show&

Jones, M., Robson, D., Whitfield, S., & Gray, R. (2010). Does psychopharmacology training enhance the knowledge of mental health nurses who prescribe? *Journal of Psychiatric and Mental Health Nursing, 17*, 804–812. Retrieved from http://onlinelibrary.wiley.com/doi/10.1111/j.1365–2850.2010.01583.x/full

Kutchins, H., & Kirk, H. (1997). *Making us crazy. DSM: The psychiatric Bible and the creation of mental disorders.* New York, NY: Simon and Shuster.

Latter, S., Maben, J., Myall, M., & Young, A. (2007). Perceptions and practice of concordance in nurses prescribing consultations: Findings from a national questionnaire survey and case studies of practice in England. *International Journal of Nursing Studies, 44*, 9–18. doi: 10.1016/j.ijnurstu.2005.11.005

Latter, S., Sibley, A., Skinner, T. C., Cradock, S., Zinken, K. M., Lussier, M.-T., ... Roberge, D. (2010). The impact of an intervention for nurse prescribers on consultations to promote patient medicine-taking in diabetes: A mixed methods study. *International Journal of Nursing Studies, 47*, 1126–1138. doi: 10.1016/j.ijnurstu.2010.02.004

Lavelle, S., & Tusaie, K. (2011). Reflections on forced medications. *Issues in Mental Health Nursing, 32*, 274–278.

Lynch, J., Goodhart, F., Saunders, Y., & O Connor, S. J. (2010). Screening for psychological distress in patients with lung cancer: Results of a clinical audit evaluating the use of the patient Distress Thermometer. *Support Care Cancer, 19*(2):193–202. doi: 10.1007/s00520–009-0799–8

Mahone, I. H., Farrell, S., Hinton, I., Johnson, R., Moody, D., Rifkin, K.,... Barker, M. R. (2011). Shared decision making in mental health treatment: Qualitative findings from stakeholders focus groups. *Archives of Psychiatric Nursing, 25*, 27–36.

Manias, E. (2008). Complexities of communicating about managing medications—An important challenge for nurses: A response to Latter et al. (2007). *International Journal of Nursing Studies, 45*, 1110–1113. doi: 10.1016/j.ijnurstu.2008.03.006

Marland, G. R., & Cash, K. (2005). Medicine taking decisions: Schizophrenia in comparison to asthma and epilepsy. *Journal of Psychiatric and Mental Health Nursing, 12*, 163–72. doi: 10.1111/j.1365–2850.2004.00809.x

Marland, G., McKay, L., McCaig, M., & Snowden, A. (2011a). Medicine-taking and recovery-focused mental health practice. *British Journal of Wellbeing, 2*, 21–5.

Marland, G., McNay, L., Fleming, M., & Mccaig, M. (2011b). Using timelines as part of recovery-focused practice in psychosis. *Journal of Psychiatric and Mental Health Nursing, 18*, 869–877. Retrieved from http://onlinelibrary.wiley.com/doi/10.1111/j.1365–2850.2011.01738.x/full

Marland, G., McNay, L., & Snowden, A. (2011c). *Promoting concordance in mental health.* Salisbury, UK: Quay Books.

McCann, T. V., Clark, E., & Lu, S. (2008). The self-efficacy model of medication adherence in chronic mental illness. *Journal of Clinical Nursing, 17*, 329–340.

Mitchell, A. J. (2007). Pooled results from 38 analyses of the accuracy of distress thermometer and other ultra-short methods of detecting cancer-related mood disorders. *Journal of Clinical Oncology, 25*, 4670–4681.

Mitchell, A. J. (2010). Short screening tools for cancer-related distress: A review and diagnostic validity meta-analysis. *Journal of the National Comprehensive Cancer Network, 8*, 487–494. doi: 8/4/487 [pii]

Moncrieff, J. (2007). *The myth of the chemical cure: A critique of psychiatric drug treatment.* London, UK: Palgrave Macmillan.

National Panel for Psychiatric Mental Health Nurse Practitioner Competencies. (2003). *Psychiatric mental health nurse practitioner competencies.* Washington, DC: National Organization of Nurse Practitioner Faculty.

Nichol, J., Thompson, E. A., & Shaw, A. (2011). Beliefs, decision-making, and dialogue about complementary and alternative medicine (CAM) within families using CAM: A qualitative study. *Journal of Alternative and Complementary Medicine, 17*, 117–125.

Noble, D. (2002). The rise of computational biology. *Nature Reviews Molecular Cell Biology, 3*, 459–463.

Noble, D. (2006). *The music of life. Biology beyond the genome.* Oxford, UK: Oxford University Press.

Nursing and Midwifery Council. (2010). Standards for pre-registration nursing education: Your view counts. *British Journal of Nursing, 19*, 515. Retrieved from http://www.ncbi.nlm.nih.gov/pubmed/20505618

Peplau, H. E. (1952). *Interpersonal relations in nursing.* New York, NY: G. P. Putnam.

Porter, R. (2002). *Madness: A brief history.* Oxford, UK: Oxford University Press.

Richardson, A., Tebbit, B., Brown, V., & Sitzia, J. (2006). *Assessment of supportive and palliative care needs for adults with cancer.* London, UK: King's College.

Rosenstock, I. M. (1966). Why people use health services. *Milbank Memorial Fund Quarterly, 44*, 94–127.

Scottish Government. (2010). Rights, relationships and recovery: Refreshed action plan 2010–2011. *Nursing.* Retrieved from http://www.scotland.gov.uk/Resource/Doc/924/0097678.pdf

Shattell, M. M., McAllister, S., Hogan, B., & Thomas, S. P. (2006). "She took the time to make sure she understood": Mental health patients experiences of being understood. *Archives of Psychiatric Nursing, 20*, 234–41.

Snowden, A. (2008a). Medication management in older adults: A critique of concordance. *British Journal of Nursing, 17*, 114–120.

Snowden, A. (2008b). *Prescribing and mental health nursing.* Salisbury, UK: Quay Books.

Snowden, A. (2009). Classification of schizophrenia. Part 2: The nonsense of mental health illness. *British Journal of Nursing, 18*, 1228–1232. Retrieved from http://www.ncbi.nlm.nih.gov/pubmed/20081658

Snowden, A., White, C. A., Christie, Z., Murray, E., McGowan, C., & Scott, R. (2011a). The end of the algorithm: Mixed methods analysis of distress management in cancer. *RCN International Research Conference.* Harrogate, UK.

Snowden, A., White, C. A., Christie, Z., Murray, E., McGowan, C., & Scott, R. (2011b). The clinical utility of the distress thermometer: A review. *British Journal of Nursing, 20*, 220–227.

Stenner, K. L., Courtenay, M., & Carey, N. (2011). Consultations between nurse prescribers and patients with diabetes in primary care: A qualitative study of patient views. *International Journal of Nursing Studies, 48*, 37–46.

Swanson, J., & Koch, L. (2010). The role of the oncology nurse navigator in distress management of adult inpatients with cancer: A retrospective study. *Oncology Nursing Forum, 37*, 69–76.

Wills, C., & Holmes-Rovner, M. (2006). Integrating decision making and mental interventions research. *Clinical Psychology: Science and Practice, 13*, 9–25.

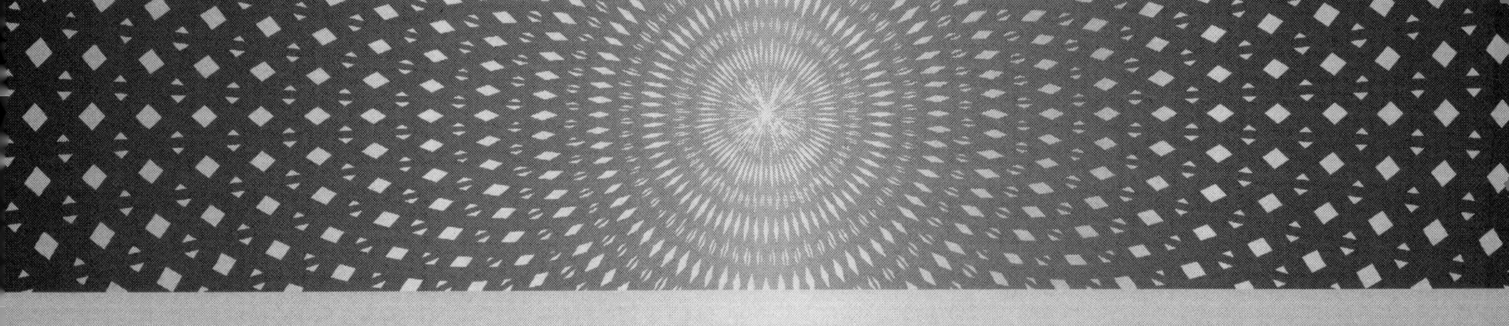

SECTION II

Foundations for Integrated Practice

CHAPTER CONTENTS

Integrative treatment is the prospective, relationship-based, client-centered, holistic approach that focuses on clients' priorities for well-being, as well as preventing, managing, and rehabilitating diseases (Deng, Weber, Sood, & Kemper, 2010). By its nature, integrative mental health treatment is broad and comprehensive, rather than reductionistic and focused on the effects of a specific treatment on a specific symptom.

This integrative approach does not consist of the haphazard selection of techniques without any overall theoretical rationale. This practice is known as syncretism, where the practitioner grabs for anything that seems to work, making no attempt to determine effectiveness. Such a lack of knowledge and skill is no better than a narrow, dogmatic approach (Lazarus, Beutler, & Norcross, 1992).

However, integrative treatment looks beyond and across the confines of a single perspective. There is the creation of a conceptual framework that synthesizes the best of several theoretical approaches under the assumption that the outcome will be richer than interventions guided by any single theory alone. By recognizing the unique contributions of each perspective, clinicians begin developing a conceptual framework that fits for themselves as well as their clients. The personal philosophical assumptions and world views of each Psychiatric Mental Health Advanced Practice Nurse (PMH-APRN) are important because these understandings influence the reality that is

CHAPTER 3

Synergy of Integrative Treatment

Kathleen R. Tusaie

perceived. Developing an integrated perspective is a lifelong process that is the product of a great deal of study, clinical practice, and theorizing.

Signs and symptoms are interpreted differently across cultures and this influences treatment approaches (Micozzi, 2011). Nursing has traditionally focused upon caring for individuals and complementary/alternative approaches use a healing approach. It is too simplistic to believe that one approach excludes another. All therapeutic approaches address some aspect of caring, curing, and healing, but the emphasis varies. For example, medicine, focused on curing, assumes all individuals with a certain diagnosis are basically the same and treatment is aimed at eliminating a single pathological process. However, complementary/alternative approaches assume all individuals are different and a unique mix of therapeutic interventions is necessary and may vary in response to the changing needs of the client. Nursing applies concepts of caring while recognizing the effectiveness of biomedical interventions for acute problems. None of these approaches are mutually exclusive and each has strengths and limitations. A holistic, integrative approach incorporates multiple explanations and treatments to maximize health.

This integrated approach to treatment represents a shift from the usual approach in Western health care. Therefore, the weaving together of psychotherapy, pharmacotherapy, and complementary/alternative approaches by Advanced Practice Psychiatric-Mental Health Nurses within the current Western health care system is a hybrid, beginning approach to integrative health care. There are several reasons this beginning shift in thinking is necessary.

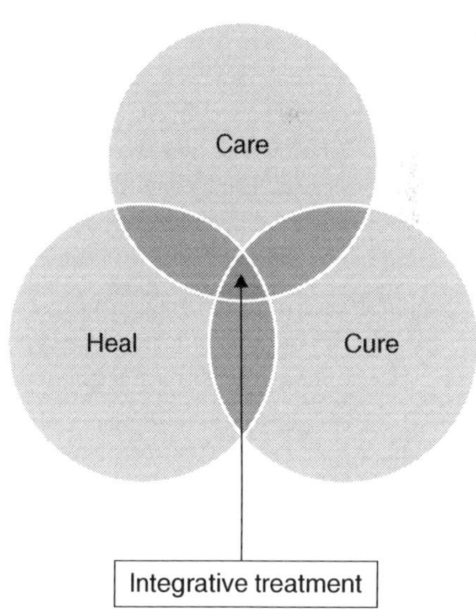

RATIONALE FOR INTEGRATED TREATMENT

First and most important, nursing practice is holistic and the phenomena of interest include not only symptoms but also health risks and health promotion. Although advanced practice focuses on a specialty area, the underlying holistic theory remains as the foundation for any intervention. Furthermore, the scope of practice in PMH-APRN is continually expanding in response to context of practice, evolution of knowledge base and the ongoing need for holistic care for clients (American Nurses Association, 2007). There have been many contextual and knowledge shifts.

One contextual shift is the increasing cost of U.S. health care in general, which is reaching a level where it will soon not be sustainable. Recent estimates show an increase from 17% of the gross domestic product (GDP) in 2009 to over 20% of the GDP in 2018, when the total cost may reach $4.35 trillion (Marshall, 2009). At the same time, effectiveness of psychopharmacology alone, the pillar of psychiatric treatment, is quite limited. It is estimated that 75% of major depressive episodes end within 6 to 15 months, but recurrence rates range from 81% to 98% within one year, and 45% within 6 years of treatment (Curry et al., 2011). Anxiety disorders are described as insidious with a chronic clinical course, low rates of recovery, and high probability of reoccurrence (Klosses & Alexopoulos, 2012). Ten years after a first psychotic episode 25% of individuals are completely recovered, 25% are improved and independent, 25% are improved but require much support, 15% are unimproved and hospitalized, and 10% are dead (Torrey, 2006). Furthermore, 80% of individuals experiencing a psychotic episode who stop their medications will relapse (National Institute of Mental Health [NIMH], 2006). This overreliance upon psychopharmacology has many consequences including failure to recognize safer and effective interventions, overestimating the value of medication to relieve suffering, and underestimating the effectiveness of psychotherapy and complementary interventions.

Furthermore, very few individuals experience only one type of psychiatric symptom. Multiple comorbidities are more the norm than the exception. Integrative treatment not only brings a greater set of interventions but an increased potential for understanding an individual's relevant experiences. An assumption of integrative care is that the wider the diagnostic lens, the more effective the diagnostic process as well as the treatment interventions. By expanding skills of PMH-APRNs to include a range of credible professional interventions and a network of referral sources, integrative practice is attainable.

Another reason integrative practice is appropriate is that psycho-physiological pathways underlying symptoms are increasingly understood to be nonlinear and multidimensional. As symptoms change in an individual there is rarely a linear pattern (Higgins, 2002). Therefore, when symptoms are acute and severity is high, a reductionist approach can effectively be applied to the symptoms. However, the acute symptoms may subside but risk return if the intervention such as psychiatric medication is removed. Along with medication, strengthening the overall system is a powerful synergistic value. For example, during a depressive episode with suicidal thoughts, antidepressants may assist in decreasing the intensity of the symptoms. However, lifestyle issues such as lack of exercise, poor nutrition, lack of sunlight as well as interpersonal conflicts and negative thinking patterns may contribute to recurrences. Therefore, psychotherapy to address these issues as well as behavior changes are necessary. If the individual is not receptive to psychotherapy or pharmacotherapy, then there are a range of other interventions available. Not all clients are willing or able to become engaged in talking therapies and/or medication. PMH-APRNs need to also think about treatment options that strengthen the individual's resilience to stressors by guiding and enhancing endogenous regulatory processes. In the ideal world, there would be systems in place and reimbursement for prevention that strengthened the individual before an acute episode, but currently research is only beginning to identify strategies to prevent recurrences.

Within this nonlinear pattern of symptom presentation, effectiveness studies have identified nonspecific elements of the helping relationship as being responsible for 75% of response to pharmacotherapy (Khan, Warner, & Brown, 2000). These nonspecific components such as hope and therapeutic alliance have been explained in detail by Hubble, Duncan, and Miller's text, *The Heart and Soul of Change: What Works in Therapy* (2006). In some studies, these nonspecific elements have been termed placebo effect. The physiology of the placebo effect is basically self-healing or nonspecific psychoneuroimmunologic stimulation activated by the context of the clinical encounter (Miller & Kaptchuk, 2008). The placebo effect has been heavily debated for years and interested readers may wish to explore the writings of Fabrizio, Wallach, Kolls, and Jonas.

Another reason that holistic, integrative thinking is important relates to the current pattern of advances in information technology. Health care information is now decentralized. There is easy access to a vast amount of health care information via Internet sources and the practitioner is not the sole information source. Of course, some of this information may be inaccurate or confusing, but access does lead to empowerment for clients. The PMH-APRN not only needs an awareness of these sources of information but also awareness of the potential influence upon a client's thinking and behavior.

For example, information on the Internet has contributed to the increased use of complementary/alternative therapies. It has been estimated that 4 in 10 Americans use complementary and alternative therapies (Institute of Medicine, 2005). However, the quality of this information varies widely and leads to potentially dangerous situations (Crone & Wise, 2000). Although the political and economic forces contributing to integration of complementary and alternative therapies vary by geographic locations, a general increase is occurring worldwide (Barrett, 2003). This shift in thinking and health care practices greatly influences client preference and adherence to treatment plans.

No matter how appropriate or cost-effective a recommended treatment is, a large percentage of outpatient clients never fill their psychotropic drug prescriptions and over 50% do not follow through with the recommended dosing pattern (Finne & Osborne, 2006; Weiden & Rao, 2005). Thus, not only is the process of reaching an agreement with a client who actively participates in treatment planning (concordance) vital, but so is offering a wide range of possible interventions.

Thomas Kuhn (1962), one of the most influential scientific philosophers of the 20th century, has stated that science does not progress via a linear accumulation of new knowledge, but undergoes periodic revolutions called paradigm shifts. These paradigm shifts do not occur easily, but only when a problem cannot be sufficiently resolved with current concepts. Shifts in thinking about health care practices do not come easily. For example, in 1911 Herrick's statement that atherosclerosis caused myocardial infarction was initially considered preposterous (Olshansky & Dossey, 2003). Perhaps this partially explains the conflicts about the need for integrative thinking and practice today.

THINKING ABOUT THE WORLD

How we think directs what we do in life as well as in clinical practice. Buck, Baldwin, and Schwartz (2005) reported that individuals who adopted mechanistic world views (all structures and functions exist as separate categories, all effects have causes that precede them) choose conventional medical treatments, while those who preferred a systems view (all structures and functions exist in context and parts interact over time), chose complementary and alternative treatments. This is a simplistic but thought provoking report.

In addition to thinking patterns, information from genomes and their derivatives are being used to make treatment decisions with the expectation of personalized treatment informed by each person's unique information (Ginsburg & Willard, 2009). At the same time, others are positing that the integration of conventional and complementary/alternative treatments is necessary for personalized treatment and this requires a shift to increasingly more complex and abstract hypotheses about how nature works and evolves (Schwartz & Schloss, 2006). These beliefs include the hypothesis that certain theories and data, by their inherent nature, cannot be visualized and may seem impossible even though they are real and termed a "mystery." The need for creativity, caring, and an exploration for discovery, not dogma, are vital for integrative treatment. Although these trends seem to be polar opposites, this is the essence of integrative treatment—applying the art and the science of advanced practice psychiatricmental health nursing. The importance of developing an awareness of your own thinking cannot be overemphasized.

TRANSDIAGNOSTIC SYNDROMES

Another result of holistic thinking is to conceptualize symptoms across diagnostic categories. There is currently no objective test to differentiate one psychiatric diagnosis from another. Signs and symptoms of psychiatric problems overlap considerably. For example, disordered mood occurs during adjustment disorders, bipolar disorder, depressive disorders, normal grief, dysthymia, and also co-occurs frequently with anxiety, many physical disorders, and substance abuse. Psychotic symptoms are experienced during mania, schizophrenia, Alzheimer's disease, and other dementias as well as during some depressions. Furthermore, disturbances of sleep, eating, and self or other directed violence characterize the behaviors of multiple diagnostic categories. Also, there are common neurobiological pathways identified in most diagnostic categories. Neurotransmitter pathways (serotonin, dopamine, norepinephrine, glutamate, gamma-aminobutyric acid), structural abnormalities identified on neuroimaging, as well as genetic predispositions cross diagnostic categories.

A clinical example of this transdiagnostic concept is that psychotropic drugs approved for treating one condition also are effective for treating other disorders. Selective serotonin reuptake inhibitors initially used for depression, now are also used for panic, social phobia, obsessive compulsive disorder (OCD), bulimia, impulse control disorders, and fibromyalgia. Anticonvulsants initially used for seizure disorders, now are found to be effective in the treatment of bipolar mania, substance abuse, impulsivity, treatment resistant anxiety, depression, and psychosis. Also atypical antipsychotics initially used for schizophrenia, now are used for bipolar mania, treatment resistant depression, OCDs, delirium, and others. These multiple efficacies indicate a shared pharmaceutical response across diagnoses. Although the concept of transdiagnostic syndromes may initially be confusing for novice PMH-APRNs, the recognition that groups of symptoms or syndromes are transdiagnostic in terms of the *Diagnostic and Statistical Manual* (DSM) is an important step in harmonizing diverse perspectives and developing the ability to provide integrative care.

The process by which integrated treatments exert efficacy across diagnostic categories has limited evidence and lacks clear answers. But, it is reasonable to use recent advances in neuroimaging as well as the time honored belief in the natural healing powers of the individual, or homeostasis. The process of neuroplasticity—synaptogenesis, dendritic spines, and neurogenesis—or modification of an individual's brain structure, may be the central process responsible for therapeutic change. This process of neuroplasticity is not a process of eliminating a specific intruding force, but more of maximizing natural healing and balance within the individual's internal environment.

The brain changes in response to external and internal stimuli including pleasant or stressful experiences and chemicals. Every encounter produces neuronal changes. These changes refurbish neurobiological structures, restoring resilience to the system that was compromised by genetic and/or environmental stressors. Perhaps by using multiple therapeutic approaches—psychotherapy, pharmacotherapy, and complementary/alternative approaches—the process of neuroplasticity may be accelerated.

EFFECTS OF INTEGRATIVE TREATMENT

Evaluating the outcomes of integrated treatment for psychiatric-mental health problems is in the beginning stages. Research for integrated approaches is broad and comprehensive, focused not only on the effects of specific treatments. However, initial studies exploring combining psychotherapy and pharmacotherapy have provided some direction for clinicians and are explored in chapters focusing upon specific syndromes.

When considering evidence to indicate additive (0.5 + 0.5 = 1.0) or synergistic (0.5 + 0.5 = 1.3) effects of integrative treatment, there are several considerations. Thase (2003) has identified statistical and pragmatic reasons why demonstration of synergy may be difficult. Use of measurements that focus only on symptom relief and not indicators of wellness do not identify higher and broader grades of response to interventions. Another problem is that the high attrition rate in studies does not allow for recognition of many who do improve and drop out. However, in one large study evaluating the combination of psychotherapy and pharmacotherapy in chronic depression, a synergistic effect was identified (Persons et al., 1996). Others have also identified the efficacy of integrating psychotherapy and pharmacotherapy (Guidi, Fava, Fava, & Papakostas, 2011). When compared to the individual effects of psychotherapy and the individual effects of pharmacotherapy, the combination resulted in more improvement than expected by an additive effect. Another recent study of individuals with bipolar illness, Systematic Treatment Enhancement Program for Bipolar Disorder (STEP-BP), identified a synergistic effect following integration of pharmacotherapy, interpersonal psychotherapy, lifestyle changes, and family sessions (NIMH, 2006). These studies demonstrate a growing trend to think about combining approaches for mental health treatment effectiveness.

Deng, Weber, Sood, and Kemper (2010) have presented a comprehensive review and suggestions for priorities in integrated health care research. They stated:

> *... it includes multidisciplinary whole system interventions, participant-centered evaluations of therapies, clinician-patient interactions, patient goals and priorities, health values and meaning, self-care, comparative effectiveness of educational and outreach strategies in promoting optimal health, environmental factors and social policies affecting health, and system factors affecting availability of resources. Research must also address patient-centered care in the context of family, culture, and community.*
>
> (Deng et al., 2010, p.144)

Priorities for research in integrated health care have been identified to include the conditions depression, anxiety, attention-deficit disorder, insomnia, and addictive disorders; therapies such as acupuncture, EEG biofeedback, and hypnosis; outcomes such as indicators of optimal functioning, satisfaction, and effects upon practitioners; epidemiological studies across the lifespan; genomic studies to investigate differences among patients with the same diagnosis; individual treatment choices by biomarkers indicative of risk, prognosis, or treatment; interventions to maximize resilience including traditional and indigenous practices; and the neurobiology of resilience and increased understanding of nonspecific placebo effects.

(pp. 155–156)

Although evidence-based practice has become popular, there are many who question the wisdom of the evidence, especially for integrated care. Failure to find effect in a randomized controlled trial cannot always be taken as lack of effectiveness. Complex interventions such as complementary and alternative approaches may best be evaluated through a circular model instead of an evidence hierarchy (Walach et al., 2006). This circular model would involve a multiplicity of methods, using different designs, counterbalancing their individual strengths and weaknesses to arrive at a pragmatic but rigorous evidence base for clinical innovation. Methods should not be viewed in terms of intrinsic worth but as valuable only in relation to the question being asked. This perspective on evidence holds the potential to bring together proponents of both traditional allopathic as well as complementary and alternative practitioners.

CONTINUUM OF TREATMENT INTERVENTIONS

When considering the use of integrated treatment, it is generally accepted to conceptualize a continuum for symptoms as well as interventions. First, the degree of risk for a disorder is determined and then progression to minimal, moderate, and severe level of symptoms in a linear or non linear fashion. The continuum of interventions begins with health promotion activities such as increasing knowledge, self-help strategies, guided self-help including lifestyle change, and over-the-counter medications or herbals. Next, the interventions move toward professional disease management with formal interventions (Figure 3-1). As the severity and number of symptoms vary in a nonlinear fashion, so do the interventions.

Psychotherapy and pharmacotherapy target different sites in the cortico-limbic pathway. Psychotherapy is believed to enhance the function of the prefrontal cortex (PFC) and then down to the limbic system in a top-down manner, while pharmacotherapy starts at the limbic system and works up to the PFC in a bottom-up pattern (Cozolino, 2002; Drevets, 2007). Many complementary/alternative therapies have multiple effects. The specifics of these interventions are explored in chapters focusing upon specific syndromes or symptom clusters.

A protocol to ensure safe and effective integration of complementary and alternative approaches within mental

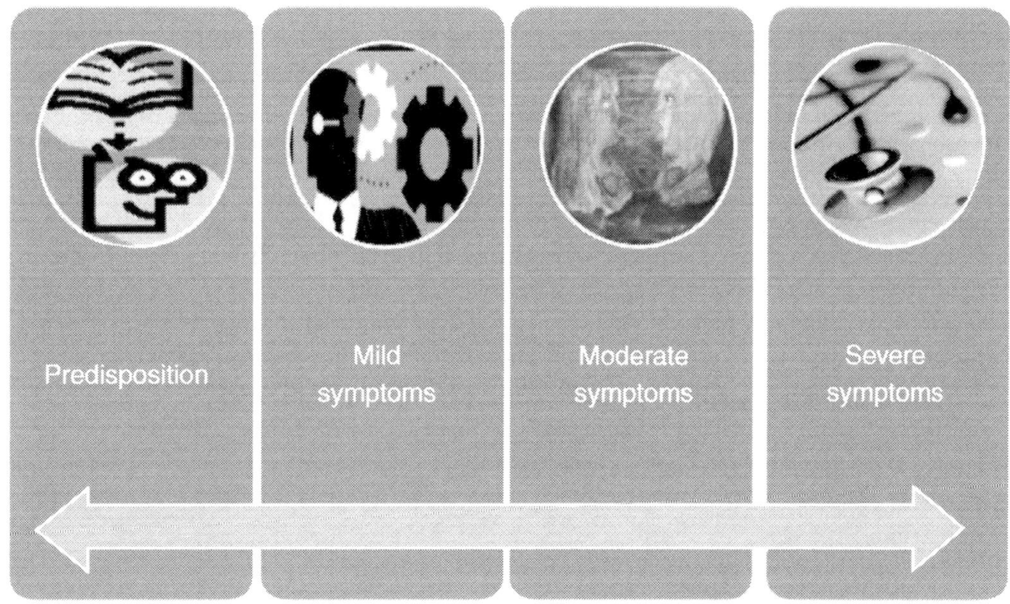

Figure 3-1 Treatment Continuum. Health Promotion to Disease Management

health care has been developed and implemented in a Dutch mental health center. See Figure 3-2 for details of this protocol.

There are many prejudices interfering with the integration of complementary and alternative approaches within mental health care. Common prejudices against complementary and alternative approaches include the following myths (1) only a few people use complementary and alternative approaches, (2) clients do not talk about using complementary/alternative approaches, (3) complementary/alternative approaches are only used if conventional approaches, do not work (4) they are not effective and (5) complementary/alternative approaches or they are not professionally respected approaches. However, the fact that clients do not discuss the use of complementary/alternative approaches, simply indicates the need for more specific questioning by mental health providers and often a good relationship between the client and the Complementary/alternative care provider is the basis for seeking this care. Furhtermore, the belief that these approaches are not effective has been dispelled by the fact that the World Health Organization has endorsed many of these practices.

Prejudices in favor of the use of complementary and alternative approaches include the belief that research is not needed, they have been used safely (bias and placebo needs identified by current standards as knowledge evolves), effects cannot be proven (science can be applied to all phenomena, the right design is needed), and natural substances are healthy (there are many toxins in nature).

To approach this issue clinically, a mental health center in the Netherlands, Lentis, formed a Center for Integrative Psychiatry (CIP) in 2006 (Hoenders et al., 2011). It consists of an outpatient clinic, a research department, an educational department, and an annual conference. Conventional psychiatric interventions as well as complementary interventions that are proven to be safe and effective are offered. Those include St. John's wort for mild-moderate depression, valerian for insomnia, relaxation for anxiety, mindfulness-based stress reduction, mindfulness-based cognitive-behavioral therapy for depression, massage for stress, anxiety, depression; exercise for anxiety, depression, insomnia; single vitamins as supplements to antidepressants (Vitamin D, folic acid); s-adenosyl methionine (SAMe) for depression; melantonin for sleep problems; inositol for depression, panic, OCD; and dietary changes for depression.

Following the identification of the complementary interventions, a protocol with an algorithm was developed. (see Figure 3-2). Complementary/alternative approaches were only offered if a conventional interventions were offered before or at least advised and if there was no danger if patient refused conventional treatment. Then treatment is provided by an external network of practitioners in conjunction with treatment at CIP. Criteria for CA providers included being members of their professional organizations with procedures for complaints and malpractice, following guidelines of their professional organizations, keeping legal files, having the office meets hygiene and privacy needs, maintaining monthly contact between CIP and provider, and agreeing to participate in evaluation.

This approach to integrative mental health is expected to not only protect against quackery, abuse, and false hope but also to add to the evidence of effectiveness. This approach has been a response to clients' needs and wishes while respecting their freedom of choice.

Chapter 6 includes discussion of complementary and alternative approaches in more detail. But if you do not have a formal protocol available in your practice, you may consider the following suggestions for selecting providers of alternative/complementary health care for yourself and/or your clients.

First, increase your knowledge base for complementary and alternative health care approaches through conferences, reading, or courses. Understand the purpose as well as adverse effects of the approaches. Be aware of the realistic outcomes of treatment. Next, shop for local providers and determine appropriate credentials (education, certification, license). This may be accomplished by talking to individuals at local support groups, health food stores, or professional organizations or schools. There are many Healing Touch Associations and the American Holistic Nurses Association (www.ahna.org/) can provide training or referral information. Once you tap into the complementary/alternative network in your area, you will find many providers. It is best to meet providers face to face, discuss their practices and beliefs, and receive their services yourself (massage, healing touch, etc.) for your own evaluation before you make a referral to clients. After meeting the practitioner, determine if you would be comfortable in a partnership with this individual and if you think the environment and cost was reasonable.

When making the referral, there are responsibilities for the PMH-APRN. First, explore the client's

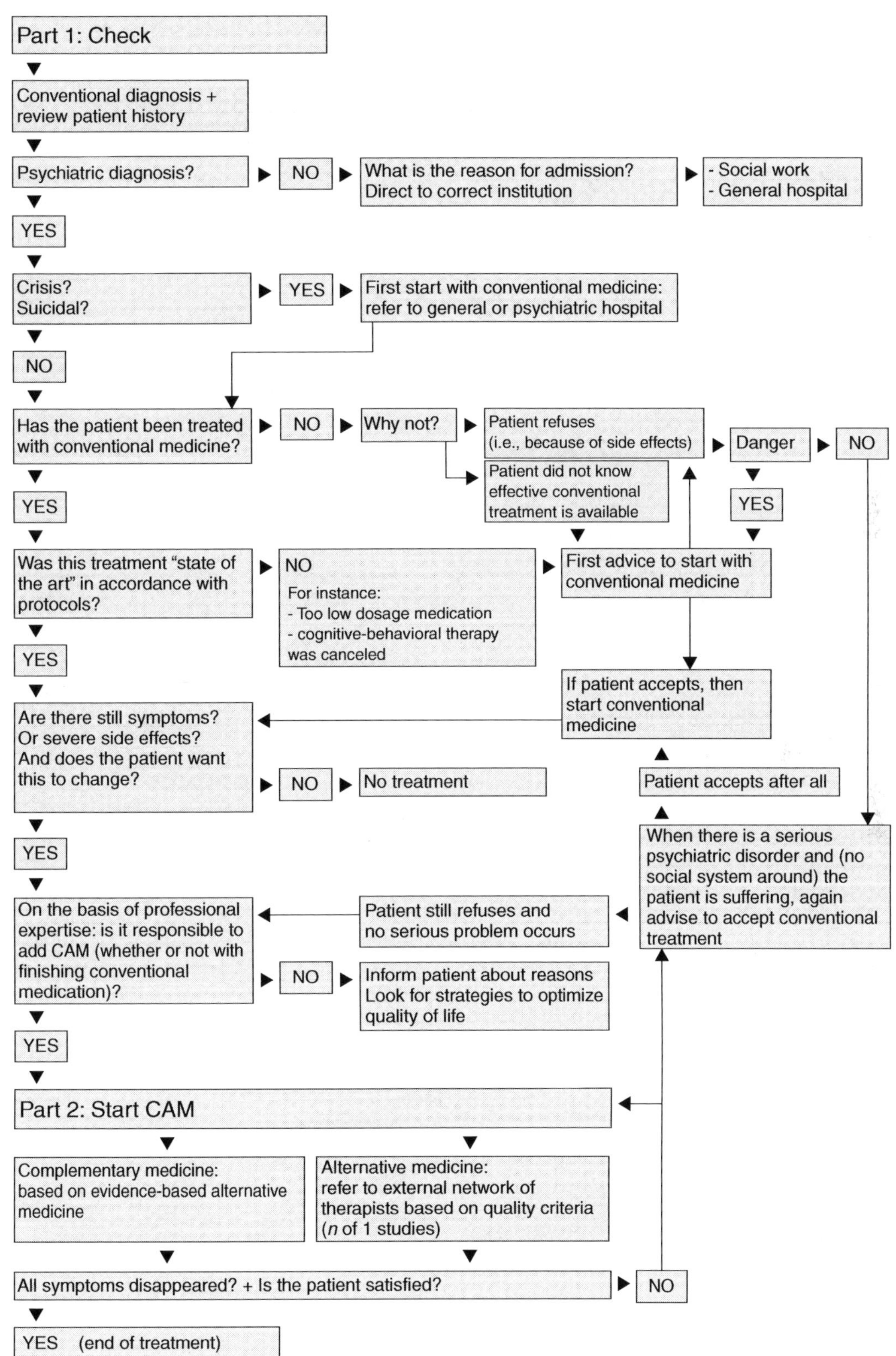

Figure 3-2 Complementary and Alternative Medicine Protocol for the Center for Integrative Psychiatry

Source: Reprinted from Hoenders et al. (2011).

understanding of his or her symptoms and expectations from the complementary/alternative provider. Then provide resources for information and discuss the evidence of effectiveness. Monitor the client's response and have the client keep a journal of subjective and objective outcomes. Advise the client about the possibility of unpleasant sensations or thoughts emerging and the importance of discussing these with the CA provider and/or you. Encourage the client not to substitute CA for conventional treatment but to integrate and discuss possible interactions or contraindications. Stress the importance of open communication among both providers, but maintain confidentiality. Some insurance plans are reimbursing for complementary/alternative approaches and the client should be assisted with exploring the possibility of reimbursement.

Currently, most nursing programs include information on alternative and complementary health care, and the increasing numbers of mental health clients seeking relief from chronic conditions with complementary and alternative approaches indicate the trend toward integrative care. With this shifting paradigm there are concomitant responsibilities for PMH-APRNs to increase their understanding and use of these approaches to maximize clients' wellness.

REFERENCES

American Nurses Association. (2007). *Psychiatric-mental health nursing: Scope and standards of practice*. Silver Springs, MD: Author.

Barrett, B. (2003). Alternative, complementary and conventional medicine: Is integration upon us? *Journal of Alternative and Complementary Medicine, 9*, 417–427.

Buck, T., Baldwin, C. M., & Schwartz, G. E. (2005). Influence of worldview on healthcare choices among persons with chronic pain. *Journal of Alternative and Complementary Medicine, 11*, 561–568.

Cozolino, L. (2002). *The neuroscience of psychotherapy: Building and rebuilding the human brain.* New York, NY: Norton.

Crone, C., & Wise, T. (2000). Complementary medicine. In P. R. Muskin (Ed.), *Complementary and alternative medicine and psychiatry* (pp. 199–240). Washington, DC: American Psychiatric Press.

Curry, J. et al (2011). Recovery and recurrence following treatment for adolescent major depression. *Archives of Psychiatric Nursing, 68*(3), 263–269.

Deng, G., Weber, W., Sood, A., & Kemper, K. (2010). Research on integrative healthcare: Context and priorities. *Explore, 6*, 143–158.

Drevets, W. (2007). Orbitofrontal cortex function and structure in depression. *Annals of the New York Academy of Sciences, 1121,* 499–527. doi:10.1196/annals.1401.029

Finne, D., & Osborne, F. (2006). Stages of change for psychiatric medication adherence and substance cessation. *Archives of Psychiatric Nursing, 20*, 166–174.

Ginsburg, G. & Willard, H. (2009). Genomic and personalized medicine: Foundations and applications. *Translational Research, 154*(6), 277-287.

Guidi, J., Fava, G., Fava, M., & Papakostas, G. (2011). Efficacy of sequential integration of psychotherapy and pharmacotherapy in major depressive disorder: A preliminary meta-analysis. *Psychological Medicine, 41*, 321–331.

Higgins, J.P. (2002). Nonlinear systems in medicine. *Yale Journal of Biological Medicine, 75*, 247–260.

Hoenders, H. J. R, , Appelo, M. T., van den Brink, E. H., Hartogs, B. M. A., & de Jong, J. T. V. M. (2011). The Dutch Complementary and Alternative Medicine (CAM) Protocol: To ensure the safe and effective use of complementary and alternative medicine within Dutch Mental Health Care. *Journal of Alternative and Complementary Medicine, 17*, 3.

Hubble, M., Duncan, B., & Miller, S. (2006). *The heart and soul of change: What works in therapy.* Washington, DC: The American Psychological Association.

Institute of Medicine. (2005). *Committee on the use of complementary and alternative medicine by the American public. Complementary and Alternative Medicine in the United States.* Washington, DC. The National Academies Press.

Khan, A., Warner, H., & Brown, W. (2000). Symptom reduction and suicide risk in patients treated with placebo in antidepressant clinical trials: An analysis of the Food and Drug Administration database. *Archives of General Psychiatry, 57*, 311–317.

Klosses, D. & Alexopoulos,G. (2012). The prognostic significance of subsyndromal symptoms emerging after remission of late life depression. *Psychological Medicine, 21*, 1–10.

Kuhn, T. (1962). *The structure of scientific revolutions*. Chicago, IL: University of Chicago Press.

Lazarus, A., Beutler, L., & Norcross, J. (1992). The future of technical eclecticism. *Psychotherapy, 29*(1), 11–20.

Marshall, E. (2009). Science and the stimulus. Medicine under the microscope. *Science, 326*, 1183–1185.

Micozzi, M. (2011). *Fundamentals of complementary and alternative medicine*. St. Louis, MO: Saunders Elsevier.

Miller, F., & Kaptchuk, T. (2008). The power of context: Reconceptualizing the placebo effect. *Journal of Social Medicine, 101*, 222–225.

National Institute of Mental Health. (2006). Early Findings from largest NIMH-funded research program on bipolar disorder begins to build evidence-base for best treatment options. *Science Update.* Retrieved from http://www.google.com/search?sourceid=navclient&aq=0h&oq=&ie=UTF-8&rlz=1T4SKPT_enUS410US411&q=nimh+step-bp+study

Olshansky, B., & Dossey, L. (2003). Retroactive prayer: A preposterous hypothesis? *British Medical Journal, 327*, 1465–1468.

Persons, J., Thase, M., & Crits-Christoph, P. (1996). The role of psychotheapy in the treatment of depression. *Archives of General Psychiatry, 53*(4), 283–290.

Schwartz, G., & Schloss, E. (2006). World hypotheses and evolution of integrative medicine: Combining categorical diagnoses and cause-effect interventions with whole systems research and nonvisualizable (seemingly impossible) healing. *Explore, 2*, 509–514.

Thase, M. (2003). Effectiveness of antidepressants: Comparative remission rates. *Journal of Clinical Psychiatry, 64* (Suppl 2), 3–7.

Torrey, E.F. (2006). *Surviving schizophrenia* (5th ed.). London, UK: Quell Publishers.

Walach, H., Falkenberg, T., Fonnebo, V., Lewith, G., & Jonas, W.(2006). Circular instead of heirarchial: Methosological principles for the evaluation of complex interventions. *BMC Medical Research Methodology, 6*(29), 1186–1471.

Weiden, P., & Rao, N. (2005). Teaching medication compliance to psychiatric residents. *Academic Psychiatry, 29*, 2.

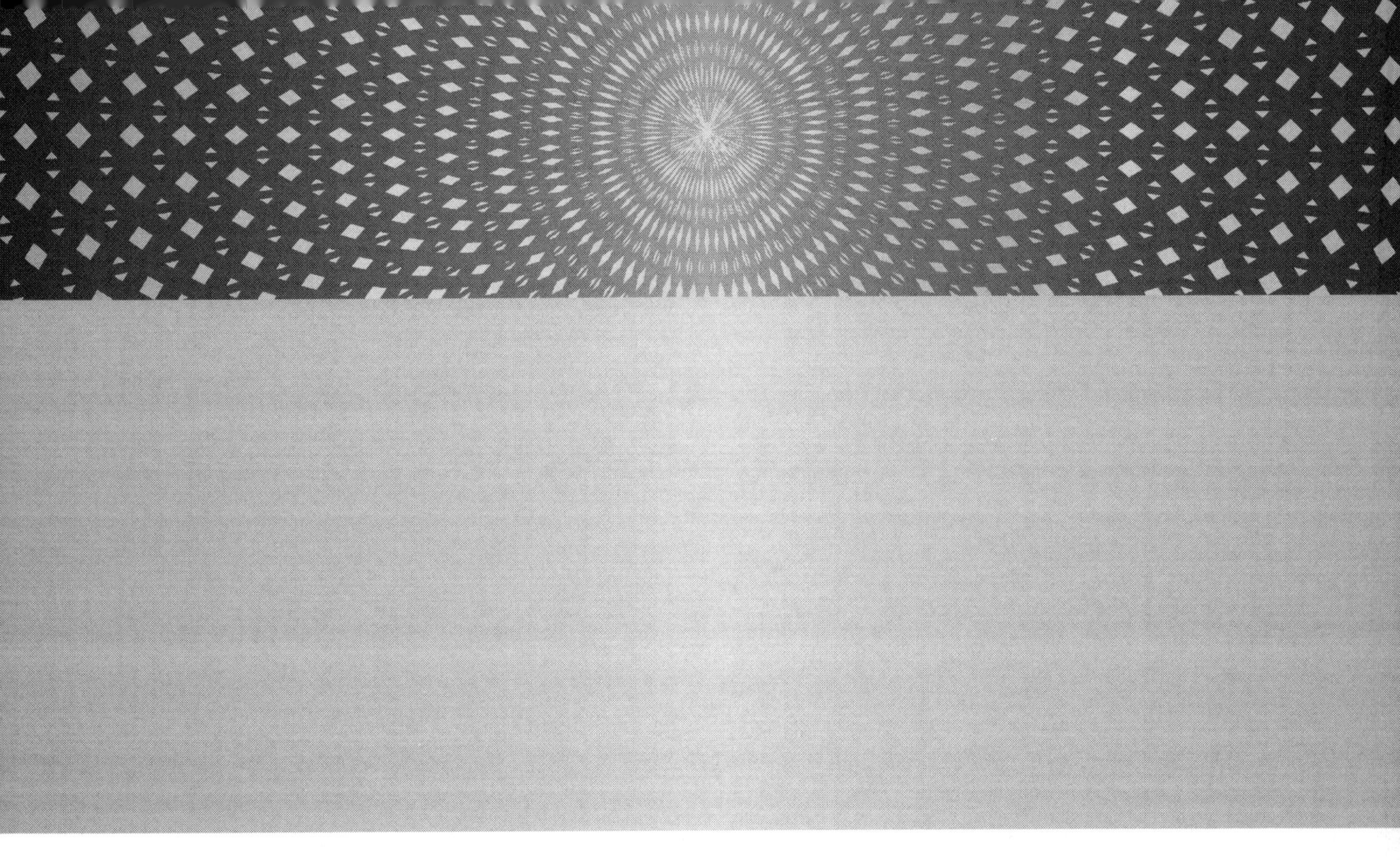

CHAPTER CONTENTS

Psychotherapy has been defined in many ways. Frank (1982) characterized psychotherapy as a practice where the clinician aims to relieve distress or disability using a particular intervention that is grounded in a defined theory. Frank goes on to explain that the clinician performing the intervention must have training in delivering this type of therapy.

This chapter presents the principles that support the fundamental models of psychotherapy. These include an array of therapy schools and intervention techniques. Each involves understandings of the mechanism of change and assumptions about the origins of the patient's psychological distress (Gurman & Messer, 2003). For example, cognitive therapies aim to change the way one thinks. The individual's distress is seen to arise from a particular pattern of thinking about self in situations and the resultant response (Beck, 1995). Cognitive techniques offer a system for practicing new thought patterns in response to affectively charged situations. The mechanism of change operates on the assumption that once maladaptive cognitive patterns are identified, new patterns of thinking can be developed, become ingrained in one's response network, and then be more readily used in situations demanding a response (Hazlett-Stevens & Craske, 2002). These new patterns of thinking will yield a more adaptive response since the individual takes in information about situations without a negative or restricting cognitive bias.

Contrast this framework with a behavioral approach that proposes that change is brought about by altering

CHAPTER 4

Overview of Psychotherapy

Kathleen R. Delaney and Ricardo Broach

the reinforcement pattern for a particular behavior generating problems for the individual. The assumption is that a behavior that is reinforced is more likely to occur (Hebert, 1981). In therapy the troublesome behavior is isolated along with its stimulus and reinforcer. Clients are then provided techniques for decoupling this stimulus-response or response-reinforcer pattern. For instance, they might be guided through mindfully suppressing their usual response to an anxiolytic stimulus by relaxing or shifting attention away from the situation. Armed with an alternative response, clients might be encouraged to either intentionally envision a triggering situation or become aware when they are in a situation that stimulates a troublesome (conditioned) response. The focus of change is on extinguishing the troublesome stimulus-response pattern. This explanation of two therapy schools illustrates how different assumptions about behavior and the mechanisms of change usher in specific techniques to target relief of the distress.

In this chapter, for each model the implicit or explicit assumptions around the cause of a client's distress, the rationale for why a method should relieve it, and the techniques used to put the intervention in motion are presented. For example, the therapy might employ a teaching-coaching method, a supportive-interpersonal process, or a person-centered approach. In Frank's (1971) view all share a common element in that the techniques transmit the therapist's influence in focusing the patient on a particular strategy to relieve distress. In the process of enacting this process element, therapists are implicitly or explicating weaving in their view of the problem as well as the accompanying theory of why the problem has occurred.

There exist some 150 to 250 schools of psychotherapy (www.goodtherapy.org/types-of-therapy.html). In spite of this plurality, it is increasingly popular to view the various therapies as basically operating in a similar manner, the so-called common factors approach (see Exhibit 4-1). While acknowledging the ascendency of the common factors approach, in this chapter we emphasize the basic differences in how therapy is approached depending on the model employed. In line with this goal, we provide an overview of four major therapy models: dynamic, cognitive, interpersonal, and behavioral, including the so-called third generation, mindfulness-based behavioral therapies. For each school of therapy the emphasis is on the proposed process of change (i.e., theoretically why patients improve), what mental functions are to change, how that change is possible, and what select therapy techniques promote the desired change.

DYNAMIC THERAPY

Psychodynamic psychiatry is often associated with a psychoanalytic approach. This representation is misguided since the techniques and schools of psychoanalytic therapy have broadened beyond traditional Freudian

EXHIBIT 4-1: COMMON FACTORS APPROACH TO PSYCHOTHERAPY

The notion that basic elements operate in all forms of psychotherapy is now depicted as the common factors approach. These common factors are framed as the extent to which these elements of therapy influence its outcomes. The common factors idea emerged from integrated research reviews of psychotherapy, which illustrated there was little difference in the outcomes of various schools of therapy (Luborsky et al., 2002). In line with this idea, common factors of therapy were isolated. A popular model maintains that client outcomes could be attributed to four common factors that therapy models share: client and extra therapeutic effects (such as the client's social support system), client-therapist relationship factors, hope/expectancy, and finally, the model or technique (Hubble, Duncan, & Miller, 1999). Thus, while students become acquainted with the various schools of therapy and the accompanying techniques, they should also keep in mind that the relationship factors, how one forms an alliance and how hope is restored, are powerful moderators of therapy outcomes regardless of the technique (behavioral, cognitive, dynamic) used (Norcross, 2002; Perraud et al., 2006).

methods. One way to organize the numerous variations that operate on the basic assumptions of a psychoanalytic approach (though not necessarily the techniques) is to consider them dynamic therapies (Gabbard, 2005). In typifying this model of therapy, the term dynamic indicates a common thread operating with a psychodynamic or dynamic model,[1] that is, a view of symptoms and behaviors as reflections of an unconscious process. In a classic psychoanalytic *conflict model*, the unconscious process is depicted as the client's need to keep an idea and associated affect out of awareness, a feat accomplished by employing a variety of defense mechanisms, particularly repression (Wolitzky, 2005). In line with this thinking, the troublesome behaviors that prompt clients to seek treatment are viewed as a reflection of an unconscious process.

Variations of psychoanalytic treatment have branched from this conflict model, the foremost being a *deficit model* where symptoms/behaviors are seen as a reflection of weak or absent psychic structures, ones that allow a person to feel whole or secure in a variety of situations (Gabbard, 2005). Defenses and how they unconsciously operate are core ideas of psychoanalytic psychiatry within both the conflict and deficit model. Our broader concern is the entire dynamic school of therapy, which encompasses not only psychoanalysis but psychoanalytically informed psychotherapy, and dynamic supportive therapy (Wolitzky, 2005) (see Figure 4-1). We clarify the distinction between these variations within the dynamic school by explaining how dynamic-oriented therapists use a particular lens (seeing behavior as a reflection of an unconscious process) but approach other elements of therapy quite differently. Specifically, these therapists emphasize transference/resistance and a reliance on the leverage of the therapeutic relationship differently.

PSYCHOANALYTIC PSYCHIATRY

While there are several variations of psychoanalytic psychiatry (e.g., Jungian, Kohutian) they share a common point of origin, that is, the work of Freud. For the last 100 years, the ideas of Freud have undergone interpretation and modification. Most readers know Freud's theory of psychosexual development, for example, oral, anal, and phallic phases, and how conflict at any one of these stages gives rise to anxiety and behaviors typical of arrested development. While grounded in Freudian theory, Melanie Klein introduced a different notion of how the infant proceeds through psychic development, one strongly influenced by interactions with the maternal figure (the object) and the infant's experiences that allow early (primitive) fantasies to be worked through and overtaken by more realistic representations of nurturing figures (Segal, 1973). There are many variations on Freudian thought; this chapter is limited to the explanation of traditional psychoanalysis explicated in the Freudian school and its elements are drawn from a chapter by Wolitzky (2005).

Wolitzky (2005) traces Freud's interest in the unconscious to his work with individuals racked by intense emotions, ones that surfaced as physical symptoms, for example, paralysis, blindness, convulsions. Using hypnosis, Freud then moved to placing his hands on the

[1] As Gabbard notes, these terms are used interchangeably. For the purposes of this chapter, the term dynamic will be used.

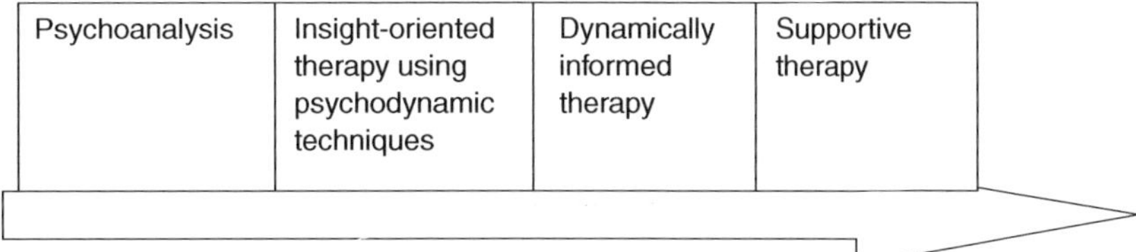

Figure 4-1 Continuum of Dynamic Therapy

patient's forehead and, with the use of pressure, attempted to help the individual remember the experience associated with the onset of symptoms (Wolitzky, 2005). These early interventions gave way to Freud's belief in free associations and a theory of mind encompassing the drives, conflicts, and defenses that were manifest in behavior. In Freud's early approach, he uncovered patients' thinking until they arrived at the core conflict, which often uncovered the memory or experience the patient had been attempting to repress. The core principles of Freudian psychiatry are summarized by Wolitzky:

- Psychic determinism (all mental phenomena have causes)
- The existence of the unconscious
- Motivation for behavior is to maximize pleasure/minimize pain or avoid excessive stimulation
- Inner conflict is inevitable given the existence of drives
- Behavior is viewed in terms of psychosexual stages, coping, and defense mechanisms
- The organization of the tripartite apparatus (id, ego, and superego)

Traditional analytic methods operate within a structure where clients free associate (lying on a couch facing away from the therapist promotes the process) and via interpretation, particularly of the transference/resistance, clients eventually arrive at insights into their difficulties. While working with clients exhibiting conversion-like symptoms, Freud initially postulated that with this insight came a cathartic release of affect and as the blocked wish or memory was reabsorbed, symptoms disappeared (Breur & Freud, 1895). Wolitzky points out that as Freud's theory of intrapsychic conflict came into prominence, psychoanalysis became focused on helping clients understand how they played out past conflicts (related to important phases of psychosexual development) in the present; particularly in response to the therapist. This introduced transference and countertransference, phenomena that continue to be viewed as fundamental processes in many therapy relationships (see Exhibit 4-2).

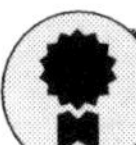

EXHIBIT 4-2: TRANSFERENCE

Transference originated with Freud, who came to see the phenomena as a tool of the analytic process, useful in examining how the client's relationships with important early figures were reenacted in the therapy relationship (Joseph, 1985). In various forms, the idea of transference arises in psychodynamic therapy, thought of as the client's patterns of expectations with significant others, developed over time, that become mobilized in response to situations that resemble the original condition (Basch, 1980). For example, a client who had been repeatedly disappointed in his bids for parental attention comes into therapy, and after some time, may begin to interpret behaviors of the therapist as failing to acknowledge what he is saying about his life. The client then begins to feel both disappointed and ashamed at exposing these needs to the therapist. The client's negative responses towards the therapist may have more to do with these childhood experiences (and attendant emotions) than the actual behavior of the therapist. Should the therapist fail to recognize this transference, but instead see the client's negativity as a sign of his or her failing (countertransference), the clinician may begin to defend his or her actions and thus fail to respond to the client's deeper conflict. Gallop and O'Brien (2003) argue that concepts such as transference are particularly valuable to psychiatric nurses who interact with clients with the aim of developing a meaningful sense of the client. This empathic position necessitates understanding how the client's response is colored by past experiences as well as their contemporary need for support.

When the examination of transference became the centerpiece of the therapeutic process, client improvement was no longer defined in terms of the cathartic release but a slightly different process: "As the patient gradually reduces the neurotic vicious cycle that characterizes his or her prior adaptive efforts, he or she will experience this change as involving an expanded sense of personal agency or freedom" (Wolitzky, 2005, p. 38). Thus, as the client's formerly unconscious conflict is viewed in the light of current reality and gradually resolved, the individual's responses (particularly in interpersonal interactions) are no longer dominated by the festering unrealistic wishes but now approached in a more reality oriented, adaptive manner. This basic understanding of traditional psychoanalytic therapy captures the essence of how the therapist works with an unconscious process to bring about change.

The interested student might explore other versions of psychoanalytic therapy and note differences in how symptoms are interpreted, the techniques to address them, and the underlying healing process. For instance, Kohut, originally a disciple of Freud, maintained the Freudian notion that turmoil operated at the unconscious level and was played out in a repetitive pattern of maladaptive interpersonal interactions. However, Kohut's methods operate from a deficit model, particularly with the concept that patients' problems in living were best understood as a lack of psychic structure needed to maintain a healthy sense of self. In Kohut's view these structural deficits arose from early relationships with key figures that had failed to help the infant tame the primitive (early) wish to be the center of the interpersonal universe (Wolf, 1988). Indeed, at two years old the toddler operates from developmentally appropriate narcissism, expecting the mother to respond to his/her wishes/needs as readily as their hand moves when they want to reach out and grab an object.

In Kohut's view the taming of this primitive narcissism gave way to a realistic view of the self in the world, with caregivers helping the toddler establish relationships and activities that sustained a balanced sense of self or self-esteem (Elson, 1987). Sometimes, however, these early wishes are maintained, albeit unconsciously, and the client strives to reexperience that sense of being held as perfect or experience the therapist as an all-knowing person capable of enacting this omnipotent role (Wolf, 1988). In Kohutian therapy a transference is seen to evolve, one grounded in the client's mirroring (the need to be positively regarded by the therapist) or idealizing needs (the need to see the therapist as calm, strong, wise). Here the process of change rests not with exploring the transference, but via transmuting internalization; a process where the functions supplied by the therapist (observing, affirming, clarifying, balancing) gradually become absorbed by the client as self functions (Kohut, 1984).

Elson (1988), a Kohutian therapist, tells a story of a client she had seen for some time who needed considerable help to buffer intense emotions and summon a sense of adequacy when confronted by challenges. In therapy the client displayed progress in taking on these self-functions (particularly emotional regulation). When Elson is about to leave on vacation she voices her concern that the client may be impacted by the loss of structure therapy provides. The client responds: "That's okay; I will keep an eye on myself for a while." Elson used this vignette to illustrate that the patient had, to some degree, internalized the affirming, supportive, and regulation functions provided in therapy. Kohut's idea of the cohesive self and the surrounding of experiences needed to sustain cohesion are valuable concepts for viewing the instances when patients report they are "falling apart." Kohut and others such as Winnicott, Klein, and Hartmann are considered to have proposed variations on traditional psychoanalytic therapy.

How do therapists formulate a sense of this unconscious process if they do not use psychoanalytic techniques? Gabbard (2005) explains that dynamically informed therapists draw upon an in-depth assessment of the patient to organize case conceptualizations and the accompanying goals of therapy. A dynamic assessment is one that considers not just symptoms and behaviors but the client's life history, experiences the client defines as critical, and elements of the client's internal world such as dreams, hopes, fears, and self-definitions (Gabbard, 2005). Interestingly, these elements of the dynamic formulation are seen as components of nursing's therapy framework and assessment (Bjorklund, 2008; Wheeler, 2008a). Dynamically informed therapies include a wide range of relational approaches (Curtis & Hirsch, 2003) and methods to examine key elements such as defenses and transference. One exemplar of a dynamically informed therapy was developed by Basch (1988).

In Basch's classic book, *Understanding Psychotherapy,* the influence of Kohut, attachment theory, and a psychoanalytically informed developmental theory are evident. Basch weaves together these theories to develop a therapy that seeks to restore a client's sense of competence and esteem, a process he depicts as reengaging with the developmental spiral. He strongly endorses a client's affect as the gateway to their inner conflicts and encourages therapists to follow both affect shifts and the client's attempts to defend against experiencing affect. Using a series of case examples, Basch explains how he used empathic immersion into clients' stories to arrive at formulations of their difficulties, particularly how anxiety-avoidance influenced their approaches to decisions and negatively impacted on a sense of competency. In Basch's model, the therapist suggests to clients when and how these unconscious defenses arise and how they block decisions that would lead to flexible and adaptive functioning. Thus, Basch's therapy system is clearly rooted in dynamic principles, such as developing a dynamic formulation of the client's difficulties, a developmental view of structure building, and a sense of the prominent defenses. But the techniques used to uncover the core difficulty and encourage functioning rely on an active therapist, support, and an interpretive approach aimed at fostering the client's insight.

Gabbard's (2005) supportive therapy (see Figure 4-1) is categorized as dynamic, which may seem contrary to the popular conception of supportive therapy as "empathic common sense." There is debate in the literature as to exactly what techniques define supportive therapy (Douglas, 2008). However, for the purpose of this discussion, we place supportive therapy on the dynamic continuum, recognizing that when one supports a client in therapy it should be planned with an understanding of exactly what emotional and mental functions need support (Schlesinger, 1969). In line with this thinking, when Misch (2000) outlines the basic strategies of dynamic supportive therapy, first on his list is the need for a formulation, the therapist's theory of what is "wrong" with the client. This case formulation is a roadmap of how the client's issues reflect how he/she thinks, believes, and acts; a self system built over the years via interactions with significant others and defining experiences (McWilliams, 1999).

Several elements of Misch's (2000) dynamic supportive framework fit with a commonsense notion of how one is supportive, including the amount of guidance that is offered, the importance of the alliance, and providing a sense of safety and containment. Misch also includes the psychodynamic idea that in supportive therapy the clinician is lending psychic structure to the patient, functions such as problem-solving skills, affect modulation strategies, and impulse control. Misch's framework instructs that supportive therapy is not a "kind" shoulder but interventions based on a theory of therapy (what supports the patient needs, why they are needed, and how the therapist will supply them). Also critical is the therapist's understanding of how the treatment process relates to its outcomes; for example, improved daily functioning, decreased impulse control, and improved stress inoculation. Supportive therapy fits well with the nursing paradigm; the approach aligns with the idea of assessing the level and extent of patient's needs and targeting interventions based on both the individual's narrative and need for external resources/structure (Wheeler, 2008).

COGNITIVE THERAPY

Most psychiatric nurses have used basic cognitive strategies; for example, pointing out to depressed clients instances of their negative cognitive bias or guiding the anxious client to question unrealistic fears. Psychiatric nurses are accustomed to using protocols that are based on cognitive approaches, often labeled as cognitive-behavioral interventions (CBT). The term CBT reflects that cognitive and behavioral interventions are somewhat reciprocal, changes in thinking will foster behavior change, and improved behaviors will influence thinking (Knapp & Beck, 2008). Rachman (1997) believes that a merger of the cognitive and behavioral schools evolved as cognitive therapists began to employ behavioral techniques, particularly in the treatment of panic disorder. It is also logical to connect these two forms of treatment since often cognitive interventions target thinking as well as the behaviors, or as is common, the same intervention affects thoughts as well as behaviors. In this section, the focus is on the cognitive component of CBT and the assumptions, structure, and proposed mechanisms of cognitive techniques.

While Aaron Beck is thought of as the father of cognitive therapy, other important theories emerged in the 20th century that laid the foundation for his innovations, particularly social learning theory. Social learning theorists detoured from the prevailing behaviorist approach to psychological issues and declared explanations for human behaviors were more than stimulus-response sequences (Miller & Dollard, 1941). They maintained that we learn how to think about social situations by *observing* how others think and behave. As social learning theory evolved, additional concepts were added to the model, particularly the concept of triadic reciprocal determinism, that is, the influence of cognitions, behavior, and environment on behavior (Bandura, 1989). This concept of social cognitive theory held that it is not just the unconscious or stimuli that prompt behavior but also the input of expectations (cognitive factors), one's own *self-efficacy beliefs* (behavioral influence), and environmental factors, such as encouragement (Bandura, 2004). These threads come into play in interventions such as motivational interviewing (see Exhibit 4-3).

Against this theoretical background cognitive therapy was launched, a treatment paradigm that postulated psychological distress should be examined in light of how

EXHIBIT 4-3: MOTIVATIONAL INTERVIEWING

Motivational interviewing is a counseling approach that has been studied extensively and is quickly acquiring evidence supporting its effectiveness (Rubak, Sandbaek, Lauritzen, & Christensen, 2005). Designed in the 1990s to address issues of clients with alcohol use, the techniques aim to engage the client's motivational system by a negotiation-type process. The client is first guided to articulate the costs and benefits of change (Treasure, 2004). The stance of the therapist is critical in motivational interviewing; it is nonconfrontational yet focused on helping clients think differently about their current behaviors and see the potential benefits of change. The therapist accomplishes this exploration of change via four central interaction principles, (a) use of empathy to convey understanding of the client's perspective, (b) helping clients see the discrepancy between how they are currently living and how they want their lives to be, (c) accepting a client's reluctance to change as natural, and (d) supporting self-efficacy (Miller & Rollnick, 2002). Motivational interviewing is successful in prompting positive change because once clients reach an image of how they would like to be seen by others, the therapeutic techniques support and encourage a client's own motivation and encourage small steps towards change (Treasure, 2004). Motivational interviewing is applicable to a wide range of treatment and health promotion issues that psychiatric nurses address (Levensky, Forcehimes, O'Donohue, & Beitz, 2007).

clients take in and process information. When Beck introduced cognitive therapies he hypothesized that at the core of psychiatric syndromes such as anxiety and depression was a systematic bias in thinking, particularly the way situations were interpreted (Hollon & Beck, 1994). He found that by helping patients uncover these biases and practice alternative ways of thinking, patients' symptoms improved and, with training in cognitive reframing skills, the improvements were sustained. Beck's daughter (1995) detailed how psychiatric disorders such as depression and anxiety, while not caused by the way one thinks, were maintained by thinking patterns and self-defeating core beliefs. In cognitive therapy this faulty thinking is explored and replaced with alternative positive ways to interpret a situation.

To begin the reframing process, the cognitive therapist works with clients to raise their awareness of the cognitions, perceptions, beliefs, and attributions that come up in response to particular stimuli (Beck, 1995). To aide in this process, clients are often instructed to write down thoughts around a troubling situation or what they were thinking when a distressing mood overtakes them. Here the individual gains practice in bringing thoughts (and the accompanying assumptions and beliefs) into awareness and also how thoughts are related to a mood or emotional response (Greenberg & Padesky, 1995). In conducting cognitive therapy, the therapist builds a cognitive conceptualization of the person's difficulties, and how patterns of thought contribute to dysfunction, and in the process translates problems into cognitive terms (Beck, 1995) (see Case Example, Exhibit 4-4).

The cognitive conceptualization of a person's difficulties includes the notion of self schema and core beliefs. Self schemas are internal representations; images of the self one holds in his or her head. These schemas are a compilation of early interpersonal experiences and important events that create assumptions about the self, which in turn guide how one interprets and negotiates interpersonal relationships (Moretti, Feldman, & Shaw, 1990). Beck (1995) believes these self schemas contain core beliefs that are associated with either unloveablity or helplessness; a sense that one is helpless to change their circumstances or that one is unlikeable or bound to be rejected. In cognitive therapy the clinician does not probe for these core beliefs but in the course of sessions, recognizes how they are operating in the client's responses and behaviors. The therapist integrates these emerging core beliefs into his or her cognitive conceptualization of the patient's difficulties, a conceptualization that is shared with the client as therapy proceeds (Beck, 1995).

Clients improve via a cognitive approach because with awareness of thinking, emotional patterns, and alternative ways of responding, they can begin to change the way they think and respond to situations (Hazlett-Stevens & Craske, 2002). Negative thoughts and patterns are seen to maintain disorders, such as depression and anxiety, and thus changing this pattern should alter the depressive or anxious affect. In addition, responses once

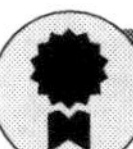

EXHIBIT 4-4: CASE EXAMPLE: COGNITIVE MODEL

Mr. S., a 55-year-old gentleman, is referred by his primary care physician due to problems with sleeping, increasing social withdrawal, a general feeling of sadness, and a pervasive sense of guilt. He presents as a sad but articulate individual who describes his increasing sense that life is slipping away. With his children grown and his job offering dwindling possibilities, he senses that he is "closing shop" on life. After hearing the client's narrative, a cognitive therapist would begin to discuss how Mr. S. might view his current situation and mood in cognitive terms. Understanding how Mr. S.'s problems began and were maintained, the therapist begins to explore the dysfunctional thoughts and beliefs that are associated with the problem and the depressed feelings accompanying these thoughts. The therapist then begins to map out with Mr. S. how he came to see his life in these terms. She understands that, from his father, Mr. S. learned to value productivity and sees anything less as moral laziness. Now, Mr. S. interprets his slowing business life as a moral failure and an indication of his incompetence. The therapist asks Mr. S. to examine how he feels when he becomes occupied with these thoughts. In doing so she begins to build the association between Mr. S.'s beliefs, interpretation of his situation, and his dysphoric feelings. Via these activities the client and therapist are beginning to work within a cognitive conceptualization of Mr. S.'s depression (Beck, 1995).

driven by dysfunctional thought patterns are now open to choice. Underneath the cognitive model is the fundamental believe that individuals have the ability to access the content and process of their thinking, see how thinking is tied to emotional and behavioral patterns, and intentionally modify their cognitive and behavioral responses to situations (Beck & Dozois, 2011).

In coaching the client on methods to forge alternative responses to situations, the cognitive therapist is also supporting a process that encourages new connections between neuronal pathways that coordinate information, emotions, and response patterns (Lemerise & Arsenio, 2000). Thus, with cognitive reframing exercises therapists are helping individuals change patterns of thinking and responding, and in a sense, their neuronal wiring. New thinking patterns are firing new neuronal connectivity. Researchers are beginning to use Functional Magnetic Imaging to illustrate the neuronal changes that follow cognitive work (Porto et al., 2009). These studies, conducted on participants in cognitive treatment, indicate that post-treatment changes in brain activity can be detected, particularly in regions involved with cognitive processing and cognitive-emotional balance (Porto et al., 2009). For instance, following cognitive therapy for anxiety, individuals demonstrated decreased activation of areas that hold contextual associations (stimulus-response) as well as reduced activity in areas of the brain that hold catastrophic thoughts (Paquette et al., 2003).

To accomplish these positive changes, the cognitive therapist establishes a treatment regime that is prescriptive in both content and structure. Beck (1995) describes these session parameters, which include how the treatment is initiated, how the assessment proceeds, and how a cognitive approach to problems is explained to the client. Cognitive therapy sessions also proceed in defined segments beginning with an evaluation of the patient's mood since last session, setting an agenda for the current meeting, review of homework, discussion of new issues, and then a plan for between-session activities and upcoming homework (Beck, 1995). The defined structure is believed to focus clients on selecting goals and solving problems (within a cognitive conceptualization of their issues), a process that brings about the experience of improved coping and growing mastery of problems (Reinecke & Freeman, 2005). Similar to brief psychodynamic methods, this structure is altered in brief forms of cognitive therapy. (See Exhibit 4-5.)

The client-therapist relationship is a critical component of cognitive therapy and intentionally structured to build a sense of teamwork. To build this type of relationship, the therapist fosters a collaborative atmosphere, that the client and therapist are together exploring events, testing out hypotheses about why events occurred, and formulating possible solutions (Newman, 1998). As Newman points out, this relationship structure empowers patients to take charge of problems. It also builds essential self-efficacy experiences in framing issues and developing solutions, skills clients will carry with them once therapy has ended. Cognitive-behavioral approaches are common with many types of therapies and interventions

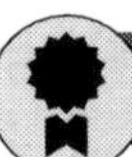

EXHIBIT 4-5: BRIEF THERAPIES: ADAPTION OF THE VARIOUS MODELS

Many of the therapies discussed in this chapter are seen as amenable to be delivered as a brief model. For instance, cognitive interventions fit well within brief models because by nature the therapy is structured and focused on specific client issues. In general, brief cognitive therapy aims at changing an element of a client's distress that is seen as adaptive to change; that is, the cognitive processes that accompany maladaptive responses. Short-term cognitive therapy typically occurs within 10 sessions. Its various models are supported by research that demonstrates it is as effective as treatments with longer protocols (Hazlett-Stevens & Craske, 2002). Proponents believe that the short cognitive models actually encourage learning and the more rapid results promote involvement. Brief psychodynamic therapy models have also been developed. These brief models continue to recognize the basic drive structure and its modifications by various defenses (Messer & Warren, 1995). As depicted in the Drive Structural Model, the therapist uses active, frequent confrontational techniques to break through resistances and come to core unconscious issues (Messer & Warren, 1995). Due to the intense nature of such therapy, it is seen as suitable for persons with milder conditions, such as adjustment disorders or for individuals dealing with personality issues such as avoidant and dependent traits.

and thus psychiatric mental health advanced practice registered nurses (PMH-APRNs) will invariably draw upon them in working with clients. APRNs who wish to develop expertise in CBT will find numerous venues for additional training, such as the instruction and certification which is available from the Academy of Cognitive Therapy.

INTERPERSONAL THERAPY

Interpersonal psychotherapy (IPT) is grounded in the assumption that specific mental health issues, such as depression, are sustained by the client's interpersonal interactions and relationship patterns. Interpersonal therapy has its roots in the work of Harry Stack Sullivan, who elucidated the connection between psychiatric disorders and interpersonal issues. Sullivan believed that interpersonal interactions shaped key aspects of personality, particularly one's view of the acceptable and unacceptable aspects of self (Sullivan, 1953). His interpersonal therapy aimed to help patients develop insight and a more realistic view of self in interpersonal relationships. Sullivan's framework holds particular significance to psychiatric nursing because of its influence on Peplau's theory of nurse-patient relationships and the centrality of anxiety in patients' pathological behaviors (Peplau, 1965).

In this review we focus on the principles of IPT set down by Myrna Weissman and Gerald Klerman as they developed IPT treatment for depression (Klerman, Weissman, Rounsaville, & Chevron, 1984). Similar to CBT, interpersonal therapy is focused and structured but, in contrast to cognitive therapy, the IPT therapist uses specific methods to examine the patterns in relationships that sustain difficulties. To elaborate the principles, underlying assumptions, and techniques of IPT, we focus on its application in the treatment of depression in both adults and adolescents; however, interpersonal therapy has a wider reach and has been modified for several other applications such as IPT tailored for persons with bulimia nervosa (Fairburn, 1998) and for depression in HIV-positive individuals (Swartz & Markowitz, 1998).

An important assumption of IPT is the association between depressive symptoms and current interpersonal difficulties (Weissman & Markowitz, 1998). In line with this assumption, IPT assessment sessions are focused on identifying depressive symptoms and the effects of these depressive symptoms on interpersonal relationships. The therapist probes to identify both the satisfying and unsatisfying aspects of current relationships, any changes in relationships proximal to the onset of depressive symptoms, as well as the relationship changes the client desires (Weissman & Markowitz, 1998). Therapists might also investigate the cultural and societal influences that cultivate role expectations, which then become intertwined with relationship factors that in turn promote depression, particularly in women (Crowe & Luty, 2005a). In these initial IPT sessions, the client is assigned the sick role both to alleviate the individual from a sense of current social obligations and to solidify that the client's job is to focus on the work of treatment (Barry, 2008). Similar to

CBT, during this initial phase, the therapist is educating the client about depression and its association to how the client interacts within interpersonal relationships.

In the middle phases of treatment the therapist and client develop strategies to address the relationship areas that have been affected by depression, plan for how the client might develop new relational patterns, and explore reactions to what is being lost in the relationships the client is leaving behind (Barry, 2008). The focus is on the here and now, what occurred between sessions, and how new strategies are working. In this middle phase the client and therapist may focus on specific areas such as role disputes or interpersonal deficits, including the client's own social or relationship skills. While the focus is on current relationships, the clients may also explore their core beliefs about self and the role they should be playing in relationships (Crowe & Luty, 2005b). Crowe and Luty (2005a) illustrate this phenomenon with a case study involving a client whose belief that she must be selfless and put the needs of others first resulted in an "ideal" standard, one the client believed she was always falling short of. This core belief spun out to a conviction that the client could not express her true feelings, and a sense of meaninglessness in relationships that compounded her depression and in turn affected relationships.

In IPT the structure of sessions and the client-therapist relationship is prescribed. The IPT therapist is instructed to convey a hopeful stance emphasizing that change is possible and that with the depression lifting, options for change will become more readily apparent (Weissman & Markowitz, 1998). The number (between 14 and 16) and phases of the sessions (assessment, middle, and final) were initially set down in an IPT manual (Klerman et al., 1984). We have already described the assessment and middle sessions. In the final phase the therapist attempts to consolidate gains, reviews the client's progress in developing new relationship strategies, and moves through the process of termination.

Recognizing the interpersonal aspects of adolescent turmoil, the IPT protocol has also been modified for treatment of teens with depressive symptoms (Mufson, Dorta, Moreau, & Weissman, 2004). Mufson and Moreau (1998) noted that adolescents often flounder in open-ended therapies because they are unsure of what they should be talking about or how to focus a session. IPT-A addresses these issues by employing a defined 12-week structure; adolescents thus know what they should do and what they can expect. This structure also addresses several issues particular to depressed teens and their reluctance to seek treatment (Draucker, 2005), as well as their preference for action over verbal communication (Mufson & Moreau, 1998). It also offers a platform for the interpersonal issues that are often at the core of the adolescent's difficulty (Mufson & Moreau, 1998). IPT-A has impressive outcomes and is included in the National Registry of Evidence Based Programs and Practices (http://www.nrepp.samhsa.gov/ViewIntervention.aspx?id=198samhsa.gov/ViewIntervention.aspx?id=198).

Interpersonal therapy is particularly suited to psychiatric nursing practice since therapists use their interpersonal skills in enacting the interventions (Crowe & Luty, 2005a). In addition, the goals of IPT align with three themes of nursing: the holistic model, the importance of interpersonal relationships, and the search for authentic relationships (Barry, 2008). The core work of IPT, examining the mutual influence of relationships and self, also fits with the specialty since the crux of psychiatric nursing is the interpersonal interaction process (McCabe, 2002). There are of course important differences between the process of developing an interpersonal relationship and initiating IPT therapy, particularly that employing the techniques of IPT therapy demand conscious application of a specific protocol by a clinician trained in the method.

BEHAVIOR THERAPIES

Behavioral therapy seeks to change a person's observable actions and responses; in so doing, behavioral therapists attempt to reduce the dysfunction in a person's life and increase the quality of life (Sadock & Sadock, 2007). The roots of this approach stretch back to actions in Roman times of Pliny the Elder, who put spiders in the drinks of alcohol abusers in an early form of aversive conditioning. As a school of planned change based in scientific principles, behavioral therapy dates back less than a century (Maultsby & Wirga, 1998). Yet in this brief span of time, three waves of behavior therapy have been developed.

The first wave started with the original works of Pavlov (1849–1936), who demonstrated a dog could be conditioned to salivate to the sound of a bell by first pairing a bell with food. Another pioneer of behaviorism was John B. Watson (1878–1958), well-known for his work with Little Albert in 1920. He enthusiastically adopted Pavlov's work with conditioning as the basis for behavior psychology (Maultsby & Wirga, 1998) and brought about the radical behavioralism movement. This school of psychology was an extreme departure from the then-popular introspective methods of data gathering that therapists had adopted.

Edward Thorndike (1874–1949) built upon Pavlov's work by exploring how reward motivates behavior.

Thorndike's most famous student, B.F. Skinner (1904–1990), developed Thorndike's reward learning theory and was committed to Watson's radical behaviorism. Skinner only dealt with behavioral responses and did not deal with emotions, which he saw as behavioral reflexes similar to drives. Skinner sought to map most human responses in terms of reinforcement patterns for behavior, specifically how particular responses were encouraged by both positive and negative reinforcers (the withdrawal of negative consequences). It bears noting that Skinner studied animal, non-human, subjects and did advise his findings be extrapolated to human beings (Maultsby & Wirga, 1998).

The second wave started with the work of E. Hobart Mowrer, who provided the corrective influence to the first wave's exclusive emphasis on only behavior with his two-factor learning approach that challenged the prevailing belief that only observable behavior merits scientific study. Due to Mowrer's work, behavior psychology opened up to the possibility that human beings possess the capacity for imagination and self-talk, elements which could be powerful factors in behaviors (Maultsby & Wirga, 1998).

As the century progressed, the field of behavior therapy gained strength from unlikely partners, psychoanalysts, some of whom were dissatisfied with the poor outcomes their interventions were yielding. A notable follower of Freud, Joseph Wolpe receives credit for the behavior technique known as systematic desensitization, a combination of deep muscular relaxation combined with emotive imagery. In systematic desensitization, the client is led through a series of mental and physical exercises where the individual learns to dampen his or her customary response to an anxiolytic stimulus. This new approach did not attend to unconscious motives, conflict, or deficit models of psychodynamics, but focused purely on behaviors. Working independently of Wolpe, the renowned psychologist Albert Ellis developed an approach he named Rational Emotive Behavior Therapy (REBT). From his work comes the now famous ABC Model. The ABC model starts with an **A**ctivating event that filters through a person's **B**eliefs and leads to **C**onsequences in behaviors and feelings (Maultsby & Wirga, 1998).

Ellis's work paved the way for the highly researched and acclaimed methods developed by Aaron Beck, known as Cognitive Behavior Therapy, which is treated elsewhere in this chapter. The field of psychology classifies the methods of Ellis and Beck as the second generation of behavior therapies (Hayes, 2004). More recently, a third wave of behavior models were developed within behavior psychology from scholars, scientists, and clinicians such as Steven Hayes, Marsha Linehan, and Jon Kabat-Zinn. This new wave includes therapies such as Acceptance and Commitment Therapy (ACT), Dialectical Behavior Therapy (DBT), Mindfulness Therapy, and Mindfulness-Based Stress Reduction (Hayes, 2004). With this brief overview of the history of behavior therapy as a context, we now describe the theoretical assumptions of each "wave," particularly how behavioral techniques are purported to relieve the patient's distress. Following this discussion, the techniques of each wave will be discussed including the rationale for why these particular behavioral methods should relieve distress.

THEORETICAL BASIS UNDERLYING CHANGE

The first wave of behavioral therapy, radical behavioralism, holds that change flows from two dynamics (attraction and aversion) underlying all behavior in response to a stimulus. Simply put, people do more of what they find pleasant and less of what they find unpleasant. Behavior therapy seeks to reinforce desired behaviors and extinguish undesired behaviors. Parents know this as reward and punishment. In contrast to psychodynamic methods, with a behavioral approach no need exists to delve into the conscious, subconscious, and unconscious mind (as the psychodynamic therapists do). By analyzing what a person likes and dislikes, the radical behavior therapist charts a course toward the goal of changing the target behavior by constructing a system of rewards and punishments. In a strict behaviorist view, people learn behaviors and they will change their behaviors when enough attraction or aversion builds around the targeted behavior.

Many behavioral therapists believe the field encompasses a range of techniques from the earliest behaviorists to the most recent developments in the field (such as ACT), recognizing how one perspective piggybacks onto another (Hayes, 2004). Others point out that the therapeutic results touted by the champions of CBT or REBT come early in the therapeutic process, where CBT and REBT place emphasis on behavior change rather than discovery and change of cognitions. They question if the field of behavior therapy abandoned the purely behavioral perspective too quickly in favor of the combined behavioral-cognitive approach (Freij & Masri, 2008). They hold that the majority of therapeutic change comes from targeting specific behaviors and working toward change through a schedule of activities. This approach encompasses the schools known as Behavior Activation Therapy (BAT) and the brief solution focused schools (Dobson et al., 2008; Freij & Masri, 2008; Martell, Dimidjian, & Herman-Dunn, 2010). Their rallying cry "Do one thing different" reflects their belief that a change in one behavior will have a ripple effect through a person's life (O'Hanlon, 2000). Similar principles permeate the Brief Solution Focused school, that is, if it isn't broken, don't fix it; if it's working, do more of the same; if it isn't working, stop doing it (Erford, Eaves, Bryant, & Young, 2009).

In this more pristine behavioral perspective, depression and anxiety occur when a person experiences an aversive situation and begins to develop new behaviors to avoid the aversive situation. Often this means a person will isolate, withdraw from social contact, and cease to do pleasurable activities. This results in a deficit of positive rewards that previously reinforced acceptable behaviors such as social contact, fulfilling work responsibilities, and so on. To overcome depression, a person learns to analyze how their new avoiding behaviors reinforce the depression and then schedule behaviors that increase pleasure and return a person to regular social contact. Feelings and cognitions do not enter into the analysis of the behaviors (Martell et al., 2010). Those familiar with the slogans of the Alcoholics Anonymous (AA) movement might describe this approach as "Suit Up and Show Up" or "Act As If." The defenders of pure behaviorism may not use the vocabulary of radical behavioralism such as "operant conditioning," or "conditioned and unconditioned stimuli," yet they operate out of the same underlying theory that all behaviors move toward that perceived as pleasant and avoid that perceived as unpleasant: attraction and aversion.

The second wave of behavior therapy, CBT and REBT, overlaps with the first wave of radical behaviorism. Based on the pioneering work of Mowrer mentioned above, these branches of psychology came to understand that the thoughts, beliefs, and values of a person need to be included as subject matter for the therapeutic process. This belief finds early expression in the King James translation of the Book of Proverbs 23:7 "as a man thinketh in his heart, so is he." The Greek stoic philosopher Epictetus provides further basis for the theory of change proposed by CBT with his observation that people are not disturbed by things that happen but by the view they take of things that happen. The purists in the field of cognitive therapy hold that the dynamics underlying all mental health problems can be found in the dysfunctional or distorted cognitive schema of the client that lead to maladaptive behaviors. Simply put, to change a person's behavior, change the way the person thinks. Purists from the radical behaviorism school counter with change the behavior, and the beliefs will change. The second wave of behavior therapy lets go of this "either/or" dichotomy in favor of a "both/and" approach.

The third group of behavior therapies includes mindfulness approaches, which are derived from the traditions of various world religions (Tolle, 2004). Through mindfulness a person gains an awareness of his or her particular thoughts and behaviors set in the broader context of his or her life. The primary dynamic of change in this third wave of therapies is based on the belief that behaviors and thoughts must be changed in order to relieve distress or disability. Thus, the third wave therapies seek to change the person's *relationship* to his or her thoughts and behaviors (Hayes & Plumb, 2007). First and second wave therapies focus on behaviors and thoughts and struggle to change them. Third wave therapies see this focus and struggle as perpetuating the problems. Instead of struggling to change, third wave therapies encourage clients to accept themselves as they are in the present moment set in the larger context of their lives. This acceptance then frees clients to refocus on their deeper values in the larger context of their lives and commit to those values. This commitment to deeper, broader values leads to relief of the distress or disability (Luoma, Hayes, & Walser, 2007).

Luoma et al. (2007) outline six core therapeutic processes of mindfulness therapies that lead to the overall goal of psychological flexibility. These six core processes counteract six dysfunctions that create psychological inflexibility. As clients become involved in the therapeutic processes, they change their relationship to themselves in the current context of their lives. The six dysfunctions are: dominance of the conceptualized past and future with limited self knowledge; lack of values; inaction; attachment to the conceptualized self; cognitive fusion; and experiential avoidance (Luoma et al., 2007, p. 12). Clients counteract these dysfunctions through developing new attitudes and behaviors: being present to the moment; defining their values and directions; committing to new actions; seeing self as the context (standard) for knowing themselves; learning to recognize and defuse (separate from) their belief patterns; and accepting themselves in the present moment (Luoma et al., 2007, p. 20).

Hayes and Smith (2005) use the metaphor of the Chinese finger trap to illustrate the theory. In this game, children stick their forefingers into both ends of a simple woven straw tube and then try to extract their fingers. The harder they pull, the tighter the tube squeezes their fingers. When the child relaxes and stops trying so hard to extricate their fingers, the tube "magically" releases their fingers. It is this change in the child's *relationship* to the tube that brings about the freedom from the problem.

In a similar way, when individuals stop struggling so hard to change their thoughts and behaviors, they gain an awareness of the dynamics of the context of their lives.

A change in their *relationship* to the problem occurs. Then they discover their deeper values, and commit to living their lives out of those values even if they do not emotionally feel like it in the moment (Hayes, 2004). Using an acronym from the phrase **A**cceptance and **C**ommitment **T**herapy, Hayes and Smith (2005) call their mindfulness approach ACT, which illustrates how this third wave of mindfulness approaches belongs to the action focused behavior therapy field. Other leaders in the third wave mindfulness approach use a variety of names and acronyms (Kabat-Zinn, 1990; Dimeff, Koerner, & Linnehan, 2007; Williams, Teasdale, Segal, & Kabat-Zinn, 2007).

TECHNIQUES OF BEHAVIOR THERAPIES

Based on the underlying principles of attraction-aversion or reinforcement-extinction, the first wave, radical behavioralism, employs many techniques familiar to parents, teachers, and health care professionals. These techniques focus on positive reinforcement, negative reinforcement, punishment, or a combination of all three. Positive reinforcement encourages the repetition of a desired behavior. Negative reinforcement, often misunderstood and confused with punishment, promotes the desired behavior by removing a negative stimulus. Punishment seeks to extinguish an undesired behavior through applying an unpleasant stimulus or removing a reward.

Among the positive reinforcement techniques, four stand out: The Premack Principle, behavior charts, token economy, and behavioral contracting. All of these involve stating the desired behavior in positive, descriptive terms. For example, instead of "He will stop jumping out of his chair," the behavior target would be "He will stay seated for up to 15 minutes." Other than the Premack Principle, the other three techniques listed reward the positive behavior with a chart marking progress, tokens rewarding behaviors, and contracts with rewards and consequences spelled out. The Premack Principle uses one preferred behavior to reward a less preferred target behavior. Most people do this automatically even though they do not call it the Premack Principle: "I will reward myself with a bowl of ice cream after I finish writing this chapter."

Five punishment techniques well known and often used both in real life and in behavior therapy are punishment, extinction, time-out, response-cost, and overcorrection. For example, in grade school the teacher might remove the privilege of recess from the rambunctious child (punishment), simply ignore the wiggly antics of another (extinction), place another child out in the hall for a few minutes (time-out), and finally use overcorrection when telling a child to write 200 times "I will not blurt out an answer in class."

BAT uses the acronym ACTIVATE (*A*ssess, *C*ounter, *T*ime, *I*nclude, *V*alidate, *A*ssign, *T*roubleshoot, *E*ncourage) to guide therapist and client in the steps of BAT (Martell et al., 2010). First, the therapist and client assess the client's behaviors to understand the patterns. Second, they counter avoidance behaviors that block the new behavior. Third, they take time to be very specific in the changes expected and the results from the change. Fourth, they include ways to monitor the activity plan. Fifth, they validate the client's efforts toward change, no matter how small or incremental. Sixth, they assign further activities as the therapy progresses. Seventh, they troubleshoot problems that arise along the way. Finally, the therapist encourages the client throughout the process, offering positive rewards.

Brief Solution Focused Therapy (O'Hanlon, 2000) uses five main techniques. First, the therapist teaches the client how to use scaling or ratings of the intensity of the problem and the attraction to change. Second, the therapist and client look for exceptions where the problem does not happen. Third, the therapist coaches the client to do what is called problem-free talk so as not to reinforce the problem. A fourth technique, called "the miracle question," invites clients to imagine what life would be like if "a miracle happened and the problem disappeared." Finally, a technique called "flagging the minefield" tries to anticipate where hidden bombs might disrupt the march toward the solution (Erford et al., 2009).

The methods of behavior therapies overlap in various patterns. CBT and REBT use many of the techniques from the first wave schools of strict behaviorism. However, drawing upon the framework of the second wave, cognitions and emotions receive more attention through techniques such as identifying and counteracting distorted cognitions, problem solving, and thought stopping (McKay, Davis, & Fanning, 2007). Prolonged Exposure (PE) (Foa, Rothbaum, & Furr, 2003) and Stress Inoculation Therapy (Meichenbaum, 1996) include techniques of attraction–aversion and reward–punishment to help clients change their behaviors around the stressors or targeted behaviors. Each adds techniques from cognitive therapy wherein clients seek to change their cognitions around those same stressors or targeted behaviors. Graded hierarchies of approach to painful stimuli are created and then clients, either in vivo or in imagination, expose themselves to the painful stimuli. They thereby learn to develop new behaviors or extinguish old ones. Two behavior skills, deep breathing and progressive muscle relaxation, help clients tolerate the exposure and develop the ability to learn new behavioral responses to stressful stimuli. These two skills have become part of many different forms of therapy.

The techniques of the third wave of behavior therapies help clients develop mindfulness or awareness of themselves. Clients learn to keep themselves in the present moment through awareness of their breathing. They learn to observe their thoughts as clouds passing across the sky or leaves floating in a river. They track the feelings connected to thoughts by listening to their bodily sensations. The client learns to become an observer involved in and yet detached from the thoughts, emotions, and bodily sensations that constitute the context of the present moment. Therapists engage clients in values clarification exercises to help clients focus on what is important and valuable to the client in the context of their own lives. Finally, the therapist and client collaborate on establishing new behaviors that express the client's values more authentically (Luoma et al., 2007).

Thus the three waves of behavior therapy often are used together. A clear example of how these approaches blend, blur, and borrow can be seen in DBT (Linehan, 1993; McKay et al., 2007). This form of therapy teaches distress tolerance skills which reflect the PE and stress inoculation techniques. Clients learn basic mindfulness skills of self-observation of breath, thoughts, emotions, and bodily sensations. They acquire new behaviors of interpersonal skills with elements of BAT and brief solution focused techniques. Throughout the process, clients are encouraged to engage in behaviors opposite (dialectical) to their usual ways of behaving that are problematic. As stated at the outset of this section, behavior therapy seeks to change a person's observable actions and responses. In so doing, behavioral therapy attempts to reduce the dysfunction in a person's life and increase the quality of life (Sadock & Sadock, 2007).

CORE COMPETENCIES, PSYCHOTHERAPY, AND PMH ADVANCED PRACTICE

NURSING

The role of PMH-APRN is rapidly changing (Delaney, 2011). The explosion of neuroscience has brought greater understanding to mental illness and with it a new perspective on treatment and recovery (Martin, 2002). While not without controversy, psychotropic medications are increasingly used as the first line treatment for mental distress (Mojtabai & Olfson, 2010). Though relationship-based psychotherapy has been and will continue to be a major component of the work of PMH-APRNs, there is increasing recognition of their role in providing the full scope of mental health services, including diagnosis/management and prescribing (Hanrahan, Delaney, & Merwin, 2010). A major change is also occurring in the certification and licensure of APRNs, one that moves PMH-APRNs to a life span nurse practitioner (NP) role (Delaney, 2009).

The driver of this change is the APRN Consensus Model. The consensus model is a decade-long initiative of national groups who license, educate, and certify APRNs in the United States (APRN Consensus Work Group, 2008). The impetus for the consensus model was the lack of uniformity among states on licensing criteria and the variation in graduate education nursing curriculums that produced the APRN work force. In response, the architects of the model isolated four roles (clinical nurse specialist [CNS], NP, midwife, and certified nurse anesthetist) and six populations, PMH being one of them. In line with this model, future graduates of PMH-APRN programs will be educated in a life span curriculum. In 2010, the two major U.S. psychiatric nursing organizations, American Psychiatric Nurses Association (APNA) and International Society of Psychiatric Nurses (ISPN), endorsed the APRN model and the PMHNP as the entry role for all advanced practice in psychiatric nursing (Farley-Toombs, 2011).

The implications for PMH nursing education is significant, the foremost being that PMH-APRNs will be prepared in a life-span curriculum, one that aligns with the core competencies outlined by the National Association of Nurse Practitioner Faculties (NONPF) (National Panel for PMHNP Competencies, 2003). In this document, conducting individual, family, and group psychotherapy is one of the core PMHNP competencies. PMH-APRN graduate programs have focused for three decades on these forms of therapy within the CNS role partially because this training was a certification requirement. At the current time the family therapy focus of PMH-APRN programs seems caught in the shifting focus away from traditional family therapy approaches (Goldenberg & Goldenberg, 2008) and toward family education models (e.g., Gross & Grady, 2002) and family-centered approaches (Tyler & Horner, 2008). Interested students will find the basics of group therapy in Yalom's classic text (Yalom & Lesczc, 2005), which continues to be used in PMH-APRN graduate programs (Wheeler & Delaney, 2008).

The issue of teaching psychotherapy across the life span is a bit more complex. Therapeutic techniques, such as ones employed in cognitive treatment, can be effectively tailored to both younger populations (Benjamin et al., 2011) and older adults (Serfaty et al., 2009;

Stanley et al., 2009). In addition, for each population there are specific evidence-based therapies that address particular, age-bound disorders, such as attention deficit problems (Kaiser & Pfiffner, 2011) and syndromes such as late-life depression (Andreescu & Reynolds, 2011). Focusing on age-specific issues within disorders is yielding important differences in the neurobiology of symptoms and comorbidities (Andreescu et al., 2011), which should lead to innovation in effective therapies. In the future, PMH-APRNs will be challenged to combine their nursing perspective on holistic, relationship-centered care with age-specific evidence-based therapies.

CONCLUSION

Each of the therapies described in this chapter lend useful concepts to a clinician's understanding of a client's emotional/mental distress and possible ways to address it. While biological psychiatry and psychopharmacology is in ascendency, psychiatric nurses should not lose sight that key developmental events and clients' interpersonal relationships influence their current experience of life events. Psychiatric APRNs also approach therapy within a context of our professional values. Nursing has particular respect for the impact of early relationships on the formation of self structure, as evidenced by the inclusion of attachment theory and a developmental interpersonal framework (Siegel, 1999) in most graduate curriculums. Psychiatric nurses also recognize how Peplau's theory influences their practice, particularly her emphasis on the use of empathy, the formation of a relationship, and seeking to understand a person's meaning system (Delaney & Handrup, 2011).

Psychiatric nurses believe in the person's capacity to heal. Every interaction is grounded in the deep belief that greater mental health and a meaningful life are within a person's reach. The psychiatric nursing approach to assessment includes the traditional data gathering techniques, but also regard the assessment as the building block of the alliance, and this process concludes with a formulation of the developmental and interpersonal dynamics at play, the client's goals, and the techniques that can be called upon to reach those goals (Bjorklund, 2008). Psychiatric nurses use all of these elements to build an intentional theory of therapy with clients based on knowing what the person wants, a formulation of what is blocking that person's progress to a meaningful life, and a relationship-based method aimed at relieving the distress and inviting awareness of new ways of thinking and coping.

REFERENCES

Andreescu, C., & Reynolds, C. F. (2011). Late-life depression: Evidence based treatment and promising new directions for research and clinical practice. *Psychiatric Clinics of North America, 34,* 335–355.

Andreescu, C., Wu, M., Butters, M. A., Figurski, J., Reynolds, C. F., & Aizenstein, H. J. (2011). The default mode network in late-life anxious depression. *American Journal of Geriatric Psychiatry, 19,* 980–983.

APRN Consensus Work Group and APRN Joint Dialogue Group. (2008). Consensus model for APRN regulation: Licensure, accreditation, certification and education. Retrieved from www.ncsbn.org/Consensus_Model_for_APRN_Regulation_July_2008.pdf

Basch, M. F. (1980). *Doing psychotherapy.* New York, NY: Basic Books.

Basch, M. F. (1988). *Understanding psychotherapy.* New York, NY: Basic Books.

Bandura, A. (1989). Social cognitive theory. In R. Vasta (Ed.), *Annals of child development. Vol. 6. Six theories of child development* (pp. 1–60). Greenwich, CT: JAI Press.

Bandura, A. (2004). Swimming against the mainstream: The early years from chilly tributary to transformative mainstream. *Behavior Research and Therapy, 42,* 613–630.

Barry, P. D. (2008). Interpersonal psychotherapy. In K. Wheeler (Ed.), *Psychotherapy for the advanced practice nurse* (pp. 203–221). St. Louis, MO: Mosby.

Beck, A. T., & Dozois, D. J. A. (2011). Cognitive therapy: Current status and future directions. *Annual Review of Medicine, 62,* 397–409.

Beck, J. S. (1995). *Cognitive therapy: Basics and beyond.* New York, NY: Guilford.

Benjamin, C. L., Puleo, C. M., Settipani, C. A., Brodman, D. M., Edmunds, J. M., Cummings, C. M.,...Philip, C. K. (2011). History of cognitive-behavioral therapy in youth. *Child and Adolescent Psychiatric Clinics of North America, 20,* 179–190.

Bjorklund, P. (2008). Assessment and diagnosis. In K. Wheeler (Ed.), *Psychotherapy for the advanced practice nurse* (pp. 81–114). St. Louis, MO: Mosby.

Breur, J., & Freud, S. (1895). *Studies on hysteria. The definitive edition.* New York, NY: Basic Books.

Crowe, M., & Luty, S. (2005a). Interpersonal psychotherapy: An effective psychotherapeutic intervention for mental health nursing practice. *International Journal of Mental Health Nursing, 14,* 126–133.

Crowe, M., & Luty, S. (2005b). Recovery from depression: A discourse analysis of interpersonal psychotherapy. *Nursing Inquiry, 12,* 43–50.

Curtis, R. C., & Hirsch, I. (2003). Relational approaches to psychoanalytic psychotherapy. In A. S. Gurman & S. B. Messer (Eds.), *Essential psychotherapy* (pp. 69–106). New York, NY: Guilford.

Delaney, K. R. (2009). Looking 10 years back and 5 years ahead: Framing the clinical nurse specialist debate for our students. *Archives of Psychiatric Nursing, 23,* 454–456.

Delaney, K. R. (2011). Psychiatric mental health nursing: Why 2011 brings a pivotal moment. *Journal of Nursing Education and Practice, 1,* 61–72. doi:10.5430/jnep.v1n1px

Delaney, K. R., & Handrup, C. (2011). Psychiatric mental health nursing's psychotherapy role: Are we letting it slip away? *Archives of Psychiatric Nursing, 25*, 303–305.

Dimeff, L. A., Koerner, K., & Linehan, M. M. (Eds.). (2007). *Dialectical behavior therapy in clinical practice: Applications across disorders and settings*. New York, NY: Guilford.

Dobson, K. S., Hollon, S. D., Dimidjian, S., Schmaling, K. B., Kohlenberg, R. J., Gallop, R. J.,...Jacobson, N. S. (2008). Randomized trial of behavioral activation, cognitive therapy, and antidepressant medication in the prevention of relapse and recurrence in major depression. *Journal of Consulting and Clinical Psychology, 76*, 468–477.

Douglas, C. J. (2008). Teaching supportive psychotherapy to psychiatric residents. *American Journal of Psychiatry, 165*, 445–452.

Draucker, C. B. (2005). Processes of mental health service use by adolescents with depression. *Journal of Nursing Scholarship, 37*, 155–162.

Elson, M. (Ed.). (1987). *The kohut seminars*. New York, NY: Norton.

Elson, M. (1988). *Self-psychology in clinical social work*. New York, NY: Norton.

Erford, B. T., Eaves, S. H., Bryant, E., & Young, K. (2009). *35 techniques every counselor should know*. Columbus, OH: Pearson Merrill Prentice Hall.

Fairburn, G. C. (1998). Interpersonal psychotherapy for Bulimia Nervosa. In J. C. Markowitz (Ed.), *Interpersonal psychotherapy* (pp. 99–128). Washington, DC: American Psychiatric Press.

Farley-Toombs, C. (2011). Shaping the future of PMH-APRN practice through engagement. *Journal of the American Psychiatric Nurses Association, 17*, 250–252.

Foa, E. B., Rothbaum, B. O., & Furr, J. M. (2003). Augmenting exposure therapy with other CBT procedures. *Psychiatric Annals, 33*, 47–53.

Frank, J. D. (1971). Therapeutic factors in psychotherapy. *American Journal of Psychotherapy, 25*, 350–361.

Frank J. D. (1982). Therapeutic components shared by all psychotherapies. In J. H. Harvey & M. M. Parks (Eds.), *Psychotherapy research and behavior change* (pp. 9–37). Washington, DC: American Psychological Association.

Freij, K., & Masri, N. (2008). The brief behavioral activation treatment for depression: A psychiatric pilot study. *Nordic Psychology, 60*, 129–140.

Gabbard, G. A. (2005). *Psychodynamic psychiatry in clinical practice* (4th ed.). Washington, DC: American Psychiatric Press.

Gallop, R., & O'Brien, L. (2003). Re-establishing psychodynamic theory as foundational knowledge for psychiatric/mental health nursing. *Issues in Mental Health Nursing, 24*, 213–227.

Goldenberg, H., &, Goldenberg, I. (2008). *Family therapy: An overview* (7th ed.). Florence, KY: Brooks/Cole Publishing.

Greenberg, D., & Padesky, C. A. (1995). *Mind over mood: Change how you feel by changing how you think*. New York, NY: Guilford.

Gross, D., & Grady, J. (2002). Group-based parent training for preventing mental health disorders in children. *Issues in Mental Health Nursing, 23*, 367–383.

Gurman, A. S., & Messer, S. B. (2003). Contemporary issues in the theory and practice of psychotherapy: A framework for comparative study. In A. S. Gurman & S. B. Messer (Eds.), *Essential psychotherapy* (pp. 1–24). New York, NY: Guilford.

Hanrahan, N., Delaney, K. R., & Merwin, E. (2010). Health care reform and the federal transformation initiatives: Capitalizing on the potential of advanced practice psychiatric nurses. *Policy, Politics and Nursing Practice, 11*(3), 235–244.

Hayes, S. C. (2004). Acceptance and commitment therapy and the new behavior therapies: Mindfulness, acceptance, and relationship. In S. C. Hayes, V. M. Folette, & M. M. Linehan (Eds.), *Mindfulness and acceptance: Expanding the cognitive-behavioral tradition* (pp. 1–29). New York, NY: Guilford.

Hayes, S. C., & Plumb, J. C. (2007). Mindfulness from the bottom up: Providing an inductive framework for understanding mindfulness processes and their application to human suffering. *Psychological Inquiry, 18*, 242–248.

Hayes, S. C., & Smith, S. (2005). *Get out of your mind and into your life: The new acceptance & commitment therapy*. New York, NY: New Harbinger Publishers.

Hazlett-Stevens, H., & Craske, M. G. (2002). Brief cognitive-behavioral therapy: Definition and scientific foundations. In F. W. Bond & W. Dryden (Eds.), *Handbook of brief cognitive therapy* (pp. 1–20). New York, NY: John Wiley & Sons.

Hebert, M. (1981). *Behavioral treatment of problem children: A practice manual*. New York, NY: Grune & Stratton.

Hollon, S. D., & Beck, A. T. (1994). Cognitive and cognitive-behavioral therapies. In A. E. Bergin & S. L. Garfield (Eds.), *Handbook of psychotherapy and behavior change* (4th ed., pp. 428–466). Oxford, UK: John Wiley & Sons.

Hubble, M. A., Duncan, B. L., & Miller, S. D. (1999). *The heart and soul of change: What works in therapy*. Washington, DC: American Psychological Association.

Joseph, B. (1985). Transference: The total situation. *International Journal of Psychoanalysis, 66*, 447–454.

Kabat-Zinn, J. (1990). *Full catastrophe living: Using the wisdom of your body and mind to face stress, pain, and illness*. New York, NY: Delacorte.

Kaiser, N. M., & Pfiffner, L. J. (2011). Evidence-based psychosocial treatments for childhood ADHD. *Psychiatric Annals, 41*, 9–15.

Klerman, G. L., Weissman, M. M., Rounsaville, B. J., & Chevron, E. S. (1984). *Interpersonal psychotherapy of depression*. New York, NY: Basic Books.

Knapp, P., & Beck, A. T. (2008). Cognitive therapy: Foundations, conceptual models, applications and research. *Review of Brazilian Psychiatry, 20*, S54–64.

Kohut, H. (1984). *How does analysis cure?* Chicago, IL: University of Chicago Press.

Lemerise, E. A., & Arsenio, W. F. (2000). An integrated model of emotion processing and cognition in social information processing. *Child Development, 71*, 107–118.

Levensky, E. R., Forcehimes, A., O'Donohue, W. T., & Beitz, K. (2007). Motivational interviewing: An evidence-based approach to counseling helps patients follow treatment recommendations. *American Journal of Nursing, 107*, 50–58.

Linehan, M. (1993). *Cognitive-behavioral treatment of borderline personality disorder*. New York, NY: Guilford.

Luborsky, L., Rosenthal, R., Diguer, L., Andrusyna, T. P., Berman, J. S., Levitt, J. T.,...Krause, E. D. (2002). The Dodo bird verdict is alive and well—mostly. *Clinical Psychology: Science and Practice, 9*, 2–12.

Luoma, J. B., Hayes, S. C., & Walser, R. D. (2007). *Learning ACT: An acceptance and commitment therapy skills-training manual for therapists*. Oakland, CA: New Harbinger.

Martell, C. R., Dimidjian, S., & Herman-Dunn, R. (2010). *Behavioral activation for depression: A clinician's guide*. New York, NY: Guilford.

Martin, J. P. (2002). The integration of Neurology, Psychiatry, and Neuroscience in the 21st century. *American Journal of Psychiatry, 159,* 695–704.

Maultsby Jr., M. C., & Wirga, M. (1998). Behavior therapy. In H. Freidman, R. Schwarzer, R. C. Silver, D. Spiegel, N. E. Adler, R. D. Parke, & C. Peterson (Eds.), *Encyclopedia of mental health, Three-volume set* (pp. 1–18). New York, NY: Academic Press. Retrieved from www.arcobem.com/publications

McCabe, S. (2002). The nature of psychiatric nursing: The intersection of paradigm, evolution, and history. *Archives of Psychiatric Nursing, 16,* 51–60.

McKay, M., Davis, M., & Fanning, P. (2007). *Thoughts and feelings: Taking control of your moods and life* (3rd ed.). Oakland, CA: New Harbinger.

McWilliams, N. (1999). *Psychoanalytic case formulations*. New York, NY: Guilford.

Meichenbaum, D. (1996). Stress inoculation training for coping with stressors. *Clinical Psychologist, 49,* 4–7.

Messer, S. B., & Warren, C. S. (1995). Models of brief psychodynamic therapy: A comparative approach. New York, NY: Guilford.

Miller, N. E., & Dollard, J. (1941). *Social learning and imitation*. New Haven, CT: Yale University Press.

Miller, W. R., & Rollnick, S. (2002). *Motivational interviewing: Preparing people for change*. New York, NY: Guilford.

Misch, D. A. (2000). Brief strategies of dynamic supportive therapy. *Journal of Psychotherapy and Practice Research, 9,* 173–189.

Mojtabai, R., & Olfson, M. (2010). National trends in psychotropic medication polypharmacy in office-based psychiatry. *Archives of General Psychiatry, 67,* 26–36.

Moretti, M. M., Feldman, L., & Shaw, B. F. (1990). Cognitive therapy: Current practice and future directions. In R. A. Wells & V. J. Giannetti (Eds.), *The Comprehensive handbook of the brief psychotherapies* (pp. 217–237). New York, NY: Plenum Press.

Mufson, L., Dorta, K. P., Moreau, D., & Weissman, M. M. (2004). *Interpersonal psychotherapy for depressed adolescents* (2nd ed.). New York, NY: Guilford.

Mufson, L., & Moreau, D. (1998). Interpersonal psychotherapy for adolescent depression. In J. C. Markowitz (Ed.), *Interpersonal psychotherapy* (pp. 35–66). Washington, DC: American Psychiatric Press.

National Panel for Psychiatric Mental Health NP Competencies. (2003). *Psychiatric-mental health nurse practitioner competencies*. Washington, DC: National Organization of Nurse Practitioner Faculties.

Newman, C. F. (1998). The therapeutic relationship and alliance in short-term cognitive therapy. In J. D. Safran & J. C. Muran (Eds.), *The therapeutic alliance in brief psychotherapy* (pp. 95–122). Washington, DC: American Psychological Association.

Norcross, J. C. (Ed.). (2002). *Psychotherapy relationships that work: Therapists contributions and responsiveness to patients*. New York, NY: Oxford University Press.

O'Hanlon, B. (2000). *Do one thing different: Ten simple ways to change your life*. New York, NY: Harper Paperbacks.

Paquette, V., Levesque, J., Mensour, B., Leroux, J. M., Beaudoin, G., Bourgouin, P., ... Beauregard M. (2003). Change the mind and you change the brain: Effects of cognitive behavior therapy on the neural correlates of spider phobia. *Neuroimage, 18,* 401–409.

Peplau, H. (1965). Interpersonal relationships: The purpose and characteristics of professional nursing. In A. W. O'Toole & S. R. Welt (Eds.), *Interpersonal theory in nursing practice. Selected works of Hildegard E. Peplau* (pp. 42–55). New York, NY: Springer Publishing.

Perraud, S., Delaney, K. R., Carlson-Sabelli, L., Johnson, M. E., Shephard, R., & Paun, O. (2006). Advanced practice psychiatric mental health nursing, finding our core: The therapeutic relationship in the 21st century. *Perspectives in Psychiatric Care, 42,* 215–226.

Porto, P. R., Oliveira, L., Mari, J., Volchan, E., Figueira, I., & Ventura, P. (2009). Does cognitive behavioral therapy change the brain? A systematic review of neuroimaging in anxiety disorders. *Journal of Neuropsychiatry and Clinical Neuroscience, 21,* 114–125.

Rachman, S. (1997). The evolution of cognitive behaviour therapy. In D. Clark, C. G. Fairburn, & M. G. Gelder (Eds.), *Science and practice of cognitive behaviour therapy* (pp. 1–26). Oxford, UK: Oxford University Press.

Reinecke, M. A., & Freeman, A. (2005). Cognitive therapy. In A. S. Gurman & S. B. Messer (Eds.), *Essential psychotherapy* (pp. 224–271). New York, NY: Guilford.

Rubak, S., Sandbaek, A., Lauritzen, T., & Christensen, B. (2005). Motivational interviewing: A systematic review and meta-analysis. *British Journal of General Practice, 55,* 305–312.

Sadock, B. J., & Sadock, V. A. (2007). *Synopsis of psychiatry: Behavioral sciences/clinical psychiatry* (10th ed.). Philadelphia, PA: Lippincott Williams & Wilkins.

Schlesinger, H. (1969). Diagnosis and prescription of psychotherapy. *Bulletin of the Menninger Clinic, 33,* 269–278.

Segal, H. (1973). *Introduction to the work of Melanie Klein*. New York, NY: Basic Books.

Serfaty, M. A., Haworth, D., Blanchard, M., Buszewicz, M., Murad, S., & King, M. (2009). Clinical effectiveness of individual cognitive behavioral therapy for depressed older people in primary care: A randomized controlled trial. *Archives of General Psychiatry, 66,* 1332–1340.

Siegel, D. (1999). *The developing mind: How relationships and the brain shape who we are*. New York, NY: Guildford.

Stanley, M. A., Wilson, N. L., Novy, D. M., Rhoades, H. M., Wagener, P. D., Greisinger, A. J., ... Kunik, M. E. (2009). Cognitive behavior therapy for generalized anxiety disorders among older adults in primary care: A randomized clinical trial. *JAMA, 301,* 1460–1476.

Sullivan, H. (1953). *The interpersonal theory of psychiatry*. New York, NY: Norton.

Swartz, H. A., & Markowitz, J. C. (1998). Interpersonal psychotherapy for the treatment of depression in HIV-positive men and women. In J. C. Markowitz (Ed.), *Interpersonal psychotherapy* (pp. 129–156). Washington, DC: American Psychiatric Press.

Tolle, E. (2004). *The power of now: A guide to spiritual enlightenment*. Novota, CA: New World Library.

Treasure, J. (2004). Motivational interviewing. *Advances in Psychiatric Treatment, 10,* 331–337.

Tyler, D. O., & Horner, S. D. (2008). Family-centered collaborative negotiation: A model for facilitating behavior change in primary care. *Journal of the American Academy of Nurse Practitioners, 20,* 194–203.

Weissman, M. M., & Markowitz, J. C. (1998). An overview of interpersonal therapy. In J. C. Markowitz (Ed.), *Interpersonal psychotherapy* (pp. 1–34). Washington, DC: American Psychiatric Press.

Wheeler, K. (2008a). The nurse psychotherapist and a framework for practice. In K. Wheeler (Ed.), *Psychotherapy for the advanced practice nurse* (pp. 3–26). St. Louis, MO: Mosby.

Wheeler, K. (Ed.). (2008b). *Psychotherapy for the advanced practice nurse.* St. Louis, MO: Mosby.

Wheeler, K., & Delaney, K. R. (2008). Challenges and realities of teaching psychotherapy: A survey of psychiatric mental health nursing graduate programs. *Perspectives in Psychiatric Care, 44,* 72–80.

Williams, M., Teasdale, J., Segal, Z., & Kabat-Zinn, J. (2007). *The mindful way through depression: Freeing yourself from chronic unhappiness.* New York, NY: Guilford.

Wolf, E. S. (1988). *Treating the self: Elements of clinical self-psychology.* New York, NY: Guilford.

Wolitzky, D. L. (2005). The theory and practice of traditional psychotherapy. In A. S. Gurman & S. B. Messer (Eds.), *Essential psychotherapy* (pp. 24–69). New York, NY: Guilford.

Yalom, I., & Lesczc, M. (2005). *Theory and practice of group psychotherapy* (5th ed.). New York, NY: Basic Books.

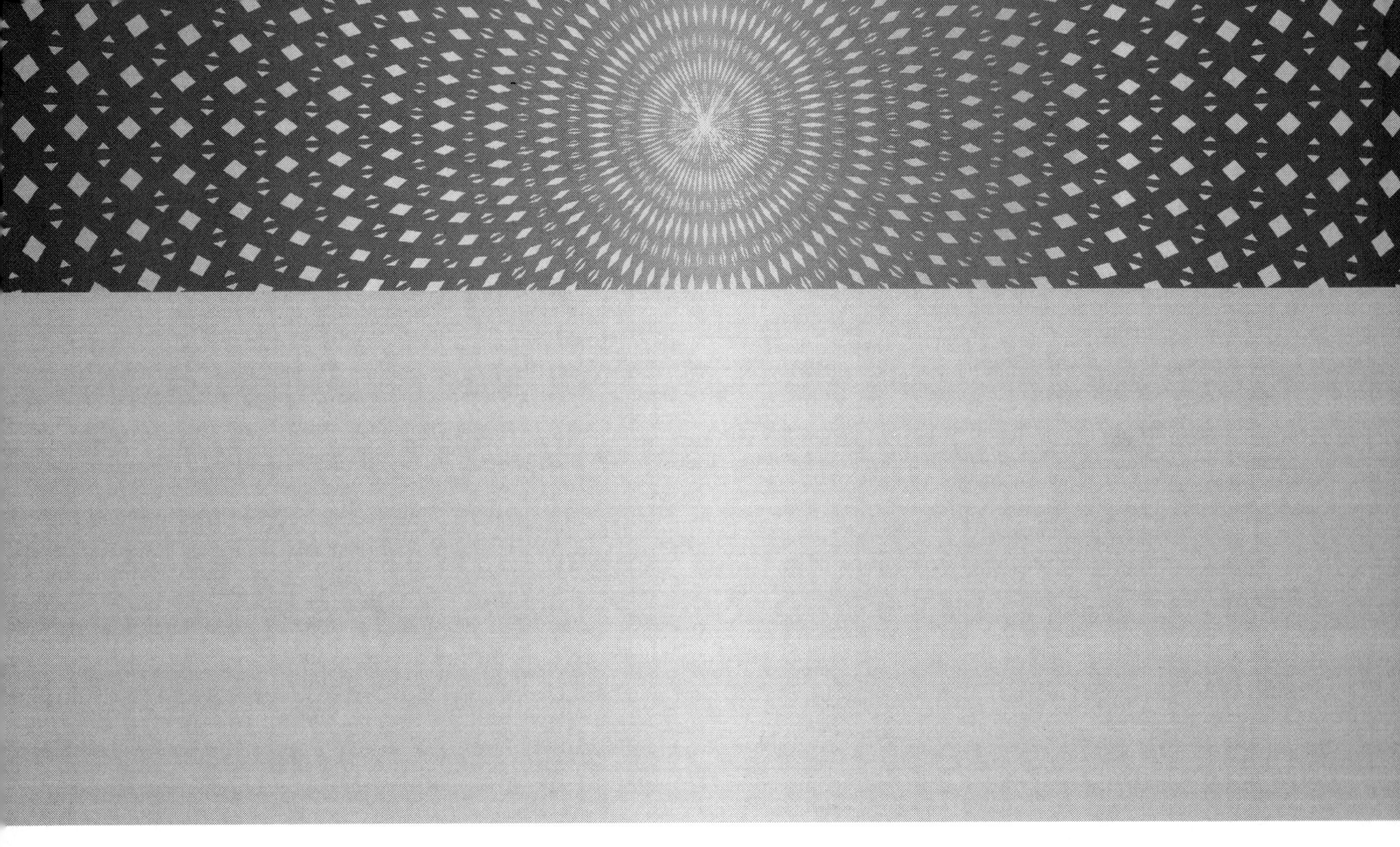

CHAPTER CONTENTS

Psychopharmacology is a science concerned with the discovery of receptors that psychotropic drugs bind to, the levels these drugs achieve in the brain, and the benefits they offer individuals in reducing the dysfunction caused by mental disorders. Essential information is covered in this chapter providing the clinician with widely recognized pharmacological concepts related to psychotropics. This review of foundational information about psychopharmacology can be adapted to individualized mental health drug management. The chapter reviews common psychotropic drugs, namely, antipsychotics, antidepressants, anxiolytics, and bipolar drugs. These medications are widely used in the treatment of mental disorders that affect thoughts, behavior, and mood.

NEURONAL TRANSMISSION

An understanding of neuronal neurotransmission is the cornerstone of psychopharmacology. Neurons are the core components of the nervous system, which includes the brain, spinal cord, and peripheral nervous system (PNS). A typical neuron possesses a cell body with a large nucleus, dendrites, and an axon. The cell body and dendrites of the neuron make up the gray matter of the brain. The features that define a neuron are electrical excitability and the presence of synapses, which are the microscopic gaps between neurons. Information travels from one neuron to another through a chemical process involving

CHAPTER 5

Overview of Psychopharmacology

Debbie Steele and Norman L. Keltner

neurotransmitters. Neurotransmitters are chemical compounds secreted from the ends of neurons, which then cross the synaptic gap to interact with receptors on the postsynaptic neuron. Neurotransmitters, then, are chemical transmitters that serve to stimulate or inhibit neighboring neurons, thus allowing impulses to be passed from one cell to another throughout the nervous system. A shortage or excess of these neurotransmitters is thought to be responsible for mental disorders (i.e., schizophrenia, depression, anxiety, bipolar disorders).

Psychotropic drugs are designed to target the major neurotransmitter systems associated with mental disorders. These drugs work primarily by either enhancing or decreasing the neurotransmitters' capacity to bind to neuronal receptors. Each psychotropic agent modulates the action of multiple neurotransmitter systems. For example, even though antipsychotics primarily act on the dopamine (DA) system, they also act on the serotonin, norepinephrine (NE), histamine, and acetylcholine (ACh) systems. Modulation of the multiple neurotransmitter systems helps explain the effectiveness, as well as the adverse side effects associated with psychotropics.

Presently, there are up to 100 different neurotransmitters known to exist in the brain. The majority of neurotransmitters are classified as amines, amino acids, circulating hormones, and neuropeptides. Of specific interest to students of psychopharmacology are: (a) the monoamines (i.e., serotonin, DA, and NE), (b) the amino acids (i.e., gamma aminobutryic acid and glutamate), and (c) ACh. Psychotropic drugs utilized in current clinical practice target these particular neurotransmitters and ultimately effect brain activity.

DA, serotonin, and NE are well known monoamine neurotransmitters that contain one amine (NH_2) group. These neurotransmitters are all derived from amino acids, but an enzyme, decarboxylase, removes the carboxylic acid (COOH) from their structure. In the end, they still have the "amino" but not the "acid," becoming **mono**amines.

DA and NE are neurotransmitters that can be grouped together into the category called catecholamines because they share a common core biochemical structure, the catechol group. Catecholamines, which are abundant in the human body, are derived from the amino acid tyrosine. The normal synthesis of catecholamines is as follows: Tyrosine is converted to levodopa (L-dopa), which is then converted to DA. Once within the synaptic vesicles, NE is metabolized from DA.

DOPAMINE

DA is a chemical messenger that affects the brain processes that control movement, emotional response, and the capacity to feel pleasure and pain. DA is vital for performing voluntary and involuntary movements. A shortage of DA can cause a lack of controlled movements such as those experienced in Parkinson's disease. Conversely, an excess of DA can cause psychotic episodes seen in schizophrenia and severe mood disorders.

NOREPINEPHRINE

Adrenergic receptors are widely distributed in the body, and present in every major organ system. NE binds to alpha- and beta-adrenergic receptors. Therefore, NE is known as an adrenergic neurotransmitter; neurons that secrete it are noradrenergic. The primary adrenergic receptor subtypes are designated as alpha-1 (α-1), alpha-2 (α-2), beta-1 (ß-1), and beta-2 (ß-2). The physiological effects of increased adrenergic activity include tachycardia, hypertension, vasoconstriction, increased alertness, anxiety, and hyperactivity. Norephinephrine reuptake inhibitors, which increase NE, have been found effective in the treatment of depression. Conversely, drugs having antagonist effects on adrenergic receptors (i.e., propranolol) are efficacious in the treatment of hypertension, as well as anxiety disorders. Side effects of adrenergic antagonists include sedation, weight gain, tachycardia, and orthostatic hypotension (Minzenberg & Yoon, 2011).

SEROTONIN

Serotonin, or 5-hydroxytryptamine (5-HT), is derived from the amino acid tryptophan and is found in the gastrointestinal tract (90%), platelets, and the central nervous system (CNS). Synthesized in the raphe nuclei of the brain stem, CNS serotonin is implicated in the regulation of normal behaviors, such as sleep, mood, pain, appetite, peristalsis, and vasoconstriction. Several serotonin receptors have been identified, including 5-HT1, 5-HT2, 5-HT3, 5-HT4, 5-HT5, 5-HT6, and 5-HT7, some with subtypes. The role of each type of receptor varies. For example, the 5-HT1A receptors are implicated in the pathophysiology of depression, while the 5-HT2A has been implicated in psychosis (Opacka-Juffry, 2008).

GABA

Gamma-aminobutyric acid (GABA) is a potent inhibitory neurotransmitter. It is widely distributed throughout the CNS, particularly in the thalamus, a region of the brain involved with sleep processes (Martin & Dunn, 2002). GABA exerts its inhibitory effects by binding to its receptor site, initiating an increase in chloride conductance through the ion channel. Increased chloride entry at the receptor site results in hyperpolarization of the neuron, which inhibits depolarization or firing of the neuron. This process results in an anti-anxiety, anti-epileptic, and/or sedative effect.

GLUTAMATE

Glutamate is a potent excitatory neurotransmitter that potentially affects all neurons and is therefore referred to as the "master switch." The normal everyday excitation of neurons activated by glutamate is necessary for learning and memory. However, excess excitability of neurons is hypothesized to result in the neurodegeneration associated with psychiatric conditions such as Parkinson's and Alzheimer's disease. Although numerous glutamate receptors exist, N-methyl-D-aspartate (NMDA) and alpha-amino-3-hydroxy-5-methyl-4-isoxazole-propionic acid (AMPA) are of particular significance. As glutamate occupies these receptors, calcium channels are opened and the neuron is activated for neurotransmission. Excessive action of the glutamate neurotransmitter leads to excess calcium channel activity and eventually the production of free radicals. As free radicals destroy neurons, symptoms such as mania or panic may result. Chronic and progressive neuronal death or excitotoxicity results in neurodegenerative symptoms (Stahl, 2008). This process helps explain the progressive loss of functioning associated with schizophrenia, Alzheimer's, and Parkinson's disease. NMDA receptor antagonists such as memantine (Namenda) are utilized in the treatment of moderate to severe Alzheimer's disease. Memantine reduces NMDA-induced excitotoxicity, while still allowing receptor signaling for physiological activation (McKeage, 2010).

ACETYLCHOLINE

ACh, which is widely distributed in the brain and the PNS, is synthesized and released by cholinergic neurons. Two main classes of ACh receptors have been identified: the muscarinic receptors and the nicotinic receptors. ACh plays a key role in learning and memory in the CNS. Within the PNS, the cholinergic system controls such functions as salivation, gastrointestinal motility, pupil size, and mucus secretion. Increasing levels of ACh, and thus enhancing cognitive functioning, is the goal of treatment for Alzheimer's disease. The best approach for increasing ACh is through the use of acetylcholinesterase inhibitors, such as donepezil. On the other hand, anticholinergic agents, which block ACh receptors, can have a negative impact on memory and learning. Other common anticholinergic side effects include dry mouth, constipation, blurred vision, and urinary retention.

PSYCHOTROPIC DRUGS

A psychotropic is a chemical substance that crosses the blood–brain barrier and acts primarily upon the CNS, where it affects brain function, resulting in changes in thoughts, feelings, and behavior. A foundational understanding of the utility of psychotropic drugs is provided to enhance clinician efficiency and expertise. The following psychotropics are reviewed: (1) antipsychotics; (2) antidepressants; (3) anti-anxiety agents; and (4) bipolar disorder medications.

Antipsychotics are the mainstay of treatment for psychotic disorders such as schizophrenia and psychotic mood disorders. They are also widely used for a range of other indications, such as refractory depression, acute mania, delirium, personality disorders, substance-related disorders, anxiety disorders, developmental disorders, and dementias (Glick, Murray, Vasudevan, Marder, & Hu, 2001). Antipsychotics do not cure any of these disorders, except for perhaps, delirious states.

The treatment of schizophrenia is focused on the three major constellations of symptoms that characterize this disorder: (a) positive symptoms such as hallucinations, delusions, and disorganized thoughts; (b) negative symptoms such as affect flattening, apathy, and avolition; (c) cognitive deficits affecting learning, memory, and attention. Long-term administration of antipsychotics has been effective in ameliorating the positive symptoms associated with schizophrenia. Treatment of the other symptoms has remained a much more elusive challenge.

HISTORY OF ANTIPSYCHOTICS

For the past sixty years, the management of psychoses has depended heavily on a group of drugs once called neuroleptics, now referred to as antipsychotics. Chlorpromazine, the first antipsychotic, was synthesized in 1950 and utilized as a centrally acting antihistamine. In 1952, Henri Laborit, a surgeon, described how patients anesthetized with chlorpromazine appeared to become indifferent to what was going on around them. At the same time, Jean Delay and Pierre Deniker reported that chlorpromazine was beneficial in controlling psychotic agitation and mania. Chlorpromazine became widely used for many psychiatric conditions, as well as for nausea, vomiting, and itching. Within a few years of its use, it became obvious that chlorpromazine was associated with Parkinson-like side effects. As new compounds were synthesized to combat schizophrenia, it seemed that only those that produced Parkinson-like symptoms brought about benefits for psychoses. The effectiveness of this group of agents found useful in the treatment of psychoses led to the DA hypothesis of schizophrenia (Healy, 2009).

The DA hypothesis of schizophrenia has a circular explanation. Since all antipsychotics block the DA system in the brain, and antipsychotics were found to be beneficial in the treatment of schizophrenia, there must be something wrong with the DA system in the brains of individuals with schizophrenia. As a result of this hypothesis, major research was designed around the development of traditional antipsychotics that were active on the DA system. Unfortunately, the early antipsychotics elicited a host of adverse effects, specifically, extrapyramidal side effects (EPSEs), tardive dyskinesia, and hyperprolactinemia. This led to the belief that antipsychotic use and adverse neurological effects went hand in hand and were essentially inescapable. In the mid-1960s, the development of clozapine as an effective antipsychotic without adverse neurological effects was determined a huge breakthrough. However, when the risk of agranulocytosis was associated with the use of clozapine, efforts were underway to develop an antipsychotic with clozapine-like effectiveness without its risk for agranulocytosis, or the adverse neurological effects of chlorpromazine. Such efforts have been partially successful with the development of atypical or second-generation antipsychotics (SGAs) (Jindal & Keshavan, 2008). Antipsychotics, then, can be divided into two major categories: (1) typical or first-generation antipsychotics (FGAs), such as haloperidol and chlorpromazine; and (2) atypical or SGAs, such as aripiprazole, clozapine, olanzapine, quetiapine, risperidone, and ziprasidone.

TYPICAL ANTIPSYCHOTICS

The mechanism of action of all antipsychotics is the antagonism of DA (D2) receptors. With typical or FGAs, the level of D2 receptor blockade is directly related to the antipsychotic effect. Positron emission tomography (PET) studies reveal that the optimal clinical effect of DA receptor antagonists occurs between 60% and 70% of D2 receptor occupancy. Hyperprolactinemia begins to occur at about 70% occupancy and the incidence of EPSE increases above the 80% threshold.

Typical antipsychotics can be differentiated into three distinct categories based on potency, a measure of the dosage required to bring about a response. If a medication has high potency, then a small dose is needed to attain the intended response; likewise, if a medication has low potency, then a larger dose is needed to attain the intended response. For example, 2 mg of haloperidol is as effective as 100 mg of chlorpromazine in alleviating the symptoms of schizophrenia, and thus haloperidol is more potent than chlorpromazine. Perphenazine is an example of a moderate potency antipsychotic. See Table 5-1 for a list of common typical antipsychotics with DA (D2) levels of potency.

Typical antipsychotics modulate the action of several neurotransmitter systems besides DA (D2) receptors. For example, chlorpromazine and other low potency typical antipsychotics have a high potency for cholinergic muscarinic and alpha-1-adrenergic receptors. Therefore, their use is associated with classic anticholinergic side effects: dry mouth, blurred vision, constipation, and orthostatic hypotension. On the other hand, the high potency typical antipsychotics have a higher incidence of EPSE. First-line treatment of extrapyramidal symptoms is an anticholinergic such as benztropine (Cogentin). In sum, high potency antipsychotics are paired with anticholinergics, while low frequency antipsychotics cause anticholingeric side effects.

To explain the paradox, one must consider that the negotiation of voluntary and involuntary movement requires that DA and ACh be in balance. Since high potency antipsychotics block DA, but not ACh, the DA/ACh equation gets out of balance. This results in movement disorders, characterized as extrapyramidal symptoms. The use of anticholinergics such as benztropine effectively rebalances the DA/ACh equation, alleviating EPSEs. Additional information detailing extrapyramidal symptoms follows.

ADVERSE EFFECTS AND TYPICAL ANTIPSYCHOTICS

Among the adverse effects caused by traditional antipsychotics, three stand out: (a) EPSE, (b) hyperprolactinemia, and (c) increased negative symptoms. As previously mentioned, adverse effects are produced as a result of antipsychotic modulation of several neurotransmitter systems. In addition, DA neurotransmitters bind to at least seven different types of DA receptors in various parts of the brain. Four different DA tracts, with four different functions are found in the CNS. The psychotic symptoms associated with schizophrenia are alleviated by the inhibition of DA in the mesolimbic tract, which is the intended effect of antipsychotics. Unfortunately, DA reduction in other DA tracts causes disturbing events. Specifically, DA inhibition in the nigrostriatal tract causes extrapyramidal symptoms. Hyperprolactinemia is linked to DA reduction in the tuberoinfundibular tract. A reduction of DA in the mesocrotical tract results in increased negative symptoms, such as apathy, alogia, and avolition. All of these events are attributed to blockade of DA receptors.

TABLE 5-1: COMMON TYPICAL ANTIPSYCHOTICS

LOW POTENCY	MODERATE POTENCY	HIGH POTENCY
Chlorpromazine (Thorazine)	Loxapine (Loxitane)	Haloperidol (Haldol)
Thioridazine (Mellaril)	Perphenazine (Trilafon)	Fluphenazine (Prolixin)

EXTRAPYRAMIDAL SIDE EFFECTS

EPSE are primarily abnormal movement disorders related to the reduction of DA in the extrapyramidal (nigrostriatal) tract, which coordinates involuntary movement. Following is a list of the EPSEs:

1. Akathisia is an unpleasant, emotional state experienced as restlessness. The hallmark symptom can be observed as the inability to sit still. Other subjective symptoms are experienced as dysphoria, irritability, or impulsivity. Akathisia oftentimes responds to anticholinergic antidotes, or to propranolol.
2. Akinesia is a Parkinson-like symptom that is characterized by stiffness and lack of movement. A person may find it difficult to start moving, lean to one side, lean forward, or stop moving. Additional symptoms include drooling, delay in answering questions, and clumsiness.
3. Dyskinesias are abnormal movements characterized by Parkinson-like tremors, especially of the hands. Other common symptoms include pill rolling of the hands, repetitive pouting of the lips, and protrusion of the tongue. Note that dyskinesias may involve the respiratory muscles leading to episodic or periodic wheezing or shortness of breath. This symptom can be misinterpreted as asthma (Healy, 2009).
4. Dystonia is defined as a muscle spasm. Oculogyric crisis is a dramatic example involving the eyeballs rolling upward so that only the whites of the eyes can be seen. Other symptoms include difficulty speaking, clenching of the jaw, and lockjaw. Spasms can be extremely painful affecting the jaw, throat, facial muscles, limbs, or trunk.

5. Tardive dyskinesia refers to late-onset abnormal movements, particularly of the mouth and face. Symptoms involve lip-smacking, chewing movements, protrusion of the tongue, and writhing movements of the limbs and trunk. These symptoms may appear several months after the antipsychotic has been started, or after it has been stopped. Whereas the other EPSEs disappear after discontinuation of the antipsychotic, tardive dyskinesia may last for months or years after drug discontinuation. Fine vermicular movement of the tongue may be an early sign of tardive dyskinesia and if the medication is stopped at that time the full syndrome may not develop.

HYPERPROLACTINEMIA

Hyperprolactinemia and breast swelling are hormonal changes that may occur in both women and men on antipsychotics. Elevated prolactin levels occur as a result of DA antagonism in the tuberoinfundibular tract, as well as blockage of DA receptors in the anterior pituitary. Consequences of hyperprolactinemia include impotence, decreased libido, amenorrhea, galactorrhea, gynecomastia, lowered sperm count, and feminization. As one would imagine, prolactin elevation is a major drawback related to typical antipsychotic adherence.

INCREASED NEGATIVE SYMPTOMS

Demotivation or a state of indifference is associated with long-term use or high doses of traditional antipsychotics. Traditional antipsychotics can increase negative symptoms and cognitive blunting not only by DA antagonism in the mesocortical tract, but also by blocking muscarinic cholinergic receptors. Many patients prefer to use nicotine and other substances of abuse rather than endure an increase in these emotions (Stahl, 2008).

NEUROLEPTIC MALIGNANT SYNDROME

Neuroleptic malignant syndrome (NMS) is a rare but potentially fatal reaction associated with the use of antipsychotics. Although most commonly associated with high doses of antipsychotics, it may occur even at low doses in patients experiencing dehydration, exhaustion, or during exercise. Blockage of dopaminergic pathways are believed to result in the major symptoms associated with NMS, coupled with noradrenergic hyperactivity. NMS characteristics include acute onset, hyperthermia, profound mental changes (i.e., confusion, agitation), catatonia or rigidity, and autonomic symptoms (i.e., labile blood pressure [BP], diaphoresis, and tachycardia). Creatine phosphokinase (CPK) elevation and leukocytosis are blood abnormalities sometimes reported in NMS. The increase in CPK is caused by muscle rigidity and subsequent rhabdomyolysis (Keltner & Folks, 2005). Once NMS is suspected, immediate withdrawal of the antipsychotic followed by supportive care is the treatment of choice for most cases. Supportive care includes the infusion of intravenous (IV) fluids for hydration and treatment with benzodiazepines (BZDs) to manage irritability and motor excitation (Steele, Keltner, & McGuiness, 2011).

Given the numerous unacceptable side effects associated with typical antipsychotics, their use has declined significantly with the availability of the atypical agents. One typical antipsychotic in particular, haloperidol (Haldol), is still used by many clinicians for the management of schizophrenia, acute agitation, and for the control of tics and vocal utterances of Tourette's disorder. In fact, Haldol is the most frequently used antipsychotic medication for delirium, due to its few anticholinergic side effects and small likelihood of causing sedation (Markowitz & Narasimhan, 2008). Haldol decanoate and Prolixin decanoate, both typical antipsychotics, are used today as injectable long-acting formulations approved for the treatment of schizophrenia.

ATYPICAL ANTIPSYCHOTICS

The primary difference between typical and atypical antipsychotics is that atypicals act as DA (D2) and serotonin (5-HT2A) antagonists. 5-HT2A receptors can be found on the axon terminal of neurons that produce DA. Antagonism or blockage of 5-HT2A receptors regulates DA release in the striatal, pituitary, and neocortical regions of the brain. This mechanism counterbalances the depletion of DA caused by antipsychotics (D2 antagonism), specifically in those areas of the brain that are responsible for adverse effects, such as EPSEs (Horacek et al., 2006). Atypical antipsychotics, then, are effective in treating positive symptoms, with a decreased incidence of EPSE, hyperprolactinemia, and negative symptoms (Komossa et al., 2009a, 2009b, 2010a, 2010b).

Atypical antipsychotics also can be differentiated from typicals based on their affinity and dissociation rate at both DA and serotonin receptors. The "Fast-Off" Theory helps explain the improved side effect profile of atypical antipsychotics. As mentioned previously, both typical and atypical antipsychotics attach to D2 receptors; however, they differ in how fast and how frequently they come on and off these receptors. Atypical antipsychotics tend to have "rapid dissociation," meaning they dissociate from D2 receptors after a brief period of time. Conversely, typical antipsychotics have a more long-lasting blockade on D2 receptors. In other words, the effects of atypical antipsychotics on D2 receptors are much more transient than those of typicals. For example, clozapine, a drug with a fast dissociation, goes on and off the D2 receptor 100 times more frequently than haloperidol (Kapur & Seeman, 2001). As antipsychotics go on and off the D2 receptor rapidly, endogenous DA is allowed to bind to and release from the same receptors. This dynamic process seems to explain how atypicals are effective in producing an antipsychotic effect without the robust extrapyramidal symptoms and hyperprolactinemia associated with the atypicals (Horacek et al., 2006; Seeman, 2002; Steele, Dowben, Vance, & Keltner, 2011).

INDIVIDUAL ATYPICAL ANTIPSYCHOTICS

No two atypical antipsychotics have exactly the same pharmacological profiles, even though some of their binding properties at DA and serotonin receptors overlap. Noting differences between the atypical antipsychotics allows the prescriber to match the best antipsychotic agent to the uniqueness of the individual patient. The most common and newest atypical antipsychotics are reviewed. Clozapine is discussed first due to its role in the advent of atypical antipsychotics.

Clozapine

Clozapine (Clozaril) is considered the "gold standard" for efficacy in schizophrenia. It has Food and Drug Administration (FDA) indications for patients with schizophrenia or schizoaffective disorder who are at chronic risk for reexperiencing suicidal behavior. It offers many clinical advantages over typical antipsychotics, including its efficacy in treatment-refractory schizophrenia, and a low propensity for EPSEs or hyperprolactinemia at even very high dosages (Jindal & Keshavan, 2008). The use of clozapine requires organized monitoring and management of risks associated with agranulocytosis, myocarditis, seizures, and metabolic side effects (Mauri et al., 2007). Due to these life-threatening and potentially fatal complications, clozapine is not considered to be a first-line treatment, but rather is prescribed when other antipsychotics fail.

The implementation of mandatory hematologic monitoring has diminished the risks of agranulocytosis associated with clozapine. All patients taking clozapine must be registered and monitored based on a standard algorithm. In short, the following parameters must be followed to protect patients on clozapine: (a) White blood cells (WBC) must be over 3,500/mm^3 and the absolute neutrophil count (ANC) above 2,000/mm^3 prior to initiating therapy; (b) weekly monitoring for six months, then biweekly; (c) stop clozapine if WBC drops below 3,000/mm^3 or the ANC drops below 1,500/mm^3; (d) rechallenge once original parameters are met and no infection develops; and (e) permanently discontinue clozapine if WBC drops below 2,000/mm^3 and ANC drops below 1,000/mm^3. In general, agranulocytosis is closely linked to the early administration of clozapine, with risks decreasing over time.

Aripiprazole

Aripiprazole (Abilify) represents a new generation of antipsychotics that are known as dopamine partial agonists (DPAs). Aripiprazole functions as a partial agonist at the DA (D2) and the serotonin (5-HT1A) receptors, and as an antagonist at serotonin 5-HT2A receptors. DPAs reduce DA hyperactivity in the mesolimbic region to a degree sufficient to alleviate psychotic symptoms, while also stabilizing DA in the nigrostriatal system to a degree sufficient to prevent the occurrence of EPSE. In other words, D2 partial agonists bind in an intermediate fashion to the D2 receptor, providing a balance between agonist and antagonist actions (Stahl, 2008). Theoretically, the unique actions of a partial agonist make DA available at a consistent level to the four dopaminergic pathways. In this way, EPSEs are minimized. Abilify is indicated for: (a) an add-on treatment to an antidepressant for adults with major depressive disorder; (b) bipolar 1 disorder in adults and in pediatric patients (ages 10–17); (c) schizophrenia in adults and in adolescents (ages 13–17); and (d) irritability associated with Autistic Disorder (ages 6–17). Abilify is available in multiple forms: tablet, oral disintegrating, oral solution, and injection.

Olanzapine

Olanzapine (Zyprexa) is a popular atypical antipsychotic indicated for the treatment of schizophrenia and bipolar 1 disorder in adults and adolescents (ages 13–17). Although effective for mood and cognitive symptoms, its use is associated with significant weight gain and other cardiometabolic risk factors (Stahl, 2008). Multiple formulations are available for acute and maintenance therapy. Zyprexa IntraMuscular is available for the treatment of acute agitation. Zydis is an orally disintegrating alternative to the Zyprexa tablet. Symbyax is an olanzapine/fluoxetine combination approved for use in adults for short-term: (a) treatment of depressive episodes associated with bipolar 1 disorder; and (b) treatment of resistant depression.

Quetiapine

Quetiapine (Seroquel) was the first atypical antipsychotic found effective as a monotherapy for the treatment of the depressed phase of bipolar disorder. Similar to the other atypicals, quetiapine is also indicated for schizophrenia and bipolar mania in adults and adolescents (ages 13–17). However, one dimension of quetiapine stands out from the others; the sedating H1-antihistamine actions relieve insomnia when administered at bedtime. Due to its anxiolytic and sedative effect, it has the potential of becoming a drug of abuse (Keltner & Vance, 2008). Quetiapine can cause metabolic symptoms such as weight gain, hyperlipidemia, and insulin resistance. Seroquel tabs and Seroquel XR (extended release) are available.

Risperidone

Risperidone (Risperdal) is an older atypical antipsychotic indicated for treatment of: (a) schizophrenia in adults and adolescents (aged 13–17); (b) bipolar 1 disorder in adults and children and adolescents (aged 10–17); and irritability associated with autistic disorder in children and adolescents (aged 5–16) years. Because risperidone is efficacious and has FDA approval for childhood disorders, it is one of the most frequently prescribed antipsychotics. However, when used in high doses, risperidone is known to cause both EPSEs and hyperprolactinemia (Stahl, 2008). Risperidone is available as tablets, an oral solution, ampules, and the M-TAB disintegrating tablets. Risperdal Consta, an injectable, long-acting form given every 2 weeks has been found to be effective for schizoaffective disorder as monotherapy, and as an adjunct to mood stabilizers and/or antidepressant therapy in adults. Paliperidone (Invega) is a metabolite of risperidone with a similar mechanism of action, but has less alpha-1 antagonist effects (Stahl, 2008).

Ziprasidone

Ziprasidone (Geodon) is a highly effective atypical antipsychotic available as a capsule or injection for the acute and maintenance treatment of schizophrenia and bipolar 1 disorder in adults. Early concerns that Geodon had the capacity to prolong the QTc interval have been dispelled and routine EKGs are generally not recommended. However, Geodon should not be given to individuals receiving other drugs known to lengthen the QTc interval (Stahl, 2008). Ziprasidone is the only atypical antipsychotic that functions as an antagonist at the 5-HT1D receptors and as an agonist at the 5-HT1A receptors, contributing to its favorable effects at decreasing anxiety and depressive symptoms, as well as improving negative symptoms (Stahl, 2008).

THE NEWEST ATYPICAL ANTIPSYCHOTICS

The three newest FDA approved antipsychotics are asenapine, iloperidone, and lurasidone. Asenapine (Saphris), in a sublingual tablet form, is indicated for the treatment of schizophrenia and bipolar mania. It binds with high affinity and specificity to DA, serotonin, NE, and histamine receptors, but with minimal affinity for muscarinic receptors. Asenapine has been shown to bind to 5-HT2A receptors more intensely than to DA (D2) receptors. This receptor binding profile is targeted to treat the negative symptoms associated with schizophrenia.

Iloperidone (Fanapt) acts as a broad spectrum DA, serotonin, and NE receptor antagonist. It has a high affinity for 5-HT2 receptors and alpha-1-adrenoceptors, with a moderate affinity for D2 receptors. Low binding affinity for histamine suggests a decreased propensity to cause sedation and weight gain. Iloperidone must be titrated slowly from a low starting dose to avoid orthostatic hypotension due to its alpha-adrenergic blocking properties.

Lurasidone (Latuda) is the newest atypical antipsychotic approved by the FDA for treatment of schizophrenia in 2010. Lurasidone is unique because it has the highest affinity of any atypical for the 5-HT7 receptor. Antagonism of the 5-HT7 receptor theoretically can improve memory and mood symptoms. Additionally, lurasidone has strong antagonistic properties for 5-HT1A and alpha-2C-adrenergic receptors, which hypothetically improve cognition and negative symptoms (Ehret, Sopko, & Lemieux, 2010). In sum, the side effect profile of these new antipsychotics appear to mimic other atypicals, but in different frequencies (Roman, 2011).

ADVERSE EFFECTS AND ATYPICAL ANTIPSYCHOTICS

Atypical antipsychotics modulate other neurotransmitters besides DA and serotonin to some degree or another. For example, clozapine also acts as an antagonist at adrenergic, cholinergic, and histaminergic receptors. Antipsychotic activity on the various neurotransmitter systems largely determines the drug's side effect profile. See Table 5-2 for a list of common antipsychotics with occurrence rates of expected side effects.

CARDIOMETABOLIC SYNDROME

Atypical antipsychotics are significantly associated with cardiometabolic adverse effects. These effects include weight gain, obesity, hypertension, lipid and glucose abnormalities, metabolic syndrome, and related cardiovascular disorders. The mechanisms and pathways underlying cardiometabolic adverse effects associated with antipsychotics are not completely understood. For example, regarding weight gain, data have been inconclusive whether antipsychotics increase appetite, decrease activity, or decrease metabolism. Blocking serotonin 5-HT2C receptors appears to make weight gain more likely, as do actions on the hormone leptin. In addition, alpha-adrenergic neurotransmitters, cannaboid receptors, as well as satiety hormones and peptides are currently being studied related to their link to the cardiometabolic adverse effects of antipsychotics (Correll, Lencz, & Malhotra, 2010; Healy, 2009). Metabolic changes associated with atypical medications increase the lifelong risk of morbidity and mortality. Ziprasidone and aripiprazole seem to be the first-line treatments for avoidance of weight gain and cardiometabolic risks (Stahl, 2008). Regardless of which atypical antipsychotic is used, regular health screens including weight, body mass index (BMI), BP, fasting blood glucose, and triglyceride levels are important components of medical supervision and follow-up. See Exhibit 5-1 for an example of a cardiometabolic screening chart.

Each antipsychotic presents its own challenges in terms of balancing effectiveness with safety and tolerability. It is important for clinicians to measure and, where necessary, treat side effects to improve patients' well-being. Formal assessment and management of side effects is essential to improve the quality of care and reduce the risk of early mortality.

NEW DEVELOPMENTS

Antipsychotics are not clean drugs that only modulate specific receptors. The use of antipsychotics entails a difficult trade-off between the benefits of alleviating psychotic symptoms and the risk of disturbing adverse events. Although atypical antipsychotics appear to produce a milder side effect profile compared to typicals,

TABLE 5-2: COMMON ANTIPSYCHOTIC DRUGS

ANTIPSYCHOTICS	DOSAGE RANGE	SEDATION	ORTHOSTATIC HYPOTENSION	EPSE	WEIGHT GAIN	ANTI-ACH EFFECTS
COMMON TYPICALS (FGA)						
Haloperidol (Haldol)	2–40 mg	low	low	+++++		+
Fluphenazine (Prolixin)	3–45 mg	low	mid	+++++		++
COMMON ATYPICALS (SGA)						
Clozapine (Clozaril)	300–900 mg	high	high	0	+++	+++++
Risperidone (Risperdal)	4–16 mg	low	mid	+	++	+
Olanzapine (Zyprexa)	5–20 mg	mid	low	+/0	+++	+
Quetiapine (Seroquel)	150–600 mg	mid	mid	+/0	++	+
Ziprasidone (Geodon)	60–160 mg	low	mid	+/0	+/0	++
Aripiprazole (Abilify)	15–30 mg	low	low	+	+/0	+
Paliperidone (Invega)	3–12 mg	low	mid	+	++	+

Sedative effects r/t antagonism of M1-muscarinic, H1-histaminic, and alpha-1-adrenergic receptors.

Orthostatic hypotension r/t antagonism of alpha-1- and beta-adrenergic receptors.

Anti-ACh effects include dry mouth, blurred vision, urinary retention, constipation.

0 = none; + = very low; ++ = low; +++ = moderate; +++ = high; +++++ = very high.

Adapted from Preston (2011); Stahl (2008).

EXHIBIT 5-1: CARDIOMETABOLIC FLOWCHART

PATIENT'S NAME	BASELINE	VISIT 1	VISIT 2
Weight	_____	_____	_____
BMI	_____	_____	_____
BP	_____	_____	_____
Fasting glucose	_____	_____	_____
Fasting triglycerides	_____	_____	_____

their use is problematic when it comes to long-term cardiometabolic adverse effects.

Several new developments are changing the landscape of antipsychotic choice. The older typical antipsychotics are available at a much lower cost than the atypicals. For example, typical antipsychotics can cost less than $30 a month, while brand name atypicals can cost over $500 a month (Consumer Reports Best Buy Drugs, 2009). In light of the depressed economy in America, new paradigms are needed to manage mental health patients. One suggestion is the use of typical antipsychotics at low doses, enough to show improvement of positive symptoms without worsening of negative symptoms. In order to make prudent antipsychotic choices for mental health patients, it is important to consider efficacy, side effect profile, cost, and individual response and preference.

ANTIDEPRESSANTS

Depression is the most prevalent mental disorder in the Western world. The monoamine theory purports that a deficiency of neurotransmission within the CNS, specifically that of the serotonin, NE, and DA systems, is the leading cause of depression. While the precise mechanism of action of antidepressants is unknown, it is suggested that they restore normal levels of neurotransmitters by blocking the reuptake of these substances from the synapse in the CNS.

The pharmacology of antidepressant agents is primarily centered on altering the concentration of the monoamine neurotransmitters serotonin and NE, with a few drugs effecting DA levels. The ratio of serotonin to NE reuptake inhibition varies from antidepressant to antidepressant. Conventional antidepressant therapies include selective monoamine reuptake inhibitors, noradrenergic and specific serotonergic antidepressants (NaSSAs), tricyclics (TCAs), and monoamine oxidase inhibitors (MAOIs), all of which aim to enhance monoaminergic neurotransmission. However, the use of these agents presents clear disadvantages, including a delay in the alleviation of depressive symptoms and numerous adverse effects.

Antidepressant agents have been approved by the FDA to treat a host of mental disorders besides depression, such as: (1) generalized anxiety disorders (GADs), (2) panic disorder, (3) post-traumatic stress disorder (PTSD), (4) obsessive-compulsive disorder, (5) social phobia, and (6) bulimia nervosa. Selective serotonin reuptake inhibitors (SSRIs) and serotonin-norepinephrine reuptake inhibitors (SNRIs) are considered first line treatments for the listed anxiety disorders due to the poor adverse event profiles associated with BZDs, TCAs, and hydroxyzine. In particular, BZDs have a high potential for dependency and withdrawal issues. The TCAs have the potential for fatalities in the case of overdose. SSRIs and SNRIs are generally well tolerated, with little potential for dependency. In addition, they are relatively safe in overdose (Carter & McCormack, 2009).

Antidepressants have many off-label uses including migraine prophylaxis, treatment of chronic pain, and fibromyalgia. Whether a given antidepressant is used for depression or for an anxiety disorder, the mechanism of action, side effect profile, and unique characteristics will essentially be the same. For example, the lag time to clinical effectiveness for the SSRIs is 2 to 4 weeks regardless of whether major depression or GAD is being treated. See Table 5-3 for a list of antidepressant categories with generic and brand names.

SELECTIVE MONOAMINE REUPTAKE INHIBITORS

The most commonly prescribed antidepressants are selective monoamine reuptake inhibitors (Drug Topics Staff, 2009). At present there are four different, distinct categories including: (1) SSRIs; (2) SNRIs; (3) norepinephrine reuptake inhibitors (NRIs); and (4) norepinephrine dopamine reuptake inhibitors (NDRIs). Each category will be discussed separately.

Selective Serotonin Reuptake Inhibitors

SSRIs are used widely for the treatment of depression and anxiety disorders (see Table 5-4). They are known to inhibit neuronal uptake of serotonin and to a lesser degree, NE and DA. In general, the SSRIs have very low or weak affinity for alpha- and beta-adrenergic, DA, histamine, and muscarinic receptors. By way of explanation, after serotonin is released into the synapse between the nerve cells, SSRIs prevent the serotonin from being reabsorbed back into the releasing neuron. This process

TABLE 5-3: LIST OF ANTIDEPRESSANT CATEGORIES WITH GENERIC AND BRAND NAMES

SSRIs	SNRIs	TCAs	OTHERS
Citalopram (Celexa)	Desvenlafaxine (Pristiq)	Amitriptyline (Elavil)	Bupropion (Wellbutrin)
Escitalopram (Lexapro)	Duloxetine (Cymbalta)	Amoxapine (Asendin)	Mirtazapine (Remeron)
Fluoxetine (Prozac)	Venlafaxine (Effexor)	Clomipramine (Anafranil)	Olanzapine/fluoxetine (Symbyax)
Fluvoxamine (Luvox)		Desipramine (Norpramin)	Vilazodone (Viibryd)
Paroxetine (Paxil)		Doxepin (Sinequan)	
Sertraline (Zoloft)		Imipramine (Tofranil)	
		Maprotiline (Ludiomil)	
		Nortriptyline (Pamelor)	
		Protriptyline (Vivactil)	

TABLE 5-4: INDICATIONS FOR SPECIFIC SSRIs

SSRIs	FDA INDICATIONS
Citalopram (Celexa)	Depression Panic Disorder
Escitalopram (Lexapro)	Depression Generalized Anxiety Disorder Panic Disorder Obsessive Compulsive Disorder Social Phobia
Fluoxetine (Prozac, Prozac Weekly)	Depression Obsessive Compulsive Disorder Bulimia Nervosa
Paroxetine (Paxil)	Depression Generalized Anxiety Disorder Panic Disorder Post-traumatic Stress Disorder Obsessive Compulsive Disorder Social Phobia
Sertraline (Zoloft)	Depression Obsessive Compulsive Disorder Panic Disorder Post-traumatic Stress Disorder Social Phobia Premenstrual Dysphoric Disorder

allows the serotonin to remain in the synapse for continued action on the receiving neuron, boosting the availability of serotonin in the brain. Stahl (1998) points out that, initially, the reuptake blockade occurs in the raphe nuclei. As serotonin levels rise around the soma of the neuron, the autoreceptors in that area (5-HT1A) become desensitized to serotonin and cease to function normally. Because the neuron's feedback system is turned off, serotonin levels continue to build up within the synaptic gap. All the while, serotonin continues to be released from the presynaptic neuron into the synaptic gap. In addition, desensitization of postsynaptic serotonin receptors is facilitated by the build-up of serotonin. Stahl suggests this sequence of events may elucidate the delay observed in the therapeutic response to SSRIs. When patients initially start antidepressants, there is commonly a delay in full response for up to 2 weeks. This dynamic seems to ring true for all of the antidepressants that inhibit the reuptake of monoamines.

Adverse Effects of SSRIs

Even though the SSRIs have become a mainstay of treatment for depression and anxiety, they have certain limitations, including the development of some specific adverse events that have a negative impact on patients' quality of life. Compared with the TCAs, SSRIs provide a better side effect profile overall (Cipriani et al., 2009; Parikh, 2009), particularly the absence of fatal cardiac events (Sicouri & Antzelevitch, 2008). However, the adverse effects associated with the SSRIs can become troubling to the point of nonadherence (Cooke & Keltner, 2008). Common symptoms involve gastrointestinal complaints (i.e., nausea and diarrhea) and neuropsychiatric complaints (e.g., insomnia and nervousness). Because serotonin is widely distributed in the stomach, gastrointestinal upset is a common adverse effect associated with elevated serotonin 5-HT3 stimulation during SSRI use (Mason, Morris, & Balcezak, 2000). Agents that block 5-HT3 such as Ondansetron (Zofran) are useful in treating the gastrointestinal side effects.

Sexual dysfunction is also very common with the use of SSRIs, with anecdotal reports suggesting that up to 60% or more of SSRI-treated patients experience some form of treatment-induced sexual dysfunction. SSRIs can affect three stages of the sexual cycle: desire, excitement, and orgasm. Damsa et al. (2004) suggest that the inhibition of DA (known as the pleasure neurotransmitter) by serotonin in the mesolimbic pathway contributes to the change in sexual function. For some men who experience premature ejaculation, use of SSRIs may actually enhance the sexual experience by prolonging the excitement stage. Other male and female disorders associated with the excitement or orgasm stages may be treated with sildenafil (Viagra) or a similar agent (Nurnberg et al., 2008). In some cases, discontinuing the SSRI may not restore normal sexual functioning immediately. Some patients report persistent sexual problems months and years after discontinuation (Csoka, Bahrick, & Mehtonen, 2008).

Special Concerns Related to SSRIs

Four important concerns related to the use of SSRIs in particular are briefly discussed in order to provide a more comprehensive appreciation of these antidepressants. These concerns involve the risk of suicide, serotonin syndrome, withdrawal or discontinuation syndrome, and apathy syndrome. Additionally, drug interactions associated with concomitant use of SSRIs is provided in Table 5-5.

Risk of Suicide

The FDA requires a Black Box Warning on antidepressant packaging inserts alerting patients to the increased risk of suicide. Since some SSRIs are approved for use with children and adolescents, the black box warning on the risk of suicidal thinking and behavior becomes of paramount concern. The use of SSRIs in a child, adolescent, or young adult must balance this risk with the clinical need. Patients of all ages who are started on antidepressant therapy should be monitored very carefully and observed closely for clinical worsening, suicidality, or unusual changes in behavior. Fluoxetine is the treatment of choice for individuals under the age of 24, as this is the only SSRI which has demonstrated clinical effectiveness in this patient population (Reeves & Ladner, 2010; Stone, 2010).

Serotonin Syndrome

Serotonin syndrome is a potentially life threatening condition associated with excess stimulation of central and PNS serotonergic receptors. It is known to primarily occur when serotonergic agents increase serotonin neurotransmission through inhibition of serotonin reuptake or direct agonism of serotonin receptors, most often the result of overdose of serotonergic agents or complex interactions between medications that modulate the serotonin system (Steele et al., 2011). Serotonin syndrome is characterized by an acute onset, hyperthermia, myoclonus and hyperreflexia, profound mental changes, psychotic symptoms, and autonomic signs such as labile BP, diaphoresis, and tachycardia.

Serotonin syndrome can develop from SSRI monotherapy, but most often is the result of drug interactions. Drug combinations necessitating caution include SSRIs or SNRIs combined with MAOIs, TCAs, lithium, levodopa, meperidine, amphetamine, tramadol, triptans

TABLE 5-5: SSRI DRUG INTERACTIONS

DRUG	INTERACTIONS ASSOCIATED WITH CONCOMITANT USE OF SSRIs
Antiepileptics	Use cautiously in patients who have epilepsy due to the risk of lowered seizure threshold.
NSAIDs	Use cautiously in patients who have an increased risk of gastrointestinal bleeding.
Warfarin	SSRIs may potentiate the effects of warfarin so monitoring of INR is required.
Lithium	Monitor patient for increased risk of lithium toxicity and serotonin syndrome.
TCAs	SSRIs may potentiate the effects of TCAs and increase the risk of serotonin syndrome. Carefully monitor the patient for adverse affects and consider lowering the TCA dose.
MAOIs	Concomitant use is contraindicated. Use caution when switching from one class to another.
St. John's wort	Patients should not be treated with antidepressants due to risk of serotonin syndrome.
Tramadol	Carefully monitor the patient for serotonin toxicity and increased risk of epilepsy.
Pimozide	Concomitant use is contraindicated due to risk of ventricular arrhythmias.

NSAIDs = Nonsteroidal anti-inflammatory drugs; INR = International normalized ratio.

Source: Adapted from Stone (2010).

(drugs used to treat migraine headaches) (Weitzel & Jiwanlala, 2001).

Withdrawal or Discontinuation Syndrome

Withdrawal or discontinuation syndrome is associated with antidepressants, particularly SSRIs. Withdrawal symptoms can occur when antidepressants are abruptly withdrawn or the dose drastically reduced. In some cases, abruptly stopping an antidepressant can result in "rebound" hypomania or mania. Patients who abruptly stop antidepressant agents with anticholinergic properties may experience nausea, vomiting, abdominal cramping, sweating, headache, and muscle spasms. Other common symptoms associated with serotonergic antidepressant withdrawal include dizziness, weakness, nausea, headache, lethargy, insomnia, anxiety, poor concentration, and paresthesias. These symptoms can persist for several weeks. Therefore, patients who are prescribed SSRIs should be fully informed of the risks associated with abrupt withdrawal as soon as treatment begins. Furthermore, withdrawal of an SSRI should take place with slow dose tapering over a period of weeks, and the patient advised to consult his or her prescriber if he or she has symptoms of withdrawal (Howland, 2010a; Inott, 2009; Stone, 2010).

Apathy Syndrome

It has been reported for over the past decade that the use of SSRIs may be responsible for the emergence of apathy syndrome (Lee & Keltner, 2005). The feeling of apathy is reported by patients to be an overwhelming lack of interest. Frontal lobe dysfunction, induced by SSRIs, may be responsible for the apathy seen. Prolonged and excessive serotonin in the synapse may lead to a decrease in transmission of DA in the frontal lobe. A decrease of DA is one of the potential causes of the apathy syndrome associated with parkinsonism. Additionally, high serotonin may cause a decrease in ACh, and vice versa, which can cause an increase in DA function thereafter. The relationship between serotonin and NE is another possible mechanism. Presently, the exact mechanism responsible for the apathy is yet to be decided (Wongpakaran, Reekum, Wongpakaran, & Clarke, 2007).

Serotonin-Norepinephrine Reuptake Inhibitors

Desvenlafaxine, duloxetine, and venlafaxine are selective serotonin and NRIs (or SNRIs), meaning they inhibit the reuptake of both serotonin and NE. Effexor XR (venlafaxine) and Cymbalta (duloxetine) are two of the top selling medications in America (Drug Topics Staff, 2009). Similar to the SSRIs, SNRIs are indicated for the treatment of depression, anxiety disorders, pain disorders, and fibromyalgia (see Table 5-6). These agents are considered to have a milder side effects profile compared to the TCAs due to their weak affinity for muscarinic, histaminic, and adrenergic receptors. However, SNRIs are not without their share of adverse effects including drowsiness, dry mouth, dizziness, constipation, nervousness, sweating, and anorexia.

Duloxetine (Cymbalta) is indicated for depression, GAD, fibromyalgia, and pain disorders. Duloxetine is a potent and selective inhibitor of serotonin and NE, and a weak inhibitor of DA reuptake. It has a low affinity for alpha-1- and alpha-2-adrenergic, histamine H1, muscarinic, cholinergic, opioid, and GABA receptors. Duloxetine is a substrate for CYPIA2 and CYP2D6 (cytochrome P-450) and a moderate inhibitor of CYP2D6. Therefore, caution should be exercised when coadministering duloxetine with TCAs. Duloxetine is used with relatively high frequency to treat diabetic neuropathy.

Venlafaxine (Effexor XR) is indicated for depression and anxiety disorders. It increases serotonin at lower dosages, NE at mid-range doses, and DA at even higher dosages (Lee & Keltner, 2006). Effexor XR is associated with sustained hypertension that appears to be dose-related. Regular monitoring of BP is recommended. Clinically relevant increases in serum cholesterol have been reported with the use of Effexor, therefore, measurement of serum cholesterol levels should be considered during long-term treatment (www.drugs.com/effexor.html). Venlafaxine is not a potent inhibitor of CYP enzymes and, coupled with its low protein binding (23%), produces relatively few drug-drug interactions.

TABLE 5-6: SNRIs AND THEIR INDICATIONS

SNRIs	FDA INDICATIONS
Desvenlafaxine (Pristiq)	Depression
Duloxetine (Cymbalta)	Depression Generalized Anxiety Disorder Diabetic Peripheral Neuropathic Pain Fibromyalgia Chronic Musculosketetal Pain
Venlafaxine (Effexor XR)	Depression Generalized Anxiety Disorder Social Phobia Panic Disorder

Desvenlafaxine (Pristiq) is the newest SNRI on the market indicated for the treatment of major depressive disorder. Desvenlafaxine is an active metabolite of the older agent venlafaxine and shares similar levels of efficacy, with a similar side effect profile. Patients receiving Pristiq should have regular monitoring of BP and lipids. Pristiq extended release tablet is administered once daily.

Norepinephrine Dopamine Reuptake Inhibitors

NDRIs are inhibitors of the neuronal uptake of NE and DA, but not inhibitors of the reuptake of serotonin. Bupropion is the only NDRI that has wide usage. Wellbutrin SR and Wellbutrin XL offer a true change in treatment strategy for patients not responding to the serotonin-enhancing agents. Unlike serotonergic agents, they do not induce sexual dysfunction. Although bupropion is contraindicated in patients with seizure disorders, it is considered a safer choice than the TCAs. Due to its impact on the adrenergic system, insomnia and agitation can develop. Bupropion marketed as Zyban is the trade name of a smoking cessation agent. Theoretically, Zyban's ability to increase DA counteracts the craving associated with withdrawal from nicotine (Keltner & Grant, 2008).

Noradrenergic and Specific Serotonergic Antidepressants

NaSSAs are unique in their mechanism for enhancing serotonin and NE neurotransmission. Rather than inhibiting the reuptake of serotonin or NE like SSRIs, NaSSAs are antagonists of adrenergic and specific serotonin receptors.

Mirtazapine (Remeron)

Mirtazapine (Remeron) is indicated for the treatment of patients with major depression. It has a distinct mechanism of action that is postulated to allow for a more rapid therapeutic response than other antidepressants (Croom, Perry, & Plosker, 2009). It is an antagonist of presynaptic alpha-2 adrenoceptors and postsynaptic serotonin 5-HT2 and 5-HT3 receptors. The blockage of alpha-2 receptors results in the synthesis and release of more serotonin and NE. The blockage of 5-HT2A and 5-HT3 receptors helps counterbalance the adverse effects associated with the other antidepressants. For example, with SSRI use, 5-HT2A activity is enhanced, resulting in diminished DA release and the accompanying sexual dysfunction. Furthermore, SSRIs use activates 5-HT3, which causes gastrointestinal upset and vomiting. In a systematic review and meta-analysis, Watanabe et al. (2010) reported that mirtazapine is less likely to cause sexual dysfunction and gastric upset, and more likely to cause weight gain and somnolence in comparison with SSRIs. Mirtazapine is a potent antagonist of histamine (H1) receptors, a property that is associated with its prominent sedative effects. Antagonism of alpha-1 adrenoceptors is associated with the occasional orthostatic hypotension and dizziness reported.

Mirtazapine is available as an orally disintegrating tablet as Remeron SolTab. Beyond its antidepressive effects, mirtazapine has been useful in treating people with SSRI-induced sexual dysfunction and in treating individuals who are experiencing insomnia (at a dosage < 15 mg). Paradoxically, as mirtazapine dosage increases, its sedating effects decline. This seemingly contradictory effect is thought to be caused by the NE elevating properties overwhelming the H1 blocking effect. Patients who receive this drug should also be warned about the slight risk of developing agranulocytosis, and are advised to contact their clinician if they experience any signs of infection.

Newer Antidepressants

Vilazodone (Viibryd) is the newest FDA approved antidepressant on the market, released in 2011. Similar to the SSRIs, vilazodone potently and selectively inhibits reuptake of serotonin. However, it is also a partial agonist of serotonergic 5-HT1A receptors. Vilazodone does not bind to NE or DA reuptake sites. Prescribing Viibryd is made convenient due to the availability of a Patient Starter Kit that contains a blister card with 30 tablets. Patients are started on 10 mg a day for 1 week, 20 mg a day for 1 week, and then a 40 mg maintenance dose.

SSRI/Antipsychotic Combination

Symbyax, a combination of fluoxetine and olanzapine, is indicated for acute treatment of depressive episodes associated with bipolar 1 disorder and treatment resistant depression in adult patients. It is an option for individuals who do not respond to two separate trials of different antidepressants of adequate dose and duration in the current episode. Dosage is once daily in the evening, generally beginning with 6 mg/20 mg (www.symbyax.com/Pages/index.aspx).

Tricyclic Antidepressants

TCAs were discovered in 1957 and found to be effective in the treatment of severe depression. TCAs, thus named because of their three-ringed molecular structure, work by blocking the serotonin and NE reuptake pumps on the presynaptic neurons. Increasing levels of NE and serotonin at the synaptic gap result in the antidepressant effects observed with this class of drugs. Some TCAs are more efficient at blocking the reuptake of serotonin and some are more efficient at blocking the reupake of NE. Evidence indicates that the secondary amine TCAs, such as desipramine, may have greater activity in blocking the reuptake of NE. Tertiary amine TCAs, such as amitriptyline, may have greater effect on serotonin reuptake (see Table 5-7). TCAs also have some anticholinergic, antihistaminic, and alpha-1-adrenergic blocking properties, which may explain their adverse effect profile (Lovatt, 2011). Anticholinergic effects occur when muscarinic ACh receptors are blocked in certain cranial nerves. Table 5-8 outlines the cranial nerve and the anticholinergic response. Histamine antagonism results in drowsiness and weight gain. When alpha-1 receptors are blocked, blood vessels lose their ability to constrict, leading to hypotension and dizziness.

In time, the adverse effect profile of the TCAs led to the development of newer antidepressants with milder side effects (i.e., SSRIs). Historically, TCAs have been widely believed to induce more side effects than SSRIs. However, Rief et al. (2009) completed a meta-analysis on both drug classes, finding that this difference was not observed. While the efficacy of TCAs and SSRIs are similar, the lethality of TCAs in overdose is a huge concern. In fact, TCAs are lethal in only eight times the average daily dose (Lovatt, 2011). The SSRIs have a low risk of toxicity in overdose. Therefore, if a patient is identified as being at risk for suicide then an antidepressant with a low risk of toxicity in overdose should be prescribed (Stone, 2010). Since TCAs are considered to be potentially hazardous to patients who are suicidal, mental health providers must be judicious when prescribing TCAs for a severely depressed patient. Another major concern related to TCAs is the potential for lethal cardiac arrhythmias and seizures caused by the disruption of sodium channels when these drugs are taken in very high doses (Stahl, 1998).

TABLE 5-7: PREDOMINANT MONOAMINERGIC ENHANCING PROPERTIES OF COMMON TCAs

SEROTONERGIC TCAs	ADRENERGIC TCAs
Amitriptyline (Elavil, Endep)	Desipramine (Norpramin)
Clomipramine (Anafranil)	Nortriptyline (Pamelor, Aventyl)
Imipramine (Tofranil)	Protriptyline (Vivactil)

Monoamine Oxidase Inhibitors

MAOIs are older antidepressants that are rarely prescribed due to the risk of serious and sometimes fatal reactions. As the name implies, MAOIs work by blocking (inhibiting) the degradation (oxidation) of the monoamines (serotonin, NE, DA). By blocking the metabolism of these neurotransmitters, a buildup occurs in the presynaptic axon terminal coupled with an increase in the synaptic gap. This increase of serotonin, NE, and DA alleviates depressive symptoms.

The buildup of monoamines in the presynaptic axon terminal can be released like a dam when certain foods or drugs are ingested. The dumping of the monoamines causes serious events, such as severe hypertension, CNS excitability, and even death. Agents that should be avoided include: (a) sympathomimetics (drugs that stimulate adrenergic receptors); (b) serotonergic drugs (i.e., SSRIs); (c) some CNS drugs (i.e., meperidine); and (d) foods that contain tyramine (i.e., cheese). Please refer to a pharmacology textbook for a complete list of substances that must be avoided.

Phenelzine (Nardil) and tranylcypromine (Parnate) are non-selective MAOIs in that they inhibit both MAO-A (which metabolizes NE and 5-HT) and MAO-B (which metabolizes DA). Moclobemide (Manerix) is a selective inhibitor of just MAO-A and is also known as a reversible inhibitor of monoamine oxidase A (RIMA). Thus, it enhances the availability of serotonin and NE. Selegiline (Emsam) is selective for MAO-B, enhancing the availability of DA. Emsam is formulated as a daily slow-releasing transdermal patch. Since the stomach is bypassed, there is less need for dietary restrictions except when higher dosages are given (Bristol-Myers Squibb, 2006).

TABLE 5-8: ANTICHOLINERGIC EFFECTS ON CRANIAL NERVES

CRANIAL NERVE	MUSCARINIC ANTAGONISM
Cranial Nerve III	(Oculomotor) = mydriasis and blurred vision
Cranial Nerve VII	(Facial) = dry mouth, decreased respiratory secretions, and decreased tearing
Cranial Nerve IX	(Glossopharyngeal) = dry mouth and decreased respiratory secretions
Cranial Nerve X	(Vagus) = constipation, urinary hesitancy, and increased heart rate

ANTI-ANXIETY AGENTS

The most common anxiety disorders can be classified into several categories including: (a) GAD, (b) social anxiety disorder or social phobia, (c) panic disorder with or without agoraphobia, (d) obsessive-compulsive disorder, and (e) PTSD. Antidepressants and anti-anxiety agents are useful in alleviating the symptoms associated with these disorders. Antidepressants, particularly SSRIs and SNRIs, are the first line treatment for chronic anxiety disorders. Often, an SSRI/SNRI and a BZD both will be prescribed initially, with the goal of weaning off the BZDs and maintaining the antidepressant. Refer to the antidepressant section for further information on anxiety disorders.

Benzodiazepines

BZDs were first introduced into the market 50 years ago, acting as anxiolytics, hypnotics, sedatives, amnestics, antiepileptics, and muscle relaxants. BZDs exert their effects by increasing the inhibitory effects of the neurotransmitter GABA. GABA modulates the frequency of opening of the inhibitory chloride channel. As more chloride is drawn into the neuron, the neuron becomes hyperpolarized, slowing neuronal firing. BZDs act primarily on GABA receptors, causing the chloride channel to open more frequently than when GABA alone is present. Thus, BZDs act as GABA agonists, yielding an anxiolytic action.

There are three primary types of GABA receptors, classified as GABA A, B, and C. Each type has its own unique structural and functional characteristics. $GABA_A$ and $GABA_C$ receptors cause inhibition by increasing chloride entry, whereas $GABA_B$ receptors cause inhibition by increasing potassium release from neurons. BZDs act primarily on the $GABA_A$ subtype, inducing sedation, hypnosis, and decreased anxiety. The three subunits of $GABA_A$ include alpha (α), beta (ß), and gamma (γ). There are also variations among these subunits, for example, α1, α2, α3, β2, γ1, γ2, each mediating specific effects. For example, sedation is mediated by the alpha-1 subunit, whereas anxiety is mediated by the alpha-2 and alpha-3 subunits (Stahl, 2008).

BZDs are typically divided into three groups based on their duration of action: less than 12 hours for short-acting BZDs, 12 to 24 hours for intermediate-acting BZDs, and more than 24 hours for long-acting BZDs (see Table 5-9). The different durations of action are largely due to the pharmacological activity of one or more metabolites associated with each BZD. BZD metabolism involves two main pathways: oxidation (Phase 1) and glucuronidation (Phase 2). Those BZDs which first undergo oxidation, mainly by action of CYP450, generate active metabolites which have then to be glucuronidated in order to be excreted. Thus, their duration of action is typically very long. On the contrary, direct glucuronidation of the drug produces inactive,

TABLE 5-9: COMMONLY USED BENZODIAZEPINES

BENZODIAZEPINES	USUAL DAILY DOSE	HALF-LIFE (HR)	ANXIOLYTIC EFFECT	SEDATIVE EFFECT
Short-Acting				
Triazolam (Halcion)	0.125–0.5 mg[b]	1.5–5	+	+++++
Intermediate				
Alprazolam (Xanax)	0.75–4.0 mg[a]	12–15	+++	+
Lorazepam (Ativan)	2–6 mg[a]	10–20	+++++	+++
Oxazepam (Serax)	30–60 mg[a]	5–20	+++	+
Temazepam (Restoril)	10–60 mg[b]	10–15	+	+++++
Long-Acting				
Chlordiazepoxide (Librium)	15–100 mg[a]	5–30	+++	++
Clonazepam (Klonopin)	0.5–10 mg[a]	18–60	+++	+
Diazepam (Valium)	4–40 mg[a]	20–80	+++++	+++

[a] In divided dosage.

[b] Used as a sedative.

+ = mild effect; ++ = moderate effect; +++ = strong effect.

Source: Adapted from Keltner & Folks (2005).

rapidly excreted metabolites. The BZDs that are mainly glucuronidated generally have a short duration of action (Mandrioli, Mercolini, & Raggi, 2008).

Shorter-acting BZDs are usually prescribed for the treatment of sleep disturbances such as insomnia, promoting rapid sleep with limited somnolence the following morning. BZDs such as temazepam (Restoril) and triazolam (Halcion) act as sedatives used in the treatment of insomnia. Intermediate- and long-acting BZDs are generally prescribed for anxiety-related disorders to manage symptoms (Mandrioli et al., 2008).

BZDs may be prescribed as an adjuvant for depressive or antipsychotic therapies. BZDs are the treatment of choice for agitation associated with acute psychotic episodes. Lorazepam and alprazolam are the most frequent BZDs used for this purpose (Thomas et al., 2009). When switching a patient from a sedating antipsychotic to a nonsedating antipsychotic, BZD are useful during the transition period to prevent agitation and rebound insomnia (Stahl, 2008). As BZDs appear to enhance the action of SSRIs, concomitant use of a long acting BZD with an SSRI may be beneficial in the treatment of protracted depression (Morishita, Sawamura, & Ishigooka, 2009).

BZD metabolism is altered as a result of the aging process or liver damage for those agents relying on Phase 1 enzymes. The elimination half-life of some BZDs increases threefold to fourfold in the elderly and/or hepatically compromised individuals as a result of declining oxidative capabilities in the liver. Therefore, oxazepam and lorazepam, two common BZDs that are directly glucuronidated without active metabolites, are the agents of choice in these vulnerable populations (Keltner & Folks, 2005). In addition, for the elderly and debilitated patients, it is recommended that the dosage be limited to the smallest effective amount to preclude development of ataxia or over sedation.

BZDs are the drugs of choice for the management of alcohol withdrawal. Alcohol and BZDs share similar pharmacodynamic properties, namely, they both act as GABA agonists. In effect, BZD use in alcohol withdrawal serves as a substitute of sufficient quantity to suppress symptoms. BZDs not only ameliorate the symptoms of alcohol withdrawal, but prevent seizure activity and delirium tremens. Long-acting BZDs such as diazepam (Valium), chlordiazepoxide (Librium), and clonazepam (Klonopin) enable once-daily dosing and contribute to an overall smooth withdrawal course with minimal breakthrough or rebound symptoms. However, lorazepam (Ativan), an intermediate BZD, may be preferred due to its ease of metabolism and elimination in cases involving the elderly or those with marked liver disease. BZDs are administered by mouth, if possible, on an as needed basis (Keltner & Folks, 2005; Riddle, Bush, Tittle, & Dilkhush, 2010).

Abuse, Dependence, and Withdrawal

Some clinicians are reluctant to prescribe BZDs for anxiety disorders due to risk of tolerance, dependence, and withdrawal reactions. Tolerance refers to the loss of response to the effects of BZDs after repeated, prolonged use. Tolerance, simply put, means the person no longer experiences the same effect at the same dosage. Therefore, more is required to achieve the same anxiolytic effect. Tolerance develops rather quickly; tolerance related to sedation occurs within weeks, while tolerance to anxiolytic properties takes months (Ashton, 2000; Juergens, 2010).

Use of BZDs may lead to the development of physical and psychological dependence. The risk of dependence increases with dose and duration of treatment. It is also greater in predisposed patients with a history of alcohol or drug abuse. Based on *DSM-IV-TR* criteria, a person who shows three or more of the following behaviors is most likely dependent on BZDs:

1. Tolerance to BZD therapy
2. Has withdrawal symptoms when BZDs are not used
3. Takes other drugs to help relieve withdrawal symptoms
4. Takes larger amounts of BZDs than planned or prescribed and for longer periods of time
5. Has a persistent desire to or unsuccessful attempts to quit
6. Is spending a lot of time and effort to obtain, use, and recover from BZD use
7. Gives up or reduces social or recreational activities
8. Misses work
9. Continues to use BZDs regardless of negative consequences (APA, 2000).

Once physical dependence has developed, abrupt termination of BZDs will be accompanied by withdrawal symptoms such as headaches, muscle pain, extreme anxiety, tension, restlessness, confusion, and irritability. For patients who are taking short-acting BZD as a sleeping aid, sudden withdrawal will result in insomnia. In cases where frequent, high doses of BZDs have been used for a prolonged period of time, abrupt termination may precipitate severe reactions including derealization; depersonalization; numbness or tingling of the extremities; hallucinations; seizures; and heightened sensitivity to light, noise, and physical contact (www.drugs.com/pro/lorazepam.html). While tolerance to chronic BZD use appears to result from desensitization of GABA receptors, sensitization of excitatory glutaminergic receptors is associated with BZD withdrawal symptoms. Rapid or abrupt withdrawal of the BZD, once tolerance has developed, results is underactivity of inhibitory GABA functions and a surge in excitatory nervous activity, giving rise to many of the BZD withdrawal symptoms (Ashton, 2005). Since abrupt withdrawal can cause seizures, individuals dependent on BZDs should become drug free if possible, but only under the care of a trained professional. As a general rule of thumb, withdrawal reactions are minimized by the intermittent use of time-limited, low dosages with gradual withdrawal.

Adverse Effects

The most common acute side effects of BZDs are related to mental alertness, anterograde amnesia, and impaired performance. Patients must be advised to use caution when driving or operating hazardous machinery. Further, some people experience paradoxical reactions and actually develop anxiety, insomnia, hyperactivity, and aggressive behavior related to BZD use. See Exhibit 5-2 for a list of common side effects of BZD.

Overdose

BZDs have a wide therapeutic index and overdose most frequently occurs in combination with alcohol or other CNS depressants, resulting in potentially fatal respiratory depression. Flumazenil (Romazicon) injectable is the treatment of choice for BZD overdose. Romazicon is a BZD receptor antagonist, competitively inhibiting the activity on the GABA/BZD receptor complex. Recommended dosage is 0.2 mg/minute titration rate to slowly awaken the patient over 5 to 10 minutes, while reducing the risk of CNS excitation (i.e., confusion and agitation) on emergence. In cases of overdose where the patient is BZD dependent, Romazicon has been shown to precipitate withdrawal seizures. In such cases, the benefits of using Romazicon must outweigh the risks of precipitated seizures (www.drugs.com/pro/romazicon.html).

EXHIBIT 5-2: COMMON SIDE EFFECTS OF BZDs

- Drowsiness
- Light-headedness
- Lassitude
- Decreased reaction time
- Dysarthria
- Ataxia
- Sexual dysfunction
- Weight gain
- Skin reactions
- Headache
- Confusion
- Depression

Source: Keltner & Folks (2005); Charlson, Degenhardt, McLaren, Hall, & Lynskey (2009).

Common BZDs

Alprazolam is an intermediate-acting BZD, commonly marketed as Xanax. An extended-release form is available as Xanax XR. Its main therapeutic uses include the treatment of panic disorder, with or without agoraphobia, and the short-term treatment of severe acute anxiety. Doses are usually 0.25–0.5 mg three times a day, with a total maximum of 4 mg (Mandrioli et al., 2008).

Lorazepam, marketed as Ativan, is an intermediate-acting BZD. The usual dose is 2–6 mg/day for anxiety and 1–2 mg at bedtime for insomnia with anxiety. Its relatively potent amnesic effect, together with its anxiolytic and sedative properties, makes lorazepam useful as a premedication before a general anesthetic. It can also be injected intramuscularly to treat acute anxiety and agitation or IV for status epilepticus. Lorazepam is metabolized by glucuronidation, thus it is less likely to accumulate and to cause adverse effects in the elderly than other BZDs, which require hepatic oxidation.

Oxazepam (Serax) is used to relieve the symptoms of anxiety and of alcohol withdrawal at daily doses of 30-60 mg or more in divided doses. Oxazepam is an intermediate-acting BZD, with a half life of 5 to 20 hours. Like lorazepam, it undergoes inactivation via Phase 2 glucuronidation, making it a safer option to use with the elderly.

Diazepam (Valium) was the second BZD introduced onto the market (after chlordiazepoxide) and is still one of the most widely used BZDs in the world. It is used for the treatment of anxiety, seizures, including status epilepticus (IV), and for preoperative anesthesia induction.

Midazolam (Versed) is a short-acting BZD used mainly for its action as a sedative before anesthesia (2.5 mg in one dose) or for sedation of intensive care patients. It can also be used for the treatment of status epilepticus.

Other Anxiety Agents

Buspirone (Buspar), a 5-HT1A partial agonist, has been shown to be effective in the treatment of anxiety disorders. Buspirone was the first available, long-term, anxiety alternative to the BZDs. Substantially different from the BZDs, buspirone has an anxiolytic effect, yet without the sedation and potential for abuse. Buspirone has a slow onset of action (2 to 4 weeks), similar to the SSRIs.

Clonidine (Catapres) is a presynaptic alpha-2 receptor agonist that can be used for anxiety disorders such as GAD, panic disorder, PTSD, and social phobia. Stimulation of presynaptic alpha-2 receptors reduces the firing rate of adrenergic neurons in the brain and thus, reduces plasma concentrations of NE. Reduction of autonomic symptoms leads to management of hyperarousal, exaggerated startle response, insomnia, vivid nightmares, tachycardia, and agitation. In addition, clonidine is effective in reducing autonomic symptoms associated with opioid, alcohol, BZD, and nicotine withdrawal states. After chronic use, abruptly stopping clonidine can cause rebound anxiety, restlessness, sweating, tremors, abdominal pain, heart palpitations, headache, and hypertension (Howland, 2010b).

Barbiturates

The barbiturates are a group of CNS depressants with potent sedative-hypnotic properties. Barbiturates are known to have a relatively small therapeutic index, meaning that approximately 10 times the therapeutic dose can often be fatal. Similar to the BZDs, barbiturates carry a high potential for abuse, tolerance, dependence, and withdrawal reactions. However, due to the lack of safety of the barbiturates in overdose, BZDs are the preferred agents. Still, some barbiturates are occasionally used for their hypnotic properties, particularly amobarbital, pentobarbital, phenobarbital, and ecobarbital.

BIPOLAR DISORDER MEDICATIONS

Mood stabilizers are recognized as the treatment of choice for bipolar disorder, although the FDA has not officially recognized the term and no consensus definition is accepted among clinicians. So then, what defines a mood stabilizer? To define the term one must understand the complexity of bipolar disorder, which features a shift in polarity between mania and major depression, in both the acute and chronic course. Therefore, the ideal mood stabilizer would have an effect upon depressive and manic phases of bipolar disorder, both for acute and maintenance treatment. Lithium is the only agent that seems to meet the full criteria of a mood stabilizer. However, in practice the anticonvulsants such as valproate, carbamazepine, and lamotrigine are also considered mood stabilizers, while the atypical antipsychotics are increasingly being placed in the same frame. See Table 5-10 for a list of medications and their specific utility in the treatment of bipolar disorder.

The manic phase of bipolar disorder is characterized by grandiosity, elevated mood, hyperactivity, irritability, pressured speech, reduced need for sleep, flight of ideas, impulsivity, and agitation. The depressive phase typically reflects the classic symptoms of unipolar depression such as sadness, anhedonia, hypersomnia, weight gain, fatigue, indecisiveness, and suicidality. In addition, psychosis may be present in severe manic and severe depressive episodes. Depressive symptoms are by far more prevalent than manic symptoms, meaning that bipolar depression carries a much higher illness burden (McIntyre & Cha, 2011). Mood stabilizers and antipsychotics, then, are prescribed to stabilize the individual between these two emotional extremes.

Lithium

Lithium is the benchmark treatment for acute mania and is said to be the gold standard for bipolar disorder. For over half a century, lithium has outperformed all other agents in the long-term maintenance and prophylaxis of bipolar disorder. Due to its efficacy, lithium use is predicted to reduce the risk of suicidality in bipolar disorder by up to 80% (Malhi, Adams, & Berk, 2009). In the treatment of acute mania, lithium combined with an atypical antipsychotic appears to be most effective due to lithium's relatively slow onset of action (6–10 days). The other benefit of dual therapy is attributed to the therapeutic sedative effect of the antipsychotic, which has an immediate action on the manic symptoms (Malhi, Adams, Cahill, Dodd, & Berk, 2009).

Lithium is a naturally occurring salt that can be found on the Periodic Table, in the same column as sodium and potassium. Lithium alters sodium transport in nerve and muscle cells and effects a shift toward neuronal metabolism of catecholamines, but the specific mechanism of lithium action is unknown. Lithium is known to have a narrow therapeutic index; serum levels above 1.5 mEq/L can be toxic and should be avoided. Recommended serum lithium levels are 0.6 to 1.2 mEq/L. Lithium levels below 2.0 mEq/L may cause early lithium toxicity, characterized by diarrhea, vomiting, drowsiness, muscular weakness, and lack of coordination. At levels above 2.0 mEq/L, ataxia, tinnitus, blurred vision, and a large output of dilute

TABLE 5-10: DRUGS USED TO TREAT BIPOLAR DISORDER

TREATMENT	ACUTE MANIA	BIPOLAR DEPRESSION	MAINTENANCE
Lithium (Eskalith)	+++	++	+++
Anticonvulsants			
Divalproex (Depakote)	+++	++	+++
Carbamazepine (Tegretol)	++	+	+
Lamotrigine (Lamictal)		+	+++
Oxcarbazepine (Trileptal)	+		+
Antipsychotics			
Quetiapine (Seroquel)	+++	+++	+
Olanzapine (Zyprexa)	+++	+	+
Risperidone (Risperdal)	+++		+
Aripiprazole (Abilify)	+++	+	++
Ziprasidone (Geodon)	+++		+

Note: + = weak evidence; ++ = moderate evidence; +++ = strong evidence.
Source: Adapted from Malhi, Adams, Cahill, Dodd, & Berk (2009).

urine may be seen. Serum lithium levels above 3.0 mEq/L may produce a complex clinical picture, involving multiple organ systems (www.drugs.com/pro/lithium.html).

Safe, efficacious use of lithium requires careful monitoring and individuals should be informed about signs of potential toxicity. Interestingly and perhaps unfortunately, common side effects overlap with the early signs of toxicity (see Table 5-11). For example, diarrhea may be a side effect or the manifestation of mild toxicity. Therefore, serum levels should be determined twice per week during the acute phase until the patient has been stabilized. During maintenance therapy, lithium serum levels should be monitored at least every 2 months. Lithium should generally not be given to patients with significant renal or cardiovascular disease, severe dehydration, or sodium depletion.

TABLE 5-11: ADVERSE EFFECTS OF LITHIUM

LITHIUM SIDE EFFECTS	LITHIUM TOXICITY
Fine tremor	Coarse tremor
Diarrhea	Increasing diarrhea
Nausea and vomiting	Vomiting
Weight gain	Anorexia
Polyuria, polydipsia	Polyuria, polydipsia
Edema	Renal failure
Fatigue	Weakness
Vertigo	Ataxia, loss of balance
Difficulty concentrating	Disorientation
Hypothyroidism	Drowsiness
Hypermagnesemia	Blurred vision
Hypercalcemia	Tinnitus
Leukocytosis	Muscle twitching
Metallic taste, dry mouth	Irritability and agitation
Benign ECG changes	Psychosis
Rash, acne, psoriasis	Seizures
Headache	Coma

Source: Adapted from Malhi, Adams, & Berk (2009).

Anticonvulsants

Anticonvulsant drugs are widely used in the treatment of bipolar disorder. They are also efficacious in a host of other common illnesses, namely, seizure disorders, pain syndromes, alcohol and BZD withdrawal symptoms, panic and anxiety disorders, dementia, schizophrenia, and personality disorders. The valproates, including valproic acid (Depakene) and divalproex (Depakote), and other anticonvulsants such as carbamazepine (Tegretol), and lamotrigine (Lamictal) are recognized mood stabilizers. Several other anticonvulsant agents are also commonly utilized in the treatment of bipolar disorder including oxcarbazepine (Trileptal), gabapentin (Neurontin), and topiramate (Topamax) (Grunze, 2010).

The mechanism of action responsible for the clinical efficacy of anticonvulsants in bipolar disorder is not completely understood. In general, anticonvulsants are known to have more than one mechanism of action including modulation of GABAergic, glutamatergic, or dopaminergic neurotransmission, and alteration of voltage-gated ion channels or intracellular signaling pathways (Landmark, 2008).

Although anticonvulsants are frequently used in the management of bipolar disorder, none have been shown to be effective for all phases of the disorder. For instance, lamotrigine is effective for prophylaxis of depression and it likely has some efficacy for acute bipolar depression, but it has little efficacy in treating acute mania or preventing mania. The valproates and carbamazepine have been shown to have efficacy in acute mania, but their efficacy for acute bipolar depression or maintenance of mood episodes is variable.

As a general rule, the anticonvulsants utilized as mood stabilizers carry a black box warning related to hepatotoxicity and pancreatitis. Patients must be educated on the symptoms associated with these two complications, namely, nausea, vomiting, anorexia, malaise, facial edema, and abdominal pain. Anticonvulsants that are highly protein bound must be given cautiously with other CNS agents that are also highly bound. For example, concomitant use of divalproex with phenytoin, BZDs, and other anticonvulsants can cause severe CNS depression (Chateauvieux, Morceau, Dicato, & Diederich, 2010; Hirschowitz, Kolevzon, & Garakani, 2010). In addition, anticonvulsant use, particularly lamotrigine, has been associated with allergic skin reactions, including Stevens-Johnson syndrome. These adverse effects usually occur when beginning therapy and can be minimized by initiating treatment at a low dosage.

Atypical Antipsychotics

Atypical antipsychotics (i.e., aripiprazole, clozapine, olanzapine, quetiapine, risperidone, and ziprasidone) have been utilized to treat bipolar disorder with increasing frequency since the mid-1990s, even before they received FDA approval for this condition. In March 2000, olanzapine was the first atypical antipsychotic to receive FDA approval for the treatment of mania. Subsequently, most of the other atypical antipsychotics received FDA indication for the treatment of bipolar disorder.

Atypical antipsychotics provide a viable treatment option for manic and mixed episodes in either acute or maintenance phases of bipolar disorder. In addition, quetiapine, quetiapine XR, and Symbyax (olanzapine/fluoxetine combination) are FDA approved for the acute treatment of bipolar depression. There is strong evidence for antipsychotics in the treatment of bipolar disorder; however, consideration should be given to their side effect profile and drug-drug interactions when selecting an agent. The reader is asked to refer to the Antipsychotics section that discusses these drugs.

SUMMARY

The role of the psychiatric mental health nurse practitioner (PMHNP) entails an advanced knowledge of psychopharmacology as presented in this chapter. Specifically, a review of the classic categories of psychotropic drugs including their mechanism of action and other pharmacodynamic properties has been presented. When treating psychiatric disturbances, an important consideration involves balancing the benefits of medication management with adverse side effects, always with the goal of improving patient functioning.

The area of psychopharmacology continues to expand at a rapid pace that requires the PMHNP to continue to pursue the most current knowledge. Therefore, it is important to keep abreast of the large body of evidence-based data supporting the use of pharmacological treatments. Positive patient outcomes will occur as a result of psychiatric nurse practitioners' ongoing clinical experience and continuous accumulation of knowledge in the art of prescribing.

A prescription must have all of the following:

1. The name and address of the patient
2. The name, dosage, and directions (including times to be taken) for use of the medicine prescribed
3. Whether a generic equivalent is acceptable
4. The date of the order
5. The DEA number when appropriate
6. The name, address, and phone number of the prescriber
7. The indication for the medication (not always required)
8. The signature of the prescriber if the prescription is handwritten
9. The number of refills, if applicable

Of course, prescribing is the first step, followed by dispensing and administering the drug, in a multi-step process that is successful when the right patient receives the right medication in the right amount at the right time. Because it is multi-step and because of the various human factors involved, prescription errors are not uncommon. Errors occur due to poor handwriting, confusion of drugs with similar names, misunderstood abbreviations, inattention, and prescriber ignorance. Furthermore, a notion embedded in all of these potential errors is the assumption that the prescriber actually wrote the correct "thing" on the prescription. As the final point above indicates, prescriber ignorance is a cause of medication error. For example, we are familiar with a case of serotonin syndrome related to a clinician not knowing that a patient was also prescribed an MAOI. The patient died.

Most of us can remember attempting to decipher the illegible scribble of some too-busy-to-write-clearly physician. As nurse practitioners, you must be careful not to recreate the bewilderment in others that you once suffered. A personal example of poor handwriting occurred when a seizure-prone 5-year-old grandchild (NLK) was given Zyrtec instead of Zantac. A grand mal seizure followed.

In order to minimize medication errors, it may be appropriate to write both generic and brand names on the prescription. Doing so can eliminate some miscommunication between the prescriber and the pharmacist. Another way to reduce the error burden is to write the indications for the medication, when doing so will not embarrass the patient.

Inappropriate abbreviations are certainly on the radar screen today. However, you must be aware of what is and what is not acceptable. For example, one of the authors worked on a psychiatric unit when a transcribing error involving digoxin occurred. The order was written as "qd" or once daily but was transcribed as "qid" or four times per day. Though the example is dated and was caught, it was not caught in time. This patient died later in the intensive care unit.

Perhaps the best solution to medication errors caused by handwritten prescriptions is the move to E-prescribing. The typing of prescriptions into a computerized system that has a number of checks and balances may be the best guard against prescription error. Whether handwritten or electronic, it is usually good practice to complete the prescription process for one patient before seeing the next patient. As simple as these suggestions seem, following them might avert a medication error.

Finally, when discussing the art of prescribing it is important to recognize that you may work for an agency that has a formulary. The practical implication of this fact is that you are limited in what you can prescribe. For instance, some health organizations have citalopram (Celexa) on their formulary but not escitalopram (Lexapro). While the difference in these two drugs might seem slight, some patients do better on escitalopram so this becomes a limitation. Other factors that the patient-centered clinician will consider are the financial implications for a given patient. Some medications may not be covered and brand name drugs might exact a higher out-of-pocket cost than the patient can comfortably bear.

In conclusion, writing a prescription correctly incorporates all of the above information in addition to a thorough grounding in the basics of psychopharmacology discussed in this and other chapters. With careful attention to this process, the patient will receive the intended benefit and outcome.

ANNOTATED BIBLIOGRAPHY RELATED TO PSYCHIATRIC DRUG-DRUG INTERACTIONS

There are a number of resources for helping the clinician understand, avoid, and deal with drug interactions.

Concise Guide to Drug Interaction Principles for Medical Practice (2003) by K. L. Cozza, S. C. Armstrong, and J. R. Oesterheld.
The authors developed this small, pocket-size book that is a treasure trove of helpful and important information. It has helped us understand cytochrome P450 enzymes and P-glycoprotein related interactions much better than any other source. Additionally, these authors also have a companion Pocket Guide entitled *Drug Interaction Principles* that is a very manageable size and can easily be slipped into a shirt pocket. Also, there are newer versions of these books with a changed order of authorship.

The Cytochrome P450 System (2001) by K. L. Cozza and S. C. Armstrong
The authors wrote what might be considered classic at this point. It does a wonderful job of elucidating this system of metabolizing enzymes.

"Psychiatric Drug-Drug Interactions: A Review" (2010) by N. L. Keltner and R. L. Moore
The authors collaborated to write what might be labeled as drug-drug interactions lite, but one of us (NLK) attempted to summarize key issues and points of drug-drug interactions in a few pages. We think it is a helpful resource.

"Guide to Psychiatric Drug Interactions" (2009) by S. H. Preskorn and D. Flockhart
The authors have compiled an excellent manuscript with 28 full pages devoted to text and tables. If you have a color printer, it is worth the extra effort to use it because there are some very nice and colorful charts that make the information stand out.

"Clinical Manual of Drug Interaction Principles for Medical Practice" (2008) by G. H. Wynn, J. R. Oesterhold, R. L. Cozza, and S. C. Armstrong
In this relatively lengthy (30 pages) article, the authors do a wonderful job of summarizing psychotropic drug-drug

interactions; 24 pages are dedicated to references and tables.

REFERENCES

American Psychiatric Association. (2000). *Diagnostic and statistical manual of mental disorders* (4th ed.). Washington, DC: Author.

Ashton, C. H. (2000). *Benzodiazepines: How they work and how to withdraw.* New Castle, UK: University of Newcastle.

Ashton, H. (2005). The diagnosis and management of benzodiazepine dependence. *Current Opinion in Psychiatry, 18,* 249–255.

Bristol-Myers Squibb. (2006). *Ensam package insert.* Princeton, NJ: Bristol-Meyers Squibb Com.

Carter, N., & McCormack, P. (2009). Duloxetine: A review of its use in the treatment of generalized anxiety disorder. *CNS Drugs, 23*(6), 523–541.

Charlson, F., Degenhardt, L., McLaren, J., Hall, W., & Lynskey, M. (2009). A systematic review of research examining benzodiazepine-related mortality. *Pharmacoepidemiology and Drug Safety, 18,* 93–103.

Chateauvieux, S., Morceau, F., Dicato, M., & Diederich, M. (2010). Molecular and therapeutic potential and toxicity of valproic acid. *Journal of Biomedicine & Biotechnology, 2010,* pii: 479364. Retrieved from www.ncbi.nlm.nih.gov/pmc/articles/PMC2926634/?tool=pmcentrez

Cipriani, A., Furukawa, T. A., Salanti, G., Geddes, J. R., Higgins, J. P., Churchill, R.,...Barbui, C. (2009). Comparative efficacy and acceptability of 12 new-generation antidepressants: A multiple-treatments meta-analysis. *Lancet, 373,* 746–758.

Consumer Reports Best Buy Drugs. (2009). *Treating schizophrenia and bipolar disorder: The antipsychotics—comparing effectiveness, safety, and price.* Yonkers, NY: Consumer Reports Best Buy Drugs. Retrieved from www.consumerreports.org/health/resources/pdf/best-buy-drugs/Antipsychs-2pager-FINAL.pdf

Cooke, B. B., & Keltner, N. L. (2008). Traumatic brain injury-war related: Part II. *Perspectives in Psychiatric Care, 44(1),* 54–57.

Correll, C., Lencz, T., & Malhotra, A. (2010). Antipsychotic drugs and obesity. *Trends in Molecular Medicine, 17,* 97–107.

Cozza, K. L., & Armstrong, S. C. (2001). *The Cytochrome P450 system.* Washington, DC: American Psychiatric Publishing.

Cozza, K. L., Armstrong, S. C., & Oesterheld, J. R. (2003). *Concise guide to drug interaction principles for medical practice.* Washington, DC: American Psychiatric Publishing.

Croom, K. F., Perry, C. M., & Plosker, G. L. (2009). Mirtazapine: A review of its use in major depression and other psychiatric disorders. *CNS Drugs, 23(5),* 427–452.

Csoka, A. B., Bahrick, A., & Mehtonen, O. P. (2008). Persistent sexual dysfunction after discontinuation of selective serotonin reuptake inhibitors. *Journal of Sexual Medicine, 5,* 227–233.

Damsa, C., Bumb, A., Bianchi-Demicheli, F., Vidailhet, P., Sterck, R., Andreoli, A.,...Beyenburg, S. (2004). "Dopamine-dependent" side effects of selective serotonin reuptake inhibitors: A clinical review. *Journal of Clinical Psychiatry, 65,* 1064–1068.

Drug Topics Staff. (2009). *Pharmacy facts and figures.* Retrieved from http://drugtopics.modernmedicine.com/Pharmacy+Facts+&+Figures

Ehret, M., Sopko, M., & Lemieux, T. (2010). Focus on lurasidone: A new atypical antipsychotic for the treatment of schizophrenia. *Formulary, 45,* 313–317.

Glick I., Murray S., Vasudevan P., Marder S., & Hu R. (2001). Treatment with atypical antipsychotics: New indications and new populations. *Journal of Psychiatric Residency, 35,* 187–191.

Grunze, H. C. (2010). Anticonvulsants in bipolar disorder. *Journal of Mental Health, 19*(2), 127–141.

Healy, D. (2009). *Psychiatric drugs explained,* (5th ed.). Edinburgh, TX: Elsevier.

Hirschowitz, J., Kolevzon, A., & Garakani, A. (2010). The pharmacological treatment of bipolar disorder: The question of modern advances. *Harvard Review of Psychiatry, 18,* 266–278.

Horacek, J., Bubenikova-Valesova, V., Kopecek, M., Palenicek, T., Dockery, C., Mohr, P.,...Hoschl, C. (2006). Mechanism of action of atypical antipsychotic drugs and the neurobiology of schizophrenia. *CNS Drugs, 20*(5), 389–409.

Howland, R. H. (2010a). Potential adverse effects of discontinuing psychotropic drugs: Part 1: Adrenergic, cholinergic, and histamine drugs. *Journal of Psychosocial Nursing and Mental Health Services, 48*(6), 11–14.

Howland, R. H. (2010b). Potential adverse effects of discontinuing psychotropic drugs: Part 2: antidepressant drugs. *Journal of Psychosocial Nursing and Mental Health Services, 48*(7), 9–12.

Inott, T. J. (2009). The dark side of SSRIs: Selective serotonin reuptake inhibitors. *Nursing, 39*(8), 31–33.

Jindal, R., & Keshavan, M. (2008). Classifying antipsychotic agents: Need for new terminology, *CNS Drugs, 22*(12), 1047–1059.

Juergens, S. M. (2010). *Understanding benzodiazepines.* Retrieved from www.csam-asam.org/pdf/misc/Juergens.pdf

Kapur, S., & Seeman, P. (2001). Does fast dissociation from the dopamine D2 receptor explain the action of atypical antipsychotics: A new hypothesis. *American Journal of Psychiatry, 158*(3), 360–369.

Keltner, N. L., & Folks, D. G. (2005). *Psychotropic drugs* (4th ed.). St. Louis, MO: Mosby.

Keltner, N. L., & Grant, J. S. (2008). Irreversible lithium-induced neuropathy: Two cases. *Perspectives in Psychiatric Care, 44(4),* 290–293.

Keltner, N. L., & Moore, R. L. (2010). Psychiatric drug-drug interactions: A review. *Perspectives in Psychiatric Care, 46,* 244–251.

Keltner, N. L., & Vance, D. E. (2008). Incarcerated care and quetiapine abuse. *Perspectives in Psychiatric Care, 44*(3), 202–206.

Komossa, K., Rummel-Kluge, C., Hunger, H., Schmid, F., Schwarz, S., Duggan, L.,...Leucht, S. (2010a). Olanzapine versus other atypical antipsychotics for schizophrenia. *Cochrane Database of Systematic Reviews, 3,* CD006654. Retrieved from http://onlinelibrary.wiley.com/o/cochrane/clsysrev/articles/CD006654/frame.html

Komossa, K., Rummel-Kluge, C., Hunger, H., Schwarz, S., Bhoopathi, P. S., Kissling, W.,...Leucht, S. (2009a). Ziprasidone versus other atypical antipsychotics for schizophrenia. *Cochrane Database of Systematic Reviews, 4,* CD006627. Retrieved from http://onlinelibrary.wiley.com/o/cochrane/clsysrev/articles/CD006627/frame.html

Komossa, K., Rummel-Kluge, C., Schmid, F., Hunger, H., Schwarz, S., El-Sayeh, H.G.,...Leucht, S. (2009b). Aripiprazole versus other atypical antipsychotics for schizophrenia. *Cochrane Database of Systematic Reviews, 4,* CD006569. Retrieved from http://onlinelibrary.wiley.com/o/cochrane/clsysrev/articles/CD006569/frame.html

Komossa, K., Rummel-Kluge, C., Schmid, F., Hunger, H., Schwarz, S., Srisurapanont, M.,...Leucht, S. (2010b). Quetiapine versus other atypical antipsychotics for schizophrenia. *Cochrane Database of Systematic Reviews, 1,* CD006625. Retrieved from http://onlinelibrary.wiley.com/o/cochrane/clsysrev/articles/CD006625/frame.html

Landmark, C. J. (2008). Antiepileptic drugs in non-epilepsy disorders. *CNS Drugs, 22*(1), 27–47.

Lee, S. I., & Keltner, N. L. (2005). Antidepressant apathy syndrome. *Perspectives in Psychiatric Care, 41(4)*, 188–192.

Lee, S. I., & Keltner, N. L. (2006). Serotonin and norepinephrine reuptake inhibitors (SNRIs): Venlafaxine and duloxetine. *Perspectives in Psychiatric Care, 42*(2), 144–148.

Lovatt, P. (2011). Tricyclic antidepressants: Pharmacological profile. *Nurse Prescribing, 9*, 38–41.

Malhi, G., Adams, D., & Berk, M. (2009). Is lithium in a class of its own? A brief profile of its clinical use. *Australian and New Zealand Journal of Psychiatry, 43*, 1096–1104.

Malhi, G., Adams, D., Cahill, C., Dodd, S., & Berk, M. (2009). The management of individuals with bipolar disorder: A review of the evidence and its integration into clinical practice. *Drugs, 69*(15), 2063–2101.

Mandrioli, R., Mercolini, L., & Raggi, M. (2008). Benzodiazepine metabolism: An analytical perspective. *Current Drug Metabolism, 9*(8), 827–844.

Markowitz, J., & Narasimhan, M. (2008). Delirium and antipsychotics: A systematic review of epidemiology and somatic treatment options. *Psychiatry, 5*(10), 29–36.

Martin, I.L. & Dunn, S.M., (2002). GABA receptors. *Tocris Reviews. 20*, 1–8.

Mason, P. J., Morris, V. A., & Balcezak, T. J. (2000). Serotonin syndrome: Presentation of 2 cases and review of the literature. *Medicine, 79*, 201–209.

Mauri, M. C., Volonteri, L. S., Colasanti, A., Fiorentini, A., De Gaspari, I. F., & Bareggi, S. R. (2007). Clinical pharmacokinetics of atypical antipsychotics: A critical review of the relationship between plasma concentrations and clinical response. *Clinical Pharmacokinetics, 46*(5), 359–388.

McIntyre, R., & Cha, D. (2011). Novel treatment avenues for bipolar depression: Going beyond Lithium. *Psychiatric Times, 28*(4). Retrieved from http://www.psychiatrictimes.com/bipolar-disorder/content/article/10168/1846994#

McKeage, K. (2010). Spotlight on memantine in moderate to severe Alzheimer's disease. *Drugs and Aging, 27*(2), 177–179.

Minzenberg, M., & Yoon, J. (2011). An index of relative central a-adrenergic receptor antagonism by antipsychotic medications. *Experimental and Clinical Psychopharmacology, 19*(1), 31–39.

Morishita, S., Sawamura, J., & Ishigooka, J. (2009). Characteristics associated with response to clonazepam augmentation therapy in patients with protracted depression. *International Medical Journal, 16*(1), 9–12.

Nurnberg, H. G., Hensley, P. L., Heiman, J. R., Croft, H. A., Debattista, C., & Paine, S. (2008). Sildenafil treatment of women with antidepressant-associated sexual dysfunction: A randomised controlled trial. *JAMA, 300*, 395–404.

Opacka-Juffry, J. (2008). The role of serotonin as a neurotransmitter in health and illness: A review. *British Journal of Neuroscience Nursing, 4*(6), 272–279.

Parikh, S. V. (2009). Antidepressants are not all created equal. *Lancet, 373*, 700–701.

Preskorn, S. H., & Flockhart, D. (2009). 2010 Guide to psychiatric drug interactions. *Primary Psychiatry, 16*, 45–74.

Preston, J. (2011). *Quick reference to psychotropic medications.* Retrieved from http://www.psyd-fx.com/Quick_Reference_bw_2011.pdf

Reeves, R. R., & Ladner, M. E. (2010). Antidepressant-induced suicidality: An update. *CNS Neuroscience & Therapeutics, 16*, 227–234.

Riddle, E., Bush, J., Tittle, M., & Dilkhush, D. (2010). Alcohol withdrawal: Development of a standing order set. *Critical Care Nurse, 30*, 38–47. doi: 10.4037/ccn2010862

Rief, W., Nestoriuc, Y., Lilienfeld-Toal, A., Dogan, I., Schreiber, S., Hofmann, S.,…Avorn J. (2009). Differences in adverse effect reporting in placebo groups in SSRI and tricyclic antidepressant trials: A systematic review and meta-analysis. *Drug Safety, 32*(11), 1041–1056.

Roman, M. (2011). Atypical antipsychotics: The two new arrivals. *Issues in Mental Health Nursing, 32*, 85–86.

Sandson, N. B., Armstrong, S. C., & Cozza, K. L. (2005). Med-Psych drug-drug interactions update: An overview of psychotropic drug-drug interactions. *Psychosomatics, 46*, 464–494.

Seeman, P. (2002). Atypical antipsychotics: Mechanism of action. *Canadian Journal of Psychiatry, 47*, 27–38.

Sicouri, S., & Antzelevitch, C. (2008). Sudden cardiac death secondary to antidepressant and antipsychotic drugs. *Expert Opinion on Drug Safety, 7*(2), 181–194.

Stahl, S. M. (1998). Basic psychopharmacology of antidepressants, part 1: Antidepressants have several distinct mechanisms of action. *Journal of Clinical Psychiatry, 59*, 5–14.

Stahl, S. M. (2008). *Stahl's essential psychopharmacology: Neuroscientific basis and practical applications* (3rd ed.). New York, NY: Cambridge University Press.

Steele, D., Dowben, J., Vance, D., & Keltner, N. (2011). Biological perspectives: Antipsychotics and the "fast-off" theory. *Perspectives in Psychiatric Care, 47*, 160–162.

Steele, D., Keltner, N., & McGuiness, T. (2011). Biological perspectives: Are neuroleptic malignant syndrome and serotonin syndrome the same syndrome? *Perspectives in Psychiatric Care, 47*, 58–62.

Stone, M. (2010). Selective serotonin reuptake inhibitors. *Nurse Prescribing, 8*(4), 173–177.

Thomas, P., Alptekin, K., Gheorghe, M., Mauri, M., Olivares, J., & Riedel, M. (2009). Management of patients presenting with acute psychotic episodes of schizophrenia. *CNS Drugs, 23*(3), 193–212.

Watanabe, N., Omori, I., Nakagawa, A., Cipriani, A., Barbui, C., McGuire, H.,… (2010). Safety reporting and adverse-event profile of mirtazapine described in randomized controlled trials in comparison with other classes of antidepressants in the acute-phase treatment of adults with depression: Systematic review and meta-analysis. *CNS Drugs, 24*(1), 35–53.

Weitzel, C., & Jiwanlal, S. (2001). The darker side of SSRIs. *RN, 64*(8), 43–48.

Wongpakaran, N., Reekum, R., Wongpakaran, T., & Clarke, D. (2007). Selective serotonin reuptake inhibitor use associates with apathy among depressed elderly: A case-control study. *Annuals of General Psychiatry, 6*(7), 7.

Wynn, G. H., Oesterhold, J. R., Cozza, R. L., & Armstrong, S. C. (2008). Clinical manual of drug interaction principles for medical practice. Washington, DC: American Psychiatric Publishing.

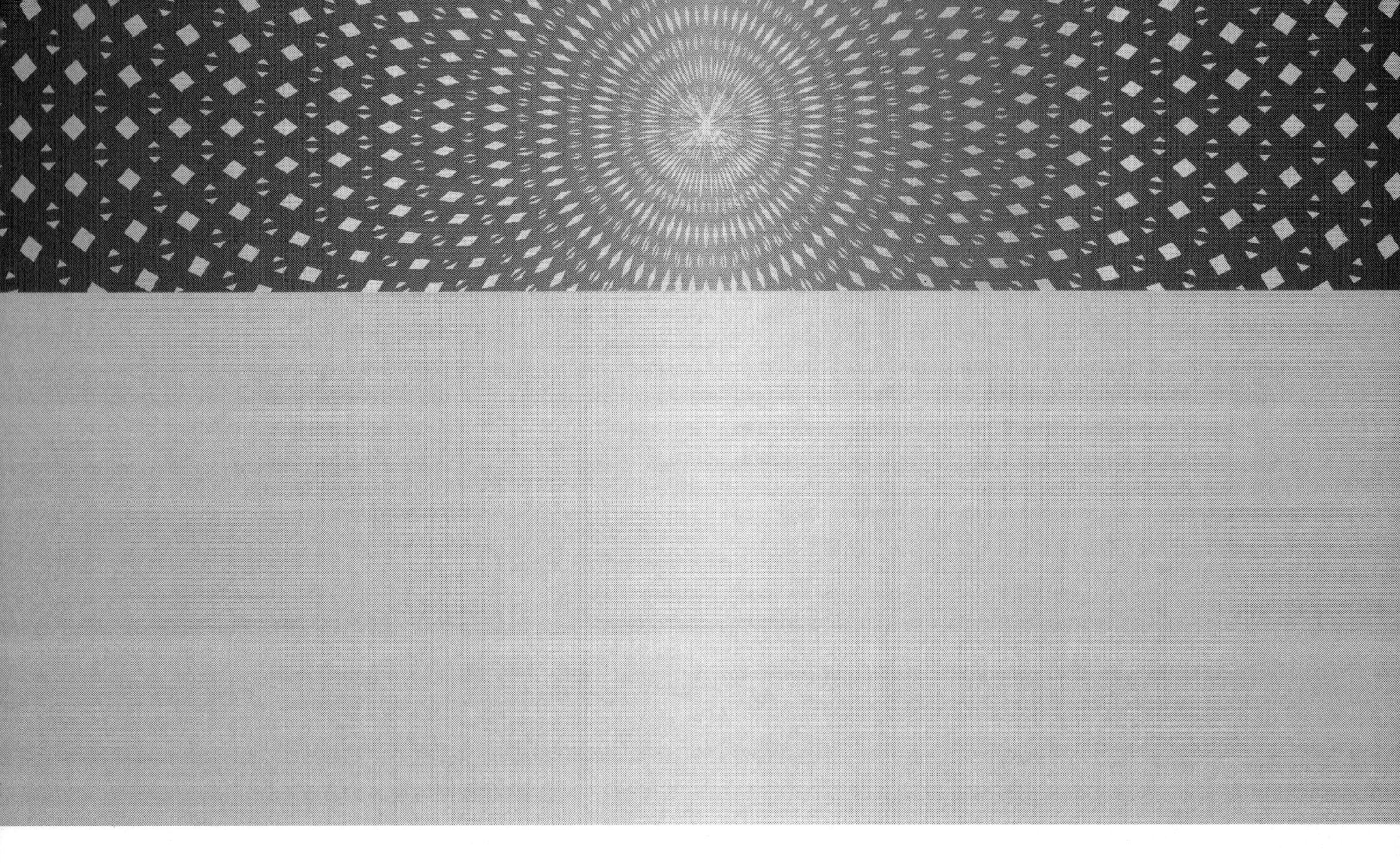

CHAPTER CONTENTS

The definition of complementary and alternative approaches in health care is broad. The National Center for Complementary and Alternative Medicine (NCCAM) at the National Institute of Health (NIH) defines Complementary and Alternative Medicine (CAM) as "a group of diverse medical and health care systems, practices, and products that are not generally considered part of conventional medicine as practiced by holders of MD (medical doctor) or DO (doctor of osteopathy) degrees and by their allied health professionals such as physical therapists, psychologists, and registered nurses."The boundaries between CAM and conventional medicine are not absolute, and specific CAM practices may, over time, become widely accepted" (NCCAM, 2012). In addition to definitions, another way to frame the differences between allopathic, approaches and alternative/complementary approaches is in terms of the general philosophical underpinnings of each. Stated simply, medical interventions involve working against natural forces and eliminating causative agents, while complimentary/alternative approaches work with the forces of nature and seek harmony and balance.

The 2007 National Health Interview Survey (NHIS), which included a comprehensive survey of CAM use by Americans, showed that approximately 38% of U.S. adults use CAM. To clarify the terms, complementary refers to adding another intervention to the medical (allopathic) model, and the term alternative refers to using an intervention in place of or without medical (allopathic) interventions.

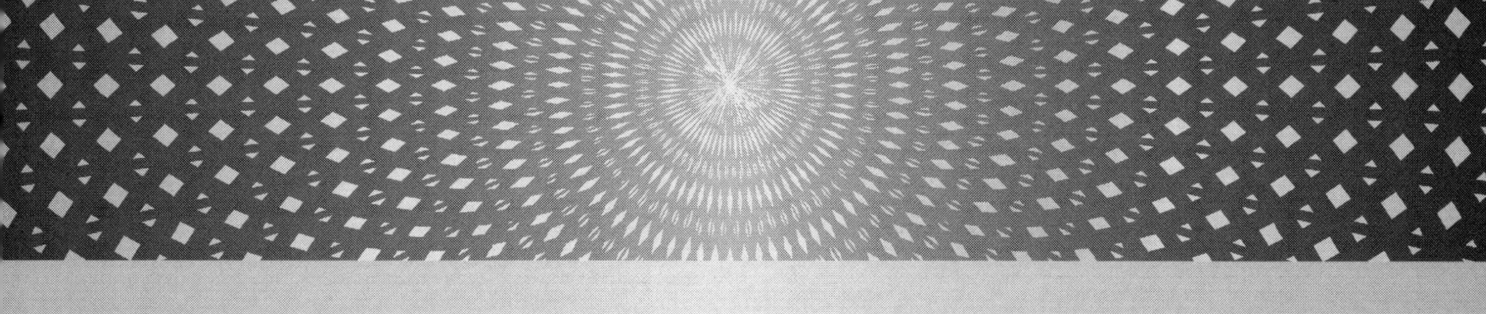

CHAPTER 6

Overview of Complementary/ Alternative Approaches

Kathleen R. Tusaie

Complementary and alternative approaches have been in existence since people began caring for each other; they also vary by cultures. Allopathic approaches have often been referred to as scientific or evidence-based and complementary/alternative approaches as unscientific. Although allopathic medicine emphasizes objectivism, reductionism, and physically measurable approaches and data, it is recognized that this is not the only way of "knowing" (Carper, 1978). When an alternative intervention alone or added to an allopathic treatment results in a physiologic or clinical change that cannot be explained by the medical model, the reality cannot be denied; rather, the explanatory models may need to be modified.

The NCCAM groups alternative and complementary practices into broad categories, such as natural products, mind-body, manipulative, and energy practices as described in Exhibit 6-1. Although these categories are not formally defined, they are useful for discussing CAM practices. Some CAM practices may fit into more than one category.

TYPES OF COMPLEMENTARY/ALTERNATIVE INTERVENTIONS

NATURAL PRODUCTS

Natural products include a variety of herbal medicines (also known as botanicals), vitamins, minerals, and other "natural products." Many are sold over the counter as dietary supplements. CAM "natural products" also include *probiotics*, that is, live microorganisms (usually bacteria) that are similar to microorganisms normally found in the human digestive tract and that may have beneficial effects. Probiotics are available in foods (e.g., yogurts) or as dietary supplements. They are not the same thing as *prebiotics*—nondigestible food ingredients that selectively stimulate the growth and/or activity of microorganisms already present in the body.

Herbals

The use of herbal or botanical medicines reflect some of the first attempts to improve the human condition. Evidence of this early use of herbs includes the mummified prehistoric "ice man" found in the Italian Alps in 1991 with pouches of medicinal herbs. During the last decade, there has been a significant increase in the consumption of herbal remedies in North America and Europe, with Germany and France leading the world in sales (Capasso, Gaginella, Grandolini, & Izzo, 2003). The 2007 National Health Interview Survey found that 17.7% of American adults had used a nonvitamin/nonmineral natural product. Next to prayer, these products were the most popular form of CAM among both adults and children. The most commonly used product among adults was fish oil/omega-3s (reported by 37.4% of all adults who said they used natural products); popular products for children included echinacea (37.2%)

EXHIBIT 6-1: TYPES OF COMPLEMENTARY/ ALTERNATIVE INTERVENTIONS

Natural Products
Mind-Body Practices
Manipulative, Body-Based Practices
Energy Approaches
Others

and fish oil/omega-3s (30.5%) (Barnes, Powell-Grina, McFann, & Nahin, 2004).

Recent reports have stated that as many as 16% of prescription drug users in the United States consume herbal supplements (Kaufman et al., 2002). However, less than half of these clients disclose herbal supplement use to health care providers and many prescribers are unaware of the potential effects, side effects, and potential interactions of herbals (Klepser et al., 2000; NCCAM, 2011). This sets the stage for potential herb-prescription interactions, which may be harmful. Although used for centuries, natural does not mean safe. The vast majority of these herbal products are unlicensed and not required to demonstrate efficacy, safety, or quality (De Smet, 2002). Herbal medicines often are mixtures of more than one active ingredient. With multiple active compounds, the likelihood of herb-prescription drug interactions is quite high. Herbal supplements have been associated with adverse events that include all levels of severity, organ systems, and age groups (Palmer et al., 2003).

Perhaps one reason people may feel attracted to the use of herbals is the perceived connection to the natural world. There is an increasing interest in our industrialized world to reconnect with the ecological substratum or to be "green." Most indigenous peoples have well-established beliefs that the natural world is powerful and they have respect for the medicinal plants they harvest. Although many humans have disconnected from the plant world, at the biological level, the connection has not been severed. Biomedical science has confirmed what traditional healers know instinctively—that humans and plants are very similar and interdependent. The structure of chlorophyll in green plants and hemoglobin found in human red blood cells (RBC) is almost identical (Libster, 2002). Chlorophyllin is sold in health food stores to decrease constipation, decrease odor from colostomy, and increase wound healing. Chlorophyll is involved in photosynthesis, the process that ultimately produces oxygen that is fundamental to human life. Also, about one fourth of all conventional drugs contain at least one active ingredient derived from plants with the remaining chemicals artificially synthesized.

An integrative approach by Psychiatric-Mental Health Advanced Practice Nurses (PMH-APRNs) involves first learning about herbs, understanding the client's interest and use of herbs, then educating or counseling with the client about effects and potential adverse effects. This approach includes integration of a scientific model with an interpersonal caring model to provide holistic care.

The herbs most commonly used for mental health reasons are presented along with their expected actions, potential adverse effects, and possible interactions with prescription drugs. Although most PMH-APRNs prescribe prescription medications, because no organization or government body certifies the labeling of herbal preparations, it is wise not to "prescribe" herbals, but to educate and discuss options for use with clients. If you are making a referral to an herbalist, be sure the individual has had formal preparation in herbology and is capable of evaluating individuals before combining various herbs for therapeutic effect.

Herbs are marketed in the United States as dietary supplements. In the United States, herbalists are not permitted to advertise or diagnosis or treat any disease. In 2007, the Federal Drug Administration (FDA) passed the Current Good Manufacturing Practice Act (CGMP). This act was an attempt to protect consumers by requiring label disclosure of the identity, purity, strength, and composition of the contents as well as the need to report adverse advents to the FDA. Companies that supply standardized extracts offer the greatest degree of quality control and thus the highest quality products.

There are several reliable resources for information on herbals. The World Health Organization (WHO) has published *Guidelines for the Assessment of Herbal Medicines* (1991), which established standards for determining safety, quality, and efficacy of herbal preparations and the development of pharmacopoeia monographs. The WHO also publishes *Monographs on Selected Medicinal Plants* (1999). Baseline standards for quality, safety, and efficacy including dosing are provided. The *PDR for Nonprescription Drugs, Dietary Supplements, and Herbals* (Murray, 2011) contains over 700 herbal monographs for the treatment of medical conditions. The *PDR for Herbal Medicines, PDRHM* (Thompson Healthcare, 2007) also provides excellent information on herbals. These publications validate the growing use of herbs and medicinal plants as official medicines.

Medicinal herbs can be purchased without a prescription in a wide variety of places including local grocery stores, drug stores, and on the Internet. This availability and increased consumer interest has led to a need for increased knowledge among clients and practitioners. This is particularly important for psychiatric health care professionals because the second fastest growing populations to utilize medicinal herbals are those with symptoms of depression and anxiety (Roy-Byrne et al., 2005), and there are multiple herbs claiming to alleviate these symptoms.

For example, the current edition of the PDRHM has listed well over 40 herbs for the treatment of anxiety and 12 for the treatment of depression. With the exception of St. John's wort for depression; there is minimal research available on other psychotropic herbs. However, based on the available research, the German Regulator Authority (Commission E), the current expert on herbal medication and an organization comparable to the U.S. FDA, has approved only 15 of these herbs as valid in the PDRHM. The most common of these herbs are discussed.

In general, herbals act similarly to conventional pharmaceuticals in that the action depends upon their chemical components. However, their effects are usually slower in onset than pharmaceuticals. Although active compounds of each plant are being identified, many herbs produce actions not consistent with the allopathic medical model. Herbs seem to impact homeostatic control mechanisms to facilitate normalization of body processes. The whole plant contains hundreds of compounds and it is difficult to know if the preparation contains only one part or the whole plant. Therefore, the mechanism of action desired is to correct an underlying cause of illness and not to eliminate a specific symptom as in the medical model. The uniqueness of each individual is important as is adaption of the herbs for each specific situation. This also results in research difficulties—if investigating one specific active component of the herb results will differ from the whole plant effects. This is further complicated by the growth conditions for the plant, stage of plant development at harvest, as well as the type of manufacturing process influencing potency. Without knowing the amounts of active ingredients administered, it is impossible to compare results of clinical trials or determine if an effect is reproducible.

There are other potential flaws of randomized trials (RCT) of botanicals. Morris and Tangney (2011) described in detail possible explanations for the null findings of RCTs of vitamin supplements. Treatment may not have proven to be effective in trials of Vitamin E, B vitamins, and docosa-hexaenoic acid (a component of fish oil) to improve cognition because nutrient intake among the participants was already at optimal levels.

A basic principle of nutrition is that nutrients have a nonlinear, inverted U-shaped association with optimum physiological function. Very low levels in diet or tissues result in poor function or even death. But optimal functioning occurs over a wide range of levels and becomes toxic only at extreme high levels. Consideration of nutrient level is critically important in research studies, but the usual hypothesis is that nutrient supplementation is effective no matter what the pre-intervention nutrient status. Insufficient nutrient intake can influence brain function. Deficiencies in niacin, thiamine, vitamin B_{12}, vitamin D, and folate are known to have adverse psychiatric effects (Fernstrom, 2000). Although the NCCAM is increasing the research studies of nutrients, there is a need for more refined and perhaps alternatively designed studies.

Taking nutritional supplements is generally considered a positive practice. However, several recent studies have reported that individuals using dietary supplements have decreased motivation to stop smoking and develop an illusion of invulnerability or psychological license to smoke more (Chiou, 2011). This effect occurs when individuals believe they have made a positive health behavior change (taking supplement), and then feel licensed or empowered to act in ways counterproductive to maintaining health. These researchers are now exploring what interventions might cancel out this effect. Therefore, the use of supplements is quite an individualized, complex health practice.

Types of Herbal Products

Many forms of herbs are available. While herbalists prefer the whole plant, capsules and tablets are the most popular forms used. Teas are available in loose or tea bag form. When steeped in boiling water, fragrant, aromatic flavor and medicinal properties are released. Herbal teas are used as an alternative to caffeinated teas, to increase digestion (peppermint, spearmint, rosehips, lemon grass, anise) or for medicinal purposes (chamomile for improving sleep or peppermint and chamomile for upset stomach). Extracts and tinctures contain alcohol and have an indefinite shelf life. Salves, balms, and ointments have been used for years for skin irritation and insect or snake bites. These are made with vegetable oil or petroleum jelly and often contain aloe, marigold, chamomile, comfrey, or St. John's wort.

General Rules for Safe Use

Medicinal herbs should be taken only when needed and never during pregnancy or breastfeeding. Before using any herb, learn as much as you can about it from reliable sources. Dosing is largely based on those traditionally used in Europe or anecdotal information. But in general, start with less than the recommended dosage listed on the bottle and monitor progress. Younger than 12, over 60 years, and underweight individuals are more at risk for toxicity. Herbs may interact with each other as well as prescription drugs. So, start with a single herb and work with a professional (herbologist, Doctor of Neuropathy, Doctor of Osteopathy) for the safest and most effective results.

General Mechanism of Herb-Drug Interactions

Herb-drug interactions are based upon the same pharmacokinetic and pharmacodynamic mechanisms as drug-drug interactions. Much of the available information about interactions between herbal products and prescribed drugs is from case reports with some clinical studies now appearing in the literature. Altered drug concentrations by coadministered herbs may be attributed to the induction or inhibition of hepatic and intestinal drug-metabolizing enzymes (cytochrome P450) and/or drug transporters such as P-glycoprotein (Zhou et al., 2003). Long-term use of St. John's wort induced hepatic CYP3A4 and other CYP enzymes involved in drug metabolism. Echinacea acts as a modulator by inducing hepatic CYP3A4 and inhibiting intestinal CYP3A4. Kava inhibits all CYP activities. In contrast, others including green tea, ginko, garlic, saw palmetto, and Siberian ginseng did not affect CYP activities in normal volunteers.

In addition to the CYP enzymes, P-glycoprotein in the intestine, liver, and kidney plays an important role in absorption, distribution, and excretion of drugs (Lin & Yamazaki, 2003). It limits cellular transport from the intestinal lumen into epithelial cells and also enhances the excretion of drugs out of hepatocytes and renal tubules into adjacent luminal spaces. These pharmacodynamic interactions may be additive or synergetic, whereby the herbal product potentiates the action of the prescribed drug or antagonistic and the herbal product reduces the availability of the prescribed drug, thus reducing the pharmacological effect. The specific herbals will be described including actions, adverse effects, and interactions.

SPECIFIC HERBS AND NUTRIENTS COMMONLY SUGGESTED FOR MENTAL HEALTH

St. John's Wort (*Hypericum perforatum*)

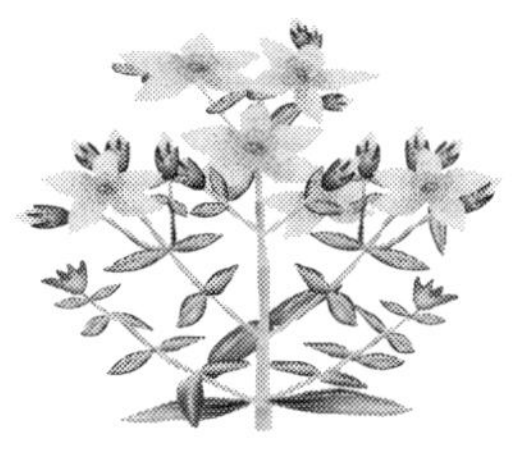

This herb has been used to treat nervous and psychiatric disorders, especially depressed mood. It has recently been reported to be less effective than previously believed for moderate and severe depression (Shelton et al., 2001; Werneke, Horn, & Taylor, 2004). However, it is difficult to compare across studies due to differences in dosage, levels of depression, and measurement tools. It may be used for individuals experiencing mild depressive symptoms and those who fear the side effects of pharmaceutical drugs, experience no relief from therapy, and have a desire for easy access without professional involvement.

The exact mechanism of action is unclear, but believed to involve inhibition of monoamine oxidase (MAO) and stimulation of serotonin, dopamine, and gamma-aminobutyric acid (GABA). It could be that several mechanisms are responsible for the therapeutic actions and this is the reason for fewer side effects. Usual dose for adults is initially 900 mg tablets qd. If there is no improvement in 4 weeks, consider augmenting or switching treatment. Side effects include headache, fatigue, restlessness, gastrointestinal (GI) complaints (nausea, diarrhea, dry mouth, constipation), photosensitivity, and pruritis.

Interactions with prescription drugs include decreasing effectiveness of immunosuppressants, antineoplastic agents, anticoagulants, oral contraceptives, and alprazolam. Watch for signs of prescription drug toxicity if St. John's wort is abruptly discontinued. It should not be taken with prescribed antidepressants, especially MAO inhibitors. There is an increased risk of serotonin syndrome if taken concomitantly with selective serotonin reuptake inhibitors (SSRIs) or Buspar (Dresser, Schwarz, Wilkinson, & Kim, 2003). It increases effects of other herbs with sedative effects such as calamus, California poppy, chamomile, kava, lemon balm, sage, sassafras, siberian ginseng, valerian, wild carrot, and wild lettuce.

Kava (*Piper methysticum*)

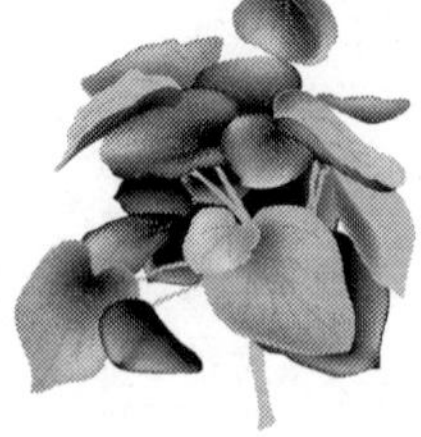

The dried rhizome and root of this perennial shrub of the black pepper family produces the commonly used kava. Throughout the South Pacific Islands, it has been traditionally used as a beverage similar to the use of wine in Europe. It has been used to reduce anxiety and promote sleep and some herbalists consider it to be an aphrodisiac.

This herb contains seven major and minor active compounds. Kava effects MAO-B and the limbic system to produce calming effects. It also inhibits voltage-gated calcium and sodium channels to produce anticonvulsant and skeletal muscle relaxant effects. Usual dose for anxiety is 50–70 mg of pure kava three times a day.

A few small studies compared kava with placebo, and kava extract might be an effective symptomatic treatment for anxiety although, at present, the size of the effect seems to be small. Kava potentiates effects of alcohol and there is some evidence that use beyond 3 months may produce addiction. It also produces mild euphoria, fluent speech, and increased sensitivity to sounds.

It may cause mild GI disturbances, mouth numbness, increased RBC count, rash, and increased high-density lipoprotein (HDL) cholesterol. In 2002, the FDA issued a warning about potential liver damage related to the use of kava containing dietary supplements. Although the WHO has identified only certain preparations of kava as harmful, kava has been banned in various European markets. There is no clarity about the safety beginning with the kava farmer and ending with the consumer (Teschke & Schulze, 2010). Rigorous trials with large sample sizes are needed to clarify the existing uncertainties. Particularly long-term safety studies of kava are needed.

Valerian (*Valeriana officinalis*)

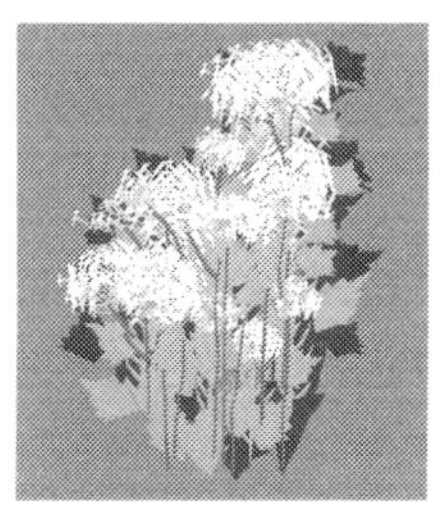

This tall perennial herb has been used since the Middle Ages for its calming effects. It has multiple active chemicals with the most potent in the root. It inhibits the enzymes responsible for breaking down GABA, thus inducing higher levels of this natural relaxant. There was only one small study available that compared valerian to valium and indicated similar symptom relief. However, there are no larger studies available (Miyasaka, Atallah, & Soares, 2011).

The usual dose to enhance sleep is 400–800 mg of root up to 2 hours before bedtime. It may take up to 2 to 4 weeks of use to notice improvement in sleep pattern and quality. Valerian tea is also gaining in popularity with taking 1 cup two or three times a day and one at bedtime.

Valerian may cause additive effects with alcohol, benzodiazepines, and other sedatives. It may also cause morning headaches, GI complaints, restlessness, and rebound anxiety if abruptly stopped after prolonged use. It also potentiates action of other sedating herbs such as catnip, hops, kava, and passion flower.

Gingko (*Gingko biloba*)

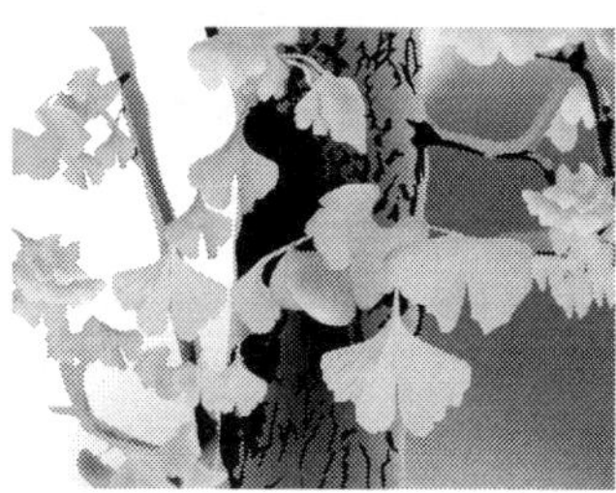

This herb is derived from the world's oldest tree, over two hundred million years old. It's leaves and seeds are used for medicinal purposes. It has been used for neuroprotection and regenerative effects on circulation. Memory and concentration problems, confusion, depression, dizziness, tinnitus, and headache are usual indications for use. The flavonoids in gingko are considered antioxidants that serve as free radical scavengers. Free radicals can damage the lining of blood vessels, cause lipid oxidation, and interfere with many cellular processes. Other modes of action are thought to be increasing blood supply by dilating vessels, reducing blood viscosity, and modification of the neurotransmitter system.

Results from recent studies are contradictory regarding cognition, activities of daily living, and mood. One reported very large positive treatment effects and others reported no difference between ginko (EGb761) and placebo. Usual dosage was 40–80 mg tablets three times a day. Therefore, there are no significant differences between ginko and placebo in the proportion of participants experiencing adverse events. Headache and bleeding have been reported.

Ginseng (*Panax ginseng, Asian ginseng*)

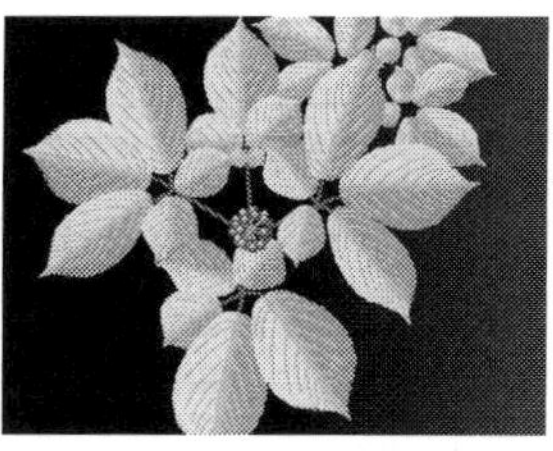

This herb is a small perennial with a single stem and a few leaves depending upon the age of the plant. Roots are used for medicinal purposes. It has been used in the East as a tonic that strengthens the "qi." It is used to promote health, increase sexual potency, and longevity rather than cure disease. Its mode of action is thought to be ginsenosides that produce immunomodulation effects including increased natural-killer cells, stimulation of interferon production, and ribonucleic acid (RNA) synthesis. Ginseng is usually taken for 15 to 20 days in two doses of 0.5–1.0 g of the root. For an individual recovering from sickness, it is taken continuously.

Ginseng inhibits CYP 3A4 and drugs that are metabolized by this enzyme must be avoided to prevent toxicity. Adverse reactions include dizziness, nervousness, changes in blood pressure, diarrhea, and vaginal bleeding.

American ginseng is considered a yin tonic and is more cooling than Asian ginseng. There are early findings that American ginseng may improve memory. After 2 weeks use of HT1001, a standardized proprietary North American ginseng (*Panax quinquefolius*) extract in healthy volunteers, memory significantly improved (Sutherland et al., 2010). However, there are no consistent large effect results supporting therapeutic benefits of Asian or American ginsing at this time.

S-Adenosyl Methionine (SAMe)

This is a naturally occurring molecule (not an herb) that decreases with human aging. It has been tested for over 25 years as a potential antidepressant. SAMe's mechanism of action is related to the process of methylation (Stahl, 2008). SAMe is formed from an essential amino acid, methionine, which is found in fish, meat, and dairy products. Methionine combining with adenosine triphosphate (ATP) forms SAMe. Next, it donates a methyl group in the Central nervous system (CNS) for methyl acceptor molecules including serotonin and dopamine. Then, it breaks down to form homocysteine. Remethylation or converting homocystine back to methionine requires vitamin B12 and folic acid. Transsulfulfuration, converting homocystine into glutathione, an antioxidant, can also occur. This process requires vitamin B6 and assists with maintaining cartilage.

There are several possible explanations how these processes provide antidepressant action. SAMe may increase the production of serotonin and dopamine or increase the number or receptivity of receptors. Lower levels of SAMe have been reported in cerebrospinal fluid of individuals who are depressed compared to non-depressed controls. Pilot studies have identified administration of SAMe to be as or more effective than TCAs but with fewer side effects (Pancheri, Scapicchio, & Chiaie, 2002). However, the studies are of short duration (30 days) and usually small sample size. There have been no studies to compare effectiveness with SSRIs. SAMe has been studied in the treatment of fibromyalgia, chronic fatigue, arthritis and migraine (McEnany, 1999). Therefore, although SAMe appears to be effective with rapid onset and few side effects, it is not yet recommended as an antidepressant due to unknown long-term effects. Side effects include nausea and GI disturbances. There have also been documented cases of switching from depression to mania during treatment. Dosage is recommended to start at 200 mg twice a day and increase at weekly intervals but not to exceed 1,600 mg per day. During intravenous administration of SAMe improvement (50% decrease) of severe depressive symptoms was noted in 4 to 7 days.

Although studies have been published since the 1980s, SAMe is not regulated by the FDA and is not currently recommended for use within the American Psychiatric Association Guidelines for treatment of Major Depression (2011). However, it has been suggested that it may be useful as an adjunct to standard antidepressant therapy (Davis, Charney, Coyle, & Nemeroff, 2003).

Omega-3 Fatty Acids

These fatty acids are selectively concentrated in synaptic neuronal membranes and help regulate receptor activity and signal transduction. Fish and seafood are the richest dietary sources. In addition to seafood, the precursor a-linolenic acid is found in mungo bean, flaxseed, and canola oil. Omega-3 supplements from fish oil are regarded as safe for consumption by the U.S. FDA and are considered nutrients.

The mechanism that impacts psychiatric problems includes increasing serotonin levels, altering dopamine functions, regulating of corticotrophin-releasing factor, inhibiting of protein kinase C, suppressing of second messengers, increasing synaptic formation, preventing of neuronal apoptosis, improving cerebral blood flow, regulating gene expression, and enzyme action resulting in decreased inflammatory response (Freeman et al., 2006). The effectiveness of these mechanisms by omega-3 fatty acids have been tested in the treatment of depression, schizophrenia, dementia, impulsivity (borderline personality disorder), attention deficit/hyperactive disorder, and learning disabilities.

As an adjunctive treatment for mood disorders in Major Depression as well as Bipolar Disorder, omega-3 fatty acids eicosapentaenoic acid (EPA), docosahexaenoic acid (DHA), or combinations (not DHA alone) have demonstrated statistically significant improvement in mood. The usual dose is 1.0–9.6 g per day. Overall, there are minimal side effects. However, at excessive doses, GI side effects and alteration of glucose metabolism in diabetics have been reported. There has been one case of induced hypomania, and interactions with anticoagulants may result in excessive bleeding (Montgomery & Richardson, 2008).

Although omega-3 fatty acids failed to alleviate the positive and negative symptoms of schizophrenia or the development of dementia, they did decrease triglyceride levels that were elevated by individuals taking antipsychotic medications. Therefore, prevention and/or treatment of antipsychotic side effects, metabolic syndrome, and cardiac prms, may be an appropriate use of omega-3 fatty acids (Gammack, Van Niekerk, & Dangour, 2011).

Decreased hostility and impulsivity was demonstrated in studies where subjects were children with Attention Deficit Disorder, adults with Borderline Personality Disorder, and felony convicted prisoners. Usual dosage was 1 g per day. Several studies added vitamin E and evening primrose. No adverse effects were reported.

Because omega-3 fatty acids have been shown to lower triglycerides and inhibit platelet aggregation and cardiac arrhythmias, the American Psychiatric Association has recommended that all adults should eat fish at least twice a week and individuals with symptoms of mood disturbances, impulsivity, or psychotic symptoms should consume 1 g EPA + DHA per day. Larger doses may be useful for individuals with mood disorders (1–9 g/d) (Freeman et al., 2006).

Folate

This is one of the 13 essential vitamins and assists in the synthesis of neurotransmitters. Dihydrofolate is obtained from dietary intake of green vegetables, yeast, liver, kidney, and egg yolk. Folic acid is the synthetic form contained in supplements and also available in high doses by prescription (Deplin). (Stahl, 2008). Several trials using methyl folate as adjunctive treatment with an antidepressant demonstrated a reduction in depressive symptoms. However, it is currently unclear if this is the case for individuals with normal folate levels as well as those with folate deficiency (Taylor, Carney, Geddes, & Goodwin, 2011).

Vitamin D

This is a fat soluble vitamin which is created by sun exposure. Vitamin D deficiency symptoms are depression, chronic fatigue, weight loss, diabetes, heart disease, stroke, and osteoporosis. Vitamin D has a significant biochemistry in the brain. Vitamin D is involved in the biosynthesis of neurotrophic factors, synthesis of nitric oxide synthase, and increased glutathione levels—all suggesting an important role for vitamin D in brain function and production of monoamines (serotonin, dopamine, norepinephrine).

Low vitamin D is a widespread problem in the United States (Holick, 2006). Due to tall buildings, pollution, and mostly indoor work, many people have decreased sunlight exposure. In the Third National Health and Nutrition Examination Survey (NHANES III) (Ganji Milone, Cody, McCarty, & Wang, 2010), 70% of participants had suboptimal levels of vitamin D. Furthermore, various studies have linked vitamin D deficiency to depression.

Serum 25(OH) D levels should be obtained when deficiency is suspected. Judicial exposure to sunlight, oral vitamin D, or both, aimed at restoring circulating levels of 25(OH) D to between 50–80 ng/mL, is the treatment of choice for vitamin D deficiency. Cholecalciferol is the preferred oral preparation of vitamin D. Oral doses ranging between 700–2,000 IU/day are adjusted to sustain circulating 25(OH) D concentrations (Institute of Medicine, 2010).

Therefore, individuals with depressive symptoms and low exposure to sunlight should be assessed for vitamin D deficiency (Zitterman, 2003). Supplements of vitamin D and sunlight exposure can correct this deficiency that may contribute to mood disorders (Heaney, Davies, Chen, Holick, & Barger-Lux, 2003; Holick, 2006; Vieth, 1999).

MIND-BODY INTERVENTIONS

Mind-body practices focus on the interactions among the brain, mind, body, and behavior, with the intent to use the mind to modulate (affect) physical functioning and promote health. All of the major body systems maintain direct, two-way communication with the brain. Furthermore, the brain continuously regulates activity to optimize the body's ability to respond to environmental and internal challenges. Many CAM practices embody this concept—in different ways. The body's major systems—the autonomic, endocrine, immune, and neuropeptide systems—are communication channels whereby the person's thoughts and images activate the genetic material and cellular structures to reorganize according to new information, to help a person move toward healing (Dossey et al., 1995). The brain continuously receives, integrates, and interprets many streams of information. As the information and its meaning are neurally represented, dedicated neural circuits respond to perceived risks and opportunities by altering internal physiology. These alterations are intended to maximize ability to adjust to environmental changes. Unusual stressors or chronic exposure to stressful situations may lead to neuronal changes that eventually become maladaptive. These changes can be magnified by existing biological vulnerabilities, including psychiatric illness. The autonomic nervous system may produce relaxation (parasympathetic) or activation (sympathetic). The clinical effects of mental processes on physiology are profound and emphasize the concept of mind-body connections.

EXHIBIT 6-2: "I AM RELAXED"... DEEP BREATHING AND RELAXATION EXERCISE

1. Sit comfortably and quietly.
2. Tell yourself that you are going to use the next 5, 10, or 20 minutes to rebalance, to heal, to relax yourself.
3. Surrender the weight of your body, allowing the chair, or floor, to support you.
4. Close your eyes, gently cutting out visual stimulation and distraction.
5. As you inhale, repeat to yourself: "I AM."
6. As you exhale, say... "RELAXED."
7. Continue to breathe normally not trying to change your breath in any way. Just watch it happening and continue to repeat: "I AM" with inhalation;..."RELAXED" with exhalation.
8. As your mind begins to wander, gently bring it back to the awareness of your breath and your statement "I AM RELAXED." Be compassionate and loving with your "leaping frog" mind, which wants to be anywhere but here.
9. Continue doing this for as long as you have established.
10. To conclude, discontinue the phrase and slowly stretch your hands and feet, your arms and legs, then your whole body.
11. Open your eyes a sliver at a time—like the sun coming up in the morning.
12. Continue on your way.

Source: From the U.S. Department of Health and Human Services, National Institute of Mental Health, Division of Communications and Education–*Plain Talk* series, Ruth Kay, Editor.

RELAXATION RESPONSE

The process of activating the relaxation response can be developed through multiple practices. The practices to be presented include deep breathing, progressive relaxation, imagery, meditation, hypnotherapy, yoga, and tai chi.

Deep-breathing exercises, progressive relaxation, and imagery are often combined and used to bring about a desired physical response such as stress reduction and relaxation (see Exhibit 6-2). When physical relaxation develops, there is a message to the mind and emotions to relax and a circular process develops. Any of various techniques (such as a series of verbal suggestions) used to guide another person or oneself in imagining sensations—especially in visualizing an image in the mind—can lead to the relaxation response. Benson (1971) has described this as The Relaxation Response, and it can be viewed at www.relaxationresponse.org/

Part of the relaxation response is deep, slow breathing, while shallow breathing that is high in the chest is referred to as fight-or-flight breathing. Breathing from the abdomen or deep breathing assists an individual to become centered in the moment and raises levels of blood oxygen, stimulating a relaxation response. Breathing those slow abdominal breaths during crisis can strip the situation of its destructive anxiety. This is a simple, mobile technique for intervening in the mind-body cycle.

During the stress response, blood flow leaves the hands and feet resulting in cooler temperature. During the relaxation response, vessels in the hands and feet expand resulting in increased warmth. Biofeedback cards that change color with temperature are a simple but effective method to measure degree of relaxation during practice.

Nancy Zi observes that most people are "shallow breathers"—they use only the narrow top portion of the lung surface for oxygen exchange. Our breath literally stops at the diaphragm. To find out if you're a shallow breather, try Zi's simple test: Put your palms against your lower abdomen and blow out all the air. Now, take a big breath. If your abdomen expands when you inhale and air seems to flow in deeply to the pit of your stomach, you're on the right track. For more information see www.theartofbreathing.com/

Progressive Muscle Relaxation

The following exercise was developed by Jacobson (1942) and has been widely used. Deep breathing and relaxation are basic steps for visualization. Many individuals are too physically tense to even attempt to visualize and it is useful to use a relaxation exercise first.

Preparation

1. Make yourself as comfortable as possible in a seated position
2. Try and sit up straight with good posture with your hands resting in your lap
3. Remove your glasses if you wear them, some people prefer to remove their contact lenses

Tensing and Relaxing Specific Muscle Groups

- **Relaxation of the feet and calves:**
  - Flex your feet (pull toes toward the knees)
  - Contract calf muscles and muscles of lower leg
  - Feel the tension build and hold the tension
  - Take a deep breath
  - As you exhale say the word "RELAX" and let the tension go
- **Relaxation of the knees and upper thighs:**
  - Straighten your knees and squeeze your legs together
  - Contract your thigh muscles and all the muscles of your legs
  - Hold the tension as it builds
  - Take a deep breath, as you exhale say the word "RELAX" and let the tension go
- **Relaxation of the hips and buttocks**
  - Tense the buttock muscles by squeezing them inward and upward
  - Feel the tension build and hold the tension
  - Take a deep breath, as you exhale say the word "RELAX" and let the tension go
- **Relaxation of the abdomen**
  - Observe your abdomen rising and falling with each breath
  - Inhale and press your navel toward the spine then tense the abdomen
  - Feel the tension build and hold the tension
  - Take a deep breath
  - As you exhale say the word "RELAX" and let the tension go
- **Relaxation of the upper back**
  - Draw the shoulder blades together to the midline of the body
  - Contract the muscles across the upper back
  - Feel the tension build and hold the tension
  - Take a deep breath
  - As you exhale say the word "RELAX" and let the tension go
- **Relaxation of the arms and palms of the hands**
  - Turn palms face down and make a tight fist in each hand
  - Raise and stretch both arms with fists
  - Feel the tension build and hold the tension
  - Take a deep breath
  - As you exhale say the word "RELAX" and let the tension go
- **Relaxation of the chin, neck, and shoulders**
  - Drop your chin to your chest
  - Draw your shoulders up toward your ears
  - Feel the tension build and hold the tension
  - Take a deep breath
  - As you exhale say the word "RELAX" and let the tension go
- **Relaxation of the jaw and facial muscles**
  - Clench your teeth together
  - Tense the muscles in the back of your jaw
  - Turn the corners of your mouth into a tight smile
  - Wrinkle the bridge of your nose and squeeze your eyes shut
  - Tense all facial muscles in toward the center of your face
  - Feel the tension build and hold the tension
  - Take a deep breath
  - As you exhale say the word "RELAX" and let the tension go
- **Relaxation of the forehead**
  - Raise eyebrows up and tense the muscles across the forehead and scalp
  - Feel the tension build and hold the tension
  - Take a deep breath
  - As you exhale say the word "RELAX" and let the tension go
- **Body awareness**
  - Focus on relaxation flowing from the crown of your head
  - Over your face
  - Down the back of your neck and shoulders
  - Down your body through your arms and hands
  - Over your chest and abdomen
  - Flowing through your hips and buttocks
  - Into your thighs, your knees, and calves
  - And finally into your ankles and feet
  - Continue to deep breathe for several minutes in silence and enjoy the relaxation

Imagery/Visualization

Many techniques combine breathing exercises and visualization. Visualization is experienced, not deduced. It causes an emotional-physiological response that involves the whole being. Each image a person chooses to concentrate upon has a specific effect that is inseparable from the nature of the object-image. Edmund Jacobson (1942) identified that when a person imagines running, measurable contractions take place in the muscles associated with running. Later, it was demonstrated that an individual could voluntarily increase the number of lymphocytes and alter the responsiveness of the immune system by employing a relaxation/imagery technique. This immunomodulation has been expanded and validated by many others (Locke, 1983; Ader et al., 1991).

These effects of visualization and mind-body connections were expanded and labeled Psychoneuroimmunology (PNI). Complementary/alternative interventions for heart disease (Ornish, 1990), cancer (Simonton et al., 1978; Spiegel, 2001), and an appreciation for transpersonal healing (Dossey, 1989) led the way for the now generally accepted importance of mindfulness (Kabat-Zinn, 1990) in healing as well as in mental health nursing (Bebbe, 2010; Tusaie-Edds, 2009).

Biochemist Candace Pert (1986) identified neuropeptides, which dramatically opened the doors between mind and body. Pert and her associates have identified over 50 neuropeptides, conveyors of emotions, scattered throughout the body. For example, insulin, which was previously believed to be a hormone produced by one gland, is a neuropeptide which is created, stored, and has a heavy concentration in receptor sites in the limbic system. The brain as well as the pancreas has the ability to produce insulin. Emotions are not just in the head but are in the body as well. There is an incredible communication system between mind and body, and indicating how emotions can be manifested throughout the body (gut reaction). This is a brief review (not comprehensive), designed to provide an appreciation of the mind-body connection and the use of imagery (see Exhibit 6-3). Now, some specific directions for using imagery as part of PMH-APRN practice will be provided.

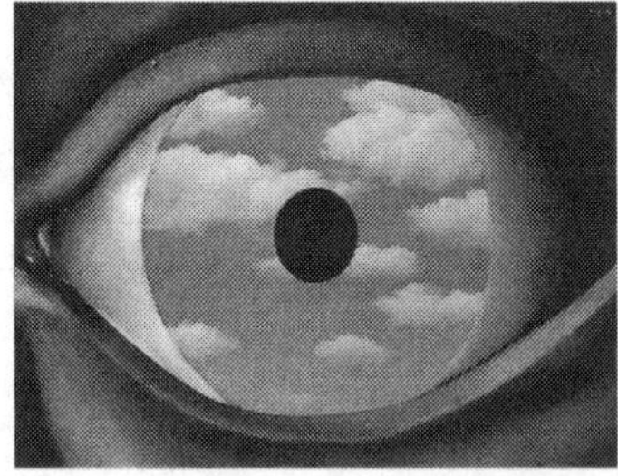

The False Mirror (*Le Faux Miroir*), painting by Renée Magritte (1928). The Museum of Modern Art (MOMA). © 2012 C. Herscovici, Brussels / Artists Rights Society (ARS), New York.

Designing Imagery

Common goals for the use of imagery include increasing relaxation to improve coping with daily stressors or pain, enhancing immune system function, or any behavior change. There are basically two types of imagery—guided and unguided. Guided imagery, using recordings, leads the individual to expand his or her ideas of imagery and recordings also are convenient. The use of guided imagery may help individuals to understand imagery and then serve as a springboard for creating their own imagery. Guided imagery is also helpful for the PMH-APRN who has not facilitated imagery long enough to feel comfortable without using a script. However, using recordings encourages a sense of outer control and may at times stunt self growth and expression. After practice, the imagery needs to become a natural process.

One beginning exercise that has been used for individuals with anxiety as well as eating disorders, but which may be beneficial for most people, is to develop an awareness of body sensations. This is often a goal of mind-body therapies. Most individuals are unaware of their bodies. For example, until I started swimming classes, I was not aware of my habit of holding my breath when anxious and the need for practicing deep breathing. The following exercise is used widely and generally found to be very helpful by clients:

Stop activities and focus upon your breathing. Focus on each part of your body beginning at your head and moving down to your toes...what is tight, heavy, relaxed, warm....take a slow, deep breath and pretend that tension and worries are floating out with each exhale and peacefulness and safety in with each inhale. Count to 4 and breathe in...now out to a count of 4...notice what shape and color those worries are as they float away...be aware of that gentle warmth and peacefulness as it spreads down from your head to your toes and enjoy for a few seconds or perhaps all the time in the world....then, when ready return to your activities.

Another guided imagery exercise focusing upon relaxation can use the image of the ocean wave. Of course the client must feel comfortable by water and not frightened by the ocean.

Imagine lying on the beach, enjoying the gentle warmth of the sand and hearing the waves. As you continue to enjoy, it is almost as if the warmth of the sun moves up from your feet through your body and up to your head. As that gentleness resides there, be aware of the ebb and flow of your energy, knowing that as it leaves, it will return and enjoying that rhythm and that knowing...always flowing, always present within you...whenever and wherever you need it...for whatever goal is secretly most important to you...knowing it

EXHIBIT 6-3: GENERAL CONSIDERATIONS FOR ALL TYPES OF IMAGERY

1. Preparation
   a. Become personally experienced with imagery before using it with a client or refer to a practitioner with this experience.
   b. Complete an assessment. Explore the imagery already taking place concerning health, values, and current issues. Any guided imagery must be syntonic with each person's values and core beliefs. For example, someone who abhors violence may not be comfortable with a war type approach to "destroying" or killing unpleasant thoughts or cancer cells. Taming or cleansing the invaders or teaching the lymphocites to act differently may be more acceptable.
   c. Discuss expected outcomes and goals for the experience (use measurable outcomes—quantify—lump in throat 8 on scale of 1–10 and after exercise was rated a 2). Create a blueprint.
   d. Review any past experiences the client has had with visualization.
   e. Make the environment and client as comfortable as possible (quiet, low lighting, no telephone interruptions, comfortable chair, no alcohol or other substances to avoid state dependent learning or sleep). If there are disturbances (grass cutting or talking outside), suggest that the sounds around are unimportant and simply add to the feeling of safety and relaxation.
   f. Music or scents may be used during the 10–15 minute sessions.
   g. Assure client that there are no right or wrong responses, but you do know there will be a change in sensations in some way.
   h. Discuss safety in terms of client having control to stop procedure if they wish by raising a hand.
   i. Set up a "yes set"—"you know that I have been using visualization for myself and clients for over 10 years.... You know that I am a PMH-APRN and you are safe in this office.... You know that we have been having therapy sessions for 3 weeks now and feel comfortable with each other."
2. During the session
   a. Start with a brief relaxation exercise.
   b. Use body mirroring techniques.
   c. Use positive language (aware of softening or relaxing, NOT decreased pain or discomfort).
   d. Follow cues from client during exercise—flushing, eyelid fluttering, deeper or audible breathing, crying, difficulty swallowing, and so on—and encourage comfort and safety.
   e. When guiding the imagery, use words to involve all senses—visual, aural, tactile, olfactory, proprioceptive, and kinesthetic.
   f. Speak in calm monotone.
3. Ending the session
   a. "When you are ready, take a few minutes, allow the image to fade, move your body, and open your eyes."
   b. Process the experience.
   c. Discuss practice and logging experiences before next appointment. Imagery becomes more effective with practice.

is all up to you to use in whatever way is best and most helpful right now. Now, feeling energized yet calm, continue your day.

Other scripts where the PMH-APRN guides the client may include a path in the woods, exploration of the rooms of a house, the building of a shield or bubble to protect oneself or taking on the identify of a mythical figure such as Wonder Woman. I had one client who experienced panic and anxiety which she had been controlling with smoking marijuana. She wanted to change that habit because she was now a mother. Along with the use of an SSRI, she also created an image of herself as having the powers of Wonder Woman whenever she rubbed her wrists together. She was able to use this simple image at social events and work to handle stress successfully.

> Author's Note: It is difficult to cite the individuals who originally developed these scripts because I have been using visualization and hypnotherapy as part of my practice for over 20 years. Therefore, these scripts are now intertwined with my ongoing clinical practice and are modified and shifted for each individual or group. My original training was in Ericksonian hypnotherapy and neurolinguistic programming.

When working with individuals experiencing anxiety, visualization can be very helpful to facilitate relaxation and a sense of self-control. When working with individuals who are depressed, be careful not to encourage withdrawal, and if active psychosis is present, it is wise not to use visualization.

There are many commercially produced recordings for relaxation or breathing exercises which can be used. Andrew Weil has excellent recordings for breathing and visualization as does Larry LeShane and Jeanne Achterberg. Dossey and colleagues in Holistic Nursing (1995) provide many excellent scripts of guided imagery for specific problems.

Another technique for teaching relaxation is the use of interactive computer games incorporating biofeedback (Tusaie, 2011). To date, the evidence base of studies evaluating games is limited and only a few health games have been subject to rigorous evaluation. However, the Robert Wood Johnson Foundation has funded Health Games Research projects that are exploring various game design elements contributing to efficacy. See www.healthgamesresearch.org/ for more details. There is great promise in channeling these hours of game playing to address mental health promotion issues.

Hypnosis

An altered state of consciousness—not unconsciousness or sleep—defines the hypnotic state. During this state there is a marked receptiveness to ideas and understandings and an increased willingness to respond either positively or negatively to those ideas (Rossi, 1989). The state of hypnotic trance is similar to daydreaming or being totally immersed in a good book or movie. But hypnosis is actually a heightened state of concentration. The aim is to focus the mind to eliminate distractions and make someone more open to suggestions, such as those that promote the aims of treatment. As an isolated experience, hypnotic trance has no meaning. It attains significance only in relation to the individual's perceptive and cognitive capabilities as they are used within the context of the primary treatment strategies. A deeper level of hypnotic trance is referred to as somnambulism and there are changes in perception, senses, body posture, and thoughts regarded as hypnotic phenomena.

Trance induction is a ceremony which facilitates transformation from usual to a special awareness. It is usually induced by a practitioner, but self-hypnosis can be learned. Although it is similar to relaxation and visualization, the nature of the experience is more self-analytical. It should only be used by professionals who are licensed by a national organization. Usually if someone refers to themselves as a hypnotist, it is a lay person who is self-trained and should be avoided.

Hypnosis may be used as part of psychotherapy or as part of a medical procedure—to alleviate anxiety and pain or depression (Alladin & Alibhai, 2007; Spiegel, 2007). It can be used to facilitate behavior change and is often used for smoking cessation and weight loss and is appropriate as an adjunctive treatment strategy in psychiatric-mental health nursing practice (Barabasz, 2007; Green & Lynn, 2000; Mottern, 2010; Zahourek, 2002). Hypnosis can facilitate and accelerate a variety of primary treatment strategies (Smith, 2006; Walters, 1998).

However, the use of hypnosis has been controversial partially due to misuse by charlatans. Its origins have been traced to Dr. Mesmer, who was quite a showman using lights and a pendulum for the induction procedure. Furthermore, hypnosis is not congruent with the dominant medical model—it is effective by maximizing an individual's potentials, not eliminating a causative agent.

Meditation

This is a conscious mental process using certain techniques—such as focusing attention or maintaining a specific posture—to suspend the stream of thoughts and relax the body and mind. Meditation has the ability to calm the mind, in a natural way. Human beings have been using the power of meditation effectively for thousands of years and continue to use it today, to reduce stress and experience a more peaceful existence.

There are dozens or more specific styles of meditation or contemplative practice. People may mean different things when they use the word, *meditation*. Meditation has been practiced since antiquity as a component of numerous religious traditions and in monastic settings. In the Eastern spiritual traditions such as Hinduism and Buddhism, meditation is more commonly a practice engaged in by many if not most believers.

When describing meditation, three main criteria are considered essential to any meditation practice: the use of a defined technique, logic relaxation, and a self-induced state or mode. Other criteria deemed important, but not essential, involve a state of psychophysical relaxation, the use of a self-focus skill or anchor, the presence of a state of suspension of logical thought processes, a religious/spiritual/philosophical context, or a state of mental silence. Oftentimes, in the West, meditation is classified in three broad categories: concentrative, mindfulness, and active meditation (Naranjo & Orenstein, 1972).

An individual can focus intensively on one particular object (so-called *concentrative mediation*), on all mental events that enter the field of awareness (so-called *mindfulness meditation*), or both specific focal points and the field of awareness. Other typologies have also been proposed, and some techniques shift among major categories. Evidence from neuroimaging studies suggests that major categories of meditation, defined by how they direct attention, appear to generate different brainwave patterns. Some evidence also suggests that using different focus objects may generate different brainwave patterns (Bond et al., 2009).

In *concentration meditation*, the meditator holds attention on a particular object while consistently bringing the mind back to concentrate on the chosen object. In *mindfulness meditation*, the subject sits comfortably, in silence, centering attention by focusing mental awareness on an object or process (either the breathing process, a sound, a mantra koan or riddle evoking questions, a visualization, or an exercise) and then consciously is encouraged to scan their thoughts in an open focus, shifting freely from one perception to the next (Kutz et al., 1985). No thought, image, or sensation is considered an intrusion. The meditator, with a "no effort" attitude, is asked to remain in the here and now. Using the focus as an "anchor" (Segal et al., 2002) brings the subject constantly back to the present, avoiding cognitive analysis or fantasy regarding the contents of awareness, and increasing tolerance and relaxation of secondary thought processes. Mindfulness meditation has become very popular in health care and many programs developed for prevention or treatment of disorders. Mindfulness or being in the "here-and-now" has long been an important aspect of psychotherapy sessions. But the use of mindfulness meditation training is now being applied to the prevention of relapse in depression stress reduction, and many other applications in psychiatric-mental health nursing (Tusaie & Edds, 2010; O'Haver-Day & Harlon-Doutsch, 2004).

Dynamic or *movement meditation* involves a great deal of movement and activity as in Sufi dancing, walking the labyrinth Osho Dynamic Meditation, or a variation of this technique. Dynamic meditation involves stages of jumping and moving, then yelling various sounds before becoming silent and relaxed. See the following website for more information: www.osho.com/Main.cfm?Area=Meditation

Yoga

The various styles of yoga used for health purposes typically combine physical postures, breathing techniques, and meditation or relaxation. The heart of any yoga practice is the performance of yoga poses (called asanas), each of which has specific physical and mental benefits. People use yoga as part of a general health regimen, and also for a variety of health conditions. It was developed in India. Recently, an increase in GABA during yoga postures has been identified. This has been superior to other forms of exercise in decreasing anxiety and increasing mood (Streeter et al., 2010).

Tai Chi Chuan

Tai chi is sometimes described as "meditation in motion" because it promotes serenity through gentle movements—connecting the mind and body. Originally developed in ancient China for self-defense, tai chi evolved into a graceful form of exercise that's now used for stress reduction and to help with a variety of other health conditions. Tai chi, also called tai chi chuan, is a noncompetitive, self-paced system of gentle physical exercise and stretching. To do tai chi, you perform a series of postures or movements in a slow, graceful manner. Each posture flows into the next without pause, ensuring that your body is in constant motion. Tai chi not only contributes to general well-being, but also to psychological health and fall prevention in the elderly (Barclay & Lie, 2011).

Tai chi has many different styles, such as yang and wu. Each style may have its own subtle emphasis on various tai chi principles and methods. There are also

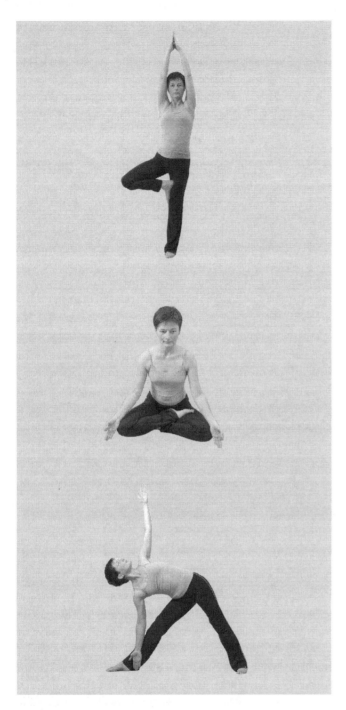

Selected Yoga Positions. Reprinted from *Yoga for Nurses* by Ingrid Kollak with permission of Demos Health Publishing. Copyright 2009.

variations within each style. Some may focus on health maintenance, while others focus on the martial arts aspect of tai chi. The result of all this variation is that there are more than 100 possible postures, many named after animals. Tai chi is often practiced by groups in a park setting.

Author's Note: When I was traveling in China and visiting various health care facilities, I participated in morning tai chi exercises led by the medical director and staff of the hospital for all patients who could walk. Following the exercise, I questioned the medical director as to the evidence that this exercise was effective in improving health. He smiled tolerantly and stated that the evidence is in the improvement of the patients.

MANIPULATIVE AND BODY-BASED PRACTICES

Manipulative and body-based practices focus primarily on the structures and systems of the body, including the bones and joints, soft tissues, and circulatory and lymphatic systems. Acupuncture, spinal manipulation, and massage fall within this category.

Acupuncture

This is a family of procedures involving the stimulation of specific points on the body using a variety of techniques, such as penetrating the skin with needles that are then manipulated by hand or by electrical stimulation. It is one of the key components of traditional Chinese medicine and is believed to be effective by manipulating qi or body energy (NCCAM, 2011).

Acupoints reside along more than a dozen major meridians. There are 12 pairs of regular meridians that are systematically distributed over both sides of the body, and two major extra meridians running along the midlines of the abdomen and back. Along these meridians, more than 300 acupoints are identified, each having its own therapeutic action. The point Shenmen (HT 7), located on the medial end of the transverse crease of the wrist, can induce relaxation.

In acupuncture clinics, the practitioner first selects appropriate acupoints along different meridians based on identified health problems. Then very fine and thin needles are inserted into these acupoints. The needles are made of stainless steel and vary in length from half an inch to 3 inches. The choice of needle is usually determined by the location of the acupoint and the effects being sought. If the point is correctly located and the required depth reached, the patient will usually experience a feeling of soreness, heaviness, numbness, and distention. The manipulator will simultaneously feel that the needle is tightened.

The needles are usually left in situ for 15 to 30 minutes. During this time the needles may be manipulated to achieve the effect of tonifying the qi. Needle manipulations generally involve lifting, thrusting, twisting, and rotating, according to treatment specifications for the health problem. Needling may also be activated by electrical stimulation, a procedure usually called electro-acupuncture, in which manipulations are attained through varying frequencies and voltages.

Treatment protocols, frequency, and duration are a matter of professional judgment of the practitioner, in consultation with the patient. A common course of treatment may initially involve between 10 and 15 treatments spaced at approximately weekly intervals, and spread out to monthly later in a program. A video of an acupuncture session may be viewed at the following web page: nccam.nih.gov/news/multimedia/

Acupuncture in mental health treatment has been discussed for depression, anxiety, insomnia, and addictions. A Cochrane review, containing 30 studies with 2,812 participants included in the meta-analysis, found an additive effect when acupuncture was combined with medication in the treatment of depression, but there was a high risk of bias in the majority of trials. However, there was insufficient evidence of a consistent beneficial effect from acupuncture compared with a wait list control or sham acupuncture control. Although there was insufficient evidence to recommend the use of acupuncture for depression, it may be considered when the client expressed an interest and when medication and psychotherapy produce inadequate results (Smith, Hay, & Macpherson, 2010).

For treatment of insomnia, acupuncture has been reported to produce superior outcomes to Western medications and produced additive effects with herbs or Western medications (Cao, Pan, & Liu, 2009). Positive findings are also reported for acupuncture in the treatment of generalized anxiety disorder but there is currently insufficient research evidence for firm conclusions to be drawn. No trials of acupuncture for other anxiety disorders were located (Pilkington, Kukerd, Rampes, Cummings, & Richardson, 2007). There is some limited evidence in favor of auricular (ear) acupuncture in perioperative anxiety and during drug withdrawal and recovery (Lu et al., 2009). Overall, the promising findings indicate that further research is warranted in the form of well designed, adequately powered studies.

Emotional Freedom Technique (Tapping)

This is a controversial variation of acupressure using the acupoints along meridians. Callahan (1999) first described this procedure to treat phobias. Callahan labeled the technique as Thought Field Therapy and claimed that a blockage or disruption of energy flow results in negative emotions that are the cause of all psychological disorders, including phobia. Callahan proposed that a brief treatment procedure involving tapping may be successfully used to treat almost any emotional disorder. There are a variety of these procedures, each tailored to a specific problem. Following a diagnosis, the procedure involves tapping on specific meridian points on one's body while focusing on the source of the distressing situation and using deep breathing and self-talk. The tapping is purported to create energy, thereby restoring the energy flow and eliminating or reducing negative emotions.

There are multiple sites/videos/online coaching and workshops available on the Internet to demonstrate tapping. However, the evidence that tapping on acupoints relieves anxiety and other emotional disorders is supported only by testimonials. Furthermore, one well designed study (Waite & Holder, 2003) reported that the effectiveness of tapping was most likely due to other factors (therapeutic relationship, deep breathing, distraction) rather than tapping points along meridians. However, no adverse effects have ever been reported and chronic anxiety is quite complex and difficult to treat. Therefore, tapping has been added to the armamentarium of many PMH-APRN practitioners.

Somatic Psychotherapy

Somatic mental health practitioners tend to bring body, body processes, and body experience into the foreground of therapy practice. Wilhelm Reich was the first person to bring body awareness systematically into psychoanalysis, and also the first psychotherapist to touch clients physically, working with their bodies (Boadella, 1985). Reich was a significant influence in the founding of Body Psychotherapy or Somatic Psychology. Several types of body-oriented psychotherapies trace their origins back to Reich, though there have been many subsequent developments and other influences are of particular interest in trauma work. Somatic awareness can supplement cognitive and psychodynamic approaches and often assists clients in renegotiating their traumatic experiences.

There is increasing use of body-oriented therapeutic techniques within mainstream psychology (like eye movement desensitization and reprocessing [EMDR] and mindfulness practice) and psychoanalysis has recognized the use of somatic resonance, embodied trauma, and similar concepts, for many years. The primary relationship addressed in somatic psychotherapy is the person's relation to and empathy with their own felt body. It is based on a belief, grounded in ancient principles of vitalism, that energy will bring healing to the affected parts if sufficient awareness is directed there.

There are a broad range of techniques. Examples include Feldenkrais Method, Alexander Technique, Rolfing, and Trager Psychophysical Integration. Moshe Feldenkrais established the Feldenkrais Guild (www.feldenkrais.com/) in 1977 to be a professional organization of practitioners and teachers of the Feldenkrais Method. Specific movement sequences are used to bring attention to parts of the self that are out of awareness and uninvolved in functional actions.

The Alexander Technique Index (www.mouritz.co.uk/) provides a wealth of resources and links on the Alexander Technique. The techniques developed by F. M. Alexander focus on how we use our bodies and provide directions to maintain health.

Rolfing or Structural Integration is a body-based practice that uses deep tissue fascial manipulation and movement education. The goal is to encourage health and relieve stress by bringing the body into proper alignment with gravity. A 10-session sequence of structural, fascial, and educational goals was developed by Dr. Ida Rolf. The Guild for Structural Integration (www.rolfguild.org/) is dedicated to Dr. Rolf's work.

Trager psychophysical integration (www.trager.com/) is the approach to movement education, created and developed over a period of 65 years by Milton Trager. Utilizing gentle, nonintrusive, natural movements, the Trager Approach helps release deep-seated physical and mental patterns and facilitates deep relaxation, increased physical mobility, and mental clarity.

Massage

The term massage therapy encompasses many different techniques. In general, therapists press, rub, and otherwise manipulate the muscles and other soft tissues of the body. People use massage for a variety of health-related purposes, including to relieve pain, rehabilitate sports injuries, reduce stress, increase relaxation, address anxiety and depression, and aid general well-being.

Dance Therapy

Dance also reflects something of this approach and is considered a study and practice within the field of somatic psychology. Based in the belief that the body, the mind, and the spirit are interconnected, dance/movement therapy is defined by the American Dance Therapy Association as "the psychotherapeutic use of movement as a process that furthers the emotional, cognitive, social, and physical integration of the individual" (www.adta.org/).

Aromatherapy

The use of essential oils extracted from plants for treating problems and promoting healing is the definition of aromatherapy. There is minimal research to provide evidence of effectiveness, but aromatherapy is widely used with expanding training programs, especially in Europe. There are also no legal requirements for labeling or ensuring contents. Contents may include mixtures of over 100 compounds and are used for various effects—calming, anti-infection, antihistamine, immunostimulant, expectorant, antiseptic, and others. Essential oils may be purchased in many commercial settings. Side effects may include dermal toxicity, photosensitivity, allergic reactions, problems with internal use, and liver toxicity (Franchomme & Penoel, 1990).

A wide variety of techniques are used in somatic psychotherapy including sound (music), touch, mirroring, scents (aromatherapy), movement, and breath. An individual records life experience during pre- and nonverbal periods differently than during a verbal and personal narrative period. Furthermore, somatic changes occur without conscious awareness. Therefore, somatic approaches work with the client's implicit knowing of these early experiences as well as the body sensations related to peptides and emotions. This understanding of consciousness, communication, and mind-body language challenges some traditional applications of the talking cure. There is minimal scientific evidence for the effectiveness of these approaches at this time, but specific use of these approaches will be presented in chapters addressing specific symptom clusters.

Other Techniques

EMDR is a form of psychotherapy that was developed by Francine Shapiro (2002) to resolve the development of trauma-related disorders.

EMDR integrates elements of effective psychodynamic, imaginal exposure, cognitive therapy, interpersonal, experiential, physiological, and somatic therapies. It also uses the unique element of bilateral stimulation (e.g., eye movements, tones, or tapping). According to Francine Shapiro's theory, when a traumatic or distressing experience occurs, it may overwhelm usual ways of coping and the memory of the event is inadequately processed; the memory is dysfunctionally stored in an isolated memory network.

EMDR uses a structured eight-phase approach and addresses the past, present, and future aspects of the dysfunctionally stored memory. During the processing phases of EMDR, the client attends to the disturbing memory in multiple brief sets of about 15 to 30 seconds, while simultaneously focusing on the dual attention stimulus (e.g., therapist-directed lateral eye movement, alternate hand-tapping, or bilateral auditory tones). Following each set of such dual attention, the client is asked what associative information was elicited during the procedure. This new material usually becomes the focus of the next set. This process of alternating dual attention and personal association is repeated many times during the session.

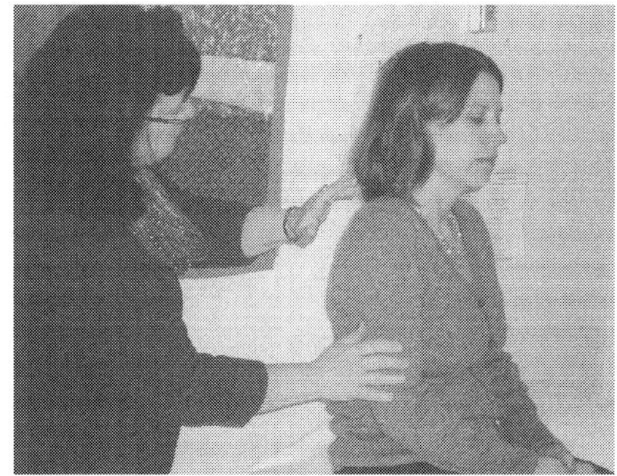

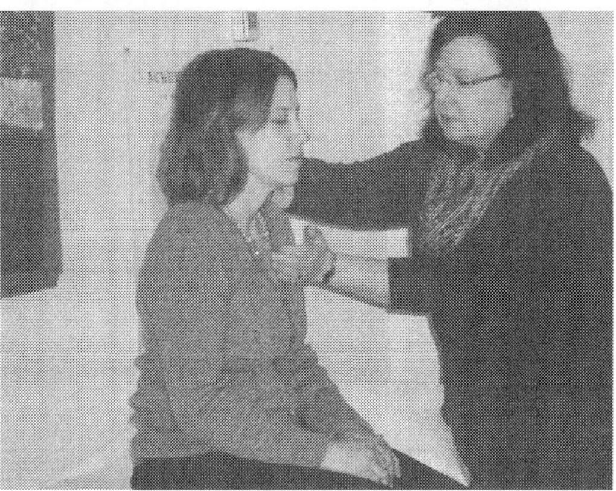

> Author's Note: There are two main perspectives on EMDR therapy. First, Shapiro proposed that although a number of different processes underlie EMDR, the eye movements add to the therapy's effectiveness by evoking neurological and physiological changes that may aid in the processing of the trauma memories being treated. The other perspective is that the eye movements are an epiphenomenon, unnecessary, and that EMDR is simply a form of desensitization (Davidson & Parker, 2001).

Although EMDR is used by many practitioners who have been certified in its use and most insurance carriers will reimburse for sessions, it remains somewhat controversial and is usually taught in post-master's continuing education workshops.

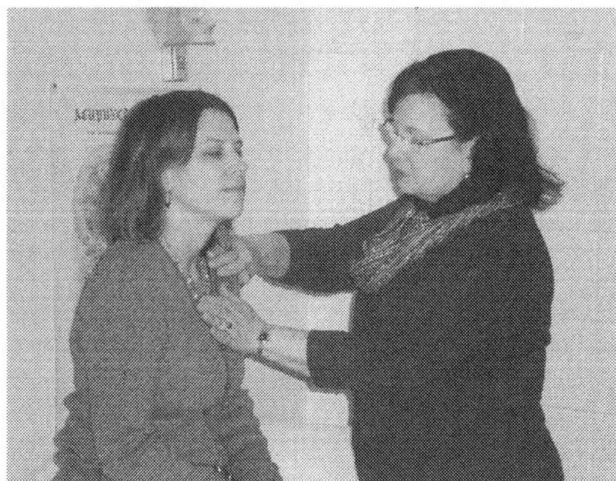

ENERGY WORK

Some CAM practices involve manipulation of energy fields to affect health. Such fields may be characterized as veritable (measurable) or putative (yet to be measured). Practices based on veritable forms of energy include those involving electromagnetic fields (e.g., magnet therapy and light therapy). Practices based on putative energy fields (also called biofields) generally reflect the concept that human beings are infused with subtle forms of energy. Qigong, Reiki, reflexology, acupressure, shiatsu massage, therapeutic touch (TT), and healing touch (HT) are examples of techniques using the concept of universal energy (Figure 6-1). Practitioners seek to transmit a universal energy to a person, either from a distance or by placing their hands on or near that person. The explanation for the healing effects is based on electromagnetic concepts, quantum physics, and transpersonal psychology.

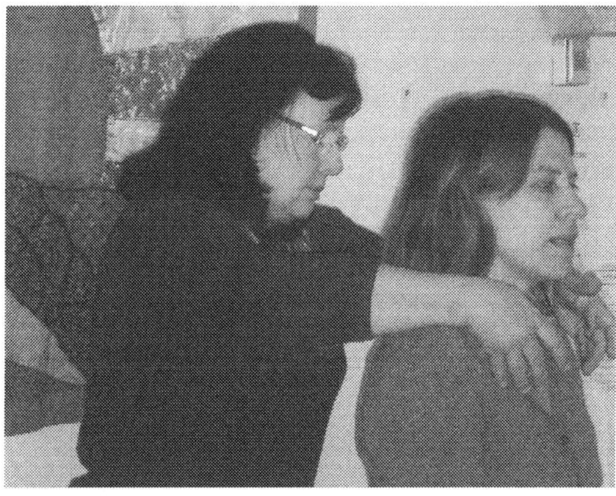

Figure 6-1 Annette Mitzel, DNP, CNS, HTCP, Delivering Healing Touch at The University of Akron's Center for Community Health

Kirlian photography refers to a form of photogram made with voltage. It is named after Semyon Kirlian, who in 1939 discovered that if an object on a photographic plate is connected to a source of voltage, an image is produced on the photographic plate. This may be considered visualization of the human aura (McCarron-Benson, 1989).

HT and TT are the approaches most commonly used by nurses. TT refers to the Krieger-Kuntz Method and HT refers to approaches taught in the American Holistic Nurses Association's Certificate Program in Healing Touch.

A session involves the following steps:

1. The practitioner centers self through meditation or other techniques focusing upon one's own state.
2. A client's or recipient's energy is assessed by passing hands over the entire body (not touching) to feel for differences in the space around the body. Ideally, the space feels even, almost like a gentle, steady breeze. A block or obstruction is apparent to the experienced practitioner.
3. For treatment, the practitioner again places their hands in the body's space to "fluff" or move the energy to become as smooth as possible.
4. During this process, the recipient may talk about problems/concerns.
5. This process is temporary, but for healing to occur, an individual needs to learn to interpret their own sensations and use strategies such as meditation, psychotherapy, biofeedback, and others to increase self-understanding and coping.

Although energy work remains controversial and the research is not well established, it is widely used by nurses and many hospitals include HT or TT as part of standard protocols.

Traditional Healers

Practices of traditional healers can also be considered a form of CAM. Traditional healers use approaches based on indigenous theories, beliefs, and experiences handed down from generation to generation. A familiar example in the United States is the Native American healer/medicine man.

Alternative Medical Systems

There are complete systems of theory and practice that have evolved over time in different cultures and apart from conventional or Western medicine. Examples of ancient whole medical systems include Ayurvedic medicine and traditional Chinese medicine.

Ayurvedic Medicine

Based in India, Ayurvedic medicine is a sophisticated, holistic system of natural health care practiced for over 2,500 years. It focuses upon the whole organism and its relation to the external world to reestablish and maintain a harmonious balance within the body and between the body, mind, and environment. Therapies include herbs, massage, yoga, and purging.

Traditional Chinese Medicine

Yin and yang, qi, essence, and spirit are the basic concepts of traditional Chinese medicine. Yin and yang express the concept that everything exists in opposing but complementary, dynamic phenomena (light & dark; hot & cold). Qi (pronounced chee) is a subtle material within the body that causes most physiological functions and maintains health and vitality (Johnke, Larkey, Rogers, & Lin, 2010). Although it is sometimes referred to as energy, this is not the meaning in Chinese medicine; it is believed to be an actual material present throughout the body. This is not consistent with the biomedical beliefs about the body. When combined with essence and spirit, these are considered the three treasures of Chinese medicine. Essence is the gift from one's parents and is the fundamental source of physiological functioning. It is replenished with food and rest and the body's reproductive abilities. Spirit is the alert radiant aspect of humans demonstrated by clear thinking and a luster in the eyes and face when healthy.

The approach to treatment involves treating the pathological condition with opposing measures to return balance. Techniques used include acupuncture, moxibustion, cupping, massage, herbals, and qigong (Johnke et al., 2010). Acupuncture was discussed under manipulative and body-based practices. Moxibustion is the burning of the dried and powered leaves of *Artemsia vulgaris,* either on or in proximity to the skin with the purpose of moving qi. Cupping involves using a small glass cup to induce a vacuum on the skin surface for the purpose of increasing circulation of blood and lymph to a specific area. Qigong is the practice of moving qi through exercises, breathing, and meditation. There are specific qigong practices that are prescribed for specific problems.

Homeopathy and Naturopathy

More modern systems that have developed in the past few centuries include homeopathy and naturopathy, which originated in Europe. Homeopathy seeks to stimulate the body's ability to heal itself by giving very small doses of highly diluted substances that in larger doses would produce illness or symptoms (an approach called "like cures like"). *The Homeopathic Pharmacopoeia of the United States* (American Institute of Homeopathy, 1979)

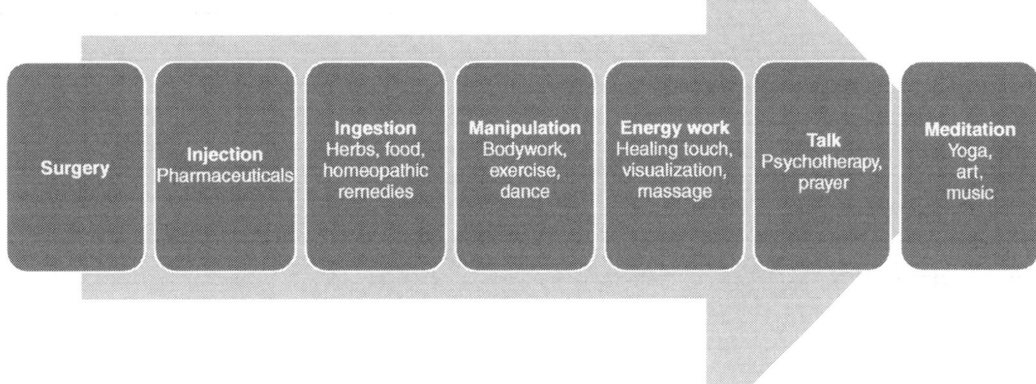

Figure 6-2 More to Less Invasive Therapeutic Interventions

is the standard for preparation of homeopathic medicines and contains over 2,000 remedies. Naturopathy is based upon the concept of vitalism—life is more than biochemical processes and constantly strives for health. Symptoms represent a constructive phenomenon that is the best response given the circumstances. The aim of treatment is to support the body's ability to heal itself through the use of dietary and lifestyle changes, together with CAM therapies such as herbs, massage, and joint manipulation.

Another method of classification for therapeutic interventions is to consider the degree of invasiveness to the client (Figure 6-2; Micozzi, 2010).

PRACTICE GUIDELINES

When considering using complementary and/or alternative treatment, be aware of the appropriate steps that are necessary. Although each state has its own nurse practice act and licensure requirements which need to be followed, these considerations may be helpful when considering the addition of a complementary/alternative technique to your practice.

1. Identify the benefit for the client.
2. Check state and federal regulations to ensure this practice is not constrained.
3. Review standards and scope of practice from psychiatric-mental health and advanced practice nursing organizations for compliance.
4. Review methods you used to gain knowledge and competence in the technique.
5. What is the evidence-base?
6. Demonstrate competence in the technique.
7. Is this a reasonable and prudent technique when considering your education in a role as well as a specialty?
8. Will you accept accountability as well as liability for the outcome? (Check with liability insurance carrier also.)
9. How will you maintain competence?

It is important to remember that our own perspectives may interfere with understanding approaches to health care from other cultures. There are many ways to conceptualize health, symptoms, and interventions. Furthermore, if there is a lack of understanding of the philosophies underlying a technique, there may be unconditional acceptance of techniques that are not clearly understood. Therefore, it is important to understand the background and philosophies underlying complementary and alternative approaches before accepting or recommending them to clients.

RESOURCES

TRAINING AND INFORMATION ON NATURAL PRODUCTS

Herb Net lists schools and universities offering training in herbology and naturopathy: www.herbnet.com/university_p2.htm

American Herbalists Guild offers certification: www.americanherbalist.com

European Herbal & Traditional Medicine Practitioners Association: http://ehtpa.eu

American Herb Association: www.ahaherb.org

American Herbal Products Association: www.ahpa.org

American Association of Oriental Medicine: www.aaom.org
For herbalists interested in the use of Chinese herbal remedies.

TRAINING AND INFORMATION ABOUT RELAXATION AND IMAGERY

Relaxation and imagery may be self-taught with the use of recordings or books or be taught by a trained professional.

American Holistic Nurses Association: www.ahna.org

Simonton Cancer Center: www.simontoncenter.com

Mind–Body Healing: www.wholeness.com

National Institutes of Health Center for Complementary and Alternative Medicine: http://nccam.nih.gov

TRAINING AND INFORMATION ABOUT HYPONOSIS

Although there are many opportunities for training in hypnosis, it is important to use professionally licensed, not just certified in hypnosis, trainers. The following organizations provide excellent opportunities for learning hypnotherapy.

American Society for Clinical Hypnosis is for licensed health care professionals and provides educational opportunities and publishes the *American Journal of Clinical Hypnosis*: www.asch.net

Society for Clinical and Experimental Hypnosis is an international organization for licensed health care professionals and publishes *The International Journal of Clinical and Experimental Hypnosi*s: http://ijceh.com/content/view/20/71/

TRAINING AND INFORMATION ON YOGA AND TAI CHI

Yoga and tai chi can be self-taught or taught by a qualified instructor. There are no ratings for levels of instructors but someone with excellent training (ask where they have trained and what they learned) and knowledge about what goes on inside the person during the form and the breathing exercises are the best teachers.

Himalayan Institute of Yoga Science and Philosophy, Box 400, Honesdale, PA 18431, 800-822-4547

The International Association of Yoga Therapists, 109 Hillside Avenue Mill Valley, CA 94941, 415-383-4587

T'ai Chi Magazine, Wayfarer Publications, 2601 Silver Ridge Ave., Los Angeles, CA 90039: www.taichinetwork.org/
This online community offers a way to easily connect teachers with students and to find studios, classes, and other resources.

TRAINING AND INFORMATION ON ACUPUNCTURE

Schools offer a certificate or doctorate in acupuncture and generally take 3 to 4 years to complete coursework and clinical practice. In states where acupuncture requires a license, the practitioner must have graduated from an accredited program, passed a state license exam, and/or earned national certification administered by the National Certification Commission for Acupuncture and Oriental Medicine (NCCAOM). Some health insurance companies will reimburse for acupuncture treatments.

Some states offer their own guidelines and acupuncture licensing distributors. Therefore, each state's department of health is responsible for overseeing state authorities, to make sure the licenses of acupuncturists are thorough and credible throughout the United States. Also, state requirements differ per state. Some require 300 hours of coursework and clinical practice in acupuncture, some require passing an examination, and some require both. Some states require nonphysician acupuncturists to be supervised by a physician. To identify the educational requirements for acupuncture certification in your state, visit Acupuncture.com/Statelaws

For a list of schools of acupuncture accredited by the National Certification Commission for Acupuncture and Oriental Medicine (NCCAOM), see www.naturalhealers.com/acaomacc.shtml
NCCAOM Certification Examination: www.nccaom.org/applicants 904-598-1005

TRAINING AND INFORMATION ON EMDR

EMDR International Association: www.emdria.org/displaycommon.cfm?an=1&subarticlenbr=43

David Baldwin's trauma website also has reviews of EMDR research articles: www.traumapages.com/s/emdr-refs.php

Journal of EMDR Practice and Research: www.springerpub.com/product/19333196

REFERENCES

American Institute of Homeopathy Committee on Pharmacopeia (1897). *The Homeopathic Pharmacopeia of the United States.* Retrieved from https:// www.hpus.com/online_database/register_action.php on June 19, 2012.

American Psychiatric Association (2011). *Guidelines for Treatment of Major Depression.* Washington, DC: American Psychiatric Publishing.

Ader, R., Felton D., & Cohen, N. (1991). *Psychoneuroimmunology* (2nd ed.). San Diego, CA : Academic Press.

Alladin, A., & Alibhai, A. (2007). Cognitive hypnotherapy for depression: An empirical investigation. *International Journal of Clinical and Experimental Hypnosis, 55*, 147–166.

Barabasz, M. (2007). Efficacy of hypnotherapy in the treatment of eating disorders. *International Journal of Clinical and Experimental Hypnosis, 55*(3), 318–335.

Barclay, L., & Lie, D. (2011). T'ai Chi may prevent falls, improve mental health in elderly. Medscape News. Retrieved from http://medscape.org/viewarticle/742923?src=cmemp

Barnes, P., Powell-Grina, E., McFann, K., & Nahin, R. (2004). Complementary and alternative medicine use among adults: United States, 2002. *Center for Disease Control Vital and Health Statistics,* 343. Retrieved from www.cdc.gov/nchs/data/ad/ad343.pdf

Bebbe, L. (2010). Bringing adjuctive treatment into the mainstream. *Journal of Psychosocial Nursing and Mental health Services, 48*(10), 2–3.

Benson, H. (1971). A wakeful hypometabolic state. *American Journal of Psychology, 221*(3), 795–799.

Boadella, D. (1985). *Wilhelm Reich:The evolution of his work.* London: Arkana-Routledge & Kegan Paul. ISBN 1-85063-034-8.

Bond, K., Ospina, M., Hooton, N., Bialy, L., Dryden, D., Buscemi, N.,... Carlson, L. (2009). Defining a complex intervention:The development of demarcation criteria for meditation. *Psychology of Religion and Spirituality, 1*(12), 1129–1371.

Callahan, R. (1999). *A Thought Field Therapy (TFT) algorithm for trauma: A reproducible experiment in psychotherapy.* Paper presented at the 105th Annual Convention of the American Psychological Association, Chicago, IL.

Cao, H., Pan, X., & Liu, J. (2009). Acupuncture for insomnia: A systematic review of randomized controlled trials. *Journal of Alternative and Complementary Medicine, 11*, 1171–1186.

Capasso, F., Gaginella, T., Grandolini, G., & Izzo, A. (2003). *Phytotherapy. A quick reference to herbal medicine.* Berlin, Germany: Springer-Verlag.

Carper, B. (1978). Fundamental ways of knowing in nursing. *Advances in Nursing Science, 1*(1), 13–24.

Chiou, W., Wan, C., Wu, W., & Lee, K. (2011). A randomized experiment to examine unintended consequences of dietary supplement use among daily smokers taking supplements reduces self-regulation of smoking. *Addiction 106/2*: doi 10.1111/j.1360-0443, 2011.03545.

Davidson, P. R., & Parker, K. C. (2001). Eye movement desensitization and reprocessing (EMDR): A meta-analysis. *Journal of Consulting and Clinical Psychology, 69(2)*, 305–16. doi:10.1037/0022-006X.69.2.305. PMID 11393607.

Davis, K., Charney, D., Coyle, J., & Nemeroff, C. (2003). *Neuropsychopharmacology: The fifth generation of progress.* New York, NY: Lippincott, Williams & Wilkins.

De Smet, P. (2002). Herbal remedies. *New England Journal of Medicine, 347*, 2046–2056.

Dossey, L. (1989). *Recovering the soul: A scientific and spiritual search.* New York, NY: Bantam Books.

Dossey, B., & Keegan, L. (2012). *Holistic Nursing.* Gaithersburg, Maryland: Aspen Publishers, Inc.

Dresser, G., Schwarz, U., Wilkinson, G., & Kim, R. (2003). Coordinate induction of both cytochrome P4503A and MDR1 by St. John's Wort in healthy subjects. *Clinical Pharmacology Therapeutics, 73*, 41–50.

Fernstrom, J. (2000). Can nutrient supplements modify brain function? *American Journal of Clinical Nutrition, 71*, 1669s–1675s.

Franchomme, P., & Penoel, D. (1990). *Aromatherapy extractions.* Limoges, France: Roger Jallois.

Freeman, M., Hibbeln, J., Wisner, K., Davis, J., Mischoulon, D., Peet, M.,...Stoll, A. (2006). Omega-3 fatty acids: Evidence basis for treatment and future research in psychiatry. *Journal of Clinical Psychiatry, 67*(12), 1954–1967.

Gammack, L., Van Niekerk, J., & Dangour, A. (2011). Omega 3 fatty acids for the prevention of dementia. *Cochrane Database of Systematic Reviews*, Art. no.: CD005379.pub2. doi: 10.1002/14651858

Ganji, V., Milone, C., Cody, M. M., McCarty, F., & Wang, Y. T. (2010). Serum vitamin D concentrations are related to depression in young adult US population: the Third National Health and Nutrition Examination Survey. *Internal Archives of Medicine, 3*, 29.

Green, J., & Lynn, S. (2000). Hypnosis and suggestion-based approaches to smoking cessation: An examination of the evidence. *International Journal of Clinical and Experimental Hypnosis, 48*(2), 195–224.

Heaney, R. P., Davies, K. M., Chen, T. C., Holick, M. F., & Barger-Lux, M. J. (2003). Human serum 25 hydroxycholecalciferol response to extended oral dosing with cholecalciferol. *American Journal of Clinical Nutrition, 77*, 204–210.

Holick, M. (2006). High prevalence of vitamin D inadequacy and implications for health. *Mayo Clinic Proceedings, 81*, 353–373.

Institute of Medicine. (2010). *Dietary reference intakes for calcium and vitamin D.* Consensus report released November 30, 2010. Washington, DC: Author.

Jacobson, E. (1942). *Progressive relaxation.* Chicago, IL: University of Chicago Press.

Johnke, R., Larkey, L., Rogers, C., & Lin, F. (2010). A comprehensive review of the health benefits of Qigong and Tai Chi. *American Journal of Health Promotion, 24*(16), 1–25.

Kabat-Zinn, J. (1990). *Full catastrophe living: Using the wisdom of your body and mind to face stress, pain, and illness.* New York, NY: Delta Trade Paperbacks.

Kaufman, D. W., Kelly, J. P., Rosenberg, L., Anderson, T. E., & Mitchell, A. (2002). Recent patterns of medication use in the ambulatory adult population of the United States: The Slone survey. *Journal of the American Medical Association, 287*, 337–344.

Klepser, T., Doucette, W., Horton, M. R., Buys, L. M., Ernst, M. E., Ford, J. K.,...Klepser, M. E. (2000). Assessment of patients perceptions and beliefs regarding herbal therapies. *Pharmacotherapy, 20*, 83–87.

Libster, M. (2002). *Delmar's integrative herb guide for nurses*. Albany, NY: Delmar.

Lin, J., & Yamazaki, M. (2003). Role of P-glycoprotein in pharmacokinetics: Clinical implications. *Clinical Pharmacokinetics, 42,* 59–98.

Locke, S. (1983). *Mind and Immunity*. New York: Praeger Publishers.

Lu, L., Liu, Y., Zhu, W., Shi, J., Ling, W., & Kosten, T. (2009). Traditional medicine in the treatment of drug addition. *American Journal of Drug and Alcohol Abuse, 35*(1), 1–11.

McCarron-Benson, J. (1989). In D. Laycock, D. Vernon, C. Groves, & S. Brown (Eds.), *Skeptical—A handbook of pseudoscience and the paranormal* (p. 11). Canberra, Australia: Imagecraft. ISBN 0–7316-5794–2.

McEnany, G. (1999). Herbal psychotropics. Part 1: Focus on St. John's Wort and SAMe. *Journal of the American Psychiatric Nurses Association, 5*(6), 192–196.

Micozzi, M. (2010). *Fundamentals of complementary and alternative medicine*. Philadelphia, PA: Saunders.

Miyasaka, L., Atallah, A., & Soares, B. (2011). Valerian for anxiety disorder. *Cochrane database of Systematic Reviews*. Issue 4. Art. no.: CD004515.pub.2. doi:10.1002/14651858

Montgomery, P., & Richardson, A. (2008). Omega-3 fatty acids for bipolar disorder. *Cochrane Database of Systematic Reviews.* Issue 2. Art. no.: CD005169.pub2. doi:10.1002/14651858

Morris, M., & Tangney, C. (2011). A potential design flaw of randomized trials of vitamin supplements. *Journal of the American Medical Association, 305*(11), 1348–1349.

Mottern, R. (2010). Using hypnosis as adjunct care in mental health nursing. *Journal of Psychosocial Mental Health Service, 48*(10), 41–44.

Murray, L. (2011) *PDR for Nonprescription drugs, dietary supplements and herbals*. Montvale, NJ: Thompson Healthcare.

Naranjo, C., & Orenstein, R. (1972). *On the psychology of meditation.* New York, NY: Julian Press.

NCCAM. (2011). *Meditation: An introduction, uses of meditation for health in US*. Bethesda, MD: Author. Retrieved from www.nccam.nih.gov

National Center for Complementary and Alternative medicine at The National Institutes of Health, What is complementary and alternative medicine. Retrieved June 19, 2012 from http://ncaam.nih.gov/health/whatiscam.

O'Hover Day, P., & Horton-Deutsh, S. (2004). Using mindfulness-based therapy interventions in psychiatric nursing practice-Part II: Mindfulness-based approaches for all phases of psychotherapy-a clinical case study. *Archives of Psychiatric Nursing, 18*(5), 170–177.

Ornish, D. (1990). *Dr. Dean Ornish's program for reversing heart disease.* New York, NY: Random House.

Palmer, M., Haller, C., McKinney, P. E., Klein-Schwartz, W., Tschirgi, A., Smolinske, S. C.,...Landzberg, B. R. (2003). Adverse events associated with dietary supplements: An observational study. *Lancet, 361,* 101–106.

Pancheri, P., Scapicchio. P., & Chiaie, R.D. (2002). A doubleblind, randomized parallel-group, efficacy and safety study of intramuscular *S*-adenosyl-L-methionine1,4-butanedisulphonate (SAMe) versus imipramine in patients with major depressive disorder. *International Journal of Neuropsychopharmacology, 5,* 287–294.

Pert, C. (1986). The wisdom of the receptors: Neuropeptides, the emotions, and bodymind. *Advances, 3*(3), 8–16.

Pilkington, K., Kukerd, G., Rampes, H., Cummings, M., & Richardson, J. (2007). Acupuncture for anxiety and anxiety disorders: A systematic literature review. *Acupuncture Medicine, 25*(1–2), 1–10.

Rossi, E. (1989). *Milton H. Erickson: The collected papers of Milton H. Erickson on hypnosis, Volume I: The nature of hypnosis*. Irvington, NY: Irvington Publishers, Inc.

Roy-Byrne, P., Bystritsky, A., Russo, J. (2005). Use of herbal medications in primary care patients with mood and anxiety disorders. *Psychosomatics, 46,* 117–122.

Segal, Z., Williams, J., & Teasdale, J. (2002). *Mindfulness-based cognitive therapy for depression*. New York, NY: Guilford Press.

Shapiro, F. (2002). *EMDR as an integrative psychotherapy approach: Experts of diverse orientations explore the paradigm prism*. Washington, DC: American Psychological Association.

Shelton, R.C., Keller, M.B., Gelenberg, A., Dunner, D.L., Hirschfeld, R., Thase, M.E.,...Halbreich, U. (2001). Effectiveness of St. John's wort in major depression: A randomized controlled trial. *Journal of the American Medical Association, 285,* 1978–1986.

Simonton, C., Matthews-Simonton, S., & Creighton, J. (1978). *Getting well again: A step by step self-help guide to overcoming cancer for patients and their families*. Los Angles: JP Tarcher Inc.

Smith, C., Hay, P., & Macpherson, H. (2010). Acupuncture for depression. *Cochrane Database Systematic Review,* Issue 1. Art. no.: CD004046.

Smith, G. (2006). Effect of nurse-led gut-directed hypnotherapy upon health-related quality of life in patients with irritable bowel syndrome. *Journal of Clinical Nursing, 15*(6), 678–684.

Spiegel, D. (2001). Mind matters: Coping and cancer progression. *Journal of Psychosomatic Disease, 50*(5), 287–290.

Spiegel, D. (2007). The mind prepared: Hypnosis in surgery. *Journal of the National Cancer Institute, 99*(17), 1280–1281.

Stahl, S. (2008). *Stahl's essential psychopharmacology. Neuroscientific basis and practical applications* (3rd ed.). Cambridge, UK: University Press.

Streeter, C. C., Whitfield, T. H., Owen, L., Rein, T., Karri, S. K., Yakhkind, A., Perlmutter, R., Prescot., A.,...Jensen. J. E. (2010). Effects of yoga versus walking on mood, anxiety, and brain GABA levels: A randomized controlled MRS study. *Journal of Alternative and Complementary Medicine, 16*(11), 1145–1152. doi:10.1089/acm.2010.0007

Sutherland, S., Purdon, S., Lai, C., Wang, L., Liu, G., & Shan, J. (2010). Memory enhancement from two weeks exposure to North American ginseng extract HT1001 in young and middle aged healthy adults. *The Open Nutraceuticals Journal, 3,* 20–24.

Taylor, M., Carney, S., Geddes, J., & Goodwin, G. (2011). Folate for depressive disorders. *Cochrane Databse of Systematic Reviews,* Issue 2. Art. no.: doi: 10.1002/14651858.CD003390

Teschke, R., & Schulze, J. (2010). Risk of kava hepatotoxicity and the FDA consumer advisory. *Journal of the American Medical Association, 304*(19), 2174–2175.

Thompson Healthcare (2007). *Physicians Desk Reference for Herbal Medicines* (4th ed.). Montvale, NJ: Author.

Tusaie, K. (2011). *Translating research on gaming and resilience into adolescent mental health promotion.* Paper presented at *American Psychiatric Nurses Association Conference,* Louisville, KY.

Tusaie, K., & Edds, K. (2009). Understanding and integrating mindfulness into psychiatric nursing practice. *Archives of Psychiatric Nursing, 23*(5), 359–365.

U.S. Food and Drug Administration, Center for Food Safety and Applied Nutrition, Office of Nutritional Products, Labeling, and Dietary Supplements. Letter regarding health claim for omega-3 fatty acids. ? Retrieved from (www.cfsan.fda.gov/~dms/ds-ltr11.html).

U.S. Government Accountability Office. New drug approval: FDA needs to enhance its oversight of drugs approved on the basis of surrogate endpoints. Washington, DC: Author. Retrieved from www.gao.gov/products/GAO-09-866

Vieth, R. (1999). Vitamin D supplementation, 25-hydroxyvitamin D concentration, and safety. *American Journal of Clinical Nutrition. 69,* 842–856.

Waite, W., & Holder, M. (2003). Emotional freedom technique. The scientific review of mental health practice, *2*(1), 20–26. Retrieved from www.srmhp.org/0201/emotional-freedom=technique.html

Walters, K. (1998). A holistic approach to meeting students' needs: Using hypnotherapy techniques to assist students in managing their health. *Journal of School Nursing, 14*(4), 44–48.

Werneke, U., Horn, O., & Taylor, D. (2004). How effective is St. John's Wort? The evidence revisited. *Journal of Clinical Psychiatry, 65*(5), 611–615.

World health Organization (WHO) (1991). Guidelines for Assessment of herbal medicines. Retrieved from: http// whqlib-doc.who.int/hq/1991/who_TRM91.4.pdf

World Health Organization (1999). *Monographs on Selected Medicinal Plants.* (vol. 1) Geneva: World health Organization Press.

Zahourek, R. (2002). Utilizing Ericksonian hypnosis in psychiatric-mental health nursing practice. *Perspectives in Psychiatric Care, 38*(1), 15–22.

Zhou, S., Gao, Y., Jiang, W., Huang, M., Xu, A., & Paxton, J. (2003). Interactions of herbs with cytochrome P450. *Drug Metabolism Review, 35,* 35–98.

Zittermann, A. (2003). Vitamin D in preventive medicine: Are we ignoring the evidence? *British Journal of Nutrition, 89,* 552–572.

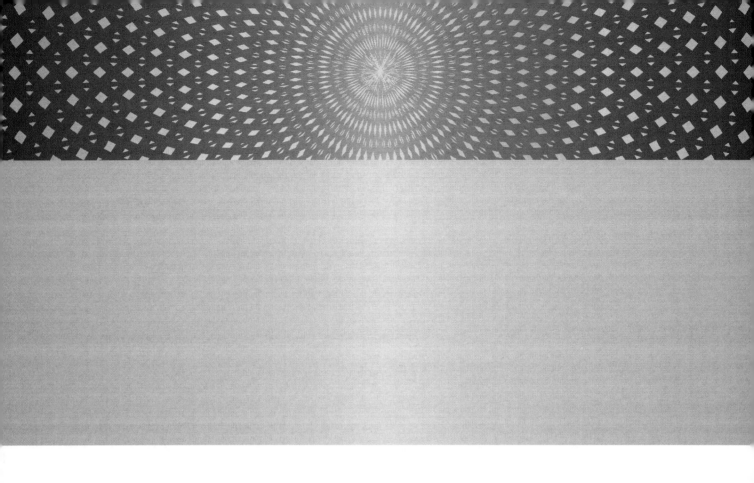

CHAPTER CONTENTS

OVERVIEW

Working with clients is dynamic and challenging. Although there are many variations of psychiatric-mental health problems, there are specific core issues to be considered for all clients. These include the overall purpose of treatment, your theory base and resources, a client's perspective and resources, and stages of treatment. These issues will be explored by describing process as well as content of treatment. Process involves both relationship issues (building the relationship, empathy, instilling hope) and interview techniques (open-ended questions, clarification, gates, shared decision making). Content, on the other hand, includes what you ask about and the details of what you hear. This chapter will provide an overview of treatment in general, or the big picture.

First, it is important to remember that all treatment has the purpose of assisting clients to bring about change in thought processes, mood, or behavior. See Figure 7-1 for a description of this generic change process. Clients are approximately 70% responsible for change and the PMH-APRN (Psychiatric Mental Health Advanced Practice Nurse) is only 30% responsible. Clients will take what they believe to be useful from each session and discard the rest (Duncan, Miller, Wampold, & Hubble, 2010). Generic factors that contribute to effective change and are common to any type of treatment include an empathetic therapeutic relationship characterized by mutual

CHAPTER 7

Stages of Treatment

Kathleen R. Tusaie

respect and trust, hope, a high degree of involvement, awareness of motivation, and common goals.

As you and the client first meet, it is the beginning of an ongoing process of mutual discovery—as if you were an explorer and a travel guide. Preparing for the interview is important for the PMH-APRN as well as the client. Self-care in terms of adequate rest, exercise, and time to be relaxed and thoughtful before a session leads to more comfort and the ability to be engaged in the interview process. Also, becoming familiar with the required forms and having resources readily available is important. These resources may be telephone numbers for referrals, emergency protocols, and reference materials (books, computer programs, or apps). Making the physical environment safe and as comfortable as possible is also helpful. Always have access to the exit door, the ability to see a clock, and avoid having a large desk between you and the client. Using the same office space that you have personalized is ideal although not always possible. Also, remembering that the foundation of all therapeutic sessions is the relationship, and that the ability to actively listen is in itself therapeutic, increases a sense of self-efficacy in the beginning PMH-APRN.

Building a therapeutic relationship is perhaps the most difficult but most basic aspect of treatment. Some describe the importance of empathy or caring about the client while maintaining your own perspective. Cozolino (2002) has posited that empathetic connections actually stimulate neurochemical brain changes that enhance

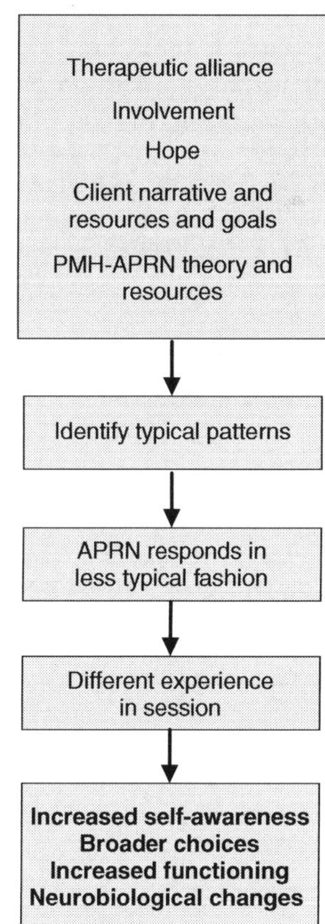

Figure 7-1 Model of Generic Change Process

learning and increase plasticity. Furthermore, neurobiologically, mirror genes have been identified that are believed to predict the degree of our ability to understand

and care about others (Dobbs, 2006). This caring relationship has even been described as the need to love our clients (Sleeth, 2010). But a therapeutic relationship differs from a personal caring/loving relationship and does require boundaries as defined by professional ethics. The caring requires a balance with a sense of curiosity about how the individual functions and what changes are needed. An ability to function on multiple levels simultaneously is needed—jumping in the relationship to feel and connect, then jumping out to observe and organize data for diagnostic and planning purposes. Expert PMH-APRNs have developed this skill through years of clinical practice and knowledge building.

One common difficulty in beginning PMH-APRNs is the desire to "fix" the client without an appreciation of the client's narrative and the PMH-APRN's own difficulty in bearing witness to suffering. This is the client's journey and we are only resources. Freud has labeled these tendencies countertransference, and it is important to use supervision or peer collaboration to identify these tendencies during clinical practice and to work through your own emotionally charged issues. Some signs that indicate significant countertransference include being late for sessions or cutting the time short, becoming drowsy during sessions, behaving seductively or overly cold or harsh, arguing with the client, dreaming about the client, or generally noting a very strong emotional reaction or total lack of any emotions. A PMH-APRN is much more than a prescriber or a diagnostician. Remembering and respecting therapeutic use of self is a necessary component of any treatment.

Awareness of one's own thinking and recognizing one's own motivations (centering or grounding) is an ongoing process. Some PMH-APRNs use supervision as part of this process, others are involved in therapy relationships as a client themselves, and many practice meditation to facilitate self-understanding. Education in mindfulness-meditation has been reported to significantly improve empathy, and decrease feelings of burnout in clinicians (Krasner et al., 2009). This centering of self or grounding process allows more openness to clients' needs which translates into more effective treatment outcomes.

TECHNIQUES FOR DEVELOPING THERAPEUTIC RELATIONSHIPS

Although the development of empathy and caring can be esoterically described in great detail, the realistic question remains about how to accomplish this within the limits of time and expected productivity in the clinical world. In addition to basic philosophical positions of valuing others, an ability to recognize strengths as well as symptoms, a sense of curiosity, and creativity, there are specific techniques that can put relationship building on fast forward. These include intentional use of your body as well as words, and are referred to as mirroring or pacing (see Exhibit 7-1).

First, the concept of joining with or pacing a client is useful. Although this is natural for many PMH-APRNs, this strategy can be maximized by awareness of the technique. Pacing or mirroring involves assuming a similar body posture as well as language of the client. This is not mimicking the individual, but a more casual and respectful approach. For example, if a client sits with legs crossed and arms crossed across chest, it is assumed much anxiety or resistance is present—almost a self-hug or self-protective armor. To verbally address this moves from an unconscious body language to a cognitive language, which may prove uncomfortable for the client, especially in the initial sessions. So, you assume a similar position, with legs crossed and perhaps hands together in your lap as you continue to talk. The client begins to feel more comfortable without ever verbally addressing this. Gradually through the session, you uncross your legs and loosen the connection between your hands and the client begins to follow. This example shows pacing in terms of using your body position as the client was using his or her body, as well as the route of communication being nonverbal following the client's route of communication. Leading or changing the pace of the communication (uncrossing legs and hands) is a very respectful, subtle, and effective strategy for setting the tone of safety in the session.

While the body language is paced, so is the verbal language or words used. Be alert to the language. For example, if a client refers to a depressed mood as the blues, there is no need to explain the difference between the blues and actual clinical depression while you are building trust and listening to the client tell their story. Use a simple reflection with their language—"You have

EXHIBIT 7-1: COMMUNICATION TECHNIQUES FOR BUILDING EMPATHY

- Simple reflections (affective, content)
- Summarizing (affective, content)
- Nonverbals (mirroring, pacing, nodding)
- Minimal verbalizations
- Silence

been feeling blue." Listen carefully and do not persist in using technical terms or interpretations to increase your own safety or to attempt to impress the client with your knowledge. Also, having patience to listen and attend to the client without yet forming a response is necessary. The development of a connection with the client is most important now.

Ways of perceiving the world and a client's problems is also revealed by the use of visual, kinesthetic, auditory, or more abstract descriptors. By recognizing and reflecting similar language, relationship building and a sense of being understood is quickly facilitated (Lankton & Bandler, 2003). For example, if a client states, "I can't see a future for myself," this is visual and you may respond, "It's difficult to visualize change for yourself. When did this start?" Use of words that are visual include colors (feeling blue), light, or seeing. Auditory descriptors include hearing (Do you hear me?) and reference to sounds such as screaming. Kinesthetic descriptors may involve movement (slowed down, racing), or feelings (closed in, far away). Practicing language pacing is very useful and later becomes automatic.

Once again, the PMH-APRN is observing and joining simultaneously. Observing therapy sessions or practicing with simulations are helpful for beginners. If there is an excess of question asking it may be related to the PMH-APRN's anxiety level, voyeurism, or desire for all the details, sadism, or the desire to see pain in the client, and/or lack of engagement of client and/or PMH-APRN.

Specific communication techniques to use during the initial sessions have been described by Shea (1998). The most important is the use of simple reflections or observations without interpretations. Examples of simple reflections are:

1. Reflect affect: "You seem to have difficulty talking about that.... You appear sad.... You sound angry.... You seem upset."
2. Reflect content: "Sounds like your husband is both your main support and your main problem.... Sounds as if you have a busy schedule."

Shea suggests the use of three simple reflections during the first 15 minutes of a session and then one every 20 minutes. Moyers, Miller, and Hendrickson (2005) encourage the use of two reflective statements to each question. This use of reflection not only builds empathy but also avoids the trap of the client being a passive recipient with the PMH-APRN doing all the work.

Another therapeutic communication technique useful in developing empathy and providing feedback to the client that they are being heard is to summarize affect or content without interpretation. Examples include:

1. Summarizing affect: "Sounds like you are having mixed feelings—sadness, fear, anger toward many people."
2. Summarizing content: "So, you are saying that your current depression is related to the death of your wife, your job change, as well as your family history of depression?"

Another useful therapeutic technique is to simply nod or use minimal verbalization such as "uh huh, okay, I see," or to be silent and observe for a few minutes. In the initial session, it is important not to rush implied understanding or intimacy. These communication techniques assist in creating a session that is more of a collaborative

EXHIBIT 7-2: CASE EXAMPLES

USING VIDEO AS A THERAPEUTIC INTERVENTION

Viewing the video recording with clients is also quite a learning experience when appropriately timed in treatment. For example, one young man who had difficulty maintaining relationships was unable to appreciate his role in this issue and would project all blame onto his ability to choose appropriate friends or lovers. After working with him for about 6 months using psychotherapy as well as antidepressants, we taped a session. After viewing a brief videotape of himself in a session, he was surprised to recognize the intensity of his anger and his aggressive body language. This was the beginning of his own recognition of need to change his style of interacting and he began to explore internal sources of his anger and fear.

CLIENT'S USE OF PHOTOGRAPHY AS SELF-THERAPY

A professional photographer, Donald Woodman, was in treatment with the same therapist for a long period of time. He then asked his therapist if he could photograph the therapist during sessions to demonstrate the client's perspective on treatment and impressions of the therapist. These photographs are quite interesting. You may wish to view his work at http://donaldwoodman.com/gallery/the-therapist-2

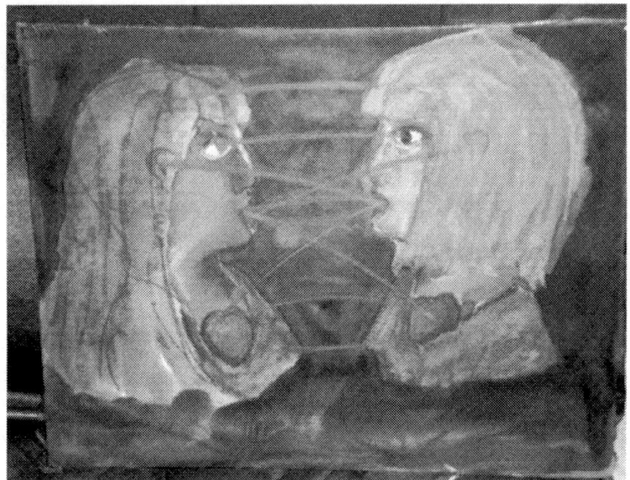

Figure 7-2 Oil Painting Created by Client and Presented to PMH-APRN During Termination of Treatment

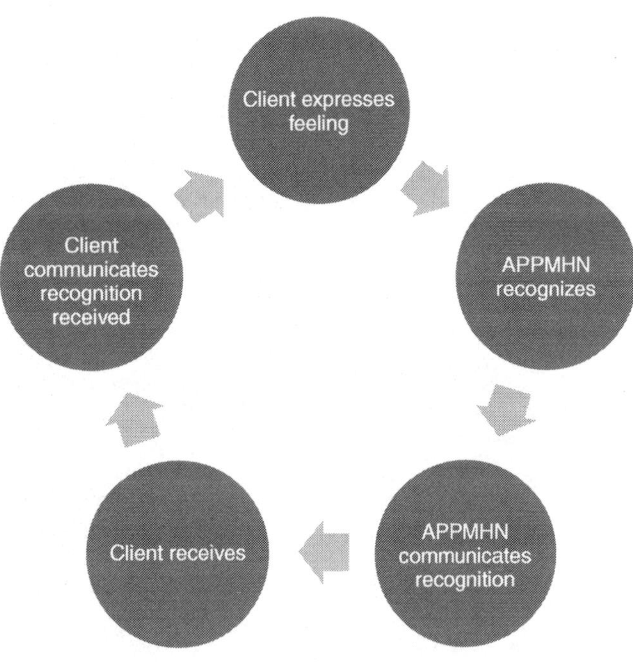

Figure 7-3 Empathy Cycle

Source: Adapted from Shea (1998).

discussion than an interrogation. Satisfaction surveys of clients have reported one of the most important factors in treatment is the belief that the professional listens and understands them (Duncan et al., 2010). Building the therapeutic alliance is an ongoing process during all sessions. However, if not initiated during the first session, it is unlikely that the client will return.

In addition to the client returning, there are strategies for evaluating the development of empathy in the session (Shea, 1998). First, at the end of the session, be aware of your own reactions. Do you think of the client as a real individual who is in pain? What is your mood? Was the session more of a conversation than your reading questions from a checklist or the computer? Second, explore the client's reactions. Ask how they now make sense of everything. And if the client is fairly high functioning, ask what you can do to help them with this. Finally, ask what they think about working together. Figure 7-2 is an original oil painting demonstrating the client's sense of connectedness with the PMH-APRN during therapy. Also, discussing sessions with peers or supervisors is helpful. Viewing your session on a videotape is always enlightening even if somewhat intimidating.

Building empathy serves many purposes. It creates a sense of safety in the relationship, thus decreasing anxiety and thus promoting neuronal changes and the ability to learn and change. Empathy also provides emotional proximity or warmth and facilitates engagement in the treatment process by both the client and the PMH-APRN. See Figure 7-3 for a description of the cycle of empathy between client and PMH-APRN.

INSTILLING HOPE

During the initial sessions, clients will also be evaluating you. Questions such as "Can this person help me? Are they competent?" will be present whether or not the words are spoken. As the session progresses the process will answer these questions for the client. As their anxiety decreases, they will notice what you ask and how you obtain information. When it is a positive session they will think that you are interested, understand their feelings and issues, and are thorough. These thoughts, of course, assist in developing hope that they can change and improve.

An additional source of evaluation has been clients looking up the clinician online. So, having a website as well as being aware of what is out there on the web about you is important.

To instill hope, you must be hopeful. For example, if you are working with an individual experiencing chronic auditory hallucinations and multiple hospitalizations, and your goal is to eliminate the hallucinations, it would be very difficult to be hopeful. However, if your mutually developed goal is to develop strategies to cope with and decrease intensity of the hallucinations, there is hope for change. If you are treating a 20-year-old individual who is self-injuring and has a history of severe childhood abuse, if you believe that the personality is formed by age 7 and the trauma is irreversible, there is minimal hope. However, if you believe that individuals are resilient and do have the capacity to change, there is hope.

It is vital to be aware of your own thinking about pathology and human functioning as well as have a sensitivity to your own reactions. Perhaps at one point in your career you enjoyed working with children who had been abused, but now you have your own child and find yourself becoming too sympathetic and emotional, believing that a child is doomed or starting to want to adopt every child. Then it becomes time to become more self-reflective and consider changing your focus of practice. There are multiple roles and specialties in Advanced Practice Psychiatric Mental Health Nursing and your effectiveness and interest may shift several times in your career. Professional flexibility and creativity are born of self-understanding and practice.

COMMUNICATION STRATEGIES TO FOLLOW UP ON LEADS AND INSTILL HOPE

- Clarification
- Open-ended questions
- Exploring feelings
- Broad openings
- Normalizing
- Giving recognition/positive affirmations

Often, the very issues that need to be explored in treatment are those that increase the client's anxiety. Therefore, skill is required in assisting the client to face those aspects that are causing difficulties with minimal damage to the client's self-esteem and avoidance of an adversial position (Wachtel, 2011). This has been termed gentle inquiry or exploration and clarification.

Following statements of the reason for seeking treatment, decisions are made as to where to focus the discussion. The focus is determined by the purpose of the session. For example, during the initial session, if the client begins to talk in great detail and length about childhood trauma, it is best to refocus upon the current symptoms because treatment decisions will need to be made. Exploration of the problem may involve *simple clarification* by such statements as "Tell me more about your experience of depression." Open-ended statements to clarify information are often gentle commands. "Tell me about the consequences of your depression." *Open-ended questions* or gentle commands set the tone for a nonjudgmental environment where clients can explore their problems in more depth. Open-ended questions cannot be answered by a simple yes or no and usually expand the information flow.

Exploring feelings is another technique to gain more information. When a client is providing only detailed information as if telling a story from the past, it is useful to switch to feelings. One way would be to ask, "How did that feel when you were divorced?" or bring it to the here-and-now by asking, "How does it feel to talk about the divorce now?" If the opposite occurs, too much emotional intensity and difficulty obtaining information, switch to more detailed logical content. For example, "I can see this is very emotional for you and it is important to express your feelings, but now we need to focus on some information so we can decide what may be most helpful treatment for you—so take a deep breath . . . "

Some clients are ready to work, and following *broad openings* such as "What brings you here today?" may help them begin to discuss their issues in depth. Others have more ambivalence about sharing and changing and require more help getting the session underway. Open-ended questions like "Tell me what has been going on for you in the past few weeks?" or, if an adolescent, "I understand your parents think you need to be here, but what are your thoughts on why they want you in treatment?" Or if the client is very anxious and uncomfortable, beginning with a broad focus by discussing his or her life in general may lead to a later problem focus.

Normalizing situations and reactions are also helpful in gathering more information without threatening or shutting down the interview flow (Shea, 1998). This technique involves phrasing a question so that the client realizes he or she is not the only person with the problem or behavior. For example, "Many people tell me that when they are extremely anxious, their thoughts sound like voices in their head—has this ever happened to you?" Or, "Sometimes when people are very unhappy and angry with their spouses, they will become romantically involved with someone else—have you ever done that?"

Giving recognition or positive affirmations is basically attributing interesting, positive qualities to clients. Avoid using "I" statements because this implies judgment. Instead, use "you" statements. For example, consider a mother who is voluntarily seeking treatment following an incident of hitting her baby. "You are concerned about being a good mother" instead of "You are afraid you will hurt your baby." Remember that the affirmation is not an end point but part of the process of gathering information. Follow-up to an affirmation may include questions such as "How did you" or "What did you . . . ?" Sometimes, simply showing up for treatment may be a focus . . ." Despite your depression, you made this appointment on time . . . How did you accomplish this?" Using these interventions assist the PMH-APRN as well as the client to have a balanced, accepting view—competencies as well as problems present are recognized. Carl Rogers (1961) has referred to this approach as "prizing" the client.

CLIENT RESOURCES

Individualized treatment takes into consideration what is being observed as well as heard and reacted to during the session. This results in focusing the session in the appropriate direction. Although, approximate time limits for obtaining content has been posited, there will be individual differences. For example, an individual who is concerned about having Alzheimer's disease will require more time with the mental status exam and include details about activities of daily living in more detail. An adolescent who has been bullied at school will need to discuss friendships and school environment in detail. An individual who expresses current suicidal ideation needs a focus upon the here-and-now, including risk and protective factors, with minimal attention to developmental history and family history. As clients becomes less organized, the PMH-APRN becomes more directive. Although the interview has a general outlined format, it is dynamic and changes for each client.

Not only client's feelings and thoughts about themselves, but also their worldview and thoughts and feelings about others around them is important to assess. Specific interviewing techniques for symptom clusters can be seen in this text as well as in Carlat's *The Psychiatric Interview* (2005), Shea's *Psychiatric Interviewing: The Art of Understanding* (1998), and Zuckerman's *The Clinician's Thesaurus 2010*.

PMH-APRN RESOURCES

Self-awareness or self-understanding is an ongoing process. There are many reasons that nurses decide to be an advanced practice psychiatric mental health nurse. The pat answer is "to help people," but there is much more involved in the decision. Some were trained by their family of origin to be rescuers and mediate the family dynamics. Others are drawn to closeness, but want only minimal emotional risk while also being in control. It can feel good to know you can influence others' lives by what you say and do. And a few others admit that they thought with proper education and training, they could resolve their own issues. Our transitions from novice to expert are related to how we think and process what is going on, not so much what we say aloud or do. It is useful to be involved yourself as a client in the psychotherapy process to facilitate self-understanding as well as clinical skills—an exercise in practicing what we preach.

Being involved in supervision assists not only the novice, but all levels of PMH-APRNs. This may be during graduate, post master's, or doctorate studies, with a peer group or an individual. Development of communities of practice have been described recently as the most effective manner of learning (Wenger, McDermott, & Snyder, 2002). The experience of seeing how peers do things, as well as discussing and sharing information, removes the heirarchial situation and provides horizontal learning. It is important to take responsibility for your own continued learning and an effective community of practice encourages learning beyond your comfort zone. Furthermore, a community of practice holds the potential to counteract the aloneness of many outpatient practices.

The community of practice may involve self-report, audio or videotape, live observation, or simulation of sessions. Trust and goodwill within the group should counter the vulnerability felt by the individual. However, there needs to be a sense of direction and preparedness. For example, if using a tape, specific segments should be identified pre-session and an awareness of one's own strengths and weaknesses identified before the session. Although several different profession's functions overlap with PMH-APRN, it is ideal to have at least one PMH-APRN in the community of practice in order to pass on and safeguard the unique aspects of our profession.

Not only ongoing supervision, but also the resources and willingness to debrief following emotional or difficult interactions is important for self-care. Vicarious traumatization is always a possibility. Although most PMH-APRNs like to consider themselves resilient, we all need help sometimes.

SKILL AND KNOWLEDGE

Benner's model of skill acquisition (Benner, 2000) can be applied to the PMH-APRN. Before starting graduate school, many students were practicing at an expert level as a registered nurse (RN). Therefore, it is anxiety producing to return to a novice level in the graduate student or PMH-APRN role. By reviewing Benner's stages, it serves as a reminder of the process of learning the skills of a PMH-APRN and an awareness of setting realistic goals for self

EXHIBIT 7-3: BENNER'S STAGES OF CLINICAL SKILLS (BENNER, 1982)

Novice—no experience, governed by rules, regulations
Advanced beginner—recognizes meaningful aspects of situations, able to make judgements
Competent—2–3 years experience, coordinates complex care
Proficient—3–5 years experience, sees situations as whole, sees long-term goals
Expert—Performance is fluid, flexible, and efficient, uses intuition

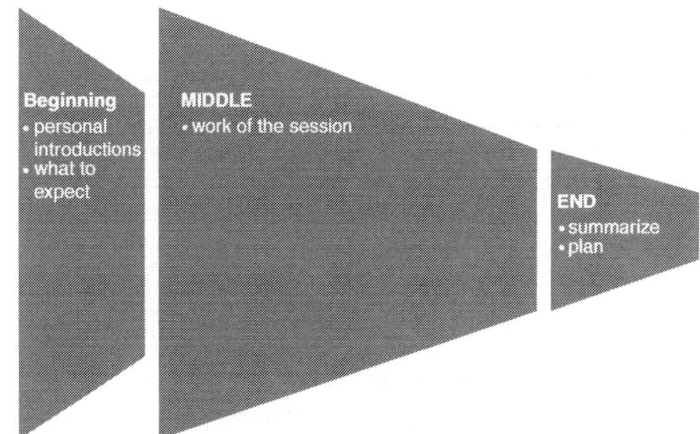

Figure 7-4 Sections of Each Session

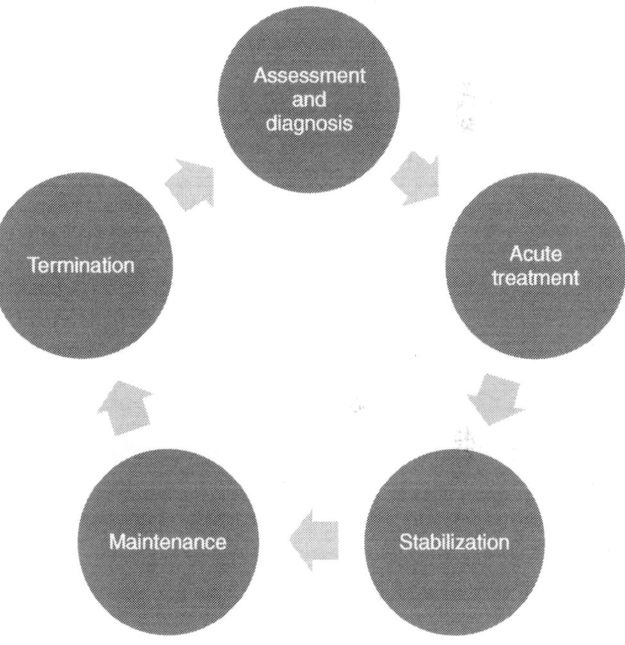

Figure 7-5 Stages of Treatment

(see Exhibit 7-3). For example, when prescribing, choose one or two drugs from each class to use and expand later. With psychotherapy, use the basic therapeutic communication techniques and combine with one specific therapy, such as cognitive behavioral therapy (CBT) on an individual basis. Later, expand to groups and additional therapies as you become competent in CBT.

The PMH-APRN works with clients to facilitate change in thought processes, mood, or behavior.

IDENTIFYING STAGES OF TREATMENT

Each session has a beginning, a middle, and an end as demonstrated in Figure 7-4. The beginning is very brief and sets the stage for this session. This introduction involves a brief explanation of the session, "Hello, I am Dr. Susan Brown. I am an advanced practice psychiatric nurse. During the next hour, I will be asking some questions to understand you and your issues better. I may need to interrupt you from time to time so I can make things more clear and I will also be taking notes from time to time so I remember information. Would you like to be addressed as Joe or Mr. Green?"

The middle is the work to achieve the goals of the session. The end is the summary and planning for the next session. It is important to attend to timing with the majority of the session being in the middle. Often, a clock is placed across the room so the PMH-APRN can look at the time as the session progresses. It is also appropriate to set limits on time by stating, "we have 10 minutes remaining, let's summarize the main points and plan for next week now." Statements encouraging the client to think about the session when summarizing are most useful—for example, "What stands out for you from our session today?" or "What is most important for you from our session?" If a client is too distressed or disorganized to summarize, you may state the major themes.

The interventions shift with the stage of treatment. These stages include assessment and diagnosis, acute treatment, stabilization/maintenance, and finally termination as illustrated in Figure 7-5. Although stages will be described as discrete in this text, there is often overlap among stages. These generic stages of treatment have specific goals which require individualized, integrated interventions for clients.

ASSESSMENT AND DIAGNOSIS

The following are general goals for the assessment process (Shea, 1998):

- To engage self and the client in the process
- To develop empathy and understanding of the client
- To collect a valid database
- To identify patterns and, develop a diagnosis and case formulation
- To instill hope and decrease anxiety

As empathy and understanding build between the client and PMH-APRN, a safe environment is created and clinical validity is now an important concept to consider. This refers to collecting data that are accurate. Of course, there are many factors that contribute to accuracy. First of all, there are multiple true interpretations of situations. In the classic Japanese movie, *Rashomon*, the story of a murder is told through the eyes and memories of several observers. Although the same events are described, the descriptions are tremendously different. Rather than thinking one is right and another wrong, we assume that each person's perception represents an equally valid, integral part of the situation. These varying interpretations may be due to natural defense mechanisms, poor memory, hidden agendas, as well as deceit. For example, if an individual's goal is to obtain disability, the representation of strengths may be limited while symptoms are exaggerated. Furthermore, Wachtel (2011) has stated that it is often the client's framing of the truth and the meaning attributed that creates problems. The process of therapy often provides a different frame which is less negative. So, it is likely that perceptions of data will be shifting as treatment progresses.

Furthermore, the manner in which the PMH-APRN asks questions will also contribute to a valid database. A technique, the *behavioral incident*, used during interviews was developed by Pascal (1983) and further described by Shea (1998). This technique is simply not asking opinions, but instead is asking specific details. For example, instead of asking a closed question eliciting an opinion, such as "Is your family fairly supportive?" ask details such as, "Who is supportive? What do they do to support you? When are they available?" Another option for questioning in the behavioral incident is to ask for specific and concrete information such as, "What happened next? What did you do or think? What was the weapon involved?"

This type of data gathering avoids the problem of leading the client and not wanting to hear about sensitive problems such as stating "You have never been suicidal, have you?" Therefore, it is not only the client but also the PMH-APRN who contributes to a valid database, which is needed for diagnostics, case formulations, and treatment planning.

TRANSITIONING TO NEW TOPICS

Transitioning from one topic to another gracefully is a skill. Shea refers to these transitions as "gates." There are several types of gates. First, the client may spontaneously move to a new content area and this is called a *spontaneous gate*. Following this shift, the PMH-APRN may refocus by asking, "That is interesting, but could we return to the topic of self-destructive thoughts now?" Or explore the new area with comments such as "Tell me more about that" or "go on."

A *natural gate* involves the PMH-APRN cueing off the client statements and making a bridge to the new content. For example, the client states that she has difficulty falling asleep and the PMH-APRN asks, "What have you tried to help with falling asleep, have you used any drugs or alcohol as a nightcap?" thus making a natural transition to the area of substance use.

A *referred gate* is the return to a new area of discussion by referring back to a previous statement made by the client. For example, "Earlier, when we discussed your work, you said you were having difficulty remembering details. Tell me more about that."

A *phantom gate* occurs when the PMH-APRN asks a question totally out of context and this interrupts the information flow. This should generally be avoided. However, sometimes this is necessary when your evaluation is 1 hour and you recognize lack of information in a specific important area. If this situation develops in an interview, it is best to be honest. For example, "We only have 10 minutes remaining and I need to ask some specific questions now. Have you ever been treated for a psychiatric problem?" Another instance of using a phantom gate may be the need to focus a wandering interview.

Implied gates join similar regions and can provide expansion. For example, a woman is discussing her daughter's pregnancy and the PMH-APRN states, "What were your pregnancies like?" Using these concepts of gates for transition of content areas leads to a smooth conversation and collection of needed data.

Often, databases are pre-printed forms or computerized and unique to each facility. However, the following content is present in diagnostic assessments:

- Identifying data
- Chief complaint/presenting problem
- History of present problem and treatment

- Past problems—psychiatric, medical, substances and treatment
- Review of systems/physical examination
- Family history (genogram)
- Personal development (birth, childhood, adolescence, adulthood)
- Adulthood (occupation history, relationships, military, education, religion, social supports, legal history, living situation, abuse history, self-care ability)
- Values
- Mental status exam
- Risk formulation
- Diagnostic and statistical (*DSM*) diagnosis
- Case formulation
- Initial plan for treatment

(Adapted from Carlat (2005); Sadock & Sadock (2007)).

Presenting Problem

This refers to the client's own words about his or her reasons for seeking help. It is best to use verbatim quotes for this section.

History of Present Problem

This section provides a chronological picture leading up to his or her current status. Asking "why now?" will assist with a more defined understanding of the client's priorities. What has been happening over the past couple of weeks? When did the symptoms start or shift? What were triggering events? What was the life situation when symptoms began? How did this all begin? How old were you when you first experienced symptoms? Attempt to obtain premorbid level of functioning. If the client is unable to share this information, seek out other informants such as family members or friends following the client's permission.

Also, asking about what self-help or professional help with this problem has been attempted is important.

Past Problems

Obtain treatment history including hospitalizations for psychiatric, medical, or substance use. Names of providers and previous medications and other treatment modalities including complementary/alternative. Include who, what, where, when, and why. Release of information to obtain past records for more details is also important.

Review of Systems/Physical Exam

This is a screening for medical illness as well as possible medical causes of the psychiatric problems. If the client has recently had a physical exam, obtain these records. For a brief review of systems, start with general questions such as, "On a scale of 1–10 with 10 being the most healthy overall, where do you rate yourself?" Describe sleep, including dreams, and eating patterns. Then progress from head to toe to screen for problems. Headaches or seizures? Vision or hearing problems? Smelling, taste, or throat problems? Thyroid problems? Problems with your breathing or lungs such as asthma, pneumonia, or coughing? Heart problems? Stomach problems or constipation or diarrhea? Problems with urination? Joint problems or difficulty walking? Any difficulties with sexual functioning or menstrual periods? Might you be pregnant? When was your last period?

To further evaluate sexual issues in a non-threatening manner, I often use the following question: "I always ask these questions of all clients and if you are uncomfortable in answering, let me know. Are you satisfied with your sexual functioning? Sometimes people have sex against their will. Have you ever been forced to have sex? Do you have any reason to believe that you are at risk for HIV—injected drugs, sex with many different partners, sex with another man or sex with a man who sleeps with other men or injects drugs."

Family History

This history is obtained to determine inherited risk of certain disorders as well as to begin the social history. Using a genogram is an organized and efficient way to record data. Tell the client that you would like to draw a diagram to better understand his or her family. Use squares for males and circles for females. Include age, if dead, include year, age, and cause (put X through square or circle), presence of psychiatric problem, substance abuse, and major medical problems, occupation/education, nationality, and status of relationship (close, estranged). See Exhibit 7-4 for example of a genogram.

PERSONAL DEVELOPMENTAL HISTORY

An appreciation of the client's past and relationship to current issues is now explored. The amount of detail is usually determined by the available time in the session. Some agencies have this information prepared in question format and the client completes it before the session on paper and pencil or computer.

The general areas include **perinatal** (full-term or premature birth, issues in pregnancy, drugs mother took during pregnancy, birth complications or defects); **childhood** (if not discussed with genogram, what parents did for a living, who was in the home, what discipline, favorite family saying, earliest memory, any abuse, who you were closest to, describe personality); **education/work** (highest level of schooling, did you enjoy it, what grades, best friend, what kind of work, how do you get along with other workers, any military involvement); **relationships** (when began dating, men/women or both, anything about sexual life or desires that makes you uncomfortable, ever forced to have sex, first important romantic relationship, current partner and how it is going, relationship with family, friends, leisure activities, current living arrangement). Legal history includes arrests as well as charges and jail time. This provides possible information about antisocial traits as well as a litigious personality. **Coping/stress tolerance** (what is the most difficult situation before current problem and how did you get through it).

VALUES/ASPIRATIONS

An individual's belief system can have a profound impact upon functioning as well as acceptance and participation in treatment. The question, "What do you think you will be doing 5 years from now and what would you like to be doing?" provides insight into the client's perception of his or her future. Other values may include spirituality, attitudes toward work, money, play, children, family, community, and cultural issues (Sadock & Sadock, 2007). Often, this information emerges during history taking.

To begin to understand the client's spirituality, it may be as simple as asking about religion such as church involvement or a more in-depth assessment of

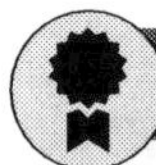

EXHIBIT 7-4: GENOGRAM

The genogram is a structural assessment tool to outline the family's internal and external structures. During the assessment process, it is a quick method to record basic structure and family history of illnesses. The genogram can concisely record important information about family history (McGuinness, Noonan, & Dyer, 2009).

Constructing the genogram can initially be used as an engagement tool and later be used in sessions to provide rich information about relationships, health, occupations, religion, and overall family functioning while increasing the client's understanding of multiple generational influences. It was first developed by Murray Bowen and widely used in all specialities today.

Start by asking concrete, non-threatening questions about names, ages, health, and occupations to maximize comfort with this assessment. Avoid discussion that is hurtful or blaming during this process.

Although there is some difference in the symbols used by different authors. The following are usually accepted:

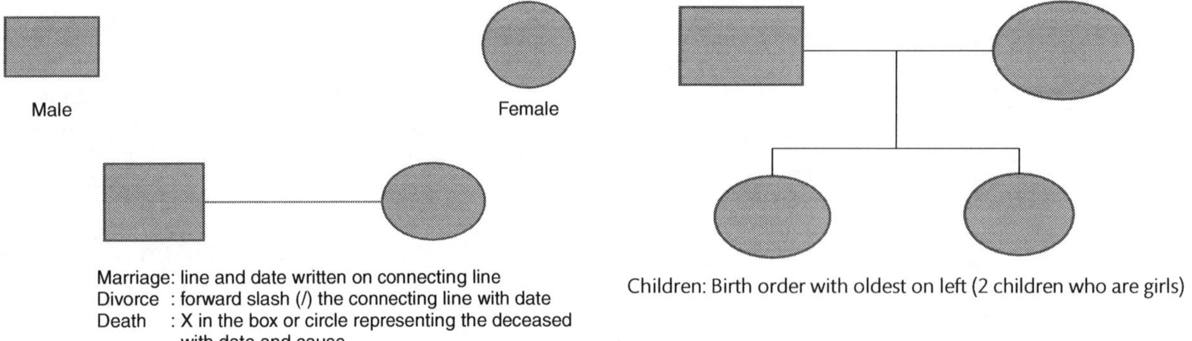

When hand drawing, divide the paper into thirds horizontally for a three-generation genogram. Begin on the left with the husband. As much or as little detail as you wish may be included. There are also several computer programs that may be purchased for drawing genograms.

The genogram can be expanded with other facts as well as symbols to indicate relationships such as very close, poor, conflicted, distant, or estranged, cut off, as described by McGoldrick, Gerson, and Shellenberger (1999). As there are many blended families today, a genogram can become quite complicated, so consider the primary purpose and focus of this tool when using it in assessment and therapy.

(Continued)

EXHIBIT 7-4: GENOGRAM (*Continued*)

BASIC, INITIAL 3-GENERATION GENOGRAM

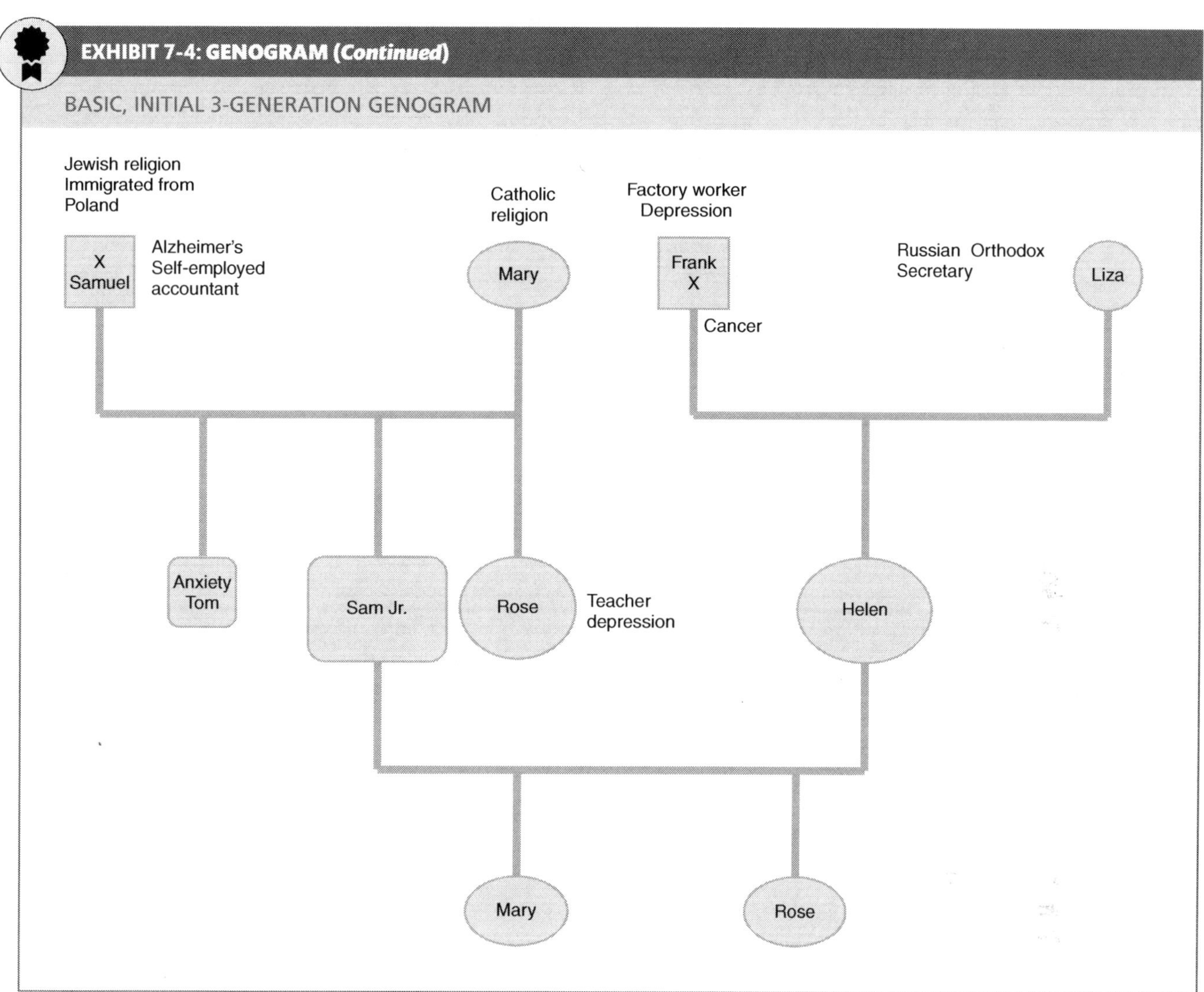

spirituality. A scale that can be downloaded to measure spiritual wellness can be found at www.elliottingersoll.com/Spiritual_Wellness_Test.html

Mental Status Examination

A Mental Status Examination (MSE) is an evaluation of the client's current status through direct observation. It includes **appearance, behavior, speech, affect, thought process, thought content,** and **cognitive examination**. MSE assists with accurate diagnosis as well as baseline information. The skilled PMH-APRN will have been evaluating mental status throughout the process of history taking and then focus upon specific areas at the end of the interview.

Appearance may be described under MSE or in the identifying data section. Statements about appearance should include description of hair (color, long, short, styled, messy, oily), facial hair, eyes (downcast, good eye contact, piercing look), body (thin, emaciated, average build, obese), movements (any abnormal movements, jittery, wringing hands, slumped posture, restless), and clothing (clean, disheveled, jeans and polished loafers, miniskirt and textured black nylons, appropriate for weather). Also any scars or bruising or tattoos should be noted here or on the Review of Systems/physical examination. It is important to be objective and not record your opinions about appearance. Also, any communication barriers such as vision or hearing impairments, unfamiliarity with English or English as a second language, or cultural issues interfering with communication. This description provides a vivid picture of the client for anyone reading your report as well as a baseline for future comparison.

Behavior in the interview will include how the client relates to you during the interview—friendly to cooperative, attentive, preoccupied, calm, very happy, and hostile, and also the overall behavior—pacing about the room, unable to sit, hypervigilant, watchful or indifferent, or almost motionless. If a child, the description may include many out-of-chairs instances investigating all the contents of the room or rearranging furniture, and temper tantrums. Also include any mannerisms, such as twisting hair, rocking, lip smacking, grunting sounds, or movements that indicate symptoms such as athetoid, serpentine, gross tremors, intention tremors, and waxy flexibility. Also include any difficulties with balance or coordination.

Speech is important to describe because it is a reflection of thought processes. Using verbatim quotes is useful. Rate (rapid, slow), volume (loud, whispered, spoke to self under breath), latency of response (halting, delayed, rushed, verbose), any difficulty finding or confusing words, rhyming, joking, and echolalia. For a child, underdeveloped vocabulary for age, or difficulty comprehending or expressing oral language.

Affect refers to your observations of the client's feelings (similar to today's weather) and mood is the more long-term subjective report by the client (similar to climate). Qualities of affect to be reported include stability, appropriateness, range, and intensity. Stability ranges from stable (normal) to labile, which would be alternating from one extreme to the opposite such as laughing to sobbing. Appropriateness to content of the conversation is important to note because inappropriateness of affect may indicate pathology, or mild inappropriateness may also be a defense mechanism to hide feelings such as denial rather than pathology. A full range of affect is normal and expected to shift in response to content of conversation, thoughts, and situations. A constricted affect often reflects depression, while a flat or blunted affect may also be present.

Thought processes refers to the way ideas and associations are put together. This can range from logical and organized to illogical and even incomprehensible. The most frequently described disorders of thought processes include circumstantiality (overinclusion of trivial details that avoid getting to the point), loose associations or derailment (breakdown of logical connections between ideas and goals of conversation), tangentiality (responses to questions approach the topic but do not answer the question), flight of ideas (a succession of rapid, multiple ideas that shift abruptly), perseveration (repition of out of context words and phrases), clang association (thoughts are associated by their sound rather than meaning, rhyming), neologism (invention of new words), and thought blocking (sudden break in flow of ideas).

Thought content refers to unusual or dangerous ideas as well as themes that were present during the interview and relate to the diagnosis. Examples include delusions (ideas about the world that are not based in reality), obsessions (ideas that are intrusive and repetitive), compulsions (behaviors that are done in repetitive manner), phobias (fears of objects or situations), suicide, and homicide. Eliciting disturbances of thought content and more details are provided in chapters focusing on specific syndromes.

Cognitive examination includes assessment of brain function and includes level of awakeness, attention, and concentration, memory, judgment, and insight. This is merely a screening of cognitive function and if indicated, a referral for more specific neuropsychological testing may be appropriate. Another important factor in cognitive function is level of intelligence. If an individual has not completed high school, they often score poorly in this area even if there is no organic impairment. However, if the client has completed high school, a quick screen for level of intelligence is the Wilson Rapid Approximate Intelligence Test (Wilson, 1967) described by Carlat (2005). If the client can calculate 2 × 48, it is unlikely they are in borderline or retarded range and if they cannot calculate 2 × 24 they are likely to meet criteria for mental retardation and should be referred for further testing.

The level of awakeness is initially assessed and may range from hyperalert, fully alert, to drowsy or comatose. If the client keeps falling asleep during the interview, it is unwise to continue the interview at this time, but important to describe and record this. Attention and concentration may be assessed by the digit span test (numbers to remember) or to subtract 7 from 100 until told to stop. However, recent studies have proven these to be of questionable value. Therefore, the most reasonable way to assess attention and concentration is to observe throughout the interview, the client's ability to focus and respond or the degree of distractability.

Short-term and long-term memory are assessed by orientation, three object recall, recall of remote personal events, and recall of general cultural events. Orientation may be determined by specifically asking, "What is your name? What is this place? What is this city? What is the date?" However, memory is often determined during the process of history taking and introductions. Often, questions such as asking about finding the office, or client reports of a family history of Alzheimer's can transition into talking about memory. Long-term memory can be assessed during history taking or also asking specific questions such as "who were the last three presidents' or 'who freed the slaves.' If you feel it is necessary to ask the specific questions following the history, use a statement such as, "Now, let's switch over to some specific questions to check memory...."

Judgement and insight can also be determined throughout the interview. The old question, "If you found a stamped envelope on the sidewalk, what would you do?" is truly not useful. More appropriate to be aware of how the client determined they needed help, and what other attempts they made to feel better. Are they aware of consequences of behaviors, did they make arrangements for sick leave and other basic needs? Insight refers to awareness of their problems and understanding of possible treatments. There may be complete denial or there may be intellectual understanding but no behavioral follow through.

USING SELF-REPORT QUESTIONNAIRES

Many settings use forms completed by the client or relative prior to the interview to provide information for the history as well as review of systems. These may be computerized or simply written responses. This approach decreases the time needed for the initial interview and also provides a resource from which specific areas may be more closely explored during the interview. Also, standard self-report screening tools such as those for depression and anxiety may also be completed before the interview and then used as reference points during the interview. (See chapters on specific syndromes for specific names of self-report questionnaires.)

To maintain a balance between eliciting pathology as well as strengths, self-report questionnaires that identify coping strategies and resilience may also be used. See *Positive Psychological Assessment* by Lopez and Snyder (2003) for specific models and measures.

SYNTHESIZING INFORMATION

Now, taking what you have heard, what you have observed, as well as your reactions, it is time to synthesize your understanding of the client's presentation and collaboratively develop a case conceptualization and *DSM* diagnosis.

Intuitive, gut-level responses to clients often represent spontaneous responses to the client and are mirrors of the client's psychopathology and feelings. These reactions are a tip-off to client's behaviors that may be sparking such a reaction in others. See Shea (1998) for more information on intuitive reactions to clients as informing this synthesis of information.

RISK FORMULATION

Because safety is always a primary concern, it is vital to create an analysis of the client's risk to self and/or others. This generally refers to potential for suicide or homicide or injury. Although predictions are difficult, clinical judgment can be applied and a three-pronged approach is the most efficient and reliable method of analysis (Shea, 2002). Simply using the client's statements is NOT adequate. The first and most important consideration is the mental status of the client. An individual who is not based in reality due to mental illness or substance use is always considered at a higher risk level. Next, risk and protective factors are elicited and considered. And finally, the ideation or verbalizations of the individual are taken into account. A low, moderate, or high risk for self or other directed violence is then determined and documented. See chapters on specific syndromes, especially Chapter 15 on self-directed injury and Chapter 16 on other-directed violence, for more details.

DIAGNOSIS (*DSM*)

The *DSM* uses clinical descriptions of symptoms, not etiology or theory. It is the currently accepted diagnostic method for most insurance and provider records in the United States. The International Classification of Disorders (ICD) is used more internationally, but they are similar and often compared in charts. The *DSM* remains controversial because it is primarily the categorical, medical model approach. The *DSM* has evolved over many revisions (which continue) by groups of clinical experts and may be explored in more depth at this website www.dsm5.org/Pages/Default.aspx or also through reviewing the *DSM* manual or software, which is necessary for all PMH-APRN practices.

CASE FORMULATION

A case formulation is a hypothesis or clinical judgement about the causes, precipitants, and maintaining influences of a person's psychological, interpersonal, and behavioral problems and their strengths (Eells, 2007). The content of this hypothesis may vary widely depending upon the the theory of development and psychopathology underlying the PMH-APRN's thinking. The identification of these patterns can be made from several different perspectives. Psychodynamic approaches include primarily unconscious mental processes and conflicts. Defense mechanisms and coping styles are commonly described.

Both the use of defense mechanisms and coping strategies are used to manage demands on an individual and to decrease levels of anxiety. The primary difference between coping styles and defense mechanisms is that coping is conscious and defense mechanisms are unconscious. Through use of a self-report measure and/or analysis of the client's history and interactive style during the session, both primary coping and defense mechanisms may be identified. Although both are dynamic, a pattern of using several can be seen. Table 7-1 provides definitions of commonly used defense mechanisms. All defense mechanisms are actually based on repression (withholding an idea or feeling from consciousness) and many do overlap. An attempt to correlate specific defense mechanisms to level of functioning was proposed in the *DSM IV-TR* (American Psychiatric Association, 1994), as a Defensive Functioning Scale, but was not finalized. Coping styles may be described as primarily behavioral (approach or avoidance) or cognitive (approach or avoidance) (Lazarus, 1991). See Table 7-2 for examples of the coping styles.

Cognitive therapy formulations focus on maladaptive/illogical thoughts and beliefs about the self and others and the world in general. While a behavioral formulation addresses a person's learning history and an analysis of environmental reinforcers and stimulus-response pairings. Stage of change and biological considerations such as genetics or other physiological factors may also be included. However, as integration of the various psychotherapies increases (Norcross, Hedges, & Prochaska, 2002), case formulations also become more integrative. As a hypothesis, the case formulation is also subject to revision as treatment progresses and additional information emerges.

The case formulation contains descriptive information which summarizes demographics, presenting problem, and history (see Exhibit 7-5). It also contains personal meaning for the client, which is how the client interpreted and experienced the descriptive information. The formulation may be in a narrative form or a graphical representation.

In addition to a case formulation, there may be a focus on a specific symptom or disorder or a specific situation. Thus identifying causes, precipitants, and maintaining forces for that specific symptom or situation. These formulations mutually inform each other and may

TABLE 7-1: SELECTED DEFENSE MECHANISMS WITH DEFINITIONS

HIGH ADAPTION OR MATURE DEFENSES	DEFINITION
Altruism	Constructive, gratifying service to others
Humor	Using comedy to express feelings without discomfort to self or others
Sublimation	Channel instincts to socially acceptable action
LOWER ADAPTIVE/IMMATURE/NEUROTIC DEFENSES	**DEFINITION**
Dissociation	Absence of conscious awareness of behaviors or stimuli, or the coexistence of separate mental systems or identities
Reaction formation	Transforming an unacceptable impulse into the opposite
Rationalization	Explaining to justify behavior, beliefs
Intellectualization	Excessive use of intellectual processes to avoid feelings or experiences
Regression	Return to an earlier stage of functioning
Somatization	Converting psychological conflicts into bodily symptoms
Blocking	Temporarily inhibiting thinking
Passive-aggressive behavior	Expressing aggression through passivity (failure, illness that affects others)
Denial	Avoiding some painful aspect of reality
Distortion	Reshaping external reality (hallucinations, delusions)
Projection	Reacting to unacceptable impulses/thoughts as if outside oneself

Source: Adapted from Sadock & Sadock (2010).

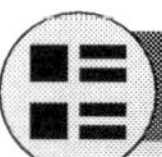

TABLE 7-2: WAYS OF COPING (WITH EXAMPLES)

COPING STYLE	EXAMPLE
Cognitive Approach	Thinking about ways to approach a problem, examining possible solutions, locating evidence
Cognitive Avoidance	"I'll think about that tomorrow"
Behavioral Approach	Trying different activities
Behavioral Avoidance	Going dancing to avoid a problem, relocating to avoid a problem neighbor

EXHIBIT 7-5: CONTENT OF AN INTEGRATED CASE FORMULATION

- Current symptoms and problems
- Possible nonpsychological explanations
- Antecedent learning experiences or vulnerabilities
- A mechanism explaining the problem plus a possible alternative explanation
- Adaptive features of the individual
- Application to treatment

be graphically represented as a chain of events to be discussed with the client and/or family.

A case formulation provides a link between theory and an individual case. It fills a conceptual vacuum created by the use of a purely descriptive *DSM* diagnosis. Making a diagnosis does not mean you understand the client. The case formulation demands that the PMH-APRN analyzes the data collected and demonstrates an understanding of the complexity involved. It also assists in translating a diagnosis into a plan for treatment and direction for the choice of specific interventions.

TREATMENT PLAN

The process of reaching concordance for the treatment plan between the PMH-APRN and client is discussed in detail in Chapter 2. Basically, the focus of the plan needs to be on what is possible and changeable, rather than what is intractable and impossible (see Exhibit 7-6). Even small changes are important. Once a small change takes place, people feel more optimistic and a bit more confident about tackling further change. Milton Erickson

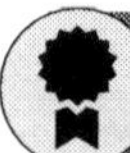

EXHIBIT 7-6: GENERIC CONSIDERATIONS FOR TREATMENT PLAN

Inpatient-outpatient
Individual-group therapy
Medication and psychotherapy
Medication alone
Psychotherapy alone
One provider
Multiple providers (split treatment)
Further testing
Self-help
Alternative strategies

used the metaphor of a snowball rolling down a mountain. Once the ball gets rolling, just stay out of the way. In addition to this process, content of the plan requires some basic yet very complicated decisions. Clients present in varying stages of acuity but the first consideration is always safety.

Next, what are the primary and secondary problems and what type of interventions are most effective and practical for this client? What are the expected outcomes of treatment? The best available evidence provides direction for these choices and is discussed for specific syndromes in this text. Next, what is practical and acceptable depending upon the resources of the client as well as the PMH-APRN?

Interventions may be delivered by one or multiple clinicians. Frequently in agencies, PMH-APRNs are placed in the role of diagnostician and prescriber, while psychotherapy is provided by a social worker or counselor. This type of delivery system is termed split treatment, collaborative treatment, divided treatment, parallel treatment, shared treatment, or triangulated treatment. When the PMH-APRN is in this role, the decision becomes one of sequencing. Is this client most appropriate for starting medication and psychotherapy simultaneously and are the resources and motivation available? Often, during the acute phase of symptoms, when functioning is impaired, medication and therapy focused upon the effects of the medication provided by the PMH-APRN are most appropriate. As acuity and somatic symptoms begin to decrease, the psychotherapy increases to focus on issues in the environment/relationship or thought patterns, and the client may now add on another clinician for psychotherapy. However, some clients may experience enough relief that they do not become involved with more intensive psychotherapy.

When treatment starts with psychotherapy alone, it is important to discuss options with the client. This includes

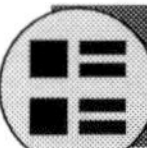

TABLE 7-3: ADVANTAGES AND DISADVANTAGES OF SPLIT TREATMENT DELIVERY (MORE THAN ONE PROVIDER)

ADVANTAGES	DISADVANTAGES
• Client has more time with providers	• Client exploits interdisciplinary tensions
• Provider vacations can be staggered to avoid sense of abandonment	• Negative transference after another provider added (she doesn't like me)
• Enhanced professional support for providers	• Provider miscommunication or missing data and poor clinical decisions
• Wider range of interventions/education for client	• Competency concerns of other provider, if unknown to each other
• Cost-effective	

Source: Adapted from Thase, Riba, & Safer (2003).

length of treatment, options for additional types of treatment, and awareness of triggers that require medication.

Of course, as the number of providers working with a client increase, there is a need for communicating and coordinating goals (see Table 7-3). If more than one provider is the treatment delivery of choice for a client, this is ideal. However, this decision may not be client-centered, but driven by cost, available resources, and agency policies, thus leading to ethical and legal concerns.

In some settings, especially private practice, delivery of all treatment may be by the PMH-APRN. The flexibility to use all or part of a session for medication issues, psychotherapy focusing on relationships or situations, or to use complementary/alternative approaches provides the flexibility to meet the changing needs of the client and/or family.

COMPARISON OF INDIVIDUAL AND GROUP THERAPY

Another decision involves the delivery of interventions through individual sessions with a client, to include the family or significant others, or in a group format. Once again, the available resources as well as acceptability are important factors. For example, in inpatient units, group therapy sessions are usually scheduled and all clients are expected to participate when able. However, it takes quite a bit of work to organize and maintain an outpatient group and clients often have concerns about confidentiality. Reimbursement and attendance are also often issues. If working with children, family is always involved and often psychoeducation or solution-focused family sessions with adult clients are used.

There is evidence for the effectiveness of group therapy for most disorders as well as specific problems. Types or goals of groups range from structured activity, to psychoeducational support and psychotherapy. Less structured groups have lower activity by the facilitator. However, some specific issues that would identify clients NOT appropriate for group therapy would include simple refusal by client, major difficulties with disclosure, suspiciousness, fear of being recognized in the community, a history of impulsive unpredictable behavior, or acute crisis.

The role of the PMH-APRN as a group facilitator is to promote therapeutic group factors in contrast to the client-centered goals of individual therapy. Yalom's (2005) curative factors include the following:

- Interpersonal learning
- Catharsis
- Group cohesiveness
- Self-understanding
- Development of socialising techniques
- Existential factors
- Universality
- Instillation of hope
- Altruism
- Corrective family reenactment
- Guidance
- Identification/imitative behavior

Summarizing, the assessment includes a brief summary of diagnostic impressions and case formulation and asking a client's current concerns/questions. Then, briefly agreeing to the timing of the next session and an overview of the treatment plan.

FURTHER TESTING/REFERRALS

Following a thorough history, conducting a comprehensive mental status examination, and performing a focused physical examination can identify areas that may need further diagnostic assessment. This may include blood work, neuroimaging, and tests of electrophysiology, or psychological testing. When deciding upon which test to order, consider ease of obtaining, costs, and clinical implications of abnormal findings.

In clinical practice, baseline screening tests often include a complete blood cell (CBC) count; serum chemistry; kidney function tests, such as blood urea nitrogen (BUN) and creatinine; levels of thyroid-stimulating hormone (TSH), vitamin B_{12}, and folate; anerythrocyte sedimentation rate (ESR); levels of substances in the urine and serum (i.e., toxicology); and syphilis serologies. Liver function tests (LFTs) are also frequently obtained, especially in patients with known liver disease, and those at high risk for liver dysfunction (e.g., secondary to alcohol abuse), or in those taking medications that are potentially hepatotoxic (Wiechers, Smith, & Stern, 2010). Additional screening tests may be added on the basis of complaints or findings during the assessment. Neuropsychological testing is often ordered to identify cognitive deficits, to differentiate dementia from depression or to identify learning disorders. Testing for level of intelligence as well as personality characteristics is also common. Baseline testing for specific syndromes will be discussed in later chapters.

ACUTE TREATMENT

Goals of acute treatment are to bring about change in the target symptoms and provide safety. The target symptoms are those that are most distressing or most important to the client. Outpatient appointments are usually scheduled weekly and if a risk to self or others, inpatient treatment may be necessary. Initiation of acute treatment for specific syndromes is discussed in detail in following chapters. Many agencies now have computerized plans with specific interventions for client problems but it is important to remember to individualize treatment.

THERAPEUTIC COMMUNICATION TECHNIQUES

In addition to the communication techniques previously discussed, now additional approaches such as interpretation and gentle confrontation are added to facilitate self-examination and the change process. Clarification gently moves toward *interpretation* and *confrontation*. For example, a client who is emerging from a depressive episode states that he feels lonely. During a discussion about his lonely feelings, the PMH-APRN asks "What do you think keeps things going this way?"With further elaboration, the client recognizes that he has been extremely negative and avoidant, often not answering the telephone and refusing invitations to socialize. Of course, this behavior can be attributed to the depression and not a source of guilt. But also, a recognition that he has the ability to change his behavior and influence his lonely feelings (self-efficacy) will emerge. Cozolino (2002) has stated that this attention to self-awareness or bringing unconscious material to awareness facilitates neuronal growth in new directions and the integration of top-down and right-left processing results in broader choices for the client.

Also during this stage of treatment, issues surrounding medication may be explored. For example, the client has developed a pattern of "forgetting" her medication several times a week. Exploring this pattern of forgetting may be facilitated by a gentle confrontation such as, "Let's talk about taking medication every day. What does that mean when someone needs medication on a daily basis?" Issues around being labeled sick, lack of money, identification with helplessness, anger, or side effects may now be processed.

Another form of confrontation may involve pointing out and exploring behaviors during the sessions. For example, "You have told me that your father was often angry and irritated with you and I notice that you easily become angry during our appointments. I wonder if you are trying to have me understand your experiences by having me in a similar experience?" This attributes a purpose to the anger in a manner that is not adversarial while encouraging more discussion and self-awareness. Also it is important to continue building upon strengths using recognition and positive affirmations while reframing, offering information, and problem solving.

STABILIZATION/MAINTENANCE

Now that the initial discomfort is relieved, the challenge becomes how to maintain the improvement. We all have difficulty maintaining change, as evidenced by the multitude of weight loss plans, reminders from our dentists for check-ups, or even reminders such as oil lights in our cars. During this stage of treatment, focus moves to potential or actual side effects of treatment and strategies to minimize these problems. Cost becomes an issue for many clients and must be addressed. Conditions that have triggered or maintained the client's symptoms are now also addressed and may include interpersonal conflicts, illogical thoughts, stressful work, lifestyle issues such as lack of exercise and poor eating habits, or simply lack of structure. Shifting to a more psychoeducational approach for prevention strategies, combined with discussions about relapse possibilities while including significant others, is also appropriate. When involving significant others, this may result in identifying the need for treatment of others in the client's environment.

During stabilization, shifts to groups, more self-help, and extended time between appointments is often appropriate. However, attention to the process of relationship building cannot be ignored. Before shifting timing or structure of treatment, these changes must be discussed and processed to avoid feelings of rejection and premature discontinuation of treatment.

TERMINATION

Termination of treatment is usually discussed during the first few sessions as part of treatment planning and often in response to client questions such as, "How long will I need to take these medications?" or "How long until I feel better?" It may have included a specific time limit ("four sessions and then we will reevaluate") or specific goals ("when you are able to sleep through the night, return to work or school, or symptoms are gone"). In some cases of serious and persistent mental illness, treatment, especially pharmacotherapy, may continue indefinitely.

Another consideration is sequencing of termination if involved in more than one treatment modality. Often, psychotherapy is time-limited and pharmacotherapy continues for 9 months to a year. It is important to appreciate the anxiety associated with termination and to gradually discontinue treatment when appropriate, one modality at a time. Usually, there are agreed upon check-ups after a month, then every 2 or 3 months. Final termination is not really final, with the PMH-APRN discussing the option of a client calling for a follow-up in the future or in case of relapse. Thoughtful termination involves discussions about triggers, early symptoms, and appropriate actions.

During termination, continued use of clinical supervision assists in avoiding boundary violations due to strong transference and countertransference. During this time there is an increased risk of accepting expensive gifts, and emotional or sexual involvement. Issues such as hugging, answering personal questions, and accepting small gifts should be discussed in supervision. These are complicated issues after being involved in a therapeutic relationship over time. Termination is an important part of treatment and contributes to decisions for future treatment.

REFERENCES

American Psychiatric Association. (1994). *Diagnostic and statistical manual of mental disorders* (4th ed.). Washington, DC: Author.

Benner, P. (1982). From novice to expert. *American Journal of Nursing, 82*(3), 402–407.

Benner, P. (2000). The wisdom of practice. *American Journal of Nursing, 100*(10), 99–102.

Carlat, D. (2005). *The psychiatric interview* (2nd ed.). Philadelphia, PA: Lippincott Williams & Wilkins.

Cozolino, L. (2002). *The neuroscience of psychotherapy*. New York, NY: Norton.

Dobbs, D. (2006). A revealing reflection. *Scientific American Mind, 17*, 22–27.

Duncan, B., Miller, S., Wampold, B., & Hubble, M. (2010). *The heart and soul of change* (2nd ed.). Washington, DC: American Psychological Association.

Eells, T. (Ed.) (2007). *Handbook of psychotherapy case formulation* (2nd ed.). New York, NY: Guilford.

Krasner, M. S., Epstein, R. M., Beckman, H., Suchman, A. L., Chapman, B., Mooney, C. J., & Quill, T. E. (2009). Association of an educational program in mindfulness with burnout, empathy, and attitudes among primary care physicians. *Journal of the American Medical Association, 302*(12), 1284–1293.

Lankton, S., & Bandler, L. (2003). *Practical magic: A translation of basic neuro-linguistic programming into clinical psychotherapy*. Wales, UK & Williston, VT: Crown House.

Lazarus, R. (1991). *Emotion and adaptation*. New York, NY: Oxford University Press.

Lopez, S. & Snyder, C. (2003). *Positive Psychological Assessment: A handbook of models and measures*. Washington, DC: American Psychological Association (Electronic version published 2011).

McGoldrick, M., Gerson, R., & Shellenberger, S. (1999). *Genograms in family assessment*. New York, NY: Norton.

McGuinness, T., Noonan, P., & Dyer, J. (2009). Family history as a tool for psychiatric nurses. *Archives of Psychiatric Nursing, 19*(3), 116–124.

Moyers, T., Miller, W., & Hendrickson, S. (2005). How does motivational interviewing work? Therapist interpersonal skill predicts client involvement within sessions. *Journal of Consulting and Clinical Psychology, 73*, 590–598.

Norcross, J., Hedges, M., & Castle, P. (2002). Psychologists conducting psychotherapy: A study of division 29 membership. *Psychotherapy: Theory, Research, Practice, and Training, 39*(1), 97–102.

Pascal, G. R. (1983). *The practical art of diagnostic interviewing*. Homewood, IL: Dow Jones-Irwin.

Rogers, C. (1961). *On becoming a person*. Boston, MA: Houghton Mifflin.

Sadock, B., & Sadock, V. (2007). *Kaplan & Sadock's synopsis of psychiatry* (10th ed.). Philadelphia, PA: Lippincott Williams & Wilkins.

Sadock, B. & Sadock, V. (2010). *Kaplan and Sadock's pocket handbook of clinical psychiatry*. Philadelphia, PA: Lippincott, Williams, & Wilkins.

Shea, S. (1998). *Psychiatric interviewing: The art of understanding* (2nd ed.). Philadelphia, PA: Saunders.

Shea, S. (2002). *The practical art of suicide assessment*. Hoboken, NJ: Wiley.

Sleeth, D. B. (2010). Integral Love: The role of love in clinical practice as a rite of passage. *Journal of Humanistic Psychology, 50*(4), 471–494.

Thase, M., Riba, M., & Safer, D. (2003). *Integrating psychotherapy and pharmacotherapy*. New York, NY: Norton.

Wachtel, P. (2011). *Therapeutic communication* (2nd ed.). New York, NY: Guilford.

Wenger, E., McDermott, R., & Snyder, W. (2002). *Communities of practice: A guide to managing knowledge*. Boston, MA: Harvard Business School Press.

Wiechers, I., Smith, F., & Stern, T. (2010). A guide to judicious use of laboratory tests and diagnostic procedures in psychiatric practice. *Psychiatric Times, 27*(5), 48–51.

Wilson, I. (1967). Rapid approximate intelligence test. *American Journal of Psychiatry, 123*, 1289–1290.

Yalom, I. (2005). *The theory and practice of group psychotherapy* (5th ed.). New York, NY: Basic Books.

Zuckerman, E. (2010). *Clinician's thesauraus, 7th Edition: The guide to conducting interviews and writing psychological reports*. New York, NY: Guilford Press.

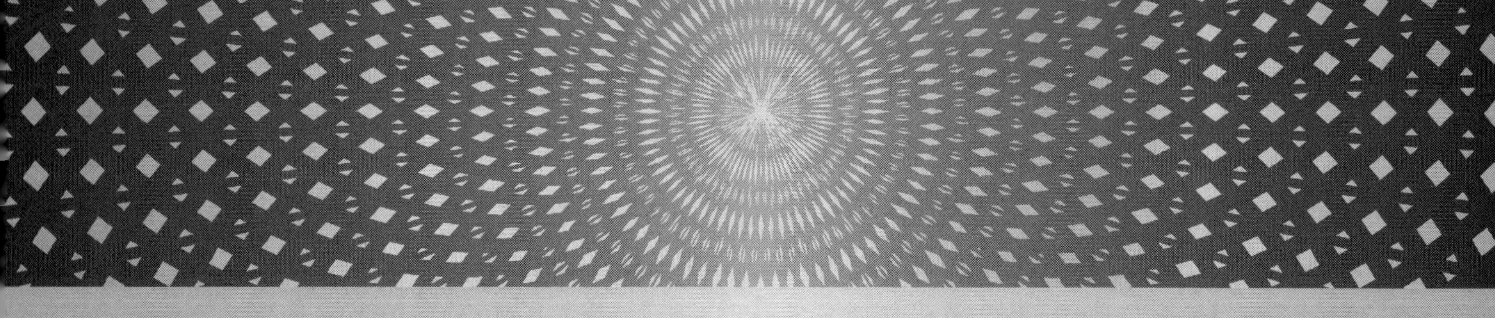

SECTION III

Integrative Management of Specific Syndromes

CHAPTER CONTENTS

OVERVIEW

Mood disorders are a unique and broad diagnostic category used by traditional as well as current diagnostic classifications (Faravelli, Ravaldi, & Truglia, 2005). Mood refers to an individual's sustained feeling tone that is experienced internally and prevails over time, while affect refers to the observed expression of the feeling state (Yudofsky & Hales, 2004). Mood is central to health and well-being and is important to our everyday lives of perceiving, evaluating, appraising, understanding, and acting in the world. Periods of mood shifting to sadness are considered normal and often vary with the cultural expectations of emotional expression. However, a persistent depressed mood is problematic and can occur at any age from a wide range of causes. This change from normal sadness to depression is described in terms of duration, possible shifts to higher than normal energy levels, and the severity of associated symptoms including disturbance of appetite, sleep, psychomotor activity (increased or decreased), loss of pleasure, cognitive impairment resulting in difficulty concentrating, and negative self-thoughts often including suicidal considerations (American Psychiatric Association [APA], 1994). Psychotic symptoms and catatonia may or may not be present.

Community studies show a continuous dimension of mood disturbance severity with a large number of people experiencing a few symptoms of mild to moderate severity, as well as a smaller number of those with increased

CHAPTER 8

Integrative Management of Disordered Mood

Kathleen R. Tusaie

severity of multiple symptoms. It is important to consider those with subclinical depressive symptoms because they are at higher risk for future clinical depression and suicide than the general population and usually not in treatment (Goldberg, 2000; Jorm & Griffiths, 2006). Over one million people die by suicide worldwide each year and that averages out to about one person dying by suicide every 40 seconds (Center for Disease Control and Prevention, 2010). Furthermore, 90% of individuals who die by suicide have a mood disorder. When an individual experiences changes in mood that result in impaired functioning in relationships, work, leisure activities, or educational pursuits, interventions are needed.

Although symptoms of mood disorders are generally related to emotions, bodily symptoms are very common in depressed persons. Vegetative symptoms form an integral part of diagnostic criteria for depression, including rumination about fatigue, weight loss, and pain ("somatic depression" or "masked depression"). These physical complaints occur frequently among the elderly who are depressed as well as certain cultures (Ballas & Staab, 2003; Suen & Tusaie, 2004). Children and adolescents with vague physical symptoms without identifiable cause may be showing the first signs of depression. These symptoms may involve any organ in the body, and often extensive medical work-ups take place with no positive findings. Headaches, stomach aches, generalized aches and pains, and symptoms affecting multiple organs are common complaints. Persistence of these symptoms may make the clients move from one medical facility to another at the cost of their time, energy, and resources. Up to 76% of individuals hospitalized for depression in the United States report multiple pain symptoms (Fava, 2003).

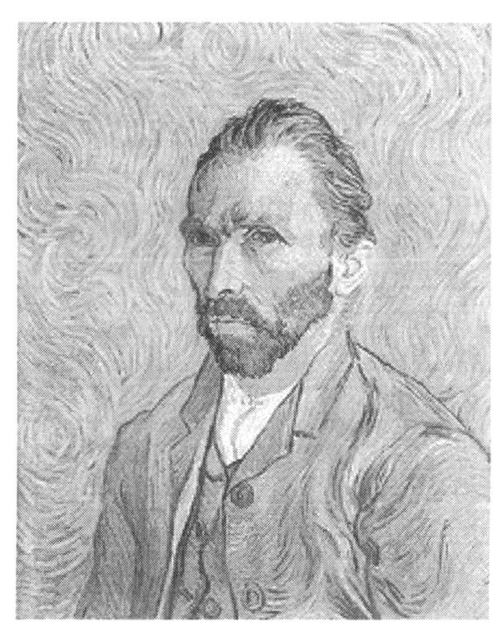

Vincent van Gogh's 1889 *Self Portrait* suggests the artist's mood and affect in the time leading up to his suicide. *Source*: Musée d'Orsay, Paris, http://www.ibiblio.org/wm/paint/auth/gogh/self/

To further complicate the presentation of mood disturbances, there is often the coexistence of another psychiatric disorder such as anxiety or other chronic and persistent psychiatric disorders. Medical problems or substances used by the client may also be responsible for the disturbed mood. But whatever the cause or causes of the mood disturbance, there is much suffering involved.

Children of depressed parents are at a significantly higher risk of developing a depressive disorder than the general population and rates of divorce for depressed persons are higher than the general population (Wade & Kendler, 2000). In addition to individual and family suffering, the economic burden of mood disorders is quite large (Greenberg, Leong, Birnbaum, & Robinson, 2003). This burden is related to cost of treatment, lost earnings due to suicide, absenteeism, and accidents. Therefore, mood disorders are a burden for individuals, families, employers, third-party payors, caregivers, and society in general.

Although disturbance of mood is a universal experience, culture can influence the language used to describe moods. For example, in Latino and Mediterranean cultures depression is reported as "nerves" and headaches. Weakness, tiredness, or imbalance are often the complaints in Chinese and other Asian cultures. Problems of the heart is the usual complaint of depressed mood in Middle Eastern cultures and experiencing a broken heart in Hopi culture (Arnault, Sakamoto, & Marwaki, 2005; Shin, 2010). Furthermore, the Men's Health and Aging Study from National Institute of Mental Health (Guilford-Blake, 2010) has reported that older men do not use red flag words such as blue or sad but discuss depression in terms of lost productivity. Older Hispanic men linked decreased productivity to inability to care for family members while white non-Hispanic older men linked productivity to individual functioning.

> *I am now the most miserable man living. If what I feel were equally distributed to the whole human family, there would be not one cheerful face on earth. Whether I shall ever be better, I cannot tell. I awfully forebode I shall not. To remain as I am is impossible. I must die or be better it appears to me.*
>
> Abraham Lincoln (Basler, 1953).

The World Health Organization measures the suffering of populations based upon time lived with disability or Disability-Adjusted Life Years (DALY). The largest cause of DALYs worldwide is the mood disorder, Major Depression. At any point in time, approximately 5% to 10% of the world's population is suffering from a mood disorder. The lifetime risk of developing a mood disorder is 10% to 20% in females and about half that in males (Murray & Lopez, 1996). These gender differences emerge over a lifetime, with childhood depression more common in boys than girls, but prevalence in children is only about 2.8% with rates increasing when based upon interviews only with children and not their parents. Then during adolescence (>13 years), depression is more common in girls and the overall prevalence rate spikes up to about 14% (Lewinsohn & Essau, 2002). During adulthood (18+) there is about a 16.6% prevalence rate. Fifty percent of children and adolescents in the United States have recalled depressive symptoms between a 1-week and 6-month period. Furthermore, the rates of depression in the elderly have been estimated to be 17% to 34%, which exceeds the general adult rate. The International Consortium in Psychiatric Epidemiology has predicted this prevalence rate for mood disorders will progressively increase during the next 20 years (Murray & Lopez, 1996).

The high global prevalence, associated disability, cost, and mortality make mood disorders a major health issue, imposing quite a burden on the community. The importance of early identification of mood disordered versus normal mood fluctuations is crucial for the appropriate interventions to be initiated.

SPECTRUM OF MOODS

Mood may be described according to discrete symptoms as in the *Diagnostic and Statistical Manual* (*DSM*) (APA, 1994). When an individual experiences symptoms above the normal with elevated, expansive, or irritable mood, or below the normal with depression and loss of interest or pleasure, a disorder may exist. If the symptoms are less severe, the terms hypomania and dysthymia are used. Hypomania also requires a duration of at least 2 years. Another way to describe mood is to consider a continuum in which an individual moves into, between, and among these different overlapping types of mood. Thinking of mood on a continuum allows the description of an individual's mood to be more realistic than attempts to fit individuals into the discrete categories. This approach refines the description of moods further to include temperament as (hyperthymic, depressive, or mixed temperament) as illustrated in Figure 8-1.

ETIOLOGY

Mood disorders are complex and multi-causal. As far back as Greek antiquity, a biological nature to mood disorders was discussed. Today, the Diathesis-Stress Model is the generally accepted explanation. This model hypothesizes that individuals have a genetic predisposition (diathesis) which is activated by stress, often involving loss. First, the genetic predisposition information will be presented followed by information about the experience of stress.

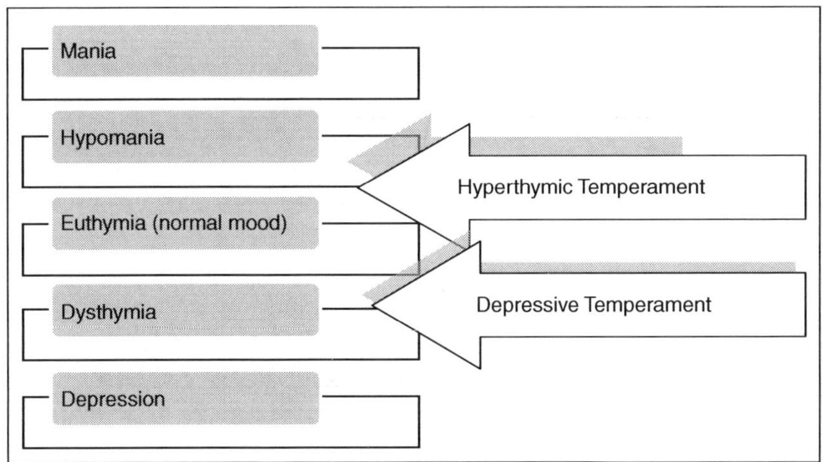

Figure 8-1 The Mood Spectrum

DIATHESIS

The monoamine hypothesis posits that depression is the result of deficiency in one or more of the three monoamines, serotonin (5-HT), norepinephrine (NE), and dopamine (DA), leading to up-regulation of postsynaptic receptors in the brain. Depending upon which monoamine pathways and receptors are affected, the specific symptom profile of an individual's depression will emerge. The genetic work surrounding the serotonin transporter gene 5-HTT by molecular biologists has been in the spotlight of research for some time and has generated the serotonin hypothesis to partially explain the diathesis.

Although the specifics of this model remain unclear, there have been some recent illuminating research findings in molecular biology and brain imaging (Martinowich & Lu, 2008). The serotonin transporter promoter is called the 5-HTTLPR. The promoter region of a gene is the on and off switch. Unless a gene is needed in a cell type, this switch is usually turned off. Structural variations in the 5-HTTLPR are inherited. One variation is the short allele (s), named for the shorter length when compared to the normal unmutated versions. Another variation is the long allele (l) named for the longer than normal length. These variations have proven to be important.

If an individual carries at least one short allele, the risk of developing depression increases. And the risk increases if the individual carries both short alleles. However, not every individual at risk develops a mood disorder. There must also be increased stress levels for the disordered mood to develop.

Imaging studies have identified one structural and one functional brain difference between depressed and nondepressed individuals, which correlates to the serotonin findings. Individuals with depression have a measurable shrinkage in the area of the anterior cingulate cortex associated with a reduction in gray matter. The functional difference involves the affective circuit between the amygdala and the anterior cingulate.

The amygadala can process both positive and negative emotions. Individuals with short alleles show similar responses to positive, nonstressful emotions as controls. But, responses to negative emotions are processed very differently in the individual with a short allele genotype. Healthy short allele carriers had decreased signal processing similar to individuals who were depressed. Although this information is beginning to explain vulnerability, the role stress plays in triggering the disorder in susceptible individuals remains unclear.

Hormonal Changes and Depression

The hormonal changes of puberty, the menstrual cycle, the postpartum period, and menopause may trigger depression in women with a genetic or other vulnerability (Steiner, Dunn, & Born, 2003). This is related to the interaction of estrogen with the monoamines, gamma-aminobutyric acid (GABA), and glutamate. These are multiple, complex interactions with estrogen specifically having a profound influence on serotonergic functions.

STRESS

Resilience

As research into positive coping with stress increases, interest in resilience or the ability to adapt well in the face of adversity (Tusaie & Dyer, 2004) has been explored in the development and treatment of depression. Resilient reactions to stress are associated with an ability to keep the hypothalamic-pituitary-adrenocortical (HPA) system and noradrenergic activity within an optimal range during stress exposure, and terminate the stress response once the stressor is no longer present (Southwick, Vythillingham, & Charney, 2005). There is controversy surrounding the genetic predisposition for this ability as well as the ability to learn this response. Predictors of a resilient response to stress vary across developmental stages but generally include perceived social support (family and friends) and a sense of connectedness, optimism, and cognitive flexibility (Herman et al., 2011; Tusaie, Puskar, & Sereika, 2007; Ozbay et al., 2007).

The broaden-and-build theory posits the upward spiral of positive emotions counters the downward spirals of negativity experienced during depressive moods. So that by facilitating the development of positive emotions there is a building of durable personal resources, which triggers further well-being and exerts a countervailing force on the depressive experience (Garland et al., 2010). So, it is not only the genetic predisposition and stressors experienced that explain the development of mood disorders but also the protective factors and resources within and around the individual that contribute to etiology.

Evolutionary Explanation

Another existentially based possible explanation for depressive episodes is related to evolution (Andrews & Thompson, 2009). If depression is a disorder, then evolution has made a mistake because depression is almost as prevalent as the common cold. Depression leads people to stop having sex and consider suicide, actions not conducive to continuation of the race. The alternate explanation is that depression has a purpose. Like fever helping the immune system fight off infection, perhaps depression has a purpose. Is this an adaptation or an accident of evolution? Perhaps the decrease in pleasurable experience and lack of motivation reduce thinking about and learning from the current stressor. If depression did not exist, if we did not react to stressors and trauma with rumination, then we would be less likely to solve our predicaments. Wisdom isn't cheap and it develops with painful experiences. Although this thinking about depression is quite controversial, perhaps it is a reflection of the variable range of symptoms involved in mood disorders and our attempts to understand them.

Stressful Life Events

Another important path of research regarding stress triggering mood disorders is the exploration of life events. Several studies identified the experience of four severe stressful life events (death of close relative, assault, serious marital problems, and divorce) predicting depression in vulnerable individuals (Kendler & Gardner, 2010). Trauma in early life also partially predicted depression. Childhood sexual or physical abuse has been associated with persistent hypothalamic-pituitary-adrenocortical hyperactivity in adulthood, which is consistent with depression (Heim et al., 2000).

Another path to partially explain depression involves the subjective experience of stress. Cognitive models propose that it is not the level of the stressor but the perception of the event, or attribution style, that determines the level of stress experienced. However, there is much controversy surrounding the actual causal relationship between life events and depressive symptoms (Kendler & Gardner, 2010).

Interpersonal Relationships

Joiner and Coyne (1999) and Joiner and Timmons (2010) have eloquently explored the dynamic nature of interpersonal relationships and depression. Stable individual characteristics that predate a depressive episode are believed to increase risk for depression. These characteristics include low level of social skills, excessive reassurance seeking, negative speech content, aversive feedback-seeking behavior, less facial animation, and fewer nonverbal gestures. These characteristics are likely to have a negative influence on others and thereby decrease social support and exposure to pleasurable experiences.

Consequences of Depression

Depression has its own effects upon stress reactivity. Neurotransmitters are sensitized and lower the threshold for new episodes, leading to lower levels of stressor to trigger episodes. Negative cognitions increase with each episode, thus increasing negative ruminations. These ruminations lead to poor concentration and poor decision making. Women may be unable to provide appropriate parenting skills, which leads to increased stress with oppositional, critical children. Furthermore, depressed individuals tend to be attracted to individuals with unstable, dysfunctional lives. Subsequently, these relationships lead to chaotic lives and increased stressors.

Polarity and Etiology

When an individual's experience of depression includes polarity, there are some differences in etiology to consider. A range of studies suggest strong genetic contributions because the likelihood of developing a mood disorder with polarity is 7 times more likely among relatives (Walters, G. & Wellcome Trust Case Control Consortium, 2007). Attempts to identify actual genes involved, such as linkage to X-chromosome, to color blindness, to 4, 11, 18, and others, has been inclusive. This may be due to the faulty assumption that there is one gene when most likely there is a complex, multiple gene interaction with environmental factors.

Although genetics play a role in development of polarity, stressful life events are also believed to be involved, especially with the occurrence of mania. Disruptions in social zeitgebers (social demands or tasks that set the biological clock by environmental events) lead to instability in circadian rhythms which may trigger mania (Ehlers, Frank, & Kupfer, 1988). Severe social rhythm disruptions such as returning from international trips, moving, or losing a job have been reported to be associated with episodes of mania (Malkoff-Schwartz et al., 1998). However, association does not prove causality. But social rhythm disruptions partially explain the disturbance of circadian rhythms in individuals who experience some degree of polarity.

SUMMARY

The stress/diathesis model of depression is only partially understood, but it provides a basic framework for expanding understanding of the etiology of mood disturbances. There are multiple complex interrelationships among molecules, multigenerational genes and relationships, environments, cognitions, and behaviors. It is unlikely that one treatment approach, such as relieving depressive symptoms with medications, would be adequate to address these interrelationships. It is important to understand the client's thinking about the cause of their mood disorder and then offer additional or alternative theory and evidence-based explanations to facilitate a sense of cognitive control as well as realistic treatment planning. Therefore, Psychiatric Mental Health Advanced Practice Nurses (PMH-APRN) need to develop their own cohesive model or models of explanation to lay the framework for an integrated approach to treating mood disturbances.

SHARED DECISION MAKING/ACHIEVING CONCORDANCE

In addition to the basic skills of knowing how to maintain a positive therapeutic alliance and having communication skills including active listening, there are additional considerations specific to working with individuals experiencing mood disorders. As the client has moved into a type of hibernation, there is frequently the absence of interpersonal warmth and much difficulty in connecting interpersonally. In fact, Joiner and Coyne (1999) have suggested that the depressive symptoms are contagious. So, you may initially experience discomfort and desire to help the client but then may move to frustration and irritability with the difficulty of the interview flow. The opposite reaction is experienced with an individual in a hypomanic or manic state. Quantum Field Theory (2006) may be the best explanation for this interactional influence between and among individuals. In other words, thoughts are energy and this energy can influence one another. An awareness of your own countertransference reactions will assist with building a positive therapeutic relationship as well as the diagnostic process.

Even though it may be difficult, the process of collaboratively setting goals and treatment strategies with clients who have a mood disturbance is especially important for several reasons. First, this process directs the client to the future. This future orientation is vital for identifying reasons to live and weakening suicidal thoughts. Also, lack of self-worth is often a component of the mood disorder syndrome and inquiring into the client's goals and collaboratively working on strategies implicity suggests the client's hopes, dreams, and desires are worthy of attention and possibly attainable. This process then begins to undermine the client's negative self beliefs. Finally, by actively eliciting the client's involvement, isolation is decreased and the client begins to have an appreciation for their ability to affect those around them as well as to bring about change (Mackrill, 2010). Of course, the severity of the symptoms must be considered when eliciting and expecting involvement by the client. A severely depressed individual may only be able to participate minimally during the first few sessions and then gradually increase participation as the depression begins to lift. And if the individual is on the other side of the spectrum, mania or hypomania, limit-setting on involvement may be necessary until the client is more stable. The PMH-APRN does not act as a technician with preset approaches and expectations, but as a professional with a theory base and appreciation of their own style combined with ongoing reflection and adjustment with each client.

BEARING WITNESS TO SUFFERING

Clients who are deeply depressed often complain and focus upon negatives. It is important to show genuine caring and interest combined with the ability to bear witness to their suffering. Often, the desire to be a PMH-APRN involves wanting to help others. However, the need to assist individuals with change cannot move forward until their suffering is first acknowledged. This is accomplished with several strategies. First, listen and reflect initially on a basic and then a complex level as the treatment progresses. During the sessions, reflections should be interspersed every 5 to 20 minutes with one or two empathetic statements during the first 5 to 10 minutes of the initial session (Shea, 1998). Also, clients who are depressed often cry. Shea (1998) suggests allowing the client to cry briefly and using statements such as "You seem sad now. ... It's all right to cry... it's our bodies' way of telling us we are hurting... maybe you can tell me more about what is hurting you" and offer a tissue.

However, if the crying becomes profuse, you may need to gently redirect by stating, "you are having a difficult time but it is important that we continue talking...perhaps you can take a few minutes and collect yourself."

To maintain safety and acceptance in the therapeutic relationship, it is important to have the ability to manage the client's emotional reactions, such as crying, as well as your reaction to the client. Your actions also serve as a model for the client's future application. If you become over-solicitous and sympathetic, this will increase the sense of powerlessness felt by the client. If you immediately redirect the crying, this will shut down the interview and result in a guarded, unsafe relationship.

So, the question becomes how to recognize and manage your reactions. First, it is important to be aware of your own thoughts and experiences with crying. When do you cry and what is the meaning? Does crying represent weakness or a natural healthy outlet? What experiences have you had with others crying? You may choose to discuss this with a peer, supervisor, your own therapist, or explore on your own. Some people think of brief periods of sadness and crying as "homework." This involves being in touch with their own areas of sadness and eliciting this emotion by thinking about past losses and crying.

Another approach to reflect upon your own reactions is to use visualization related to the client session. Find a quiet, peaceful place, close your eyes, and take a few deep breaths. Then think of your greatest fear related to a client crying. Picture the scene in great detail and notice the feelings that arise in you. Hold that for a few minutes. Then yawn and move around and open your eyes. Next, write down what you have pictured. Realistically, what parts of this scene are likely to occur and what parts probably won't happen? Then think about what parts were created mostly out of your feelings? Compare the lists. Next, close your eyes, take a few deep breaths, and imagine your client crying and your interventions in a realistic manner. Hold on to this briefly, then smile and move around after opening your eyes. As you become aware of your own history and emotions, you become less reactive and more able to bear witness to suffering and to be helpful to clients.

ASSESSMENT

The primary purpose of assessment is to make a diagnosis and case conceptualization to assist in the choice of treatments, as well as to make a prognosis to anticipate the course of the illness. Be curious as to the experience for this client while also considering diagnostic criteria. The assessment involves present status and presenting complaint, and history including physical status. The components of the assessment are presented in more detail in Chapter 7 while this chapter will focus upon the unique aspects of assessing an individual with a mood disorder.

The major task when assessing a client's mood is to differentiate between normal fluctuations of mood and affect and clinical syndromes. Determination of the symptom severity, safety, as well as available strengths within the individual and environment are identified. This is achieved only when viewed as a process of understanding the person within the context of his or her life and using a systematic assessment process. Developing and maintaining the therapeutic, trusting relationship is necessary for collection of a valid database. This dual process results in the collaborative development of a diagnosis as well as a case conceptualization leading to a plan for treatment.

SUICIDAL AND HOMICIDAL THOUGHTS

Another important topic is suicidal and homicidal thoughts. This must be addressed and considered with every client but especially with individuals with mood disorders. These topics are addressed in depth in Chapters 15 and 16.

DIAGNOSIS

Signs

A clinical interview is the primary method of diagnosing mood disorders. Before any words are spoken, signs of depression will be seen and felt by the PMH-APRN. Although mood disorders are experienced and presented in ways unique to each individual and each developmental stage, there are similarities in presentation. Facial expressions and gestures are usually limited. Nutritional status may be reflected in a person's weight. Personal hygiene may be lacking with an unkempt appearance including dirty nails, messy clothing, and hair. An emptiness in an individual's eyes and lack of eye contact are also often present. As the individual walks into your office, there is a slowness of movement and overall lack of responsiveness. The opposite may be true with hypomania or mania. This may involve the client dressing in a flamboyant or seductive manner with excessive jewelry and makeup, while being overly friendly and talkative. Of course, it is important to be alert to social and professional norms as to not be judgmental. Another possible presentation of depressive symptoms is the individual who is agitated. There is constant movement, an inability to sit still, and distressed facial expression. As discussed in Chapter 7, there are other important observations of posture and movements during every clinical session.

The mental status exam begins with your first observation. As the interview continues, be careful to avoid broad general questions or there may be false positives. For example, by asking "Have you been depressed?" the client may think he or she is mostly tired and has back pain, but is not depressed. So, ask specific questions to elicit symptoms, review a self-report questionnaire, or use a structured interview form. At the same time, there must be empathetic statements to facilitate building of the relationship. The skilled PMH-APRN operates on multiple levels with the depressed client—jumping into the relationship to understand the subjective experience of the client, jumping back to recognize symptoms and signs, while also considering safety issues.

Children

In infants, Failure to Thrive (FTT) has many similarities to depression and is believed to be one manifestation of depression in infancy. FTT involves weight below the 3rd percentile, on body charts, psychomotor delay, iron deficiency, behavioral problems, and feeding problems with no identified disease process (Krugman & Dubowitz, 2003).

In the structured assessment, *DSM* criteria for depressive episodes are often used either by asking a set of predetermined questions (Structured Clinical Interview for *DSM-IV*) or less structured questions while keeping the criteria in mind. When assessing children, it is important to use multiple sources of information. Children are likely to know more about their internal subjective states while teachers and parents might be better reporters of observed symptoms. Furthermore, there are very small correlations between parents', children's, and teachers' reports so all three are needed for the best picture. Self-rating and clinician rating scales can also assist not only with assessment but also with the responses to treatment.

Because mood is subjective and reports retrospective, researchers are working to develop more accurate techniques for reporting mood changes. Wenze and Miller (2010) are using Ecological Momentary Assessment (EMA), which is basically intensive sampling of current emotional experience while engaged in normal activities in natural environments. This may involve questionnaires or biological and physiological measurements, which are self-administered, automated, or clinician administered. Initial data suggest that EMA is feasible and highly promising for data collection in mood disorders. Although EMA is not commonly used in clinical settings, the strategy of keeping a daily log of moods experienced by self-rating is a common practice. An example of a mood log may be downloaded at www.psychiatry24x7.com/bgdisplay.jhtml?itemname=mooddiary

SYMPTOMS/QUESTIONNAIRES

Self-rating questionnaires are especially useful for clients with depressed mood because they often are slowed in their thinking and responses. The paper and pencil questionnaire may be completed prior to or during the appointment and then reviewed, discussed, and interpreted during the session. Most questionnaires take approximately 5 to 10 minutes to complete. Of course, the client's ability to read, write, and comprehend must be determined in terms of physical and cognitive abilities as well as intellectual limitations before providing the questionnaire. It is also important to assess the reliability and validity of any questionnaire before using it. Computer-based questionnaires have been reported to provide more valid data from adolescents than written responses or face-to-face interviews. Commonly used clinical measures for assessing mood disturbances will be discussed and presented in Table 8-1. with information on reliability, validity, and availability.

Adults

There are several self-rating and clinician-rating forms for assessing disordered moods. *The Hamilton Depression Rating Scale* (*HAM-D*) provides a semi-structured interview format that has been used for the assessment of adult depression for more than 40 years. It was developed primarily to determine the effects of treatment with the first generation antidepressants (Hamilton, 1960) and became

TABLE 8-1: MEASURES COMMONLY USED FOR SCREENING OF MOOD DISTURBANCES ACROSS THE LIFE SPAN

NAME	AGE APPROPRIATENESS	PUBLIC DOMAIN
Hamilton Depression Rating Scale (HAM-D)	adults	Yes
Montgomery-Asberg Depression Rating Scale (MADRS)	adults	Yes
Zung Self-Rating Depression Screening tool (ZSDS)	adults	Yes
Inventory of Depressive Symptoms (IDS) Quick Inventory of Depressive Symptoms (QIDS)	adults	Yes
Mood Disorder Questionnaire (mania)	adults	Yes
Young Mania Rating Scale (degree of mania)	adults	Yes
Geriatric Depression Scale	60+	Yes
Cornell Scale for Depression in Dementia	60+	Yes
Beck Depression Inventory II (BDI)	14+ Questionable for elderly	No
Reynolds Adolescent Depression Scale (RADS)	13–18	No
Bipolarity Index	15+	Yes
Children's Depression Inventory (CDI)	7–17	No
Reynolds Child Depression Scale (RCDS)	8–12	No
Young Mania Rating Scale-Parent Version	7–18	Yes

the gold standard for measuring depressive symptoms, especially during drug studies. It is currently the most frequently used form for rating depressive symptoms (Williams, 2001). The clinician rates 21 symptom groupings on a scale from 0 (not present) to 4 (severe) at the time of the interview. There is no available self-rating version of the HAM-D. Scores range from 0 to 23 indicating severity of symptoms. Cronbach's alpha has ranged between 0.46 and 0.97. However, the HAM-D has been increasingly criticized for lack of interrater reliability and lack of any organizing framework. These weaknesses have led to poor replication across samples and reliance upon clinician's level of clinical expertise for valid results (Bagby, Ryder, Schuller, & Marshall, 2004). (The instrument and instructions for use may be downloaded at http://mentalhealthnurse.co.uk/more_info.asp?current_id=191) To address some of the limitations of the HAM-D, additional scales have been developed.

The Montgomery-Åsberg Depression Rating Scale (MADRS) is a semi-structured clinician rated interviewing form closely correlated to the HAM-D (r = .62). It has an expanded scoring scale of 7 points for each of the 10 items to be more sensitive to changes in depressive symptoms during treatment (Montgomery & Asberg, 1979). The instrument as well as a detailed comparison to the HAM-D may be downloaded at www.psych-world.com/madrs.htm

Another rating scale closely correlated (r = .69) to the HAM-D is the *Zung Self-Rating Depression Screening Tool (ZSDS)* (Zung, 1965). This quick self-report questionnaire is sensitive to identifying affective as well as somatic symptoms associated with depression. It consists of 10 statements with half framed positively and half negative statements. It is widely used for self-scoring and is on multiple websites, with the caution that results are not diagnostic and do not replace a professional examination. ZSDS tool with scoring may be downloaded at http://thewayup.com/newsletter/zung.htm

The next instrument developed was the *Inventory of Depressive Symptoms*. The Inventory of Depressive Symptoms (IDS) and the Quick Inventory of Depressive Symptomatology (QIDS) are both available in clinician-rated and self-rated versions (Rush et al., 1986; Rush, Gullion, Basco, Jarrett, & Trivedi, 1996). Both are written at the sixth-grade level of reading and designed for screening as well as determining the severity of symptoms related to mood disturbances. The IDS consists of 30 items while the QIDS was shortened to only 16 items for clinical convenience. The QIDS covers only the nine diagnostic symptom domains used by the *DSM-IV* (APA, 1994) to diagnose major depressive episode while the IDS also contains questions to address atypical and associated symptoms of depression. Both versions have demonstrated reliability and validity with clinical adult samples. Cronbach's alpha was 0.94 for both self and clinician rated versions of IDS (Rush et al., 1996; Rush, Carmody, & Reimitz, 2000), and both versions of the QIDS reported a Cronbach's alpha of 0.85 (Trivedi et al., 2004). These questionnaires have not yet demonstrated appropriateness for children/adolescents nor the elderly. The instruments as well as extensive information on development, scoring, and interpretation can be downloaded at www.ids-qids.org

The World Health Organization Collaborating Center in Mental Health has developed another self-report scale, the *Major Depression Inventory (MDI)*, using the International Coding Diagnostics (ICD)-10 and *DSM* criteria for Major Depression as the framework for questions. It consists of 11 items rated on a 7-point Likert scale from all the time to none of the time. The MDI is reliable and valid with a Cronbach's alpha of 0.89 and correlates strongly with other measures of depression, as well as with diagnosis from a clinical interview (Cuijpers, Dekker, Noteboom, Smits, & Peen, 2007). Scoring indicates the level of depression as well as a cutoff score for clinical diagnosis. The MDI may be downloaded at http://mentalhealthnurse.co.uk/more_info.asp?current_id=191

The Beck Depression Inventory Second Edition (BDI-II) is a 21-item self-report instrument intended to assess the existence and severity of symptoms of depression as listed in the APA's *Diagnostic and Statistical Manual of Mental Disorders–Fourth Edition (DSM-IV;* APA, 1994). This new revised edition replaces the BDI and the BDI-1A. When presented with the BDI-II, a patient is asked to consider each statement as it relates to the way they have felt for the past 2 weeks. Each of the 21 items corresponding to a symptom of depression is summed to give a single score for the BDI-II. There is a 4-point scale for each item ranging from 0 to 3. Total score of 0 to 13 is considered minimal range, 14 to 19 is mild, 20 to 28 is moderate, and 29 to 63 is severe (Beck, Ward, Mendelson, Mock, & Erhbaugh, 1961).

The BDI has been used for 35 years to identify and assess depressive symptoms, and has been reported to be highly reliable regardless of the population. It has a high coefficient alpha (.80), its construct validity has been established, and it is able to differentiate depressed from nondepressed patients. For the BDI-II, the coefficient alphas (.92 for outpatients and .93 for the college students) were higher than those for the BDI-1A (.86). The correlations for the corrected item total were significant at a .05 level (with a Bonferroni adjustment), for both the outpatient and the college student samples. Test-retest reliability was studied using the responses of 26 outpatients who were tested at first and second therapy sessions 1 week apart. There was a correlation of .93, which was significant at $p < .001$. The scale is reported to be appropriate for individuals 14 years old and up. (Beck & Steer, 1984). However, Sharp and Lipsky (2002) report that psychometric data on the BDI are mixed so the BDI may not be the best screening measure for elderly patients. Furthermore, the authors warn against the use of this instrument as a sole diagnostic measure, as depressive symptoms may be part of other primary diagnostic disorders. Harcourt Assessment, Inc., administers the rights for the Beck scales under contract from Dr. Beck. This tool can be purchased from them.

Older Adults

Scales specifically for adults over 60 years include the *Geriatric Depression Scale* long and short form and the *Cornell Scale for Depression in Dementia*. Elderly individuals require screening for cognitive impairment before administering a self-report questionnaire. A Folstein Mini Mental Status Exam (MMSE) of 15 or less usually excludes the use of self-report (Folstein, Folstein, & McHugh, 1975). Depressive symptoms seen more frequently in the elderly than other age groups include decreased ability for self-care, irritability, psychomotor retardation and "pseudodementia." Depression is rarely the only illness an older adult is experiencing. Multiple physical complaints without any identifiable cause are also often present. Also, approximately 50% of individuals with Alzheimer's disease or Parkinson's disease also develop a depressive disorder and their caretakers are at increased risk for depression (Butler & Lewis, 1995). Furthermore, 25% of adults with heart disease or diabetes also have depression. Medical illness is associated with increased rates of depression and depression is associated with poorer physical health and total health care costs (Kessler & Merikangas, 2004).

The original *Geriatric Depression Scale (GDS)* (Brink et al., 1982) is now shortened to 15 items framed from the past week and responses are only yes or no. Fewer questions and less response options (than 4–7 point scale) allow for easier comprehension. Both the original and the short form have demonstrated robust reliability and validity with an average Cronbach's alpha of 0.9 (Sheikh & Yesauage, 1986). The GDS with information about the development and scoring, as well as the opportunity to blog about use of the scale, can be viewed and downloaded at www.stanford.edu~yesavage/Testing.htm

If the client is cognitively or visually impaired, the use of a semi-structured interview with the Hamilton Depression Scale or the Cornell Scale for Depression in Dementia (Alexopoulos, Abrams, Young, & Shamoian, 1988) is indicated. The caregiver is the most appropriate respondent. The Cornell Scale consists of 19 items rated on a 4-point scale from the past week. Responses are totaled and a sum over 12 indicates depression and further assessment is needed. This scale has been translated to several languages and consistently demonstrates test-retest reliability and validity with a Cronbach's alpha of .86. The Cornell Scale for Depression in Dementia with instructions may be downloaded at http://scalesandmeasures.net/files/files/The%20Cornell%20Scale%20for%20Depression%20in%20Dementia.pdf.

Children and Adolescents

There are few developmental differences in the symptoms of depression but the expression of the symptoms does have developmental variation. During infancy, brief expressions of sadness usually appear in the last quarter of the first year and are seen as crying, brief withdrawal, and brief anger. During early childhood, withdrawal over losses due to death or loss of a treasured object are expected. Middle childhood often involves loss of self-esteem over failures in addition to the sadness of loss. Children in hospitals or institutions may experience some of the emotions that accompany death or separation and mimic a grief reaction. When the sadness persists and is combined with other symptoms, criteria for a disorder are met. In addition to sadness, the child may have temper tantrums in increased number and severity and physical symptoms such as constipation, enuresis, encopresis, and nightmares. There may also be brief thoughts of suicide, apathy, boredom, low self-esteem, irritability, and physical symptoms such as headaches and stomach aches. Social withdrawal, loss of interest, and psychotic symptoms (hallucinations and delusions) may also be present. Due to limited language abilities of children, it is vital to include others, parents, siblings, and teachers during the assessment process. When gathering information from a variety of settings and people involved with the child, it is recommended to value all information equally.

There are several structured interviews for assessing mood disorders in children. *Diagnostic Interview for Children and Adolescents* (*DICA*) (Reich, 2000) and *Children's Interview for Psychiatric Symptoms* (*CHIPS*) (Weller Fristad, Rooney, & Schecter, 2000) are appropriate for age 6 and over. Both interview tools have good interrater reliability and moderate reliability. The *Schedule for Affective Disorders and Schizophrenia for School Age Children (K-SADS)* (Kaufman et al., 1997) is widely used with children as young as 8 and has adequate reliability and validity. Finally, there are measures created to evaluate mood disturbances in very young preschool children. Pictorial instruments such as the *Preschool Symptom Self-Report* (*PRESS*) (Martini, Strayhorn, & Puig-Antich, 1990) and the *Dominic-R* and the *Terry Questionnaires* (Valla, Bergeron, & Smolla, 2000). The *Berkeley Puppet Interview* (*BPI*) (Measelle, Ablow, Cowan, & Cowan, 1998) uses puppets to assess perceptions of academic and social competence, peer acceptance, anxiety, and depression in very young children.

The self-report questionnaire, *Children's Depression Inventory* (*CDI*), was developed by Kovacs (1992) to assist in identifying symptoms of depression in children age 7 to 17 years. The original form had 27 items and the revised version has 10 items. Each item has three possible responses and the child chooses the statement best describing them over the past 2 weeks. The scales include anhedonia, negative self-image, ineffectiveness, interpersonal problems, and negative mood. The CDI has demonstrated reliability and validity with Cronbach's alpha of 0.89 and test-retest correlation of 0.83. It is written at the first grade level and takes approximately 5 to 15 minutes to complete. It may be purchased at www.mhs.com and completed in paper and pencil, online, or software format. Teacher rating, parent rating, as well as child rating forms are available.

Another self-report questionnaire for children and adolescents is the *Center for Epidemiological Studies Depression Scale for Children* (*CES-DC*). This scale addresses the behavioral and cognitive components of depression and also adds a dimension for happiness. It has demonstrated poor reliability and validity and is not recommended for clinical use (Faulstich, Carey, Ruggiero, Enyart, & Gresham, 1986). The CES-DC may be viewed at www.brightfutures.org/mentalhealth/pdf/professionals/bridges/ces_dc.pdf

The *Reynolds Child Depression Scale* (Reynolds & Mazza, 1998) is a 30-item self-report for children in grades 3 through 6. It is widely used in research and is a reliable and valid measure for clinical identification of depression in children. Cronbach's alpha is 0.88. The items are based on *DSM* criteria for depression and rated on a 4-point Likert scale, almost never to all the time. The last item is five smiley faces rated from sad to happy. The Reynolds Child Depression Scale may be purchased at www.parinc.com

Developmental brain changes and social pressures during adolescence lead to displays of emotion ranging from overt anger to extreme sadness. So parents experience difficulty in knowing when moodiness is normal or when it is actually a symptom of mood disorders. The criteria for diagnosis are the same as adults but the evaluation of severity of symptoms, with a duration of 2 weeks or longer and difficulties in several areas of functioning (home, school, and friends) would indicate need for further assessment. Often during adolescence, depression is associated with substance abuse, and behavioral problems involving high risk behaviors such as reckless driving, shoplifting, fighting, sexual acting out, or apathy. Ghost driving, or standing on the front or top of a moving car, has caused so many head injuries and deaths in adolescents that the Center for Disease Control and Prevention (CDC) is now counting and reporting these incidents. Additional signs that professional help may be needed include dramatic changes in overall appearance such as style of dressing, multiple body piercings, bright hair color changes, change in peer group, lying, threats of suicide, decline in school performance and hesitancy attending school, excessive worries, and persistent fear of being different from peers. Physical symptoms may include recurrent headache, chronic fatigue, and abdominal pain. Furthermore, a family history of alcoholism and/or depression also increases the risk of a disorder. During adolescence, the prevalence of mood disorders increases significantly from childhood and subsequent episodes are common.

The screening questionnaires for adolescent mood disorders often have false positives, which are detected during follow-up clinical interviews (Roberts, Lewinsohn, & Seeley, 1991). Screenings are meant only to alert professionals, not make a diagnosis, and therefore should not be used alone for diagnostic purposes. The most commonly used screening for adolescent mood disorder is the CDI and the *Reynolds Adolescent Depression Scale (RADS)* (Reynolds, 1986).

The RADS is a 30-item self-report questionnaire with four domains—dysphoric mood, anhedonia/negative affect, negative self-evaluation, and somatic complaints. It is based upon the *DSM-IV* and the ICD 10, written at the 3rd-grade reading level, and takes approximately 5 to 10 minutes to complete. Scores for each subscale and a total score are made. The RADS has demonstrated strong reliability and validity with a Cronbach's alpha of .93 (Reynolds & Mazza, 1998). It may be purchased through Sigma Assessments at www.sigmaassessmentsystems.com

HISTORY OF MOOD DISORDER SYMPTOMS

As the recognition and understanding of mood disorders grow, it becomes clear that for many people depression is not only an acute, self-limiting episode but more of a lifelong illness that changes in terms of intensity and duration of symptoms. The process of subthreshold stimulation of neurons, kindling, may explain the recurrent nature of depression. Between episodes of depression, an individual's mood may appear normal, but there are subthreshold neuron changes which create a likelihood of another episode of depression. Just as tire tracks in a dirt road become deeper with each passing of a vehicle, it becomes more difficult to drive in another path (Frank et al., 2005).

In addition to repeated episodes, the scar hypothesis indicates permanent personality or temperament changes, including cognitive shifts, may occur as a result of depressive episodes. This has been especially explored in adolescents revealing increased shyness and decreased social skills following a depressive episode. However, this is controversial due to brain plasticity, especially if the adolescent received therapy and there is a greater likelihood of being resilient. So then the question becomes one of the type of thinking and mood that was present before the initial episode. In other words, what is the normal mood for this individual?

Understanding the course of the mood disorder involves an appreciation of more than the current status of the client. Tracking the history of the client's moods including contextual information (family, friends, life events) will contribute to increased understanding for both clinician and client, formation of an accurate diagnosis, case conceptualization, treatment plan, and evaluation of response to treatment.

When tracking an individual's mood results in evidence of shifts from depression to mania, this is considered bipolar illness (manic-depressive illness). When the shifts are less severe, perhaps from depression to hypomania, this is considered Bipolar II. Therefore, tracking past symptoms will assist with a more complete understanding of the diagnostic options. There are several scales commonly used for identifying symptoms of mania.

The *Mood Disorder Questionnaire (MDQ)* (Hirschfeld et al., 2000) is a simple self-report questionnaire developed by a group of experts and validated in psychiatric and community samples. It has a sensitivity of 0.281 and specificity of 0.972. The MDQ has been widely promoted as a screening self-report tool for bipolar disorder to avoid under recognition of bipolar disorder, especially with depressed individuals. It appears in multiple websites including many pharmacological sponsored sites also discussing use of their drugs for treatment. A recent study (Zimmerman et al., 2010) has reported that using the MDQ is as likely to identify borderline personality disorder as bipolar disorder and thus, there should be more caution with its use. As with all screening tools, there will be false positives and a diagnosis does require a clinical workup. Use of the MDQ will identify the clinician to the presence of mood swings, which is quite important in determining treatment (download, with scoring information: www.dbsalliance.org/pdfs/MDQ.pdf)

The *Young Mania Rating Scale* was first published in 1978 to assess the severity of mania symptoms in adults with a diagnosis of bipolar illness. It is clinician administered and evaluates 12 areas (elevated mood, increased energy, activity, sleep, irritability, speech rate & amount, thought disorder, content, aggressive, disruptive behavior, appearance, and insight) and each is rated for level of severity. It has demonstrated high interrater reliability (0.93) and has been widely used and translated into several languages (www.atlantapsychiatry.com/forms/ymrs.pdf)

In 2002, it was modified for pediatric use and information obtained from parents or teachers (Gracious, Youngstrom, Fiadling, & Calabrese, 2002). The parent version of the Young Mania Rating Scale (P-YMRS) has also been widely used and has demonstrated a Cronbach's alpha of 0.75 (www.healthyplace.com/images/stories/bipolar/p-ymrs.pdf)

Beck Cognition Checklist for Mania (CCL-M) was developed in 2003 by Dr. Aaron Beck to detect prodromal thought patterns for mania. There are seven subscales: Myself (which measures exaggerated self importance), relationships, spending, excitement, frustrations, activity, and Past/future, which deals with hyperpositive memories and expectations. It is not in the public domain at this time.

Another structured instrument is the *Bipolarity Index* (Sachs et al., 2003), which conceives of bipolarity as a spectrum along which affective illness may fall. There are five subsets, each scored from 0 to 20, with 0 indicating no evidence of bipolarity and 20 indicating most convincing evidence of bipolarity. Individuals 15 years old and up are appropriate for this index. It is part of the Systematic Treatment Enhancement Program for Bipolar Disorder study (STEP-BD), the largest treatment study to date of bipolar disorder. The Bipolarity Index may be downloaded at www.psycheducation.org/depression/STEPBipolarityIndex.htm.

In children it is often difficult to differentiate bipolar illness from Attention Deficit Disorder and this will be discussed in Chapter 14, Integrative Management of Disordered Attention. In adolescents, depression is often characterized by irritability and associated with risky behaviors such as substance abuse, sexual activity, and excessive risk taking. Recent research has suggested risky behaviors preceed depression, which contradicts the previous belief that risky behaviors followed depression and were attempts to alter discomfort.

The dilemma now is to determine if the shifts are more in terms of mood or affect. When using *DSM* criteria this would be a diagnostic issue between Bipolar 1, 2, not otherwise specified (NOS), cyclothymia, or borderline personality disorder. However, this becomes complicated because often there is both dysregulation of affect as well as mood swings present. The main differentiation is in the history of the symptoms and often including a significant other in the interview will add to this differentiation.

In bipolar disorder, there are defined episodes with periods of euthymia without functional impairment. The mood shifts are sustained and move from mania to crashing depression without external causes. There is usually a family history of mood disorder. In contrast, borderline personality disorder involves a consistent lifetime pattern in thinking, relating, and acting. This enduring pattern includes a chronic sense of emptiness and extreme fear of abandonment. The moods are not sustained and may shift in minutes or hours and are usually in response to a real or perceived interpersonal rejection. This affective instability or roller-coaster ride is often characterized by anxiety, anger, and a sense of desperation. As the client's history is explored there is frequently childhood sexual abuse present. Thus it is important to use the client's life as the context for the diagnosis and not simply a cross-sectional perspective.

Another context to consider when evaluating mood swings is your own bias. Often, individuals with bipolar illness are more likeable than borderline personality disorders, easier to treat, and it is easier to understand the illness due to the extensive research available. Therefore, diagnostic decisions may be influenced.

A seasonal pattern in mood may be noted, usually with depression evolving as there is less sunlight and colder weather. This pattern is only identified by a longitudinal pattern over several years. As the pattern of mood shifts is identified, the treatment becomes more refined and effective.

Mood swings in children becomes even more controversial in terms of diagnosis. During the past 15 years the diagnosis of bipolar disorder in children has increased fourfold in the United States (Tusaie, 2010). This pattern has led to close examination of the diagnostic practices and the strong recommendation by *DSM-5* contributors to apply the same criteria to children as adults. Also, more appropriate diagnoses such as severe temper dysregulation are proposed. Thus, it becomes clearer that there is a spectrum of polarity across several *DSM* diagnostic categories.

Self-Evaluation

There is an ever-expanding source of opportunities for self-evaluation of mood disorders in lay literature and on the web. This process of self-evaluation of a mood disorder with a screening tool is controversial for several reasons. Screening tools are not diagnostic and often have false positive results. This may result in unnecessary angst and inappropriate treatment. However, when considering the high morbidity and mortality associated with mood disorders and high rate of untreated individuals who are suffering, promotion of mental health through screening seems reasonable. The Columbia Teen Screen Program (http://teenscreen.org) is one such screening for adolescents. This program is monitored through Columbia University and not only offers online screening but also professional consultation and monitored blogs. There has been a backlash against mental health screening for children and adolescents because some people believe it is backed by pharmaceutical companies wanting to sell their products. However, checklists and self-report scales abound online as well as in lay literature.

Another possibility for screening lies with primary care providers, especially for the elderly. PMH-APRNs may be involved in consultation with primary care providers (PCP) or receiving or initiating referrals. This is an important collaboration due to the high rate of psychiatric problems in individuals who visit primary care providers. Furthermore, a large percentage of individuals who die by suicide had visited their PCP within the previous month (Juurlink, 2004).

COMORBIDITY

Comorbidity refers to the co-occurrence of two or more distinct disorders during a specified time period. Comorbidity rates in children with depression are as high as 95% (Sorensen, Nissen, Mors, & Thomsen, 2005). Substance abuse is often a comorbid problem with disturbed mood and should always be assessed. The substance may produce direct physiological effects that produce the mood disturbances or intoxication or withdrawal may also be responsible. Anxiety disorders, eating disorders, attention deficit hyperactivity disorder, and general health problems are also frequently present. Comorbidity is usually associated with poor response to treatment and increased mortality, especially in bipolar illness. Therefore, when comorbid conditions are identified in the assessment, the severity of the disorder is definitely increased. Comorbidity will be discussed in more detail in Chapters 17 and 18.

Medical disorders often associated with depression include:

- Focal lesions such as stroke, tumor, epilepsy
- Focal degenerative diseases such as Parkinson's, Huntington's, Pick's, Wilson's disease, and carbon monoxide exposure
- Diffuse diseases such as Alzheimer's, AIDS, dementia, multiple sclerosis
- Endocrine disorders such as hypo- or hyperthyroidism, Cushing's and Addison's disease, diabetes
- Inflammatory diseases such as systemic lupus, neurosyphillis, AIDS
- Tuberculosis, mononucleosis, Sjogren's syndrome, chronic fatigue syndrome
- Metabolic disorders such as uremia, porphyria, vitamin deficiencies
- Miscellaneous disorders such as migraines, medication side effects, chronic pain syndromes, sleep apnea, cancer, and heart disease
- Mild traumatic brain injury

(Gotlib & Hammen, 2010)

INSOMNIA

Insomnia is often part of and/or a prodromal symptom of depression or mania. It will become very important to have a complete assessment of sleep disturbance when beginning to manage mood disorders. Insomnia is also classified as a primary disorder in the ICD and may be independent of any other diagnosis. Sleep disturbances will be addressed in Chapter 11. It is generally accepted clinical practice to treat sleep disturbance and not wait for this to remit as the depression lifts.

COLLABORATIVE CASE CONCEPTUALIZATION

A case conceptualization is basically a melding of the client's thinking about his or her symptoms and the PMH-APRN's thinking about the symptoms. Because each has a unique frame of reference, discussion and negotiation is needed to develop a mutually acceptable framework and narrative. This is a process of seeking and using information from the client to reconcile differences between personal experiences and empirical models of mood disorders. Of course, before this can happen the PMH-APRN must have a clear understanding of theoretical and empirical models of mood disorders. If using a cognitive framework, Kuyken, Padesky, and Dudley's book *Collaborative Case Conceptualization* (2009) provides an in-depth description and clinical examples. See Figure 8-2 for illustration of a descriptive case conceptualization.

As discussed in Chapter 7, developing a case conceptualization is dynamic and evolves during therapy from a descriptive level to a more explanatory and preventive level. In mood disorders, there are often common themes of hopelessness, difficulty regulating emotions, and a history of unstable interpersonal relationships, which may include trauma, negative self-beliefs, and recent major life stressors. A descriptive case conceptualization is simply an organized, theory-based manner of describing the presenting symptoms. This would involve mapping out the current life situation, thoughts, moods, physical reactions, and behaviors.

An integrated approach to collaborative case conceptualization involves describing the Diathesis-Stress Model combined with the Cognitive Behavioral Model. An example of a discussion of a case conceptualization with a client follows: "After talking it seems that both of your parents have experienced depression and this has given you a certain neurological makeup that makes you more likely to be depressed when stressed [diathesis]. You have experienced recent stressful events—a divorce and death of a close friend this year. So you have been feeling sad and nervous and lonely, thinking you are never going to be able to have a close relationship. As a result of all of this you are now having difficulty sleeping, avoiding talking to people at work, and not enjoying anything right now. Let's draw this out to see how everything relates." Be careful not to provide too much detail and overwhelm the client. Give this broad type of description and then in future sessions focus in on mutually agreed upon areas.

As therapy progresses, a deeper exploration of thought patterns and relationships to feelings, bodily states, and behavior develops. Then as automatic thoughts are identified, strategies to shift negative patterns are practiced. Finally, the conceptualization moves to explanations such as core beliefs about self or schemas and strategies to prevent relapse are explored. These preventive strategies are basically building protective factors and decreasing risk factors.

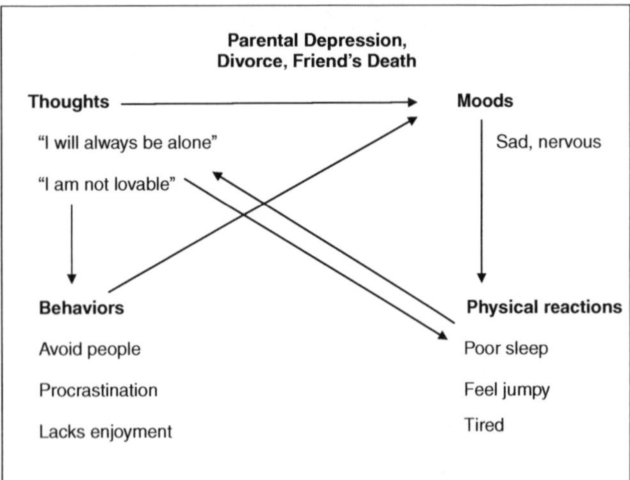

Figure 8-2 Descriptive Conceptualization

The skill level and available time of the PMH-APRN as well as the courage, emotional strength, and desires of the client will determine the level of conceptualization explored. This work may continue over several episodes of treatment or be an ongoing process over extended periods of time. However, clients may also find adequate relief with the basic descriptive conceptualizations and not desire further exploration.

In addition to a case conceptualization, a five-axis *DSM* diagnosis is made. The *DSM* (APA, 2004) provides organization of signs and symptoms for each diagnostic category, as well as decision trees starting with presenting symptom to assist with the diagnostic process. Of course, this is the diagnostic system most accepted in the United States. Internationally, the ICD-10 is used.

EXPECTED OUTCOMES

Although specific treatment outcomes are collaboratively decided as discussed in Chapter 2, there are some generic expectations for outcomes when working with individuals with mood disorders.

- Development of a therapeutic relationship
- Provision of safety without injury to self or others
- Maintenance of physical health
- Alleviation of mood disturbance
- Return to effective functional level
- Recognition of signs and symptoms of mood disturbance
- Grieve losses in an appropriate manner
- Improve strategies to develop/maintain positive interpersonal relationships
- Expand coping skills
- Develop plan to deal with symptoms and decrease/prevent relapse

TREATMENT

After developing the collaborative case conceptualization (descriptive) and *DSM* diagnosis, it is now appropriate to consider initiating treatment. The overriding goals of treatment are to decrease intensity and number of symptoms, modify risk factors, and increase protective factors. There is a large buffet of possible interventions available for treatment of mood disorders. The possible treatment modalities include self-help, guided self-help, psychotherapy, pharmacotherapy, alternative/complementary approaches, bright light therapy, electroconvulsive therapy (ECT), transcranial magnetic stimulation (TMS), and vagal nerve stimulation (VNS). These interventions may be used individually or in various combinations. See Figure 8-3 for a decision tree to direct initiation of treatment.

RESPONSE

A large percentage of individuals with mood disorders never receive any treatment and of those who do and follow treatment plans, only about one third fully recover, one third have a moderate response, and one third do not respond (Rush, 2007). Furthermore, as has been previously noted, with each episode, there is an increased likelihood of recurrence with a 50% chance after the first episode, 70% after the second episode, and 90% after three episodes (Judd et al., 2000).

Although the brain changes that correspond with clinical improvement are only speculative, baseline predictors of treatment response have been discussed. Hypermetabolism in the rostral (pregenual) cingulate has been identified with treatment responders and hypo metabolism in nonresponders (Yudofsky & Hales, 2004). These findings suggest that physiologic differences in various subgroups of mood disordered individuals may be important in understanding response to different treatments.

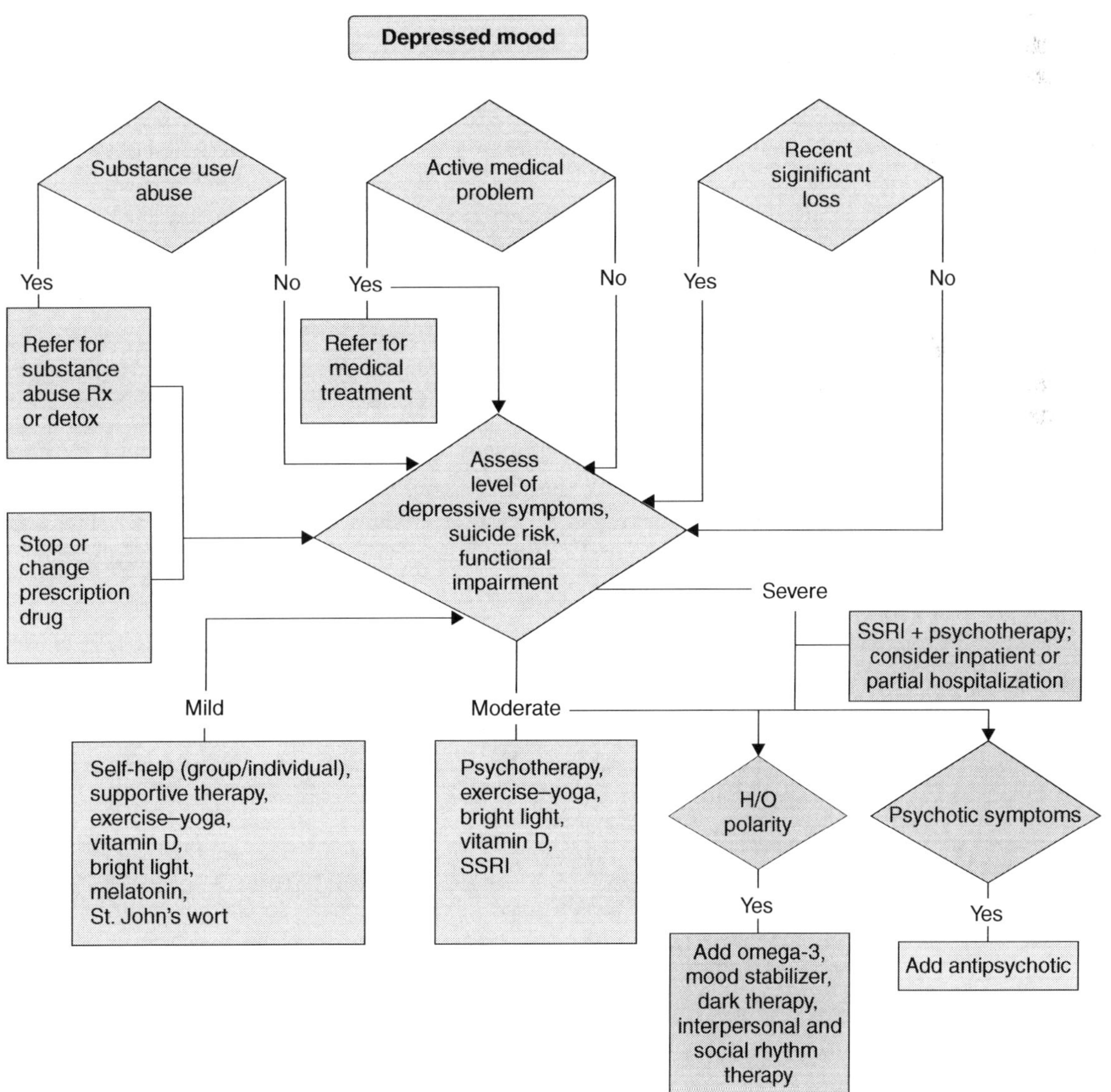

Figure 8-3 Initiation of Treatment for Individual Experiencing Depressed Mood

Attempts to identify which interventions are most effective with specific subgroups of depressive symptoms have been inconclusive. Adults between 25 and 65 seem to have the best response to antidepressants, while those younger and older have the least evidence of proven benefit. In general, more vegetative symptoms such as anhedonia, sleep disturbance, and psychomotor retardation/agitation respond best to psychopharmacology and more interpersonal symptoms respond best to psychotherapy. However, the most recent studies have identified *level of symptoms* and not type of symptoms as being most important in choosing interventions. Furthermore, for moderate to severe symptoms, best results have been reported with integrated strategies including psychotherapy, psychopharmacology, and some complementary/alternative strategies.

Due to the changing and continuing nature of mood disturbances, a MacArthur Foundation Task Force (Frank et al., 1991) recommended that change points be described with the following terms: *episode, remission, response, relapse,* and *recurrence.* See Figure 8-4 for an illustration of these change points in the course of treatment.

An *episode* is described as having a certain number of symptoms over a defined time period and usually follows *DSM* criteria. A *remission* is the point when an episode ends. If the criteria are no longer met, it is a full remission and if minimal symptoms remain it is a partial remission. This may or may not be related to an intervention. *Response* indicates approximately 50% decrease in symptoms after an intervention. The client is better but not well. These terms are used during the acute phase of the illness. *Remission* is the absence of symptoms for several months and *recovery* is defined as full remission that lasts for 6 to 12 months. Full remission and recovery is the goal of treatment but often difficult to attain. One reason is that only one third of clients follow through with treatment plans. Furthermore, Sequenced Treatment Alternatives to Relieve Depression (STAR-D) has found only one third of clients remit on their first treatment and only two thirds ever remit (Rush, 2007).

Relapse is the return of symptoms after a response, usually within 4 to 6 months. So, the use of these terms implies that relapse is a continuation of the episode. Even if some of the symptoms of depressed mood improve, there remains much anxiety and dysfunction (anxious responder). Or the mood improves but a general lack of motivation and fatigue, insomnia, and multiple physical complaints persist (apathetic responder). These partial responders are most likely to have a chronic course.

In contrast, *recurrence* is a new episode after recovery from a previous episode. There is an assumption that symptoms have been gone and a state of wellness is present and then the symptoms reoccur and a new episode emerges.

Concern about satisfaction with and effectiveness of treatment for mood disorders has also moved into the lay literature. The 2010 July issue of *Consumer Reports* described results of a survey of their readers currently in treatment for depression and or anxiety, which revealed best perceived results from drugs and talk therapy combined over a minimum of seven sessions. Also, the website Patients Like Me (www.patientslikeme.com/) has a community for individuals experiencing depressed moods. On this website, individuals in treatment report details of their treatment effectiveness, which is then summarized by the software.

INITIATING TREATMENT

Active Medical Problem

Initially, three contributing or causative conditions must be evaluated. First, the possibility of a currently active medical problem requires exploration. There are multiple medical conditions presenting with depression. The relationship between mood disturbances and medical disorders is discussed in detail in Chapter 18. This can be determined by obtaining medical records from the past year and/or performing a physical exam and basic laboratory tests. Often, physical exams are not performed by the PMH-APRN and more often are referred to a primary

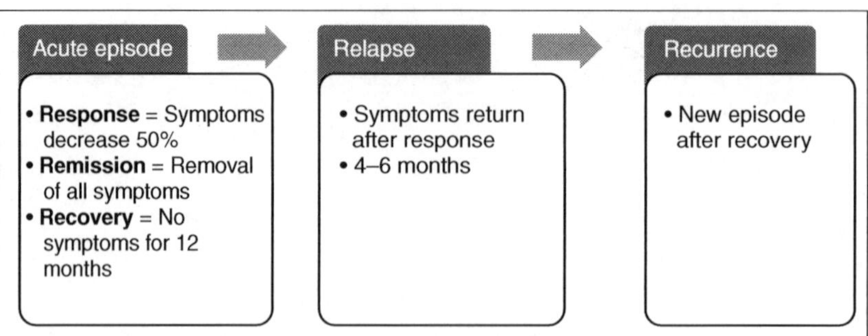

Figure 8-4 Change Points in Mood Disorders

care provider. The lab tests often include complete blood count, chemistry panel including electrolytes, vitamin B_{12} level, thyroid stimulating hormone to rule out hypothyroidism, cortisol level to rule out Cushing's disease, vitamin D level, iron level, lipid profile, and blood sugar for baseline information. Hormonal disturbances, especially during perimenapause and menopause, often contribute to the mood disturbance. Another consideration is sleep apnea. Any individual with periods of apnea followed by snoring and daytime sleepiness should be referred for a sleep study. Sleep apnea contributes to fatigue, depression, and anxiety as well as cardiovascular problems. It is wise to develop a working relationship with several primary care providers to facilitate referrals and case consultations.

If an active medical condition is present, referral for treatment is necessary. If the level of psychiatric symptoms and risk are low, it is best to wait to see if treatment of the medical problem resolves the mood disturbance while providing support to the client. However, if the psychiatric symptoms are moderate to severe, both conditions should be treated in a coordinated fashion with cross communication.

Prescription Drugs

Next, a review of all prescription and street drugs being used requires exploration. Street drugs and effects on mood and other psychiatric symptoms will be presented in Chapter 17. There are common prescription drugs contributing to mood disorders, including the following:

- Flunarizine
- Corticosteroids
- Digoxin
- Minor tranquilizers (benzodiazepines)
- Interferon
- Amantadine
- Isocarboxazid
- Levetiracetam
- Oral contraceptives (conflicting evidence)
- Reserpine
- Reglan

The initial approach is to wait to see if shifting the offending drug resolves the mood disorder while providing support to the client. During the 4 weeks of watchful waiting, client should be seen weekly and supportive psychotherapy provided (Nash, 2008).

Recreational Drugs

Street drugs, alcohol, and other abused substances may be responsible for the mood disturbance. A urine screening and blood sample may be ordered to screen for chemicals present. Individuals with an addiction issue are well known to minimize their use. Laboratory tests may reveal thiamine deficiency or liver abnormalities as reflected in the gamma-glutamyl transpeptidase, (GTP) results. If the level of psychiatric symptoms and the risk are low, treatment should focus upon promotion of sobriety using Motivational Interviewing (see Chapters 4 and 17) and referral to Alcoholic Anonymous or other appropriate self-help program. The client requires monitoring for withdrawal and may require referral for detoxification and/or rehabilitation. If the mood disturbance has a moderate to high level of severity and risk, then treatment for both the substance abuse and mood disorder should be initiated. When considering treatment involving psychotropic medication, consideration of liver function is important to avoid toxicity.

Now, the decision becomes what to treat first. Of course, this is a shared decision between PMH-APRN and client if the risk and severity are low to moderate. However, if the risk is high, severity high, and especially if psychosis is present, benevolence or providing safety for the client guides decision making about treatment initiation (Lavelle & Tusaie, 2011).

DETERMINE SEVERITY OF SYMPTOMS AND LEVEL OF RISK

After identifying the signs and symptoms, severity of the symptoms and safety is determined. Severity and safety will determine the initial setting appropriate for treatment—outpatient, partial hospitalization, or inpatient. Severity of symptoms is determined after gathering data from several sources:

- Scores on self-report instruments
- Observations during the session and mental status
- Global Assessment of Functioning score (*DSM* Axis V)
- Risk and protective factors

Severity and risk are usually rated as low, moderate, or high. Factors that increase severity include:

- Psychotic symptoms
- Symptoms of comorbidity, especially recent onset of illness, anhendonia, impulsivity, hopelessness, high anxiety and panic, global insomnia, and command hallucinations
- Alcohol/substance abuse, current or past
- Suicidal behavior including prior attempts, aborted attempts or self-injurious behavior
- History of or current abuse/neglect
- Family history of suicide attempts or psychiatric hospitalizations

- Triggering events leading to humiliation, shame, decreased productivity, or perceived burden to others
- Chronic medical illness with pain
- Access to firearms

(Adapted from Suicide Prevention Resource Center, 2006)

Although protective factors are important to identify and enhance, if risk is high they may not counteract the high risk present. So, when determining level of severity and risk, mental status is the most important variable. The presence of altered mental status as in intoxication, psychosis, dementia, or delirium, combined with a lethal suicide attempt, strong intent, or suicidal rehearsal would indicate the need for inpatient treatment. Protective factors include both internal and external variables including:

- History of resilient outcomes to stressors
- Religious beliefs that instill hope
- Absence of psychosis with logical thinking
- Strong social support as perceived by client
- Responsibility to significant others or pets
- Positive therapeutic relationships
- Cognitive flexibility

Determining level of risk is a clinical judgment and not based strictly on scores or presence of a symptom or protective factor. The judgment is based upon a holistic assessment combined with the PMH-APRN's expertise and intuition as well as available treatment resources and client preferences. When this judgment is difficult, it is wise to consult with a peer by bringing them briefly into the session for a second opinion as well as consulting with significant others of the client for additional information as well as validation.

A moderate severity/risk level may involve multiple risk factors and few protective factors, but minimal or absent suicidal thinking/behaviors. Treatment setting may be outpatient or partial hospitalization. While low severity/risk includes risk factors that are modifiable, mild symptoms and strong protective factors present. Treatment is outpatient. So, when making initial treatment decisions with the client experiencing a mood disturbance, the concept of stepped care is relevant.

Stepped Care

You have completed the intake, including history, mental status, and physical evaluation. You have developed a collaborative descriptive case conceptualization and *DSM* diagnosis. Now, you begin treatment. Stepped care is where clients with less severe symptoms are first presented with the simplest interventions and then proceed to more complex interventions only if necessary. Even before an individual with mood dysregulation seeks professional help, there are usually informal self-help activities. These may include increased physical and social activity, reading self-help books or websites, drinking alcohol to relax, and taking vitamins or other herbal preparations over the counter (OTC), vacations, or time off work. Self-help is more common in those with few or low severity symptoms and these activities decrease as severity of symptoms increase. An Overlapping Waves of Action Model has been developed by Jorm and Griffiths (2006) for treatment of mood disorders.

The first wave involves preclinical or low levels of symptoms and interventions include increased use of self-help strategies such as physical exercise, enjoyable activities, and seeking support from friends and family. As symptoms become more severe, the first wave of self-help activities diminishes in importance. The second wave involves use of self-help not in the usual everyday activities such as OTC drugs (St. John's wort, omega-3 fatty acids, valerian, SAMe, sleep aids) and changes to diet. As symptoms reach a moderate to severe level, professional help is usually necessary and involves guided self-help, psychotherapy, prescription medication, bright light therapy, hospitalization, ECT, TMS, or vagal nerve stimulation. Therefore, when a client presents for treatment of a mood disorder, it is important to question what self-help strategies have been attempted.

LOW SEVERITY/LOW RISK

Guided Self-Help and Psychotherapy

Initial treatment with individuals experiencing low level symptoms and low risk involve guided self-help strategies combined with psychotherapy. Recent studies have reported that antidepressant medications are not effective with low level symptoms of mood disorders but increase in effectiveness with moderate to severe symptoms. The strategies will evolve from the collaborative case conceptualization. If the conceptualization primarily identified a distorted thinking pattern that led to the disordered mood, then the guided self-help strategies may include recommending a self-help method such as reading a book (bibliotherapy) and then discussing the content in sessions. Several self-help books for mood disorders have a cognitive-behavioral framework including *The Feeling Good Handbook or Workbook* (Burns, 1999) and *Mind Over Mood* (Greenberger & Padesky, 1995).

Age appropriate websites that offer self-help for adolescents who are computer literate and have access to the Internet include an Australian program, *The Mood Gym* (www.moodgym.anu.edu.au/welcome). Using web-based programs are especially effective for adolescents due to the fact that the majority of adolescents use computers on a daily basis. Although there is controversy surrounding computer use, it seems that excessive length of use is associated with pathology but moderate use facilitates learning and is an excellent medium for connecting with adolescents. These programs may be accessed together during a session or independently and then discussed in session. Computer programs such as *Beating the Blues* (www.beatingtheblues.co.uk/) and teaching cognitive behavioral therapy (CBT) skills have also been used successfully as an adjunct to therapy for adults with low to moderate symptoms (Foroushani, Schinerder, & Assareh, 2011; Kaltenthaler et al., 2002).

In addition to bibliotherapy and computer programs, reducing self-help strategies that increase depression and fatigue need to be addressed. For example, the use of alcohol and marijuana initially bring relief but then will increase depression and sleep disturbance. Amphetamines initially increase energy, but then delete serotonin and lead to a crash in mood. The use of sugars and fats to self-soothe leads to a roller-coaster mood. A balanced diet with more protein will lead to a more stable mood. Also the use of caffeine for energy will also lead to agitation, sleep disturbance, and depression.

Next, scheduling pleasurable activities and increasing physical activity are appropriate. Having the client keep a log of daily activities will identify areas requiring adjustment. If the client is unable to follow through with this, something as simple as drawing a circle and dividing into percentages of the day sleeping, working, and so on, will provide direction for strategies. Although these strategies sound simple, the anxiety and difficulties associated with change cannot be minimized. Symptoms of mood disorder often slow down all activities and if changes are not very small and attainable, the client will be unable or unwilling to follow through and move deeper into the depressed mood. Sometimes, the act of attending a scheduled appointment is the only achievement. So, be in touch with your expectations and once again your ability to bear witness to the client's suffering while celebrating small steps toward goals.

Exercise and pleasurable activities at any level are associated with better physical and mental health for both genders, especially older adults (Kurtze, Rangul, Hustvedt, & Flanders, 2008). Activity facilitates feeling better for several reasons. First, it is a distraction from negative ruminations and it provides an opportunity to experience success and pleasure. Furthermore, various cascades of brain chemicals are stimulated resulting in increased attention, processing, and memory as well as up-regulation of neurotrophic factors involved in the action of antidepressants and feel-good chemicals such as endocannabinoids and endorphins. Jacobson, Martell, and Dimidjian (2001) published an updated version of the work of earlier research related to the centrality of activity in treating depression.

Although aerobic exercise seems to have the greatest positive influence on mental health, this is often an unrealistic expectation. Movement ranges from rapid motions of dance, sports, or aerobics to the careful, slow movements of yoga or tai chi. Using computer games such as Wii to increase activity are also gaining use. It is important to choose activities that are attractive and physically possible for clients. Simple walking on a daily basis is safe, flexible, and inexpensive. Furthermore, the APA Guidelines for Treatment of Major Depression (2010) can be viewed at www.psych.org/

The guidelines have included exercise for any level of depressive symptoms. Encouraging a gradual increase in a walking pace to 3.5 miles per hour resulting in a 2-mile walk over 35 minutes meets the suggested activity level of the American College of Sports Medicine and the American Heart Association.

Readiness for Change

An individual experiencing a mood disturbance usually experiences difficulty with change and getting started. Of course, if the client immediately follows through with the plan for change, celebrate and move on to other issues. However, remember to not minimize the anxiety and ambivalence associated with change. There are several strategies to assist with change. First, using Motivational Interviewing techniques are helpful—discussing the pros and cons of the activity; encouraging change talk; managing resistance; negotiating a plan with incremental, achievable steps; affirming strengths; and reinforcing any change (Rosengren, 2009). When developing a plan for change, the use of relaxation exercises and visualization of the desired change can be effective, for example, "See yourself walking along enjoying the gentle breeze and knowing your body is healing...enjoying all the sights, sounds, and aromas, and feel the muscles of your body reacting, and so on." Relaxation exercises are discussed in more detail in Chapter 6, Overview of Complementary/Alternative Approaches. Another effective intervention is the use of Eye Movement Desensitization Reprogramming (EMDR) to encourage recognition of one's own resources, small behavior changes, and then future visions (Shapiro, 2009). The training, skill level, and resourcefulness of the PMH-APRN, combined with the therapeutic relationship and client's wishes will determine ability to make changes. To appreciate the difficulty of change, take a few minutes and think about a New Year's resolution or a long-time goal of your own to change a specific behavior. What interfered with goal attainment and what facilitated change?

Interpersonal Issues

The collaborative conceptualization often has identified problems with relationships or bereavement as prominent. If the symptoms and risk are low to moderate, the initial treatment is usually interpersonal psychotherapy (Frank et al., 2005). This is an important consideration in choosing the therapy approach. The current thinking about kindling indicates that an initial depressive episode may bring about changes to neurotransmitters in the limbic system that make the individual more prone to depressive episodes, so that even small stressors can lead to depressive episodes. Addressing marital problems, parenting difficulties, and even the broader context of stress and depression has been helpful in decreasing the level of stress. Humiliating events such as partner infidelity, marital discord, and abuse have resulted in six-fold increase in diagnosis of depression after controlling for family history of depression (Cano & O'Leary, 2000). Therefore, the importance of identifying and shifting interpersonal stressors is vital for recovery as well as relapse prevention. Another approach has combined Behavioral Marital Therapy with Cognitive Therapy with excellent results (Bodenmann, 2007). This approach involves teaching the spouse of the depressed individual basic cognitive therapy techniques to assist the client in processing events differently. When compared to cognitive therapy alone, both approaches decreased depressive symptoms but only the combination decreased both depressive symptoms and marital discord. Furthermore, if the client believes that the marital problems have caused the depression, the client is more likely to be engaged in treatment and the approach is more likely to be successful. When working with couples, the interventions require a balance among focusing upon cognition, behavior, and affect (Baucom & Epstein, 1991).

The specific interventions are again focused upon a recognition of the couple's patterns. For example, if there is a pattern of selective attention to negative aspects of the relationship, interventions assist with development of a more balanced recognition of the relationship. Or there may be negative attributions to behavior such as "he doesn't love me any more" when in reality, the lack of attention to spouse is related to the depressive illness. So then the approach would include education and consideration of alternate explanations for behavior. Then a move toward understanding future expectations and acceptance of the positive as well as negative aspects is facilitated.

So, in addition to education about depression, there is a need for the couple to share thoughts and feelings with each other as well, and to problem-solve and develop strategies for change. Using structured approaches may be helpful when working with couples. Dr. Gottman has a program developed from extensive research and offers many useful worksheets for sessions as well as self-help for couples (http://gottman.com)

Parental depression as well as behavior problems in the children were significantly decreased. This outcome demonstrates the importance of a collaborative case conceptualization for effective treatment strategies.

If a child is the identified client, the approach always involves the family and outcomes are usually focused upon school performance, family functioning, and peer relationships. Once an assessment of self-competence is completed and the reality of the belief identified, then the strategies can move forward. If the perception of low competence is reality based, then skill building is developed. If this is not reality based, then therapy can focus upon more realistic self-appraisal. Prepubertal children tend to respond best to play therapy. Paper, pencil, crayons, scissors, tape, a doll family or figures, and two or three toy cars are adequate. Patterns of repetitive, reckless activity and issues of loss and retrieval should be noted. Displaced aggression may be acted out and later allowed to express feelings and to cope with them. Play therapy may be individual or with a group and provides children with an opportunity to experience success (Schaefer, 2003).

A recent study exploring effectiveness of a hands-on coaching approach involving parents and depressed children (3 to 7 years old) has also been very promising. In Parent-Child Interaction Therapy–Emotion Development (PCIT-ED), parents were taught and practiced positive play with their child. Results included decreased disruptive behavior and increased ability to manage emotions (Luby, Lenze, & Tillman, 2011). Group therapy focusing upon insight and social skills is useful in assisting the child to express feelings in a safe and supportive environment while enhancing social skills. Of course, this type of group requires an energetic and empathetic clinician. Children and adolescents require shorter sessions than adults and ongoing family contact is necessary.

CBT is best with adolescents who have low intensity and low risk symptoms. The format is somewhat modified with more active involvement by the PMH-APRN, who moves among the roles of teacher, confidant, role model, collaborator, and expert (Reinecke, Datillo, & Freeman, 2003). If using CBT with children, metaphors, stories, and play are usually used (Nelson & Tusaie, 2011).

If the loss involves death of a loved one, the focus of the therapy is grief work and the prevention of complicated grief. This is considered a specialized type of interpersonal therapy. The severity of symptoms wax and wane as ocean waves during grief and may move across the levels of severity. The bereavement period is not time limited. Certain aspects may continue indefinitely for otherwise high functioning individuals. Grief becomes circumscribed and submerged but will reemerge in response to certain triggers—anniversary dates, memories, and so on. Although many symptoms overlap with depression, the individual usually has positive thoughts coesisting with the negative ones. Complicated grief refers to normal bereavement moving into depression and inability to function. Therapy focusing upon the relationship with the individual who has died and the recognition that the relationship is not lost, but shifted. The ability to remember and internalize those memories is a continued relationship and often helpful to grieving individuals.

Responses to death are colored by developmental level. Children may not display grief reactions, but throw themselves into excessive activity, play grief games, or regress in eating, sleep, or bowel or bladder functions. Children may withdraw, become overly mature, or refuse to go to school. Children's coping strategies need to be respected, but also, they must be encouraged to talk and assisted to understand that the death was not their fault. Adolescent reactions may be as diversified as adults with stoicism, behavior problems, somatic complaints, erratic moods, and sexual acting out. Children, adolescents, and adults need rituals to assist with their grief. The funeral as well as more private rituals may be helpful. See *Good Grief Rituals: Tools for Healing* (Childs-Gowell, 1995) for an expanded description of grief rituals.

Group therapy has been effective for many individuals but holds several practical issues in an outpatient practice. First, there is minimal flexibility around time and length of sessions. Often, individuals with low-level symptoms are continuing to work or attend school and may require more flexibility in scheduling. Second, the skill of the PMH-APRN in facilitating cohesion and other therapeutic factors is required. It is inappropriate to use individual therapy techniques within the group sessions. Also, if everyone in the group is experiencing a mood disorder, it takes a competent, strong facilitator to move the group beyond the contagious sadness and negativity. The advantages of group therapy include the ability to provide treatment in a cost-effective manner as well as the experience of curative factors not present in individual therapy (Yalom & Leszcz, 2005).

COMPLEMENTARY/ALTERNATIVE APPROACHES

Several complementary and alternative strategies have been helpful with individuals experiencing a mood disturbance. Chronotherapeutics, changes in diet, herbals, and healing touch will be discussed.

Chronotherapeutics

Chronobiology is the science of rhythms. Daily (circadian), monthly, tidal, and seasonal rhythms manifest themselves at every hierarchical level from the general population (more auto accidents at night), to the individual sleep-wake cycle to each organ, cell, and molecule. Dysregulation of these rhythms, as in jet lag or shift work, does not necessarily cause psychopathology, but a regular rhythm is necessary for restful sleep, daytime alertness, adequate stable mood, cognition, and neurobehavioral functioning. Any misalignment of sleep and rhythms brings a propensity for mood fluctuation, especially in vulnerable individuals. An example of dysregulation is the increased incidence of depressive episodes after a westward flight and manic episodes after flying east (Jauhar & Weller, 1982).

Bright light therapy has been used successfully with mood disorders that have a seasonal pattern. Seasonal depression usually starts around October and remits in early spring (Lam, et al., 2006). Bright light therapy may be used alone or in combination with other approaches. If the case conceptualization has identified a predominant seasonal pattern, therapy is also needed to assist with understanding and coping with the symptoms. If mood symptoms are moderate or severe, bright light therapy can also be combined with prescription antidepressants as well as psychotherapy. In locations with very low amounts of sunlight, bright light therapy has been used as an adjunctive treatment with mood disorders without seasonal patterns. Bright lights are full spectrum, high intensity (6,000 to 10,000 lux) light boxes used for 15 to 30 minutes in the morning and are more effective than non-bright lights (Golden et al., 2005). The mechanism of treatment effectiveness is believed to be the influence upon circadian rhythms. Circadian rhythms are the physical, mental, and behavioral changes that occur over the course of a day in response to light and darkness. Special nonimaging cells in the retina contain melantopsin which is sensitive to blue light and influences these daily rhythms (Gooley, et al., 2010). Side effects of bright light therapy include headache and difficulty falling asleep. These side effects may be modified by decreasing length of time of exposure to the light. There are multiple online sites to purchase light therapy boxes and some PMH-APRNs have the light box in their office for clients to use during morning sessions. Although there are no Food and Drug Administration (FDA) approved light boxes, partial or full insurance reimbursement is now common if the appropriate diagnostic code for mood or circadian rhythm disorder is listed with the prescription.

In addition to light therapy, wake therapy, dark therapy, and melantonin also are based upon chronobiology. One night of sleep deprivation has resulted in significant mood improvement in 60% of individuals with a mood disturbance (Wirz-Justice, Benedetti, & Terman, 2009). Dark therapy, which involves keeping an individual who is in a manic episode within a dark room during the night, and wearing sunglasses during the day, has been reported to improve symptoms and stop cycling (Phelps, 2008).

Melatonin is a hormone secreted by the pineal gland and is a signal of darkness as of night length. If rhythms are dysregulated as in depression, melatonin may be secreted at the wrong time. An evening dose of melatonin ranging from 1 mg–6 mg may synchronize circadian rhythms and promote sleep. Melatonin is widely available OTC as well as in drinks. Melatonin agonists, Rozerem and Tasimelton (completed phase-3 clinical trials) are available with prescription. Another melatonin agonist, agomelantine, is available in the European Union and has an additional antidepressant effect. A treatment manual, *Chronotherapeutics for Affective Disorders: A Clinician's Manual for Light and Wake Therapy* by Wirz-Justice, Benedetti, and Terman (2009) provides clinical guidelines in more detail.

Nutritional Issues

We are aware of the correlation between what we eat and how we feel. Several studies have identified a strong correlation between mood disorders and obesity. It is not clear if depressive symptoms lead to poor choices in eating habits and decreased exercise, if poor choices and obesity lead to depressive symptoms, or if the obesity is a side effect of antidepressants, or perhaps a combination of all of these. Self-soothing with food, especially carbohydrates and dark chocolate, is a well known pattern in depressed individuals. Issues in disordered eating will be discussed in depth in Chapter 12.

There are multiple anecdotal reports of individuals with mood disorders making poor dietary choices. One young woman had been eating only corn chips, cheese dip, coffee, and soft drinks for almost a year. Once her depression began to lift, a focus of several therapy sessions was to explore the pros and cons of changing her eating patterns and then to develop a simple plan for doing this. As her dietary choices began to shift, she lost over 50 pounds and began exercising. A portion of therapy should always assess eating habits and gradual changing to a well balanced diet. Joining Weight Watchers in person or online or Overeaters Anonymous (OA) may also be helpful. Tufts University has a website, navigator.tufts.edu, that is also useful for information about an appropriately balanced diet.

Other nutritional concerns with depression include levels of vitamin D and folate. Vitamin D deficiency is related to not only dietary intake but also lack of sunlight. Following a blood level, supplements should be ordered. Low folate levels also contribute to depressive symptoms and have been reported to interfere with the effectiveness of antidepressant drugs.

Herbals used in mood disorders include St John's wort, SAMe, and omega-3 fatty acids. St. John's wort is widely used to treat low-severity and low-risk symptoms of mood disorders. See Chapter 6 for more information.

Healing Touch has been used adjunctively to treat the symptoms of mood disturbances. As previously discussed, many individuals with symptoms of depression also have pain or other somatic symptoms. Healing touch has been proven to bring about not only more relaxation and symptom relief but also release of "muscle memories" and the facilitation of psychotherapy explorations. There are many anecdotal case reports about effectiveness. One client, who had been experiencing severe headaches and had been unable to discuss anything but the headaches in sessions, was soon able to discuss interpersonal stressors and begin working toward management of the headaches after several healing touch sessions.

As the symptoms of the mood disturbance increase or decrease in intensity and number, the risk as well as approach must vary. A general rule is that more severity requires more structured, behavioral, and psychopharmacy approaches and as symptoms decrease, the talking, cognitive, and self-help components are enhanced.

MODERATE SEVERITY AND RISK

As the severity of symptoms and the risk for self or other-directed violence increases, self-help treatment strategies become less important. Generally, psychopharmacotherapy and psychotherapy are now needed. Due to side effect profiles, selective serotonin reuptake inhibitors (SSRIs) currently dominate the treatment of mood disorders. Clients are seen a minimum of once weekly outpatient and may require partial hospitalization and crisis services. If safety is not an issue, psychotherapy based on the case conceptualization is usually initiated first for approximately four sessions. If safety is a concern, then both psychotherapy and pharmacotherapy are initiated.

Another important variable at this point is the presence of affective or mood instability, which will influence both the choice of psychotherapy as well as the drug of choice. See Tables 8-2 and 8-3 for information on antidepressants commonly used. Although all the antidepressants have basically a similar effect upon symptoms of depression, the choice of the drug to initiate treatment is based upon the following factors:

- Client preference
- Effectiveness
- The side effect profile (including half-life as risk for discontinuation syndrome)
- History of past response pattern
- Family history of response
- Type of symptoms experienced and neurotransmitter specificity of drug
- Safety (potential for overdose)
- Comorbid conditions
- Half-life
- Cost

TRANSCRANIAL MAGNETIC STIMULATION

TMS is an alternative to antidepressant therapy and is most effective for those depressed individuals who are younger adults and less treatment resistant, while other forms of brain stimulation are reserved for treatment-resistant, severely ill individuals. There are anecdotal reports of TMS being effective for individuals with mild to moderate affective instability (Schuttor, 2009). Meta-analysis of studies of TMS have shown significant results with a moderate to large effect size (Herrmann & Ebmeier, 2006).

TMS is delivered outpatient by placing an electromagnetic coil over the left dorsolateral prefrontal cortex and creating a rapidly changing magnetic field that induces an electric current. This is similar to a magnetic resonance imaging machine (MRI). Due to the localized effect, there are none of the cognitive side effects of ECT and the client is alert and awake, not requiring any medication or anesthesia. The treatment is experienced as a mild scalp tingling. The treatment takes less than an hour and acute treatment involves daily administration for 4 to 6 weeks. The treatment is very expensive and insurance reimbursement is often difficult to obtain.

If instability of affect and/or mood are identified, treatment choices are somewhat different and focus upon stabilization of mood. Psychopharmacotherapy starts with a mood stabilizing medication. However, polarity may be identified only after an antidepressant has been ordered and induced mania symptoms (antidepressant-induced mania) (Daray, Thommi, & Ghaemi, 2010).

The challenege is to effectively treat or prevent manic, mixed, or depressive episodes without triggering episodes of the opposite polarity. Approximately 60% to 70% of individuals show a remission of mania symptoms with lithium and it has been estimated to decrease hospitalization rates by 82% (Keck et al., 1998). However, the side effect profile is quite harsh and has shifted prescribers to use divalproex sodium, Tegretol, and lamotrigine for mania and maintenance treatment. However, these drugs are only minimally effective with depressive episodes. As a result, many prescribers add antidepressants to a mood stabilizer. When used alone antidepressants can induce mania, but there is less evidence that this happens when used in combination with a mood stabilizer. Atypical antipsychotics have also been proven to be effective in treating mania and maintenance, but also carry a potential for serious side effects. Seroquel (quetiapine) is being used to treat all stages of polarity including maintenance.

Childhood and adolescent polarity is characterized by lengthy episodes, a high rate of psychosis, and a highly recurrent course. A mood stabilizing agent and/or an atypical antipsychotic is usually initiated. Often, attention deficit hyperactivity disorder (ADHD) or anxiety disorders are also present. But treatment of comorbid conditions is initiated only after the child's mood has stabilized (Kowatch et al., 2005).

PSYCHOTHERAPY

The type of psychotherapy is determined by the case conceptualization developed and the mental status of the client, in addition to preference of the client and the skills of the PMH-APRN. However, a hybrid type of therapy (Miklowitz, Goodwin, Bauer, & Geddes, 2008) including the most effective factors in treatment of individuals with polarity has been reported to include:

- Education about symptoms for client and significant others
- Education about medications and side effects
- Focus upon resolving interpersonal issues
- Coping with the stigma of a chronic mental illness
- Regulation of sleep-wake cycles
- Specific strategies for education have included individual approaches involving increased awareness of the symptoms, by keeping a self-rated mood chart to include low moods as well as high and "normal" moods throughout the week and consequences. Another important aspect

TABLE 8-2: MEDICATIONS COMMONLY USED FOR INITIAL TREATMENT OF MOOD DISORDERS

CLASS	INITIAL DOSE	THERAPEUTIC DOSE	COMMON SIDE EFFECTS	MANAGEMENT OF SIDE EFFECTS
SSRIs				
Citalopram (Celexa)	10–20 mg	20–40 mg	Activation & nausea, Moderate sedation Sexual Weight gain Cardiac changes >40mg	Wait, take with food Take at hs or switch Decrease dose, add bupropion or sildenafil Add exercise & diet changes or switch
S-citalopram (Lexapro)	5–10 mg	10–30 mg	Activation, insomnia, & nausea Mild sedation Sexual Mild weight gain	Same as above
Fluoxetine (Prozac, Prozac weekly, Serafem)	5–10 mg	10–60 mg	Strong activation Insomnia, myoclonus, nausea Sexual Rare increase of suicidal ideation	Wait, take with food Take in morning Reduce dose, in a few weeks, switch or add trazadone or benzodiazepines for sleep Add bupropion, sildenafil, vardenafil, or tadalafil Switch, closely monitor, add therapy
Fluvoxamine (Luvox, Luvox CR)	25–50 mg	100–300 mg	Mild activation Strong sedation & fatigue Sexual	Wait, take with food Take at hs, decrease dose, in few weeks switch
Paroxetine (Paxil, Paxil CR)	10–20 mg Child: 5 mg	20–60 mg	Mild activation Sedation Sexual Weight gain	Wait, take with food Take at hs Same as above Add exercise & diet changes or switch
Sertraline (Zoloft)	25–50 mg	50–200 mg	Mild activation Moderate sedation Insomnia Sexual	Wait, take with food Reduce dose Take at hs, switch if persists a couple weeks Same as above
SNRIs				
Venlafaxine (Effexor, Effexor XR)	25–37.5 mg Child: 12.5 mg	150–300 mg	Headache, nervousness, insomnia, sedation, Hypertension Sexual dysfunction Hyponatremia	Wait, short-term benzo use, reduce dose, or add trazodone for sleep After several weeks, if persists, switch to sildenafil, vardenafil, or tadalafil
Duloxetine (Cymbalta)	10–20 mg Child: not established	60–120 mg	Nausea, diarrhea Dry mouth, constipation Sexual dysfunction Insomnia, sedation, dizziness Hypomania, possible weight gain Sweating, urinary retention	Wait, increase fiber Decrease dose, sildenafil, vardenafil, or tadalafil Trazadone, mirtazapine for sleep Switch if persists several weeks
Desvenlafexine (Pristiq)	50 mg Child: not established	50–400 mg	Same as venalafexine but less intense Weight gain unusual	

(*Continued*)

TABLE 8-2: MEDICATIONS COMMONLY USED FOR INITIAL TREATMENT OF MOOD DISORDERS (*Continued*)

CLASS	INITIAL DOSE	THERAPEUTIC DOSE	COMMON SIDE EFFECTS	MANAGEMENT OF SIDE EFFECTS
Mood Stabilizers				
Carbamazepine (Tegretol, Carbatrol, Equetro)	200 mg	400–1,200 mg	Sedation, dizziness, confusion, nausea, diarrhea, transient leukopenia, rare aplastic anemia, rash & Stevens-Johnson syndrome, hyponatremia, weight gain	Take at hs; use extended release, decrease dose; switch drug
Lamotrigine (Lamictal)	25 mg	100–200 mg	Sedation, fatigue, dizziness, nausea, rare rash & Stevens-Johnson syndrome, non-viral encephalitis rare	Take at hs, reduce dose If rash widespread, or purpuricor on neck or face, and abnormal CBC, discontinue drug if abnormal liver function, urea= d/c
Lithium (Escalith, Lithobid)	300 mg	600 mg–1,800 mg	Ataxia, delirium, tremor, memory problems, diabetes, diarrhea, nausea, unsteady gait, weight gain, rash, alopecia, leukocytosis, lithium toxicity, renal impairment, arrhythmia,	Obtain baseline labs, electrocardiogram (EKG) Lower dose, check therapeutic blood levels, take with food, controlled release, If toxic stop drug Many drug interactions
Oxcarbazepine (Trileptal)	600 mg	1,200–2,400 mg	Sedation, unsteady gait, headache, confusion, nausea, abnormal vision, hyponatremia, weight gain	Take at hs Switch drug
Valproate (Depakote, Depakote ER, Depakene)	250–500 mg	500–1,000 mg	Sedation, tremor, dizziness, headache, weight gain, diarrhea, alopecia, rare pancreatitis, liver failure	Baseline date, check blood levels, take at hs, lower dose, use extended release Propranolol for tremor, zinc & selenium for alopecia Switch drug

CBC = complete blood count.

of education and awareness involves discussion of the client's and family's reactions to the symptoms and treatment. For example, the enjoyment of hypomania in self as well as by others. "I don't want medication to dull my creativity. …He is so much fun sometimes…" It is important to explore these thoughts in detail and to discuss possible effects of treatment. There is a growing interest in the positive aspects of bipolar illness and literature has identified spirituality, empathy, creativity, and resilience as being enhanced in some individuals with bipolar illness (Galvez, Thommi, & Ghaemi, 2011). So, it seems that part of coping with stigma, as well as understanding effects of medication, needs to include the aspects of bipolar illness that are perceived as positive and develop treatment strategies that minimize the reduction of these positive experiences.

Another approach to treatment of bipolarity is Interpersonal and Social Rhythm Therapy (IPSRT), which emphasizes the importance of social and circadian rhythm dysregulation in the onset of manic episodes. When this approach was studied with individuals already experiencing at least one manic episode and included family education and assistance with regulation of events, there were longer periods of remission and less severe depressive episodes (Frank et al., 2005). Regulation of sleep-wake cycles and CBT-Insomnia will be discussed in Chapter 11, Integrative Management of Sleep Disturbances.

Group therapy using these approaches combined with medications for individuals and/or families with bipolar illness have resulted in decreased social isolation, increased consistency in medication use, the ability

TABLE 8-3: ADDITIONAL ANTIDEPRESSANTS

	INITIAL DOSE	THERAPEUTIC DOSE
TCAs		
Amitriptyline (Elavil, Endep)	25–50 mg	100–300 mg
Amoxapine (Ascendin)	50–100 mg	150–400 mg
Clomipramine (Anafranil)	25–50 mg	100–250 mg
Desipramine (Norpramine)	25–50 mg	100–300 mg
Doxepin (Sinequan, Adapin)*	25–50 mg	100–300 mg
Imipramine (Tofranil)	25–50 mg	100–300 mg
Maprotiline (Ludiomil)	25–50 mg	100–225 mg
Nortriptyline (Aventyl, Pamelor)	10–25 mg	50–150 mg
Protriptyline (Vivactil)	10 mg	15–60 mg
Trimipramine (Surmontil)	25–50 mg	100–300 mg
Others		
Bupropion (Wellbutrin)	100–150 mg	300–450 mg
Mirtazapine (Remeron)	15–30 mg	15–60 mg
Nefazodone (Serzone)	50 mg	400–600 mg
Trazadone (Desyrel)*	50 mg	150–400 mg
MAOI		
Isocarboxazid (Marplan)	10–20 mg	30–60 mg
Phenelzine (Nardil)	15–30 mg	30–90 mg
Selegiline (Eldepryl)	10 mg	20–60 mg
Selegiline transdermal (Emsam patch)	6 mg	6–12 mg
Tranylcypromine (Parnate)	10–20 mg	30–60 mg

*Used as hypnotics.

to recognize oncoming episodes, and support against stigma, with longevity of these effects.

If the bipolarity symptoms are less severe and more related to affect shifts, the treatment starts with psychotherapy using a skill-building approach, Dialectical Behavior Therapy (DBT). This is a broad-based CBT approach that is prescriptive and available in a manual with multiple handouts (Linehan, 1993). The focus of this approach is for the client to learn to tolerate more distress and regulate his or her affect. The *DSM* diagnosis for these individuals is usually Borderline Personality Disorder, which carries quite a heavy load of stigma. As this diagnosis has moved into lay literature and media in a negative fashion, it may be best to avoid the use of this diagnosis with clients and instead use terms such as "affect dysregulation" or "bipolarity spectrum." There are also several books available to coach partners through living with individuals who experience affect dysregulation such as *I Hate You Don't Leave Me* by Kreisman & Straus and the *Stop Walking on Eggshells Workbook* by Kreger with Shirley. Furthermore, mood stabilizers as well as omega-3 fatty acids have been helpful to individuals with affective dysregulation. Although lithium has the most evidence for maintaining mood stability, its popularity is decreasing due to the narrow therapeutic window and side effect profile. Lamictal is also being used increasingly.

With bipolarity an important factor in effective treatment is a long-term trusting relationship. There is currently no cure, but a consistent relationship with a clinician allows the flexibility of a range of approaches necessary for the client's coping and functioning at an acceptable level. Rarely is an individual with polarity able to function with only one medication and one type of therapy. Furthermore, the insecure interpersonal attachments and anxiety associated with aloneness experienced by individuals with affective instability is somewhat decreased by the trusting long-term relationship with an individual clinician or a therapy group. As this anxiety decreases, learning coping skills becomes more possible. Both psychotherapy and medications are necessary during the various phases of treatment with medications being more effective as the symptoms increase in severity.

HIGH LEVEL OF SEVERITY OF SYMPTOMS AND RISK

When severity of symptoms is high and the risk for injury to self and/or others is also high, hospitalization must be a consideration. At this stage, the focus of treatment is safety and symptom reduction. Psychopharmacotherapy is the primary treatment strategy. Psychotherapy is supportive for both the client and the significant others and focuses upon the understanding and relief of symptoms.

As severity decreases, psychotherapy becomes more active. If psychosis is present, an antipsychotic is initiated also. A benzodiazepam is usually ordered for catatonia. If the client has responded well to ECT in the past, this is a consideration. Vagus Nerve Stimulation is also a consideration.

ELECTROCONVULSIVE THERAPY

ECT is the oldest of all biologic treatments for psychopathology and the most controversial. It's effectiveness in severe depression has been estimated to be 70% to 90% remission rates in clinical trials and 30% to 47% in community samples (Prudic, Olfsan, Marcus, Fuller, & Sackeim, 2004). However, there is a high relapse rate in 6 months for those who responded acutely. Often, antidepressants are ordered after ECT series to assist in relapse prevention. Although the short-term effectiveness of ECT is well documented, many individuals consider it to be barbaric and the FDA classification is class III, high risk.

ECT is not used as a first-line treatment, but for those who have failed multiple antidepressant and combined treatment therapies and have high level severity and risk. Individuals with medical contradictions for medication are also appropriate for ECT. Cognitive side effects include post-ECT confusion and anterograde and retrograde memory deficits, with a few patients complaining of long-term deficits.

ECT is administered on an inpatient or outpatient basis using a short-term anesthesia, muscle relaxant to prevent fractured bones, and electroencephalogram (EEG) monitoring. Electrodes are placed either bilaterally on the forehead or unilaterally over the nondominant hemisphere to minimize confusion. The therapeutic action is related to induction of sufficient seizure activity (grand mal pattern) for a duration of 20 seconds. The dose of electricity used is also adjusted with higher doses associated with more confusion but better antidepressant effects. There is usually a series of six to 12 treatments delivered two to three times a week. The exact neurobiological action is unknown but believed to be related to changes in multiple neuropeptides and upregulation of brain-derived neurotropic factor (BDNF), giving rise to formation of new cells in the hippocampus. The hippocampus is important for emotions, learning, and memory.

VAGAL NERVE STIMULATION

VNS is a well-established treatment for medically refractory partial-onset seizures, but has only recently been approved for treatment of drug-resistant depressive disorders. The vagus nerve has afferent fibers carrying information to the brain from the head, neck, and thorax. It has sensory afferent connections in the nucleus tractus solitarious to many brain areas (forebrain and locus coeruleus). Thus, incoming sensory connections of the vagus nerve provide direct projections to areas of the brain involved in psychiatric disorders (Bolwig, 2003).

A pulse generating device surgically implanted in the patient's chest, like a cardiac pacemaker, with a wire attached to the left vagus nerve delivers the VNS. Side effects include hoarseness, cough, and mild shortness of breath. Efficacy increases over 1 year and shows a 27% response rate as compared to 13% in treatment as usual (George et al., 2005).

VNS is most appropriate for those people who are severely and chronically treatment resistant. However, it is not widely used due to need for surgical implantation, high cost, minimal data on effectiveness in depression, and uncertain insurance payment.

ACUTE FOLLOW-UP/CONTINUATION

During the initial 2 to 4 weeks of treatment, clients should be seen weekly. If a response of beginning decrease in presenting symptoms is noted, continue the treatment for at least 4 to 9 months. There is usually a quicker response to medications than therapy. If there is not an adequate response, consider augmenting or changing the treatment. Remember to follow the case conceptualization.

For example, if the treatment has been medication only, add psychotherapy to assist with decreasing stress levels. If the type of therapy has been supportive, switch to a more dynamic approach using CBT, interpersonal psychotherapy (IPT), or solution-focused psychodynamic therapy.

If there has been no response or inadequate response to trials of two different SSRIs, then switch to another class of drugs. The switch follows the symptom profile, ordering the drug that addresses the symptom profile. Of course, the dosage of the initial drug should be maximized as well as the duration before any other changes are made. Stahl (2008) suggests a symptom-based algorithm for choosing the antidepressant. For example, if lack of sleep is a problem, use a drug that effects serotonin, GABA, or histamine, which would include a sedating antidepressant such as trazadone or a hypnotic such as eszopicione. Another strategy to improve sleep is to stop an activating antidepressant. Sometimes, switching the preparation of the medication may also help. If concentration and fatigue are problematic use drugs that effect NE and/or DA, which may include switching to a norepinephrine dopamine reuptake inhibitor (NDRI), an NE reuptake inhibitor (NRI) such as Strattera, serotonin norepinephrine reuptake inhibitor (SNRI) such as Effexor, Cymbalta, or Pristiq, or a monoamine oxidase inhibitor (MAOI) such as Parnate, Marplan, or Nardil. Augmenting drugs that affect NE and DA include modafinil, stimulants, serotonin-dopamine antagonists (SDA), lithium, thyroid hormone, L-methylfolate (MTHF), and serotonin 1A agonists.

If two medications from the same class have been tried, such as two different SSRIs, then switch to a different class, such as SNRI. If during the first 2 to 4 weeks, new or increased symptoms develop, such as mania or increased suicidality, a different class of drug and more protective treatment such as partial hospitalization or inpatient treatment may be required. If mania develops, of course the antidepressant is stopped and a mood stabilizer initiated. Usual continuation period is 4 to 9 months. During the continuation period, the medication dosage is kept at the same level unless side effects or relapse develop.

Sequenced Treatment Alternatives to Relieve Depression (STAR-D) (Trivedi et al., 2006) has recommended the following options if response to initial treatment is ineffective:

1. Augment the first antidepressant with psychotherapy or another class of medication
2. Change to a different antidepressant or psychotherapy
3. Discontinue the first antidepressant and add psychotherapy
4. Switch to another antidepressant
5. Augment with another class of medication

During the continuation phase, psychotherapy moves toward understanding and modifying triggers and risk factors while building up protective, coping strategies. Focus of sessions continue to follow the case conceptualization but now move to another level. Focus of sessions may include fear of never fully recovering from the depression, loss of former self in terms of fun, sex drive, feeling attractive, or thinking quickly. Other losses may involve relationships, employment, and other lost opportunities. The frequency of sessions is decreased as negotiated between PMH-APRN and client.

Also during this phase of treatment, the PMH-APRN expands thinking as a preventionist—not only preventing a relapse in the client, but also preventing or identifying symptoms in children and significant others of the client is needed. This may be accomplished by gentle questioning about interpersonal relationships as well as requests for adjunct sessions including children or significant others for screening. As the acute symptoms have decreased, other strategies may be introduced such as self-help readings, group therapy, planned activity, or complementary alternative approaches such as healing touch for general well-being.

There is ongoing assessment of symptom severity and number including the emergence of new symptoms such as substance abuse, medical problems, or an additional psychiatric disorder such as anxiety or shift to mania. It is important to use the same evaluation format as during treatment initiation for consistency. This may include repeating the same self-evaluation form or structured interview at regular intervals. The emergence of side effects must also be assessed. More than simply asking "Are you having any side effects?" is necessary. There are standardized questionnaires and structured interviews available. Potential danger to self and others requires continuing assessment. Satisfaction with treatment and adherence to the plan also needs attention, as does functioning level.

MANAGING SIDE EFFECTS

The theoretical framework as well as clinical training of the PMH-APRN often determines the type of psychotherapy offered and implemented. Although this is expected, there is a need to be aware of the changing needs of the client and your expectations. For example, if you are skilled in psychodynamic therapy, but your client's anxiety reaches intolerable levels during sessions, the client will most likely discontinue treatment. So knowing when to offer supportive therapy, education, symptom relief, behavioral strategies, interpersonal strategies, or combined psychotherapy with medications in response to the client's status and desires is important. The issue of sequencing is quite individualized. Once the distressing symptoms have been minimized, clients may wish to only continue medication or to discontinue all treatment.

PHARMACOTHERAPY

Side effects of medications may include serotonin syndrome, antidepressant discontinuation syndrome, hypnotranemia, sexual side effects, weight gain, and tachyphylaxis or pooping out. If the client is experiencing distressing side effects and the decision is to switch or stop antidepressants, there is a risk of serotonin syndrome as well as discontinuation symptoms. Serotonin syndrome may be triggered by administering too-high doses of any drug blocking reuptake of serotonin (especially in the elderly) or by combining drugs with the same action, such as an SSRI with a MAOI. Symptoms of serotonin syndrome include hyperthymia, coma, seizures, brain damage, and death. Treatment is prevention by careful prescribing and if serotonin syndrome does develop, stop the medication and provide supportive treatment usually on an inpatient basis.

Risk factors for developing antidepressant discontinuation syndrome (ADS) include abrupt discontinuation of antidepressant, shorter half-life antidepressants, intermittent nonadherence, use of a "drug holiday," younger age including children, female gender, a breast-fed infant of a mother who is on an antidepressant, a history of ADS, more than 4 to 6 weeks of taking antidepressants, switches between generic formulations of antidepressants (variation in bioequivalence), and history of early adverse reactions during initiation of the antidepressant (Muzina, 2010). ADS rates are as low as 0% with fluoxetine (long half-life) and up to 78% with venlafaxine XR (short half-life). There are also fewer reports of ADS with bupropion, mirtazapine, MAOIs, and nefazodone.

Symptoms of ADS are related to rapid depletion of tryptophan, the essential amino acid precursor for synthesis of 5-HT, and complex interactions among serotonin, NE, and cholinergic systems combined with genetic factors influencing the individual's metabolism of drugs (Blier & Tremblay, 2006). Symptoms vary among clients but generally include the "FINISH" syndrome: flu-like symptoms, insomnia, nausea, imbalance, sensory disturbance, and hyperarousal (anxiety/agitation) (Berber, 1998). ADS symptoms are similar with SSRIs and SNRIs but anticholinergic effects (hallucinations, delirium, abdominal cramping, and diarrhea) may also occur with tricyclic antidepressants (TCAs).

For mild ADS symptoms, providing support and education combined with sedative-hypnotics for sleep or a benzodiazepine for anxiety over 10 days usually leads to resolution of the symptoms. For more severe ADS, or when ongoing antidepressant use is indicated, restarting the antidepressant at the previous dose resolves the symptoms in 24 hours. Another strategy is to restart the antidepressant at the previous dose plus fluoxetine 5–20 mg. Then begin tapering the original antidepressant by 50% every 5 days until stopped. One week later, reduce fluoxetine to 10 mg/day for 5 days and then discontinue. Of course, there is the danger of serotonin syndrome, but several case studies using this strategy have proven to be safe with close follow-up safe with close follow-up (Benazzi, 1998). Remember, psychopharmacotherapy is only partially based upon evidence and is truly more of an art of balancing the client's needs/reactions with the currently available evidence.

Another infrequent but potentially dangerous side effect associated with antidepressants, carbamazepine, lamotrigine, valproic acid, and lithium is hyponatremia. Most clients experiencing hyponatremia were older than 40 years and taking concomitant medications (Madhusoodanan, Bogunovic, Brenner, & Gupta, 2003). Symptoms include lethargy, confusion, and weakness. Treatment involves withdrawal of the drug, fluid restriction, and administration of saline which reverses the electrolyte disturbance.

Another side effect that may develop later in treatment is tachyphylaxis, "pooping out," or apathy. There is controversy if this is a tolerance to the medication or lack of initial recovery from the episode. After several months of continuing on the drug, the client begins to feel apathetic and "flat" with lack of interest or motivation. This effect has been reported for antidepressants as well as with lithium. Treatment has included adding psychotherapy as well as increasing dose of the medication or switching to another class or adding buproprion. Tachyphylaxis may occur in spite of the best of current treatment with medication as well as psychotherapy. If this proves to be true, other interventions involving primary prevention gain importance.

Sexual side effects and weight gain are frequent reasons for clients discontinuing the medication. Approximately 30% to 40% of individuals taking SSRIs experience sexual side effects. Sexual dysfunction can develop as part of a psychiatric disorder, a physical disorder, can be drug-induced, or related to relationship problems. Common medical causes of sexual dysfunction in women include diabetes, hypertension, stroke, urinary incontinence, and urinary tract infections.

Because sexual side effects are so common with SSRIs, it is important to obtain baseline information with questions related to interest, arousal (erectile function in men, lubrication and feelings in women), and orgasm. Although the research is scant, MAOIs have the highest rate of sexual side effects, then TCAs. Of the SSRIs, paroxetine (Paxil) causes the highest level of sexual side effects followed by fluioxetine (Prozac), citalopram (Celexa), sertraline (Zoloft), fluvoxamine (Luvox), and escitalopram (Lexapro) (Keltner, McAfee, & Taylor, 2002).

General treatment strategies include decreasing the dose, waiting, switching, transient discontinuation, and antidotes (Verma & Asghar-Ali, 2006). Often, SSRIs show a flat dose-response curve, meaning that the doses above typical range are not associated with increased efficacy, only more side effects. Therefore, it is hoped that lowering the dose will maintain efficacy while reducing side effects. There have been some antidotal reports of clients accommodating or naturally reducing the intensity of these side effects after 4 to 6 weeks. Switching to bupropion (Wellbutrin) or nefazodone (Dutonin) has resulted in fewer sexual side effects. Of course, when switching antidepressants, there is always the danger of inducing relapse. Another strategy may be to take a drug holiday and discontinue the drug for 1 day. Antidotes used but with minimal data of effectiveness published include bupropion (Wellbutrin) for decreased libido and orgasmic problems, cyproheptadine (an antihistamine), amantadine for anorgasmia, or stimulants. For erectile dysfunction, yohimbine, sildenafil (Viagra), or tadalafil (Cialis) have been effective. Gingko biloba has also been anecdotally reported to relieve sexual dysfunction. Regardless of the level of evidence available, when sexual dysfunction is related to antidepressant treatment, both general strategies and antidotes should be considered on an individual basis. It is also important to review all medications the client is using when considering sexual side effects. See exhibit 8-1 for a list of nonpsychotic prescription medications that may cause sexual dysfunction. As studies in this area hopefully increase, each can be informative and evaluated as to where or how it fits into the current body of evidence relating to treatment of sexual side effects.

Weight gain is a common side effect of antidepressants. Although some individuals develop carbohydrate craving and greatly increased appetite, others state they are eating the same but gaining weight. Switching the antidepressant often helps. Paxil has been reported to be the worst offender. Some prescribers order antidepressants with Topamax as a mood stabilizer as well as an appetite suppressant. Bupropion (Wellbutrin) or low dose stimulants have also been used in the same manner. Regular exercise and well balanced healthy diet are also important factors.

EXHIBIT 8-1: NONPSYCHOTROPIC PRESCRIPTION MEDICATIONS CAUSING SEXUAL DYSFUNCTION

Anabolic steroids	Lipid-lowering agents
Anticholinergics	Methyldopa
Antihistamines	Narcotics
Antihypertensives	Oral contraceptives
Chemotherapeutic agents	

MAINTENANCE

Because mood disorders are often recurrent or chronic, long-term treatment is often necessary. This may involve only medication and supportive therapy with the understanding that therapy may become more intensive as needed. The frequency of sessions may be extended out to initially monthly and then every 3 months. With individuals who are stable on medication, medication groups have been used to maximize resources, especially in community mental health settings. There is no evidence that long-term use of antidepressants or mood stabilizers have negative effects on organs or physiology, but it is important to continue periodic monitoring during maintenance. However, the atypical antipsychotics have a more serious risk of long-term negative effects and suggested monitoring will be discussed in more detail in Chapters 5 and 10.

Another possibility is therapy only. In this case, medications are gradually tapered while sessions focus on current functioning and symptom level and building prevention strategies. Segal and associates (2002) have published an eight-session program for preventing relapse of depression, *Mindfulness-Based Cognitive Therapy*. This type of approach is often used in Partial Hospitalization programs and then the individual moves into supportive or self-help strategies. This program is more a class than therapy and usually has at least 12 clients. Aims of the class include helping individuals with a history of depression to prevent reoccurrences, and to become more aware of bodily sensations, feelings, and thoughts in the moment, to develop mindful acceptance of unwanted feelings, and to choose the most skillful, alternative responses to unpleasant thoughts, feelings, and sensations. Psychoeducation not only increases skills but brings a sense of cognitive control to counteract hopelessness and negativity.

Other clients will discontinue therapy and only use treatment if another episode occurs. With clients who are discontinuing all treatment, a discussion about prodromal signs and symptoms combined with probability of relapse and a plan for reentering treatment is necessary. If clients simply stop attending sessions, follow-up by telephone or letter is appropriate. Hopefully, individuals will learn prodromal symptoms and engage in treatment to prevent or decrease the intensity of another episode. The strength of a therapeutic relationship holds the potential for the client to return when needed.

PRIMARY PREVENTION

Although most health care resources are directed toward treatment, this has not been proven effective in decreasing the prevalence of mood disorders. The literature is growing not only for preventing relapse, but also for preventing the first episode of a mood disorder through universal prevention programs. Prevention programs for youth have a cognitive-behavioral approach with training in coping, problem solving, social skills, and communication. A list of prevention programs proven to be effective are available at the Substance Abuse and Mental Health Services Administration (SAMSHA) (www.samhsa.gov/prevention/)

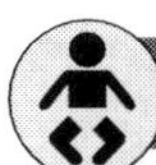

PEDIATRIC POINTERS

Behavior activation (BA) and Antidepressant-Induced Mania (AIM), occur in approximately 8% to 17% of preadolescent children treated with SSRIs and 2% to 3% of adolescents treated with SSRIs. At high risk for these side effects are children with anxiety disorders, mental retardation, autism spectrum disorders, and tic disorders (Safer & Zito, 2006). BA may occur any time in treatment but is usually in the first 2 to 3 weeks. Withdrawl of the SSRI usually results in baseline symptoms. There are controversial findings about suicidal ideation and BA, but the FDA issued a "black box" warning for increased suicidal ideation in 2004.

Although BA and mania are similar, the distinguishing symptoms are the decreased need for sleep and grandiosity seen in mania (Reinblatt DosReis, Walkup, & Riddle, 2009). There are several studies demonstrating a high rate of association between AIM and suicidal ideation, but there is much controversy around the cause. Questions continue as to the presence of bipolar illness with activation of mania or if it is simply a side effect.

Whatever the cause of BA and AIM, it is more common in children and adolescents. Therefore, frequent, careful monitoring after initiating and during SSRI treatment, as well as therapy to improve coping skills, are a necessity when treating depression in children and adolescents.

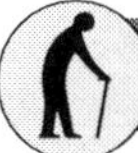

AGING ALERTS

Major depression beginning after the age of 50 often has a higher incidence of structural brain lesions including strokes as well as subcortical and periventricular white matter changes (Yudofsky & Hales, 2004). Furthermore, mild cognitive impairment and co-occurring depression are often an early sign of Alzheimer's disease.

The clinical presentation of depression in older adults often is comorbid with physical illness and when compared to middle-aged adults, there is less guilt, more often a weight loss than gain, and more rumination about death. Treatment is basically the same with lower dosages of medications usually needed and an emphasis upon self-efficacy, activities, and social involvement in psychotherapy. Usual treatment is with the primary care provider and there is a risk of under-treatment in terms of medication dosing as well as lack of psychotherapy. The MacArthur Foundation has published an initiative covering the diagnosis and treatment of depression in primary care (available at www.depression-primarycare.org).

RESOURCES

TREATMENT GUIDELINES FOR CHILDREN AND ADOLESCENTS

Specific guidelines for treating depression in children and adolescents have been developed by several organizations:

American Academy of Child and Adolescent Psychiatry. *Practice parameter for the assessment and treatment of children and adolescents with depressive disorders*. Retrieved from www.aacap.org/galleries/PracticeParameters/Vol%2046%20Nov%202007.pdf

Texas Children's Medication Algorithm: www.ncbi.nlm.nih.gov/pubmed/17513980

National Institute for Clinical Excellence in the United Kingdom: www.nice.org.uk

FOR CLIENTS

BOOKS

The Bipolar Workbook: Tools for Controlling Your Mood Swings (2006) by M. Basco

The Feeling Good Handbook (1999) by D. Burns

The Hypomanic Edge: The Link Between (A Little) Craziness and (A Lot of) Success in America (2005) by J. Gartner

I Hate You Don't Leave Me: Understanding the Borderline Personality (1989) by J. Kreisman, and H. Straus

Stop Walking on Eggshells Workbook: Taking Your Life Back When Someone You Care About Has Borderline Personality Disorder (1998) by P. Mason, and R. Kreger

WEBSITES

American Foundation for Suicide Prevention (AFSP): www.afsp.org

BP Magazine: www.bphope.com/

Depression and Bipolar Support Alliance: www.dbsalliance.org

National Alliance for the Mentally Ill (NAMI): www.nami.org

National Institute of Mental Health website for best practices and clinical trials: www.nimh.nih.gov/trials/index.shtml

REFERENCES

Alexopoulos, G. A., Abrams, R. C., Young, R. C., & Shamoian, C. A. (1988). Cornell scale for depression in dementia. *Biological Psychiatry, 23*, 271–284.

American Psychiatric Association. (1994). *Diagnostic and statistical manual of mental disorders*, (4th ed.). Washington, DC: Author.

American Psychiatric Association. (2010). *Practice guidelines for the Treatment of patients with major depressive disorder* (3rd ed.). Arlington, VA: Author

Andrews, P., & Thompson, J. (2009). The bright side of being blue: Depression as an adaptation for analyzing complex problems. *Psychological Review, 116*(3), 620–654.

Arnault, D., Sakamoto, S., & Mariwaki, A. (2005). Association between negative self-descriptives and depressive symptomatology: Does culture make a difference? *Archives of Psychiatric Nursing, 19*(2), 93–100.

Bagby, R. M., Ryder, H. A., Schuller, D. R., & Marshall, M. (2004). The Hamilton Depression Scale: Has the gold standard become a lead weight? *American Journal of Psychiatry, 161*, 2163–2167.

Ballas, C. A., & Staab, J. P. (2003). Medically unexplained physical symptoms: Toward an alternative paradigm for diagnosis and treatment, *CNS Spectrum, 8*(12), 21–26.

Basco, M. (2006). *The bipolar workbook: tools for controlling your mood swings*. New York, NY: Guilford Press.

Basler, R. (1953). *The Collected Works of Abraham Lincoln*. Washington, DC: The Abraham Lincoln Association.

Baucom, D., & Epstein, N. (1991). Will the real cognitive-behavioral therapy please stand up? *Journal of Family Psychology, 4*(4), 394–401.

Beck, A. (1991). Cognitive therapy: A 30-year retrospective. *American Psychologist, 46*(4), 368–375.

Beck, A. T., & Steer, R. A. (1984). Internal consistencies of the original and revised Beck Depression Inventory. *Journal of Clinical Psychology. 40*(6), 1365–1367.

Beck, A. T., Ward, C. H., Mendelson, M., Mock, J., & Erbaugh, J. (1961). An inventory for measuring depression. *Archives of General Psychiatry, 4*, 561–571.

Benazzi, F. (1998). SSRI discontinuation syndrome treated with fluoxetine. *International Journal of Geriatric Psychiatry, 13*(6), 421–422.

Berber, M. (1998). FINISH: Remembering the discontinuation syndrome. *Journal of Clinical Psychiatry, 59*(5), 255.

Blier, P. & Tremblay, P. (2006), Physiologic mechanisms underlying the antidepressant discontinuation syndrome. *Journal of Clinical Psychiatry, 67*, Supplement 4, 8–13.

Bodenmann, G. (2007). Improving in marital distress prevention programs and marital therapy: Dyadic coping and the 3-phase method in working with couples. In L. VanderCreek & J. Allen (Eds.), *Innovations in clinical practice: Focus on group and family therapy* (pp. 235–252). Sarasota, FL: Professional Resources Press.

Bolwig, T. (2003). Putative common pathways in therapeutic brain stimulation for affective disorders. *CNS Spectrums, 8*(7), 490–495.

Brink, T. L., Yesavage, J. A., Lump, O., Heersema, P., Adey, M. B., & Rose, T. L. (1982). Screening test for geriatric depression. *Clinical Geronotologist, 1*, 37–44.

Burns, D. (1999). *The Feeling Good Handbook*. London, UK: Plume.

Butler, R. N., & Lewis, M. I. (1995). Late-life depression: When and how to intervene. *Geriatrics, 50*, 44–55.

Cano, A., & O'Leary, K. (2000). Infidelity and separations precipitate major depressive episodes and symptoms of nonspecific anxiety. *Journal of Consulting and Clinical Psychology, 68,* 774–781.

Centers for Disease Control and Prevention (CDC), Web-based Injury Statistics Query and Reporting System (WISQARS). (2010). National Center for Injury Prevention and Control, CDC. Retrived from www.cdc.gov/injury/wisqars/index.html

Childs-Gowell, E. (1995). *Good grief rituals: Tools for healing.* Barrytown, NY: Station Hill.

Consumer Reports. (2010). Depression and anxiety: Readers reveal the therapists and drugs that help. *Consumer Reports* magazine, July, pp. 5–12.

Cuijpers, P., Dekker, J., Noteboom, A., Smits, N., & Peen, J. (2007). Sensitivity and specificity of the Major Depression Inventory in outpatients, *BMC Psychiatry, 7,* 39.

Daray, F., Thommi, B., & Ghaemi, N. (2010). The pharmacogenetics of antidepressant-induced mania: A systematic review and meta analysis. *Bipolar Disorders, 12*(7), 702–706.

Ehlers, C., Frank, E., & Kupfer, D. (1988). Social zeitgebers and biological rhythms: A unified approach to understanding the etiology of depression. *Archives of General Psychiatry. 45*(10), 948–952.

Faulstich, M. E., Carey, M. P., Ruggiero, L., Entart, P., & Gresham, F. (1986). Assessment of depression in childhood and adolescence: An evaluation of the Center for Epidemiological Studies Depression Scale for Children (CES-DC). *American Journal of Psychiatry, 143*(8), 1024–1027.

Fava, M. (2003). Depression with physical symptoms: Treating to remission. *Journal of Clinical Psychiatry, 64*(Suppl. 7), 24–28.

Folstein, M., Folstein, S., & McHugh, P. (1975). Mini-Mental State. A practical method for grading the cognitive status of patients for the clinician. *Journal of Psychiatric Research, 12,* 189–198.

Foroushani, P. S., Schneider, J., & Assareh, N. (2011). A meta-review of effectiveness of computerized CBT in treating depression. *BMC Psychiatry, 11*(131).

Frank, E., Kupfer, D., Thase, M. E., Mallinger, A., Swartz, H., Fagiolini, A.,...Monk, T. (2005). Two-year outcomes for interpersonal and social rhythm therapy in individuals with bipolar I disorder. *Archives of General Psychiatry, 62*(9), 996–1004.

Frank, E., Prien, R., Jarrett, R., Keller, M., Kupfer, D., Lavori, P.,...Weissman, M. M. (1991). Conceptualization and rationale for consensus definitions of terms in major depressive disorders: Remission, recovery, relapse, and recurrence. *Archives of General Psychiatry, 48,* 851–855.

Galvez, J., Thommi, S., & Ghaemi, N. (2011). Positive aspects of mental illness: A review of bipolar disorder. *Journal of Affective Disorders, 128,* 185–190.

Garland, E., Fredrickson, B., Kring, A., Johnson, D., Meyer, P., & Penn, D. (2010). Upward spirals of positive emotions counter downward spirals of negativity: Insights from the broaden-and-build theory and affective neuroscience on the treatment of emotion dysfunctions and deficits in psychopathology. *Clinical Psychology Review, 30,* 849–864.

Gartner, J. (2005). *The hypomanic edge: the link between (a little) craziness and (a lot of) success in America.* New York, NY: Simon & Schuster.

George, M., Rush, A., Marangell, J., Sackeim, H., Brannan, S., Davis, S.,...Goodnick, P. (2005). A one-year comparison of vagus nerve stimulation with treatment as usual for treatment-resistant depression. *Biological Psychiatry, 58*(5), 364–373.

Goldberg, D. (2000). Plato versus Aristotle: Categorical and dimensional models for common mental disorders. *Comprehensive Psychiatry, 41,* 8–13.

Golden, R. N., Gaynes, B. N., Ekstrom, R. D., Hamer, R. M., Jacobsen, F. M., Suppes, T.,...Nemeroff, C. B. (2005). The efficacy of light therapy in the treatment of mood disorders: A review and meta-analysis of the evidence. *American Journal of Psychiatry, 162*(4), 656–662.

Gooley, J., Rajaratnam, S., Brainard, G., Kronauer, R. E., Czeisler, C. A., & Lockley, S. W. (2010). Intensity and duration of light exposure affects circadian rhythm. *Science Translational Medicine, 2*(31), 1–9.

Gotlib, I., & Hammen, C. (2010). *Handbook of Depression* (2nd ed.). New York, NY: Guilford.

Gracious, B., Youngstrom, E. A., Fiadling, R. L., & Calabrese, J. R. (2002). Discriminative validity of the parent version of the Young Mania Rating Scale. *Journal of the American Academy of Child and Adolescent Psychiatry, 41*(11), 1350–1359.

Greenberg, P., Leong, S., Birnbaum, H., & Robinson, R. (2003). The Economic Burden of Depression. *Journal of Clinical Psychiatry, 64*(Suppl. 7), 17–23.

Greenberger, D., & Padesky, C. (1995). *Mind Over Mood.* New York, NY & London, UK: Guilford.

Guilford-Blake, R. (2010, April). Some men talk about depression differently: Older men should be encouraged to talk about changes in work, health, and family context. *Clinical Psychiatry News,* p. 17.

Hamilton, M. (1960). A rating scale for depression. *Journal of Neurology, Neurosurgery, & Psychiatry, 23,* 56–62.

Heim, C., Newport, D. J., Heit, S., Graham, Y. P., Wilcox, M., Bonsall, R.,...Nemeroff, C. B. (2000). Pituitary-adrenal and autonomic responses to stress in women after sexual and physical abuse in childhood. *Journal of the American Medical Association, 284*(5), 592–597.

Herman, H., Stewart, D., Diaz-Granados, S., Berger, E., Jackson, B., & Yuen, T. (2011). What is resilience? *Canadian Journal of Psychiatry, 56*(5), 258–265.

Herrmann, L., & Ebmeier, K. (2006). Factors modifying the efficacy of transcranial magnetic stimulation in the treatment of depression: A review. *Journal of Clinical Psychiatry, 67*(12), 1870–1876.

Hirschfeld, R. M. A., Williams, J. B. W., Spitzer, R. L., Calabrese, J. R., Flynn, L., Keck, P. E.,...Zajecka, J. (2000). Development and validation of a screening instrument for bipolar spectrum disorder: The mood disorder questionnaire. *American Journal of Psychiatry, 157,* 1873–1875.

Jacobson, N., Martell, C., & Dimidjian, S. (2001). Behavioral activation treatment for depression: Returning to contextual roots. *Clinical Psychology: Science and Practice, 8,* 255–270.

Jauhar, P., & Weller, M. (1982). Psychiatric morbidity and time zone changes: A study of patients from Heathrow airport. *British Journal of Psychiatry, 140,* 231–235.

Joiner, T., & Coyne, J. (1999). *The interactional nature of depression.* Washington, DC: American Psychological Association.

Joiner, T., & Timmons, K. (2010). Depression in its interpersonal context. In I. Gottlieb & C. Hammen (Eds.), *Handbook of depression* (pp. 322–335). New York, NY: Guilford.

Jorm, A. F., & Griffiths, K. (2006). Population promotion of informal self-help strategies for early intervention against depression and anxiety. *Psychological Medicine, 36,* 3–6.

Judd, L. L., Paulus, M. J., Schettler, P. J., Akiskal, H. S., Endicott, J., Leon, A. C.,...Keller, M. B. (2000). Does incomplete recovery from first lifetime major depressive episode herald a chronic course of illness? *American Journal of Psychiatry, 157,* 1501–1504.

Juurlink, D., Herrman, J. P., Szalai, J., Kopp, B., & Redelmeir, D. (2004). Medical illness and risk of suicide in the elderly. *Archives of Internal Medicine, 164*(11), 1179–1184.

Kaltenthaler, E., Schackley, P., Stevens, K., Beverly, C., Parry, G., & Chilcott, J. (2002). A systematic review and economic evaluation of computerized cognitive behavioral therapy for depression and anxiety. *Health Technology Assessment, 6*, 1–89.

Kaufman, J., Birmaher, B., Brent, D., Rao, U., Flynn, C., Moreci, P.,... Ryan, N. (1997). Schedule for affective disorders and schizophrenia for school-aged children present and life time version (K-SADS-PL): Initial reliability and validity data. *Journal of the American Academy of Child and Adolescent Psychiatry, 36*, 980–988.

Keck, P. E., McElroy, S. L., Strakowski, S. M., West, S. A., Sax, K. W., Hawkins, J. M.,... Haggard, P. (1998). 12- month outcome of patients with bipolar disorder following hospitalization for a manic or mixed episode. *American Journal of Psychiatry, 155*, 646–652.

Keltner, N., McAfee, K., & Taylor, C. (2002). Mechanisms and treatments of SSRI-Induced sexual dysfunction. *Perspectives in Psychiatric Care, 38*(3), 111–116.

Kendler, K. S., & Gardner, C. O. (2010). Dependent stressful life events and prior depressive episodes in the prediction of major depression: The problem of causal inference. *Archives of General Psychiatry, 67*(11), 1120–1127.

Kessler, R., & Merikangas, K. (2004). The National Comorbidity Survey Replication (NCS-R): Background and aims. *International Journal of Methods in Psychiatric Research, 13*, 60–68.

Kovacs, M. (1992). *Children's Depression Inventory*. North Tonawanda, NY: Multi-Health System.

Kowatch, R., Fristad, M., Birmaher, B., Wagner, K., Findling, R., & Hellander, M. (2005). Treatment guidelines for children and adolescents with bipolar disorder. *Journal of the American Academy of Child and Adolescent Psychiatry, 44*(3), 213–235.

Kreger, R., & Shirley, J. (2002). *The stop walking on eggshells workbook*. Oakland, CA: Harbinger Press.

Kreisman, J., & Straus, H. (1989). *I hate you don't leave me: Understanding the borderline personality disorder.* New York, NY: Harper Collins.

Krugman, S., & Dubowitz, H. (2003). Failure to thrive. *American Family Physician, 68*(5), 879–884.

Kurtze, N., Rangul, V., Hustvedt, B., & Flanders, W. (2008). Reliability and validity of self-reported physical activity in the Nord-Trondelag Health Study – Hunt 1. *Scandinavian Journal of Public Health, 36*(1), 52–61.

Kuyken, W., Padesky, C., & Dudley, R. (2009). *Collaborative case conceptualization*. New York, NY & London, UK: Guilford Press.

Lam, R. W., Levitt, A. J., Levitan, R. D., Enns, M. W., Morehouse, R., Michalak, E. E., & Tam, E. M. (2006). The Can-SAD study: A randomized controlled trial of the effectiveness of light therapy and fluoxetine in patients with winter seasonal affective disorder. *American Journal of Psychiatry, 163*(5), 805–812.

Lavelle, S., & Tusaie, K. (2011). Reflections on forced medications. *Issues in Mental Health Nursing, 32*, 274–278.

Lewinsohn, P., & Essau, C. (2002). Depression in adolescents. In I. Gotleib & C. Hammen (Eds.), *Handbook of depression* (pp. 541–559). New York, NY: Guilford.

Linehan, M. (1993). *Skills training manual for borderline personality disordeer*. New York, NY: Guilford.

Luby, J., Lenze, S., & Tillman, R. (2011). A novel intervention for preschool depression: Findings from a randomized controlled trial. *Journal of Child Psychology and Psychiatry, 53*(3), 313–322. doi 10.1111/j 1496–2011.02483.x

Mackrill, T. (2010). Goal consensus and collaboration in psychotherapy: An existential rationale. *Journal of Humanistic Psychology, 50*(1), 96–107.

Madhusoodanan, S., Bogunovic, O., Brenner, R., & Gupta, S. (2003). Hyponatremia secondary to antipsychotics, mood stabilizers, and anxiolytics. *Psychiatric Annals, 33*(5), 310–315.

Malkoff-Schwartz, S., Frank, E., Anderson, B., Sherrill, J. T., Siegel, L., Patterson, D., & Kupfer, D. J. (1998). Stressful life events and social rhythm disruption in the onset of mania and depressive bipolar episodes: A preliminary investigation. *Archives of General Psychiatry, 55*(8), 702–707.

Martini, D., Strayhorn, J., & Puig-Antich, J. (1990). A symptom self-report measure for preschool children. *Journal of the American Academy of Child and Adolescent Psychiatry, 29*, 594–600.

Martinowich, K., & Lu, B. (2008). Interaction between BDNF and serotonin: Role in mood disorders. *Neuropsychopharmacology, 33*, 73–83.

Mason, P., & Kreger, R. (1998). *Stop walking on eggshells workbook: taking your life back when someone you care about has borderline personality disorder.* Oakland, CA: New Harbinger Publishers.

Measelle, J. R., Ablow, J. C., Cowan, P. A., & Cowan, C. (1998). Assessing young children's views of their academic, social, and emotional lives: An evaluation of the self-perception scale of the Burkley Puppet Interview. *Child Development, 69*(6), 1556–1576.

Miklowitz, D., Goodwin, G., Bauer, M., & Geddes, J. (2008). Common and specific elements of psychosocial treatment for bipolar disorder: A survey of clinicians participating in randomized trials. *Journal of Psychiatric Practice, 14*, 1–9.

Montgomery, S. A., & Asberg, M. (1979). A new depression scale designed to be sensitive to change. *British Journal of Psychiatry, 134*, 382–389.

Murray, C., & Lopez, A. D. (1996). *The global burden of disease*. Cambridge, MA: Harvard University Press.

Muzina, D. (2010). Discontinuing an antidepressant. *Current Psychiatry, 9*(3), 51–61.

Nash, M. (2008). Substance induced mood disorders. *E-medicine Medscape*, Art. no. 286885.

Nelson, A., & Tusaie, K. (2011). Developmentally sensitive cognitive behavioral therapy: Guides from pedagogy. *Archives of Psychiatric Nursing, 25*(6), 485–487.

Ozbay, F., Johnson, D., Dimoulas, E., Morgan, C. A., Charney, D., & Southwick, S. (2007). Social support and resilience to stress: From neurobiology to clinical practice. *Psychiatry, 4*(5), 35–40.

Phelps, J. (2008). Dark therapy for bipolar disorder using amber lens for blue light blockade. *Medical Hypotheses, 70*, 224–229.

Prudic, J., Olfsan, M., Marcus, C., Fuller, R., & Sackeim, H. (2004). Effectiveness of electroconvulsive therapy. *Biological Psychiatry, 55*, 300–312.

Quantum Field Theory. (2006). Stanford Encyclopedia of Philosophy. Retrieved from http://Plato.stanford.edu/entries/quantum-field-theory

Reich, W. (2000). Diagnostic interview for children and adolescents (DICA). *Journal of the American Academy of Child and Adolescent Psychiatry, 39*, 59–66.

Reinblatt, S., DosReis, S., Walkup, J., & Riddle, M. (2009). Activation adverse events induced by selective serotonin reuptake inhibitors in children and adolescents. *Journal of Child and Adolescent Psychopharmacology, 19*(2), 119–126.

Reinecke, M., Datillo, F., & Freeman, A. (2003). *Cognitive behavioral therapy with children and adolescents*. New York, NY: Guilford Press.

Reynolds, W. M. (1986) *Reynolds adolescent depression scale*. Odessa, FL: Psychological Assessment Resources.

Reynolds, W., & Mazza, J. (1998). Reliability and validity of the Reynolds depression scale with young adolescents. *Journal of School Psychology, 36*(3), 295–312.

Roberts, R., Lewinsohn, P., & Seeley, P. (1991). Screening for adolescent depression: A comparison of depression scales. *Journal of the American Academy of Child and Adolescent Psychiatrists, 30*(1), 58–66.

Rosengren, D. (2009). *Building motivational interviewing skills: A practitioner workbook*. New York, NY: Guilford.

Rush, A. (2007). STAR-D: What have we learned? *American Journal of Psychiatry, 164*(2), 201–204.

Rush, A. J., Carmody, T., & Reimitz, P. E. (2000). The inventory of depressive symptomatology (IDS): Clinician (IDS-C) and self-report (IDS-SR) ratings of depressive symptoms. *International Journal of Methods in Psychiatric Research, 9*, 45–59.

Rush, A. J., Giles, D. E., Schlesser, M. A., Fulton, C. L., Weissenburger, J. E., & Burns, C. T. (1986). The inventory of depressive symptomatology (IDS): Preliminary findings. *Psychiatry Research, 18*, 65–87.

Rush, A. J., Gullion, C. M., Basco, M. R., Jarrett, R. B., & Trivedi, M. H. (1996). The inventory of depressive symptomatology (IDS): Psychometric properties. *Psychological Medicine, 26*, 477–486.

Sachs, G. S., Thase, M. E., Otto, M. W., Bauer, M., Miklowitz, D., Wisniewski, S. R.,... Rosenbaum, J. F. (2003). Rationale, design, and methods of the systematic treatment enhancement program for bipolar disorder (STEP-BD). *Biological Psychiatry, 53*(11),1028–1042.

Safer, D., & Zito, J. (2006). Treatment-emergent adverse events from selective serotonin reuptake inhibitors by age group: Children versus adolescents. *Journal of Child and Adolescent Psychopharmacology, 16*(1–2), 159–169.

Sanders, M., & McFarland, M. (2000). Treatment of depressed mothers with disruptive children: A controlled evaluation of cognitive-behavioral family intervention. *Behavior Therapy, 31*, 89–112.

Schaefer, C. (2003). *Foundations of play therapy*. Hoboken, NJ: Wiley.

Schuttor, D. (2009). Antidepressant efficacy of high-frequency transcranial magnetic stimulation over the left dorsolateral prefrontal cortex in double-blind sham-controlled designs: A meta-analysis. *Psychological Medicine, 39*, 65–75.

Segal, Z., Williams, M., and Teasdale, J. (2002). *Mindfulness-based cognitive therapy for depression*. NY: The Guilford Press.

Shapiro, R. (Ed.). (2009). *EMDR solutions II: For depression, eating disorders, performance, and more*. New York, NY: Norton.

Sharp, L. K., & Lipsky, M. S. (2002). Screening for depression across the lifespan: A review of measures for use in primary care settings. *American Family Physician, 66*(6), 1001–1008.

Shea, S. C. (1998). *Psychiatric interviewing: The art of understanding* (2nd ed.). Philadelphia, PA: Saunders.

Sheikh, J. I., & Yesavage, J. A. (1986). Geriatric depression scale: Recent evidence and development of a shorter version. *Clinical Gerontologist, 5*, 165–173.

Shin, J. (2010). Understanding the experience and manifestations of depression among Korean immigrants in New York City. *Journal of Transcultural Nursing, 21*(1), 73–80.

Sorensen, M., Nissen, J., Mors, O., & Thomsen, P. (2005). Age and gender difference in depressive symptomatology and comorbidity: An incident sample of psychiatrically admitted children. *Journal of Affective Disorders, 84*, 85–91.

Southwick, S. M., Vythillingham, M., & Charney, D. S. (2005). The psychobiology of depression and resilience to stress: Implications for prevention and treatment. *Annual Review of Clinical Psychology, 1*, 255–291.

Stahl, S. (2008). *Essential Psychopharmacology*. New York, NY: Cambridge University Press.

Steiner, M., Dunn, E., & Born, L. (2003). Hormones and mood: From menarche to menopause and beyond. *Journal of Affective Disorders, 74*, 67–83.

Suen, L.W., & Tusaie, K. (2004). Is somatization a significant depressive symptom in older Taiwanese Americans? *Geriatric Nursing, 25*(3), 157–163.

Suicide Prevention Resource Center. (2012). Best practices registry. Retrieved June 2, 2012, from www.sprc.org/bpr

Trivedi, M. H., Rush, A. J., Ibrahim, H. M., Carmody, T. J., Biggs, M. M., Suppes, T.,... Kashner, T. M. (2004) The inventory of depressive symptomatology, clinician rating (IDS-C) and self-report (IDS-SR), the quick inventory of depressive symtomatology, clinician rating (QIDS-C) and self-report (QIDS-SR) in public sector patients with mood disorders: A psychometric evaluation. *Psychological Medicine, 34*, 73–82.

Trivedi, M., Rush, A., Wisniewski, S., Nierenberg, A., Warden, D.,... Fava, M. (2006). Evaluation of outcomes with citalopram for depression using measurement-based care in STAR-D: Implications for clinical practice. *American Journal of Psychiatry, 163*(1), 28–40.

Tusaie, K. (2010). Is the tail wagging the dog in pediatric bipolar disorder? *Archives of Psychiatric Nursing, 24*(6), 438–439.

Tusaie, K., & Dyer, J. (2004). Resilience: A historical review of the construct. *Holistic Nursing Practice, 18*(1), 3–9.

Tusaie, K., Puskar, K., & Sereika, S. (2007). A predictive and moderating model of psychosocial resilience in adolescents. *Journal of Nursing Scholarship, 39*(1), 54–60.

Valla, J., Bergeron, L., & Smolla, N. (2000). The Dominic-R: A pictorial interview for 6- to 11-year-old children. *Journal of the American Academy of Child and Adolescent Psychiatry, 39*, 85–93.

Verma, N., & Asghar-Ali, A. (2006). Female sexual dysfunction: Don't assume it's a side effect. *Current Psychiatry, 5*(7), 47–57.

Wade, T., & Kendler, K. (2000). The relationship between social support and major depression: Cross-sectional, longitudinal, and genetic perspective. *Journal of Nervous and Mental Disease, 188*, 251–258.

Walters, G. & Wellcome Trust Case Control Consortium. (2007). Genome-wide association study of 14, 000 cases of 7 common diseases and 3,000 shared controls. *Nature, 447*(7145), 661–678.

Weller, E., Fristad, M., Rooney, M., & Schecter, J. (2000). Children's Interview for Psychiatric Symptoms (CHIPS). *Journal of the American Academy of Child and Adolescent Psychiatry, 29*, 76–84.

Wenze, S., & Miller, I. (2010). Use of ecological momentary assessment in mood disorder research. *Clinical Psychological Review, 30*(6), 794–804.

Williams J. B. (2001). Standardizing the Hamilton depression rating scale: Past, present, and future. *European Archives of Psychiatry and Clinical Neuroscience, 251*(suppl. 2):II/6-II/12.

Wirz-Justice, A., Benedetti, F., & Terman, M. (2009). *Chronotherapeutics for affective disorders: A clinician's manual for light and wake therapy*. Basel, Switzerland: Karger.

Yalom, I., & Leszcz, M. (2005). *Theory and practice of group psychotherapy*. New York, NY: Basic Books.

Yudofsky, S., & Hales, R. (2004). *Essentials of neuropsychiatry and clinical neurosciences*. Washington, DC & London, UK: American Psychiatric Publishing.

Zimmerman, M., Galione, J. N., Ruggero, C. J., Chelminski, I., Young, D., Dalrymple, K., & McGlinchey, J. B. (2010). Screening for bipolar disorder and finding borderline personality disorder. *Journal of Clinical Psychiatry, 71*, 1212–1217.

Zung, W. (1965). A self-rating depression scale. *Archives of General Psychiatry, 12*, 63–70.

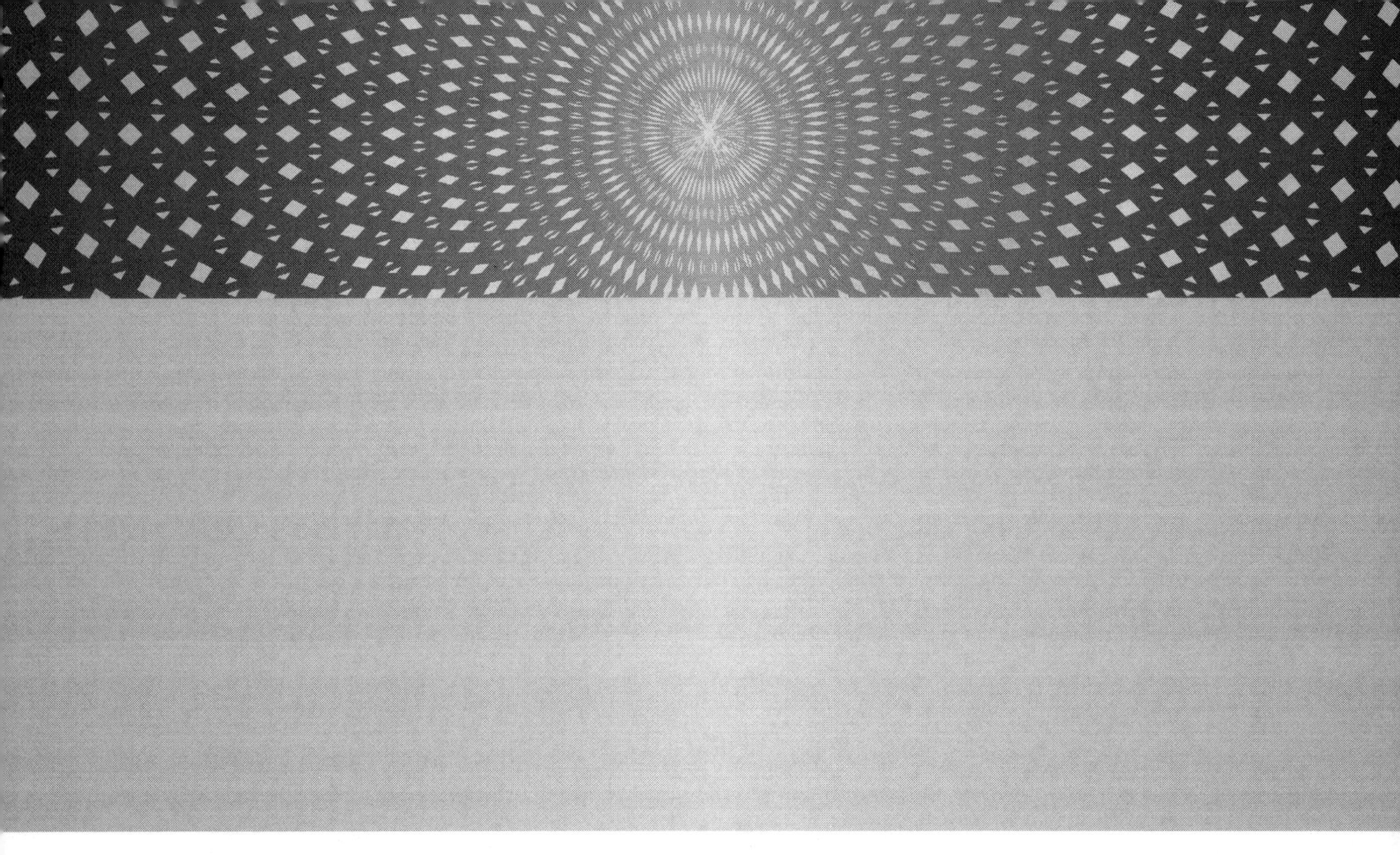

CHAPTER CONTENTS

Anxiety is a sense of distress in response to a perceived threat, either to one's physical safety or emotional well-being. In its mildest form, anxiety is motivational and adaptive, prompting action. As anxiety increases, however, one becomes less able to take in information and misperception is common. Although everyone experiences brief periods of anxiety in response to life's inevitable stressors, anxiety disorders are differentiated by the chronicity and severity of anxiety symptoms.

THE ANXIETY CYCLE

Development of anxiety may be seen as a cyclical process in which physical, psychological, and behavioral factors interact to either increase or decrease the sense of threat and consequent responses (see Figure 9-1). Since all anxiety conditions are characterized by a state of heightened arousal or fear, this model draws on theory about the acute stress response, also referred to as "fight-or-flight." However, anxiety is more complex than physiologic arousal since anxious responses are disproportionate to the nature of the threat, last longer, and are affected by complex cognitive and behavioral processes (U.S. Department of Health and Human Services [DHHS], 1999).

Anxiety begins when a stimulus triggers a sense of threat. Anxiety triggers can include external factors such as threats to safety, as well as internal factors like excessive

CHAPTER 9

Integrative Management of Anxiety

Beth Phoenix and Kathryn Johnson

self-demands or cognitive distortions. The magnitude of the anxiety response is influenced by an individual's predisposing factors, such as a genetic predisposition to excessive anxiety or altered stress responses resulting from previous trauma or abuse.

PHYSIOLOGIC RESPONSES

Threat perception begins in the brain stem where exposure to a novel stimulus triggers the release of norepinephrine from the locus ceruleus. This causes an increase in alertness, and if the stimulus is perceived to be threatening, further norepinephrine release activates the sympathetic nervous system to mobilize the body for action. Common physical manifestations of anxiety such as increased heart rate and muscle tension result from the effect of norepinephrine on nerve endings acting on the heart, blood vessels, and muscles.

Response to the perceived danger continues in the amygdala, a structure in the limbic system, where perception of the current stimulus is compared to stored information about previous threats. Neural projections from the amygdala connect to multiple brain systems involved in behavioral and physiological fear responses (DHHS, 1999). Neurotransmission to the hypothalamus begins the activation of the hypothalamic-pituitary-adrenal (HPA) axis and the release of cortisol. Information is

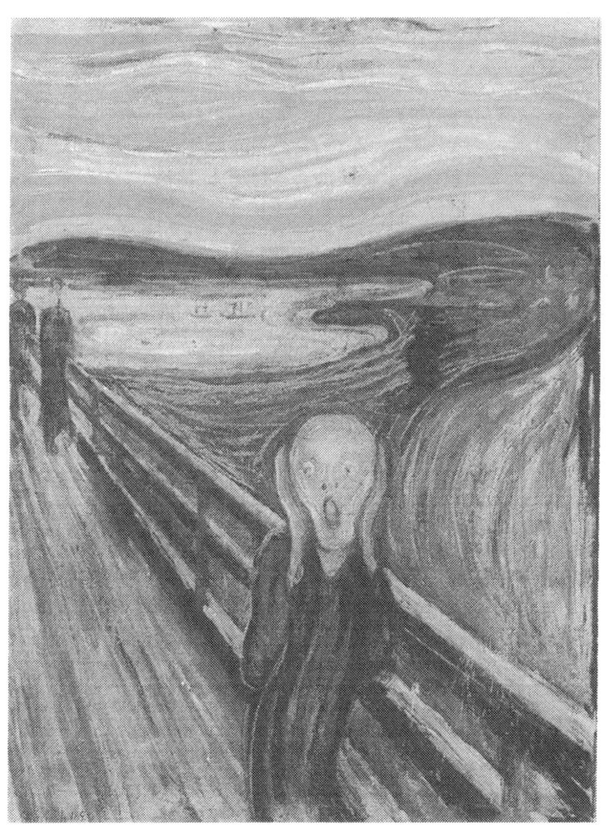

This Famous Painting Has Been Described as, "a trenchant visual expression of Munch's feeling, the product of his own anxiety and depression at the time." (Glueck, 2006). Edvard Munch, *The Scream* (1893), National Gallery, Oslo, Norway.

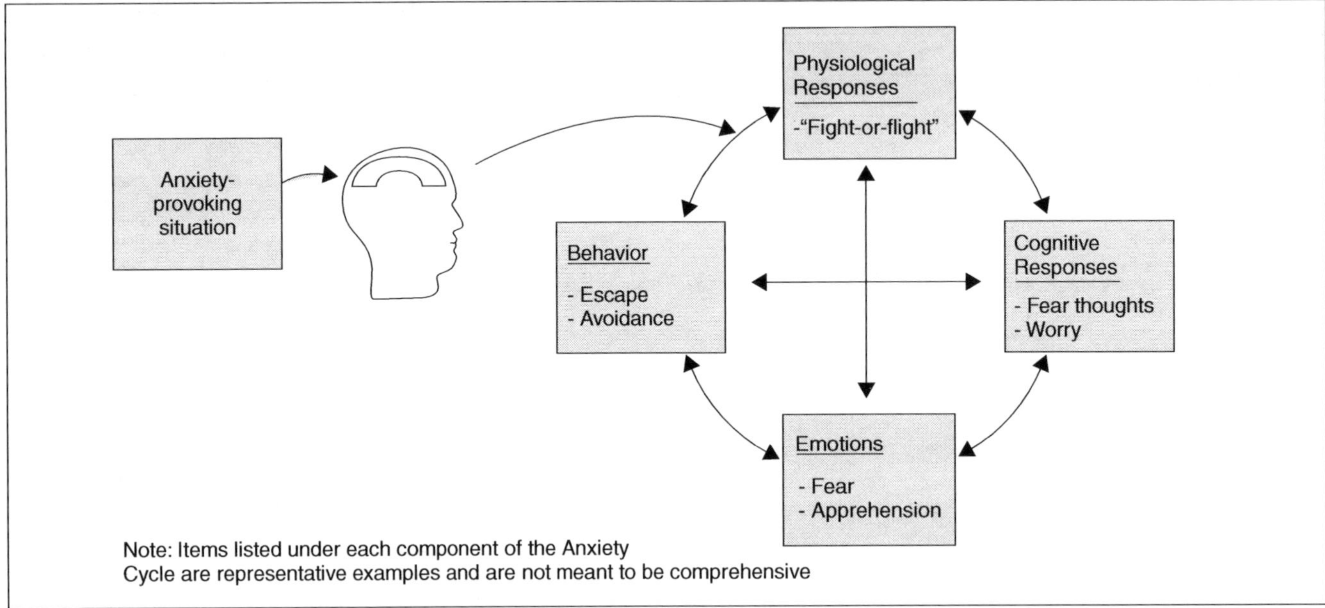

Figure 9-1 The Anxiety Cycle

then transmitted to the hippocampus, where the access to more detailed memories allows further interpretation of the situation. Evaluation of potential threats by these subcortical structures is rapid and crude—it is only when the threat message reaches the cerebral cortex that it can be fully examined and interpreted.

COGNITION

Thoughts can contribute to beginning the cycle of anxiety, and cognitive responses can either accelerate or slow down the body's response to an initial threat message. For instance, the prospect of taking an elevator may cause anxiety in someone who has claustrophobia. Thoughts such as, "What if the elevator gets stuck and I can't get out?" are likely to increase the sense of apprehension and the associated physiological response. In contrast, feedback from the cortex in the form of thoughts like, "I've never gotten stuck in an elevator before. I can practice deep breathing to keep myself calm," reduces the sense of threat and inhibits the anxiety response. Conversely, physical responses may influence cognitive processes—the chest tightness and shortness of breath experienced during a panic attack may elicit fear thoughts such as, "I'm having a heart attack! I'm about to die!"

BEHAVIORAL RESPONSES

Behavior influences thoughts and physical responses, and is influenced by them. For instance, practicing relaxation reduces sympathetic hyperarousal and decreases fear thoughts. In contrast, physiologic responses such as dry mouth and sweaty palms combined with distorted cognitions like, "Everyone thinks I'm stupid" may cause persons with social anxiety to avoid public speaking.

Different theoretical approaches may emphasize different parts of the anxiety cycle as targets for intervention. Neurobiologic theories may focus on use of medication to decrease baseline physiologic hyperarousal or stabilize hypersensitized stress response systems. Cognitive theories examine the contribution of distorted cognitions, such as overestimating danger, that contribute to anxiety. Behavioral theories identify connections between conditioned stimuli (e.g., enclosed spaces) and subsequent responses (fear), and use techniques such as exposure to correct faulty associations.

ANXIETY DISORDERS

The *Diagnostic and Statistical Manual (DSM) IV-TR* (American Psychiatric Association [APA], 2000) categories of anxiety disorders are generalized anxiety disorder (GAD), social anxiety disorder (SAD, also referred to as social phobia [SP]), specific phobia, panic disorder (PD) with and without agoraphobia, obsessive-compulsive disorder (OCD), post-traumatic stress disorder (PTSD), acute stress disorder, anxiety secondary to a general medical condition, and substance-induced anxiety disorder. Available literature on prevalence and treatment of anxiety disorders relies on this diagnostic system, so these diagnostic terms will be used throughout the chapter.

Modifications under consideration for the *DSM-5* would change this categorization in several ways: (a) agoraphobia would be a separate diagnosis rather than merely an associated feature of PD; (b) obsessive-compulsive and related disorders would be a separate diagnostic category; (c) PSTD would be included in a new category, "Trauma- and Stressor-Related Disorders" (APA, "*DSM-5* Development," n.d.). Since diagnostic nomenclature is in the process of change, and because many symptoms and symptom clusters are found in multiple anxiety disorders, this chapter will broadly examine anxiety-related conditions with a focus on key symptom profiles.

Ataque de nervios ("attack of nerves"), a transient response to a severe psychosocial stressor characterized by impulsive and dramatic behaviors such as screaming uncontrollably, crying, trembling and nervousness, and breaking things, commonly includes or co-occurs with anxiety symptoms (Hinton, Chong, Pollack, Barlow, & McNally, 2008). *Ataque de nervios* is categorized by the *DSM-IV-TR* as a culture-bound syndrome that occurs in Latino cultures and is not considered an anxiety disorder, but is mentioned here because of the prominence of anxious symptoms.

PREVALENCE AND IMPACT OF ANXIETY CONDITIONS

Anxiety disorders are among the most common psychiatric disorders—epidemiological data show a lifetime prevalence rate of 28.8% for the anxiety disorders as a group (Kessler, Chiu, Merikangas, Demler, & Walters, 2005). Anxiety symptoms typically begin in childhood—the National Comorbidity Study Replication found the median age at onset of anxiety disorders was 11 years, in contrast to 30 years for mood disorders (Kessler et al., 2005a). Despite this high prevalence, treatment rates for anxiety disorders are low, typically in the range of 30% to 40% for both children and adults (Bienvenu & Ginsburg, 2007).

Anxiety disorders show clear gender differences. Data from the Collaborative Psychiatric Epidemiology Studies (CPES) indicate that women's prevalence rates are 70% to 80% higher than men's for anxiety disorders in general. Women are more likely to suffer from each of the anxiety disorders except for SAD, which shows no differences in gender distribution. In addition to greater prevalence, anxiety disorders are also more disabling in women (McLean, Asnaani, Litz, & Hofmann, 2011). As with depression, hormonal influences and greater exposure to psychosocial stressors such as poverty and discrimination may contribute to women's greater illness burden from anxiety.

Anxiety disorders are highly comorbid conditions that can be debilitating, especially when they coexist with other psychiatric disorders. Anxiety disorders, particularly GAD, commonly co-occur with other anxiety disorders (Woodman, 1997). Mood and substance abuse disorders are the most common comorbid disorders with generalized anxiety (Davidson, 2009), and the presence of alcohol dependence is particularly high in persons with social anxiety (Boschloo et al., 2011). Mood disorders are further discussed in Chapter 8, and substance abuse with psychiatric syndromes is addressed in depth in Chapter 17.

The cost of anxiety to society in the form of lost wages and productivity, misdiagnosis, and inappropriate use of medical services is high. DuPont et al. (1996) found that in 1990 the annual overall cost burden of anxiety disorders in the United States was estimated to be $47 billion. Due to the frequency of somatic symptoms associated with the disorder, patients suffering from GAD are high utilizers of primary care services. Patients suffering from GAD who present to primary care providers are not often accurately diagnosed, and consequently rarely receive appropriate treatment from their primary care providers or referrals to mental health specialists (Wittchen et al., 2001). Patients with PD often present in emergency settings—as many as 25% of patients who present to hospital emergency rooms with chest pain and shortness of breath are actually having a panic attack (Huffman & Pollack, 2003).

In addition to presentations of anxiety symptoms being misdiagnosed as other medical conditions, severe and persistent anxiety itself may lead to additional medical sequelae. In their most severe form, anxiety disorders have multiple health consequences and can be life-threatening. Anxiety has been associated with inflammation and hypercoagulable states in people who do not have preexisting cardiovascular disease (Pitsavos et al., 2006). Even brief periods of severe stress may lead to hemoconcentration with increases in blood viscosity and serum lipid concentrations (Geiser et al., 2008; Muldoon et al., 1995). Men who experienced high levels of anxiety were at increased risk of altered cardiac autonomic function, a risk factor for sudden cardiac death (Kawachi, Sparrow, Vokonas, & Weiss, 1995).

Anxiety disorders also increase mortality from suicide. Using data from the National Epidemiologic Survey on Alcohol and Related Conditions Wave 2,

Nepon, Belik, Bolton, and Sareen (2010) interviewed over 34,000 individuals who met *DSM-IV* criteria for an anxiety disorder, mood disorder, or personality disorder to determine the risk factors for suicide. They noted that over 70% of persons reporting a lifetime history of suicide attempts had an anxiety disorder, and that PD and PTSD were found to be independent risk factors for suicide (Nepon et al., 2010).

TYPES OF ANXIETY PROBLEMS

Although there is considerable overlap in anxiety symptoms across disorders, characteristic differences in symptom profiles are the basis for diagnostic classification.

Generalized Anxiety

Excessive worrying and nonspecific physical tension are hallmark symptoms of generalized anxiety. Generalized anxiety sufferers feel on edge and are unable to fully relax. Physical symptoms such as muscle and jaw tension are not unusual. Generalized anxiety rarely presents in children and adolescents, is more prominent in women than men, and increases with age (Wittchen, Zhao, Kessler, & Eaton, 1994). Lifetime prevalence rate for GAD is estimated to be 5% (Kessler et al., 2005b), and may be as high as 9% in geriatric populations (Schoevers, Beekman, Deeg, Jonker, & van Tilburg, 2003). Generalized anxiety commonly presents in the context of a mood disorder, prompting some to suggest that this type of excessive anxiety "commonly represents a state of incomplete recovery from any number of anxiety and affective disorders," which may portend relapse of a major depressive episode (Stahl, 2003, p. 298).

Social Anxiety

Social anxiety or SP is a common anxiety condition that manifests as intense discomfort when the person perceives being the focus of attention. SAD is one of the most common anxiety disorders, with a lifetime prevalence of 12% of the U.S. population. Social anxiety commonly presents during adolescence, but symptoms go beyond the feeling of awkwardness and self-consciousness that is common during the teen years.

Compared to generalized anxiety, social anxiety appears to be slightly less prevalent in older populations, but this may be due to the fact that elderly people are more likely to be homebound and less socially active in general. Loss of hearing and visual acuity may also contribute to a decline in social confidence. It has been suggested that the disorder may be more common in seniors who have experienced the loss of a spouse. Common fears for this population include eating in front of strangers and for men, difficulty urinating in public bathrooms (Bassil, Ghandour, & Grossberg, 2011; Cairney et al., 2007).

Just as age influences presentation of symptoms, culture may also play a role. This is particularly striking with the core symptoms of SAD. Caucasian populations who suffer from SAD experience an intense fear of being scrutinized and judged. By contrast, Japanese and Korean populations may fear bringing shame and embarrassment on another person. This emphasizes the need to define social anxiety in relation to a particular reference group since similar social behavior may be perceived differently by different sociocultural groups (Hofmann, Asnaani, & Hinton, 2010).

Many people with social anxiety use alcohol or other substances to cope with embarrassment from what they perceive as intense scrutiny, which may become problematic. Fear of being assertive and avoidance of situations in which performance will be judged can prevent the person from accomplishing educational, career, and interpersonal goals. In its most severe form, social anxiety can lead to extreme isolation.

Specific Phobia

Simple (or specific) phobias, defined as persistent intense irrational fears of an object or situation, are the most common anxiety disorders—as many as 25% of the population meets criteria for the disorder at some point during their lifetime (Sadock & Sadock, 2003). Phobias are common in children and become less frequent in adulthood (Kim et al., 2010). Specific phobias are often exaggerated responses to things that could potentially be harmful, including spiders, heights, and flying. The person may experience anything from mild anxiety to panic attacks when faced with the object or situation.

Panic

Panic attacks represent a particularly severe form of anxiety, which may lead to avoidance and isolation as the person attempts to thwart another attack by avoiding any situations that they may connect with a previous attack. Symptoms such as rapid heart rate and chest pressure or overt pain may be confused with myocardial infarction, leading the person to seek emergency room services. Ringing in the ears, hyperventilation and subsequent dizziness, paresthesias, and sweaty palms are not uncommon. Many panic sufferers experience intense cognitive distortions during an attack, such as a sense that they are "losing control" or fear that they are going crazy. A sense of "impending doom" is also quite common. Panic attacks may be linked to a particular stimulus but often occur without warning.

Traumatic Stress

Traumatic experience has long been understood as a precipitant to anxiety symptoms. What is now identified as PTSD was earlier identified as "shell shock" and "battle fatigue" and thought to be caused by exposure to the violence of war. Classic post-traumatic symptoms are now recognized in civilian populations of all ages as well, and may be caused by severe emotional, sexual, or physical trauma. The persistent state of autonomic hyperarousal caused by the perceived need to be constantly vigilant for threats leads to anxiety symptoms such as hypervigilance, exaggerated startle response, sleep disturbances, irritability, and somatic complaints. PTSD symptoms also include avoidance or dissociative symptoms such as depersonalization, derealization, and avoiding reminders of the traumatic experience; and chronic reexperiencing of the traumatic event(s) in the form of intrusive memories, nightmares, and flashbacks.

Obsessive-Compulsive Disorder

Obsessive-compulsive disorder (OCD) causes an individual to experience intrusive, repetitive, ego-dystonic thoughts. Obsessive thoughts may be experienced without associated behavior, or the person may try to dissipate the anxiety by completing a compulsive ritual. Rituals may include such things as religious scrupulosity, ordering objects in the physical environment, hand washing, and checking or counting behaviors. Phobias about germs are not uncommon and the person may feel compelled to avoid touching objects, even to the point of wearing gloves to ward off contamination. The momentary relief the person experiences in response to following through with a compulsion quickly dissipates, leading to the need to begin the process all over again. In severe forms of the disorder, completing compulsive rituals may preclude the individual from being able to attend to other activities in his or her life. Obsessions and compulsive rituals often cause the individual much shame and embarrassment. Many people with OCD are able to hide their symptoms and choose to suffer in silence rather than risk potential ridicule, thus delaying diagnosis and treatment.

ETIOLOGY OF ANXIETY DISORDERS

As with other psychiatric disorders, the etiology of anxiety disorders appears to be due to a combination of psychological traits, life stressors, and genetic vulnerability. Anxiety is multi-dimensional, and has been studied from a variety of perspectives including evolutionary, physiological, cognitive, and behavioral (Corr, 2011). Psychological and neurobiological perspectives explicate different aspects of the experience of anxiety, identify different risk factors, and provide the basis for a range of treatment approaches.

PSYCHOLOGICAL VIEWS OF ANXIETY

Psychological theories of anxiety identify cognitive, behavioral, and psychodynamic factors.

Cognitive

The way people perceive and interpret actual or potential stressors plays a significant role in the development of anxiety. Negative cognitive biases lead to misinterpreting neutral stimuli as threatening and overestimating the degree of threat. Anxious individuals may also underestimate their ability to cope with stressful situations due to negative self-appraisals. Perception of *uncontrollability*, and a sense of helplessness related to a perceived inability to predict or control events, is implicated in a variety of anxiety conditions including traumatic stress (Allen, 2001). Childhood experiences of parental loss or parental unresponsiveness disrupt attachment and have been implicated in the development of anxiety disorders that persist into adulthood.

Behavioral

Behavioral theories of anxiety focus on classical conditioning and social learning. In *classical conditioning*, neutral stimuli acquire the ability to evoke a fear response when they are frequently associated with a frightening stimulus. For instance, an adolescent who has witnessed domestic violence that is usually preceded by loud arguments may become highly anxious whenever she hears yelling, even in benign contexts such as cheering at sports events. Parental anxiety may lead to anxiety in a child through *social learning* as the child is repeatedly exposed to parents' worrying or fearful responses to stress.

Psychodynamic

Psychodynamic perspectives generally view anxiety as a result of unresolved conflicts, often having to do with expression of anger or unsolved issues in intimate relationships. In terms of unconscious processes, anxiety arises when the ego experiences discord between the demands of the id and the superego. As the id demands gratification of primitive impulses, the superego insists on ideals of morality. For instance, a man whose religion demands marital fidelity in thought as well as actions might become anxious if an attractive co-worker became flirtatious.

PHYSIOLOGIC FACTORS

In 1915, physiologist Walter Cannon described the concept of a person's ability to react to perceived danger as "fight-or-flight," and later described the body's complex system of feedback mechanisms to maintain equilibrium in the presence of stressors as "homeostasis" (Cannon, 1932). Hans Selye later identified universal stages of coping with physical and psychological stress as the "General Adaptation Syndrome," demonstrating that what begins as compensatory reactions in the HPA axis may lead to dysregulation and disease states in the presence of prolonged activation. (See Figure 9-2.) Building on the work of Cannon and Selye, McEwen and Stellar (1993) coined the concept of "allostatic load" to describe the tipping point at which the neuroendocrine system can no longer maintain stability.

Anxiety disorders have been the focus of much research and debate over the last decade. Recent studies on the neuroanatomy and physiology of anxiety disorders implicate interactions between the amygdala and prefrontal cortical structures (Shin & Liberzon, 2010). Exaggerated amygdala response combined with insufficient cortical and hypothalamic structure reaction is postulated as causing hyperarousal conditions.

Gene studies have shown high expression of N-Methyl-D-aspartate (NMDA) receptors in the hippocampus, leading to speculation that disruption of noradrenergic and glutamatergic neurotransmission may prevent or reverse memory consolidation (Garakani, Mathew, & Charney, 2006). Results however, have been inconclusive. Serotonin neuron subtypes which project to the cortex, hypothalamus, hippocampus, and amygdala have also been implicated in learned helplessness conditions (Hammack, Cooper, & Lezak, 2012; Martin, Ressler, Binder, & Nemeroff, 2009).

OCD models show additional distinct brain structure involvement from other anxiety disorders. Fronto-striatal circuitry is clearly implicated in ritualized behavior. Numerous studies have demonstrated that the orbitofrontal cortex, anterior cingulate cortex, and striatal regions are hyperreactive in persons with OCD, and quiet following treatment (Menzies et al., 2008). Hyperactivity of these regions distinguishes OCD from other anxiety disorders. Furthermore, brain imaging studies of people with OCD demonstrate amygdalar hyporeactivity when exposed to nonspecific threat images (Cannistraro et al., 2004).

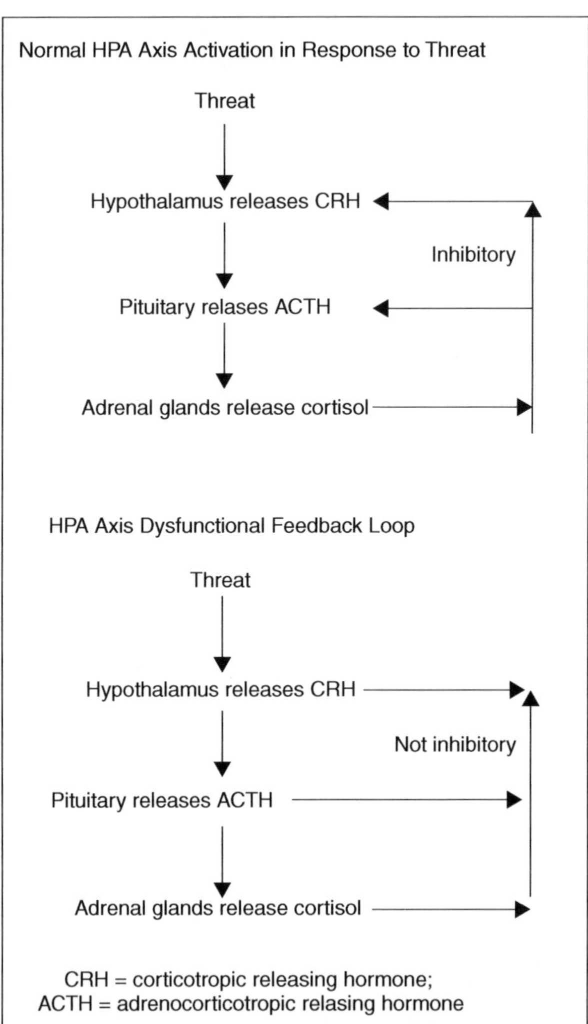

Figure 9-2 Normal and Dysfuntional HPA Axis Response

GENETIC FACTORS

It has long been clear that anxiety disorders run in families, and twin and family studies indicate a genetic component. In particular, risk for developing PD, GAD, phobia, and OCD appears to be under significant genetic influence (Hettema, Neale, & Kendler, 2001). Recent genetic research (Donner et al., 2008) has identified specific genes that are statistically associated with anxiety disorders.

ASSESSMENT

There are a variety of screening and diagnostic instruments in common use for clinical assessment of anxiety. See Exhibit 9-1 for an overview of commonly used assessment tools. In the clinical interview, areas for assessment include the chief complaint, history of the present symptoms,

EXHIBIT 9-1: ANXIETY ASSESSMENT TOOLS

INSTRUMENT/REFERENCE	DESCRIPTION
Diagnostic Assessments	
Anxiety Disorders Interview Schedule for *DSM-IV* (ADIS-IV) Brown, DiNardo, and Barlow (1994)	Semi-structured interview to assess for presence of *DSM-IV* anxiety disorders. Screens for mood and somatoform disorders, psychotic symptoms, and substance use.
Structured Clinical Interview for *DSM-IV* Axis I disorders (SCID-I) First, Spitzer, Gibbon, and Williams (1995)	Structured interview that includes modules for each *DSM-IV-TR* Axis I diagnosis. Scoring protocol to ensure valid and reliable diagnosis.
General Anxiety	
Anxiety Sensitivity Index (ASI) Reiss, Peterson, Gursky, and McNally (1986)	Self-report questionnaire (16 items) that measures fear of anxiety sensations (belief that these symptoms have harmful physical or psychological consequences).
Beck Anxiety Inventory (BAI) Beck, Epstein, Brown, and Steer (1988)	Self-report questionnaire (21 items) that measures the degree to which an individual has experienced a range of anxiety symptoms in the previous 2 weeks.
Hamilton Anxiety Scale (Ham-A) Hamilton (1959)	Semi-structured assessment scale widely used in treatment outcome studies of anxiety. 14 items assessing clusters of common anxiety symptoms. Public domain.
Depression Anxiety Stress Scale (DASS 21) Lovibond and Lovibond (1995)	Self-report questionnaire (21 items) that measures symptoms in past week related to negative emotional states including anxiety.
Penn State Worry Questionnaire (PSWQ) Meyer, Miller, Metzger, and Borkovec (1990)	Questionnaire (16 items) that assesses characteristics of pathological worry.
Spielberger State-Trait Anxiety Inventory (STAI) Spielberger (1983)	Self-report questionnaire (40 items) that measures the degree to which individuals exhibit state (momentary) and trait (stable) characteristics of anxiety.
Social Anxiety	
Social Phobia and Anxiety Scale (SPAS) Turner, Beidel, Dancu, and Stanley (1989)	Self-report questionnaire (45 items) with two subscales: social phobia and agoraphobia.
Social Interaction Anxiety Scale (SIAS) Mattick and Clark (1998)	Assesses fear of general social interaction.
Liebowitz Social Anxiety Scale (LSAS) Liebowitz (1987)	Self-report questionnaire assessing fear of performance and social situations. Also available as a structured interview.
Panic	
Discomfort Intolerance Scale (DIS) Schmidt, Richey, and Fitzpatrick (2006)	Self-report questionnaire (5 items) that assesses the ability to tolerate bodily sensations.
Obsessive-Compulsive	
Children's Yale-Brown Obsessive-Compulsive Scale (CY-BOCS) Scahill et al. (1997)	Semi-structured interview. Obsessions and compulsions assessed separately; interview also yields an overall severity scale. Can be completed by the child, parents, or both working together.
Yale-Brown Obsessive-Compulsive Scale (Y-BOCS) Goodman et al. (1989)	Semi-structured interview that measures presence of obsessions and compulsions and their frequency and degree of associated distress.

(Continued)

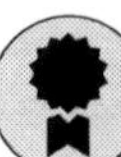

EXHIBIT 9-1: ANXIETY ASSESSMENT TOOLS (*Continued*)

INSTRUMENT/REFERENCE	DESCRIPTION
Obsessive-Compulsive Inventory–Revised (OCI-R) Foa et al. (2002)	Self-report questionnaire (18 items) that assesses symptoms of OCD including washing, checking, ordering, obsessing, hoarding, and neutralizing.

Traumatic Stress

The *National Center for PTSD* has a listing of over 50 tools for assessing trauma exposure and traumatic stress in children and adults at www.ptsd.va.gov/professional/pages/assessments/all_measures.asp. Listing includes links to information about each tool and instructions for how to obtain it. The **Traumatic Events Screening Inventory—Child** (TESI-C), **Combat Exposure Scale,** and **Primary Care PTSD Screen** (PC-PTSD) are available online. The *FAQs About PTSD Assessment: For Professionals* page (www.ptsd.va.gov/professional/pages/faq-ptsd-professionals.asp) discusses considerations in selecting the most appropriate assessment instrument for the needs of one's practice.

psychiatric and medical history, social and developmental history, and the mental status examination.

CHIEF COMPLAINT

The chief complaint may refer to emotional ("I feel so wound up") or cognitive ("I can't stop worrying") aspects of anxiety, but are also likely to focus on somatic manifestations such as gastrointestinal (GI) disturbances, muscle tension, or headaches. Since chronic hyperarousal and worry may preclude restful sleep, sleep problems may be a presenting complaint.

HISTORICAL DATA

History of Present Illness

In addition to determining onset and course of anxiety symptoms, it is important to identify stressors that may be related to onset or exacerbation of anxiety. Assessment of how symptoms are affecting the client's life should include information about common behavioral responses such as avoidance of anxiety-provoking situations and how this may impact the patient's functioning.

Psychiatric History

Since persons with anxiety disorders may suffer for a long time before presenting for mental health treatment, it is important to ask about onset of anxiety symptoms. Ask about any hospitalizations, suicide attempts, or other self-harm behaviors. Discussion of previous therapy and medication trials should include assessment of side effects and perception of benefit.

Medical History

Given the frequency with which anxiety disorders present with somatic symptoms, a thorough medical history is especially important. This should include discussion of surgeries, hospitalizations, current medical problems, and treatment. Information should be obtained about medical conditions that may present with anxiety symptoms. Medical history should also include questions about head injury with loss of consciousness, seizures, syncope, arrhythmia, or structural heart defect. These symptoms may offer clues as to current diagnoses, and the presence of these disorders provides guidance about medication selection.

Social and Developmental History

Since problems with anxiety often begin in childhood, the personal history provides important assessment information. A history of separation anxiety or school refusal, age-inappropriate fears or excessive worry during childhood suggests early onset and chronicity of anxiety problems. Assessment of previous abuse or trauma is important to identify risk factors for post-traumatic stress. Discussion of these sensitive issues should be conducted when rapport has been established and the patient should be observed for indications of excessive distress.

Substance Use History

Information about current and previous substance use/abuse is important in the assessment of the client with severe anxiety. Current use of prescribed, over-the-counter or recreational drug use is necessary to identify possible chemical precipitants to anxiety symptoms

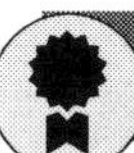

EXHIBIT 9-2: MEDICAL MIMICS OF ANXIETY DISORDERS

Medications, Herbal Supplements

Antidepressants
Antipsychotics
Antihypertensives Stimulants
Decongestants
Bronchodilators
Caffeine
St. John's wort
Yohimbine
Ma huang (ephedra)
Alcohol (withdrawal)
Benzodiazepines (withdrawal)
Antihistamines (particularly in children)

Illicit Substances

Cocaine, methamphetamine
Ecstasy
Cannabis
"Spice" (salvia)
Lysergic acid diethylamide (LSD)

Illnesses

Hyperthyroidism
Myocardial infarction
Mitral valve prolapse
Paroxysmal supraventricular tachycardia
Anemia
Orthostatic hypotension
Hypoglycemia
Asthma, chronic obstructive pulmonary disease (COPD)
Pheochromocytoma

(see Exhibit 9-2). Information about use of coffee, soda, or energy drinks is important since caffeine is a common trigger for anxiety symptoms. Since the anxiolytic properties of alcohol may be especially reinforcing for patients experiencing discomfort from anxiety, assessment of alcohol use should include specific questions about amount and frequency.

Family History

Family psychiatric history, treatment, and medical history should be documented. Some clients will not be aware of family members who have a psychiatric diagnosis, but asking about family members who are "nervous" or excessive worriers may elicit information suggestive of family history of anxiety. Asking about a family history of substance abuse or violence toward self and others is important as these behaviors may be indicative of mood or anxiety disorders. Inquiring about family cardiac history, syncope, or sudden death will provide further information about a client risk factors for side effects from medications.

MENTAL STATUS EXAMINATION

General Appearance and Behavior

The examiner may perceive a general sense of acute discomfort as the client enters the interview room. Other manifestations of anxiety, such as furrowed brows, dry mouth, and fidgeting, may be apparent. The client may display hypervigilance, manifested by tense body posture and constant scanning of their environment.

Mood and Affect

Clients may describe their mood using such adjectives as "tense," "worried," or "edgy." Affect may be congruent to mood or incongruent (e.g., a client who describes his or her mood as "fine" but is frowning and appears tense). Anxious clients may have a full range of affect, or may seem constricted or even flat. Chronic sympathetic hyperarousal may present as irritability or anger.

Speech

Speech may have normal rate and rhythm or have unusual prosody and flow. A person experiencing significant anxiety often speaks with notable pressure and/or loud volume. Conversely, children and adolescents who are oppositional, defiant, or guarded may display a paucity of spontaneous speech, giving monosyllabic answers to questions.

Thought Process and Content

Thought process may be linear, goal directed, and easily followed. The person experiencing acute distress may become circumstantial or even tangential. Elderly people in particular may be perseverative. Thought content may be ruminative or focus on specific or general worries. The person may ask for constant reassurance. Intrusive thoughts or memories may be experienced during the mental status exam, and should be noted. Obsessive thoughts may be reported, as may ideas of reference ("The people on the bus think, 'That girl is stuck-up' when they see me.") Thoughts about self-harm, hopelessness, and helplessness should also be evaluated. People experiencing distress may experience vague suicidal ideation (e.g., "I don't want to live like this"), but deny having a plan or intent to harm themselves. Clients with post-traumatic stress may experience a level of mistrust that may present as general suspiciousness or even frank paranoia.

Perceptual Disturbance

Hallucinations are not common in persons with anxiety disorders, although auditory or visual hallucinations related to traumatic experience will sometimes be experienced by persons with post-traumatic stress. Careful assessment of such perceptual anomalies will help to determine if they are related to psychosis or are better understood as a post-traumatic flashback.

Cognitive Functions

Concentration may be significantly affected by anxiety, and impaired concentration may be reflected in difficulties with immediate recall and short-term memory. Anxiety may also interfere with memory recall.

Insight and Judgment

These may be intact, or may be significantly affected by anxiety symptoms. For instance, a person with post-traumatic stress who is anxious and mistrustful may understand that this is a misperception related to past trauma. In contrast, another person with PTSD symptoms may firmly believe that others intend to harm them, despite lack of evidence to support this belief.

CONCORDANCE AND TREATMENT PLANNING

Perhaps more than with any other psychiatric condition, successfully engaging the client with severe anxiety depends on the clinician being able to establish a sense of safety and respect. According to Shea (1998, p. 28), the goal is for the client "to come away with the feeling that the clinician is not going to pass judgment on him." Simply put, the client must perceive that the PMH-APRN understands their emotional perspective and accepts them unconditionally. This is particularly salient for clients with social anxiety, whose condition is characterized by fear of being judged. Respect can be conveyed by the simple act of asking how the client prefers to be addressed. Positioning oneself across from the client without a desk in between or offering the person a cup of coffee or tea (ideally decaffeinated!) before beginning the interview can set a tone of mutual respect without hierarchy and can be particularly comforting to an anxious person.

It is important to provide clients with psychoeducation tailored to their cultures and levels of health literacy that communicates basic concepts about the physiologic basis for anxiety symptoms, and that covers the role of thought and behavior patterns in exacerbating or relieving anxiety. Clients who have been referred for mental health treatment after presenting in other settings for somatic complaints may feel the validity of their complaints has been dismissed—"They think it's all in my head." Such clients benefit from reassurance that physical discomfort related to anxiety does indeed have a physiologic basis.

Psychoeducation is particularly important for persons with post-traumatic stress, who may be disturbed by the intensity and unpredictability of symptoms such as intrusive memories, sleep disturbance, and hyperresponsiveness to innocuous stimuli. Understanding of how these responses are triggered makes them easier to predict, and therefore less disconcerting. Similarly, awareness of the physiologic basis for these responses can decrease self-blame (Phoenix, 2007).

Experienced nurses understand that human beings are far more complex than a label or diagnostic category, and that regardless of the nurse's theoretical orientation, there is no set "recipe" for treatment. The range of evidence-based treatments and self-care options available to the client should be explained and the client's preferences considered in selecting treatments. Since treatments for anxiety may involve asking clients to replace behaviors that have short-term effectiveness in reducing distress, such as avoidance or use of alcohol, it is important to respect client decisions about how much discomfort they are willing to tolerate. The essence of the nurse-client relationship is always "doing with," not "doing to."

Behavioral therapies which involve exposure and re-experiencing of distressing stimuli are widely used as part of the healing process for anxiety conditions. Clients with hypervigilance related to traumatic stress may be fearful that they will miss signs of danger as this symptom is reduced by medication. The PMH-APRN can enhance client confidence in the effectiveness of such treatment modalities through judiciously sharing research findings demonstrating his or her efficacy, but it is often the sense of safety provided by the client-nurse relationship that allows the client to tolerate the treatment.

EXPECTED OUTCOMES

The process of collaboratively deciding on specific treatment outcomes is discussed in Chapter 2. Some general outcomes that would be desired in working with clients with anxiety conditions are listed below, as well as outcomes specific to particular anxiety problems.

- Development of a therapeutic relationship
- Provision of safety without injury to self or others
- Maintain or improve physical health
- Return to effective functional level
- Recognition of anxiety symptoms
- Expand coping skills
- Reduce use of ineffective or harmful responses to anxiety (e.g., substance misuse)
- Develop plan to deal with symptoms and decrease/prevent relapse

Generalized anxiety

- Decrease time spent worrying
- Lower baseline level of sympathetic arousal
- Improve sleep

Social anxiety

- Improve social and occupational functioning
- Decrease avoidance of situations involving performance

Phobia

- Ability to tolerate feared object or situation
- Decrease escape or avoidance behavior

Panic

- Identify panic triggers
- Reduce baseline level of sympathetic arousal
- Decrease frequency and severity of panic attacks
- Use coping strategies to minimize distress during panic attacks
- Decrease escape or avoidance behavior

Post-traumatic stress

- Insure current safety
- Decrease escape or avoidance behavior
- Reduce baseline level of sympathetic arousal
- Reduce intrusive memories and flashbacks
- Improve sleep
- Develop a coherent trauma narrative

Obsessions and compulsions

- Identify triggers for OC symptoms
- Use coping strategies
- Reduce amount of time/energy spent on obsessions and compulsive rituals

TREATMENT INITIATION

Clients suffering from anxiety generally present for treatment when their symptoms are impacting their work or personal lives and they have been unsuccessful at controlling them using their usual coping skills. Despite agreeing to a psychiatric evaluation, many people continue to have ambivalence about treatment, and particularly about taking medications. They may feel ashamed or weak that they are unable to control their symptoms. They may have misperceptions about medications used to treat anxiety, thinking that all medications have the potential for addiction. Some individuals have been in psychotherapy or tried medications in the past and have had side effects or other negative experiences with treatment. Family members, significant others, or friends may have negative views of psychiatric treatment and influence the individual's thinking. Finally, because anxiety and mood disorders frequently run in families, individuals may fear that if they allow themselves to take medication, they will become like some other family member who has long-standing dysfunction as a result of their disorder or treatment.

Before suggesting any treatment for an individual with anxiety, the PMH-APRN should explore the individual's thoughts about treatment. What is the individual's goal for being in treatment? Is he or she willing to be in psychotherapy? What are the individual's time and financial resources? Is there anything in particular he or she would like to have happen? Is there anything he or she would consider "a deal breaker"? For example, some patients may say, "I won't take anything that will likely cause weight gain," or, "I won't take anything that may cause sexual side effects."

It is important to determine what has been used to ameliorate symptoms in the past. What medication(s) has the individual or a family member or friend tried, and what has their experience been? Many clients have misinformation about medications and it will be critical to elucidate any misperceptions and to educate them about medication options, potential risks, and benefits. However, even when a client has misperceptions about risks of a given medication or medication class, it is crucial to be sensitive to their values and concerns. Be clear that although all medications may cause side effects, you will make every attempt to select a medication that has the best chance of giving them symptom relief with the least likelihood of causing serious side effects.

It is important to be clear, however, that the more disabling, distressing, or even life-threatening the person's symptoms, the more imperative that a medication intervention work as quickly as possible. Therefore, severe psychiatric symptoms justify selecting a medication that has a greater possibility of high side effect burden if it also offers a greater probability of symptom relief. When symptoms are mild-moderate, however, the potential side effect risks of this same medication may be unacceptable and use of a medication that has lower chance of serious side effects, even though response data are less robust, may be more reasonable.

Finally, before suggesting a medication to any client, clinicians should ask themselves if faced with a similar scenario, despite the risk of serious side effects, would they be willing to take this medication or prescribe it to a loved one? Assuming the answer is "yes," sharing this with the client may go a long way in ameliorating mistrust.

PSYCHOTHERAPY

COGNITIVE BEHAVIORAL THERAPIES

Cognitive Behavioral Therapy (CBT) is the best-studied form of psychotherapy for treating anxiety disorders, and there is strong evidence that cognitive-behavioral and behavioral approaches are effective in treating a range of anxiety conditions across the life span (Butler, Chapman, Forman, & Beck, 2006; Roth & Fonagy, 2005; Silverman, Pina, & Viswesvaran, 2008). Different combinations of cognitive and behavioral techniques that target the most prominent symptoms are used to treat specific anxiety disorders. However, relaxation training is commonly used across anxiety conditions to reduce the chronic sympathetic hyperarousal that is implicated in so many anxiety symptoms. See Exhibit 9-3 for a summary of psychotherapeutic techniques used to treat anxiety conditions.

Cognitive therapy is a highly structured, skill-building, goal-oriented therapy designed to help the client examine faulty thinking patterns (called *irrational thoughts* or *cognitive distortions*) that are thought to give rise to dysfunctional behavior and emotional distress. Clients are assisted to examine their thoughts and identify distorted cognitions. They are then challenged and assisted to replace irrational thoughts with more accurate beliefs. This process is referred to as *cognitive restructuring*.

A tenet of behavioral therapy is that phobias are based on faulty threat assessments which trigger fear and subsequent avoidant behaviors. In therapy, clients are exposed, either gradually and in small doses (systematic desensitization) or all at once (flooding or massed exposure), to stimuli that represent the objects of their fears. Often, relaxation may be practiced in conjunction with exposure. By repeatedly being exposed to an anxiety-provoking stimulus in situations where there is no danger, the faulty association between the feared object and the sense of threat is overridden and the person becomes desensitized to the stimulus. For persons with social anxiety, exposure therapy might involve practicing public speaking—Toastmasters (www.toastmasters.org) is a great resource.

OTHER PSYCHOTHERAPIES

Although there is currently little evidence to support the use of psychodynamic therapy in treating anxiety (Roth & Fonagy, 2005), this approach may be useful when anxiety results from subconscious conflicts or from frightening unconscious meanings associated with real-life stressors. The evidence base for supportive or nondirective therapies is similarly limited. Interpersonal therapy techniques, such as assertiveness training, may

EXHIBIT 9-3: THERAPIES COMMONLY USED TO TREAT ANXIETY

Psychotherapies

1. Cognitive and behavioral therapies including:
    - Relaxation training
    - Cognitive restructuring
    - Exposure (phobic avoidance)
        - Gradual desensitization
        - Flooding
    - Exposure with response prevention (compulsive rituals)
    - Thought-stopping (worry, obsessive or intrusive thoughts)
    - Worry scheduling (worry)
2. Interpersonal therapy:
    - Assertiveness training
3. Psychodynamic therapy
4. Mindfulness-based psychotherapy

Other therapeutic approaches

1. EMDR (traumatic stress)
2. Plant-based remedies
3. Computer-based CBT
4. Bibliotherapy
5. Exercise
6. Yoga
7. Massage

be useful for clients whose anxiety interferes with interpersonal functioning. Use of mindfulness practices, such as Mindfulness-Based Stress Reduction, appears to have some promise for treating anxiety symptoms (Rapgay, Bystritsky, Dafter, & Spearman, 2011; Vøllestad, Sivertsen, & Nielsen, 2011). Further study is needed to clarify the extent to which mindfulness *per se* contributes to treatment effects.

EYE MOVEMENT DESENSITIZATION AND REPROCESSING

Eye Movement Desensitization and Reprocessing (EMDR) has been widely employed and studied in the treatment of post-traumatic stress. EMDR combines imaginal exposure (summoning memories of a traumatic situation) and cognitive restructuring with induction of saccadic eye movements seen in rapid eye movement (REM) sleep as the client follows the therapist's rhythmic finger movements. Although there is a significant evidence base demonstrating the effectiveness of EMDR, it remains unclear whether the induced eye movements play a significant role in treatment outcome (Seidler & Wagner, 2006). It has been suggested that the eye movements help ground the client in the present reality of the therapy session, diminishing the sense of threat, or that eye movements compete with traumatic memories for cognitive resources, thus decreasing the vividness of the sensory response.

MEDICATIONS

BENZODIAZEPINES

Benzodiazepines, while controversial, remain an important component of a large medication arsenal available in the treatment of anxiety disorders. All benzodiazepines are effective in treating acute and chronic anxiety; however, the most robust support for their use appears to be in treating GAD, SAD, and PD (Ravindran & Stein, 2010). Data examining use in OCD and PTSD have been mixed, with some studies finding that alprazolam has been useful in addressing nonspecific anxiety, but has little effect on specific PTSD symptoms or sleep (Braun, Greenberg, Dasberg, & Lerer, 1990; Cates, Bishop, Davis, Lowe, & Woolley, 2004).

All benzodiazepines work by binding to γ-Aminobutyric acid (GABA) A and B receptors, thus enhancing the inhibitory effect of this neurotransmitter. Alprazolam, however, is the exception of the group, as in addition it appears to have the unique ability to cause down-regulation of beta-adrenergic receptors, possibly causing antidepressant activity as well. $GABA_A$ receptor binding is responsible for the anxiolytic, sedative, and anticonvulsant effects, while $GABA_B$ receptor binding leads to muscle relaxant effects. Therefore, the non-benzodiazepine hypnotics zolpidem, eszopaclone, and zaleplon, which bind specifically to $GABA_A$ receptors, do not have muscle relaxant properties. Compared to other medications used to treat anxiety, benzodiazepines have a rapid onset of action. They are inexpensive and are relatively safe in overdose. They are not without side effects, however. Excess sedation, dizziness, ataxia, anterograde amnesia, and dysphoria are not uncommon, and can be especially problematic in elderly patients and with higher dosing in all age groups. These side effects can usually be addressed by careful selection of a particular benzodiazepine and by lowering the dose of the given medication.

Consideration must also be given to half life, onset of action, and cytochrome P450 interactions. Onset of action for all of the benzodiazepines appears to be mediated by lipophilic properties, that is, the higher lipophilic drugs more readily cross the blood-brain barrier, giving rise to rapid onset of action. This is particularly significant when treating elderly patients who have a higher ratio of fatty tissue to lean body mass. It is important to recognize, however, that while highly lipophilic drugs turn on their effect rapidly, they also turn off their effect rapidly as they leave the brain and are stored in the body's fatty tissue. Lipophilic properties must also be considered in decision making about route of administration. Although a highly lipophilic drug may work quickly via oral administration, that same drug may exhibit slow rate of effectiveness when given intramuscularly. Furthermore, onset and duration of effectiveness may have very little relationship to overall half-life of the drug. With the exception of lorazepam and oxazepam, all of the benzodiazepines undergo oxidative metabolism and can give rise to pharmacokinetic interactions with other drugs.

Tolerance may occur with any of the benzodiazepines. Data about tolerance have been mixed, however, and many long-term follow-up studies have shown little evidence of tolerance while noting that the majority of patients maintained treatment gains (Curtis et al., 1993; Worthington et al., 1998). More recent studies examining the short- and long-term effects of combining a benzodiazepine with a selective serotonergic reuptake inhibitor (SSRI) have demonstrated earlier benefit as compared to using an SSRI alone; however, this advantage was not sustained in the long run, suggesting that while benzodiazepines may be a reasonable "bridge" medication while waiting for benefit from an antidepressant, many patients will not derive continued benefit over taking the SSRI alone (Goddard et al., 2001). Risk factors for benzodiazepine tolerance and abuse include a history of substance abuse, particularly in those with a history of alcohol or benzodiazepine abuse. Use in this population should be minimized if used at all.

In general, benzodiazepines should be used for as short a time period as possible, and in the lowest dose that affords adequate symptom control. It is important for the PMH-APRN to discuss the purpose, potential risks and benefits, and expected course of using a benzodiazepine when starting it with an SSRI. Scheduled dosing is beneficial in preventing breakthrough symptoms. The benzodiazepine taper should only occur once the patient has adequate anxiolytic benefit from client's antidepressant, and this may take 6 to 8 weeks to achieve. Patients who have taken a benzodiazepine on a daily basis for more than a month should be advised on how to taper off the medication.

Common symptoms of benzodiazepine withdrawal include increased anxiety, palpitations, clammy hands, and sweating. In severe withdrawal the person may experience extreme sensitivity to light and sound. And although rare, seizures can occur if a benzodiazepine is discontinued abruptly. It is important to note that while withdrawal symptoms may occur within the first day or two of stopping a short half-life drug, they may not occur for a week after stopping a long half-life drug such as diazepam or clonazepam. Tapering should occur at a rate of no more than 10% of total dose/week. Clients may have much more difficulty tapering off short half-life drugs (i.e., lorazepam or alprazolam) than long half-life drugs, and for this reason, it is a common strategy to convert the client who is taking a short half-life drug onto a drug such as clonazepam to facilitate a more comfortable

TABLE 9-1: BENZODIAZEPINE DOSING AND PHARMACOKINETICS

GENERIC (BRAND) NAME	AVAILABLE FORMULATION	ANXIOLYTIC DOSE RANGE/DAY	HALF-LIFE	OXIDATION (CYP450 INTERACTIONS)	RATE OF ONSET AFTER ORAL DOSE
Chlordiazepoxide (Librium)	Capsule: 5, 10, 25 mg	15–40 mg	20–110 hrs*	yes	intermediate.
Clorazepate (Tranxene)	Tablet: 3.75, 7.5, 15 mg	15–40 mg	30–100 hrs*	yes	fast
Diazepam (Valium)	Tablet: 2, 5, 10 mg Oral solution: 5 mg/5 ml Injectable: 5 mg/5 ml	5–40 mg	30–100 hrs*	yes	fast
Clonazepam (Klonopin)	Tablet: 0.5, 1, 2 mg Wafer: 0.125, 0.25, 0.5, 1, 2 mg	0.5–4 mg	20–50 hrs*	yes	intermediate
Lorazepam (Ativan)	Tablet: 0.5, 1, 2 mg Oral solution: 2 mg/ml Injectable: 2 mg/ml, 4 mg/ml	1–6 mg	14 hrs	no	intermediate
Oxazepam (Serax)	Capsule: 10, 15, 30 mg	15–120 mg	9 hrs	no	slow-intermediate
Alprazolam (Xanax, Xanax XR)	Tablet: 0.25, 0.5, 1, 2 mg Oral solution: 1 mg/ml Disintegrating tabs: 1, 2, 3 mg XR tab: 1, 2, 3 mg	1–4 mg	14 hrs	yes	intermediate

*Includes active metabolites.

Table adapted from Schatzberg, Cole, and DeBattista (2009).

taper. Any signs of withdrawal should be evaluated and can generally be addressed by temporarily increasing the dose of the drug and tapering off more slowly. Clients who have been taking extremely high doses of benzodiazepines, however, or who have been abusing benzodiazepines and alcohol should be hospitalized for safe detoxification (Schatzberg, Cole, & DeBattista, 2010). Table 9-1 provides dosing and half-life information.

ANTIDEPRESSANTS

Owing to their safety profile, ease of dosing, and broad efficacy, the SSRIs and serotonin/norepeinephrine reuptake inhibitors (SNRIs) have emerged as the treatment of choice for anxiety disorders. Although each of the antidepressants has different Food and Drug Administration (FDA) indications (see Table 9-2), all of the SSRIs are assumed efficacious at treating all of the anxiety disorders; the SNRIs have been shown to have efficacy for all of the anxiety disorders with the exception of OCD. Mirtazapine has data to support its use in social anxiety, PTSD, and OCD (Ravindran & Stein, 2010).

Two tricyclic (TCA) antidepressants, clomipramine and imipramine, have been widely investigated in the treatment of PD. Evidence indicates that both are more effective than placebo and may be as efficacious as the SSRIs in treating panic (Mavissakalian, 2003). Clomipramine, with its potent serotonergic reuptake properties, is the only TCA indicated for the treatment of OCD. There is evidence suggesting nefazodone is helpful in PD and PTSD (Davis et al., 2004; McRae et al., 2004); however, reports about possible hepatotoxicity caused the drug to be withdrawn from the market in several countries, and even though it is still available in generic form in the United States, further studies have not been conducted. Despite efficacy, the side effect and safety profiles of each of these drugs has relegated them to third-line agents as clinicians shy away from them in favor of what they perceive are less risky choices.

Similar to those being treated for depression, individual clients may benefit or tolerate one drug over another. SSRIs and SNRIs can cause side effects such as jitteriness, headache, insomnia, somnolence, and GI disturbances early in treatment and for this reason, starting all medications at a low dose and increasing the dose slowly will be imperative. Thorough teaching about the usual course of treatment, side effects, and strategies to manage side effects is particularly important when treating clients with anxiety disorders. Clients should be reassured that most side effects are transient, but that if they do experience intolerable and/or intractable side effects, other medications can be tried. People suffering from PD, GAD, and SAD may experience relief with relatively low dose SSRIs, while those with OCD generally require higher dosing to achieve good symptom control (Simon et al., 2009).

AZAPIRONES

Buspirone is an anxiolytic medication whose putative mechanism of action is via partial agonism of the 5-HT 1A receptor. Buspirone is indicated for the treatment of

TABLE 9-2: FDA MEDICATION INDICATION FOR ANTIDEPRESSANTS

	FLUOXETINE	SERTRALINE	PAROXETINE	FLUVOXAMINE	CITALOPRAM	ESCITALOPRAM	CLOMIPRAMINE	VENLAFAXINE XR	DULOXETINE
PD	√ (adult)	√ (adult)	√ (adult)					√ (adult)	
SP		√ (adult)	√ (adult)					√ (adult)	
GAD			√ (adult)			√ (adult)		√ (adult)	√ (adult)
OCD	√ (adult, ped)	√ (adult, ped)	√ (adult, ped)	√ (adult, ped)			√ (adult, ped)		
PTSD		√ (adult)	√ (adult)						

PD = panic disorder; SP = social phobia; GAD = generalized anxiety disorder; OCD = obsessive-compulsive disorder; PTSD = post-traumatic stress disorder.

anxiety, but is not indicated for any specific anxiety disorder. Buspirone has been found to be as effective as the benzodiazepines in generalized anxiety. It has a benign side effect profile, does not cause tolerance, and is therefore not addictive. Despite efficacy and tolerability, buspirone is often overlooked in the treatment of anxiety. Because it does not cause sedation, patients who are familiar with benzodiazepines assume it does not work. Schatzberg et al. (2010) suggest that this is because the patient does not experience "the pause that refreshes" as they do when taking a benzodiazepine, and clinicians unfortunately often buy into this assumption. But for clients who are benzodiazepine-naïve, or for those who do not wish to take anything that may cause sedation or dependency, buspirone may be the ideal anxiolytic. Aggressive dosing can cause headache, dizziness, and sedation. Dosing should start low (generally 5 mg bid) and increase gradually with a typical target dose between 20–30 mg bid. Optimum effect, therefore, may not occur for several weeks.

NORADRENERGIC AGENTS

Because many symptoms of anxiety result from involvement of the sympathetic nervous system, investigators have been intrigued by the potential for adrenergic blockade in ameliorating anxiety symptoms. Postsynaptic beta blockade as well as presynaptic and postsynaptic alpha blockade have all been studied. Although they do not affect psychological symptoms of anxiety, beta-blockers have been shown to stop the somatic effects (tachycardia, tremor) that commonly occur for those with performance anxiety. Students who are immobilized by the thought of having to give a presentation or to speak up in class can not only participate but also note a sense of increased confidence. The drugs have also been useful in calming tremor caused as a side effect of lithium and other medications. Trauma investigators have postulated that beta-blockers given during the period immediately following trauma may block consolidation of traumatic memory and thereby prevent the development of PTSD. Numerous trials have been conducted but results are conflicting, suggesting that larger controlled trials are needed. beta-blockers can cause bronchoconstriction and should be avoided in clients with asthma.

Alpha-blocker drugs are also useful in blocking tachycardia and sweating that commonly occur with social anxiety. The alpha-blocker prazosin has been used with success in the treatment of nightmares caused by PTSD (Taylor, Freeman, & Cates, 2008).

Caution must be used when either class of these drugs are employed as they can cause orthostatic hypotension and bradycardia. Monitoring blood pressure and pulse should be done on a regular basis. The adage "start low and go slow" is once again imperative. Finally, if the client has been taking beta-blocker medications for any length of time, they should taper off the medication slowly to avoid rebound hypertension.

ANTICONVULSANTS

None of the anticonvulsants have an FDA indication for treating anxiety. Most, however, have been used on the basis that anxiety appears to be due to dysregulation of fear circuitry involving GABA and glutamate. Despite apparent lack of robust efficacy, gabapentin is still widely used in substance abuse programs for clients who are having anxiety and insomnia related to detox from various substances. Studies investigating topiramate and lamotrigine in the treatment of PTSD have yielded mixed results. Pregabalin has been studied in the treatment of GAD and may be the most promising agent in this class. With the exception of pregabalin for the treatment of GAD, anticonvulsants do not appear to be useful in treating anxiety disorders (Ravindran & Stein, 2010).

SECOND-GENERATION ANTIPSYCHOTICS

Although off-label for this purpose, all of the second-generation antipsychotic medications (SGAs) have been used for augmentation when severe anxiety symptoms do not remit with antidepressants and/or benzodiazepines. Olanzapine, risperidone, and quetiapine are perhaps the most studied of the SGAs used for this purpose. Few double-blind placebo-controlled studies exist and most of these are underpowered, making it difficult to draw any clear conclusions. Clinicians are thus faced with anecdotal evidence and trial and error in an attempt to give their clients relief from incapacitating symptoms.

As when any drug is used without FDA approval, care should be taken to inform the patient that the drug is being used off-label. SGA metabolic guideline parameters must be strictly adhered to and documented in the patient's chart. The client's primary care provider should be informed of the rationale for use of the drug as well as results from any lab studies done. Beyond the potential metabolic side effects, clients should be informed of the remote risk of tardive dyskinesia (TD) and should be screened for involuntary movements throughout treatment. An Abnormal Involuntary Movement Scale (AIMS) test is the most thorough tool for evaluating signs of TD and should be done on an annual basis.

CLIENT SELF-MANAGEMENT

Factors such as the high prevalence of anxiety disorders, lack of access to evidence-based care, and reluctance to seek mental health treatment suggest the importance of self-help strategies in the management of anxiety. Such approaches also encourage empowerment and increase self-efficacy when successful. Clients may have tried self-help techniques before seeking treatment from an PMH-APRN, so it is important to assess what self-management efforts have been or are being used. Herbal remedies or nutritional supplements may interact with prescribed medication (e.g., the combination of St. John's wort and a SSRI increases risk for serotonin syndrome), but other self-help methods such as yoga or exercise may enhance the effect of professional interventions. PMH-APRNs can also provide useful information about the evidence base for self-management methods, since some can be not only ineffective but potentially harmful.

HERBAL REMEDIES AND NUTRITIONAL SUPPLEMENTS

Many herbs, supplements, and other complementary therapies have been proposed as potential remedies for anxiety problems, but unfortunately there is very little evidence to evaluate their usefulness. A recent comprehensive review of self-help strategies (Morgan & Jorm, 2009) identified only 12 plant-based remedies or supplements for which there was at least one randomized controlled trial evaluating their efficacy. Of these, 5-hydroxy-tryptophan, combined plant preparations, gingko biloba, inositol, kava, omega-3 fatty acids, and *Withania somnifera* had some evidence of efficacy in treating anxiety but all required more study. The available evidence indicates that St. John's wort is ineffective in the treatment of anxiety. Updated information on complementary treatments can be found on the Natural Medicines Comprehensive Database (http://naturaldatabase.therapeuticresearch.com), which has both consumer and professional versions.

Since such "natural" therapies are not patentable and therefore unlikely to be profitable, we are unlikely to see a dramatic increase in research on herbs or supplements. PMH-APRNs and their clients may have to rely on anecdotal evidence to guide use of supplements for the foreseeable future. Most such remedies are unlikely to cause harm (an exception is kava, which may cause liver damage), so as long as their use is not overly expensive and does not preclude use of other effective treatments, patient preference should be respected.

BIBLIOTHERAPY AND COMPUTER-ASSISTED CBT

Use of self-help books or workbooks, often based on a cognitive-behavioral approach to anxiety management, has strong support for its effectiveness and may in some circumstances be as effective as professional treatment (Morgan & Jorm, 2009). Since self-help books vary widely in usefulness and quality of content, Redding, Herbert, Forman, and Gaudiano (2008) evaluated 50 best-selling psychological self-help books based on criteria such as grounding in science, offering reasonable expectations, specific guidance for implementing self-help techniques, and avoidance of potentially harmful advice. Predictors of overall quality included using a cognitive-behavioral approach, being written by doctorally prepared mental health professionals, and focusing on specific problems such as panic or worry. See Client Resources at the end of this chapter for highest-ranked books on anxiety.

Computer or Internet-based interventions based on CBT have expanded rapidly in recent years and show substantial evidence of efficacy for panic, phobias, and traumatic stress (Morgan & Jorm, 2009). Several Internet-based treatments are government-funded and are widely available online. The *FearFighter* program (www.fearfighter.com/) is funded by the UK's National Health Service for its patients. *E-couch* (http://ecouch.anu.edu.au), developed by the Australian National University, is available free to people with GAD and SAD worldwide.

PHYSICAL METHODS

As would be expected given its potential to decrease sympathetic arousal, self-managed relaxation practice has a significant evidence base to support its effectiveness in a variety of anxiety disorders (Morgan & Jorm, 2009). Relaxation techniques include progressive muscle relaxation, guided imagery, and deep breathing practice. See Client Resources at the end of this chapter for websites offering scripts or audio files narrating relaxation exercises.

Although further research would help to substantiate the value of methods such as exercise, yoga, and massage, existing research evidence supports the value of these self-care strategies in managing anxiety conditions. Perhaps because of the variety of meditation approaches studied and the use of a variety of comparison conditions, the evidence for the value of meditation in managing anxiety is limited (Morgan & Jorm, 2009). However, studies that demonstrate the value of meditation in improving perception, regulating emotions, and enhancing emotional well-being suggest that meditation practice could be valuable not only in reducing anxiety symptoms but in improving overall quality of life (Parker, 2010). See Exhibit 9-4 for an account of a client's experience in learning how to manage his anxiety.

SPECIAL CONSIDERATIONS: PREVENTION

Although anxiety disorders do not typically cause as much disability as other psychiatric disorders, such as mood or psychotic disorders, they produce a high cost burden to societies due to the high prevalence and early onset of anxiety problems. Since anxiety disorders typically have their onset during childhood or adolescence, prevention efforts thus far have focused on children and youth and their parents.

Bienvenu and Ginsburg (2007) review research on populations demonstrating early symptoms of an anxiety disorder (indicated prevention) or at risk for anxiety problems (selective prevention), and universal prevention. Indicated and selective interventions have used psychoeducational and cognitive-behavioral approaches to target child characteristics such as anxiety symptoms,

EXHIBIT 9-4: THE STORY OF J.B.

I am a 49-year-old divorced man, diagnosed with attention deficit hyperactivity disorder (ADHD) and generalized anxiety disorder (GAD). It is hard for me to focus on things for very long, and when I do I become more physically tense.

I was always a sad person, having missed out on some necessary parts for emotional development as a child. I was insecure, but I projected the façade of a confident, more arrogant me to the outer world. At 46, I left my marriage of 16 years to run away from the stresses of daily life. I was stung with deep anxiety and guilt, and was engulfed in total pain.

I began reading books by Buddhist practitioners, and these helped me begin to see that I was not the only one who had ever fallen apart. Although I was reading and exploring my life in therapy, I still felt great pain. I turned to exercise to release some of my stress. I also found a Hatha yoga class that helped me to learn how to breathe deeply and pay attention to what was going on in my body, and to learn to be okay with who I am.

While practicing yoga, I also changed therapists. My new therapist saw my level of anxiety and sent me to a nurse practitioner, who prescribed a medication to help me deal with my daily stresses without being bogged down or cut off from reality. Buspirone helped me to have a layer of tolerance so that I could manage my anxiety while dealing with the daily stresses such as working long hours, responding to the needs of my children, and dealing with difficult situations and my loneliness.

Having found a level of calm in my body, I could then work toward a greater acceptance of who I was through spiritual teaching. I incorporated a daily routine of yoga and meditation and changed my diet. I began studying and practicing Buddhist philosophy in earnest. My decision to go off medication came about 18 months after I started using it. I thought I could manage stress using meditation, mindfulness, and deep breathing.

It has been months since I stopped taking medication. I'm doing great! When stress hits me, I refocus on my breath and accept the stress for what it is. If I slip, I am gentle with myself. I am now okay with my anxiety. It is a part of me.

What happens next? I don't know. I take it one day at a time…one moment at a time, in fact. I am not against using medication. If I find I cannot use breathing, meditation, and yoga to ground myself, I may need to reconsider using medication to help. I appreciate both the benefits of the medication, and the support I get from the practitioner that guides me through my use of it.

PEDIATRIC POINTERS

- Anxiety disorders often begin in childhood. Phobias, both specific and social, are particularly likely to begin before adolescence.
- As with adults, pediatric anxiety disorders are often comorbid with other psychiatric disorders such as depression and bipolar disorder. Older children and adolescents may abuse substances to self-medicate. Careful screening to rule out comorbidity must occur before starting and during treatment.
- Sudden onset of OCD symptoms may be connected to streptococcal infection. Referred to as pediatric autoimmune neuropsychiatric disorders associated with streptococcal infections (PANDAS), the disorder is postulated to cause inflammation of the basal ganglia and may respond to early treatment with antibiotics.
- Children often interpret invasive medical treatment as traumatic. This experience can lead to symptoms of PTSD.
- Preschool children can develop PTSD but because they lack sophisticated verbal skills, they are unable to describe the experience. Clinicians may need to assess for behavioral manifestations of flashbacks: constriction of play, social withdrawal, and extreme temper tantrums.
- Loss or separation from a primary attachment figure can cause lasting effects on the HPA axis.
- High levels of parental distress negatively affect the child's ability to cope with traumatic events.
- Psychotherapy is the treatment of first choice for children and adolescents with anxiety disorders. Older children and adolescents may benefit from CBT. Severe symptoms or symptoms that do not respond to psychotherapy should be treated with medications such as SSRIs.
- Potential risks of SSRI and other medication use must be weighed against potential risks of untreated anxiety symptoms and discussed with parents. Age-appropriate discussion of common side effects should also occur with the child.

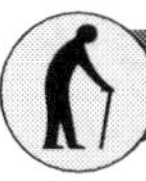

AGING ALERTS

- It is a myth that anxiety disorders drastically decline with age. However, individuals with OCD tend to be less symptomatic in older age.
- Anxiety disorders in geriatric populations may overlap with medical conditions.
- Elderly clients often express anxiety symptoms as somatic symptoms.
- As with younger populations, anxiety disorders are often comorbid with other psychiatric conditions. Social anxiety may lead to social isolation and agoraphobia and increase the risk for depressive illness. Careful screening for depression is imperative and if found, should be treated aggressively.
- GAD is the most common anxiety disorder manifesting in geriatric patients.
- Cognitive, sensory, or physical impairments may be a significant cause of anxiety in elderly persons.
- Benzodiazepines must be used in the lowest dose and for the shortest time possible, as they may lead to memory problems and falls. Adhere to "start low and go slow," but as with younger adults, treat to remission.
- New onset panic attacks are rare and may be due to side effects from medication or associated with other medical etiologies.

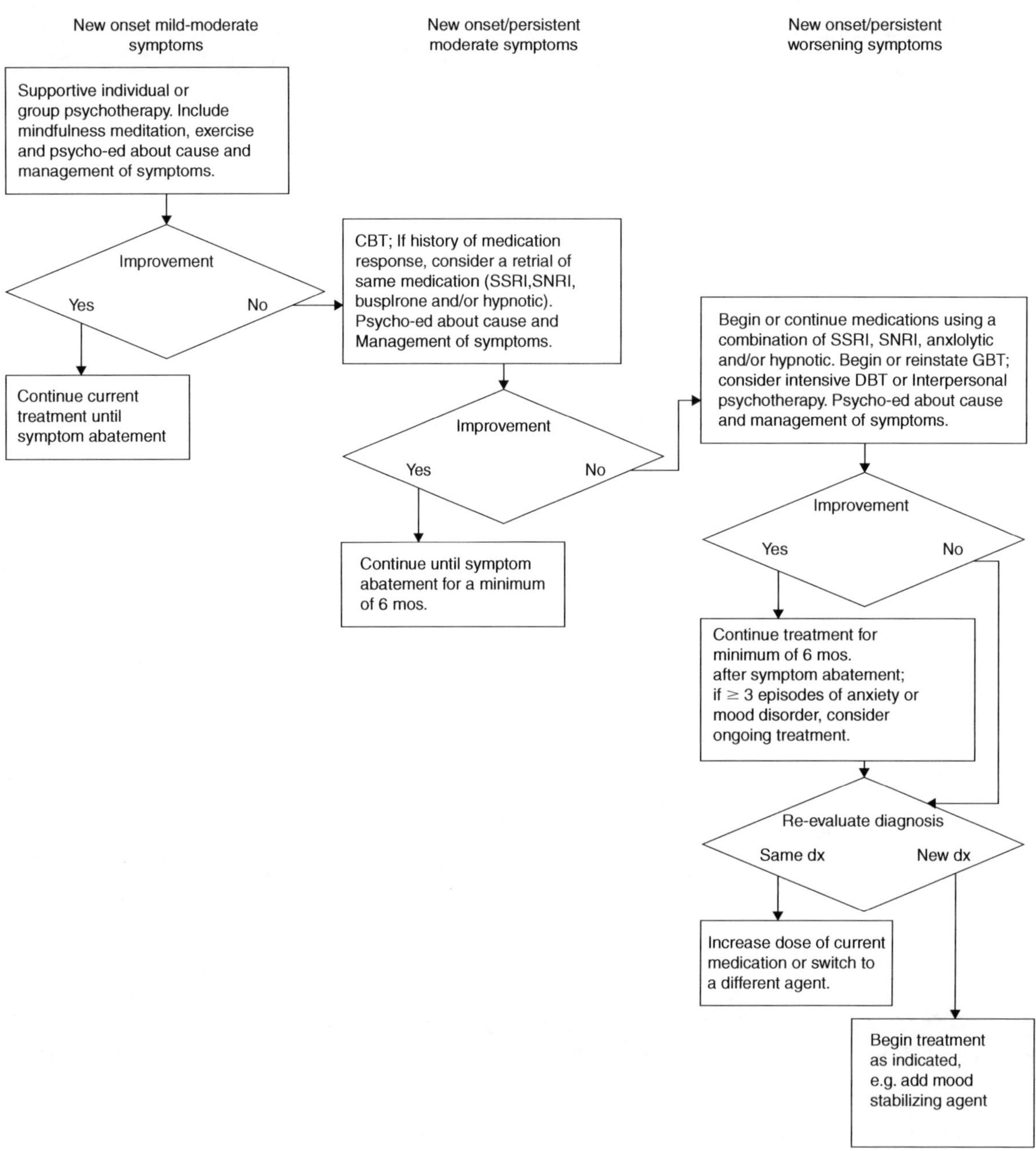

Figure 9-3 Decision Tree for Anxiety

avoidant behavior, maladaptive cognitions, and poor coping or problem-solving skills, and parent characteristics including overprotection, modeling anxiety, and criticism or conflict. These efforts have shown efficacy in reducing anxiety symptoms and related behaviors, though follow-up has not been long enough to establish the persistence of these gains in later life. An Internet-delivered intervention for college students with elevated anxiety sensitivity demonstrated significant treatment effects on anxious cognitions and depressive symptoms (Kenardy, McCafferty, & Rosa, 2006), which suggests that online interventions may be an effective and efficient means of targeting individuals at risk.

School-based universal interventions that teach coping and emotion-management skills to elementary and secondary school children have been shown to reduce the likelihood that students will develop anxiety problems (Barrett, Farrell, Ollendick, & Dadds, 2006). Bienvenu and Ginsburg (2007) recommend a larger role for education as a prevention strategy. This could take the form of a public health campaign to educate the populace about anxiety disorders, as well as educational efforts focused on primary care providers, who could play an important role in identification, initial treatment, and referral for anxiety-related problems.

CLIENT RESOURCES

BOOKS

Selections from self-help books for anxiety conditions that were ranked 70/100 or higher in "Popular Self-Help Books for Anxiety, Depression, and Trauma: How Scientifically Grounded and Useful Are They?" (2008) By R. E. Redding, J. D. Herbert, E. M. Forman, and B. A. Gaudiano

Anxiety, Phobias, and Panic (Revised) (2005) by R. Z. Peurifoy

Calming Your Anxious Mind (2003) by J. Brantley

Dying of Embarrassment (1992) by B., Markway, C. A, Pollard, T., Flynn, and C. N. Carmin

Obsessive-Compulsive Disorders: A Complete Guide to Getting Well and Staying Well (2000) by F. Penzel

The OCD Workbook: Your Guide to Breaking Free From Obsessive-Compulsive Disorder (1999) by B. M., Hyman, and C. Pedrick

Overcoming Compulsive Checking: Free Your Mind From OCD (2004) by P. R. Munford

The Shyness and Social Anxiety Workbook: Proven Techniques for Overcoming Your Fears (2000) by M. M., Antony, and R. P. Swinson

Stop Obsessing! How to Overcome Your Obsessions and Compulsion (2001) by E. B. Foa, and R. Wilson

ONLINE INFORMATION

National Institute of Mental Health:

- www.nimh.nih.gov/health/publications/anxiety-disorders/summary.shtml
- www.nimh.nih.gov/health/topics/anxiety-disorders/index.shtml
- Information in Spanish: www.nimh.nih.gov/health/publications/spanish/index-publication-all-es.shtml

National Library of Medicine MedLine Plus anxiety page: www.nlm.nih.gov/medlineplus/anxiety.html

Natural Medicines Comprehensive Database: http://naturaldatabase.therapeuticresearch.com

ORGANIZATIONS

Anxiety Disorder Association of America: www.adaa.org/

Freedom from Fear: www.freedomfromfear.org/

International OCD Foundation: www.ocfoundation.org/

Mental Health America: www.nmha.org/

National Alliance for Mental Illness: www.nami.org/

Social Phobia/Social Anxiety Association: www.socialphobia.org/

Toastmasters: www.toastmasters.org/

ONLINE CBT PROGRAMS

E-couch (http://ecouch.anu.edu.au): available free to people with general anxiety and social anxiety worldwide

FearFighter (www.fearfighter.com/): available to patients of the UK's National Health Service

RELAXATION TRAINING

AllAboutDepression.com (www.allaboutdepression.com/relax/): Audio clips narrating a variety of relaxation techniques.

Arizona State University Virtual Counseling Center (http://vcc.asu.edu/relax/index.shtml): Includes scripts and audio and video files of relaxation exercises in English, Spanish, American Sign Language, and English Sign Language.

REFERENCES

Allen, J. G. (2001). *Traumatic relationships and serious mental disorders*. Chichester, UK: Wiley.

American Psychiatric Association. (2000). *Diagnostic and Statistical Manual of mental Disorders, 4th edition, text revised.* Washington DC: American Psychiatric Association Publishing.

American Psychiatric Association. (n.d.). *DSM-5 development: Anxiety disorders*. Retrieved from www.dsm5.org/proposedrevision/Pages/AnxietyDisorders.aspx

Antony, M. M., & Swinson, R. P. (2000). *The shyness and social anxiety workbook: Proven techniques for overcoming your fears.* Oakland, CA: New Harbinger.

Barrett, P. M., Farrell, L. J., Ollendick, T. H., & Dadds, M. (2006). Long-term outcomes of an Australian universal prevention trial of anxiety and depression symptoms in children and youth: An evaluation of the FRIENDS program. *Journal of Child and Adolescent Psychology, 35*, 403–411.

Bassil, N., Ghandour, A., & Grossberg, G. (2011). How anxiety presents differently in older adults. *Current Psychiatry, 10*(3), 65–71.

Beck, A. T., Epstein, N., Brown, G., & Steer, R. (1988). An inventory for measuring clinical anxiety: Psychometric properties. *Journal of Consulting and Clinical Psychology, 56*, 893–897.

Bienvenu, O. J., & Ginsburg, G. S. (2007). Prevention of anxiety disorders. *International Review of Psychiatry, 19*(6), 647–654.

Boschloo, L., Vogelzangs, N., Smit, J. H., van den Brink, W., Veltman, D. J., Beekman, A. T., & Penninx, B. W. (2011). Comorbidity and risk indicators for alcohol use disorders among persons with anxiety and/or depressive disorders: Findings from the Netherlands study of depression and anxiety (NESDA). *Journal of Affective Disorders, 131*, 233–242.

Bourne, E. J. (2000). *The anxiety and phobia workbook* (3rd edition). Oakland, CA: New Harbinger.

Brantley, J. (2003). *Calming your anxious mind.* Oakland, CA: New Harbinger.

Braun, P., Greenberg, D., Dasberg, H., & Lerer, B. (1990). Core symptoms of posttraumatic stress disorder unimproved by alprazolam treatment. *Journal of Clinical Psychiatry, 51*(6), 236–238.

Brown, T. A., DiNardo, P. A., & Barlow, D. H. (1994). *Anxiety disorders interview schedule for DSM-IV (ADIS-IV)*. New York, NY: Graywind.

Butler, A. C., Chapman, J. E., Forman, E. M., & Beck, A. T. (2006). The empirical status of cognitive-behavioral therapy: A review of meta-analyses. *Clinical Psychology Review, 26*(1), 17–31.

Cairney, J., McCabe, L., Veldhuizen, S., Corna, L. M., Streiner, D., & Herrmann, M. (2007). Epidemiology of social phobia in later life. *American Journal of Geriatric Psychiatry, 15*(3), 224–233.

Cannistraro, P. A., Wright, C. I., Wedig, M. M., Martis, B., Shin, L. M., Wilhelm, S., & Rauch, S. L. (2004). Amygdala responses to human faces in obsessive-compulsive disorder. *Biological Psychiatry, 56*(12), 916–920.

Cannon, W. B. (1932). *The wisdom of the body*. New York, NY: Norton.

Cates, M. E., Bishop, M. H., Davis, L. L., Lowe, J. S., & Woolley, T. W. (2004). Clonazepam for treatment of sleep disturbances associated with combat-related posttraumatic stress. *Annals of Pharmacotherapy, 38*(9), 1395–1399.

Corr, P. J. (2011). Anxiety: Splitting the phenomenological atom. *Personality and Individual Differences, 50*, 889–897.

Curtis, G. C., Massana, J., Udina, C., Ayuso, J. L., Cassano, G. B., & Perugi, G. (1993). Maintenance drug therapy of panic disorder. *Journal of Psychiatric Research, 27*(1), 127–142.

Davidson, J. (2009) First-line pharmacotherapy approaches for generalized anxiety disorder. *Journal of Clinical Psychiatry, 70*(Suppl. 2), 25–31.

Davis, L. L., Jewell, M. E., Ambrose, S., Farley, J., English, B., Bartolucci, A., & Petty, F. (2004). A placebo-controlled study of nefazodone for the treatment of chronic posttraumatic stress disorder: A preliminary study. *Journal of Clinical Psychopharmacology, 24*(3), 291–297.

Donner, J., Pirkola, S., Silander, K., Kananen, L., Terwilliger, J. D., Lönnqvist, J.,... Hovatta, I. (2008). An association analysis of murine anxiety genes in humans implicates novel candidate genes for anxiety disorders. *Biological Psychiatry, 64*(8), 672–680.

DuPont, R. L., Rice, D. P., Miller, L. S., Shiraki, S. S., Rowland, C. R., & Harwood, H. J. (1996). Economic costs of anxiety disorders. *Anxiety, 2*(4), 167–172.

First, M., Spitzer, R., Gibbon, M., & Williams, J. (1995). *Structured clinical interview for DSM-IV Axis I disorders. Patient edition (SCID-I/P)*. New York, NY: Biometrics.

Foa, E. B. & Wilson, R. (2001). *Stop obsessing! How to overcome your obsessions and compulsions* (revised). New York, NY: Bantam Books.

Foa, E., Huppert, E., Leiberg, S., Langner, R., Kichic, R., Hajcak, G., & Salkovskis, P. (2002). The Obsessive-compulsive inventory: Development and validation of a short version. *Psychological Assessment, 14*(4), 485–496.

Garakani, A., Mathew, S. J., & Charney, D. (2006). Neurobiology of anxiety disorders and implications for treatment. *The Mount Sinai Journal of Medicine, 73*(7), 941–947.

Geiser, F., Meier, C., Wegener, I., Imbierowich, K., Conrad, R., Liedtke, R.,... Harbrecht, U. (2008). Association between anxiety, factors of coagulation and fibrinolysis. *Psychotherapy and Psychosomatics, 77*, 377–383.

Glueck, G. (2006, February 17). Art review: Munch was more than a scream. *The New York Times*. Retrieved from www.nytimes.com/2006/02/17/arts/design/17munc.html

Goddard, A. W., Brouette, T., Almai, A., Jetty, P., Woods, S. W., & Charney, D. (2001). Early coadministration of clonazepam with sertraline for panic disorder. *Archives of General Psychiatry, 58*(7), 681–686.

Goodman, W., Price, L., Rasmussen, S., Mazure, C., Fleischcmann, R., Hill, C.,... Charney, D. (1989). The Yale-Brown obsessive-compulsive scale: I. Development, use and reliability. *Archives of General Psychiatry, 40*, 1006–1011.

Hamilton, M. (1959). The assessment of anxiety states by rating. *British Journal of Medical Psychology*, 32, 50–55.

Hammack, S. E., Cooper, M. A., & Lezak, K. R. (2012). Overlapping neurobiology of learned helplessness and conditioned defeat: Implications for PTSD and mood disorders. *Neuropharmacology, 62*, 565–575. doi: 10.1016/j.neuropharm.2011.02.024

Hettema, J. M., Neale, M. C., & Kendler, K. S. (2001). A review and metaanalysis of the genetic epidemiology of anxiety disorders. *American Journal of Psychiatry, 158*, 1568–1578.

Hinton, D. E., Chong, R., Pollack, M. H., Barlow, D. H., & McNally, R. J. (2008). Ataque de nervios: Relationship to anxiety sensitivity and dissociation predisposition. *Depression and Anxiety, 25*(6), 489–495.

Hofmann, S. G., Asnaani, A., & Hinton, D. E. (2010). Cultural aspects of social anxiety and social anxiety disorder. *Depression and Anxiety, 27*, 1117–1127.

Huffman, J., & Pollack, M. (2003). Predicting panic disorder among patients with chest pain: An analysis of the literature. *Psychosomatics, 44*(3), 222–236.

Hyman, B. M., & Pedrick, C. (1999). *The OCD workbook: Your guide to breaking free from obsessive-compulsive disorder*. Oakland, CA: New Harbinger.

Kawachi, I., Sparrow, D., Vokonas, P. S., & Weiss, S. T. (1995). Decreased heart rate variability in men with phobic anxiety (data from the normative aging study). *American Journal of Cardiology, 75*(14), 882–885.

Kenardy, J., McCafferty, K., & Rosa, V. (2006). Internet-delivered indicated prevention for anxiety disorders: Six-month follow-up. *Clinical Psychologist, 10*(1), 39–42.

Kessler, R. C., Berglund, P., Demler, O., Jin, R., Merikangas, K. R., & Walters, E. E. (2005a). Lifetime prevalence and age-of-onset distributions of DSM-IV disorders in the National Comorbidity Survey Replication. *Archives of General Psychiatry, 62*, 593–602.

Kessler, R. C., Chiu, W. T., Merikangas, K. R., Demler, O., & Walters, E. E. (2005). Prevalence, severity, and comorbidity of 12-month DSM-IV disorders in the National Comorbidity Survey Replication. *Archives of General Psychiatry, 62*, 617–627.

Kessler, R. C., Demler, O., Frank, R. G., Olfson, M., Pincus, H. A., Walters, E. E.,... Zaslavsky, A. M. (2005b). Prevalence and treatment of mental disorders, 1990 to 2003. *New England Journal of Medicine, 352*(24), 2515–2523.

Kim, S. J., Kim, B. N., Cho, S. C., Kim, J. W., Shin, M. S., Yoo, H. J.,... Kim, H. W. (2010). The prevalence of specific phobia and associated co-morbid features in children and adolescents. *Journal of Anxiety Disorders, 24*, 629–634.

Liebowitz, M. (1987). Social phobia. *Modern Problems in Pharmacopsychiatry, 22*, 141–173.

Lovibond, S., & Lovibond, P. (1995). *Manual for the Depression Anxiety Stress Scales* (2nd ed.). Sydney, N.S.W: Psychology Foundation.

Markway, B., Pollard, C. A., Flynn, T., & Carmin, C. N. (1992). *Dying of embarrassment*. Oakland, CA: New Harbinger.

Martin, E., Ressler, K. J., Binder, E., & Nemeroff, C. B. (2009). The neurobiology of anxiety disorders: Brain imaging, genetics and psychoneuroendocrinology. *Psychiatric Clinics of North America, 32*, 549–575.

Mattick, R., & Clark, J. (1998). Development and validation of measures of social phobia scrutiny fear and social interaction anxiety. *Behaviour Research and Therapy, 36*, 455–470.

Mavissakalian, M. R. (2003). Imipramine vs. sertraline in panic disorder: 24-week treatment completers. *Annals of Clinical Psychiatry, 15*(3–4), 171–180.

McEwen, B. S., & Stellar, E. (1993). Stress and the individual: Mechanisms leading to disease. *Archives of Internal Medicine, 153*(18), 2093–2101.

McLean, C. P., Asnaani, A., Litz, B. T, & Hofmann, S. G. (2011). Gender differences in anxiety disorders: Prevalence, course of illness, comorbidity and burden of illness. *Journal of Psychiatric Research, 45*, 1027–1035.

McRae, A. L., Brady, K. T., Mellman, T. A., Sonne, S. C., Killeen, T. K., Timmerman, M. A.,... Bayles-Dazet, W. (2004). Comparison of nefazodone and sertraline for the treatment of posttraumatic stress disorder. *Depression and Anxiety, 19*(3), 190–196.

Menzies, L., Chamberlain, S. R., Laird, A. R., Thelen, S. M., Sahakian, B. J., & Bullmore, E. T. (2008). Integrating evidence from neuroimaging and neuropsychological studies of obsessive-compulsive disorder: The orbitofronto-striatal model revisited. *Neuroscience and Biobehavioral Review, 32*(3), 525–549.

Meyer, T., Miller, M., Metzger, R., & Borkovec, T. (1990). Development and validity of the Penn State Worry scale. *Behaviour Research and Therapy, 28*, 487–495.

Morgan, A. J., & Jorm, A. F. (2009). Outcomes of self-help efforts for anxiety. *Expert Review of Pharmacoeconomics and Outcomes Research, 9*(5), 445–459.

Muldoon, M. F., Herbert, T. B., Patterson, S. M., Kameneva, M., Raible, R., & Manuck, S. B. (1995). Effects of acute psychological stress on serum lipid levels, hemoconcentration, and blood viscosity. *Archives of Internal Medicine, 155*(6), 615–620.

Munford, P. R. (2004). *Overcoming compulsive checking: Free your mind from OCD*. Oakland, CA: New Harbinger.

Nepon, J., Belik, S. L., Bolton, J., & Sareen, J. (2010). The relationship between anxiety disorders and suicide attempts: Findings from the National Epidemiologic Survey on alcohol and related conditions. *Depression and Anxiety, 27*, 791–798.

Parker, J. B. (2010, Fall). Worth contemplating: Scientists and scholars examine the power of meditation. *UC Davis Magazine, 28*(1), 10.

Penzel, F. (2000). *Obsessive-compulsive disorders: A complete guide to getting well and staying well*. New York, NY: Oxford University Press.

Peurifoy, R. Z. (2005). *Anxiety, phobias, and panic (revised)*. New York, NY: Warner Books.

Phoenix, B. J. (2007). Psychoeducation for survivors of trauma. *Perspectives in Psychiatric Care, 43*(3), 123–131.

Pitsavos, C., Panagiotakos, D. B., Papangeorgiou, C., Tsetsekou, E., Soldatos, C., & Stefanadis, C. (2006). Anxiety in relation to inflammation and coagulation markers among healthy adults: The ATTICA study. *Atherosclerosis, 185*(2), 320–326.

Rapgay, L., Bystritsky, A., Dafter, R. E., & Spearman, M. (2011). New strategies for combining mindfulness with integrative cognitive behavioral therapy for the treatment of generalized anxiety disorder. *Journal of Rational Emotive and Cognitive Behavioral Therapy, 29*(2), 92–119.

Ravindran, L. N., & Stein, M. B. (2010). The pharmacologic treatment of anxiety disorders: A review of progress. *Journal of Clinical Psychiatry, 71*(7), 839–854.

Redding, R. E., Herbert, J. D., Forman, E. M., & Gaudiano, B. A. (2008). Popular self-help books for anxiety, depression, and trauma: How scientifically grounded and useful are they? *Professional Psychology: Research and Practice, 39*(5), 537–545.

Reiss, S., Peterson, R., Gursky, D., & McNally, R. (1986). Anxiety sensitivity, anxiety frequency, and the prediction of fearfulness. *Behaviour Research and Therapy, 24*, 1–8.

Roth, A., & Fonagy, P. (2005). *What works for whom? A critical review of psychotherapy research* (2nd ed.). New York, NY: Guilford Press.

Sadock, B. J., & Sadock, V. A. (2003). *Kaplan and Sadock's synopsis of psychiatry* (9th ed.). Philadelphia, PA: Lippincott Williams & Wilkins.

Scahill, L., Riddle, M. A., McSwiggin-Hardin, M., Ort, S. I., King, R. A., Goodman, W. K., ... Leckman, J. (1997). Children's Yale-Brown Obsessive-Compulsive Scale: Reliability and validity. *Journal of the American Academy of Child and Adolescent Psychiatry, 36*, 844–852.

Schatzberg, A., Cole, J. O., & DeBattista, C. (2010). *Manual of clinical psychopharmacology* (7th ed.). Washington, DC: American Psychiatric Association.

Schmidt, N. B., Richey, J., & Fitzpatrick, K. (2006). Discomfort intolerance: Development of a construct and measure relevant to panic disorder. *Journal of Anxiety Disorders, 20*, 263–280.

Schoevers, R. A., Beekman, A. T., Deeg, D. J., Jonker, C., & van Tilburg, W. (2003). Comorbidity and risk-patterns of depression, generalised anxiety disorder and mixed anxiety-depression in later life: Results from the AMSTEL study. *International Journal of Geriatric Psychiatry, 18*(11), 994–1001.

Seidler, G. H., & Wagner, F. E. (2006). Comparing the efficacy of EMDR and trauma-focused cognitive-behavioral therapy in the treatment of PTSD: A meta-analytic study. *Psychological Medicine, 36*(11), 1515–1522.

Shea, S. C. (1998). *Psychiatric interviewing: The art of understanding* (2nd ed.). Philadelphia, PA: Saunders.

Shin, L. M., & Liberzon, I. (2010). The neurocircuitry of fear, stress, and anxiety disorders. *Neuropsychopharmacology, 35*(1), 169–191.

Silverman, W. K., Pina, A. A., & Viswesvaran, C. (2008). Evidence-based psychosocial treatments for phobic and anxiety disorders in children and adolescents: A review and meta-analyses. *Journal of Clinical Child and Adolescent Psychology, 37*(1), 105–130.

Simon, N., Otto, M., Worthington, J. J., Hoge, E., Thompson, E. H., LeBeau, R. T., & Pollack, M. H. (2009). Next-step strategies for panic disorder refractory to initial pharmacotherapy: A 3-phase randomized clinical trial. *Journal of Clinical Psychiatry, 70*(11), 1563–1570.

Spielberger, C. (1983). *Manual for the State-Trait Anxiety Inventory (STAI)*. Palo Alto, CA: Consulting Psychologists Press.

Stahl, S. M. (2003). *Essential psychopharmacology: Neuroscientific basis and practical applications* (2nd ed.). New York, NY: Cambridge University Press.

Taylor, H. R., Freeman, M. K., & Cates, M. E. (2008). Prazosin for treatment of nightmares related to posttraumatic stress disorder. *American Journal of Health System Pharmacy, 65*(8), 716–722.

Turner, S., Beidel, D., Dancu, C., & Stanley, M. (1989). An empirically derived inventory to measure social fears and anxiety: The social phobia and anxiety inventory. *Psychological Assessment, 1*, 35–40.

U.S. Department of Health and Human Services. (1999). *Mental health: A report of the surgeon general*. Rockville, MD: U.S. Department of Health and Human Services, Substance Abuse and Mental Health Services Administration, Center for Mental Health Services, National Institutes of Health, National Institute of Mental Health.

Vøllestad, J., Sivertsen, B., & Nielsen, G. H. (2011). Mindfulness-based stress reduction for patients with anxiety disorders: Evaluation in a randomized controlled trial. *Behavioral Research and Therapy, 49*(4), 281–288.

Wittchen, H-U., Krause P., Hoyer, J., Beesdo, K., Jacobi, F., Hofler, M., ... Winter, S. (2001). Prevalence and correlates of GAD in primary care. *Fortschritte der Medizin, 143*, 17–25.

Wittchen, H-U., Zhao, S., Kessler, R. C., & Eaton, W.W. (1994). DSM-III-R generalized anxiety disorder in the National Comorbidity Survey. *Archives of General Psychiatry, 51*(5), 355–364.

Woodman, C. L. (1997). The natural history of generalized anxiety disorder: A review. *Medscape Psychiatry and Mental Health eJournal, 2*(3).

Worthington, J. J., Pollack, M. H., Pollack, M. H., Otto, M. W., McLean, R. Y., Moroz, G., & Rosenbaum, J. F. (1998). Long-term experience with clonazepam in patients with a primary diagnosis of panic disorder. *Psychopharmacology Bulletin, 34*(2), 199–205.

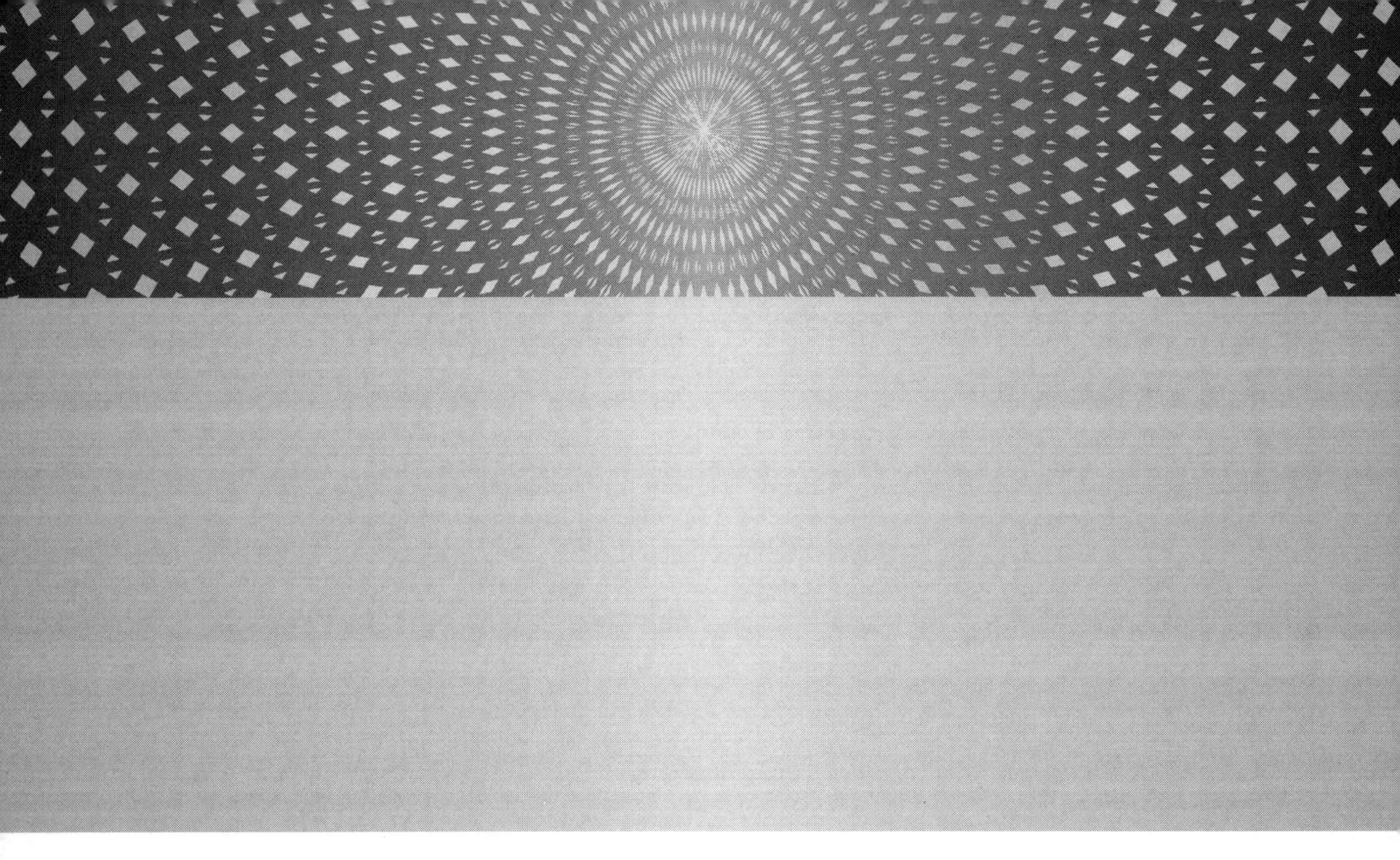

CHAPTER CONTENTS

Although there have been major advances in the understanding of the biology and functioning of the human brain, we are still limited in our ability to effectively treat the most serious and persistently mental ill. Nursing is both an art and a science that incorporates multiple realms of care, including the physical, developmental, emotional, social, psychological, cultural, and spiritual; advanced practice psychiatric mental health nurses must draw upon this nursing philosophy as well as their in-depth knowledge of mental health disorders and psychotherapeutic and psychobiologic interventions. Caring for the patient with psychosis can be a challenging yet rewarding aspect of nursing practice.

Mental health clinicians use psychosis to describe many phenomena, including: breaks with reality testing, abnormal sensations, catatonia, bizarre behaviors, and so-called formal thought disorders (Rose, Stuart, Hardy, & Loewy, 2010). Psychosis is not actually a specific disease but a symptom where the individual has a loss of contact with reality. This disruption of an individual's reality testing where the person may not distinguish internal sensory perceptions or ideas from the external reality can cause significant pain and confusion. Common symptoms of psychosis include hallucinations, delusions, trouble organizing thoughts, and hallucinations. Psychosis is a nonspecific condition and the symptoms of psychosis do not identify the exact cause of the brain condition.

Psychotic disorders of different etiologies have interested both clinicians and researchers, but for different

CHAPTER 10

Integrative Management of Psychotic Symptoms

Linda Jacobson and Marianne Tarraza

reasons. People with psychosis have been some of the most challenging for clinicians to treat due to the severity and chronicity of symptoms. One potential problematic aspect of treatment is differential diagnosis as psychosis can result from numerous etiologies and many patients have more than one risk factor (Fujii & Ahmed, 2007).

Although psychosis can be from many different causes—that is, drugs, toxins, mania, certain medical conditions—this chapter is primarily focused on the psychosis associated with severe mental illness like schizophrenia or schizoaffective disorder. Despite this focus, one does need to be careful to not automatically assume psychosis means schizophrenia. As mentioned, psychosis is a symptom of a clinical condition much like a fever may have many different explanations. An exhaustive review of the concept of schizophrenia, an in-depth comprehensive explanation on brain biology, and evolving treatment paradigm for psychosis throughout history is beyond the scope of this chapter.

Schizophrenia is a brain disease where the clinical presentation reflects impairments in areas of thinking and cognition. It is a devastating disorder for most people who are afflicted, and very costly for families and society. The impact on the individual and family is obvious but the impact on our society is immense.

The overall U.S. cost of schizophrenia in 2002 was estimated to be $62.7 billion, with $22.7 billion excess direct health care costs ($7.0 billion outpatient, $5.0 billion drugs, $2.8 billion inpatient, and $8.0 billion long-term care). The total direct non-health care excess costs, including living cost offsets, were estimated to be $7.6 billion. The total indirect excess costs were estimated to be $32.4 billion (Wu et al., 2005). It has been estimated that nearly half of all beds for mental health disorders and over one-quarter of total hospital beds are occupied by individuals with schizophrenia.

INCIDENCE-PREVALENCE

Schizophrenia is a severe form of mental illness affecting approximately 7 in 1,000 of the adult population, and most concentrated in the age group between 15 to 35 years. It is averaged that 1% of the population has this illness. Although the incidence is low (3–10,000), the prevalence is high due to chronicity—worldwide, approximately 24 million people are affected (World Health Organization, 2011).

Gender differences in the prevalence of all psychiatric disorders have long been acknowledged, but the differences in the presentation, comorbidities, and course of the treatment have also been noted. Although bipolar disorder is about equally prevalent in both genders, women are more prone to rapid mood cycling. The incidence of schizophrenia appears to be pretty balanced between men and women, but the course of schizophrenia can be quite different between the sexes.

Gender differences are highlighted in Exhibit 10-1 (Burt & Hendrick, 1997). There is evidence that schizophrenia

EXHIBIT 10-1: GENDER DIFFERENCES IN SCHIZOPHRENIA

Compared to men, women:

Are less likely to have structural brain abnormalities
Are more likely to have relatives with the illness
Are more likely to have late onset schizophrenia
Are less likely to have comorbid substance abuse
Are less likely to commit suicide
Tend to exhibit more positive and fewer negative symptoms
Tend to exhibit more affective symptoms
Tend to respond to lower doses of neuroleptics
Tend to maintain better social functioning (i.e., higher rates of employment and marriage)

can run in families. The illness may occur in only 1 percent of the general population, but it occurs in 10 percent of people who have a first-degree relative with the disorder. People who have a second-degree relative with the disease also develop schizophrenia more often than the general population. The risk is highest for an identical twin of a person with schizophrenia. He or she has a 40% to 65% chance of developing the disorder (NIMH, 2011).

HISTORY

It can be intriguing, and at times distressing, to see how individuals with psychosis have been viewed throughout time. There were times they were believed to hold special powers, or were seen as cursed or even possessed. The Greeks first coined the term paranoia, and it was used by Hippocrates to refer to a delirium or disorganized thinking. The term was abandoned, but then renewed in 1863 by Karl Kahbaum. He believed that paranoia was a persistent delusional illness that remained unchanged throughout its course (Murray & Huelskoetter, 1983).

Freud's theory of paranoia centered on the idea that delusional thinking in both sexes came from the projection and reaction formation of unacceptable homosexual wishes. Freud proposed that schizophrenia resulted from developmental fixations that produced defects in ego development. These defects contributed to the symptoms of schizophrenia (Sadock & Sadock, 2008).

H. S. Sullivan later postulated that the paranoid person suffers from a deep sense of inferiority, insecurity, and feelings of rejection. This creates a state where the person experiences feelings of loneliness and unworthiness that are intolerable. Security is obtained by the projection of these feelings and by transfer of blame onto others. Sullivan viewed schizophrenia as a disturbance in interpersonal relatedness. He saw the symptoms of schizophrenia as an adaptive means to avoid panic and disintegration of self (Sadock & Sadock, 2008).

Schizophrenia was systematically described in 1896 by Emil Kraepelin. He called the behaviors and symptoms *dementia praecox,* meaning a deteriorated, hopeless condition with poor prognosis. He emphasized the chronic and debilitating course of the illness. He divided the behaviors and symptoms into four major disease types: simple, catatonic, hebephrenic, and paranoid (Murray & Huelskoetter, 1983).

The actual term *schizophrenia* was coined on April 24, 1908, when Paul Eugen Bleuler gave a lecture at a meeting of the German Psychiatric Association in Berlin, "taking the liberty of employing the word schizophrenia for revising the Kraepelinian concept. In my opinion the breaking up or splitting of psychic functioning is an excellent symptom of the whole group" (Fusar-Poli & Politi, 2008). Many people still falsely think of schizophrenia as the splitting of the personality into two parts perpetuated in the "split personality," where Bleuler was actually emphasizing the splitting off of the mind between the functions of feeling and thinking, the disorganization of thought and emotional processes.

Well over a hundred years ago, long before computed tomography (CT) scans and MRIs, Bleuler realized that the condition was most likely a group of interrelated disease states rather than a single specific disease (he referred to a "whole group" of schizophrenias). He set up criteria of primary and secondary symptoms, criteria that are still in use today for the diagnosis of schizophrenia. The primary symptoms are denoted by the four A's: (a) autism, (b) ambivalence, (c) affective disturbance, and (d) loosening of associations. Secondary symptoms include (a) illusions, (b) delusions, (c) hallucinations, (d) symptoms related to muscular activity, (e) withdrawal, and (f) lack of touch with reality (Murray & Huelskoetter, 1983).

Historically, it had been proposed that two distinct syndromes in schizophrenia could be discerned from the phenomenological profiles. The type I, or positive syndrome was composed of florid symptoms, such as delusions, hallucinations, and disorganized thinking. The type II, or negative syndrome was characterized by deficits in cognitive, affective, and social functions, including blunting of affect and passive withdrawal (Kay, Fiszbein, & Opler, 1987).

It is important to remember that we are still very early in our understanding of the cause and treatments for psychotic diseases. In mental health, we have generations of claims and theories that did not support tenets of science and many of our patients suffered because of us. One needs only to go back to the 1970s to find hemodialysis and beta-endorphins as treatments for schizophrenia gracing the pages of our most prestigious journals (Keith, 2006).

ETIOLOGY

It is often frustrating for our patients and their families that we cannot identify a single causation of this devastating illness. They want to compare to other types of medical illness where treatment is directly connected to etiology, such as pneumonia, where the infectious agent can be identified and the appropriate antibiotic is prescribed. We are not yet there in psychiatry and certainly not in the treatment of psychosis.

It is now widely accepted that schizophrenia is a manifestation of a brain disease of perhaps many differing genetic or acquired origins. Today, we recognize the foundation of biology in causation with the impact of treatment and environment on its course. Regardless of the exact causation, the result is impairment in brain function that may produce the psychotic symptoms that can be seen in the diagnosis of the schizophrenia spectrums (Nasrallah, 1986). This multi-causal origin continues to challenge clinicians trying to offer the best symptom relief to their patient but remains an area of potential promise.

There is evidence that there are changes in brain structure in individuals with schizophrenia. Research has identified that some patients have abnormal brain morphologic structure, which is already present at the time of the first psychotic episode (Wood et al., 2006). There have been significant cortical gray matter deficits and lateral and third ventricular enlargements in patients with schizophrenia compared to control subjects (Talbot et al., 1998). However, it is unclear when these structural brain changes actually emerge and more research is indicated in this area.

Altered activation of dopamine receptors has typically been the prevailing explanation for the classic symptoms of schizophrenia. Today, it is generally believed that the dopamine hypothesis is too simplistic to explain the whole syndrome, but remains a cornerstone of the treatment paradigm. We now know that multiple neurotransmitters in the brain are involved and have a complex interplay among each other.

The dopamine hypothesis suggests that the symptoms of schizophrenia are due primarily to a functional hyperactivity in the dopamine system in limbic regions and a functional hypoactivity in frontal regions. Further suggestion is that the hyper-dopaminergic state existing in the mesolimbic pathway results in the positive symptoms and a hypo-dopaminergic state in the mesocortical pathways leads to the negative, cognitive, and affective symptoms (Citrome, 2011a, suppl). Much of the support for the dopamine hypothesis arose from the observation that the efficacy of many of the antipsychotic drugs used to treat schizophrenia was highly correlated with their ability to block dopamine (D2) receptors. Conversely, drugs that enhance dopamine transmission, such as the amphetamines, tend to worsen the symptoms of schizophrenia. Therefore, the dopamine hypothesis suggested that the abnormality in this illness might lie specifically in the D2 receptors (Andreasen & Black, 2006).

The role of serotonin has also been implicated in schizophrenia and has been the focus of many of the drug developments in the past two decades. Serotonin inhabits dopamine synthesis and therefore agents that occupy serotonin receptors may increase dopamine levels in areas that need it and improve negative symptoms (Keltner, Folks, Palmer, & Powers, 1998). Positron emission tomography (PET) has been used to measure receptor occupancy, providing an in vivo method for directly observing the mechanisms of pharmacological action.

More recently, newer "second generation" (atypical) antipsychotics have been developed that have a broader pharmacologic profile. In addition to dopamine receptor blockade, they also block serotonin type 2 (5-HT2) receptors, suggesting a role for serotonin in the pathophysiology of schizophrenia (Andreasen & Black, 2006).

The total complexity of brain neurochemistry is at its infancy state and the potential in this area offers such promise for the treatment of the seriously mentally ill. Recently attention has been given to glutamate, a ubiquitous neurotransmitter in the brain, which may have implications in the pathophysiology of schizophrenia. The first major clue that schizophrenia may be related to glutamate pathways was the observation more than 3 decades ago that phencyclidine phosphate (PCP)-induced psychosis manifests all the symptom domains of schizophrenia (positive, negative, cognitive, and formal thought disorder) (Nasrallah, 2011b, suppl).

According to the glutamate hypothesis, excessive amounts of glutamate are released and exert a neurotoxic effect that leads to the signs and symptoms of schizophrenia (Andreasen & Black, 2006). The interplay between glutamate and dopamine may hold the key to addressing more fully those symptom domains that have impacted on the functionality of patients with schizophrenia, namely negative and cognitive symptoms (Citrome, 2011a).

There is a genetic contribution to some, perhaps all, forms of schizophrenia, and a high proportion of the variance in liability to schizophrenia is due to additive genetic effects (Sadock & Sadock, 2008). Genetic contribution to liability for schizophrenia has been estimated as high as 60%, although models of genetic transmission, predisposing genes, and the link between genetic factors and the phenomenology of schizophrenia are far from being identified. Available data leave considerable room for environmental influences, as shown by concordance rates of less than 50% in monozygotic twins and lifetime risk of about 45% in children of two schizophrenic parents. Only 10% of people with schizophrenia have an affected parent. Given the heterogeneous nature of schizophrenic disorders, it is also possible that both genetic and nongenetic forms of the disorder exist (Barbato, 2011; WHO, 2011).

There is the stress model that suggests individuals may carry a genetic predisposition, but this vulnerability is not "released" unless other factors also intervene. Although most of these factors are considered environmental, most are more biological rather than psychological. This could include factors such as birth injuries, poor maternal nutrition, viral exposure, or maternal substance abuse (Andreasen & Black, 2006). The incidence of schizophrenia is increased in children whose mothers were exposed to influenza in the second trimester of pregnancy. Perinatal anoxia is also associated with the later development of schizophrenia (Knesper, Riba, & Schwenk, 1997).

Psychological stressful life events may also have a connection to the onset of relapse in a major psychotic illness. The possibility remains that types of psychological stresses at critical developmental stages could lead a *vulnerable* individual into the development of schizophrenia. There has been interest in exploring the effects of both acute and chronic stressors and the expression of illness. There have been studies that link a high frequency of independent social stressors in the 3 weeks before a psychotic relapse (Stoudemire, 1990).

As in any chronic illness model, the impact of environment, development, learning, and social dynamics can contribute to the stability or exacerbation of symptoms. There were many theories that stated schizophrenia was a result of family dynamics where the family was dysfunctional, hostile, or withholding. These theories caused more damage and created blame on many loving families. There was limited recognition of the impact on the family who was living with family member with chronic illness or that other children in the same "skewed" family had no expression of the illness.

The concept of the "schizophrenogenic mother" was finally put to rest in the 1970s (Stoudemire, 1990). There were many mothers who tormented themselves that they must have done something wrong as a parent despite having other healthy functioning children, or believed they may have ingested something during the pregnancy. They continued to blame themselves or searched every day for answers. This is an area where nursing can try to educate and repair the damage done to families.

Although the former hypothesis that schizophrenia was in some way related to parenting style has been discredited, it is true however that certain parenting and family communication styles are associated with a less favorable course and outcome of the illness. Family interactions involving high levels of expressed emotion can be detrimental to these patients (Knesper et al., 1997). Family psychoeducation becomes very important in clarifying symptom states, expectations, and communication strategies.

Even though researchers are still struggling for additional facts about the etiology and development of the schizophrenic process and diseases, we do have a sense of the emotional experience of these individuals. Many articulate patients have described their experiences, and many therapists and psychiatric nurses working closely with their patients/clients have experienced and described the feelings of these patients. The subjective experience of schizophrenia is often one of loneliness, fear, dread, depression, anxiety, and utter confusion. It is critical as an empathic, compassionate nurse to continue to strive to give nonjudgmental emotional support and care.

ASSESSMENT

STAGES OF SCHIZOPHRENIA

Although psychosis can occur with a relatively rapid onset of serious symptoms, just as often, severe mental illness can begin with gradual, more insidious onset of symptoms. This is referred to as the ***prodromal* phase** of the illness which may occur over months or even years. Parents or loved ones may describe subtle changes in behavior where the individual may have increasing isolation, withdrawal from usual activities, less affect or emotion, or strange or unusual thinking. Parents often report a disinterest in friends, perhaps giving up sports or other clubs, a decrease in grades or motivation. Clinicians in early intervention programs are trained to routinely ask referred young people "if their eyes and ears are beginning to play tricks" or if there are other subtle changes in thinking and behavior, as their potentially ominous significance may not be recognized (Maier, 2011).

The ***active* phase** of the illness is with the emergence of the psychotic symptoms which may include hallucinations, delusions, or disorganized speech and behavior. Although dated, it is still very useful when considering the common characteristics of schizophrenia to organize conceptualization around the presence of "Bleuler's Four A's." (loose associations, affect, autism, and ambivalence) (Fusar-Poli & Politi, 2008). Others have added anxiety and auditory hallucinations to this list.

Hallucinations are one of the core "positive" symptoms of schizophrenia. Although hallucinations in schizophrenia may involve different senses, such as visual or tactile, the majority of patients with hallucinations report auditory verbal hallucinations. Approximately 60% to 80% of patients with schizophrenia at some point in their illness "hear voices," making auditory hallucinations one of the most frequent and fundamentally disturbing symptoms. Patients often report hearing words, intrusive disparaging comments, fragments of conversations, multiple voices arguing, and sometimes commands urging them to act. Most often the voices are different than one's own. One in four patients will experience auditory hallucinations that are not responsive to medication treatment (Maletic, 2011).

The symptoms in this active phase are often what lead to the interaction with the health care system. As with any acute psychosis, interventions focus on safety and security in meeting the patient's physical health and safety needs. Hospitalization is often necessary for the safety of the patient or others. Crisis intervention, symptom resolution, development of a therapeutic alliance, and setting up adequate aftercare are keys to preventing further decompensation and additional relapse.

The ***residual* phase** may reflect that the active phase symptoms are absent or no longer prominent. There are often role impairment, negative symptoms, or attenuated positive symptoms. Acute-phase symptoms may reemerge during the residual phase ("acute exacerbation") (Andreasen & Black, 2006). The goals at this stage are to prevent relapse, engage the patient and family into a chronic treatment paradigm, reintegrate the patient into the community, and perhaps, give a referral to a vocational rehabilitation program.

Patients with severe and chronic mental illness often require a comprehensive system of care that incorporates inpatient acute settings, outpatient follow-up, partial day hospital program, case management services, and vocational rehabilitation programs. Long-term consistent care is desirable where both the medication and psychosocial supports and education can be provided. The most common conditions that may contribute to relapse during this residual or transition phase include: failure to take the medication, failure to connect or continue in aftercare, inadequate supports, and isolation (Maxmen & Ward, 1995).

CLINICAL ASSESSMENT

Interviewing and communication have always been primary nursing skills, but this is the core of the assessment and care with the patient with mental health concerns. This ability to listen with a "trained" ear is an art and a complex skill. Observation of behavior and affect can be instrumental in the assessment. These skills become our "equipment" when we assess not only the words, but the thoughts, actions, and feelings beneath the words.

It is not always an acute presentation to an emergency room or a hospital, in many instances, it is the primary care provider who first detects psychotic symptoms. It may present as the patient's or family's complaint but equally often as an incidental finding. Although schizophrenia is often best managed by the psychiatric team, patients with schizophrenia and other psychoses require continued care for unrelated medical conditions, and they may remain in the primary provider's care, even while specific treatment for the psychosis is carried on elsewhere. For a small number of very stable patients with psychosis, it may be desirable for the primary care provider to assume responsibility for their long-term management (Knesper et al., 1997).

Like any initial assessment, attention must be given to the pattern of onset and a thorough current physical examination be made available to help rule out medical causes of schizophrenia symptoms. There are many disorders that may masquerade as schizophrenia and psychotic symptoms can be found in many other illnesses, including substance abuse, tumors and mass lesions, infectious processes, endocrine disorders, medication adverse effects, metabolic disorders, and so on.

If unable to perform a physical exam, collaboration with the primary or other medical provider is indicated. Typical routine laboratory tests may be helpful in ruling out potential etiologies. These might entail a complete blood count, comprehensive metabolic profile, thyroid function tests, and serologic tests for evidence of an infection with syphilis or HIV. If lesions, brain injury, or other brain disorders are suspected, an MRI or CT scan might be warranted.

This careful assessment, including psychiatric and medical history, should include the family history, review of systems, and as mentioned, any pertinent physical and neurological symptoms. A full substance use history must be obtained and any information from family and others can prove to be invaluable. A drug or poisoning history is essential as there are numerous prescription and street drugs and other toxic agents that can produce psychotic features that may be misdiagnosed as schizophrenia (Nasrallah, 1986).

Although the psychiatric assessment is covered in Chapter 7, there are some unique aspects to interviewing the patient with psychotic symptoms. It is important to engage with the patient at their level of their concern whenever possible. Many times the patient may be seen at the request at others when they do not perceive any problem or the presenting complaint might be a somatic or paranoid delusion where there is lack of insight. It is important to try to find some ability to establish rapport and demonstrate a willingness to help.

When a person cannot appreciate that they have a serious psychiatric illness, a tremendous challenge to family members and caregivers follows. About one half of people living with schizophrenia, and a smaller percentage who live with bipolar disorder, have this clinical feature. Individuals with Alzheimer's disease and dementia also may have this feature. The medical term for not seeing what ails you is anosognosia, more commonly known as a lack of insight. Having a lack of awareness raises the risks of nonadherence to treatment. From the person's viewpoint, if they feel they are not ill why should they go to appointments, take medication, or engage in therapy? This can be a difficult dilemma in working with the psychotic patient (NAMI, 2011).

It may be unlikely that the presenting problem will be distress from hallucinations and the patient is asking for help to make them stop. More often, the patient presents with paranoia, referential thoughts, or delusions that suggest not to trust you or not to share what is happening to them. The patient may present with complaints about others: "people won't let up on me," "people try to get into my head or hear my thoughts," "people are trying to morph into my body." This can be challenging if the problem is seen as outside of them. The patient may be reluctant to see the problem as an illness or to start a medication.

Sometimes just simply acknowledging the mental energy required to fight these symptoms can be helpful. Think how exhausting it would be if your thoughts were not private and every time you ventured out, others could read your thoughts. You might be inclined to stay home, avoid interactions with people, or even confront them for their intrusion. Validation does not mean endorsing the symptoms, but recognizing the individual's experience and their courage can facilitate the nurse-patient relationship.

It takes a gentle approach, along with intuition of the patient's tolerance, to perhaps share that others have suffered this same experience and medication has helped. It is not helpful to confront and challenge, as this is the individual's reality and experience. There can be a joining of goals where the discussion becomes not whether the symptoms are the result of mental illness, but whether the medication can help the paranoid individual manage stress and better tolerate people.

Symptoms of psychosis might change the patient's usual style of interaction and his or her ability to comprehend. The clinician may have to structure the interview by asking more direct questions. If the patient becomes too disorganized or loose, the clinician will need to be more active and redirect. The cognitive impairments can be subtle or more obvious; they can be frustrating for both the patient and the clinician. The inability to process or recall information may require the interview be done in parts or shortened altogether.

Many patients will have normal intelligence and may have a solid fund of knowledge, but it is possible that every person who has schizophrenia has cognitive dysfunction compared to what he or she would be able to do without the disorder (Sadock & Sadock, 2008). These cognitive impairments cannot be diagnostic, but as has been stated, they will certainly impact the functional outcome and course of the illness. It is this attention to cognitive functioning that will later direct your treatment planning and thoughts about care within the home and disposition.

An inability to externalize or show emotion may also be common and is frequently seen in the mental status exam. There may be a flat or blunted affect. There may be a cold, indifferent expression where little emotion is evident. It can be unnerving when the patient appears to look through you or offer little recognition. Although this flat affect may be a symptom, it is important to assess whether the affect could be a result of severe depression.

Sorting these symptoms can be a challenge in the psychiatric interview. The negative symptoms may make engagement difficult for the patients. There may be the coexistence of post-traumatic stress syndrome (PTSS). Many studies show a significant proportion of patients with schizophrenia develop PTSS when they experience devastating psychotic episodes. The negative symptoms of PTSS, such as blunting, can be imbedded in the overall symptoms of schizophrenia (Nasrallah, 2011b).

Words are normally associated by a common idea, and the sentences flow toward a goal. In the interview with a patient with psychosis, there may be rambling, disorganized, illogical patterns of thinking. The words may not hang together, and the links to connect the ideas to logic will be missing. These can be cardinal signs of schizophrenia and they can make the interview process challenging to conduct.

Other times, the time will come to document the interview and it will be a challenge as it will be difficult to ascertain what the conversation really has been about. Despite the fact that the individual may have been quite engaging, themes or threads just won't seem to emerge. This disorganization and loose association can be very diagnostic and an important part of the assessment.

At times, the provider may feel a sense of anxiety or unease with the psychotic or acutely disturbed patient. This can be particularly useful and vital to recognize. This can be part of the diagnostic process. Anxiety helps to protect us—makes us more attentive to and observant of things we see, hear, and feel. There are those patients whose anxiety is simply broadcast into the room. The fear and paranoia of another can help one stay vigilant and prepared. It is important to listen to your "gut" and take the necessary precautions.

The patient who is potentially violent or assaultive usually has a prodromal pattern of behavior that precedes the overt aggression. It becomes imperative for the clinician to pay attention to the patient's posture, motor activity, and language. It is not uncommon to see the patient pacing and becoming increasingly restless or to even become verbally abusive. Fortunately, sudden unexpected physical assault is rare and most violence has a predictable culmination of a 30- to 60-minute period of escalation (Stoudemire, 1990).

It is critical to be mindful of one's own anxiety and how it is handled as this can certainly influence one's effectiveness with others. Although recognition of one's own anxiety is important, anxiety can become overwhelming and limit one's endeavors. The point at which anxiety ceases to be useful and becomes interfering in the therapeutic process is highly individual as we all have our own tolerance of others' distress. It may be helpful to discuss this in supervision with a peer or colleague.

There will be times the patient is uncooperative, hostile, or too paranoid to tolerate the interview. The provider must be flexible, attend to immediate medical and safety issues, but also be sensitive to the patient's capacity. Is the interview agitating the patient more or escalating the symptoms?

If the patient is hostile, maintaining physical distance by having appropriate boundaries and allowing for personal space is warranted. Asking for security or other staff to be on standby during the interview is another safety measure. The interviewer should not block them behind a desk, nor turn their back to the patient, and may want to leave the door open. There should be easy access to the exit if needed.

If at any point during the interview the patient states intent to harm themselves or another, hospitalization should be recommended. If the patient reveals they have a weapon, this should be removed and the patient informed that weapons of any kind cannot be allowed in a therapeutic setting. It has been recommended that the interviewer never accept the weapon directly but ask the patient to place the weapon on a table or desk (Stoudemire, 1990). If the patient refuses, the interview should be terminated and the appropriate safety and security staff alerted. For more on the intervention and interaction with patients with other-directed violence, please refer to Chapter 16.

Data may have to be gathered from significant others, other providers, and past medical records. Although this information is important, the provider needs to be careful to not sacrifice the relationship in the pursuit of extensive information gathering. Again, be mindful of the patient's tolerance. Many paranoid patients will not tolerate extended direct eye contact. They may require a larger berth of personal space and boundaries. It may be more comfortable for the provider to sit at an angle or to one side as opposed to directly across.

Many times the clinician may feel that the line of questioning in the psychiatric interview is awkward or embarrassing. There may be hesitation to ask questions about hearing voices or thoughts of suicide. This may be from discomfort on how to inquire, or there may be anxiety regarding the response. Simply assuming the patient seems "fine" and believing certain questions are not applicable will guarantee psychiatric problems will be overlooked. It can be very helpful to watch as many interviews as possible to learn about interview techniques. Each provider will develop their own style and comfort with the assessment interview, and hopefully, will employ a variety of questions including both open and closed types.

Exhibit 10-2 is a list of questions that may be utilized in the assessment process with an individual experiencing psychosis. Most of the questions are closed questions but more information can be gleaned by asking for

EXHIBIT 10-2: QUESTIONS FOR ASSESSMENT OF PSYCHOTIC SYMPTOMS

Do you feel as if other people can read your mind? Hear your thoughts?
Does it feel like other people can put thoughts or ideas into your head?
Do you feel that you receive special messages from other people without using words?
Have you ever had an experience where the television, radio, or newspaper was talking to you or about you?
Do you have a lot of worries or things on your mind?
Does this interfere with your ability to do your usual routine or activities?
Do you ever feel like people are out to get you or have it in for you?
Have you ever had to get physical with someone to keep them from bothering you?
Do you have any special powers, skills, or abilities?
Do you ever hear sounds or voices when you are alone or no one else is around?
Do you ever feel like your mind plays tricks on you?
Do you have a special relationship with God?

clarification or more details. The provider may follow up with, "What is the experience like for you? How do you manage it? Do you think there are other explanations that might account for this? What do you do that makes it better or worse?"

Often, one of the biggest challenges entering the health care profession is learning the language. Not only is it full of specific terms, abbreviations, and acronyms, each specialty has an additional vocabulary unique in and of itself. Psychiatry and mental health nursing is no different. In order to communicate your findings in the language of your peers, you need to understand the terminology.

Exhibit 10-3 provides a list of commonly used terms and generally agreed upon definitions in the care of psychotic patients.

ASSESSMENT SCALES

There are many psychiatric scales, exams, and rating forms that have been developed to assist health care providers in assessment, diagnosis, and evaluation of outcomes. Some instruments can be self-administered, others used as part of an interview, and still others that family members or concerned others can complete. Generally, rating scales and tools can be printed out as part of the medical record, can provide value with a longitudinal view, and can be utilized with the patient to monitor progress and affect the treatment plan. There are some scales that require additional training, some used primarily in research settings, and some that are not public domain and require purchase. There are many sites available on the Internet that can provide access to scales and rating tools, but the *Psychiatric Times* has an easy site to access where, under "resources," you can find clinical scales for several diagnoses (www.psychiatrictimes.com/features-and-resources).

Brief Psychiatric Rating Scale

The Brief Psychiatric Rating Scale (BPRS) is a widely used rating scale in psychiatry. It comprises 24 items rated from 1 (not present) to 7 (extremely severe) and includes symptoms such as somatic concern, anxiety, depressive mood, hostility, and hallucinations. The scale is used to measure the severity of psychiatric symptomology (Sadock & Sadock, 2008).

The scale is quantitative; it was constructed for the sole purpose of rating the current clinical picture. It is not a diagnostic tool. When the scale is used in repeated (weekly) ratings, each assessment must be made independently, without reference to previous interviews.

Global Assessment of Functioning Scale

The Global Assessment of Functioning Scale (GAF), which is a modified version of the Global Assessment Scale (GAS), which is a modified version of the GAS, first appeared in *Diagnostic and Statistical Manual (DSM)-III-R* in 1994. In the *DSM*, this is Axis V on the multiaxial assessment and used for reporting the clinical judgment of the individual's overall level of functioning. This scale may be particularly useful when tracking the clinical progress of the individual in global terms, using a single measure. The GAF scale is rated with respect to psychological and occupational functioning only and it is scored in real time for current functioning.

The GAF scale is a continuum rating from 1 to 100. For example, a score of 91 to 100 would reflect superior functioning in a wide range of activities, life's problems are manageable, is sought out by others because of his or her many positive qualities. A mid-range score of 51 to

EXHIBIT 10-3: COMMONLY USED TERMS IN CARE OF PSYCHOTIC PATIENT

TERM	DEFINITION
Affect	The instantaneous, observable expression of emotion. Affect differs from mood, which is the subjective experience of emotion. There is a saying, "Affect is to mood as weather is to climate." Moods are symptoms; affects are signs. Common affect descriptions might include: Patients with *blunted, flat, or constricted* affects show almost no emotional lability, appear expressionless, look dulled, and speak in a monotone. *Broad* affect is a normal range of affect. *Inappropriate* affect is incongruous with the situation: A patient smiles while hearing of the death of family pet. *Labile* affect shows a range of expression with rapid and abrupt shifts of emotion, as when a patient cries one moment and laughs the next.
Alogia	Impoverished speaking often as a result of slowed, empty thought processes; may be result of thought blocking or thought disorganization.
Ambivalence	Having two strongly opposite ideas or feelings at the same time, which may make the individual unable to respond or decide. It is best to not offer too many choices or give too many details as this creates distress.
Anhedonia	Mood where there is pervasive inability to perceive and experience pleasure in actions and events that would be normally pleasurable or satisfying for the individual or most people.
Apathy	A sense of detachment or indifference.
Autistic thinking	An individual being preoccupied with his own private world or where thoughts are derived from fantasy; individual may base his environment on internal fantasies instead of on external realities
Avolition	Lack of initiative or goals; seen as a negative symptom in schizophrenia.
Blocking	The train of thought may abruptly and unexpectedly stop. It can be important to give the individual time to respond as this slowness may not reflect absence of thought but trouble accessing.
Cataplexy	Sudden, unexpected, purposeless, generalized, and temporary loss of muscle tone.
Circumstantiality	Pattern of speech that may be filled with detours, irrelevant remarks, and excessive details, but eventually does reach its point; tangentiality is when the point isn't reached.
Clang associations	Type of language in which the sound of a word, instead of its meaning, dictates the course of subsequent associations (e.g., "ding, dong, dell…"). Rhyming and punning may be substituted for logic. For example, when asked about mood, the patient responds with "crude, that's rude, not my attitude."
Compulsions	Repeated, overtly senseless actions or rituals that are performed to prevent anxiety. Compulsions are obsessions expressed in actions or behaviors.
Concrete thinking	The inability to think abstractly, metaphorically, or hypothetically. Ideas and words are usually limited to a single meaning. Figures of speech are taken literally and nuances of language are missing. For example, "What brought you in today?" "A car."
Delusions	Fixed, blatantly false convictions deduced from incorrect inferences about external reality; they are maintained despite clear proof to the contrary.
Depersonalization	When a person perceives their body as unreal, floating, dead, or changing in size, for example, the arm may feel like wood or seem detached from the body.
Derealization	A person perceives the environment as unreal or strange. The individual feels removed from the world, as if he is viewing it on a movie screen.
Echolalia	A parrot-like, meaningless, persistent, verbal repetition of words or sounds heard by the patient.
Echopraxia	The repetitive imitation of another person's movements.
Ego-dystonic	A sign, symptom, or experience that the patient finds uncomfortable or doesn't want.
Ego-syntonic	A sign, symptom, or experience that the patient finds acceptable and consistent with his personality. Many, but not all, delusions, hallucinations, and overvalued ideas can be ego-syntonic.

(Continued)

EXHIBIT 10-3: COMMONLY USED TERMS IN CARE OF PSYCHOTIC PATIENT (*Continued*)

TERM	DEFINITION
Flight of ideas	Accelerated speech with many rapid changes in subject from understandable associations, distracting stimuli, or play on words. In flight of ideas, the connections linking thoughts may be understandable, whereas in looseness of associations (LOA) they are not.
Folie a deux	"Madness for two," when two closely related persons, usually in the same family, share the same delusions.
Hallucinations	False perceptions in the senses, hearing, seeing, touching, tasting, and smelling, based on no external reality. Differ from illusions which are false perceptions based on real stimuli. Hallucinations are disorders of perception; delusions are disorders of thinking. Delusions are always psychotic, hallucinations only sometimes.
Ideas of reference	Overvalued ideas or faulty interpretations where the patient is convinced that objects, people, or events in his immediate environment have personal significance for him or reference to self.
Illogical thinking	Conclusions that contain clear, internal contradictions or are blatantly erroneous given the initial premises.
Looseness of associations	Inability to organize thoughts logically; having or expressing thoughts that seem unrelated. Speech patterns characterized by leaps from subject to subject without clear connections or the patient's awareness of the rapid shifts.
Magical thinking	When the person is convinced that words, thoughts, feelings, or actions will produce an outcome that defies all laws of cause and effect.
Mood	Subjectively experienced feeling state. Differs from affect, which is transitory and apparent to others.
Mood-congruent	Delusions or hallucinations that are *consistent* with the patient's dominant mood. A mood-congruent delusion in mania might be, "I'm the Second Christ."
Mood-incongruent	Delusions and hallucinations that are *inconsistent* with the patient's dominant mood. Mood-incongruent delusions can be distressing, persecutory.
Neologism	Distortion of words or new words that a patient invents; may have idiosyncratic meanings to the patient.
Paranoid delusion	A delusion of persecution.
Paranoid ideation	An overvalued idea that one is being persecuted. Thinking is predominantly suspicious, but not delusional.
Perseveration	A persistent pathological repetition of speech or movement to different stimuli.
Poverty of speech	A remarkable restriction or lack of speech; answers are brief or monosyllabic or no answer is given at all.
Psychosis	A severe mental state in which the person is unable to distinguish reality from fantasy. Classic characteristics include impaired reality testing, delusions, and hallucinations
Tangentiality	A disturbance of speech where the person "goes off on a tangent." Differs from circumstantiality in that it does not return to the point.
Thought disorder	General term to describe disturbance in speech, thought content, or communication. Range can be mild to severe and may include profound delusions, looseness of associations, and so on. The term is often used synonymously with psychosis.
Word salad	Mixture of words or phrases that lack logic or understandable meaning

60 would indicate moderate symptoms (e.g., flat affect and circumstantial speech, occasional panic attacks) OR moderate difficulty in social, occupational, or school functioning (e.g., few friends, conflicts with peers or co-workers). The end of the spectrum, with a score of 0 to 10 would indicate persistent danger of severely hurting self or others (e.g., recurrent violence) OR persistent inability to maintain minimal personal hygiene, OR serious suicidal act with clear expectation of death (*DSM-IV-R*; APA 2000). It is easy to see how an individual with chronic, severe, and persistent mental illness who has significant negative symptoms and an isolated lifestyle would score in the 30s. Many times the ability to achieve a certain level of care, like admission to hospital, day program, or case management services is dependent on a certain GAF score.

Positive and Negative Syndrome Scale

The Positive and Negative Syndrome Scale (PANSS) was developed as a more rigorously and objective method for evaluating positive, negative, and other symptom dimensions in schizophrenia. The PANSS assessment is derived from behavioral information collected from a number of sources including: observations during the interview; a clinical interview; and reports by primary care or hospital staff or family members. The PANSS ratings should be based on all the information relating to a specified period, normally identified as the previous week. The PANSS constitutes four scales measuring positive and negative syndromes, their differential, and general severity of illness (Kay et al., 1987). There are 30 different symptoms rated on a scale of 1 to 7. If the item is absent it is scored as 1, increased levels of psychopathology are assigned scores from 2 (minimal) to 7 (extreme). The PANSS has become a standard tool for assessing the clinical outcome in treatment studies of schizophrenia (Kaplan & Sadock, 2008).

The Structured Clinical Interview

The Structured Clinical Interview for *DSM-IV* Axis I Disorders (SCID-I) is a semi-structured interview for making the major *DSM-IV* Axis I diagnoses, where the SCID-II is a semi-structured interview for making *DSM-IV* Axis II: Personality Disorder diagnoses. The tool is designed to be administered by a clinician or trained mental health professional. It has been valued as helping clinicians of all levels of experience improve their clinical assessment and interviewing techniques and provides extensive documentation of the diagnostic process. The SCID-I covers those *DSM-IV* diagnoses most commonly seen by clinicians and includes the diagnostic criteria for these disorders with corresponding interview questions. The SCID-I is divided into six self-contained modules that can be administered in sequence: mood episodes; psychotic symptoms; psychotic disorders; mood disorders; substance use disorders; and anxiety, adjustment, and other disorders. It can be purchased from American Psychiatric Publishing online, or more information may be obtained through the following link: www.scid4.org/faq/scidfaq.html

Calgary Depression Scale for Schizophrenia

Many of the frequently used depression scales were designed to assess depression in nonpsychotic patients. These scales contain items that do not distinguish depressed from nondepressed psychotic patients. The Calgary Depression Scale for Schizophrenia (CDSS) was designed to assess symptoms of depression in the presence of schizophrenia. It measures the severity of symptoms such as depressed mood, hopelessness, guilt, insomnia, and suicide (Addington et al., 1993). This scale is also designated for use by a trained rater. The Scale is copyrighted and the copyright is held by Dr. Donald Addington and Dr. Jean Addington. The Scale may be used free by any student or non-profit organization. Permission to use the Scale will be given to for-profit organizations upon request to Dr. Donald Addington by e-mail to addingto@ucalgary.ca or in writing.

CONCORDANCE AND SHARED DECISION MAKING

Working with a patient who is paranoid, suspicious, or actively psychotic can be challenging in the treatment process. Experienced clinicians will often attempt to leverage a patient's insight into ancillary symptoms, such as impaired sleep, anxiety, and dysphoria, to encourage a therapeutic alliance and hopefully adherence. If the patient feels his concerns are not addressed, he or she may not return. They may consider the treatment to be inadequate even though the intensity of their hallucinations and delusions may have decreased (Citrome, 2011b).

By definition, delusional ideas are not open to correction by evidence to the contrary. It is extremely important to be sensitive to the patient's fixed belief system. While not colluding, being direct and honest in acknowledging the patient's belief is warranted. Later, some gentle reality testing may be tolerated, but initial challenging and confronting is not therapeutic as the goal is to establish some rapport and a relationship.

A direct statement acknowledging the patient's belief and the physician's alternative view is preferable, combined with a recommendation for treatment. An example script can be found in *Primary Care Psychiatry*:

> *You have been experiencing some very disturbing things in the past few weeks. I know the voices sound very real to you, and the threats seem quite frightening. These experiences are very much like those we see in some types of illness within the brain itself, and I believe that is what is happening to you. These symptoms sometimes occur when there is an infection or injury involving the brain. I have performed tests for these possibilities, and you do not appear to have these problems. Instead, I believe that you have developed a problem in the chemistry of the brain. We don't know very much about why these problems occur, but there are medications that are very helpful in controlling these symptoms, and I recommend that we begin treatment with one of them." (Knesper et al., 1997)*

Educating the patient that there is hope and giving him reason to believe that he will have relief from symptoms becomes important in the engagement process. If a definitive diagnosis has been made, particularly one of schizophrenia, instilling hope is important. There are many negative beliefs and stereotypes that are associated with the illness, and it will be important to lay a foundation with expectations of remission and recovery.

Setting goals should be patient driven. Short-term goals again can be geared to their more immediate concerns of sleep, safety, and symptom reduction with longer-term goals geared toward needed social supports, recovery, and improved functioning. Outlining expectations, both for the patient and from the provider is helpful. The goals and objectives should align appropriately to the phase of illness and the individual characteristics of each patient. Having the discussion about diagnosis, prognosis, and the expected benefit of treatment is part of the decision-making process.

If the patient is too disorganized, responding to internal stimuli, or seems to be having trouble processing the interaction, it is important to keep communication simple and straightforward. Avoid lengthy, intense verbal interactions. Looking for insight or psychodynamic formulations is counterproductive at this point. Do not offer too many choices or provide too much information. It is best to ask for one task at a time, "Can you sit down now?" versus "Can you sit down, take your medications, and then we will go upstairs to the unit?" Being patient and appreciating that the patient's brain is having trouble operating efficiently can help the clinician appreciate that the patient's intent is not to be difficult or resistive.

Deciding upon the appropriate level of care can be another negotiation, always erring on the side of safety of any question. The treatment decisions will obviously depend on the setting and the environment. The acutely psychotic patient, by nature of his very symptoms, may be so ill or agitated that he cannot participate in the treatment planning process. Treatment may need to be initiated with medicating the individual against their will or even hospitalizing as an involuntary status. This can be difficult for all parties.

It is important to be familiar with the laws and standards for your state and community when providing for the safety of the patient and others when treatment is not welcomed. Most states have carefully regulated civil commitment laws with definitions of disability, inability to care for self, and presenting danger to self or others. There are many states that allow for outpatient commitment; this is generally for the severe or chronically noncompliant patient targeted at reducing hospitalizations.

The difficulty of goals not being mutually shared between providers and patients can be very challenging, both clinically and emotionally. What to do with the patient who is living on the streets after stopping his medications, despite his promising recovery and return to the workforce only months before? Does the provider force treatment against his wishes? There are many ethical, legal, and humane issues that come into play.

EXPECTED OUTCOMES

Like any disease model, the concepts of prevention and early detection suggest a better chance of a successful outcome. In many fields of medicine, early intervention definitely favors good outcomes. This is most certainly true in the treatment of schizophrenia.

Public health strategies that target identifying individuals who have developed schizophrenia as early in the course of illness as possible may improve outcomes. On average, there is a delay of 1 year between development of psychosis and initiation of treatment. There are numerous studies identifying that the longer the delay from the onset of psychosis to the onset of treatment, the worse the outcome in terms of symptom relief and return of social and vocational function (Perkins, 2011).

There has been controversy about actually treating an individual with antipsychotics before the full emergence of psychotic symptoms, but the implications of preventing an episode of psychosis are compelling. This area of early detection and treatment has been the focus of cutting-edge research and has seen the emergence of many early intervention efforts. There is a pamphlet entitled "Warning Signs of Major Mental Illnesses" which can be downloaded from the American Psychiatric Association's (APA's) website, www.healthyminds.org (Maier, 2011).

Recovery After an Initial Schizophrenia Episode (RAISE) is a National Institute of Mental Health (NIMH) research project that seeks to fundamentally change the trajectory and prognosis of schizophrenia through coordinated and aggressive treatment in the earliest stages of illness. RAISE is designed to reduce the likelihood of long-term disability that people with schizophrenia often experience. It aims to help people with the disorder lead productive, independent lives. At the same time, it aims to reduce the financial impact on the public systems often tapped to pay for the care of people with schizophrenia.

Treatment models being tested focus on intervening as soon as possible after the first episode of psychosis. Each model integrates medication, psychosocial therapies, family involvement, rehabilitation services, and supported employment. Each component is aimed at promoting symptom reduction and improving life functioning.

As schizophrenia still is believed to have many possible etiologies, it is also true that the disease has a heterogeneous outcome. There are poorer outcomes associated with the presence of premorbid symptoms, persistent negative symptoms, and even gender. The course of illness is generally more favorable in women, who tend to have a later onset of the illness, fewer negative symptoms, and a better treatment response. Early onset schizophrenia shows a male preponderance, poor outcome (chronicity), low familial predisposition for psychosis, and the presence of structural cerebral pathology (Piccinelli & Homen, 1997). The differences in gender and course of illness are a promising area in future research offering further explanation about this complex disease.

The length of time a person is ill before treatment begins has been related to the disease outcome. There is now a consensus that the duration of untreated psychosis might be crucial to success of the early stages of schizophrenia treatment. Additional first-episode research has demonstrated that the length of the prodrome, or the time before full symptoms emerge, may be related to poor outcome (MacDonald & Schulz, 2009).

Treatment of this at-risk population or early intervention in the prodromal stage continues to be an area of great debate and study. The potential objectives of pharmacotherapy at this early stage can be varied. For those individuals who are seeking help for their presenting symptoms, that is, attenuated psychotic symptoms, very low-dose antipsychotic medication can be considered for short-term symptom relief. Such a prescription would be "off-label" in terms of indication and there are only limited trial data to inform dosage (Barnes & the Schizophrenia Consensus Group of the British Association for Psychopharmacology, 2011).

In general, the dosages of antipsychotics prescribed for people with an at-risk mental state are even lower than those used in first-episode psychosis. These affected individuals tend to be exquisitely sensitive to both the therapeutic effects and adverse effects of such medication. However, individuals with an at-risk mental state are often reluctant to take medication, and frequently express a preference for psychological intervention. There is preliminary evidence that both low-dose antipsychotics and cognitive behavioral therapy (CBT) can improve presenting symptoms (Barnes & the Schizophrenia Consensus Group of the British Association for Psychopharmacology, 2011).

Another potential objective is to delay, prevent, or reduce the severity of the onset of a psychotic illness. The findings of a few clinical trials suggest that this may be possible with either low-dose antipsychotic drugs or CBT, but fall short of providing convincing evidence, as they were all modest in size. A final objective for treatment is to intervene as soon as psychosis develops, in order to improve the subsequent outcome. If subjects at high risk have already been engaged by mental health services before the onset of illness, the delay between the onset of frank psychosis and the initiation of treatment can potentially be substantially reduced (Barnes & the Schizophrenia Consensus Group of the British Association for Psychopharmacology, 2011).

It has been stated that the greatest unmet need in schizophrenia is the lack of treatments for the primary positive, negative, and cognitive symptoms, all of which account for the functional disability of schizophrenia (Nasrallah, 2011b). Persistent negative and cognitive symptoms are the real cause of long-term vocational and social disability in schizophrenia. Cognitive deficits are now recognized as a core feature of schizophrenia and include deficits in attention, learning and memory, working memory, speed of processing, and reasoning and problem solving, among others.

Cognitive impairment is a better predictor of level of function than is the severity of the psychotic symptoms. The attention to cognitive deficits has gained increased attention over the years. There is currently a great research interest in all modes of intervention around improving cognitive outcomes from therapeutic modalities, learning strategies, and drug development.

Although these are disorders that are manifested by changes in cognitive, affective, social, and perceptual domains, like many chronic illnesses, often there are remissions and exacerbations. It can be very difficult on providers and families to accept that even under the best of treatment circumstances, some mental illnesses can be extreme, progress, and be just as deadly and malignant as the most metastatic cancers. It can be devastating, frustrating, and demoralizing to see the patient and their potential continue to relapse and not respond to current-day treatments.

Psychotic illness continues to have many misconceptions and myths surrounding it. There remains much fear, stigma, and stereotyping around the concept of psychosis and this is perpetuated in the media, but at times, even with other health professionals. Nurses are in an excellent position to help educate around these disorders and to help destigmatize these ideas.

It is unfortunate that there is the widely accepted belief that persons with psychosis are dangerous. This belief was prevalent before the tragic events at Virginia Tech and Tucson, Arizona, but was reinforced by them. Clinicians know that, similar to the general population, only a small proportion of persons suffering from a psychotic illness exhibit violent behavior. In fact their illness renders them more likely to be victims than perpetrators of crime (Nasrallah, 2011b).

Homelessness is common in this population, in part because of social policy decisions and in part as a direct result of negative symptoms. Petty crime is not unusual, especially violations incidental to life on the streets, such as trespassing, defrauding an innkeeper, or urinating in public. With schizophrenia, patients are frequently the victims of robbery and assault for similar reasons (Knesper et al., 1997).

There has been much attention over the past few decades to offer a more promising and positive outlook to persons experiencing psychotic symptoms. Over a decade ago, the U.S. Surgeon General emphasized the concepts of recovery and reestablishment of a meaningful life, despite serious mental illness (Rose et al., 2010). This shift from symptom control to role, level of functioning, establishment of natural supports, and improved self-esteem is another key area where advanced practice mental health nurses can be proactive.

SUICIDE AND PSYCHOSIS

Suicide is the leading cause of premature death among people with schizophrenia. Compared with the general population, these patients have an 8.5-fold greater risk of suicide (Kasckow, Felmet, & Zisook, 2011). Suicide attempts are made by 20% to 50% of these patients, with long-term suicide rates estimated to be 10% to 13% (Sadock & Sadock, 2008). Risk factors with a strong association with later suicide include being young, male gender, and a high level of education.

Illness-related risk factors are important predictors, with number of prior suicide attempts, depressive symptoms, active hallucinations and delusions, and the presence of insight all having a strong evidential basis. A family history of suicide, and comorbid substance misuse were also positively associated with later suicide. The only consistent protective factor for suicide was delivery of and adherence to effective treatment (Hor & Taylor, 2010).

The majority of suicides for patients with schizophrenia occur within the first 10 years after illness onset and 50% occur within the first 2 years. Patients are at higher risk in the years directly following their initial diagnosis, and further, are also more likely to commit suicide within the first few weeks or months following a hospital discharge (Kasckow et al., 2011). Regardless of time in treatment, risk assessment is an ongoing process.

There is an assumption about the risk of suicide and connection to a post-psychotic depression. One theory speculates that the patient's symptoms may have improved in the hospital which consequently may have increased their sense of the seriousness and lifelong course of their illness. This has been thought of as a "demoralization syndrome" and there may be a corresponding increase in risk for suicide on discharge.

There is modest evidence suggesting that antipsychotic medications may protect against suicidal risk; the evidence appears to be most favorable for second-generation antipsychotics, particularly clozapine, which is the only medication approved by the U.S. Food and Drug Administration (FDA) for preventing suicide in patients with schizophrenia. In addition, treating depressive symptoms in patients with schizophrenia is an important component of suicide risk reduction. While selective serotonin reuptake inhibitors (SSRIs) ameliorate depressive symptoms in patients with schizophrenia, they also appear to attenuate suicidal thoughts (Kasckow et al., 2011).

It is obvious during the acute phase of the illness and the identification of the diagnosis that the risk would be high, but due to the chronicity of the disorder and the possible comorbid mood disorder vulnerability, risk must be continually assessed. Two-thirds or more of schizophrenic patients who commit suicide have seen an unsuspecting clinician within 72 hours of death (Sadock & Sadock, 2008). Prevention of suicide in schizophrenia will rely on identifying those individuals at risk, and treating comorbid depression and substance misuse, as well as providing best available treatment for symptom management.

DIAGNOSIS

Making any diagnosis is a thoughtful process and like any serious life illness, the ramifications can be life altering. Not only do the various psychotic disorders differ in their prognosis and in their therapeutic management, but making the diagnosis of schizophrenia has serious implications for the patient and the family. In mental health nursing there are not necessarily CT scans or blood tests to diagnose our patients; we must use our analytical skills to reach an acceptable diagnosis. There must be a systematic method of careful assessment and interviewing skills, and collaboration and coordination of data with others when possible. It is then when one can reach an objective diagnosis based on the information and on clinical experience. The nurse-patient relationship creates a therapeutic alliance that is critical to the success of this diagnostic process.

As reviewed, a diagnosis of schizophrenia obviously carries many implications so it is imperative that one should always be careful to gather enough data over time to reach the correct diagnosis. There are no laboratory tests yet that can confirm a diagnosis of schizophrenia, so we rely on the assessment and the presence of a constellation of symptoms and factors. Schizophrenia is often thought of as a diagnosis of exclusion because the consequences of the diagnosis are severe and can limit therapeutic options.

The *Diagnostic and Statistical Manual of Mental Disorders* is published by the APA and is the official psychiatric coding system used in the United States (Sadock & Sadock, 2008). The *DSM* defines a standard criterion for each mental health disorder and the criteria describe the features or signs and symptoms that must be present for the diagnosis to be made. Ultimately, the *DSM* is strictly a diagnostic tool and offers no information regarding particular treatments or causation.

In general, most of all the disorders must have signs and symptoms present that are sufficient to cause "clinically significant distress or impairment in social, occupational, or other important areas of functioning." There are also qualifiers that may sometimes be used, for example, mild, moderate, or severe forms of a disorder. It is an important tool for the advanced practice registered nurse (APRN) to learn the language of the *DSM* as it is the shared common language among clinicians, helps initiate a treatment pathway, and is often required by third-party payers. The fifth edition ("*DSM-5*") is currently in consultation, planning, and preparation, due for publication in May 2013.

Overall, the APA's *DSM* (*IV-R* edition) defines five subtypes of schizophrenia. For the purposes of this text, these subtypes are not broken down into further definition, but they include paranoid, disorganized, catatonic, undifferentiated, and residual type. For the diagnosis of schizophrenia, there are the expected symptoms of delusions, hallucinations, disorganized speech or behaviors, or negative symptoms, but not all of these must be present. There must be a disturbance in social or occupational functioning and the duration of symptoms must be greater than 6 months. There is the exclusion that the symptoms are not due to the effects of a substance or medical condition and there are specifics about the relationship of symptoms in the presence of a developmental disorder (APA, 2000).

There are other common conditions that include psychosis as a prime symptom from the *DSM-IV-R* (APA, 2010). These include schizoaffective disorder, delusional disorder, and brief psychotic disorder. In short, **schizoaffective disorder** has features of both schizophrenia (thought) disorder and an affective (mood) disorder. There are time frames around the duration and relationship to the mood symptoms, as well as subtypes specified as bipolar type or depressive type (APA, 2000).

Delusional disorder is characterized by the presence of nonbizarre delusions, such as those that could actually occur in real life. For example, the person who believes they are being followed or their spouse is having an affair. Again, there are seven types based on the predominant delusional theme: erotomanic, grandiose, jealous, persecutory, somatic, mixed, and unspecified type. Despite the delusion and its related implications, the individual does not have impaired functioning and they do not appear odd or bizarre.

In brief psychotic disorder, the psychotic symptoms are sudden, last for at least a day or more, but don't persist beyond a month. The symptoms are acute and the individual makes a full recovery and returns to a previous level of functioning. Like the others, this condition cannot be explained from the effects of a substance or a medical condition. There are qualifiers that would indicate if if there are stressors present or not or if the onset was within 4 weeks postpartum (APA, 2000).

DIFFERENTIAL DIAGNOSES

As the implications and consequences of the diagnosis of schizophrenia are so severe to the patient and the family, it is important to be thorough and comprehensive in reaching a diagnosis. Medical problems always lead the differential diagnoses, irrespective of the pattern of symptoms observed. Although many clinical features may suggest either a psychiatric or a medical cause of the psychosis, these are of limited reliability, and a thorough medical evaluation is required in all cases (Knesper et al., 1997).

Psychotic symptoms are found in many other illnesses, including substance abuse, toxicity from prescribed medications, infectious processes, metabolic and endocrine disorders, tumors, and so on. Please refer to Chapter 18 on common medical comorbidities, which may give insight on a psychotic disorder that was due to a general medical condition.

Substance-induced psychosis must be investigated in the differential as there have been many clients who have entered treatment quite psychotic and disorganized when the history ultimately unfolds revealing significant substance or illicit drug use. One young gentleman was admitted to the acute inpatient unit with severe agitation, confusion, disorganization, and hallucinations. On the surface it was easy to suspect schizophrenia as he was in his late teens, the right gender, and had many common symptoms. After a few days, he began to clear. His labs returned showing positive for cocaine and other drugs and high carbon monoxide. As it turned out, he had been using drugs over several days, became depressed, and tried to commit suicide in his garage with his car running. His friends had found him, brought him into the hospital but did not share the information about drug use or carbon monoxide poisoning as they didn't "want to get him in trouble."

Routine laboratory tests may be helpful in ruling out medical etiologies. Testing may include a complete blood count, urinalysis, liver enzymes, serum creatinine, blood urea nitrogen, thyroid function thyroid function tests, and serologic tests for evidence of an infection with syphilis or HIV. CT or MRI may be useful in selected patients to rule out brain disorder (e.g., tumors, strokes) during the initial workup for new onset cases (Andreasen & Black, 2006).

There are a few features that some consider in making the diagnosis of schizophrenia, differentiating it from other psychotic illnesses. One feature is that the actual course of the illness must be considered. Schizophrenia has a deteriorating course. This is not to say that the illness may not have remissions, but in general, it is a declining condition. Another general feature is that between psychotic episodes, patients with schizophrenia do not completely recover from the psychosis, while patients with a mood disorder or a psychosis from substances or general medical problems usually do (Maxmen & Ward, 1995).

The differential diagnosis of schizophrenia from other psychotic mental health disorders includes clarification from schizoaffective disorder, schizophreniform disorder, mood disorder, delusional disorder, and personality disorders.

A chief distinction from schizoaffective disorder and psychotic mood disorders is that in schizophrenia, a full depressive or manic syndrome is either absent, develops after the psychotic symptoms, or is brief relative to the duration of psychotic symptoms (Andreasen & Black, 2006). In the *DSM-IV-TR*, the duration of mood symptoms relative to schizoaffective disorder are detailed and in the International Classification of Diseases (ICD)-10 revision, schizoaffective disorder can be applied to patients who have co-occurring mood symptoms and schizophrenic-like mood-incongruent psychosis (Sadock & Sadock, 2008).

Schizophreniform disorder is usually diagnosed in patients who have the symptoms of schizophrenia but recover without residual symptoms within a 6-month period of time (Stoudemire, 1990). The *DSM-IV-TR* distinguishes this disorder from schizophrenia in that the symptoms last at least 1 month but less than 6 months. Patients with schizophreniform disorder may be further classified into those with good prognostic features and those without good prognostic features. Good prognosis features must include two or more of the following: acute onset, confusion in height of the episode, good premorbid functioning, and the absence of flat affect (APA, 2000).

Extreme elevated or depressed mood symptoms associated with mood disorder, and mood congruent delusions without a formal thought disorder may be clues to a mood disorder diagnosis. Patients with primarily a mood disorder often have normal baseline functioning and they will report previous episodes of mood symptoms of depression or mania. It is often the case there may be relatives with a mood disorder (Maxmen & Ward, 1995).

Delusional disorder and brief reactive psychosis are two other possible diagnoses to rule out. Where schizophrenia is characterized by the presence of bizarre delusions and hallucinations are common, in delusional disorder, the patient will have non-bizarre delusions that last for at least 1 month. The behavior is generally not odd or unusual, and the delusion is one that, although it is not real, it is technically possible (APA, 2000).

Patients with a brief psychotic disorder have psychotic symptoms that last at least 1 day but no more than 1 month, with gradual recovery. Remission is expected and the individual returns to premorbid level of functioning. In contrast to schizophrenia, brief psychotic disorder usually has an acute precipitant, a rapid onset, delusions and hallucinations that pertain to the stressor, and a quick and complete recovery (Maxmen & Ward, 1995).

Postpartum onset must be specified in brief reactive disorder if the symptoms had onset within 4 weeks postpartum and this should be distinguished from other postpartum conditions. Postpartum blues, which may occur in up to 80% of new mothers, lasts for a few days after delivery, and is considered normal. It is generally thought to be related to the rapidly changing hormone levels and reactions to childbirth. Symptoms that persist longer than 2 weeks should be evaluated further, but generally no treatment is required (Sadock & Sadock, 2008).

Postpartum psychosis, on the other hand, is considered a psychiatric emergency. The presence of delusions, depression, and often thoughts of harming self and/or the baby require immediate intervention. Typically there are prodromal symptoms of mood lability, insomnia, and agitation prior to the onset of the florid psychosis. Again, safety to both mom and baby are priorities (Sadock & Sadock, 2008).

Despite the criteria outlined in the *DSM-IV-TR* regarding each disorder, often the distinctions between psychotic disorders and decompensated personality patterns can be difficult to distinguish. Schizotypical, paranoid, and borderline personality disorders may present as psychosis and resemble the prodromal or acute phase of schizophrenia, but unlike schizophrenia, the psychotic symptoms remit in hours or days. Severe schizoid personality disorder may produce a schizophrenic-like social withdrawal; these patients, however, rarely become psychotic (Maxmen & Ward, 1995). Unlike schizophrenia, personality disorders have mild symptoms, history of occurring throughout a person's life, and they lack an identifiable date of onset (Sadock & Sadock, 2008).

It is always possible that the patient who imitates the symptoms of schizophrenia may have ulterior motives, either consciously or unconsciously. They may be trying to gain admission to a hospital, to qualify for some type of benefit, or to avoid some type of legal complication. These potential psychiatric disorders, which include factitious disorder with psychological symptoms and malingering, must also be ruled out. Patients with factitious disorder fake illnesses. They may undergo great pain or injury to themselves to be in the "sick role" or to receive emotional care and attention. Malingering differs from factitious disorder in that the motivation for symptoms is an external incentive where a specific goal is involved, whereas in factitious disorder, the symptoms are intentionally produced (APA, 2000).

CULTURAL CONSIDERATIONS

The nurse requires the use of strategies tailored to patient's ethnicity and cultural norms and values. The meaning of behavior varies according to the norms and rules of each culture. Cultural groups vary in the incidence and symptoms of mental illness. Although there are basic symptoms of mental illness that appear the same in all cultures, variations in the symptoms show the influence of culture (Louie, 1996). Culture, in its broadest dimensions involves shared symbols and meanings that people create in the process of social interaction. It can shape one's experiences (including the experience of schizophrenia), one's interpretations, and one's actions. It thereby orients people in their ways of thinking, feeling, and being in the world (Jenkins & Barrett, 2004).

There has always been a tension in defining the relationship between culture and mental illness. Culture may provide a framework for one's bizarre and extraordinary experiences. If the experience fits into the comfort and context of one's culture, the experience may not be as distressing as it would be to another person without the cultural context. The opposite may also be true in that the cultural influences may direct the individual with psychotic symptoms to conceal the experience from others. This can create additional isolation and present barriers to treatment.

Culture is critical in nearly every aspect of the schizophrenic illness experience; the identification, definition, and meaning of the illness during the prodromal, acute, and residual phases: the timing and type of onset; symptom formation in terms of content, form, and constellation; gender and ethnic difference; the personal experience of the schizophrenic illness, social response, support, and stigma; and perhaps, most important, the course and outcome of disorders (Jenkins & Barrett, 2004).

FAMILIES

Schizophrenia or any other mental illness not only impacts the individual but the family and other significant relationships as well. Mental illness can present a unique and heavy burden to families as there is often fear and stigma associated with it. To make matters worse, it was not all that long ago when families were often blamed and seen as contributing to the illness. Often is the case when families have developed many creative strategies where they can teach us.

It is critical to collaborate with families and check on the effects the illness has on the family. The illness may have taken a toll in many areas, whether it is resources, mental energy and reserves, or impacts on siblings, and so on. As important as it is to allow the patient to discuss their thoughts and reactions to the diagnosis, it is equally important to allow their loved ones the same opportunity.

Families may go through a grieving process and may want to share their dreams and expectations for their loved ones. Families are often not comfortable expressing their own emotions for fear of upsetting or distressing their loved ones. The parents' hopes and dreams for their child may be initially crushed. Parents and siblings may feel at a loss, isolated from their friends and their experiences. They may feel unsure how to relate to their families and friends who may be celebrating their children's successes in marriages, college, or employment. They should be offered their own support and treatment if indicated.

Family therapy, combined with antipsychotic medication, has been shown to reduce relapse rates in schizophrenia (Andreasen & Black, 2006). Providing families with an understanding of the illness, its causes, its prognosis, and the available treatment and services will benefit the patient and the long-term outcome. Educating families about precipitants, warning signs, management of stress, and medications will be an important aspect of the treatment plan.

Family psychoeducation is a method and model that acknowledges the essentially chronic nature of this disease and seeks to engage families in the rehabilitation process by creating a long-term working partnership with them (McFarlane, 2002). It combines clear, accurate information about mental illness with training in problem solving, communication skills, coping skills, and developing social supports. The goals are to markedly improve consumer outcomes and quality of life, as well as to reduce family stress and strain.

The partnership combines the complementary expertise and experience of family members, consumers, and professionals to develop coping skills that lay the foundation for recovery. The model emphasizes that families do not cause the illness, but, at times, in their efforts to respond to it, they may inadvertently exacerbate the condition. It is a strength-based philosophy. The *multi-family* model expands these concepts by engaging the patient and his family with other patients and families of similar experiences. The workbook for the model is available online at: www.nebhands.nebraska.edu/files/FamPsy_Workbook.pdf

TREATMENT

Given the advances in biological psychiatry, treatments of mental health disorders have evolved with a more holistic biopsychosocial perspective. Although psychopharmacology is a foundation of the treatment for psychotic disorders, there are other treatment modalities to be integrated for a comprehensive treatment plan. Treatment approaches will vary to some degree based on the timing and setting of the patient's presentation. Please refer to the Decision Tree for Treatment Initiation (Figure 10-1).

Acute treatment most often refers to that phase in which the patient has experienced a relapse or exacerbation of the illness, often with an increase in the positive symptoms of delusions, hallucinations, or agitated behavior. This acute treatment also applies to the person who is experiencing a first episode or receiving treatment for the first time. An exacerbation of schizophrenia may occur rapidly or it may occur gradually. Many of our medications are long acting and the patient may have stopped medications believing the lack of emerging symptoms validated the medications were not necessary, only to have the signs and symptoms reemerge slowly.

Antipsychotics are indicated early on, especially when the patient is highly agitated or experiencing great emotional turmoil. In the acute phase of the illness where psychotic symptoms are present, safety and physical needs take precedence. To provide a secure environment, a crisis unit or hospitalization may be necessary for the safety of the patient or others. Many psychotic patients may be so delusional or distraught that they will need protection from any self-destructive tendencies, that is, voices that tell them to harm themselves or to "escape" like the patient who jumped off a bridge to escape the "demons."

The goals of intervention in the acute phase of a psychotic experience are to reduce stimulation and provide a safe and structured environment where clear communication, little demand for performance, and firm limit-setting by tolerant and supportive staff can complement the use of medication in achieving a rapid resolution of symptomatic behavior. Immediate contact with the family is important in developing an alliance, providing crisis intervention to resolve stress that may have caused or been caused by the patient's relapse, and planning for future treatment (Stoudemire, 1990). Hospitalization allows monitoring of the individual's physical needs, that is, assessing for adequate hydration, nutrition, and elimination. It can be an opportunity to establish rapport and attempt to create a therapeutic alliance with the patient.

During this initial contact, it is important to not overwhelm the individual with too many choices, as ambivalence can be distressing. Be clear and direct about what are the expectations and the initial treatment goals. Set small daily goals that are realistic and can be accomplished with success, that is, shower, eat, take medication, walk the hallway, and so on.

It may be tempting to want to reason or try to rationalize with the patient about his symptoms, but this is not helpful. Providers want to provide reality testing and reassurance with the patient but to not directly confront

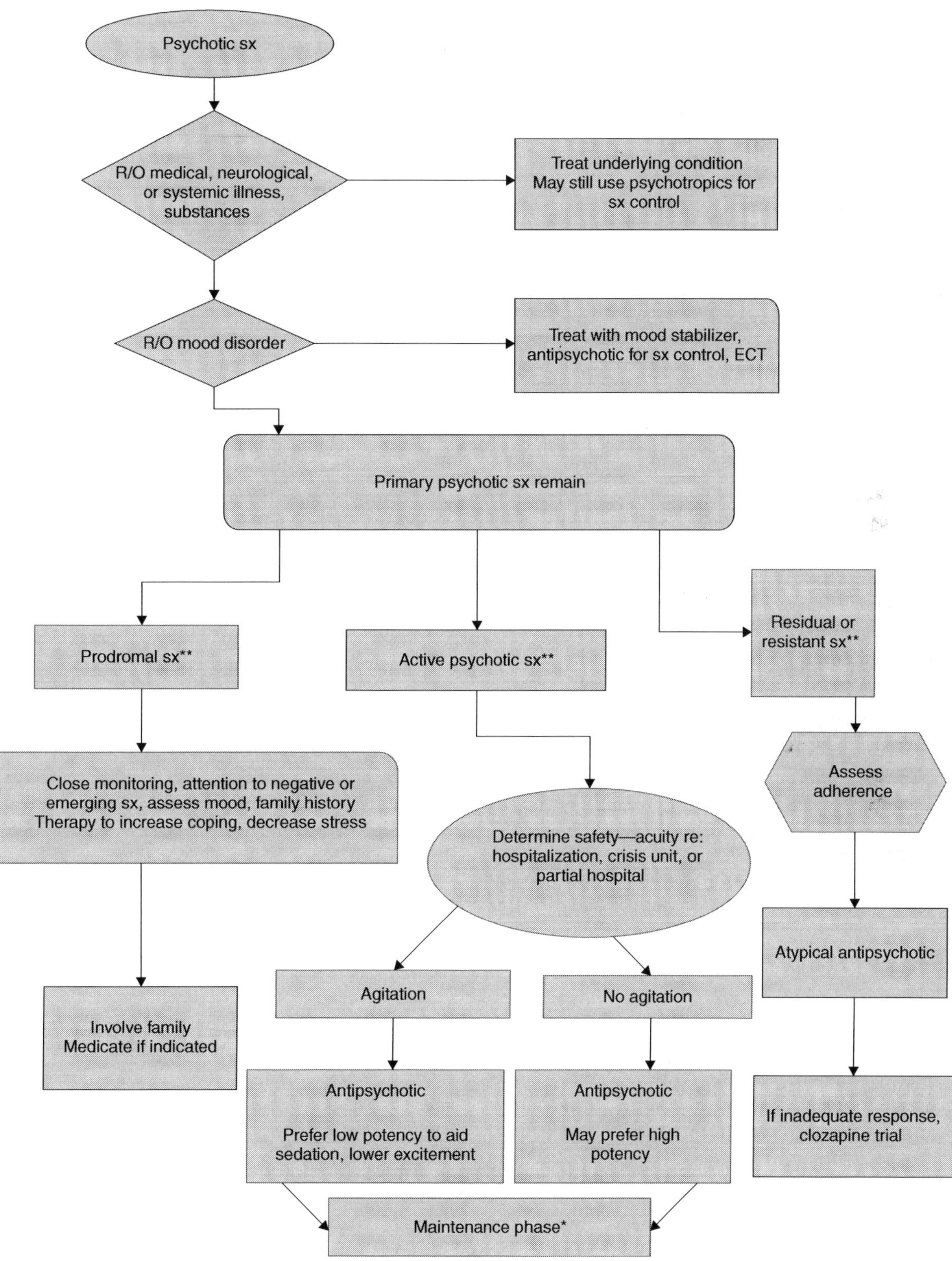

*If first episode, can decrease medication to maintenance dose after 1 year, then evaluate further necessity.
**Therapeutic interventions indicated along the continuum of care (beyond medication) include psychoeducation and support for the patient and family, therapy, and application of principles of the chronic disease model.
sx = symptom.

Figure 10-1 Decision Tree for Treatment Initiation

the symptoms. To do so may increase anxiety and escalate aggressive behaviors. It is therapeutic to be genuine, honest, and accept the reality of his experiences. For example, you might acknowledge and validate the situation, "I can understand how scary it must be for you when the voices threaten to kill you." Or, "Being responsible for the battle against evil every day must be so exhausting."

If the symptoms are more stressor related, as in a brief psychotic episode, the security of the hospital milieu itself can be very therapeutic. Medications may be indicated for only a brief period as the individual clears. For acute episodes of schizophrenia, doses in the range of 400–600 mg of chlorpromazine or its equivalent are necessary for successful treatment. Megadoses of neuroleptics (over 2,000 mg of chlorpromazine or its equivalent) do not seem to result in any greater or faster improvement of schizophrenia (Stoudemire, 1990). Identification of the triggering stress or event can be processed within the support of others in the hospital environment.

The majority of treatment occurs in the maintenance phase of the process, which is typically outpatient and centers around psychopharmacology. Medications are not given in a vacuum and the ongoing treatment relationship will impact the long-term prognosis, the rate of relapse, and long-term optimal functioning. Other treatment modalities, like psychosocial and vocational supports, will need to be combined and implemented for the best outcome. The principal goals of treatment at this stage are to prevent relapse while adjusting medication to a maintenance level and to help the patient reintegrate into the community. It is important for the clinician to attend to the major impact that an acute psychotic episode has on the family system (Stoudemire, 1990).

As stated, the mainstay of treatment for patients experiencing psychosis, particularly schizophrenia, is antipsychotic medication. Clinical expertise in choosing and managing drug therapy for an individual patient involves an understanding of the evidence regarding the options. The maintenance strategy is to find the lowest dose of antipsychotic that will protect against psychotic relapse while not interfering with the psychosocial functioning of the individual, thus reducing the risk for tardive dyskinesia (TD) (Stoudemire, 1990).

The side effect profile of the medication can be maximized or selected to the clinical need. For example, in an agitated psychotic patient, a sedating drug would be beneficial wherein a patient with pronounced psychomotor retardation, a sedating drug would not be your first choice. Choices need to be coordinated and balanced with the patient's symptom profile, their financial circumstances, and their input.

As reviewed, the probable mechanism of action of antipsychotics is their ability to block postsynaptic dopamine D2 receptors in the limbic forebrain. This blockade is thought to initiate a cascade of events responsible for both acute and chronic therapeutic actions. These drugs also block serotonergic, nonadrenergic, cholinergic, and histaminic receptors to differing degrees, accounting for the unique side effect profile of each agent (Andreasen & Black, 2006). Practitioners should identify specific target symptoms with attention always geared to safety and engagement. Symptom relief and remission are identified and defined for the individual patient.

Obviously, when prescribing medications to the psychiatric patient, the goal is to provide the right medication to the right person at the right dose. It is equally important to establish a rapport and communication with the patient about their partnership in this process. Although the provider prescribes the medication, it is the patient who must agree to take it.

Choosing the treatment that is best suited for your patient is a complex and collaborative process. The treatment agreement requires that the provider understand their patient's challenges, beliefs, barriers, and concerns. The patient-centered paradigm has seen a shift in even the way we discuss treatment planning with our patients and their families. We have moved away from *compliance* where the provider tells the patient what they must do, to use of the term, *adherence,* which suggests a more collaborative agreed upon treatment plan. There are scales that can be used to measure adherence of medications (Foster, Sheehan, & Johns, 2011).

Treatment adherence is often a problem in patients with severe and persistent mental illness. It has been reported "noncompliance is even higher among psychiatric patients especially on an outpatient basis where the noncompliance rate has been shown to average 50% and psychiatric outpatients with a diagnosis of schizophrenia have the highest noncompliance rates" (Seltzer & Hoffman, 1980). Up to half of schizophrenia patients, experience extended gaps in their treatment in a 1-year period leading to increased hospitalizations and other adverse outcomes. There have been a number of focused attempts to reduce the frequency of these gaps (Mojtabai et al., 2009).

Noncompliance is often the primary cause of rehospitalization of those who suffer from schizophrenia or the affective disorders. The reasons for not following treatment recommendations can be numerous, and not limited to: uncomfortable side effects, breakthrough symptoms, lack of insight about illness or need for treatment, ambivalence about the medications, misunderstanding of the lifelong commitment to treatment, confusion or memory issues, and financial constraints. Efforts to address and to improve patients' adherence have utilized psychosocial interventions based on motivational interviewing methods, other cognitive-behavioral approaches, psychoeducation, medication self-management, and, more recently, environmental support (Mojtabai et al., 2009).

It is imperative that the clinician try to fully understand the patient's thoughts and beliefs around their treatment to help with improved adherence as relapse can add to the severity of the illness, increase the associated risks of the disease, and worsen the prognosis. There has been much in recent literature of the "neurotoxic effects" of the presence of psychosis, and it is critical to educate the patient on the possible treatment-resistant effects that can occur from chronic relapse.

Medication adherence is both an attitude and a behavior. Without some motivation to take medication, adherence is unlikely. Yet, motivation alone does not guarantee compliance behavior (Freudenreich, Kontos, & Querques, 2011). In assessing for understanding and adherence to treatment, it can be very useful in the aspect of the interview around medications to first *ask* the patient how and what are they are taking for medications. Do not try to save time by stating, "You're still taking the Geodon?" There have been many interviews where the patient has responded that they were taking their medication to only find out later there was a great deal of miscommunication around dosages, timing, or the medication itself.

It may be highlighting the obvious, but it is worth stating often: the provider should always prescribe the simplest regimen. When taking meds once daily, nighttime is preferred. However, this is not always possible and the most successful adherence strategy is one where the patient and the provider have an open, honest dialogue in which the patient should always be encouraged to ask questions and to report side effects early. It is helpful to inquire if they think there might be any barriers or problems to anticipate with compliance.

Whereas the use of depot medications and various psychosocial interventions have been shown to improve adherence with medication treatments, the use of both remains limited (Mojtabai et al., 2009). There are intramuscular (IM) or depot forms of antipsychotics available with dosing from weekly to monthly, depending on the medication and the patient's symptoms and tolerance profile. These medications can provide an alternative for the patient who is ambivalent or disorganized to take medication on daily basis.

Some clinics schedule an "injection clinic" where patients come in at a scheduled time, which can be a social opportunity with peers. The injection clinic may also pose another opportunity for contact, engagement, and assessment of the patient. Commonly prescribed neuroleptics IM medications today still include fluphenazine (Prolixin) and haloperidol (Haldol), but Risperdal Consta and paliperidone (Invega) have become popular.

There are also long-acting antipsychotics that are available in patches and sublingual tablets. The future may bring additional formulations with more localized central nervous system (CNS) activity (i.e., intrathecal antipsychotic drug administration) to avoid organ system complications. Inhalable formulations may be around the corner and could offer quicker onset of efficacy (Nasrallah, 2010).

MEDICATIONS

There is growing evidence that guideline-conformant treatments could potentially improve patient outcomes and reduce the avertable social and health burden of psychiatric illness at minimal additional costs. However, services have been slow in adopting care practices that are consistent with the evidence-based guidelines. The individual practice styles and institutional barriers such as lack of resources all likely contribute to the slow adoption of the guideline-consistent practices (Mojtabai et al., 2009).

Clinical Practice Guidelines and treatment bundles stand to pave the way for standardized treatments that are evidence-based, taking into consideration best practice with cost considerations. This will lead to pay for performance, quality improvement, and consensus on outcome measurement. Although clinicians should consider the applicability of recommendations in clinical guidelines to each patient for whom they provide care, such recommendations should guide rather than dictate practice.

A method to evaluate the strength of the evidence found in a published guideline can help support the implementation of a specific guideline into practice. The use of the Appraisal of Guidelines for Research and Evaluation II (AGREE II) tool is an evidence review guide that qualifies the strength of the published data. The use of a measured review of the strength of data will encompass a comprehensive evaluation of publications that will help to create practice guidelines rather than mandate practice.

In 1999, the Texas Medication Algorithm Project (TMAP) published its guidelines for the treatment of schizophrenia and related disorders (Miller et al., 1999). This review was implemented in outpatient public mental health clinics in Texas with treatment focused on stages of illness and prior history of medication trial. Since then, several entities have refined and adopted these guidelines with an emphasis on current clinical evidence along with the premise that no algorithm addresses all the clinical situations that will arise in the medication management of schizophrenia. The APAs, Expert Consensus Guidelines and the Patient Outcomes Research Team (PORT) project contribute to clinical guidelines yet may be less specific with junctures related to circumstances that occur in everyday practice (Miller et al., 1999). Since the publication of the 1999 Texas Implementation of Medication Algorithms (TIMA) guidelines, a 2006 update narrows the recommendation for clozapine trials which is recommended after two failed antipsychotics and earlier if there are other risk factors (Moore et al., 2007).

In 1992, the Agency for Health Care Policy and Research (now the Agency for Healthcare Research and Quality [AHRQ]) and the NIMH funded the Schizophrenia PORT Study. The Schizophrenia PORT was one of 14 patient outcome research teams. It was created in the late 1980s in response to concerns raised about the appropriateness of care being delivered for several common medical and psychiatric conditions, including schizophrenia. The goal was to reduce variations in care by promoting the adoption of treatments supported by strong scientific evidence or "evidence-based practices." (Kreyenbuhl et al., 2010).

However, unlike TMAP, the PORT includes recommendations for adjunctive psychopharmacologic treatments as well as for antipsychotic medications. It also is inclusive of recommendations for psychosocial interventions, which are important treatments that augment gains from medication therapies. The PORT recommendations are based primarily on empirical data (Kreyenbuhl et al., 2010).

The 2003 landmark Clinical Antipsychotic Trials for Interventions Effectiveness (CATIE) reviewed antipsychotic medication efficacy, side effect profiles, and effectiveness, and added a more refined treatment review with a quasi-algorithm based on effectiveness and side effect management. This trial was an NIMH multi-centered clinical trial that added clinical consideration in treatment protocols that are not included in algorithm designs. It considered the use of antipsychotic medications for disorders in which antipsychotics are indicated such as bipolar disorder or psychotic depression. The drive toward evidence-based decision making has prompted systems to adopt guidelines with implementation plans to encourage providers to follow scientific evidence and what occurs in actual practice.

The Michigan Implementation of Medication Algorithms (MIMA) is an example of an implementation project that refined and adopted the TMAP guidelines in an effort to encourage practice in this manner. It's important to remember that algorithms are not clinical trials but are an organization of evidence that determines a roadmap to treatment. The TMAP guidelines provide specifics, whereas APA practice guidelines define steps and groupings rather than specific medications. Since the publication of both the TMAP project and the CATIE trial, there are newer agents that have been approved for the treatment of schizophrenia. These agents however are within the class of medications entitled "atypical antipsychotics" or "third-generation" antipsychotics. Newer classes and approaches to treating psychosis are on the horizon and will shape a change in the treatment of psychosis from the psychopharmacological perspective.

The six stages in the TMAP guidelines are sequenced in a manner that a clinical presentation may enter at any of the six stages depending on history and previous medication trials. This has been a debate in health care continuum mostly related to risk benefit as it relates to cost. However, second- and now third-generation antipsychotics are favored over first-generation because of the reduction in risk of TD. The TMAP guidelines did not factor in cost as an indicator in its review. As many of the atypicals are now available in generic form, the cost factor will be less of an indicator. APA guidelines include both typicals and atypicals in early steps of treatment since the method is, as noted earlier, more general than specific in its medication options.

The PORT-updated schizophrenia treatment recommendations around pharmacological treatments appear in Exhibit 10-4.

Overall, atypical antipsychotics are referred to as second- and third-generation antipsychotics and are less likely to cause TD (APA, 2006). The first second generation antipsychotic, clozapine is recommended after failure of at least two atypicals and one typical antipsychotic. This is because clozapine carries the inherent risk of agranulocytosis among other potential serious side effects. Yet, in spite of these risks, the Clinical Antipsychotic Trials of Intervention Effectiveness (CATIE) identified clozapine as the most effective treatment for chronic and treatment resistant schizophrenia (Swartz, et. al, 2008). This is because of the monitoring involved in the use of clozapine in light of the risk of agranulocytosis.

Treatment-resistant or nonresponding schizophrenia is complex and requires combining agents and/

EXHIBIT 10-4: UPDATED SCHIZOPHRENIA PORT TREATMENT RECOMMENDATIONS: PSYCHOPHARMACOLOGICAL TREATMENT RECOMMENDATIONS

ACUTE PHASE	RECOMMENDATIONS
Acute Positive Symptoms in Treatment-Responsive People With Schizophrenia: Acute Antipsychotic Treatment Medication	In people with treatment-responsive multi-episode schizophrenia who are experiencing an acute exacerbation of their illness, antipsychotic medications, other than clozapine, should be used as the first line of treatment to reduce positive psychotic symptoms. The initial choice of antipsychotic medication or the decision to switch to a new antipsychotic should be made on the basis of individual preference, prior to treatment response, and side effect experience; adherence history; relevant medical history, and risk factors; individual medication side effect profile; and long-term treatment planning.
Acute Positive Symptoms in People With First-Episode Schizophrenia: Antipsychotic Medication Choice	Antipsychotic medications, other than clozapine and olanzapine, are recommended as first-line treatment for persons with schizophrenia experiencing their first acute positive symptom episode.
MAINTENANCE PHASE	
Maintenance Pharmacotherapy in Treatment-Responsive People With Schizophrenia: Maintenance Antipsychotic Medication Treatment	People with treatment-responsive, multi-episode schizophrenia who experience acute and sustained symptom relief with an antipsychotic medication should be offered continued antipsychotic treatment in order to maintain symptom relief and to reduce the risk of relapse or worsening of positive symptoms.
Maintenance Pharmacotherapy in Treatment-Responsive People With Schizophrenia: Long-Acting Antipsychotic Medication Maintenance	Long-acting injectable (LAI) antipsychotic medication should be offered as an alternative to oral antipsychotic medication for the maintenance treatment of schizophrenia when the LAI formulation is preferred to oral preparations. The recommended dosage range for fluphenazine decanoate is 6.25–25 mg, administered every 2 weeks, and for haloperidol decanoate is 50–200 mg, administered every 4 weeks, although alternative dosages and administration intervals equivalent to the recommended dosage ranges may also be used. The recommended dosage range for risperidone long-acting injection is 25–75 mg administered every 2 weeks.
Clozapine for the Treatment of Residual Symptoms: Clozapine for Positive Symptoms in *Treatment-Resistant* Schizophrenia	Clozapine should be offered to people with schizophrenia who continue to experience persistent and clinically significant positive symptoms after 2 adequate trials of other antipsychotic agents. A trial of clozapine should last at least 8 weeks at a dosage from 300 to 800 mg/day.
OTHER	
Medication for the Treatment of Acute Agitation in Schizophrenia	An oral or intramuscular (IM) antipsychotic medication, alone or in combination with a rapid acting benzodiazepine, should be used in the pharmacological treatment of acute agitation in people with schizophrenia. If possible, the route of antipsychotic administration should correspond to the preference of the individual.
Intervention for Smoking Cessation in Schizophrenia	People with schizophrenia who want to quit or reduce cigarette smoking should be offered treatment with bupropion SR 150 mg twice daily for 10 to 12 weeks, with or without nicotine replacement therapy, to achieve short-term abstinence. This pharmacological treatment should be accompanied by a smoking cessation education or support group.

Source: Kreyenbuhl et al. (2009).

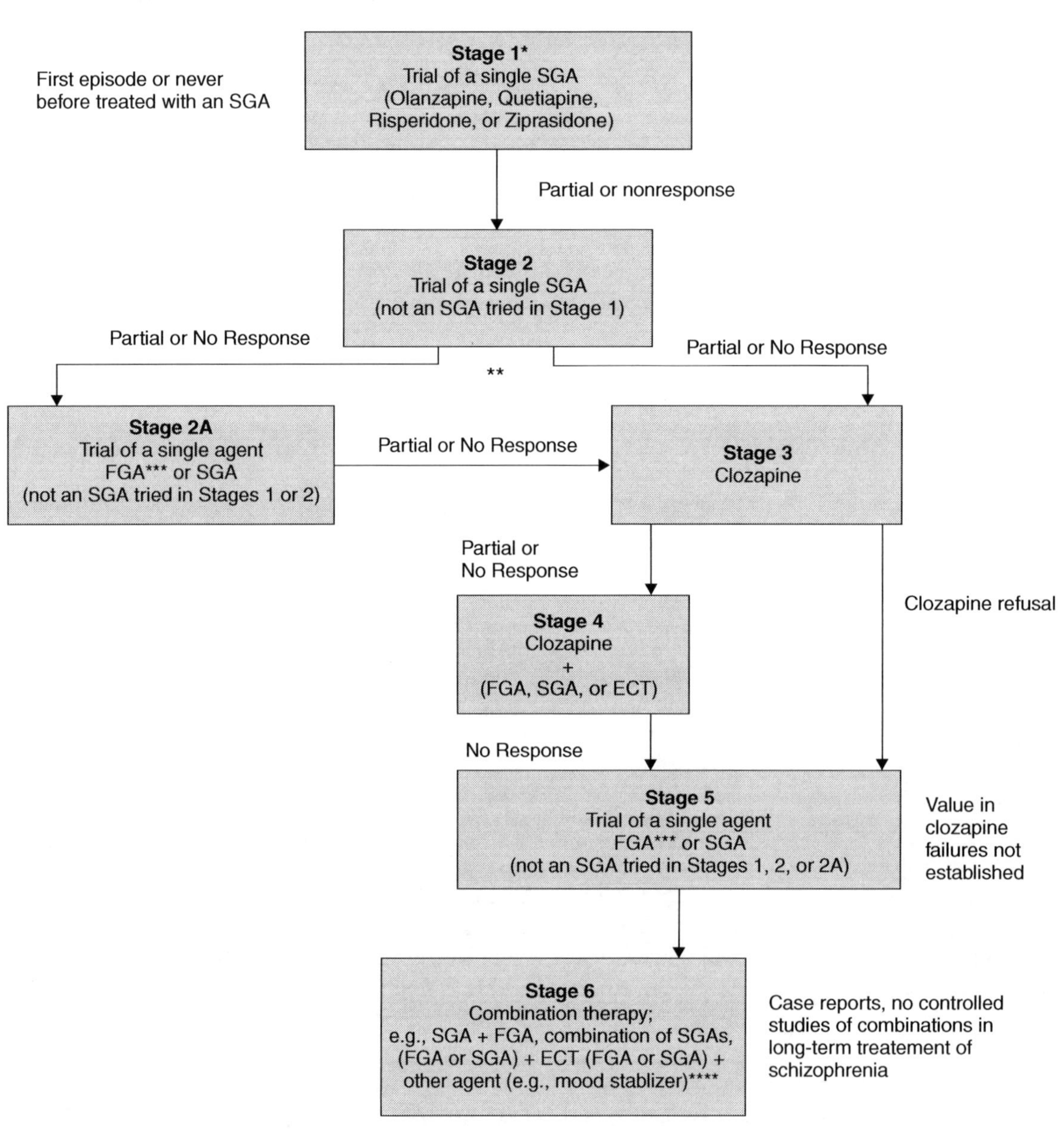

*If patient is nonadherent to medication, the clinician may use haloperidol decanoate or fluphenazine decanoate at any stage, but should carefully assess for unrecognized side effects and consider a different oral AP if side effects could be contributing to nonadherence.
** See text for discussion. Current expert opinion favors choice of clozapine.
***Assuming no history of failure on FGA.
****Whenever a second medication is added to an antipsychotic (other than clozapine) for the purpose of improving psychotic symptoms, the patient is considered to be in Stage 6. FGA = First generation AP; SGA = Second generation AP.

Figure 10-2 Algorithm for Treatment of Schizophrenia.

or inclusion of electroconvulsive therapy (ECT). The combination of specific medications otherwise considered "polypharmacy" is not widely studied. However, since this practice has become increasingly common the NIMH has recently completed an efficacy study that reviews the use of more than one antipsychotic, but at the time of this publication results are not yet available (www.clinicaltrials.gov). The inclusion of antidepressants or mood stabilizers is determined by patient presentation as it relates to clinical assessment of symptoms.

In addition to specific medication options, there are also recommendations and clinical guidelines relating to

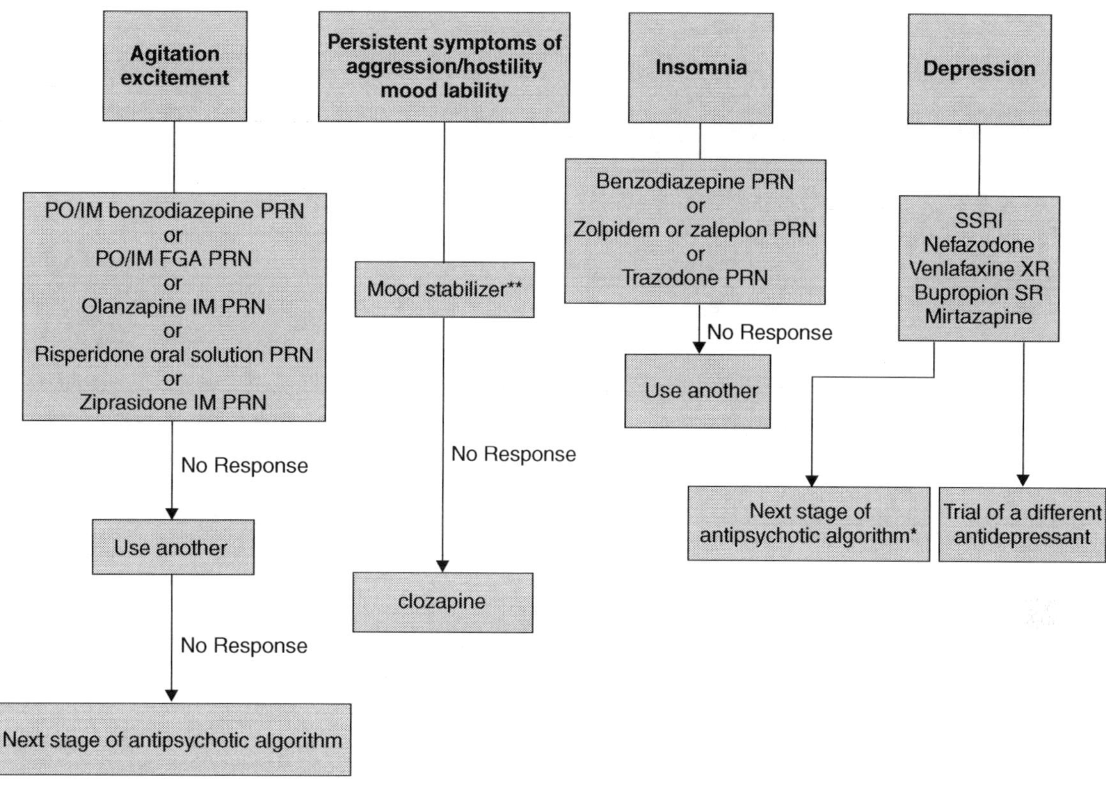

*Refer back to Figure 2, Algorithm for Treatment of Schizophrenia.
**Consider clozapine in patients with persistent suicidal behaviors or ideation.

Figure 10-3 Algorithm for Treatment of Co-existing Symptoms.

decision points in treatment. Often, adherence is a significant deterrent in remission of symptoms. An adequate trial is defined as at least 3 weeks with the exception of clozapine, which can take up to 3 months. In addition, the assessment of an adequate trial can take up to 9 weeks (Miller et al., 1999). Figure 10-2 and Figure 10.3 provide algorithms for both treatment of schizophrenia and the commonly occurring co-existing symptoms. Table 10.1 shows a list of commonly prescribed antipsychotic medications with average doses, side effect potentials and clinical tips.

Positive, negative and cognitive symptoms, as well as social functioning can present differently across the life span. The psychopharmacologic and psychosocial interventions used for an adult patient would typically not be appropriate for the pediatric patient or the senior adult with schizophrenia. Exhibit 10-5 presents some important age related considerations when prescribing to these vulnerable populations.

Treatment Resistance or Inadequate Response

Patients with treatment-resistant schizophrenia can be broadly defined to include any persons with residual symptoms that cause distress or impairment despite several treatment attempts. Unfortunately, this definition may include most of our patients with schizophrenia (Citrome, 2011b). Before considering an individual as treatment-resistant or a nonresponder, a full assessment of compounding variables must occur.

In the patient with no response to the antipsychotic, there are certain factors that must be considered. It can be helpful to start with going back over the assessment and ascertain if the diagnosis is correct. Next, the provider needs to research if the patient is actually taking the medication. There was one such patient who went to the lab weekly for his blood draws with clozapine, only to find the pills stockpiled in his drawer. It was no wonder when each week the prescriber increased the dose, there was no improvement.

It is equally important to not give up on a medication too quickly. Has there been an adequate trial period? Often, families may be so eager for improvement in their loved ones, who finally consented to medications, that expectations may need to be managed. Is the dose prescribed therapeutic? This may arise in either doses that are too high and causing side effects or

TABLE 10-1: ANTIPSYCHOTIC MEDICATIONS

GENERIC	BRAND	DOSAGE RANGE	SEDATION	EPS	*ACH EFFECTS	CLINICAL TIP
Low Potency						
chlorpromazine	Thorazine	50–1500 mg	High	Medium	High	Can ↓ BP, ↓ seizure threshold, ↑ risk photosensitivity reactions: wear sunblock
thioridazine	Mellaril	50–800 mg	High	Low	High	Can prolong QTc: get baseline EKG
clozapine	Clozaril	200–900 mg	High to Very High	Very low	High to Very High	Remember to monitor WBC 4 weeks D/C. Monitor metabolic syndrome. May need antiseizure drug if dose ↑
quetiapine	Seroquel	100–750 mg	High	Very low to low	Low	Monitor metabolic syndrome
High Potency						
perphenazine	Trilafon	8–60 mg	Medium	Medium to High	Low	Recommend sunblock
loxapine	Loxitane	50–250 mg	Low	High	Medium	
trifluoperazine	Stelazine	5–40 mg	Low	High	Low to Medium	Recommend sunblock
fluphenazine	Prolixin	2–20 mg	Low	High to Very High	Low	Recommend sunblock
thiothixene	Navane	5–60 mg	Low	Medium to High	Low	Recommend sunblock
haloperidol	Haldol	2–40 mg	Low	High to very high	Low	Carbamazepine may ↓ level
olanzapine	Zyprexa	5–20 mg	Medium	Low	Low	Monitor metabolic syndrome, may ↓ body's ability to ↓ temp
risperidone	Risperdal	2–10 mg	Low	Low	Low	Monitor metabolic syndrome
ziprasidone	Geodon	40–160 mg	Low	Very low	Low	Give with food; Monitor metabolic syndrome
aripiprazole	Abilify	10–30 mg	Low	Very low	Low	Monitor metabolic syndrome

For all antipsychotics, monitor for tardive dyskinesia and NMS, recommend avoid alcohol. Cautious use in pregnancy, risk-benefit review required, all are class C risk category except clozapine is risk category B.

These are average dose ranges: lowest dosages with elderly and children; may see higher doses in acutely ill populations.

*ACH (anticholinergic) = dry mouth, blurry vision, constipation, urinary retention, potential delirium.

doses that are too low to be of benefit. Are there other substances involved that are complicating the picture? Does the patient smoke or take other agents that impact metabolism?

The decision made to switch antipsychotics can be based on many factors. If the side effects limit dose or contribute to noncompliance, switching between classes is appropriate. Evidence has suggested that switching from

EXHIBIT 10-5: MEDICATIONS AND AGE-RELATED CONSIDERATIONS

PEDIATRIC CONSIDERATIONS	GERIATRIC CONSIDERATIONS
Second-generation antipsychotics are used as first-line therapy in most clinical situations due to decreased risk for EPS, dysphoric effects, and TD. Conventional antipsychotics are often used only on a prn or short-term basis, or in persons who do not respond or cannot tolerate novel agents. Antipsychotics are found useful for the following indications: pervasive developmental disorder (autism), schizophrenia, conduct disorders, and tic disorders. Used to reduce target symptoms such as aggression, temper tantrums, psychomotor excitement, stereotypies, and hyperactivity unresponsive to other therapy. Start doses low and increase slowly. Limit dose and duration of therapy. Assess dosage requirements and continued need for drug. Monitor for early signs of tardive dyskinesia.	Start dose low and increase slowly; elimination half-life tends to be increased in the elderly. Clearance of drugs metabolized by CYP3A4 (e.g., quetiapine, ziprasidone, haloperidol, etc.) appears to decline with age. Monitor for excessive CNS and anticholinergic effects; aim for drugs least likely to cause these effects. Elderly are more sensitive to anticholinergic SE (e.g., tachycardia, constipation, difficulty urinating, impairment in concentration & memory, delirium). Elderly are more sensitive to EPS, more vulnerable with moving, eating, and sleeping, and risk of falls. Balance need for antiparkinsonian drug with type of antipsychotic used. Caution combining with other drugs with CNS properties (sedation lasts longer in the elderly; can impair arousal levels during the day and increase risk of falls; additive effects can result in confusion, disorientation, delirium) • As most "2nd and 3rd generation" antipsychotics and some conventional agents (e.g., phenothiazines) can cause orthostatic hypotension, caution with dose titration and other hypotensive agents (fall risk). • High incidence TD in elderly with conventional antipsychotics—risk about 30% per year in persons over age 45.

Source: Bezchlibnyk-Butter & Jeffries (2007).

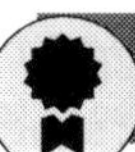

EXHIBIT 10-6: REASONS FOR SWITCHING ANTIPSYCHOTIC DRUG REGIMENS

Persistent positive symptoms—switch to a conventional or a second-generation antipsychotic.

Persistent negative symptoms—switch to a second-generation antipsychotic or lower the dose; consider aripiprazole.

Relapse despite compliance.

Noncompliance—consider a depot preparation.

Persistent extrapyramidal side effects (EPS) despite dosage decrease.

Tardive dyskinesia (TD)—clozapine and quetiapine offer minimal risk.

Persistent/chronic side effects, e.g., galactorrhea, impotence, weight gain.

Source: Bezchlibnyk-Butler & Jeffries (2007).

a conventional to a second-generation agent may result in enhanced response. Last, switching from another second-generation agent to clozapine may offer response in up to 50% of patients (Bezchlibnyk-Butler & Jeffries, 2007).

The reasons for switching may be as varied and may be summarized in Exhibit 10-6.

Like most of medicine, there is more than one option when looking at methods to switch antipsychotics:

1. Withdraw the first drug gradually and begin the second drug following a washout period—this may not be clinically practical when patient is experiencing symptoms.
2. Stop the first drug and start the second drug at its usual initial dose; increase the dose over a 2 to 4 week period—used when the patient has had a serious adverse reaction to the first drug; may result in drug withdrawal symptoms.
3. Maintain the first drug for 2 to 3 weeks while titrating the dose of the second drug; then withdraw the first drug over 1 to 2 weeks.
4. Decrease the dose of the first drug and start the second at a low dose; continue decreasing the dose of the first drug as the second one is increasing over the 2 to 4 week period (data suggest olanzapine can be started at 10 mg and maintained at this dose).
   - Be aware of additive or synergistic side effects of both drugs. When possible, avoid the ongoing use of two or more antipsychotics simultaneously.
   - Rate of switching or cross-tapering should be slower in the elderly and in young patients.

- When switching from high potency to low potency, continue the antiparkinsonian drug, if currently prescribed, until the changeover is complete to prevent the emergence of extrapyramidal side effects (EPS), and then withdraw the antiparkinsonian drug gradually.

For patients who are clear nonresponders to antipsychotics or combination drug strategies and/or pose an immediate danger, ECT may be useful, either alone or in combination with an antipsychotic (Janicak & Sadek, 1996). ECT has been studied in both acute and chronic schizophrenia. Patients with recent onset who received ECT found that the ECT was about as effective as antipsychotic medications and more effective than psychotherapy. Other studies suggested supplementing antipsychotic medication with ECT was more effective than medication alone. Antipsychotic medications should be administered during and after ECT treatment (Sadock & Sadock, 2008).

As advances occur daily in the neurosciences, there appear to be many promising treatments down the pike for patients with psychotic disorders. Research is proceeding to identify genes and single nucleotide polymorphisms that predict response to a given antipsychotic. Deep brain stimulation may also have very promising application to psychiatry. Studies suggest applications for psychosis and insights are being sought as to how deep brain stimulation can bring back to life a dormant corner of the brain or turn off a rogue neural circuit (Nasrallah, 2010).

Furthermore, evidence indicates that ailing brains can be structurally repaired. Brain disorders, such as schizophrenia, show gray and white matter deterioration and acute episodes often are associated with detrimental neuroplastic changes. Advances in neuroprotection, neurogenesis, neurotrophic factors, and antiapoptotic cascades will give psychiatric clinicians a toolbox to regenerate, reconnect, and resculpt brain regions in their patients by using specific pharmacologic agents and evidence-based psychotherapy (Nasrallah, 2010).

Since the persistent negative and cognitive symptoms are seen as the ultimate cause of long-term vocational and social disability in schizophrenia, there are collaborative efforts under way with NIMH, academic researchers, and the pharmaceutical industry to develop pharmacological agents for cognitive deficits. A standard cognitive battery for use by all investigators for drug development, as well as a list of brain receptor targets or pathways for the successful development of new cognition-enhancing drugs, was developed under the auspices of a project called the Measurement and Treatment Research to Improve Cognition in Schizophrenia (MATRICS) (www.matrics.ucla.edu). This collaboration among academia, industry, and government is a hopeful development in future treatment methods. Although no drugs have yet received FDA approval for use in schizophrenia, these cognitive enhancing agents are being investigated (Nasrallah, 2011).

Other promising pharmacological strategies target the glutamate system and are being evaluated initially as adjunctive treatment to antipsychotics in schizophrenia.

Several novel strategies show promise to prevent or treat residual symptoms. Public health efforts to reduce the duration of untreated psychosis show a potential to mitigate the severity of negative symptoms. Psychotherapeutic interventions, especially if utilized early in the course of illness, may result in improved cognitive function as well as decreased positive and negative symptoms and may even prevent neuroprogression as evaluated with brain magnetic resonance structural imaging (Perkins, 2011).

MANAGING SIDE EFFECTS

Pharmacodynamic interactions are caused by additive or competing effects of multiple drugs. The most serious of these involve medications that increase a patient's risk of serotonin syndrome or neuroleptic malignant syndrome (NMS); both are medical emergencies that require immediate hospitalization (Casher, Bostwick, & Yu, 2011). See Figure 10-4 for an overview of treating neuroleptic side effects.

NEUROLEPTIC MALIGNANT SYNDROME

NMS is a rare, yet potentially life-threatening syndrome. The pathophysiology of NMS is complex and most likely involves the relationships between multiple central and systemic pathways and neurotransmitters. It is thought that NMS may be an extreme variant of drug-induced parkinsonism or catatonia. There is compelling evidence to suggest that dopamine blockade plays a central role (Strawn, Keck, & Caroff, 2008).

Once NMS is identified, the offending medication must be discontinued. For patients presenting with mild signs and symptoms, supportive care and careful clinical monitoring may be sufficient. If the patient is agitated and sedation is desired, lorazepam 1–2 mg parenterally is a reasonable first-line NMS intervention. In advanced NMS cases with extreme hyperthermia, severe rigidity, and hypermetabolism, treatments are more aggressive. Severe hyperthermia requires volume resuscitation and

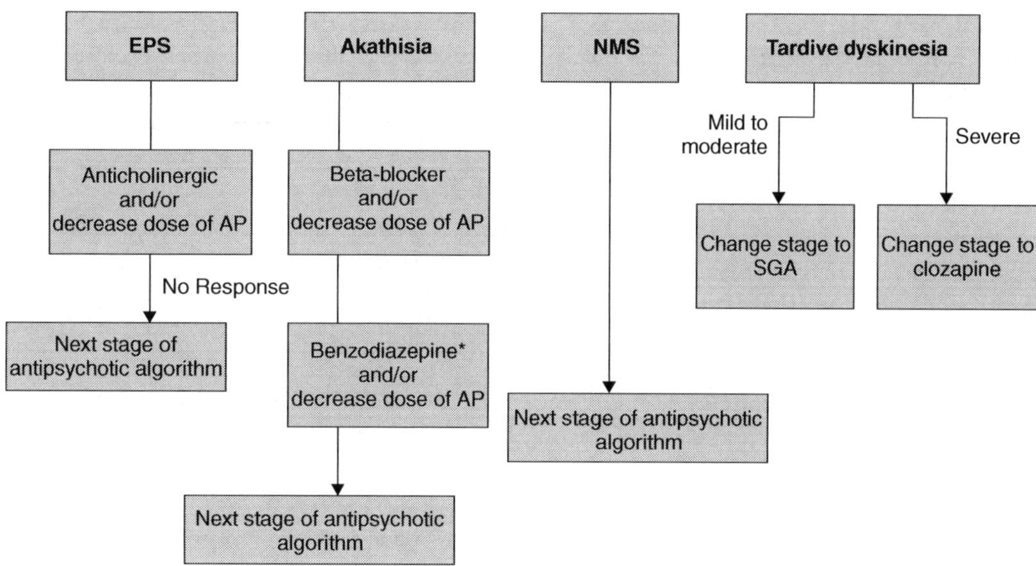

*Avoid combinations of FGA anticholinergic and benzodiazepine.

Figure 10-4 Algorithm for the Treatment of Neuroleptic Side Effects

cooling measures, intensive medical care, and careful monitoring for complications (Strawn et al., 2008).

Although the central treatment for patients with psychosis is the use of antipsychotic agents, it is understandable that there may be some misgivings about restarting such a medication after an episode with NMS. It has been estimated that up to 30% of patients may be at risk for recurrence (Strawn et al., 2008). There are guidelines to follow that may lower the risk and allow continued safe antipsychotic coverage.

It is important to document the indications for the antipsychotic medication. It is also essential to recheck the accuracy of the diagnosis of a previous NMS episode. Patients may confuse this with previous side effect reactions from the past. There should be an educational process where the risk of recurrence is reviewed with the patient and family.

In this risk analysis, other pharmacologic agents should be considered. A lower-potency antipsychotic from a different class may be a safer option. When at all possible, minimize any risk factors and permit time to pass as the body clears itself. Allow at least 2 weeks before a rechallenge and up to 4 weeks if the offending drug had been a long-acting injectable. Once rechallenge is decided, selection of low-potency, first-generation APs (FGAs) or second-generation AP (SGA) may help lower the risk. It is important to prescribe an initial test dose and monitor vital signs and neurologic status. Doses should be started low and titrated gradually. Clozapine has been associated with lower incidence of NMS (Strawn et al., 2008).

SEROTONIN SYNDROME

Serotonin syndrome occurs when an excess of serotonin builds up in the bloodstream. This condition, which once was considered rare, is now seen more frequently with the widespread use of SSRIs to treat depression, migraine, anxiety disorders, and other conditions. Many patients add to the risk unknowingly by taking over-the-counter medications, like St. John's wort, or they may even be prescribed serotonergic agents for other conditions, such as fibromyalgia, which they may not think to mention. Attention to the patient's side effects and full medication regime is essential as a single therapeutic dose of an SSRI has been noted to have caused the serotonin syndrome (Boyer & Shannon, 2005).

Serotonin syndrome came into the spotlight in 1984 with the death of an 18-year-old young woman named Libby Zion in New York City. She had presented to the hospital with fever, agitation, and jerking motions in her body. She had been taking phenelzine (an monoamine oxidase inhibitor [MAOI]) and on admission she was prescribed the drug, meperidine (painkiller and sedative) to control the shaking. Despite all the other issues that came to light with this case, education and awareness around serotonin syndrome was a positive end result.

Serotonergic drugs work by blocking the reuptake of the neurotransmitter serotonin, which results in an increase in serotonin levels. Usually, this is the intended effect, but the problem occurs when these serotonergic drugs are mixed with other drugs that can increase the CNS's serotonin activity. It is an expected, *predictable* consequence of excess serotonergic agonism of CNS receptors and peripheral serotonergic receptors (Boyer & Shannon, 2005).

There are many medications that have been associated with this condition. These medications include MAOIs, tricyclic antidepressants, SSRIs, opiate analgesics, serotomimetic drugs such as over-the-counter cough medicines, weight reduction agents, and antiemetics. There are other psychiatric medications linked including lithium, some antipsychotic medications, and herbal supplements such as St. John's wort and gingko biloba. Antimigraine medications in the triptan family, such as sumatriptan and naratriptan, have also been implicated. Drugs of abuse such as lysergic acid diethylamide (LSD), amphetamines, and cocaine have all also been connected. The combination most likely to cause serotonin syndrome is an MAOI given with an SSRI (Boyer & Shannon, 2005).

The intensity of the treatment response depends on the severity of illness. Many cases of serotonin syndrome typically resolve within 24 hours after the initiation of therapy and the discontinuation of the serotonergic drugs, but symptoms may persist in patients taking drugs with long half-lives, active metabolites, or an extended duration of action. Supportive care, comprising the administration of intravenous fluids and correction of vital signs, remains a mainstay of therapy.

Mild cases (e.g., with hyperreflexia and tremor, no fever) can usually be managed with supportive care, removal of the precipitating drugs, and treatment with benzodiazepines. Moderately ill patients should have a more aggressive approach and may benefit from the administration of 5-HT2A antagonists. Hyperthermic patients (higher than 41.1°C) are severely ill and should receive the above therapies as well as immediate sedation, neuromuscular paralysis, and orotracheal intubation (Boyer & Shannon, 2005).

The clinical manifestations of serotonin syndrome range from mild and barely perceptible to lethal. In severe cases, serotonin syndrome can progress to seizures, disseminated intravascular coagulation, renal failure, coma, and death. Patient education for both syndromes should be part of any relevant patient treatment plan.

Table 10-2 offers a comparison of serotonin syndrome and NMS.

EXTRAPYRAMIDAL SIDE EFFECTS

It is worth repeating that lack of efficacy and bothersome side effects remain the major reasons for medication nonadherence in most cases (Mojtabai et al., 2009). One major area of side effect concern with antipsychotics is extrapyramidal syndrome. This syndrome includes a variety of signs and symptoms, and results from dysfunction of the extrapyramidal system. Second-generation antipsychotics have a lower liability for EPS as compared with first-generation antipsychotics (Perkins, 2011).

The extrapyramidal systems are involved in the unconscious control of all voluntary musculature. Neuroleptics have complex effects on the extrapyramidal systems that are exacerbated by anxiety, disappear during sleep, and can be consciously controlled for a limited time with effort. EPS can be classified into those that can happen early or late in treatment (Stoudemire, 1990).

Acute dystonic reactions are one of the EPS that occurs early on in treatment. These are involuntary spasms of voluntary muscle groups that are often painful and frightening to patients. They usually occur in the upper body, such as the face, head, and neck areas, but any part of the body may be involved. Young men on high-potency neuroleptics are at the greatest risk for the development of acute dystonic reactions. Low-potency neuroleptics, especially ones that have significant anticholinergic effects, have less likelihood of inducing acute dystonic reactions.

Acute dystonic reactions tend to happen relatively early in treatment, and there is some tolerance that develops to them. The presumed mechanism of action is an imbalance induced by antipsychotic agents blocking dopamine receptors that are in balance with the cholinergic system. The use of neuroleptics with an anticholinergic agent or dopamine agonist results in the reestablishment of this dopamine-cholinergic balance. Considering the impact of such reactions on patient compliance, it is worthwhile to consider using antiparkinsonian agents in a prophylactic manner in patients who are started on neuroleptics (Stoudemire, 1990).

Akathisia, an extreme inner sense of restlessness, is a very common side effect that is also quite uncomfortable and one of the primary causes for patient initiated discontinuation of medication. It is remarkable how many schizophrenic patients will not spontaneously complain of this side effect, but will simply stop the medication. It is therefore important to inquire specifically about the presence of akathisia during follow-up visits (Preston & Johnson, 2005).

Akathisia should be immediately suspected when a patient initially responds to neuroleptic treatment and then worsens. It is not as responsive as other EPS to anticholinergic agents. Some patients with akathisia respond to the use of beta-blockers such as propranolol. The most

TABLE 10-2: COMPARISON OF SEROTONIN SYNDROME AND NEUROLEPTIC MALIGNANT SYNDROME

	SEROTONIN SYNDROME	NEUROLEPTIC MALIGNANT SYNDROME (NMS)
Etiology	Increased CNS serotonin	Proposed dopamine blockade
Medication HX	Serotonergic agent	Dopamine antagonist
Risk factors	Administration of a serotonergic agent	Agitation Dehydration Exhaustion Organic brain syndromes Higher doses Rapid titration IM injections High-potency first-generation antipsychotics (FGAs) especially haloperidol
Hallmark signs	Hyperthermia Altered muscle tone—hyperkinesia Change in mental status Autonomic instability Rhabdomyolysis, DIC	Hyperthermia Muscle rigidity—bradykinesia Delirium/Confusion Fluctuating LOC Autonomic instability Parkinsonian signs
Time frame	Rapid onset 60% within 6 hrs of initiation, dose change, or overdose	Slower onset Evolves 1–3 days
Lab findings	None definitive *Perhaps* ↑ CPK, serum aminotransferase, metabolic acidosis,	↑WBC ↑ CPK
Interventions	Discontinue offending agents Supportive treatments, i.e., fluids Control of hyperthermia Control of agitation Administration of 5-HT2A antagonists Control of autonomic instability	Discontinue the offending agent Supportive treatments, i.e., hydration, control temp Benzodiazepines Dopamine receptor agonists Dantrolene ECT
Other		NMS Information Service Hotline 1–888-NMS-TEMP

Patient Education Tips: Warn patients taking SSRIs about the possibility of serotonin syndrome, as well as the drugs that could cause it. Encourage patients to tell care providers about all the medications they're taking, including over-the-counter and illicit drugs. Caution patients to stop taking an MAO inhibitor at least 14 days before starting SSRI therapy. Educate patients about the subtle changes that could herald serotonin syndrome, that is, confusion, unusual behavior, or agitation, and contact provider as soon as possible.

HX = History; WBC = white blood cell; CPK = creatine phosphokinase.

effective treatment for akathisia is a reduction in neuroleptic dose (Stoudemire, 1990).

Akathisia should always be considered a prominent part of the differential diagnosis of excessive activity, impulsivity, or irritability in patients treated with neuroleptics (Teicher & Glod, 1990). Excessive use of caffeine (colas, coffee, tea, chocolate) may worsen anxiety and agitation and counteract the beneficial effects of antipsychotics. The additional caffeine may further agitate the patient experiencing akathisia.

Parkinsonian side effects may occur that include tremor, muscle stiffness and rigidity, shuffling gait, drooling, and bradykinesia (Sadock & Sadock, 2008). Bradykinesia is diminished spontaneous motor movements associated with reduction in spontaneous speech, general apathy, and trouble with initiation. As in Parkinson's disease, bradykinesia is accompanied by cognitive impairment or bradyphrenia (Nasrallah, 2011). Bradykinesia can be difficult to differentiate from depression and negative symptoms. Because anticholinergic agents are effective in treating bradykinesia, such symptoms should be aggressively treated with these agents (Stoudemire, 1990).

Parkinsonism can be treated with anticholinergic agents, Benadryl, and dopamine agonists. They should be withdrawn after 4 to 6 weeks to assess whether tolerance to the parkinsonian effects has developed (Sadock & Sadock, 2008). Antiparkinsonian agents may be required during the first few weeks of treatment with conventional antipsychotics and prophylactically on a temporary basis, by young males, or by individuals with a history of EPS on low doses of antipsychotics or when given "conventional" antipsychotics.

Although treatment of the EPS is important to link to adherence, there are cautions to observe with these agents. These agents should only be used for the EPS of antipsychotics as excess use of these agents may precipitate an anticholinergic (toxic) psychosis. Anticholinergic medications given to reverse EPS can significantly worsen memory and exacerbate already severe primary memory impairment. Excessive dopamine blockade (resulting from too high a dose of the antipsychotic) impairs the executive cognitive function of the prefrontal cortex. This secondary cognitive deficit can be reversed by simply lowering the antipsychotic dose (Nasrallah, 2011b).

Anticholinergics can reduce peristalsis and decrease intestinal secretions leading to constipation. It is recommended that increasing fluids and bulk (i.e., bran, salads), as well as fruit in the diet can be beneficial. If it is necessary, a bulk laxative (i.e., Metamucil) or a stool softener (e.g., docusate) can be used. In severe or chronic constipation, lactulose is effective. Constipation does need to be assessed to rule out a bowel obstruction. Please refer to Exhibit 10-7 for common side effects of antipsychotic medications.

TARDIVE DYSKINESIA

TD is generally a late onset EPS (Preston & Johnson, 2005). TD presents as an involuntary movement disorder, most often with nonrhythmic, repetitive, purposeless hyperkinetic symptoms. It usually affects orofacial and lingual musculature with chewing, bruxism, protrusion, and curling or twisting of the tongue. Lip smacking, puckering, sucking, grimacing, or pursing may be present. Eye blinking and blepharospasm could be present (Caroff, Miller, Dhopesh, & Campbell, 2011).

Choreoathetoid movements of the fingers, hands, or upper or lower extremities also are common. Severe dyskinesias can affect breathing, swallowing, or speech and can interfere with walking and activities of daily living (Caroff et al., 2011). It is difficult to sit with a patient who is writhing in pain from trunkal TD, unable to easily sit in a chair, or is self-conscious and embarrassed from the constant involuntary movements.

The neurophysiology underlying TD is not well understood so there is no uniform treatment. Although various drugs have been used to reduce TD symptoms, there is no true cure. As TD may be irreversible in most cases, treatment really starts with prevention. Preventive principles include first confirming and documenting the indication for antipsychotic use, using conservative measures for dosing and using the newer or lower potency medication choices, and informing the patient and family of the risks (Caroff et al., 2011). Monitoring and detection for TD should be present in each visit with use of standardized tools, such as the Abnormal Involuntary Movement Scale (AIMS).

In assessing for the presence of TD, diagnostic criteria have been proposed by Schooler and Kane. TD onset occurs insidiously over 3 months of antipsychotic exposure and may begin with tic-like movements or increased eye blinking. TD is often suppressed or masked by ongoing antipsychotic medication and will become noticeable when the medication has been stopped, the dose lowered, or switched to another agent. Dyskinesias

EXHIBIT 10-7: COMMON SIDE EFFECTS OF ANTIPSYCHOTICS

EXTRAPYRADIMAL SYMPTOMS (EPS)	ANTICHOLINERGIC	OTHER
Restlessness/Akathisia	Dry mouth	Sedation
Bradykinesia	Constipation	Hypotension
Parkinsonism	Urinary hesitancy	Sexual dysfunction
Acute dystonia	Blurred vision	NMS
Muscle rigidity	Delirium	Weight gain
Tremor		Blood dyscrias
Tardive dyskinesia		Jaundice-hepatotoxicity
		Metabolic syndrome
		Photosensitivity
		Seizures

increase with emotional arousal, activation, distraction, and diminish with relaxation, sleep, or volitional efforts (Caroff et al., 2011).

Once TD has been confirmed, there are various treatment decisions to consider. Initially consider tapering any anticholinergic agents unless there is acute EPS or tardive dystonia present. These medications can worsen TD but not tardive dystonia; 60% of TD cases improve after stopping the anticholinergic (Caroff et al., 2011).

The next treatment decision point would be to explore if the antipsychotic can be safely tapered, switched, or stopped. If the clinical condition does not warrant a taper, consider if there is a less potent antipsychotic choice available. Stopping the medication is an option, but there is insufficient evidence to support drug cessation or reduction as effective treatment for TD, especially when compared to the high risk of psychotic relapse after drug withdrawal (Caroff et al., 2011). Patients and families should be informed that if stopping the medication becomes the choice, initial worsening of the dyskinesia is expected as the drug not only causes the syndrome but also tends to mask it.

Other options for the stable patient are to continue on the antipsychotic with attempts to gradually lower the dose over time, informing and educating patients and families about the risks, and monitoring closely. The natural course of TD after stopping the offending drug is unclear. As mentioned, there will be an expected increase in symptoms initially and in long-term follow-up, 36% to 55% of patients showed improvement. Complete and permanent reversibility beyond withdrawal period is rare (Caroff et al., 2011).

In switching to another antipsychotic, the risk for destabilizing the patient and precipitating another psychotic episode cannot be overlooked. More potent antipsychotics, like Haldol, suppress TD in approximately 67% of patients and may need to be considered in patients with severe and disabling symptoms. Clozapine in particular has been recommended for suppressing TD, especially in cases of tardive dystonia (Caroff et al., 2011).

There has been evidence that the use of levetiracetam (Keppra) has been effective for the patient with TD. The mechanisms of its therapeutic effect are unclear but may involve reducing neuronal hypersynchrony in basal ganglia (Woods, Saksa, Baker, Cohen, & Tek, 2008). In the randomized, double-blind, placebo-controlled study, patients continuing on levetiracetam continued to improve, and patients crossed over to open-label levetiracetam improved to a similar degree as those initially assigned. The medication was also well tolerated.

All patients receiving antipsychotics should sign an informed consent form which explains the risk of TD (Preston & Johnson, 2005). Being informed extends beyond that initial visit as education around treatment, risks of nonadherence, and medications is an ongoing process. Antipsychotic therapy has been a source of litigation; it is important for the patient and family to have honest information about the risks of the medications as well as the destructive and dangerous risk of ongoing psychosis.

All medications carry risk and no antipsychotic is perfectly safe; for TD, some may be safer than others. The newer agents (i.e., clozapine, quetiapine, risperidone, and olanzapine) seem to have lower risk and are felt to have antidyskinetic effects. Again, the provider should document a baseline assessment for movement disorders, and monitor regularly (e.g., every 6–12 months) (Bezchlibnyk-Butter & Jeffries, 2007). The AIMS exam is considered the reliable tool for assessment of TD.

ABNORMAL INVOLUNTARY MOVEMENT SCALE

This scale aids in the early detection of TD as well as providing a method for ongoing surveillance. This is a checklist that takes about 10 minutes to complete and uses a 5-point rating scale for recording scores for seven body areas: face, lips, jaw, tongue, upper extremities, lower extremities, and trunk. TD is considered less risky with the use of atypical antipsychotics but the risk is still present. The AIMS is used to obtain a baseline when possible before medication is started and the exam is to be repeated no less than every 6 months while the patient is on antipsychotic medications. It was developed in the 1970s. The website (www.psychiatrictimes.com/features-and-resources) provides an instructional video on how to administer and score the AIMS. The forms can also be downloaded in pdf format. It is suggested that you download and print out the AIMS Form and the AIMS Instructions before viewing the Instructional Video so that you will be able to follow along on www.psychiatrictimes.com/clinical-scales/movement_disorders/

OTHER SIDE EFFECTS OF CONSIDERATION

The high prevalence of medical problems in patients with schizophrenia calls for integration or better coordination of mental health and general medical services.

However, coordination between various services for this patient group and other patients with severe mental disorders is often inadequate. In addition, the widespread use of the atypical or second-generation antipsychotic medications has further contributed to the medical problems of patients. There needs to be awareness for proper monitoring of metabolic parameters and interventions to reduce the risk of future comorbidities (Mojtabai et al., 2009).

As the newer atypical antipsychotics have lost some of their initial glamour with the rising link to metabolic syndrome, many clinicians have adopted the belief that atypical antipsychotics are associated with weight gain, but older neuroleptics are not. Many also believe that some atypicals are weight neutral compared with other atypicals. The evidence from the European First Episode Schizophrenia Trial (EUFEST) debunked both beliefs by finding substantial weight gain with all antipsychotic drugs, old or new, after 1 year of treatment with haloperidol and several atypicals. Neither old antipsychotics, such as haloperidol, nor metabolically "benign" atypicals, such as ziprasidone, are exceptions (Nasrallah, 2011a).

With this type of risk profile, providers find themselves facing difficult choices in terms of the treatment for schizophrenia. The older, first-generation drugs have a higher risk of movement disorders, but the newer agents have higher risk of metabolic problems of weight gain, elevated labs of blood glucose, triglycerides, and cholesterol. The CATIE study showed 43% of patients with schizophrenia met the criteria for metabolic syndrome, many of whom had hypertension as one of the criteria (Nasrallah, 2011a).

Metabolic syndrome is a name for a group of risk factors that occur together which include dyslipidemia, obesity, hypertension, and type 2 diabetes. There are identifiable risk factors for diabetes or prediabetes which are not limited to, but may include a body mass index (BMI) greater than 25 kg/m, lack of physical activity, and first-degree relatives with diabetes, certain high-risk ethnic populations, hypertension, and so on. Despite awareness of these risk factors, expert guidelines do not always agree on the screening criteria.

In 2004, the American Diabetes Association (ADA), American Association of Clinical Endocrinologists (AACE), and North American Association for the Study of Obesity (NAASO) created consensus guidelines for screening psychiatric patients receiving atypical antipsychotics. These guidelines recommend regular screening in all patients taking atypical antipsychotic for weight gain and dyslipidemia, obtaining baseline values of fasting plasma glucose, rechecking fasting plasma glucose after 3 months, and then screening annually for diabetes or prediabetes (McCarron, 2009).

For those patients not on atypicals, screening is suggested for those patients under the age of 30. It is important to regularly review the risk factors for diabetes, and in those patients over age 30, it is suggested to screen annually for prediabetes/diabetes. Screening is done most simply by ordering a fasting plasma glucose test. For those patients with risk factors for developing diabetes or prediabetes while taking an atypical antipsychotic, it is suggested to consider an atypical with a lower risk of diabetes, that is, aripiprazole or ziprasidone (McCarron, 2009).

The practitioner should monitor weight and BMI during course of treatment. Counseling around nutrition and other weight-loss strategies can be part of an effective patient visit. Motivational interviewing can be useful in looking at barriers, motivation, and readiness. Reviewing information about proper diet, exercise, and avoidance of calorie-laden beverages should be included in the visit if indicated. Many practitioners find it useful to write a prescription for activity, indicating a frequency, time, and duration matched to the patient's stamina and tolerance.

There is a new online simulation instrument that can be used to predict how body weight will change and how long it will likely take a person to reach their weight goals. The tool is meant for general research but demonstrates how diet and exercise can alter metabolism over time. It can help counter patients' expectations about weight loss as the tool shows that body-weight response to a change of energy intake is slow, with an average of about 1 year. (Developed by National Institute of Health, available at www:http://bwsimulator.niddk.nih.gov)

Many chronically mentally ill patients smoke. It is not a new insight or revelation that cigarette smoking is increased in this patient population, but the estimated prevalence of smoking in schizophrenia patients in one meta-analysis was 62% (Mojtabai et al., 2009). The increased prevalence has been a topic of interest, both in terms of physiology and in terms of treatment effects.

The reasons for this high smoking prevalence in schizophrenic patients is thought to be at least partially related to enhancement of brain dopaminergic activity, which, in turn, results in behavioral reinforcement due to the stimulant effects. Smoking stimulates dopaminergic activity in the brain by inducing its release and inhibiting its degradation.

There is also evidence that cigarette smoking can reduce deficits relative to dopamine hypofunction in the prefrontal cortex (Sagud et al., 2009).

Use of caffeine and nicotine is often linked, with smokers using more caffeine due to interacting metabolic effects. Studies of neurobiology reveal evidence of specific brain changes in schizophrenia that are impacted by nicotine and caffeine and suggest self-medication effects (Williams & Gandhi, 2008). Smoking may be an attempt by schizophrenic patients to alleviate cognitive deficits and to reduce extrapyramidal side-effects induced by antipsychotic medication (Sagud et al., 2009).

Nicotine has been linked to lowering neuroleptic levels, improving parkinsonism, and possibly improving cognition (Goff, Henderson, & Amico, 1992). Nicotine seems to improve cognitive functions critically affected in schizophrenia, in particular sustained attention, focused attention, working memory, short-term memory, and recognition memory. Nicotine not only may improve information processing, but may reduce side effects of antipsychotic medications (Cattapan-Ludewig, Ludewig, Jaquenoud-Sirot, Etzensberger, & Hasler, 2005).

Smoking status is a significant factor that should be considered in assessment of neuroleptic dose requirements and neuroleptic side effects (Goff et al., 1992). Cigarette smoke increases the activity of cytochrome P450 (CYP) 1A2 enzymes, thus decreasing the concentration of many drugs, including clozapine and olanzapine (Sagud et al., 2009). Cigarette smokers receive significantly higher neuroleptic doses because of a smoking-induced increase in neuroleptic metabolism (Goff et al., 1992).

Clearly, the clinical effects of both of these substances are important. They may complicate the interpretation of schizophrenia symptoms and antipsychotic medication side effects. Given the high frequency of smoking in schizophrenic patients, clinicians need to check smoking status in each patient. Schizophrenic patients who smoke may require higher dosages of antipsychotics than nonsmokers. Conversely, upon smoking cessation, smokers may require a reduction in the dosage of antipsychotics (Sagud et al., 2009).

There are some potentially serious additional side effects that can occur with antipsychotic medications, including agranulocytosis, possible prolongation of QTc interval, impaired temperature regulations, and thus increased risk of heat stroke or hypothermia (Preston & Johnson, 2005). There were five patients in a state institution in New England who died in the summer of 1988 during a particularly extended heat wave. Although it was felt to be preventable as there were problems with ventilation and air conditioning, all five patients were on antipsychotic medications.

Hematologic complications can be a risk with patients on antipsychotics. These blood effects may include neutropenia, agranulocytosis, eosinophilia, thrombocytopenia, purpura, and anemia. Agranulocytosis is usually most closely linked with clozapine, carbamazepine, and typical antipsychotics. In addition, many antipsychotics are associated with increased risk of seizures. Among antipsychotics, clozapine and chlorpromazine carry the highest seizure risk (Casher et al., 2011).

Hypersalivation has been a well-documented side effect of clozapine and may affect nearly 30% of the patients taking the drug. As clozapine has anticholinergic properties that would be expected to reduce secretions, this hypersalivation is considered a paradoxical effect (Lamba & Ellison, 2011). Helping the patient find practical and useful solutions will aid in compliance.

Patients who chew gum during the day will increase their swallowing unconsciously. Recommend a sugarless gum to help avoid tooth decay and gum disease (Lamba & Ellison, 2011). Many patients report the drooling is particularly worse at night and this can be both annoying and frightening. Raising the head of the bed with additional pillows or risers under the legs may help as well as putting a towel over the pillow.

There are pharmacological interventions that may be offered to the patient with hypersalivation. These rely on counteracting clozapine's secretion-inducing effects by opposing muscarinic agonism, adrenergic antagonism, or both. Antimuscarinic medications such as benztropine, trihexyphenidyl, amitriptyline, or pirenzepine often are used (Lamba & Ellison, 2011).

Many of our patients do not have connections with other health care providers. Meeting the patients' multiple needs for medical care and substance abuse treatment can be especially difficult for practitioners working in solo practices or in small, single-specialty group practices. For these practitioners, the solution to this problem calls for the establishment of more meaningful links and better coordination with other providers or agencies (Mojtabai et al., 2009).

CONCERNS IN PRESCRIBING

Polypharmacy has become more the norm than not and psychiatric patients are more likely than other individuals to have more complex medication regimens (Casher et al., 2011). It is an obvious goal to employ prescribing practices that promote improved health and functioning with minimal side effects, but this can be challenging in this population. As a provider, it is essential to consider other mediations your patients may be taking and the potential drug interactions that may occur. It is a safe practice to inquire at every visit what medications the individual is taking, any change in medications from other providers, and any over-the-counter additions or herbal supplements. Inquiring about illicit substances, alcohol, and nicotine are equally important in considering the risks of an adverse drug effect. Supplying the patient with a medication card they can keep in a purse or wallet is one suggested strategy.

Although limited data support the practice, antiepileptics commonly are combined with antipsychotics to treat patients with schizophrenia. Clinicians who prescribe carbamazepine should recognize the potential for drug-drug interactions with antipsychotics (i.e., increased metabolism of antipsychotic caused by CYP3A4 induction) (Gerst, Smith, & Patel, 2010). Lithium is also commonly used with dopamine antagonists and is typically safe and effective, yet coadministration of higher doses of the antipsychotic may result in a synergistic effect. Lithium induced neurological side effects and neuroleptic extrapyramidal symptoms can occur. In rare circumstances, encephalopathy has been reported with this combination (Sadock & Sadock, 2008).

Drug diversion and drug misuse has unfortunately become problematic throughout our country. The misuse of benzodiazepines, stimulants, and opiates may be more intuitive, but the misuse of antipsychotics seems to be an emerging trend. The misuse of anticholinergic agents has been reported for well over 50 years as psychiatric patients have been reported to increase use of anticholinergics for their movement side effects as well as hallucinogenic effects. Although clinicians try to be vigilant about patients' misuse of psychoactive substances, recent case reports have been describing abuse of antipsychotics, particularly second-generation antipsychotics (Bogart & Ott, 2011).

Most published case reports of antipsychotic abuse involve quetiapine, although olanzapine has also been described. Patients have reported abusing quetiapine for its sedative, anxiolytic, and calming effects. The methods of quetiapine misuse included ingesting pills, inhaling crushed tablets, and injecting a solution of dissolved tablets. One patient reported snorting crushed quetiapine tablets combined with cocaine for "hallucinogenic" effects. "Q-ball" refers to a combination of cocaine and quetiapine.

Quetiapine and olanzapine have been used to treat cocaine and alcohol abuse, and work perhaps by decreasing the dopamine reward system response to substance use. Quetiapine's rapid dissociation from the dopamine receptor has been theorized to contribute to the drug's abuse potential, possibly through relatively lower potency and decreased residence time at the dopamine receptor. This mechanism may contribute to the drug's lower risk of EPS, making the drug easier to tolerate (Bogart & Ott, 2011).

Although outpatient misuse is more common, this practice is becoming more frequent in correctional settings. The reasons for misuse may be the same as with patients: to treat anxiety, to promote sleep, or to "get high." The clinician now must differentiate inmates who have legitimate psychiatric symptoms that require antipsychotic treatment from those who are malingering to obtain the drug (Bogart & Ott, 2011).

No matter what the substance involved, the clinician's goal is to help the patient reduce their use and continue along the continuum for recovery. If the patient is abusing their antipsychotic, there are many other treatment options. The clinician can opt to switch to another agent with less abuse potential, can prescribe a limited amount that can be monitored more closely, can opt to try depot preparations, or can increase the follow up to assess adherence. Motivational interviewing around use and other substance use strategies may also be offered to the patient.

TREATMENT: PSYCHOSOCIAL AND OTHERS

Comprehensive care for the individual with psychosis requires integrating a variety of perspectives. As schizophrenia and other psychotic disorders most likely occur from a combination of both biological and environmental influences on brain development, it would make sense that no one single treatment should be offered. To simply think of psychosis as a biological problem is too simplistic. Like many chronic conditions, "skills" are as equally as important as the "pills."

Although antipsychotic medications are key to control of symptoms, the psychosocial and rehabilitative treatments can improve the long-term functioning and course of recovery. The practice that simply dispenses a prescription will be marginal in success for recovery and forestalling relapse. A number of psychosocial treatments are available for persons with schizophrenia, including social skills training, CBT, cognitive remediation, and social cognition training.

Before exploring each one of these approaches, it is worthy to note and recognize the work of Gerald E.

Hogarty. Hogarty was a scholar and clinician whose career was dedicated to improving the lives of persons with schizophrenia through the development and research of psychosocial treatment approaches. This interest in psychosocial approaches for schizophrenia laid the groundwork that would guide future treatment development efforts: (a) that time is a key element in understanding the role of psychosocial treatments for schizophrenia, (b) such approaches are best developed on a platform of appropriate pharmacological treatment, and (c) that effective treatment could extend far beyond the prescription of medication (Eack, Schooler, & Ganguli, 2007).

One of his earlier works was major role therapy (MRT), an early precursor to clinical case management. MRT provided an atheoretical form of compassionate care that mobilized individual social casework and vocational rehabilitation for persons with schizophrenia returning to the community after hospitalization. MRT was pragmatic; its goals were based on the observation that individuals with schizophrenia were not fulfilling major life roles, and therefore, the approach attempted to provide resources and supports to address that problem (Eack et al., 2007).

When indicated, case management can be a critical aspect of a patient's treatment plan. Many patients with schizophrenia are at an increased risk of homelessness and associated adverse social health outcomes, such as victimization and sexually transmitted diseases. These patients often need the help of a case manager to negotiate the elaborate maze of social service organizations and to obtain housing and other needed social services (Mojtabai et al., 2009). Not every community has case management services and there are often funding restrictions, but case mangers help to coordinate the overall treatment with the patient. They can be invaluable in helping with compliance with appointments, providing a glimpse at how things are in the home, and connecting to other needed resources.

The Assertive Community Treatment program (ACT) was originally developed out of Madison, Wisconsin, in the 1970s. The model was targeted for an intensive care delivery system for patients with chronic mental illness. The model is made up of a multi-disciplinary team consisting of nurses, psychiatrists, social workers, case managers, and so on. All care is managed by the team and is staffed round the clock, seven days a week. The team is mobile and responds to the needs of the patients at the time, that is, seeing the patient in their home, delivering medications daily if indicated, and accompanying to appointments. ACT programs have been shown to lower the risk of rehospitalization and relapse but they are labor intensive and expensive to administer. There have been many cuts in these types of programs (Sadock & Sadock, 2008).

As has been discussed, the patient does not experience this illness in a vacuum. The chronicity of the illness, the usual young age of onset, in addition to the financial, emotional, and social implications certainly impacts not just the patient but those who are close to him. Support and psychoeducation regarding management of the illness needs to be offered to the patient and family alike.

Another of Hogarty's major contributions to the treatment of schizophrenia was the development of family psychoeducation, a psychosocial approach now widely accepted as one of the pillars of evidence-based treatment for this population. This approach to reduce stress within the family was developed as a promising method for preventing relapse among this population. He defined the problem of relapse in schizophrenia based upon a "core psychological deficit" that was manifested by sensitivity to intense stimuli and a biological susceptibility to stress. He linked this theoretical understanding of the pathogenesis of relapse in schizophrenia to emerging evidence that stress within the family environment (particularly those environments characterized by high levels of "expressed emotion" or criticism and emotional overinvolvement) was a substantial predictor of positive symptom exacerbations (Eack et al., 2007).

Psychoeducational Multifamily Groups (PMFG) is a treatment modality designed to help individuals with mental illness attain as rich and full participation in the usual life of the community as possible. The intervention focuses on informing families and supporters about mental illness, developing coping skills, solving problems, creating social supports, and developing an alliance between consumers, practitioners, and their families or supporters. Practitioners invite five to six consumers and their families to participate in a psychoeducation group that typically meets every other week for at least 6 months. *Family* is defined as anyone committed to the care and support of the person with mental illness. Consumers often ask a close friend or neighbor to be their support person in the group. Group meetings are structured to help people develop the skills needed to handle problems posed by mental illness.

Practitioners of all mental health disciplines—psychiatrists, psychologists, social workers, nurses and nurse practitioners, counselors, occupational therapists and licensed counselors—have proven to be remarkably capable of conducting this model of treatment. There is a manual and workbook available online for interested mental health practitioners and case managers wishing to learn and apply this approach to treatment and recovery.

EXHIBIT 10-8: SAMPLE TREATMENT PLAN FOR PSYCHOSIS

PROBLEM(S) (CHECK ALL THAT APPLY)	SHORT-TERM GOAL(S) AND OBJECTIVES	TARGET DATES	TREATMENT INTERVENTIONS (METHODS/FREQUENCY)
1. Mood-thought disturbance AEB: • Hallucinations • Confusion • Paranoia • Disorganization • Grandiosity • Suspicion • Suicidal thoughts • Homicidal thoughts • Aggressive behavior • Racing thoughts • Sense of being "taken over" • Social isolation • Inability to manage ADLs • Other	1. Pt will report mood stability and thought clarity AEB: • Sleeping 6–7 hours/night • No episodes of paranoia • Keeping scheduled appointments with providers • Maintaining his schedule of meetings, school, etc. • Abstaining from alcohol/marijuana • No isolating at home or ruminating excessively about health concerns • Taking medications as prescribed and reporting any concerns or side effects to treatment team • Ability to keep weekly wellness program, i.e., walking, gym, swimming, biking, healthy food plan • Utilizing strategies for stress management, i.e., music, exercise, AA/NA meetings • Other ___________________	3–6 months	1a. Medication management and monitoring by APRN of response to medication, assessment of any side effects, etc., bi-weekly until stable, then monthly and prn. 1b. Monthly and prn visits with APRN using CBT focus to assist with reality testing, management of symptoms. 1c. Support group 2x month for problem solving, psychoeducation, crisis management prn, and support. 1d. Case management to assist in community supports/needs. 1e. Vocational services to assist in goals of part-time employment, student services.
2. Potential for health problems and ongoing health maintenance	2. Pt will: • Keep routine, scheduled annual physical exams and see PCP as indicated for any health concerns. • Monitor bowel habits and track constipation (most likely due to clozapine) • Practice safety behaviors when indicated, use seatbelt, using helmet when on bike, hydration while exercising, avoid sun and heat exposure, etc. • Other	Annual and prn	

Long-Term Goals: (Pt driven) 1. "Continue good mental health with no hospitalizations or relapses. 2. Continue to pursue my music career, wherever it takes me. 3. Maintain my sobriety"

This treatment plan, its risks, and benefits have been explained to me. I understand and consent to this treatment plan. I have been offered a copy of this plan. ___accepted ___ declined.

______________________	___________	______________________	___________
Signature of Patient	Date	Signature of Clinician	Date/Time

The website is listed: www.nebhands.nebraska.edu/files/FamPsy_Workbook.pdf

Mental health professionals have adapted learning principles to treatment environments for years. There are a few overarching tenets that led to this logical merger. The first one being that psychiatric patients, including those with psychotic disorders like schizophrenia, exhibited behavioral excesses and deficits, as well as inappropriate behaviors that could be defined. These oddities or aberrations in social behavior could result in the individual being isolated or shunned by others. Ultimately, these behaviors would cause difficulties in the larger social world and would inhibit the individual from achieving personally desirable goals (Kern, Glynn, Horan, & Marder, 2009).

So, even if the etiology of a psychiatric illness and its concomitant problems proved to be biological, humans experiencing these illnesses are still social beings and their environment plays a role in shaping their behavior. Thus, their behavior is amenable to change using learning principles. A final tenet was that although symptoms such as hallucinations, delusions, and formal thought disorder were important aspects of the illness, social skills could be taught even in persons experiencing these symptoms (Kern et al., 2009).

This observation greatly expanded the range of possible social skills training interventions to include not only primary reinforcement but also behavioral demonstrations, role-playing, prompting, coaching, modeling, shaping, secondary reinforcement, and planned generalization training through out-of-session assignments. These techniques are all critical components of any effective social skills training program (Kern et al., 2009). These principles can be incorporated into an individual therapy plan with an aim at supporting any social and independent living skills and strategies for target symptoms.

Social skills training, which focuses on initiating and maintaining interpersonal relationships to better integrate patients into their communities, has also shown not just improved relationships, but the ability to improve function in patients with schizophrenia (MacDonald & Schulz, 2009). Groups, of course, have the added advantages of offering more opportunities for observational learning as well as providing a variety of persons with whom to practice the skills. Offering social skills training in group settings can also provide opportunities to bolster social support (Kern et al., 2009).

Similar to social skills training, there has been increasing work in the area of social cognition. The social and cognitive deficits remain the largest determinants of poor functional outcome in schizophrenia. Schizophrenia patients show substantial deficits in several aspects of social cognition, with impairments in the following: *affect perception,* such as perceiving facial and vocal expressions of emotion; *social perception,* including the ability to judge social cues and nonverbal gestures; *attributional style,* which refers to the way individuals characteristically explain the causes for positive and negative events in their lives; and *theory of mind,* the ability to understand that others have mental states that differ from one's own and the capacity to make correct inferences (Kern et al., 2009).

Cognitive therapy appears to be a valuable adjunct to pharmacotherapy and standard of care for patients with acute psychosis. The challenging and testing of delusions in a nonconfrontational manner can be extremely helpful for patients. CBT targets symptoms that may lead to improvements in social functioning and quality of life.

CBT is based on a cognitive model of psychopathology that proposes that biological factors are understood to be the cause of the initial diathesis or vulnerability to develop symptoms under stress, but faulty appraisals of these experiences are hypothesized to result in the development of the complete illness syndrome (Kern et al., 2009). CBT for schizophrenia adapts cognitive restructuring techniques originally developed for treating major depression. These techniques allow one to challenge, and ultimately shape, the meaning of various negative emotions or aberrant experiences into something less threatening (MacDonald & Schulz, 2009).

With more severe disorders such as psychosis, medication is seen as a necessary but insufficient treatment, insofar as it is not expected to fully correct faulty appraisals of internal experiences. These need to be targeted directly. Perceptions of events, rather than the events themselves, are seen as the key to emotional states and are selected as targets of treatment in the cognitive therapy model of psychotic symptoms. While the original work in CBT for psychosis targeted positive symptoms, greater attention has been recently paid to applying the cognitive model of psychosis to negative symptoms (Kern et al., 2009).

Cognitive remediation targets cognitive impairments that may lead to improvements in work and social functioning. Hogarty, again, can be credited for his pioneering work in this area. He began to examine the contributions of other factors to poor social adjustment and functional recovery from schizophrenia and this led to the development of cognitive enhancing therapy (CET), a unique integrated neuro-cognitive and social-cognitive remediation program for stabilized persons with schizophrenia (Eack et al., 2007).

Hogarty felt a cognitive rehabilitation approach was needed to "jump start" the arrested cognitive development in these areas seen among persons with schizophrenia.

The focus of CET is to broadly provide patients with enriched cognitive experiences through computer training and secondary socialization opportunities. The goal is that individuals will develop the social and nonsocial cognitive abilities needed to succeed in complex interpersonal interactions (Eack et al., 2007).

Hogarty's CET includes cognitive training plus group therapy. Treatment begins with computer-based cognitive exercises that focus on attention, memory, and problem solving (Kern et al., 2009). In addition, there are 45 group sessions that target social cognitive function emphasizing experiential learning (Perkins, 2011).

In contrast to cognition-enhancing approaches, compensatory approaches aim to bypass or "compensate" for cognitive impairments. These compensatory approaches directly target functional deficits but with consideration of the cognitive impairments that may impede or restrict training success. Cognitive adaptation training (CAT) is a compensatory cognitive remediation program that uses in-home environmental supports (e.g., alarms, signs, and checklists) and structure (e.g., reorganizing placement of belongings) to facilitate independent living in the home environment. CAT has been used to improve medication and appointment adherence, grooming and hygiene, care of living space, and leisure and social activities (Kern et al., 2009).

Other areas for treatment could include vocational rehabilitation and work-related supports, self-help groups, occupational therapy involvement, and any substance abuse programming that supports patients' recovery. It is important to emphasize to patients and families that medication is still needed for the psychotic condition and most likely will enable the patient to benefit more fully from participation in any psychosocial treatment programs. Those who remain on an antipsychotic have substantially lower risk of relapse.

Consistent with the paradigm shift in schizophrenia treatment from a focus on long-term disability to one focused on optimism and recovery, the ultimate goal of the Schizophrenia PORT has been to increase the use of evidence-based treatments in order to optimize outcomes by reducing illness symptoms and the disability and burden associated with the illness (Kreyenbuhl et al., 2010). The PORT benchmarks set not only evidence-based quality indicators for pharmacological, but for psychosocial treatments of schizophrenia as well. Exhibit 10-8 is an actual sample treatment plan for an individual with any psychotic disorder. It is certainly not exhaustive of all the target symptoms that may be addressed in this condition but it was unique to this client. He would develop somatic concerns which would be an early indicator of psychosis.

Psychosocial treatments are likely more beneficial in the later stages of illness when the acute symptoms have subsided. As health care reform and budget cuts loom nationally, the long-term impact of managed care on the clinical and social outcomes of the patients with schizophrenia remains to be fully appreciated (Mojtabai et al., 2009). Exhibit 10-9 is the 2009 Updated PORT Psychosocial Treatment Recommendations.

A recovery orientation to psychiatric illness holds that individuals are more than the sum of their symptoms and that recovery involves "a redefinition of one's illness as only one aspect of a multi-dimensional sense of self, capable of identifying, choosing, and pursuing personally meaningful goals and aspiration" (Kern et al., 2009). As the clinical treatment literature in psychotic disorders continues to evolve and expand, so will approaches in developing and updating clinical pathways and treatment guidelines. Each patient is unique in their struggle but following evidence-based practice will allow us the integration of the best available evidence for treatment of psychosis.

PATIENT EDUCATION

Patient empowerment is critical for the successful management of any chronic disease and the cornerstone of empowerment is knowledge. Education must be tailored to the patient's unique learning style and be geared to the patient's ability to engage in the process. Obviously, in sitting with an acute, agitated patient, a conversation about diagnosis and expected outcomes would be inappropriate. Information may be broken down into parts and shared over time, across multiple sessions. There are some clear points that should be part of any teaching plan and they are included in Exhibit 10-10.

EXHIBIT 10-9: UPDATED SCHIZOPHRENIA PORT PSYCHOSOCIAL TREATMENT RECOMMENDATIONS: 2009

TREATMENT	RECOMMENDATIONS
Assertive Community Treatment	Systems of care serving persons with schizophrenia should include a program of assertive community treatment. This intervention should be provided to individuals who are at risk for repeated hospitalizations or have recent homelessness. The key elements of assertive community treatment include a multi-disciplinary team including a medication prescriber, a shared caseload among team members, direct service provision by team members, a high frequency of patient contact, low patient to staff ratios, and outreach to patients in the community. Assertive Community Treatment has been found to significantly reduce hospitalizations and homelessness among individuals with schizophrenia.
Supported Employment	Recommendation: Any person with schizophrenia who has the goal of employment should be offered supported employment to assist them in both obtaining and maintaining competitive employment. The key elements of supported employment include individually tailored job development, rapid job search, the availability of ongoing job supports, and the integration of vocational and mental health services.
Skills Training	Recommendation: Individuals with schizophrenia who have deficits in skills that are needed for everyday activities should be offered skills training in order to improve social interactions, independent living, and other outcomes that have clear relevance to community functioning.
Cognitive Behavioral Therapy	Recommendation: Persons with schizophrenia who have persistent psychotic symptoms while receiving adequate pharmacotherapy should be offered adjunctive cognitive behaviorally oriented psychotherapy to reduce the severity of symptoms. The therapy may be provided in either a group or an individual format and should be approximately 4 to 9 months in duration. The key elements of this intervention include the collaborative identification of target problems or symptoms and the development of specific cognitive and behavioral strategies to cope with these problems or symptoms.
Family-Based Services	Recommendation: Persons with schizophrenia who have ongoing contact with their families, including relatives and significant others, should be offered a family intervention that lasts 6 to 9 months. Interventions that last 6 to 9 months have been found to significantly reduce rates of relapse and rehospitalization. Possible benefits for patients include reduced psychiatric symptoms, improved treatment adherence, improved functional and vocational status, and greater satisfaction with treatment. Positive family outcomes include reduced family burden and increased satisfaction with family relationships.
Psychosocial Interventions for Alcohol and Substance Use Disorders	Recommendation: The key elements of treatment for alcohol or drug use disorders for persons with schizophrenia include motivational enhancement and behavioral strategies that focus on engagement in treatment, coping skills training, relapse prevention training, and its delivery in a service model that is integrated with mental health care.
Psychosocial Interventions for Weight Management	Recommendation: Individuals with schizophrenia who are overweight (BMI 25.0–29.9) or obese (BMI greater than or equal to 30.0) should be offered a psychosocial weight loss intervention that is at least 3 months in duration to promote weight loss. The key elements of psychosocial interventions for weight loss include psychoeducation focused on nutritional counseling, caloric expenditure, and portion control; behavioral self-management including motivational enhancement; goal setting; regular weigh-ins; self-monitoring of daily food and activity levels; and dietary and physical activity modifications.

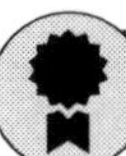

EXHIBIT 10-10: PATIENT EDUCATION POINTS

1. Diagnosis, definition of psychosis, schizophrenia
2. Establishment of a medical illness, not character or personality disorder
3. Review any common myths or incorrect beliefs about the disorder
4. Explanation of common symptoms, attention to the patients unique symptoms
5. Identification of "early warning signs" and a response plan, that is, "two nights of no sleep, call NP."
6. Strategies to deal with voices, paranoia, and so on
   May include: reality test with self or trusted others, distraction, sleep, music, and so on
7. Medications
   To include: how they work, side effects to report, compliance concerns, risks associated with relapse/nonadherence, nonaddictive, and so on
8. Cautions to consider from medications:
   - Careful in sun and heat, wear sunscreen, hats, sunglasses.
   - Avoid exposure to extreme heat and humidity as antipsychotics affect the body's ability to regulate temperature.
9. Impact of substance use on symptoms, prognosis, and medication effects
10. Importance of family support and education re: expectations
11. Resources/supports
    May include community consumer groups, NAMI, other support groups, case management services, community-based clinical teams, visiting nurse, and so on

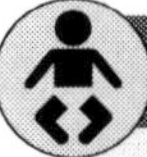

PEDIATRIC POINTERS

Childhood mental disorders are actually common. The prevalence has been estimated that 5% to 15% of children will experience a psychiatric disturbance that is sufficiently severe to require treatment or to impair their functioning during the course of a year (Andreasen & Black, 2006). Dealing with children and adolescents is a unique and challenging area of psychiatric mental health nursing. Not only does the provider need to be mindful of the common psychiatric conditions that can arise during this time, one needs to be cognizant of the appropriate maturational processes and normal growth and development. When assessing children, the clinician must have a good sense of what is normal for a given child at a given age as well as an awareness that norms may vary widely. In addition, like adults, there needs to be a keen awareness of the more common medical conditions that could mimic or pass for psychiatric illness. The need to rule out any medical conditions, any substance use, or any other organic causes still applies.

While there are some similarities in dealing with children and adults, there are some obvious differences. The type of assessment and therapy will vary depending on the age of the child. A young child most likely will not have the verbal or reasoning skills to participate in routine assessment and would respond better to play therapy versus verbal therapy. How one might engage and build rapport with a teenager would be different than establishing a relationship with a toddler. In assessing children, it is critical to have the information and involvement of others. This may include family, teachers, care providers, and other medical personnel.

Although the child may be the "identified patient," this can be a sensitive area as it may soon become clear that there are serious problems with the parents or within the family system. In this scenario, the provider should suggest treatment of the parents or family

(Continued)

PEDIATRIC POINTERS (*Continued*)

therapy. Another potential problem area is that the child is being asked to be seen at the request of the care providers or the school system and the parents do not accept or recognize a mental health disorder. This obviously requires tact and sensitivity for all in trying to help the child reach improved mental health and functioning. If a mental health disorder is present, and particularly a serious condition that may be a lifelong condition, it is a disservice to the child and family to not be honest and present unrealistic expectations. If the child has schizophrenia or bipolar disorder, they will not "outgrow" it and will need guidance for management.

Several adult disorders may have their first onset during childhood or adolescence. Common examples are schizophrenia, major depression, and bipolar disorder. Although there may be differences in presentation and the symptoms may be less than clear cut, children with these disorders meet the criteria that have been defined for adults.

Schizophrenia often presents initially during adolescence, but in rare instances the onset is during childhood. Childhood schizophrenia has been estimated to be present at a rate of .5 per 1,000. The prevalence increases after puberty, approaching adult levels in late adolescence (Stoudemire, 1990). Neurodevelopmental damage seems to be greater in childhood schizophrenia than in the adult-onset type. Most schizophrenic children show delays in language and other functions long before their psychotic symptoms (hallucinations, delusions, and disordered thinking) appear, usually at age seven or later. In the first years of life, about 30% of these children have transient symptoms of pervasive developmental disorder, such as rocking, posturing, and arm flapping (Mental Health America, 2011).

Schizophrenia in adolescence often begins insidiously; examples may be withdrawal from usual interests and friends, a change in personal hygiene, and a decrease in performance in school. There can also be the acute condition where the individual experiences the "psychotic break," but it is rare there were not hints or changes in the previous months. In adolescence, boys seem to be more vulnerable to acute dystonic reactions than adult patients, so prophylactic antiparkinsonian medication may be indicated. Weight gain may be problematic with the long-term use of the low-potency neuroleptics so parent and patient education on nutrition, activity, and monitoring of this is essential. Weight gain can impact the child's self-esteem and body image, but further, can contribute to other more chronic health conditions like diabetes, hypertension, and heart disease.

Schizophrenia may be particularly difficult to distinguish from depression and other psychiatric disorders. A challenge in assessing childhood schizophrenia involves determining the difference between normal childhood fantasies and frank delusions and hallucinations. Additionally, disorganized speech and behavior must be distinguished from abnormalities of speech and behavior that might be due to developmental slowness or mental retardation (Andreasen & Black, 2006). Visual hallucinations are more common in children than in adults. Acute hallucinations are not uncommon in children, resulting from acute phobic reactions, physical illness with fever or metabolic aberration, or medications.

Early diagnosis and medical treatment are important. Many treatments are available including medications, psychotherapies, social skills treatments, cognitive therapies, group therapies, and more. The therapy is based on the child's diagnosis and individual presenting needs. The best outcome is obtained with a treatment program that incorporates multiple methods of intervention. Hospitalization and/or long-term residential treatment may be needed. Currently, the FDA approves the use of two second-generation drugs in children ages 13 to 17, risperidone (Risperdal) and aripiprazole (Abilify).

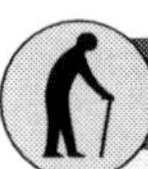

AGING ALERTS

Prevalence data for mental health disorders in elderly persons vary widely, but a conservative estimate suggests 25% have significant psychiatric symptoms (Sadock & Sadock, 2008). There is a higher risk for suicide in this population, particularly for white men older than age 65. Development of schizophrenia is rare in the patient over age 65, but psychosis can and does appear.

Although there are many patients who will achieve stability in symptoms later in life, there is a late onset schizophrenia condition. This is more common in women and can occur after age 45. The presentation is more often the paranoid type. Delusional disorder can also occur later in life and will most likely present as paranoid-persecutory type. Having worked with a woman who became convinced late in life that her husband was going to harm her, the implications of the delusion on the family was devastating. The adult children had to come to terms with their parents separating after a long and healthy marriage.

Pharmacology in the older patient requires an appreciation of the aging process, the existence of other medical conditions and medications, and the social factors related to aging. Most are familiar with the saying, "start low and go slow" with the elderly population. There are many aspects of the aging body that makes one sensitive to medications: slower metabolism, decreased receptor sensitivity, decreased bowel motility, increase in body fat relative to body water, and decreased liver and kidney clearance. Due to these changes, care must be given to risk for falls, delirium or confusion, sedation, orthostatic hypotension, constipation, and toxicity of the agents.

The older patient is often on many medications for numerous medical conditions. This can create a high-risk situation for drug-drug interactions. Doing a careful medication history and getting informed consents to coordinate care with other providers is essential. Asking the individual how they actually take their medication is important as it is not uncommon for the older adult to take their medications other than as prescribed. This may be due to side effects, beliefs about the dose being too high or too low, financial concerns, and so on. There are many examples: the woman who had a large co-pay and took her aripiprazole every other day or the gentleman who felt the Seroquel was too sedating and cut the dose in half. Verifying their regime, how they track use (use of caddy, what system to "remember," etc.), and how they maintain a current medication list are points to discuss in the visit.

SUMMARY POINTS: PSYCHOSIS

1. Psychosis is not actually a specific disease but a symptom where the individual has a loss of contact with reality.
2. Although psychosis can occur with a relatively rapid onset of serious symptoms, just as often, severe mental illness can begin with gradual, more insidious onset of symptoms.
3. Psychotic symptoms should be treated aggressively with antipsychotic treatment, regardless of the cause of the psychosis.
4. Schizophrenia is a brain disease where the clinical presentation reflects impairments in areas of thinking and cognition. It is a chronic and relapsing disorder.
5. As schizophrenia still is believed to have many possible etiologies, it is also true that the disease has a heterogeneous outcome.
6. Psychotic illness continues to have many misconceptions and myths surrounding it. There remains much fear, stigma, and stereotyping around the concept of psychosis. Nurses are in an excellent position to help educate around these disorders and to help destigmatize these ideas.
7. Suicide is the leading cause of premature death among people with schizophrenia.
8. There are no laboratory tests yet that can confirm a diagnosis of schizophrenia, so we rely on the assessment and the presence of a constellation of symptoms and factors.

9. Given the advances in biological psychiatry, treatments of mental health disorders have evolved with a more holistic biopsychosocial perspective.
10. Although psychopharmacology is a foundation of the treatment for psychotic disorders, there are other treatment modalities to be integrated for a comprehensive treatment plan.
    - It has been well demonstrated that the most effective treatment for schizophrenia involves a combination of neuroleptic medication and psychosocial treatment modalities.
11. Treatment approaches will vary to some degree based on the timing and setting of the patient's presentation.
12. An adequate trial of an antipsychotic agent should include 4 to 6 weeks of the full dose to target active symptoms with second-generation antipsychotics as the first-line therapy.
13. IM medication can be used with patients who are agitated, uncooperative, or have a history of problems with compliance.
14. Family therapy is important and families should be offered education around chronic illness management. Support may also be found through local chapters of the National Alliance on Mental Illness (NAMI), 2011.

RESOURCES TO RECOMMEND TO PATIENTS AND FAMILIES

ORGANIZATIONS

National Alliance on Mental Illness (NAMI): www.nami.org
Since its inception in 1979, NAMI has been dedicated to improving the lives of individuals and families affected by mental illness. It has established itself as the most formidable grassroots mental health advocacy organization in the country.

National Institute of Mental Health (NIMH): www.nimh.nih.gov
The mission of NIMH is to transform the understanding and treatment of mental illnesses through basic and clinical research, paving the way for prevention, recovery, and cure.

Choices in Recovery: www.choicesinrecovery.com
A website about the mental health recovery process—living a full, productive life after a diagnosis of schizophrenia, schizoaffective disorder, or bipolar 1 disorder. Advertised as "If you love or care for someone who lives with one of these conditions, we'd like to help you too."

BOOKS

How to Live With a Mentally Ill Person: A Handbook of Day-to-Day Strategies (1996) by C. Adamec and D. J. Jaffe

I Am Not Sick, I Don't Need Help! How to Help Someone With Mental Illness Accept Treatment (10th Anniversary ed.) (2010) by X. Amador

100 Questions and Answers About Schizophrenia: Painful Minds (2nd ed.) (2011) by L. E. DeLisi

Recovered, Not Cured: A Journey Through Schizophrenia (2003) by R. McLean

Surviving Schizophrenia: A Manual for Families, Consumers, and Providers (5th ed.) (2006) by E. F. Torrey

WEBSITES

www.psychiatryfindit.com
www.schizophrenia.com
www.adult-schizophrenia.com
www. treat-schizophrenia.com
www.ncbi.nlm.nih.gov/pubmed
www.micromedex.com

REFERENCES

Adamec, C., & Jaffe, D. J. (1996) *How to live with a mentally ill person: A handbook of day-to-day strategies*. Hoboken, NJ: Wiley.

Addington, D., Addington, J., & Maticka-Tyndale, E. (1993). Assessing depression in schizophrenia: The calgary depression scale. *British Journal of Psychiatry, 163*(Suppl. 22), S39–S44.

AGREE II next steps consortium. (2011). *Agree II instrument. European centre for disease prevention and control. Evidence-based methodologies for public health—how to assess the best available evidence when time is limited and there is lack of sound evidence.* Stockholm, Sweden: ECDC. Retrieved from http://www.agreetrust.org/?o=1029

Amador, X. (2010). *I am not sick, I don't need help! How to help someone with mental illness accept treatment* (10th Anniversary ed.). Peconic, NY: Vida Books.

American Psychiatric Association. (2000). *Diagnostic and statistical manual of mental disorders* (IV-R ed.). Washington, DC: Author.

American Psychiatric Association. (2006). *Practice guidelines for treating psychiatric disorders: Compendium*. Arlington, VA: Author.

Andreasen, N. C., & Black, W. (2006). *Introductory textbook of psychiatry* (4th ed.). Arlington, VA: American Psychiatric Publishing.

Barbato, A. (2011). *Nations for Mental Health. Schizophrenia and Public Health.* Retrieved from http://www.who.int/mental_health/media/en/55.pdf

Barnes, R. E., & the Schizophrenia Consensus Group of the British Association for Psychopharmacology. (2011). Evidence-based guidelines for the pharmacological treatment of schizophrenia: Recommendations from the British Association for Psychopharmacology. *Psychopharmacology, 25*(5), 567–620.

Bezchlibnyk-Butler, K. Z., & Jeffries, J. J. (2007). *Clinical handbook of psychotropic drugs* (17th ed.). Ashland, OH: Hogrefe Publishing.

Bogart, G. T., & Ott, C. A. (2011). Abuse of second generation antipsychotics: What prescribers need to know. *Current Psychiatry, 10*(5), 77–79.

Boyer, E. W., & Shannon, M. (2005). The serotonin syndrome. *New England Journal of Medicine, 352*, 1112–1120.

Burt, V., & Hendrick, V. (1997). *Concise guide to women's mental health.* Washington, DC: American Psychiatric Press.

Caroff, S. N., Miller, D. M., Dhopesh, V., & Campbell, E. C. (2011). Is there a rational management strategy for tardive dyskinesia? *Current Psychiatry, 10*(10), 23–32.

Casher, M. I., Bostwick, J., & Yu, M. (2011). How to prevent adverse drug events. *Current Psychiatry, 10*(7), 54–64.

Cattapan-Ludewig, K., Ludewig, S., Jaquenoud-Sirot, E., Etzensberger, M., & Hasler, F. (2005). Why do schizophrenic patients smoke? *Nervenarzt, 76*(3), 287–294.

Citrome, L. (2011a). Neurochemical models of schizophrenia: Transcending dopamine. *Current Psychiatry, 10*(Suppl. 9), S10–S14.

Citrome, L. (2011b). Treatment-resistant schizophrenia: What can we do about it? *Current Psychiatry, 10*(6), 53–59.

Cytochrome P450 drug interaction table. Retrieved from www.drug-interactions.com.

DeLisi, L. E. (2011). *100 questions and answers about schizophrenia: Painful minds* (2nd ed.). Sudbury, MA: Jones & Bartlett.

Eack, S. M., Schooler, N. R., & Ganguli, R. (2007). Gerald E. Hogarty (1935–2006): Combining science and humanism to improve the care of persons with schizophrenia. *Schizophrenia Bulletin, 35*(5), 1056–1062.

Foster, A., Sheehan, L., & Johns, L. (2011). Promoting treatment adherence in patients with bipolar disorder. *Current Psychiatry, 10*(7), 45–52.

Freudenreich, O., Kontos, N., & Querques, J. (2011). The ABCs of estimating adherence to antipsychotics. *Current Psychiatry, 10*(6), 90.

Fujii, D., & Ahmed, I. (2007). *The spectrum of mood disorders: Neurobiology, etiology, and pathogenesis.* New York, NY: Cambridge University Press.

Fusar-Poli, P., & Politi, P. (2008). Paul Eugen Bleuler and the birth of schizophrenia (1908). *American Journal of Psychiatry, 165*(11), 1407.

Gerst, T., Smith, T., & Patel, N. (2010). Antiepileptics for psychiatric illness: Finding the right match. *Current Psychiatry, 9*(12), 51–66.

Goff, D. C., Henderson, D. C., & Amico, E. (1992). Cigarette smoking in schizophrenia: Relationship to psychopathology and medication side effects. *American Journal of Psychiatry, 149*, 1189–1194.

Hor, K., & Taylor, M. (2010). Suicide and schizophrenia: A systematic review of rates and risk factors. *Journal of Psychopharmacology, 24*(4), 81–90.

Janicak, P. G., & Sadek, H. S. (1996). Psychopharmacotherapy for acute and recurrent psychotic disorders. *Psychiatric Annals, 26*(2), 68–77.

Jenkins, J. H., & Barrett, R. J. (2004). *Schizophrenia, culture and subjectivity: The edge of experience.* New York, NY: Cambridge University Press.

Kasckow, J., Felmet, K., & Zisook, S. (2011). Managing suicide risk in patients with schizophrenia. *CNS Drugs, 25*(2), 129–143.

Kay, S. R., Fiszbein, A., & Opler, L. A. (1987). The positive and negative syndrome scale for schizophrenia. *Schizophrenia Bulletin, 13*(2), 261–276.

Keith, S. J. (2006). Are we still talking to our patients with schizophrenia? *American Journal of Psychiatry, 163*(3), 362–364.

Keltner, N. L., Folks, D. G., Palmer, C. A., & Powers, R. E. (1998). *Psychobiological foundations of psychiatric care.* St. Louis, MO: Mosby-Year Book.

Kern, R. S., Glynn, S. M., Horan, W. P., & Marder, S. R. (2009). Psychosocial treatments to promote functional recovery in schizophrenia. *Schizophrenia Bulletin, 35*(2), 347–361.

Knesper, D. J., Riba, M. B., & Schwenk, T. L. (1997). *Primary Care Psychiatry.* Philadelphia, PA: W. B. Saunders Company.

Kreyenbuhl, J., Buchanan, R. W., Dickerson, F. B., Dixon, L. B. (2010). The Schizophrenia Patient Outcomes Research Team (PORT); updated treatment recommendations 2009. *Schizophrenia Bull, 36* (1) 94–103. Doi:10.1093/schbul/sbp130.

Lamba, G., & Ellison, J. M. (2011). Reducing clozapine induced hypersalivation. *Current Psychiatry, 10*(10), 77–78.

Louie, K. B. (1996). Cultural issues in psychiatric mental health nursing. In S. Lego (Ed.), *Psychiatric nursing: A comprehensive reference* (pp. 571–577). Philadelphia, PA: Lippincott-Raven Publishers.

MacDonald, A. W., & Schulz, S. C. (2009). What we know: Findings that every theory of schizophrenia should explain. *Schizophrenia Bulletin, 35*(3), 493–508.

Maier, J. (2011). Maine voices: Recognizing and treating mental illness may save young lives. *Portland Press Herald*, A10.

Maletic, V. (2011) Community Forum of Treating the Whole Patient: Integrating Mind, Body Connection into Mental Health Care, July 1, 2011http://www.cmellc.com/Home/TreatingtheWholePatient/articleType/ArticleView/articleId/4806/Hallucinations-in-Schizophrenia/

Maxmen, J. S., & Ward, G. (1995). *Essential psychopathology and its treatment* (2nd ed.). New York, NY: Norton.

McCarron, R. M. (2009). Diabetes screening: Which patients, what tests, and how often? *Current Psychiatry, 8*(3), 19–23.

McFarlane, W. R. (2002). *Multifamily groups in the treatment of severe psychiatric disorders.* New York, NY: Guilford.

McLean, R. (2003). *Recovered, not cured: A journey through schizophrenia.* Crows Nest, Australia: Allen & Unwin.

Mental Health America. (2011). *Schizophrenia in children.* Retrieved from http://www.nmha.org/index.cfm?objectId=C7DF8F81-1372-4D20-C84C5539FAB14576, 12/22/2011

Miller, A. L., Chiles, J. A., Chiles, J. K., Crismon, M. L., Rush, A. J., & Shon, S. P. (1999). The Texas medication algorithm project (TMAP) schizophrenia algorithms. *Journal of Clincial Psychiatry, 60*, 649–657.

Mojtabai, R., Fochtmann, L., Chang, S., Kotov, R., Craig, T. J., & Bromet, E. (2009). Unmet need for mental health care in schizophrenia: An overview of literature and new data from a first admission study. *Schizophrenia Bulletin, 35*(4), 679–695.

Moore, T. A., Buchanan, R. W., Buckley, P. F., Chiles, J. A., Conley, R. R., Crismon, M. L.,... Miller, A. L. (2007). The Texas medication algorithm project antipsychotic algorithm for schizophrenia: 2006 update. *Journal of Clinical Psychiatry, 68*(11), 1751–1762.

Murray, R. B., & Huelskoetter, M. N. (1983). *Psychiatric/mental health nursing: Giving emotional care.* Englewood Cliffs, NJ: Prentice Hall.

Nasrallah, H. A. (1986). Cerebral hemispheric asymmetries and interhemispheric integration in schizophrenia. In H. A. Nasrallah & D. R. Weinberger (Eds.), *Neurology of Schizophrenia: Handbook of Schizophrenia* (pp. 157–174). New York, NY: Elsevier.

Nasrallah, H. A. (2010). Psychiatric futurology. *Current Psychiatry, 9*(7), 9–10.

Nasrallah, H. A. (2011a). Folie en masse! it's so tempting to drink the kool-aid. *Current Psychiatry, 10*(3), 12.

Nasrallah, H. A. (2011b). The primary and secondary symptoms of schizophrenia: Current and future management. A bridge to the future; redefining the scientific paradigm in the treatment of schizophrenia. *Current Psychiatry, 10*(Suppl. 9), S4–S9.

National Alliance on Mental Illness. (2011). *Mental illness: Schizophrenia*. Arlington, TX: Author. Retrieved from http://www.nami.org/Content/NavigationMenu/Mental_Illnesses/Schizophrenia9/Anosognosia_Fact_Sheet.htm

NIMH. (2011). *Health topics*: *Schizophrenia*. Bethesda, MD: Author. Retrieved from http://www.nimh.nih.gov/health/topics/schizophrenia/raise/index.shtml

NIMH, Science Writing, Press and Dissemination Branch. (2011). Schizophrenia. Bethesda, MD: Author. Retrieved from http://www.nimh.nih.gov/health/publications/schizophrenia/complete-index.shtml

NIMH, Centre for Addiction and Mental Health (2012). Antipsychotic polypharmacy in schizophrenia. Retrieved from http:///clinicaltrials.gov/ct2/show/NCT00493233

Perkins, D.O. (2011) Efficacy of available antipsychotics in schizophrenia. *Current Psychiatry, 10*(9), S15–S19.

Piccinelli, M., & Homen, F. G. (1997). *Gender differences in the epidemiology of affective disorders and schizophrenia*. Geneva, Switzerland: World Health Organization. Retrieved from http://www.who.int/mental_health/media/en/54.pdf

Preston, J., & Johnson, J. (2005). *Clinical psychopharmacology made ridiculously simple* (5th ed.). Miami, FL: MedMaster.

Rose, D., Stuart, B., Hardy, K., & Loewy, R. (2010). Re-envisioning psychosis: A new language for clinical practice. *Current Psychiatry, 9*(10), 23–28.

Sadock, B. J., & Sadock, V. A. (2008). *Kaplan and Sadock's concise textbook of clinical psychiatry* (3rd ed.). Philadelphia, PA: Lippincott Williams & Wilkins.

Sagud, M., Mihaljević-Peles, A., Mück-Seler, D., Pivac, N., Vuksan-Cusa, B., Brataljenović, T., & Jakovljević, M. (2009). Smoking and schizophrenia. *Psychiatric Danub, 21*(3), 371–375.

Seltzer, A., & Hoffman, B. F. (1980). Drug compliance of the psychiatric patient. *Canadian Family Physician, 26*(5), 725–727.

Stoudemire, A. (1990). *Clinical psychiatry for medical students.* Philadelphia, PA: J. B. Lippincott.

Strawn, J. R., Keck, P. E., & Caroff, S. N. (2008). Neuroleptic malignant syndrome: Answers to 6 tough questions. *Current Psychiatry, 7*(1), 95–100.

Swartz, M. S., Stroup, T. S., McEvoy, J. P., Davis, S. M., Rosenheck, R. A., Keefe, R. S., Hsiao, J. K., & Lieberman, J. A., (2008). What CATIE found: Results from the schizophrenia trial. *Psychiatry Services, 59*(5), 500–506.

Talbot, J., Ballenger, J., Frances, R., Lydiard, R., Meltzer, H., Schowalter, J. E., & Tasman, A. (1998). *The yearbook of psychiatry and applied mental health.* St. Louis, MO: Mosby.

Teicher, M. H., & Glod, C. A. (1990). Neuroleptic drugs: Indications and guidelines for their rational use in children and adolescents. *Journal of Child and Adolescent Psychopharmacology, 1*(1), 33–56.

Torrey, E. F. (2006). *Surviving schizophrenia: A manual for families, consumers, and providers* (5th ed.). New York, NY: Quill (Harper Collins Publishers).

Williams, J. M., & Gandhi, K. K. (2008). Use of caffeine and nicotine in people with schizophrenia. *Current Drug Abuse Review, 1*(2), 155–161.

Wood, S. J., Berger, G. E., Lambert, M., Conus, P., Velakoulis, D., Stuart, G. W.,... Pantelis, C. (2006). Prediction of functional outcome 18 months after a first psychotic episode. *Archives of General Psychiatry, 63*, 969–976.

Woods, S. W., Saksa, J. R., Baker, C. B., Cohen, S. J., & Tek, C. (2008). Effects of levetiracetam on tardive dyskinesia: A randomized, double-blind, placebo-controlled study. *Journal of Clinical Psychiatry, 69*(4), 546–554.

World Health Organization, Mental Health: Disorders Management. (2011). Schizophrenia. Retrieved from http://www.who.int/mental_health/management/schizophrenia/en

Wu, E., Birnbaum, H. G., Shi, L., Ball, D. E., Kessler, R. C., Moulis, M., & Aggarwal, J. (2005). The economic burden of schizophrenia in the United States in 2002. *Journal of Clinical Psychiatry, 66*(9), 1122–1129.

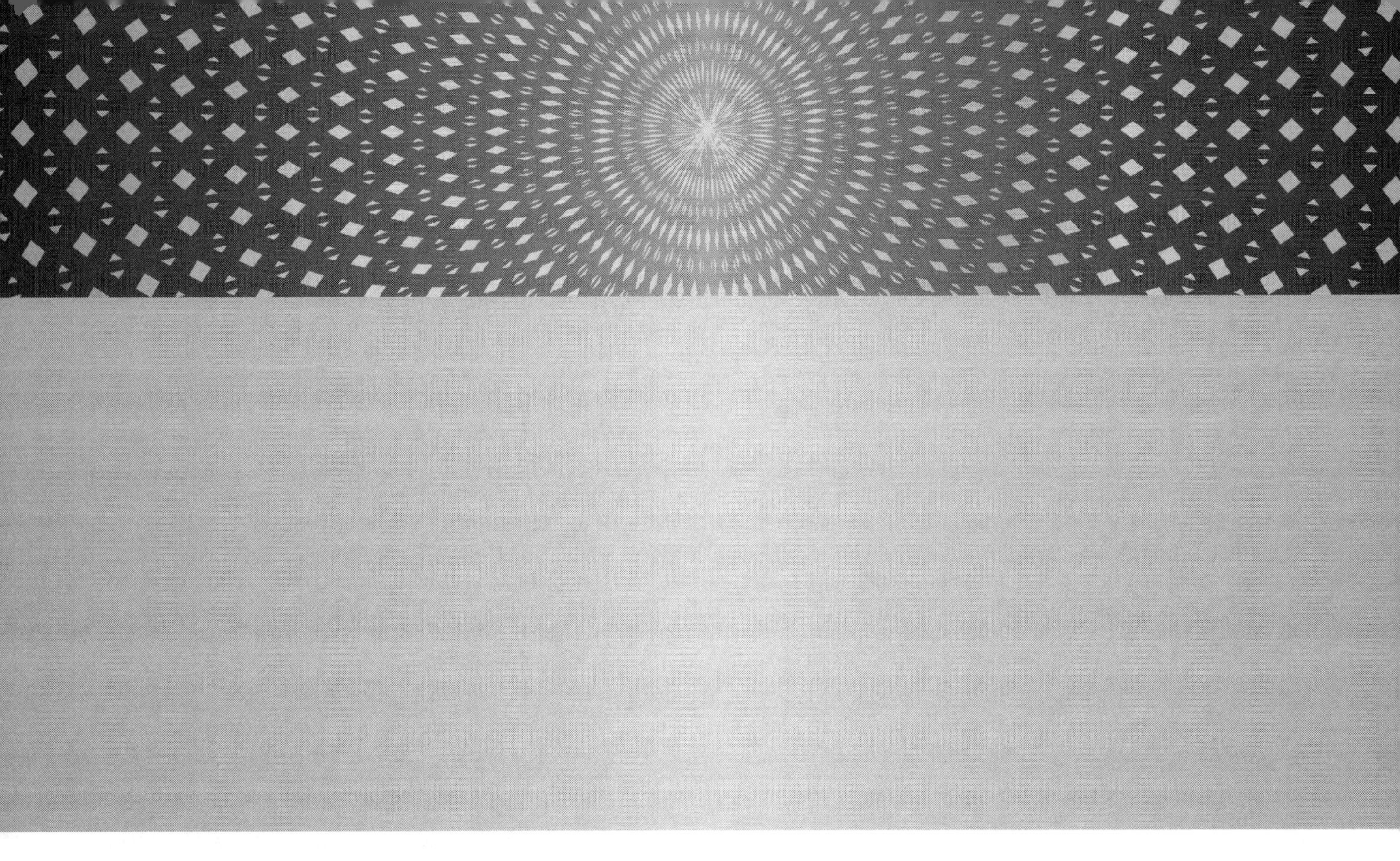

CHAPTER CONTENTS

Advanced practice psychiatric nurses (PMH-APRNs) are frequently called upon to manage the care of clients with presenting complaints of sleep disturbance or of clients other mental health issues who have comorbid sleep disturbance. The management of sleep disturbance requires basic knowledge of normal sleep, age-related changes in sleep, interrelationships of sleep with common psychiatric disorders, sleep assessment methods and findings, and recommended treatment modalities. From a holistic perspective, the relationship of a client's psychological and sleep symptoms with medical comorbidities is also relevant to comprehensive care. For example, insomnia and obstructive sleep apnea (OSA) increase the risk of hypertension, which has major implications for cardiac health. Although the underlying pathophysiology of sleep and health interactions is still emerging, it is clear that sleep is a dynamic process, with behavioral and biological aspects that both stimulate and respond to changes in health.

The science of sleep is relatively new. Polysomnography (PSG), developed in the 1970s, revolutionalized sleep science by allowing the documentation of actual electroencephalographic changes during sleep with distinction between normal and abnormal sleep patterns and events (Dement, 2011). Standardization of sleep nomenclature and dissemination of sleep education, practice guidelines, and research by professional organizations such as the American Academy of Sleep Medicine (AASM) and the Sleep Research Society (SRS) further established sleep as

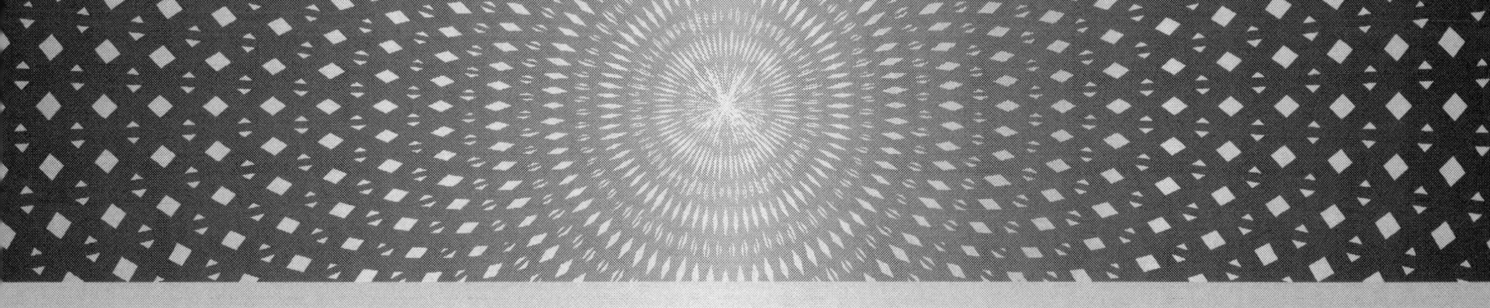

CHAPTER 11

Integrative Management of Sleep Disturbances

Carol Enderlin, Martha E. Kuhlmann, Melodee Harris, Matthew Hadley, Arlene Sullivan, Karen M. Rose, and Anita Mitchell

a health care specialty. A working knowledge of standard sleep terminology is a critical first step in analyzing current sleep literature, documenting sleep assessment data, and understanding feedback from sleep specialists to manage client care. Common terms pertaining to sleep are briefly defined in Exhibit 11-1.

NORMAL SLEEP ARCHITECTURE

Normal sleep is composed of nonrapid eye movement (NREM) and rapid eye movement (REM) sleep, which alternate in four to six 90 to 110 minute cycles per night. NREM sleep consists of progressively deepening sleep with intact muscle tone and decreasing responsiveness to stimuli across four stages. Stages 1 and 2 are considered light sleep, and Stages 3 and 4 are referred to as slow wave or deep sleep. In contrast, REM sleep includes dreaming and is characterized by variable responsiveness to stimuli with voluntary muscle paralysis. Autonomic activity during REM sleep is variable, with increased vital signs (heart rate, respiration, blood pressure increased), increased cerebral blood flow, and decreased temperature regulation. Total sleep time is composed of 75% to 80% NREM sleep (2% to 5% Stage 1 sleep, 45% to 55% Stage 2 sleep, 13% to 23% Stage 3 and 4 sleep), and 20% to 25% REM sleep in a young adult. Slow wave or deep sleep is more dominant during the initial third of the night, while REM dominates the final one third (Carskadon & Dement, 2000). Changes in sleep occur across the life span, and these changes must be considered in the assessment of potential sleep disturbance.

SLEEP ACROSS THE LIFE SPAN

Sleep is unique to individuals, although certain architectural changes are associated with advancing age. Sleep should also be considered within cultural and social contexts, such as usual sleep-wake times, family sleeping arrangements, meal patterns, and infant feeding practices (Redeker, 2011). From a developmental perspective, sleep may be divided into age groups from infancy to older adulthood.

PRETERM NEWBORN PERIOD

Preterm infants exhibit quiet sleep (corresponds to NREM sleep in adults), active sleep (corresponds to REM sleep in adults), and indeterminate sleep characterized by high voltage bursts alternating with flat electroencephalogram (EEG) periods of 10 to 20 seconds. With maturation, a pattern of lower voltage bursts alternating with rapid low-voltage waves on EEG becomes predominant and progresses to a high-voltage slow pattern by term. Sleep staging in this age group requires behavioral observations, with sleep identified by sustained eye closure and wake by open eyes, as EEG patterns are not

EXHIBIT 11-1: COMMON SLEEP TERMS AND GENERAL DEFINITIONS

SLEEP TERM	GENERAL DEFINITION
Sleep Architecture	Relative amounts of sleep stages that compose sleep and timing of sleep cycles (Berry, 2012)
Sleep (Onset) Latency	Time from lights out to first epoch of sleep (any stage) (Berry, 2012)
Wake After Sleep Onset	Wake from sleep onset during time in bed to lights on (Berry, 2012)
Arousals	In NREM sleep, a sudden shift in EEG frequency > 3 seconds including alpha, theta frequencies > 16 Hz, in REM sleep, requires concurrent increase in submental EMG of at least 1 second (Berry, 2012)
Total Sleep Time	Total minutes of NREM 1, 2, 3 and REM stages (Berry, 2012)
Sleep Efficiency	Time in bed × 100/time in bed (Berry, 2012)
Nonrapid Eye Movement (NREM) Sleep	Sleep Stages & 4 (Perlis, Jungquist, Smith, & Posner, 2005)
Rapid Eye Movement (REM) Sleep	Sleep stage characterized by fast frequency, low-voltage mixed EEG, rapid eye movements, and muscle atonia (Perlis et al., 2005)

EEG = electroencephalogram; EMG = electromyelogram; REM = rapid eye movement; NREM = nonrapid eye movement.

distinct. Specialized guidelines have been established for sleep staging in infants up to and over 2 months of age (Anders, Emde, & Parmelee, 1971; Grigg-Damberger et al., 2007; Iber, Ancoli-Israel, Chesson, & Quan, 2007).

NEWBORN PERIOD

Newborn infants sleep 16 to 20 hours daily. However, they do not have an established circadian rhythm, and therefore nighttime awakenings are common and normal, with infants waking up to feed at regular intervals. Newborn infants typically will not sleep more than 2 to 4 hours at a time. A circadian rhythm may begin by 10 to 12 weeks, with gradually increasing nighttime sleep (Galland, Taylor, Elder, & Herbison, 2011). Newborn infants generally need to awaken at night to nurse until they weigh 12 to 13 pounds. Sleep patterns alternate between light and deep sleep, and infants may awaken easily and have their sleep disrupted as they transition from deep to light sleep. Younger infants spend more time in REM sleep than older infants. During REM sleep, infants may exhibit fluttering eyelids, body movements, irregular respirations, and at times grunting or other vocalizations (Lucille Packard Children's Hospital, 2011).

INFANCY

Infant respiratory patterns are often characterized by "periodic breathing," periods of deep, rapid breathing with alternating apneic periods (Engel, 2006). Infants exhibit quiet sleep (slow, regular respirations with decreased muscle movements) and active sleep (irregular respirations, increased muscle movements, eye movements) in approximate 50 to 60 minute cycles. NREM and REM sleep are demonstrated by approximately 3 months of age (Markhov & Goldman, 2006), with increasing organization and consolidation of nighttime sleep by 5 months of age (Touchette et al., 2005). Sleeping through the night usually occurs by 9 months of age (Anders, Sadeh, & Appareddy, 1995). Infants progress from sleeping approximately 66% of the day to sleeping approximately 50% of the day with two naps by 1 year of age (Crabtree & Williams, 2009). However, these patterns may vary by infant feeding practices and family sleeping arrangements (Mindell, Sadeh, Kohyama, & How, 2009; Mindell, Sadeh, Wiegand, How, & Goh, 2010).

TODDLERHOOD

After 1 year of age, total sleep time and nocturnal sleep duration decrease up to the age of 3 years (Crabtree & Williams, 2009). Daytime napping decreases from approximately three to one nap per day during this period (Mindell et al., 2010). Sleep efficiency (time spent asleep while in bed attempting to sleep divided by the time in bed) becomes stable by approximately 5 years of age (Goodlin-Jones, Burnham, Gaylor, & Anders, 2001), REM sleep increases (Montgomery-Downs & Gozal,

2006), and napping usually ceases (Ward, Gay, Anders, Alkon, & Lee, 2008). Total sleep time and nocturnal sleep duration continue to decrease until around 7 years of age (Montgomery-Downs & Gozal, 2006). Overall, sleep pattern organization is considered a reflection of neurological development.

SCHOOL-AGE

During the school-age years, total sleep time and slow wave sleep appear to decrease, while REM sleep may slightly increase until adolescence. Sleep efficiency appears to remain unchanged until adolescence (Guillerminault, Lirisoglu, & Ohayon, 2004). Circadian patterns of sleep in school-age children advance with earlier bedtimes and wake times, with typical sleep durations of approximately 9 to 10 hours per night (Russo, Bruni, Lucidi, Ferri, & Violani, 2007). As late school-age children approach adolescence, sleep duration decreases, daytime sleepiness increases, and sleep deficits may occur (Crabtree & Williams, 2009). Bedtime routines and leisure activities such as television influence sleep in this age group (Mindell, Meltzer, Carskadon, & Chervin, 2009).

ADOLESCENCE

Adolescents experience a decrease in total sleep time to a range of 7 to 8 hours (Knutson & Lauderdale, 2009), including decreased NREM slow wave sleep and increased REM sleep (Guilleminault, Lirisoglu, & Ohayon, 2004). Circadian changes during adolescence, characterized by later bedtimes and later wake times, may reflect maturation of the suprachiasmatic nucleus (circadian pacemaker that responds to light stimulation) in response to puberty (Hagenauer, Perryman, Lee, & Carskadon, 2009). Increased daytime sleepiness in adolescence may be due to decreases in total sleep time being inadequate for restorative needs (Wolfson, Spaulding, Dandrow, & Baroni, 2007). Decreased slow wave sleep (Tarokh & Carskadon, 2010) and responsiveness to homeostatic sleep pressure following deprivation (Randler, 2008) may also be contributing factors. Allowing later school start times for adolescents has been associated with increased total sleep time, as well as improved mood and decreased daytime sleepiness (Owens, Belon, & Moss, 2010). Lifestyle factors including school, work, and social and recreational activities contribute to inadequate sleep during this developmental period (Redeker, 2011).

YOUNG AND MIDDLE-AGED ADULTHOOD

In adulthood, total sleep time, NREM slow wave sleep, REM sleep, and sleep efficiency decrease, while wake after sleep onset increases approximately 10 minutes per decade of age from 30 to 80 years (Ohayon, Carskadon, Guilleminault, & Vitiello, 2004). Napping varies, and reportedly one third of Americans nap one or more times per day. Adult sleep is strongly influenced by work, family, and childcare obligations. In women, issues related to the menstrual cycle and its cessation may also impact sleep (National Sleep Foundation, 2005).

OLDER ADULTHOOD

In healthy older adults, sleep duration remains consistent with earlier adulthood (Floyd, Medler, Aer, & Janisse, 2000). However, successful aging is associated with "normal" changes in sleep architecture (Vitiello, 2006), which are comparable for men and women from ages 61 to 102 (Ohayon et al., 2004). In healthy older adults, sleep efficiency decreases by a mean value of 3% each decade (Ohayon et al., 2004), REM sleep decreases 2% to 3% (Bliwise, 2005), and slow wave (restorative) sleep also declines (Carskadon & Dement, 2005).

FAMILIAL AND GENETIC IMPLICATIONS

The possible inheritance of sleep disorders has been explored using candidate gene and genome-wide association (GWA) studies. Genetic mutations have been associated with human sleep disorders, including fatal familial insomnia (Goldfarb et al., 1992) and familial advanced sleep phase syndrome (Jones et al., 1999). A number of genes (Circadian Locomotor Output Cycles Kaput [CLOCK], BMAL1, PER1–3, CRY1–2, and TIM) and associated polymorphisms have been suggested as contributing to sleep-wake regulation (Landolt & Dijk, 2011). Heritability of habitual bedtime has also been suggested by a GWA study based on the Framington Heart Study 100K Project (Gottlieb, O'Conner, & Wilk, 2007). Two GWA studies have identified and replicated three genomic regions associated with restless legs syndrome (RLS) (Stefansson et al., 2007; Winkelman et al., 2007), a disorder with strong familial patterns. A genetic susceptibility for narcolepsy has been strongly suggested (Chabas, Taheri, Renier, & Mignot, 2003), although specific mutations have not yet been clearly identified and replicated (Faraco & Mignot, 2011). Given the heritable aspects of many sleep disorders, a family sleep pedigree (genogram) should be routine when taking the sleep history of a client with complaints of sleep disturbance.

SLEEP DISORDERS

A classification system of sleep disorders emerged in 1979 (Association of Sleep Disorders Centers and Association for Psychophysiological Study of Sleep, 1979), and *The International Classification of Sleep Disorders Second Edition* (ICSD-2) in current use was published by the American Academy of Sleep Medicine (AASM; 2005) for diagnostic, epidemiologic, and research purposes. Sleep disorders are also described in the *International Classification of Diseases*-10 codes (ICD-10, 1992), which are used worldwide and have a planned transition date of October 1, 2013, in the United States. Due to the upcoming transition of ICD-10 codes, this chapter describes sleep disorders based on the ICSD-2 classification system.

The ICSD-2 (AASM, 2005) organizes sleep disorders by eight categories, which are further subdivided into 85 sleep disorders. Although not always in a setting where definitive diagnosis and management are possible, advanced practice psychiatric nurses should become familiar with the main categories and common sleep disorders. General definitions, diagnosis, and management of the main sleep categories and some of the most common sleep disorders are summarized in Table 11-1. Sleep disorders usually encountered in specific age groups are described later under age-related implications.

SLEEP HISTORY AND PHYSICAL

Promotion of client and public sleep education by the AASM and the National Sleep Foundation (NSF) has increased awareness of how important sleep is to health and safety. As a result, today's clients are better informed and more likely to consult health care providers about sleep issues than in the past. Health care providers are also increasingly cognizant of the need to include a sleep-related history and physical assessment in their routine practice. The ability to obtain a meaningful sleep history, administer standardized sleep measures, and perform a focused physical assessment is of paramount importance for identification, management, and referral of clients with sleep disturbance.

GENERAL SLEEP HISTORY

Optimally, the client should complete a 2-week sleep diary before visiting the health care provider for a sleep disturbance concern. If this is not possible, a sleep diary can be maintained by the client in the interim before the follow-up visit. This sleep diary or log gives the health care provider insight into the client's usual sleep pattern, sleep hygiene, and lifestyle practices. Keeping the sleep diary also promotes client self-awareness of sleep and sleep habits, and it can promote shared decision making in addressing sleep problems. A number of sleep diaries are available for use, such as through the National Heart, Lung, and Blood Institute (2005). The Pittsburgh Sleep Diary (PSD), another standardized sleep diary, collects information about sleep latency, sleep duration, sleep efficiency, as well as other factors that may influence sleep (Monk et al., 1994).

Eliciting the client's presenting concern in his or her own words is a simple way to begin the sleep history. Sleep problems may be broadly grouped to include one or more of the following: (a) symptoms of insomnia (b) symptoms experienced during sleep or nighttime awakenings, or (c) symptoms of excessive daytime sleepiness. Because the client may be unaware of some symptoms that occur during sleep (snoring, kicking, or violent behavior), a history from the bed partner can contribute important information (Malow, 2011). It is also important to question the patient about bed partner sleep habits or symptoms, such as snoring, and about pets who share the sleep environment.

When obtaining the client history, especially in psychiatric settings, it is critical to question patients about their typical 24-hour sleep pattern. It is also important to ascertain how often the client experiences partial or total sleeplessness, the total duration of periods without sleep (24 hours or longer), and self-medication measures used to combat inability to sleep. Conversely, it is important to question the client about excessive time spent sleeping, including daytime napping. Using standardized sleep assessment tools can assist the nurse to collect sleep information systematically, in a fashion that supports diagnostic reasoning and is conducive to evaluating treatment outcomes.

Several assessment tools provide helpful frameworks for obtaining a sleep history. The Brief Sleep History (Libbus, Baker, Osgood, Phillips, & Valentine, 1995), collects information about prior sleep patterns and characteristics. The Sleep Hygiene Awareness and Practices Scale (SHAPS) assesses understanding and practice of factors that may influence sleep (Lacks & Rotert, 1986). The 11-item Global Sleep Assessment Questionnaire (GSAQ) elicits information about potential sleep disorders (insomnia, excessive daytime sleepiness, OSA, RLS, periodic limb movements [PLMs] in sleep, REM

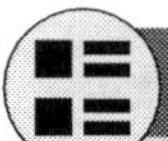

TABLE 11-1: DEFINITIONS, DIAGNOSIS, AND MANAGEMENT OF SLEEP DISORDERS

SLEEP DISORDER	DIAGNOSIS	MANAGEMENT
Circadian Rhythm Disorder "A recurrent or chronic pattern of sleep disturbance (that) may result from alterations of the circadian timing system or a misalignment between the timing of the individual's circadian rhythm of sleep propensity and the 24-hour social and physical environments" (American Academy of Sleep Medicine [AASM], 2005)	Based on patient report plus 7-day sleep diary or ACTG (Morgenthaler, Alessi, et al., 2007; Reid & Zee, 2011) Adjunct: Horne-Ostberg Morningness-Eveningness Questionnaire (Horne & Ostberg, 1976)	Behavioral Treatment: Chronotherapy Light Therapy Pharmacologic Treatment: Melatonin (Reid & Zee, 2011)
Hypersomnias of Central Origin Narcolepsy "Rapid transition from wakefulness to REM sleep" (AASM, 2005)	Based on patient-reported symptoms (AASM, 2005) Adjunct: Multiple Sleep Latency Test (Carskadon & Dement, 1982; Carskadon et al., 1986) PSG, CSF hypocretin-1 level <110 pg/mL (AASM, 2005)	Behavioral Treatment: Sleep hygiene Pharmacologic Treatment: Sodium oxybate (gamma-hydroxybutyrate [GHB]), Stimulants (Modafinil, Amodafinil, Methylphenidate, Atomoxetin, Dextroamphetamine, Methamphetamine) (Guilleminault & Cao, 2011)
Insomnia "Repeated difficulty with sleep initiation, duration, consolidation, or quality despite adequate time and opportunity for sleep" that results in some form of daytime impairment (AASM, 2005)	Based on patient-reported symptoms (AASM, 2005) Adjunct: Insomnia Severity Index (Bastian, Vallieres, & Morin, 2001) 2-Week Sleep Log/Diary (Berry, 2012) Actigraphy (Morganthaler, Alessi et al., 2007)	Cognitive Behavioral Treatment: Stimulus control, cognitive therapy, relaxation, paradoxical intention, biofeedback, sleep restriction, sleep hygiene (in multi-component therapy) (Morganthaler, Kramer et al., 2007) Pharmacologic Treatment: Specific Sleep onset insomnia: ramelteon, zaleplon Sleep maintenance insomnia: zolpidem, eszopiclone, temazepam (Schutte-Rodin et al., 2008) Pharmacologic Treatment: General Benzodiazepine receptor agonists (BxRAs), melatonin receptor agonist; some antidepressants, anxiolytics, antipsychotics, anticonvulsants, and antihistamines (Krystal, 2011; Walsh & Roth, 2011)
Parasomnias REM Sleep Behavior Disorder "Abnormal behaviors emerging during REM sleep that cause injury or sleep disruption" (AASM, 2005)	PSG recording of sustained EMG activity or intermittent loss of REM atonia or excessive phasic muscle twitch activity of submental or limb EMG during REM sleep (AASM, 2005)	Pharmacologic Treatment: Clonazepam, Melatonin, Levodopa (for Parkinson's disease) Adjunct Environmental Measures: Removal of dangerous objects from bedroom, padding around bed, window protection as needed (Mahowald & Schenck, 2011)
Sleep Related Breathing Disorders Obstructive Sleep Apnea A syndrome "characterized by repetitive episodes of complete (apnea) or partial (hypopnea) episodes of airway obstruction" (AASM, 2005)	Based on patient/partner-reported symptoms and/or PSG recordings of apneas and/or hypopneas by established criteria (AASM, 2005)	Behavioral Treatment: Weight loss, lateral recumbent position with head of bed (HOB) elevated 30 degrees for sleep, reduction of alcohol (Atwood, Strollo, & Givelber, 2011). Nasal Continuous Positive Airway Pressure (CPAP) (Buchanan & Grunstein, 2011)

(Continued)

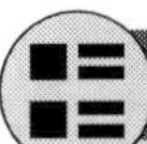

TABLE 11-1: DEFINITIONS, DIAGNOSIS, AND MANAGEMENT OF SLEEP DISORDERS (*Continued*)

SLEEP DISORDER	DIAGNOSIS	MANAGEMENT
Sleep-Related Movement Disorders *Restless Legs Syndrome* "A sensorimotor disorder characterized by a complaint of a strong, nearly irresistible, urge to move the legs" (AASM, 2005)	Based on patient-reported symptoms (AASM, 2005) Adjunct: Suggested Immobilization Test (Michaud, Paquet, Lavigne, Desautels, & Montplaisir, 2002) IRLSSG Severity Scale (IRLSSG, 2003)	Nonpharmacologic Treatment of RLS & PLM: (Mild or intermittent RLS) Stretching, heating or cooling of extremities (bath), avoidance of alcohol and caffeine, avoidance of antidepressant therapy associated with RLS, iron plus ascorbic acid as needed (Berry, 2012)
Periodic Limb Movement Disorder "Periodic episodes of repetitive, highly stereotyped, limb movements that occur during sleep," associated with reports of sleep disturbance, unrefreshing sleep, and/or excessive daytime sleepiness (AASM, 2005, p. 182)	PSG recordings of PLMs; usual onset in Stage 1 sleep, most frequent Stage 2 sleep, decreased frequency Stages 3 to 4, usually absent REM sleep.	Pharmacologic Treatment of RLS & PLM: Dopaminergic agents,* dopaminergic agonists, of RLS & PLM opioids, anticonvulsants, benzodiazepines (Montplaisir, Allen, Walters, & Ferini-Strambi, , 2011)

*Ropinirole or pramipexole are treatments of choice, taken 2 hours before symptoms for optimal effectiveness.

PLM = periodic limb movement; RLS = restless leg syndrome.

behavior disorder), daytime function, and causes of sleep disturbance (Roth et al., 2002). The Epworth Sleepiness Scale (ESS), an 8-item Likert-type scale, assesses daytime sleepiness by rating the likelihood of falling asleep in certain situations. High scores on the Epworth suggest, but are not diagnostic of, OSA or narcolepsy (Johns, 1991; 1992; 1993; 1994). The Pittsburgh Sleep Quality Index (PSQI) is a 10-item measure of global sleep quality (subjective perception of sleep as restorative) that also assesses sleep disturbance, sleep medication use, and daytime dysfunction (Buysse, Reynolds, Monk, Berman, & Kupfer, 1989).

Pediatric assessment tools include the BEARS framework (Bedtime problems, Excessive sleepiness, Awakenings, Regularity of sleep, and Sleep-disordered breathing) for general sleep assessment (Owens & Dalzell, 2005). The Pediatric Sleep Questionnaire may be used to screen for sleep-disordered breathing and sleepiness (Chervin, Hedger, Dillon, & Pituch, 2000). Last, the Children's Sleep Habits Questionnaire assesses sleep disturbance and mood in school-aged children (Owens, Spirito, & McGuinn, 2000).

Common symptoms that may suggest a sleep disorder include snoring, client-reported mood disturbance (anxiety, depression), daytime sleepiness, fatigue, and morning headache. Symptoms associated with narcolepsy include abrupt loss of muscle tone with strong emotional stimulation (cataplexy), sleep paralysis when transitioning into or out of sleep, and hallucinations at the onset or end of sleep (hypnagogic and hypnopompic hallucinations). Behavioral symptoms of a sleep disorder include purposeful but inappropriate activities when partially asleep (automatic behavior), excessive movement during sleep (parasomnia), or repetitive movements of the lower extremities during sleep (PLMs of sleep). In children, parental reports of behavioral disturbance, inattention, or hyperactivity may suggest sleep disorders (Vaughn & D'Cruz, 2011).

A review of the client's general medical and dental history is important to help identify possible risk factors for sleep disturbance, such as injuries, chronic conditions, and medications (discussed later in this chapter). For example, a history of nose trauma or mouth breathing suggests possible nasal obstruction. A history of dental malocclusion and overcrowding of the teeth and/or of early wisdom teeth removal suggests a small oral cavity with potential crowding at the base of the tongue. A history of snoring and bruxism (teeth grinding) are strongly suggestive of OSA (Cao, Guilleminault, & Kushida, 2011).

Environmental factors such as home and job demands should also be assessed, as they may precipitate or exacerbate sleep problems. For example, the stress of caring for a young child or an older family member may result in disrupted sleep. Jobs requiring night work, rotation of shifts, or travel across time zones can lead to altered circadian rhythms. The client with sleep disturbance should also be questioned about recent life stresses such as relocation, bereavement, or loss of employment.

FOCUSED PHYSICAL ASSESSMENT

During the general survey it is important to note signs that may suggest a sleep disorder. For example, a hyperalert appearance suggests insomnia, as might the sad or flattened affect characteristic of depressed mood. Dark circles under the eyes, yawning, and rubbing the face suggest daytime sleepiness, which is often associated with sleep fragmentation and disorders such as OSA or RLS. Difficulty staying attentive or awake during the interview might also suggest narcolepsy (Vaughn & D'Cruz, 2011).

A focused physical assessment should include but not necessarily be limited to measurement of height, weight, and neck circumference with calculation of body mass index (BMI). Neck circumference should be measured at the superior border of the cricothyroid membrane with the client positioned upright. A BMI exceeding 30 kg/m2 has been associated with OSA in both men and women. A neck circumference of 40 cm or greater has also been associated with OSA and demonstrated 61% sensitivity and 93% specificity (Kushida, Efron, & Guilleminault, 1997).

The upper airway structures should be examined with the client in both the seated and supine positions for narrowing of the airway or nasal obstruction. Mandibular retrognathia (abnormal posterior positioning), current malocclusion, and overcrowding of the teeth again suggest a small oral cavity with potential crowding at the base of the tongue and OSA. Macroglossia (a large tongue) also predisposes to OSA. Visualization of the oropharynx and use of either the Mallampati scale (mouth widely open, tongue protruding) or modified Mallampati technique (mouth widely open, no tongue protrusion) may be used to rate the severity of structural crowding from 1 to 4, open to hard palate visibility only (Friedman et al., 1999; Mallampati et al., 1985). Crowding of the tonsils may be evaluated with the Friedman scale rating severity from 0 to 4, absent to hypertrophied and obstructed (Friedman et al., 1999). The nose should be inspected for septal deviation, signs of trauma, or enlarged inferior nasal turbinates. The nares should be assessed for symmetry, size, and collapsibility (Cao et al., 2011).

ANALYSIS OF SLEEP SYMPTOMS AND SPECIALIZED SLEEP SCREENING

Once the general sleep history and physical assessment data have been collected and critically analyzed, the advanced practice nurse must determine if additional specialized assessment is required to guide management or support referral to a sleep specialist for further evaluation. For example, if the client or sleep partner reports a history of snoring and gasping during sleep, falling asleep unintentionally, or a history of car accidents or other accidental injuries questionnaires can be used for further assessment. These questionnaires include the Berlin, STOP (snoring, tiredness, observed apnea and high blood pressure), and BANG (body mass index, age, neck circumference, and gender). These questionnaires can be used to screen for OSA. Based on the findings of these tools, referral to a sleep specialist and a possible polysomnogram (overnight sleep study) may be arranged. If a client describes uncomfortable sensations in the legs that interfere with rest or a positive family history of RLS, screening for RLS with the Cambridge-Hopkins RLS Questionnaire (Allen, Burchell, MacDonald, Hening, & Earley, 2009) may be indicated. Even if the client's reported symptoms are consistent with insomnia, other possible underlying causes of sleep disturbance should first be considered and ruled out. Once this is done, the severity of insomnia could be assessed with the Insomnia Severity Index (Bastian, Vallieres, & Morin, 2001) to determine if referral to a behavioral sleep medicine specialist is warranted for chronic or severe insomnia symptoms or if more basic measures may reasonably be attempted for acute or less severe symptoms. Less well-defined sleep disturbances during sleep may require further evaluation by a sleep specialist and PSG to capture the occurrence within the sleep cycle and correctly diagnose the events. Non-sleep related surgeries, disorders, medications, substances, or activities may initiate or exacerbate sleep disturbance, and other tools may be used to assess pain, mood, alcohol or substance use, and activity/exercise. Referral to nonsleep specialists for other contributory factors such as worsening cognitive, pulmonary, or cardiac symptoms may also be needed, if they are suspected sources of sleep disturbance.

SPECIALIZED SLEEP SCREENING TOOLS

Creation and testing of specialized clinical assessment tools complemented technological advances in sleep measurement. Actigraphy (ACTG), usually worn on the wrist, detects motion, and the absence of motion is measured as a proxy of sleep (Tyron, 1991). More convenient and less expensive than PSG, ACTG allows monitoring of sleep in the client's home environment over an extended period of time. Actigraphy is considered valid and reliable for sleep assessment in normal healthy adults (Morgenthaler, Alessi, et al., 2007), and it provides a better measure of total sleep time than of other sleep variables, although accuracy decreases as sleep disturbance increases (Ancoli-Israel et al., 2003). Actigraphy is used for the assessment of circadian rhythm disorders, circadian rhythms, and sleep-wake patterns in adults with insomnia as well as for estimation of total sleep time in adults with OSA and in populations intolerant of PSG, such as children and elderly adults (Morgenthaler, Alessi, et al., 2007). Ankle actigraphy can also be used to assess PLMs of sleep (Kazenwadel et al., 1995; Kemlink, Pretl, Sonka, & Nevsimalova, 2008). Advanced practice psychiatric nurses can use ACTG to augment subjective sleep reports and to monitor the effectiveness of sleep treatments. Use of wrist ACTG in clients with an arteriovenus shunt or impaired lymphatic drainage of the arm should be avoided, as with any potentially constrictive devices. Actigraphy of the lower extremities may be contraindicated in clients with impaired peripheral perfusion and at increased risk of blood clot formation.

Numerous specialized tools have also been developed for screening and severity rating of such disorders as insomnia, OSA, and RLS. These tools can be helpful in narrowing the underlying causes of sleep disturbance. A brief description of some commonly used sleep screening tools is provided in Table 11-2.

REGULATION OF SLEEP

The underlying mechanisms that control sleep are extremely complex and are theorized to include

TABLE 11-2: SPECIFIC SLEEP SCREENING TOOLS

MEASURE OR TOOL	PURPOSE	DESCRIPTION	SCORE	TIME
Berlin Questionnaire (Netzer, Stoohs, Netzer, Clark & Strohl, 1999) www.swclab.com/images/PDFS/Berlin-Questionnaire.pdf	Screen & rate obstructive sleep apnea risk	Questionnaire Based on 3 categories of risk for having sleep apnea 10 items (snoring, apnea, fatigue, drowsy driving, high blood pressure, high body mass index)	High risk: 2 or more categories + Low risk: 1 or more categories +	5 min.
STOP-BANG Questionnaire (Chung & Elsaid, 2009; Chung et al., 2008).		Questionnaire Based on signs, symptoms, and risk factors 8 items (snoring, tiredness, observed apnea, high blood pressure [STOP]; body mass index, age, neck circumference, gender [BANG])	High risk: ≥3 yes answers low risk: <3 yes answers	5–10 min.
Cambridge-Hopkins Restless Legs Syndrome Questionnaire (CH-RLS-Q13) (Allen Burchell, MacDonald, Hening, & Earley, 2009)	Screen for restless legs syndrome symptoms	Questionnaire based on the symptoms of RLS 13 items (recurrent uncomfortable urge to move legs, position when experiencing urge, influence of activity on symptoms, severity of distress with symptoms, frequency of symptoms, and age of symptom onset)	Definite: numbers 1–6 (+ symptoms, urge to move, occur sitting/lying, start sitting/lying, relief on movement, timing in p.m.) Probable: all but #1 or 4	10–20 min.
Insomnia Severity Index (ISI) (Bastian, Vallieres, & Morin, 2001)	Screen & rate insomnia symptom severity	Likert-type scale rating severity of insomnia symptoms 7-item (0–4 points each) (difficulty falling asleep, staying asleep, waking up too early, satisfaction with sleep, sleep interference with function, how noticeable sleep impairment is to others, distress about sleep)	<8 = no clinical insomnia symptoms; 8–14 = subthreshold; 15–24 = moderate; 24 or > = severe	5 min.

RLS = restless leg syndrome.

homeostatic, circadian, neurological, neurochemical, and hormonal processes. The Two-Process Model of sleep proposes that sleep propensity is driven by the need for sleep, in concert with circadian cycles (Borbély, 1982). Circadian cycles are driven by the suprachaismatic nucleus (SCN) of the hypothalamus (master body clock) in approximate 24-hour patterns (Scheer & Shea, 2009) and are synchronized to environmental light exposure received via the retina (Chou et al., 2003). The SCN innervates the ventrolateral pre-optic area of the hypothalamus, which contains sleep-promoting cells, and the lateral hypothalamus, which contains wake-promoting cells (McGinty & Szymusiak, 2003). Mutually inhibitory interaction of the preoptic area sleep-promoting system with sleep-arousal (wake-promoting) systems is believed to control brain activity during the sleep-wake cycle and is known as the "flip-flop switch" model of homeostatic and circadian regulation of sleep and wake (Lu, Sherman, Devor, & Saper, 2006). This neuronal interaction results in inhibition or release of neurotransmitters that stimulate arousal and wakefulness (Fuller, Gooley, & Saper, 2006), including serotonin, norepinephrine, histamine, orexin, acetylcholine, dopamine, and glutamate (McGinty & Szymusiak, 2011). Hormones further influence arousal, including cortisol and melatonin. Cortisol is associated with arousal, rises during wake time, and is inhibited by sleep. Melatonin levels rise during the day in response to sunlight exposure, peak near the onset of sleep, promote sleep initiation and maintenance, and reach a nadir near the onset of waking (Scheer & Shea, 2009). In summary, disruption of sleep homeostasis and circadian timing, damage or degeneration of neuronal structures, and alterations in neurotransmitter or hormone production can all adversely affect sleep.

SLEEP AND COMORBID PSYCHIATRIC DISORDERS

Notably, many of the neurotransmitters that influence sleep and wake states contribute to the pathophysiology of psychiatric disorders as well. Common psychiatric disorders, associated sleep disorders, and their theorized pathophysiological interrelationships are summarized in Table 11-3.

SLEEP AND COMORBID MEDICAL DISORDERS

Research continues to discover the health implications of sleep disorders and how common medical disorders interrelate with sleep. Because nursing is holistic, advanced practice psychiatric nurses should be aware that certain medical disorders may precipitate or exacerbate sleep disturbance. Table 11-4 provides a brief description of commonly encountered sleep and comorbid medical disorders as well as their theorized pathophysiological interrelationships.

NURSING DECISION TREES

The nursing assessment of sleep complaints requires systematic incorporation of general and specific sleep tools into the decision process. When evaluating sleep disturbance it is important to note that several sleep disorders may coexist, so that consideration of one should not preclude consideration of another. Professional judgment is always required based on the individual client presentation of symptoms; however, an organized approach can provide direction for decision making. Decision trees for excessive daytime sleepiness, insomnia symptoms, and unusual behaviors during sleep are outlined in Figures 11-1, 11-2, and 11-3, and they were adapted for advanced practice psychiatric nurses from diagnostic flow charts by Vaughn and D'Cruz (2011).

SHARED DECISION MAKING AND COLLABORATIVE TREATMENT PLANNING

Because sleep is complex and biobehavioral in nature, it is important for advanced practice psychiatric nurses to recognize the importance of client and family collaboration in managing sleep disturbance. Addressing client and family learning needs about sleep regulation, factors that can negatively impact sleep, and practices that can promote healthy sleep support shared decision making and responsibility for sleep intervention. Because sleep disturbance is often chronic, it is important for clients to gain confidence in their ability to manage it effectively. Pharmacologic, nonpharmacologic, and complementary and alternative modalities of treatment are available, and they may be used singly or in combination to help clients achieve adequate and restorative sleep.

TREATMENT

Pharmacologic therapies are often used in the management of sleep disturbance comorbid with psychiatric disorders. Because many sleep and psychiatric disorders share some pathophysiological relationships, pharmacological therapies may target neurotransmitters associated

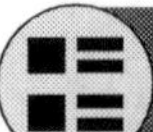

TABLE 11-3: COMMON PSYCHIATRIC DISORDERS, ASSOCIATED SLEEP DISORDERS, AND THEORIZED PATHOPHYSIOLOGY

PSYCHIATRIC DISORDER/CONDITION	SLEEP DISORDER	THEORIZED PATHOPHYSIOLOGICAL INTERRELATIONSHIPS
Anxiety Disorders: panic disorder, generalized anxiety disorder, social phobia, obsessive–compulsive disorder, post-traumatic stress disorder (PTSD)	Insomnia due to mental disorder	Anxiety-associated increase in cortical and peripheral arousal; inadequate sleep for restoration of cortical arousal (Ramsawh, Stein, & Mellman, 2011)
Mood Disorders: depression, unipolar & bipolar disorders, seasonal affective disorder	Insomnia due to mental disorder, Hypersomnia	Gamma-aminobutyric acid (GABA)-ergic inhibition of arousal due to histamine, orexin, serotonin, and noradrenalin, controlled by the pre-optic area of the brain (Krishnan & Nestler, 2008); altered levels of norepinephrine, serotonin, and dopamine (Sadock & Sadock, 2003) Decreased melatonin-cortisol ratio; delayed body rhythms (Hastings, O'Neill, & Maywood, 2007); and desynchronization of melatonin (Brown, Cardinali, & Pandi-Perumal, 2010)
Schizophrenia	Insomnia due to mental disorder, total sleeplessness Dyssomnias (inadequate sleep hygiene, irregular sleep–wake patterns) Parasomnias, OSA, Movement Disorders (RLS, PLMS)	Hyperactivity of the mesolimbic dopamine system; excitatory neurotransmitter glutamate (Goff & Coyle, 2001); susceptibility genes that target glutamatergic transmission (Harrison & Own, 2003); abnormal neuronal connectivity and integrative neuronal circuits (Davis et al., 2003; Feinberg & Guazzelli, 1999)
Substance Abuse: caffeine, amphetamines, cocaine, marijuana, nicotine, alcohol	Insomnia due to drug or substance, Sleep-disordered breathing, PLMS of sleep	Dependent upon substance; rebound or withdrawal (Conroy, Arnett, & Brower, 2010); most substances of abuse interact with the dopaminergic system (Roehrs & Roth, 2011)

OSA = obstructive sleep disorder; RLS = restless leg syndrome.

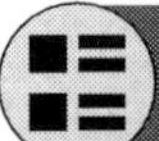

TABLE 11-4: COMMON MEDICAL DISORDERS, ASSOCIATED SLEEP DISORDERS, AND THEORIZED PATHOPHYSIOLOGY

MEDICAL DISORDER/ CONDITION	SLEEP DISORDER	THEORIZED PATHOPHYSIOLOGICAL INTERRELATIONSHIPS
Alzheimer's disease, other dementias	Circadian Rhythm Sleep Disorder, Obstructive Sleep Apnea Syndrome	Disrupted melatonin production (Wu et al., 2006; Wu & Swaab, 2005); apolipoprotein E epsilon 4–related increased risk (Kadotani et al., 2001)
Asthma, nocturnal	Insomnia	↑Anxiety secondary to dyspnea, wheezing, coughing, air hunger, chest tightness (American Academy of Sleep Medicine [AASM], 2005); nocturnal bronchoconstriction and wheezing due to circadian rhythm-related increases in parasympathetic airway tone (Raherison, Abouelfath, Le Gros, Taytard, & Molimard, 2006)
Bacterial & viral infections	Hypersomnia	Proinflammatory cytokine (IL-1β, TNF-α, and IL-6) triggering of the acute phase response to infection, including increased NREM sleep (Majde & Krueger, 2005; Opp, 2005)

(Continued)

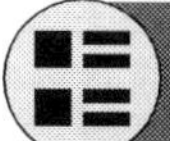

TABLE 11-4: COMMON MEDICAL DISORDERS, ASSOCIATED SLEEP DISORDERS, AND THEORIZED PATHOPHYSIOLOGY (*Continued*)

MEDICAL DISORDER/ CONDITION	SLEEP DISORDER	THEORIZED PATHOPHYSIOLOGICAL INTERRELATIONSHIPS
Cancer	Insomnia, Excessive Daytime Sleepiness	Cancer cell production & induced production of cytokines; increased cytokines (IL-1β, TNF-α, and IL-6); increased anxiety/depression & pain; hormone-blocking, steroid, & radiation therapy (Ardestani, Inserra, Solkoff, & Watson, 1999; Dunlop & Campbell, 2000)
Cardiovascular disease atherosclerosis, hypertension, coronary artery disease, congestive heart failure	Obstructive Sleep Apnea, Central Sleep Apnea, Cheyne Stokes Respirations	↑Inflammatory cytokines, adhesion molecules, WBC transmigration & endothelial attachment, ↑oxidative stress, reactive oxygen species production, gene-mediated vasoactive & inflammatory protein production (Minoguchi et al., 2005); pulmonary congestion-stimulated hyperventilation, ↓CO_2 levels below apneic threshold and post-hyperventilatory apnea (AASM, 2005)
Cerebrovascular Accident (CVA)	Central Sleep Apnea, Cheyne Stokes Respirations	Stroke lesion-related sleep disordered breathing (Rowat, Wardlaw, & Dennis, 2007); ↓CO_2 levels below apneic threshold (AASM, 2005)
Chronic Obstructive Pulmonary Disease	Insomnia, Sleep Related Hypoventilation/ Hypoxemia due to Lower Airways Obstruction	↑Anxiety secondary to respiratory distress (AASM, 2005); REM sleep-related hypoxemia (Catterall et al., 1985); and hypotonia of intercostal muscles with impaired diaphragmatic mechanical efficiency due to pulmonary hyperinflation (Douglas, 2011)
Chronic Renal Disease	Excessive Daytime Sleepiness, Insomnia, Restless Legs Syndrome, Periodic Limb Movement Disorder	Increased BUN and PLMs (Hanley, Gabor, Chan, & Pierratos, 2003); warm hemodialysis solution (Parker, Bliwise, & Rye, 2000); attenuated nocturnal melatonin (Koch et al., 2009); iron deficiency (Siddiqui, Kavanagh, Traynor, Mak, Deighan, & Geddes, 2005)
Diabetes	Obstructive Sleep Apnea, Excessive Daytime Sleepiness, Insomnia	↓Insulin sensitivity, ↓insulin production (Punjabi & Beamer, 2009)
Fibromyalgia	Insomnia	SWS and REM sleep deprivation-induced hyperalgia; high- frequency cyclic alternating pattern (CAP)-related sleep disruption in stage 2 non-REM sleep (Lentz, Landis, Rothermel, & Shaver, 1999); increased CSF substance P –related sleep arousal (Lyon, Cohen, & Quintner, 2011; Stahl, 2009); brain volume-related central pain augmentation (Wood, Glabus, Simpson, & Patterson, 2009)
Head Trauma	Narcolepsy	Brain injury (Maccario, Ruggles, & Meriwether, 1987)
Parkinson's disease, Lewy Body Dementia	REM Behavior Disorder, Narcolepsy	Neurodegenerative damage to brain regulation of sleep and arousal; behavioral, respiratory, & motor symptoms; medication side effects (Trenkwalder & Arnulf, 2011); nondopaminergic lesion to subcoeruleus nucleus in the pons that controls atonia in REM sleep (Boeve et al., 2007)

CSF = cerebrospinal fluid; IL = interleukin; NREM = nonrapid eye movement; PLMs = periodic limb movements; SWS = slow wave sleep; REM = rapid eye movement; TNF = tumor necrosis factors; WBC = white blood corpuscles.

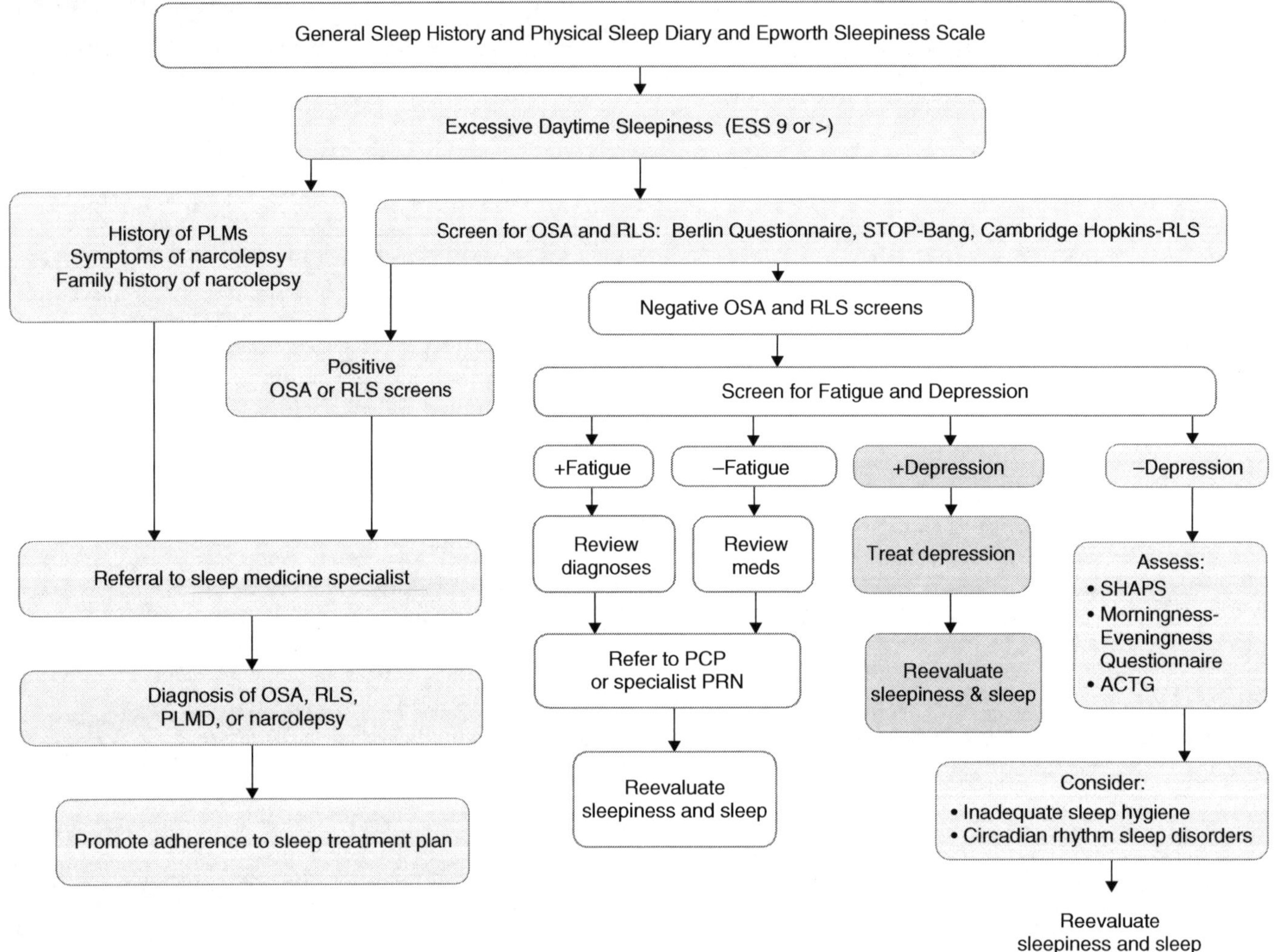

Figure 11-1 Decision Tree for Excessive Daytime Sleepiness

with both. In general, pharmacologic therapies for sleep disorders act by enhancing sleep-promoting systems, blocking wake-promoting systems, or enhancing wake-promoting systems.

Selection of sleep agents should depend not only upon the sleep problem or disorder identified, but also on the acuity of the disorder in addition to individual risks and comorbidities. For example, benzodiazepines have the potential for residual sedative and amnestic effects, rebound insomnia on discontinuation, dependence, and abuse. Consequently, the recommended use of benzodiazepines is limited to short-term insomnia. The use of alternative agents should be considered for older adults with insomnia in whom risk for falls and cognitive deficits are a concern. The use of benzodiazepines are also contraindicated in persons with OSA, substance abuse disorder, or advanced liver disease due to exacerbation of apnea, potential for abuse, and impaired hepatic metabolism (Walsh & Roth, 2011). Trazodone, the most frequently used off-label insomnia agent, has low potential for abuse and is a preferred agent for management of insomnia in patients with substance abuse disorder. However, trazodone is associated with orthostatic hypotension and should be used cautiously in patients at risk for falls, such as the elderly. Effects of trazodone are also variable due to common genetic polymorphisms that influence its metabolism (Krystal, 2011). The most commonly used medications for sleep management, their pharmacokinetics, and effects on sleep or waking are summarized in Table 11-5.

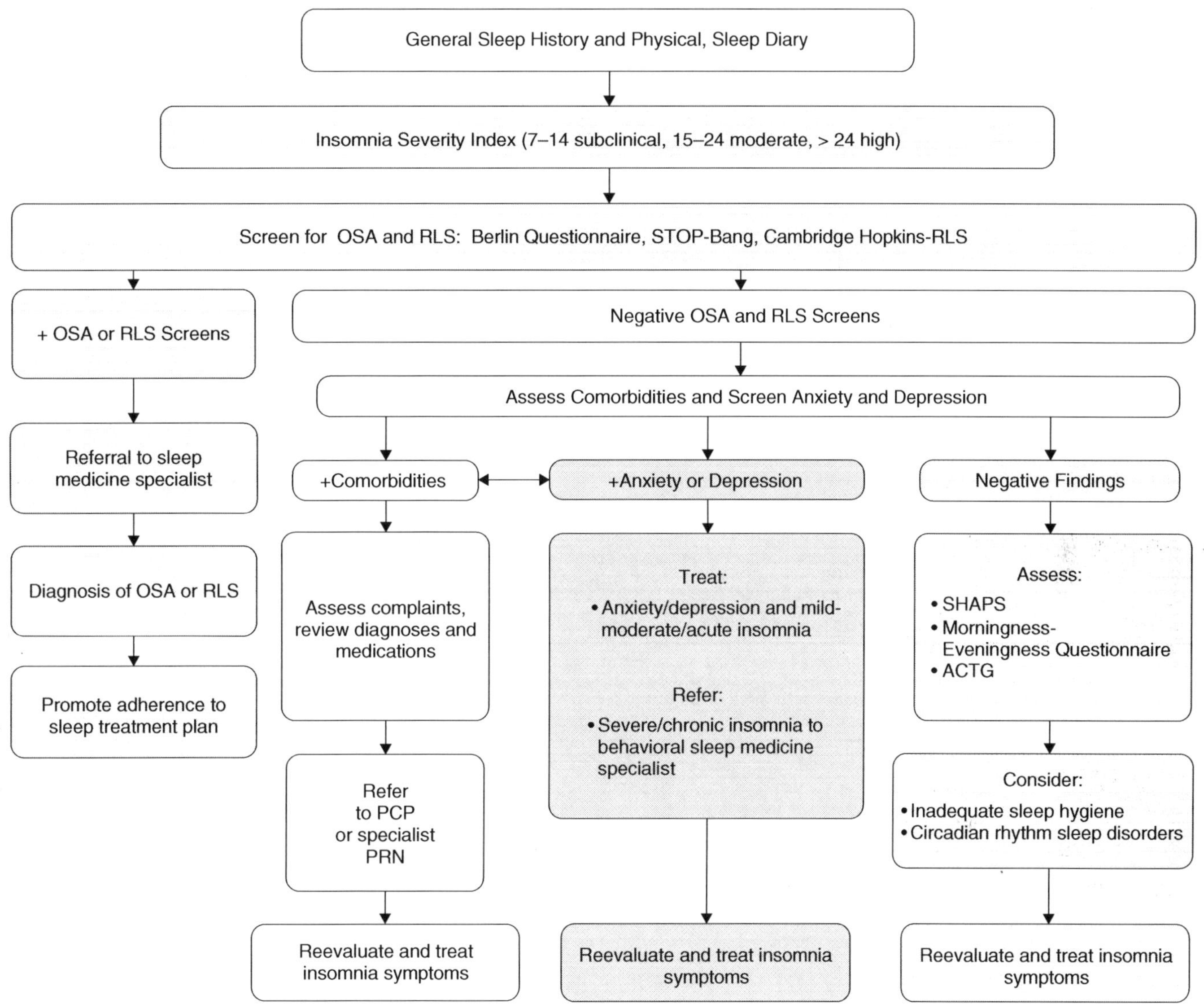

Figure 11-2 Decision Tree for Insomnia Symptoms

NONPHARMACOLOGIC TREATMENT OF SLEEP DISORDERS

In addition to pharmacologic sleep interventions, a number of nonpharmacologic interventions are available to address sleep disturbance associated with insomnia symptoms and poor sleep hygiene. Cognitive and behavioral therapies have been recognized as equivalent to pharmacologic therapy for insomnia and as more sustained in effectiveness (Rieman & Perlis, 2009; Smith et al., 2002). These therapies include a number of recognized approaches that are often combined as multi-component therapy (Bootzin, 2005). Cognitive-behavioral therapy (with/without relaxation therapy), stimulus control therapy, and relaxation therapy (progressive muscle relaxation, guided imagery) are considered effective and standard therapy modalities. Paradoxical intention, biofeedback, sleep restriction, and multi-component therapy are classified as guidelines and also considered effective. Sleep hygiene does not have a recommendation classification, but it may be included in multi-component therapy (Morgenthaler et al., 2006).

Cognitive (Restructuring) Therapy

Cognitive therapy for insomnia is based on the premise that insomniacs have sleep-related worry, which arises

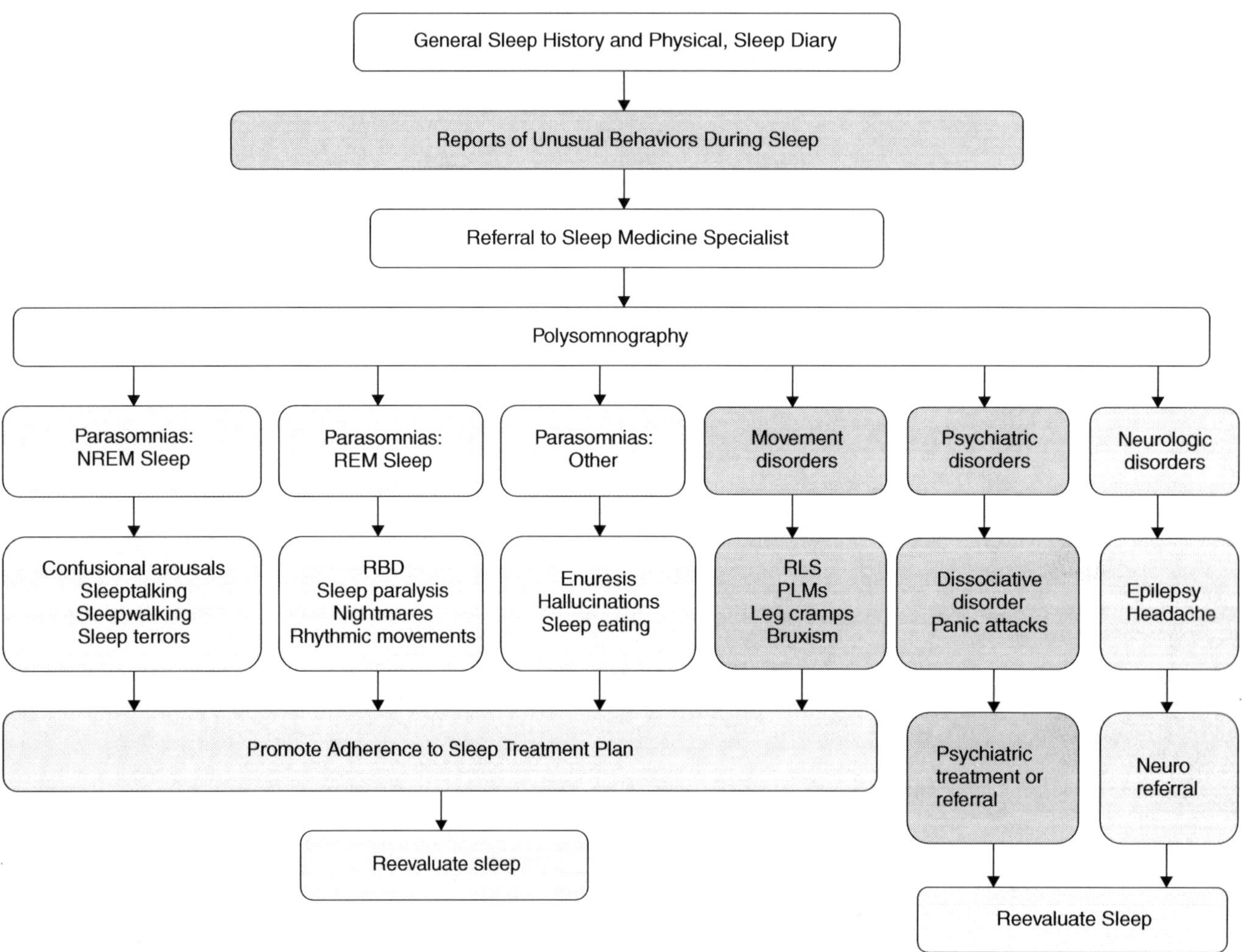

NREM = nonrapid eye movement; REM = rapid eye movement; RBD = REM behavior disorder; PLMs = periodic limb movements of sleep; RLS = restless legs syndrome.

Figure 11-3 Decision Tree for Unusual Behaviors During Sleep

from maladaptive cognitions and beliefs (catastrophic thinking) and that poor sleep will probably have devastating consequences. This method assists the patient to identify these cognitions and beliefs, critically analyze them, recognize that they may not be factual, and restructure them in a more positive light (Buysse & Perlis, 1996; Perlis & Gehrman, 2011; Schutte-Rodin, Broch, Buysse, Dorsey, & Sateia, 2008). This therapy may be administered with or without relaxation therapy (Berry, 2012).

Stimulus Control Therapy

Stimulus control is based on an operant paradigm suggesting that bed and bedroom are no longer sleep stimuli for insomniacs, but are associated with behaviors incompatible with sleep (anxiety), leading to wakefulness and arousal. The purpose of stimulus control is to reassociate the bed and bedroom with rapidly falling asleep (Bootzin, Epstein, & Ward, 1991; Bootzin & Perlis, 2011).

Relaxation Therapy

Relaxation therapy includes numerous approaches that focus on decreasing elevated levels of arousal. Progressive muscle relaxation is aimed at reducing somatic arousal, and it consists of systematic tension and relaxation of muscle groups. Guided imagery is aimed at reducing cognitive arousal and includes visualization of relaxing settings or activities (Berry, 2012; Lichstein, Taylor, McCrae, & Thomas, 2011).

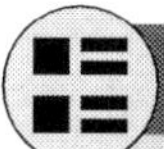

TABLE 11-5: MEDICATIONS USED TO MANAGE SLEEP DISORDERS

MEDICATION CLASSIFICATION	INDICATION	MECHANISM OF ACTION
Agents That Enhance Sleep-Promoting Systems (Walsh & Roth, 2011)		
Sedative-Hypnotics benzodiazepines: estrazolam (ProSom) flurazepam (Dalmane) flunitrazepam (Rohypnol) temazepam (Restoril) triazolam (Halcion) quazepam (Doral) Non-benzodiazepines: eszopicione (Lunesta) zaleplon (Sonata) zolpidem (Ambien) zolpidem extended release	Insomnia	Gamma-hydroxybutyrate (GABA) Inhibition GABA Inhibition
Other Medications That Enhance Sleep-Promoting Systems (Krystal, 2011)		
Anti-Anxiety buspirone (BuSpar)	Insomnia	5-HT (serotonin) antagonist
Hormone: melatonin rozerem (Ramelteon)	Insomnia	Binds at MT1 & MT2 receptors Melatonin agonist at MT1 & MT2 receptors
Agents That Block Wake-Promoting Systems (Krystal, 2011)		
Sedating Antidepressants Tricyclics: amitriptyline (Elavil) doxepin (Sinequan) trimipramine maleate (Surmontil) Other: trazodone (Desyrel) mirtazapine (Remeron)	Insomnia	Serotonin, norepinephrine, & histamine receptor blockers Antagonize norepinephrine, serotonin, & histamine receptors
Antihistamines: diphenhydramine (Benedryl, Nytol, Sleep-Eez, Sominex) Benedryl combination medications (Anacin P.M., Excedrin P.M., Tylenol P.M.) doxylamine (Unisom)	Insomnia	Antagonizes histamine H1 receptors; muscarinic cholinergic antagonism
Antipsychotics: olanzapine (Zyprexa) quetiapine (Seroquel)	Insomnia	Antagonize dopamine, histamine (H1), serotonin, muscarinic, cholinergic, & adrenergic receptors
Agents That Enhance Wake-Promoting Systems (Guilleminault & Cao, 2011)		
Stimulants: amphetamine methamphetamine methylphenidate (Ritalin) pemoline (Cylert) selegiline (Elderyl, Emsam, Zelapar) modafinil (Provigil) armodafinal (Nuvigil) Anticataplectics: venlafaxine (Effexor) atomoxetine (Strattera) fluoxetine (Prozac)	Narcolepsy	↑MAO release (dopamine, norepinephrine, & 5-HT); Similar to amphetamine, fewer peripheral side effects; Blocks MAO uptake at lower dose than amphetamine; Inhibits dopamine uptake; MAO-B inhibitor; converts to amphetamine; unknown mode of action; inhibits dopamine uptake serotonin & norepinephrine reuptake blocker Norepinephrine reuptake blocker Serotonin uptake blocker MAO uptake blockers

(Continued)

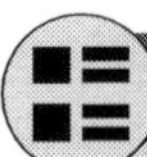

TABLE 11-5: MEDICATIONS USED TO MANAGE SLEEP DISORDERS (Continued)

MEDICATION CLASSIFICATION	INDICATION	MECHANISM OF ACTION
apo-imipramine (Protriptyline) imipramine (Tofranil) desipramine (Norpramin) clomipramine (Anafranil) Other: sodium oxybate (Xyrem) GABA (gamma hydroxybutyrate)		↑Dopamine release ↑Brain dopamine levels directly
Agents That Increase or Enhance Dopamine and Decrease Associated Symptoms (Montplaisir, Allen, Walters & Strambi, 2011)		
Dopamine agonists: pramipexole (Miripex) ropinirole (Requip)	RLS	Bind to dopamine receptors(D3) in place of dopamine and directly stimulate dopamine receptors
Dopamine precursors: Levodopa/carbidopa	RLS	↑ Available dopamine
Benzodiazepines: clonazepam (Klonopin) temazepam (Restoril) nitrazepam (Mogadon)	RLS	Depress nerve transmission in the motor cortex (decrease PLMs and PLMs-associated arousals in RLS with comorbid PLMs; given for insomnia symptoms secondary to dopaminergic agents)
Opiates: oxycodone codeine	RLS	Possible ↑opiate receptor binding and opioid levels to counterbalance endogenous opioid system dysfunction
Anticonvulsants: gabapentin (Neurontin)	RLS	↑Brain dopamine levels directly (decrease pain in RLS associated with peripheral neuropathy "neuropathic RLS")
Pediatric Agents That Enhance Sleep-Promoting Systems (Jetnalani, 2011)		
Antidepressants: Tricyclic: doxepin (Sinequan) Other: trazodone (Desyrel)	Insomnia	Antagonizes 5-HT2, norepipnephrine, & aceteylcholine, histamine 1, histamine 2, muscarinic 1 receptors Antagonizes 5-HT2, norepipnephrine, histamine
Antihistamines: hydroxyzine (Atarax)	Insomnia	Histamine antagonist
Antihypertensives: clonidine (Catapres) clonidine patch	Insomnia	Alpha-2 agonist

PLMs = periodic limb movements; RLS = restless leg syndrome.

Paradoxical Intention and Biofeedback

Paradoxical intention aims at eliminating performance anxiety by having the patient avoid any intentional effort to fall asleep (Espie, 2011). Biofeedback focuses on reducing somatic arousal by training the patient to control physiological variables using visual or auditory feedback (Berry, 2012).

Sleep Restriction

Sleep restriction is based on the premise that insomniacs spend excessive time in bed trying to sleep. The purpose of sleep restriction is to strengthen homeostatic and circadian processes, consolidate sleep, and establish sleep-wake patterns. Sleep restriction limits time in bed to reported total sleep time (Spielman, Saskin, & Thorpy, 1987). For example, if the total sleep time is 6 hours, the sleep restriction prescription limits time in bed to 6 to 6.5 hours. Wake time remains consistent, but bedtime is set 15 to 30 minutes earlier per session based on progress in improvement of sleep efficiency. Sleep restriction therapy is contraindicated in persons who require maximal vigilance to prevent accidents such as drivers and operators of heavy machinery, and in those with conditions exacerbated by sleepiness such as epilepsy, parasomnias, and sleep-disordered breathing (Epstein & Bootzin, 2002; Spielman, Yang, & Glovinsky, 2011).

Sleep Compression

Sleep compression is similar to sleep restriction, except that sleep is restricted incrementally over a period of about 5 weeks by either phase-delaying bedtime or phase-advancing wake time until the sleep efficiency goal is achieved. This technique is an alternative approach for patients who cannot tolerate the sudden reduction in total sleep time, such as older adults with serious medical comorbidities (Lichstein, Riedel, Wilson, Lester, & Aguillard, 2001; Lichstein, Thomas, & McCurry, 2011). Sleep compression is not classified as a treatment for insomnia.

Multicomponent Therapy

This consists of combinations of stimulus control, relaxation, and sleep restriction therapies, with or without cognitive therapy (Berry, 2012). Cognitive-behavioral therapy for insomnia (CBT-I) is one form of multi-component therapy, which emphasizes stimulus control and sleep restriction therapy. CBT-I is designed for patients who need intensive therapy, is delivered over 6 to 8 weeks at weekly visits, and is administered by a behavioral sleep medicine specialist. Brief behavioral treatment of insomnia (BBTI) was adapted from CBT-I as a first-line therapy for patients seen in primary care settings. BBTI is designed to be delivered over a shorter time period in fewer visits and/or in a small group format, and can be administered by master's level clinicians including nurses. BBTI is contraindicated in those for whom sleep restriction therapy is not recommended, as well as for persons with bipolar or psychotic disorders due to potential exacerbation of symptoms (Espie et al., 2007).

Sleep Hygiene Education

Sleep hygiene education is most often used in combination with other cognitive behavioral therapies to address problems with sleep initiation and maintenance. Initially developed by Hauri (1991), the purpose of sleep hygiene education is to increase knowledge of homeostatic and circadian processes, and encourage sleep-promoting behaviors. It consists of standardized recommendations regarding behavioral factors (sleep schedule, stimulants, environment, etc.) that may potentially influence sleep (Chesson et al., 1999; Posner & Gehrman, 2011). This intervention is thought to be most effective when tailored to the individual client (Perlis et al., 2005).

COMPLEMENTARY AND ALTERNATIVE MEDICINE MODALITIES

Complementary and alternative medicine (CAM) modalities were originally developed outside conventional Western medicine, and are used for symptom management of chronic conditions by many Americans (Barnes, Bloom, & Nahin, 2008). These modalities may be classified as whole-body, mind-body, and biological-based, manipulative and body-based, and meditation and movement-based.

Acupuncture is a whole-body modality that has been used successfully for insomnia symptom relief (Yeung, Chung, Leung, Zhang, & Saw, 2009). This traditional Chinese medical technique involves the insertion of special needles into specific meridians or channels of energy flow for the purpose of unblocking and restoring energy flow (National Center for Complementary and Alternative Medicine [NCCAM], 2007).

Mindfulness-based stress reduction, a mind-body modality, has been used effectively to treat insomnia symptoms (Winbush, Gross, & Kreitzer, 2007), by reducing stress through focused attention on breathing and increased awareness of the present (NCCAM, 2011). Mindfulness-based therapy for insomnia (MBTI) incorporates stimulus control, sleep restriction, and sleep hygiene with mindfulness principles such as letting go and acceptance. Its goal is to decrease night wakefulness and negative emotional response to sleep disturbance. MBTI is delivered in eight weekly sessions and one all-day retreat to small groups of six to eight participants (Ong & Manber, 2011).

Biological-based CAM sleep interventions include herbals that may be ingested, inhaled, or applied topically (Rose & Bourguignon, 2011). Orally administered valerian has been associated with symptom improvement of RLS (Cueller & Ratcliffe, 2009). Lavender oil, continuously inhaled overnight as aromatherapy (aerosolized), has been associated with improvement in insomnia symptoms (Lewith, Godfrey, & Prescott, 2005).

Massage, a manipulative and body-based modality, includes a variety of techniques that involve muscle and soft tissue manipulation (NCCAM, 2011). Studies in different populations including patients with migraines and insomnia have demonstrated sleep quality improvement using massage (Lawler & Cameron,

2006; Richards, 1998; Soden, Vincent, Craske, Lucus, & Ashley, 2004) in community-dwelling and hospitalized patients.

Tai chi and yoga both involve some form of meditation and movement (NCCAM, 2011). Tai chi, proposed to improve energy focus, flow, and balance (NCCAM, 2011), has been associated with improved subjective and objective sleep quality in older adults with sleep disturbance (Chen et al., 2009). Yoga, which stresses postures and breathing exercises to promote relaxation, has also been associated with improvement of insomnia symptoms (Khalsa, 2004).

In summary, the CAM modalities that have been investigated in research studies as sleep interventions and provide the best evidence of effectiveness include acupuncture, mindfulness meditation, massage, tai chi, and yoga (Rose & Bourguignon, 2011). Advanced practice psychiatric nurse practitioners should also be aware that many Americans take herbals, which may in themselves have sleep side effects, and which may potentially interact with pharmacologic therapies. Consequently, it is imperative that use of herbals in all forms be included when obtaining the current health history to avoid adverse medication events.

LONG-TERM MANAGEMENT OF SLEEP DISORDERS

CIRCADIAN RHYTHM DISORDERS

Long-term management of circadian rhythm disorders is aimed at the maintenance of the dark-light entrained sleep cycles established in initial therapy. Continued resolution of delayed sleep phase disorder (DSPD) depends upon adherence to good sleep hygiene practices including a set sleep-wake schedule. Light therapy (early morning exposure and evening avoidance) and melatonin may be incorporated into the plan of care. Long-term management of advanced sleep phase disorder (ASPD) requires maintenance of the established later bedtime schedule. Light therapy may be used during the evening hours to help delay sleep time, and melatonin may be given in the morning although evidence for this practice is limited. Melatonin is used for management of free running disorder (FRD) in blind or sighted persons, and light therapy may be used in sighted persons. Irregular sleep-wake rhythm (ISWR) is managed with mixed modalities including light therapy, and scheduled physical and social activities. Management of shift work disorder may include the use of a hypnotic such as zolpidem to promote daytime sleep, and use of stimulant medications such as modafinil to promote alertness during night work (Morgenthaler, Lee-Chiong, et al., 2007; Sack et al., 2007a; Sack et al., 2007b). Bright light therapy may be used to promote adjustment to night work, with use of a portable light box (bright blue or white) at the work station until 4 a.m. if possible. Light-related education for night shift workers includes wearing dark sunglasses in the morning after work and maintaining a light-tight (dark) bedroom to promote sleep. Bright light or light box exposure after 12 noon may be helpful on days off to promote wakefulness (Smith, Fogg, & Eastman, 2009). Bright light therapy is contraindicated in persons with eye disease or on photosensitizing medications. Bright lights can also induce migraines and mania (rarely) (Burgess, 2011).

NARCOLEPSY

Stimulant therapy is considered effective for long-term management of narcolepsy symptoms, and antidepressants for cataplexy, sleep paralysis, and hypnagogic hallucinations. Careful medication titration and monitoring are necessary to control symptoms and detect adverse side effects. Drug tolerance, addiction, hypertension, impaired hepatic function and psychosis may occur. Regular sleep times and two short scheduled naps per day can be helpful adjunct therapy to reduce day sleepiness and sleep episodes (Morgenthaler, Kapur et al., 2007; Rogers, 2011). Because many patients are symptomatic for years before receiving a narcolepsy diagnosis, depressive symptoms are common. Consequently, management of secondary mood symptoms and referral to support groups such as the Narcolepsy Network may be needed (Guilleminault & Cao, 2011). Advanced practice psychiatric nurses may collaborate with sleep specialists in the management of mood disturbance and promotion of positive adaptation to this challenging disorder.

INSOMNIA

Although there are a number of modalities for the management of insomnia, evidence supporting the efficacy of one method over another for long-term use is limited. Nor has the advantage of particular modalities for specific patient populations or insomnia subtypes been established. Additionally, the very nature of insomnia and its complex interrelationship with other comorbidities necessitate individualization of care. Psychological and behavioral therapies are recommended for first-line management of both primary and comorbid chronic insomnia. Stimulus reduction, relaxation training, and cognitive therapies are considered standard care, with sleep hygiene therapy as adjunct. Sleep restriction and other modalities such as paradoxical intention and biofeedback have less supportive evidence, but may be useful with particular clients (Chesson et al., 2000; Sateia, Doghramji, Hauri, & Morin, 2000; Schutte-Rodin et al., 2008).

REM BEHAVIOR DISORDER

Although there is no specific pharmacologic treatment for REM behavior disorder (RBD), melatonin given in the evening may be helpful for sleep promotion. Clonazepam may be given prior to bedtime if sleep-related injury is a concern, but must be administered with caution to clients with dementia, gait disorders, or OSA. Other interventions focus on promoting safety, and may include protection of the sleep partner with pillows or separate sleeping arrangements, mattress placement directly on the floor, and reduction of environmental breakables that could cause injury (Aurora et al., 2010). Medications associated with induction of RBD should be avoided and include clomipramine, selegiline, and phenelzine (Hoque & Chesson, 2010).

CENTRAL AND MIXED SLEEP APNEAS

Long-term management of central sleep apnea requires oversight and intermittent monitoring by a sleep-pulmonary specialist. If related to alveolar hypoventilation, such as with neuromuscular disorders, central sleep apnea may be managed with nocturnal ventilatory assistance using a nasal mask plus pressure- or volume-cycled ventilation (Shneerson & Simonds, 2002). If secondary to opioids that cannot be decreased in dosage, such as in palliative care, central sleep apnea may be managed by a sleep-pulmonary specialist with bi-level positive pressure (Alattar & Scharf, 2009). Mixed central and OSAs, as well as Cheyne-Stokes repirations, require careful individualized respiratory and pharmacologic care coordinated with medical management of the underlying pathophysiological processes (Wellman & White, 2011). As it is not uncommon for persons with degenerative neuromuscular disorders and end-of-life conditions to suffer from cormorbid depression and anxiety, advanced practice psychiatric nurses may collaborate with other health care specialists to provide supportive mental health care to these clients and their families.

OBSTRUCTIVE SLEEP APNEA

Effective long-term management of OSA includes client education and reduction of risk factors. Weight loss to a BMI of 25 kg/m2 or less, and bariatric surgery may be considered as an adjunct therapy in obese individuals in whom other methods have been unsuccessful. Avoidance of alcohol or sedatives prior to bedtime is recommended to prevent exacerbation of OSA. Positional therapy, including sleeping in a nonsupine position can be helpful as an adjunct therapy. Continuous positive airway pressure (CPAP) is used to manage moderate to severe OSA, and is more effective than oral appliances or surgery (Epstein et al., 2009). However, adherence may be challenging. This is a particular problem for smokers, who can have both chronic obstructive pulmonary disease and OSA, but who have lower compliance with CPAP than nonsmokers. Future insurance reimbursement for CPAP is anticipated to depend on demonstration of "benefit," as measured in part by adherence (Phillips & Kryger, 2011). Support including home visits and cognitive behavioral therapy have been somewhat effective in improving CPAP compliance (Haniffa, Lasserson, & Smith, 2004; Smith, Nadig, & Lasserson, 2009). A number of protocols are available to promote adherence to positive airway pressure including motivational enhancement therapy, exposure therapy for claustrophobic reactions, self-management, and CBT (Perlis, Aloia, & Kuhn, 2011). Advanced practice psychiatric nurses may collaborate with clients and sleep medicine specialists to achieve sleep goals. CAM modalities may also be used to promote adoption of positive health changes, and nonpharmacologic management of chronic pain and tension.

RLS AND PLM OF SLEEP

Management of RLS includes correction and monitoring of underlying risk factors for RLS, such as low serum ferritin (< 45–50 mcg/L). Oral iron and vitamin C supplementation are recommended to correct deficiencies (Montplaisir, Allen, Walters, & Ferini-Strambi, 2011). Pharmacologic therapy with dopamine agonists has become preferred therapy for the long-term management of RLS, due to augmentation of symptoms with levodopa. Use of other medications should be individualized based on relief of symptoms (Hening, Allen, Earley, Picchietti, & Silber, 2004). Intermittent monitoring for adverse side effects, augmentation, tolerance or development of other sleep disorders such as sleep apnea and insomnia is standard care (Chesson et al., 1999). Augmentation of RLS symptoms, a common problem with dopaminergic therapy, may be identified through recognition of an approximate 4-hour advance in the usual starting time symptoms, or a combination of changes in body parts with RLS symptoms, latency of symptom occurrence when at rest, increased severity of symptoms, and medication effect on symptoms (Garcia-Borreguero et al., 2007). If augmentation is suspected, the client should be referred back to a sleep medicine specialist for evaluation. Antihistamines and benzodiazepines have been found to exacerbate daytime RLS symptoms, and should be avoided (Allen, Lesage, & Earley, 2005). Specific medications associated with induction of RLS symptoms (escitalopram, fluoxetine, mianserin, mirtazapine, olanzapine, and tramadol) and PLMs (bupropion, citalopram, fluoxetine, paroxetine, sertraline, and venlafaxine) should also be avoided (Hoque & Chesson, 2010). Alcohol use has also been associated with increased PLMs (Aldrich & Shipley, 1993), and alcoholism with both PLMs and RLS in the presence of iron, ferritin, magnesium, and vitamin B_{12} deficiencies (Roehrs & Roth, 2011). Consequently, reduction in alcohol intake should be considered. Advanced psychiatric nurses can collaborate with sleep medicine specialists in managing depressed mood that may occur with impaired sleep, with attention to medications that might further exacerbate RLS and PLMs symptoms. They can also assess and monitor alcohol use and associated vitamin and mineral deficiencies.

AGE-RELATED SLEEP IMPLICATIONS

Pregnancy, Childbirth, and Postpartum

The first trimester of pregnancy is characterized by daytime sleepiness due to increased progesterone. Fragmentation of sleep in the first and third trimesters is also common due to pregnancy-related changes and discomforts (Hedman, Pohjasvaara, Tolonen, Suhonen-Malm, & Myllyla, 2002). Snoring frequency and severity increase during pregnancy, and OSA may develop, especially in women who are obese and/or who have a large neck circumference (Edwards, Blyton, Hennessy, & Sullivan, 2005). Sleep-disturbed breathing during pregnancy can contribute to complications such as increased maternal blood pressure and decreased uteroplacental blood flow (Guilleminault, Querra-Salva, Chowdhuri, & Poyares, 2000). Sleep disturbance due to pregnancy-related RLS is associated with decreased folate, plasma iron, hemoglobin, and mean corpuscular volume (Manconi et al., 2004). Pregnancy-associated insomnia symptoms are extremely common in pregnancy and may be related to increased metabolism and body temperature (AASM, 2005). Gastroesophageal reflux, also associated with progesterone elevation, often disrupts sleep and limits positions for sleep (Ali & Egan, 2007). During the postpartum period, new mothers commonly experience altered circadian rhythm related to infant care and feeding, which may increase fatigue (Thomas & Burr, 2006). Advanced practice psychiatric nurses should be particularly cognizant of how sleep deprivation may precipitate or exacerbate depressive symptoms in women during this vulnerable period (Wolfson, Crowley, Anwer, & Basette, 2003).

Preterm and Term Newborn Implications

Newborn infants who were born prematurely, had low Apgar scores, or have experienced illnesses such as sepsis are at greater risk for primary sleep apnea of infancy. Primary sleep apnea of infancy is classified as obstructive, central, or mixed. Obstructive apnea, characterized by thoracic movement but little or no nasal airflow, may occur with gastroesophageal reflux disease. Central apnea is caused by immature control of the respiratory system and is more common in preterm infants who weighed <1,500 grams at birth. It is characterized by absence of both thoracic movement and nasal airflow. Mixed apnea describes events that begin with either central apnea or obstructive apnea and then change to the other type. These events may occur in preterm infants or those who have experienced illness such as sepsis or hyperbilirubinemia (Poblano, Marquez, & Hernandez, 2006). Preterm infants also spend more time in REM sleep than older infants, and this stage of sleep contributes to sleep apnea. The upper airway muscles are more relaxed during REM sleep, leading to possible airway obstruction (Di Fiore, 2005). Although 98% of preterm infants are free of apneic symptoms by 40 weeks post-conceptional age, 2% continue to experience sporadic apneic episodes up to 6 months of age (AASM, 2005).

Apnea in newborn infants is exacerbated by respiratory infections such as bronchiolitis caused by the respiratory syncytial virus. Supportive respiratory care with management of associated underlying disease processes is the priority for apnea of infancy not due to immaturity (AASM, 2005).

The newborn period can be a very stressful time for parents because sleep patterns have not been established and nighttime sleep can be erratic. Even healthy newborns can exhaust their parents with difficulty going to sleep and waking up frequently at night. Parents who are frequently up at night and deprived of sleep on an ongoing basis are not only very tired, but may become anxious and depressed (Hauck, Hall, Dhaliwal, Bennett, & Wells, 2011). Exhaustion and emotional distress from frequent night awakenings are common causes of complaints to health care professionals. The implications for sleep and healthy relationships between parents and newborns are significant. One study has shown that infant-mother attachment at 12 months of age is related to night waking patterns during the first 6 months of life (Beijers, Jansen, Riksen-Walraven, & deWeerth, 2011). If the newborn infant is ill or requires a monitor for apnea events, the problems are compounded. Monitoring a newborn infant around the clock is very stressful and may precipitate additional anxiety and depression. A good family history is essential, and a sleep diary is recommended for parents who have newborns at home. Parents need practical advice on how to soothe crying infants and how to help infants develop stable sleep habits. Some good resources include the American Academy of Pediatrics (AAP) at www.aap.org/healthtopics/sleep.cfm; the Parenting Science website at www.parentingscience.com/newborn-sleep.html; Kids Health at http://kidshealth.org/parent/growth/sleep/sleepnewborn.html#; and a newborn sleep organization at http://newbornsleep.org. Sleep disruption and deprivation may be particularly stressful for new parents with a current or past history of depression, and may require psychological support to prevent induction or exacerbation of mood disturbance.

Infancy and Childhood

Since 1976, sleep scientists have systematically investigated the sleep of children, resulting in a growing awareness of how sleep disruption in childhood may adversely impact mood, behavior, and learning (Super & Johnson, 2011). The specific concerns regarding sleep for infants and children are presented in the section on pediatric pointers.

Menopause

During mid-life, women experience cessation of the menstrual cycle with accompanying changes in hormones including decreased estrogen. As a result, many women experience "hot flashes" and "night sweats," which are symptoms of a nocturnal thermoregulatory phenomenon characterized by peripheral vasodilation and diaphoresis (Freedman, 2005). These symptoms are associated with decreased subjective sleep quality (Hollander et al., 2001; Polo-Kantola, Erkkola, & Irjala, 1999), and increased nocturnal awakenings, sleep efficiency, and sleep stage changes (Woodward & Freedman, 1994). Hot flushes occur during NREM sleep and are inhibited during REM sleep. Consequently, perception of sleep quality appears to be influenced by the quantity of REM sleep experienced (Freedman & Roehrs, 2006). Although most commonly associated with menopause, women may continue to experience hot flushes for years after menopause (Barnabei et al., 2002). Hormone replacement therapy is only recommended for short-term symptom relief in women with a negative history of breast cancer or stroke. Other pharmacologic treatments include selective serotonin reuptake inhibitors such as paroxetine (Stearns, Beebe, Iyengar, & Dube, 2003), and gabapentin (Guttuso, Kurlan, McDermott, & Kieburtz, 2003). Nonpharmacologic therapies such as sleep hygiene education related to the sleep environment may be helpful (Freedman & Roehrs, 2006). Complementary and alternative therapies including relaxation and stress reduction may also be beneficial (Borelli & Ernst, 2010).

Postmenopausal women are 2.6 times more likely to have sleep-disordered breathing than their premenopausal counterparts, and 3.5 times more likely to have severe sleep-disordered breathing (Young, Finn, Austin, & Peterson, 2003). Lower levels of progesterone associated with decreased ventilator drive (Lin, Davidson & Ancoli-Israel, 2008), obesity (Young, Peppard, & Gottlieb, 2002), and visceral adiposity (Vgontzas, Bixler, & Chrousos, 2003) are believed to precipitate sleep disordered breathing in this age group. Sleep disordered breathing, hypertension, and obesity are strongly correlated in postmenopausal women, and the risk for the first two disorders is thought to be due to the third rather than to menopausal factors alone (Brown et al., 2000; Dart, Gregoire, Gutterman, & Woolf, 2003).

Older Adults

Older adults have an increased risk of several sleep disorders that are associated with medical conditions and disorders, including OSA and RLS. OSA is 1.7 to 3 times more prevalent in persons 60 years of age or older (Young et al., 2002). The major risk factor for OSA is obesity (Lee, Hagubadi, Kryger, & Moklesi, 2008), and weight gain is more strongly associated with OSA in men than in women (Newman et al., 2005). A weight gain of only 10% is associated with a six-fold increase in the odds of developing moderate to severe OSA, and sleep apnea increases the risk of developing hypertension, cardiac disease (Peppard, Young, Palta, Dempsey, & Skatrud, 2000), and diabetes (Punjabi & Beamer,

2009). Older adults may present with complaints of nocturia, disturbed sleep, and excessive daytime sleepiness (Endeshaw, 2006). They may also demonstrate impaired cognitive function and are at increased risk for injury due to drowsy driving (Ellen et al., 2006). Continuous positive airway pressure is first-line treatment for OSA, and requires long-term follow-up to establish and maintain effectiveness of therapy (Epstein et al., 2009). Older adults are also at higher risk for RLS, and it is suggested to be more prevalent in older women than in older men (Rijsman, Neven, Graffelman, Kemp, & deWeerd, 2004). In older adults this syndrome is associated with decreased sleep quality, mood, and overall quality of life (Cueller, Strumpf, & Ratliffe, 2007). Risk factors beyond familial phenotypes associated with earlier onset, include serum iron deficiency and use of selective serotonin reuptake inhibitors (Cueller & Redeker, 2011). Treatment focuses on correction of any underlying factors and medications aimed at reducing symptom severity (Cueller & Ratliffe, 2008).

Sleep disturbance is a common geriatric syndrome in older persons with mental health conditions, and occurs with depression, anxiety, substance abuse, dementia, and other neurological disorders such as Parkinson's disease (Vaz Fragoso & Gill, 2007). Older persons are also living longer with underlying psychiatric conditions that influence sleep (Crystal, Sambamoorghi, Walkup, & Akincingial, 2003).

Late life mental health conditions place older persons at risk for severe sleep disturbance. One in five older persons (26.3%) has a mental disorder, 16% have a primary mental health condition, and 3% also have dementia (Jeste et al., 1999). Because mental health disorders do not disappear with old age, conditions such as depression, bipolar disorder, and schizophrenia often worsen with chronic conditions or when superimposed on dementia. While only 1% of older adults suffer from bipolar disorder or schizophrenia (Substance Abuse and Mental Health Services Administration [SAMHSA], 2007), older adults are living longer with these debilitating conditions that are associated with sleep disturbance. Older adults experiencing the manic phase of bipolar disorder perceive a decreased need for sleep (American Psychiatric Association, 2000). Older adults with schizophrenia may demonstrate reversal of the sleep-wake cycle, long episodes of complete sleeplessness, decreased total sleep time, prolonged sleep-onset latency, and fragmented sleep (Benson & Zarcone, 2005).

Mood disorders are common in older adults, and 11% are affected by depression. Depressed older adults have delayed REM sleep; decreased deep, restorative sleep; and difficulty falling back to sleep due to sadness and worry (Benca, 2005). Poor sleep efficiency of about 73% is found in depressed older persons (Bliwise, 2005). Depression is often accompanied by anxiety, and 20% of older adults report anxiety symptoms (SAMHSA, 2007). Anxiety is characterized by nighttime panic attacks and insomnia symptoms (Brenes, Miller, Stanley, Williamson, Knudson, & McCall, 2009; Stein & Mellman, 2005). Older persons with generalized anxiety disorders (with or without depression) have more severe sleep disturbance than those without a psychiatric diagnosis (Brenes et al., 2009).

Dementia is one of the most common geropsychiatric disorders, and is associated with neurodegenerative changes resulting in fragmented sleep. Older adults with dementia are at high risk for severely disturbed sleep due to damage in the neuronal pathways that interfere with homeostatic and circadian rhythm processes (Bliwise, 2005). Older adults with dementia often present with a typical sleep pattern of nighttime wandering and daytime sleepiness, and their sleep architecture is characterized by decreased slow wave sleep and less REM (Petit, Montplaisir, & Boeve, 2005). Disturbed sleep is a common reason for institutionalization of older adults with dementia, and fragmented sleep is more severe among nursing home residents.

Parkinson's disease is most common among older adults, and is a neurodegenerative disorder caused by insufficient amounts of dopamine produced in the substantial nigra of the brain. RBD is common in older adults with Parkinson's disease, and in dementia with Lewy bodies (Petit et al., 2005; Postuma et al., 2009). Older adults with RBD awaken suddenly and act out their dreams, demonstrating a loss of muscle atonia and an increase in motor activity such as kicking and biting. Research shows that RBD may actually predict Parkinson's disease (Postuma et al., 2009). Nonpharmacological management focused on safety is recommended because pharmacological therapy can worsen associated sleep apnea and dementia (Petit et al., 2005).

Although mental health and sleep disorders are common in older adults and predict their quality of life, sleep complaints are seldom documented (Reid et al., 2006). Advanced practice psychiatric nurses must become knowledgeable and proactive in the assessment and management of sleep disturbance in older persons. Although a variety of psychotropic medications are available to treat sleep disorders and underlying mental health conditions, older persons are at risk for adverse side effects of these medications such as orthostatic hypotension, cognitive impairment, excessive daytime sleepiness, and interactions due to polypharmacy. Consequently, nonpharmacological interventions are first-line treatments for older adults with and without mental health conditions.

CONCLUSION AND DISCUSSION

In conclusion, advanced practice psychiatric nurses must be well-prepared to address the concerns of clients who present with complaints of sleep disturbance, based on current knowledge of developmental sleep changes, sleep disorders, and recommended screening, diagnostic, and management modalities. Health care provider–initiated evaluation of sleep disturbance is also critical to the treatment of all mental health conditions and disorders. Undiagnosed and poorly managed sleep symptoms often exacerbate psychiatric symptoms, may precipitate maladaptive behaviors, and can significantly reduce the effectiveness of any treatment offered. Consequently, advanced practice psychiatric nurses should incorporate the care of sleep into routine practice for all clients across the life span, from the initial interview through each follow-up encounter.

PEDIATRIC POINTERS

Behavioral insomnia of childhood is a common disorder of infancy and childhood, and is characterized by reliance on specific conditions or objects to initiate sleep (sleep-onset association type), or bedtime refusal behaviors (limit-setting type) (Mindell, Kuhn, Lewin, Meltzer, & Sadeh, 2006). Management of behavioral insomnia of childhood is primarily focused on parenting skills (Mindell et al., 2006), but may include pharmacologic therapy. Numerous protocols for managing childhood insomnia are available including unmodified and graduated extinction, extinction with parental presence, bedtime pass, "excuse me drill," and daytime correction (Perlis, Aloia, & Kuhn, 2011). Excessive daytime sleepiness may go unrecognized in children and adolescents, who demonstrate hyperactivity, impulsivity, or aggressiveness rather than classic adult symptoms (Moore et al., 2009; O'Brian et al., 2007), and poor school performance (Gozal, 1998). Excessive daytime sleepiness in toddlers and early school-age children may be associated with OSA, which is most commonly due hypertrophy of the adenoids and tonsils (Halbower & Marcus, 2003), and which usually responds to surgical management (Hoban, 2010). Nasal CPAP may also be used (AAP, 2002). Escape extinction within a multi-component behavior therapy approach can be used to promote positive airway pressure adherence in children with and without developmental disabilities (Slifer, 2011). Behaviorally induced insufficient sleep syndrome is most common in adolescents due to school and social demands (AASM, 2005), although normal developmental changes in circadian sleep patterns may also contribute to delayed sleep phase syndrome (Tarokh & Carskadon, 2010). Management of these disorders includes modification of wake-time activities, sleep hygiene education, gradual bedtime adjustment, and reduction of bedtime stimuli (Archbold, 2011). Motivational interviewing may also be used to promote healthy sleep-related behaviors in adolescents, using collaboration, evocation (assisting adolescents to identify personal motivation for change), and autonomy (emphasizing the adolescent's responsibility for changing behavior) (Gold & Dahl, 2011). RLS may become symptomatic in childhood, is described differently than by adults (bubbling, crawling, itching), and can present as behavioral or academic problems (Chervin et al., 2002). Narcolepsy, another disorder with hereditary implications, often emerges by adolescence, and requires referral to a sleep specialist for definitive diagnosis (Guilleminault & Pelayo, 2000). Both RLS and narcolepsy require specialized medication management. Childhood parasomnias arise from NREM slow wave sleep, include sleep terrors and sleep walking, are characterized

(*Continued*)

PEDIATRIC POINTERS (*Continued*)

by amnesia of the episode, and typically resolve by early school age. These are distinguishable from nightmares, also common, which arise from REM sleep and are remembered by children (Bloomfield & Shatkin, 2009; Snyder, Goodlin-Jones, Pionk, & Stein, 2010). Management recommendations for sleepwalking and sleep terrors include having the child empty his or her bladder at bedtime, and awakening the child 30 minutes prior to the anticipated episode nightly for a week to interrupt the pattern (Byars, 2011; Howard & Wong, 2001). Nurses should be alert to parental reports of children demonstrating stereotypical behaviors such as lip-smacking or hand hitting the head during episodes of sleepwalking, as these may be symptoms of nocturnal seizures and require further evaluation (Silvestri & Bromfield, 2004). Children with pervasive developmental delays may demonstrate a variety of sleep disorders, such as head-banging by those with autism. Children with attention deficit hyperactivity disorder have increased rates of PLMs of sleep and sleep-disordered breathing (AASM, 2005). Bedtime fading may be used in children with and without developmental disabilities, and includes putting the child to bed later than typical onset of sleep, eliminating daytime naps, and establishing a set sleep-wake pattern. It also includes removing the child from bed if sleep does not occur within 15 minutes and allowing engagement in regular evening activity, as well as only allowing the child to remain in bed when sleep is highly likely. This protocol is based on similar principles as stimulus control and sleep restriction therapies, and pairs bedtime stimuli with sleepiness and sleep-related behaviors (Kodak & Piazza, 2011). Awareness of sleep symptoms in children may be both a clue to possible developmental problems, as well as to possible causes for exacerbation of related behavioral symptoms. In summary, advanced practice psychiatric nurses must be knowledgeable of normal developmental changes in sleep across childhood, common sleep disorders that usually resolve during childhood, differences in the presentation of sleep disorders in children as compared to adults, and symptoms that warrant further evaluation by a sleep specialist.

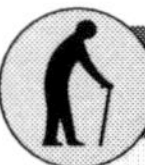

AGING ALERTS

Older persons tend to spend a longer time in bed, go to bed earlier, and awaken earlier than younger adults (Vitiello, 2006). Napping remains variable in this age group, but is common and appears to increase with age (Driscoll et al., 2008; Foley et al., 2007). Lifestyle changes such as retirement and alterations in social interactions may impact the sleep of older adults (Redeker, 2011). Grief due to bereavement, often cumulative in older adults, may also be accompanied by sleep disturbance such as insomnia (AASM, 2005). Overall, sleep disturbance in older adults appears to be associated with medical, psychiatric, and sleep disorders (Vitiello, Moe, & Prinz, 2002), rather than with advanced aging alone.

RESOURCES FOR PROFESSIONALS

SLEEP AND SLEEP PROBLEMS

American Academy of Sleep Medicine: www.aasmnet.org or www.sleepeducation.com

National Center on Sleep Disorders Research of the National Heart, Lung, and Blood Institute: www.nhlbi.nih.gov/about/ncsdr/index.htm

National Sleep Foundation: www.sleepfoundation.org or www.sleepfoundation.org/healthcare-professionals

SPECIFIC SLEEP DISORDERS

American Sleep Apnea Association: www.sleepapnea.org

Narcolepsy Network: www.narcolepsynetwork.org

Restless Legs Syndrome Foundation: www.rls.org

REFERENCES

Alattar, M. A., & Scharf, S. M. (2009). Opioid-associated central sleep apnea: A case series. *Sleep and Breathing, 13*(2), 201–206.

Aldrich, M. S., & Shipley, J. E. (1993). Alcohol use and periodic limb movements of sleep. *Alcoholism, Clinical and Experimental Research, 17*(1), 192–196.

Ali, R. A., & Egan, L. J. (2007). Gastroesophageal reflux disease in pregnancy. *Best Practice and Research Clinical Gastroenterology, 21*(5), 793–806.

Allen, R. P., Burchell, B. J., MacDonald, B., Hening, W. A., & Earley, C. J. (2009). Validation of the self-completed Cambridge-Hopkins questionnaire (CH-RLSq) for ascertainment of restless legs syndrome (RLS) in a population survey. *Sleep Medicine, 10*(10), 1097–1100.

Allen, R. P., Lesage, S., & Earley, C. J. (2005). Antihistamines and benzodiazepines exacerbate daytime restless legs syndrome (RLS) symptoms (abstract). *Sleep, 28*, A279.

American Academy of Pediatrics (AAP) Section on Pediatric Pulmonology, Subcommittee on Obstructive Sleep Apnea Syndrome. (2002). Clinical practice guideline: Diagnosis and management of childhood obstructive sleep apnea. *Pediatrics, 109*(4), 704–712.

American Academy of Sleep Medicine. (2005). *The international classification of sleep disorders: Diagnostic and coding manual* (2nd ed.). Westchester, IL: Author.

American Psychiatric Association. (2000). *Diagnostic and statistical manual of mental disorders* (Rev. ed.). Washington, DC: Author.

Ancoli-Israel, S., Cole, R., Alessi, C. A., Chambers, M., Moorcroft, W., & Pollak, C. P. (2003). The role of actigraphy in the study of sleep and circadian rhythms. *Sleep, 26*(3), 342–392.

Anders, T., Emde, R., & Parmelee, A. (1971). *A manual of standardized terminology, techniques, and criteria for scoring of stages of sleep and wakefulness in newborn infants*. Los Angeles, CA: Brain Information Service, UCLA.

Anders, T. F., Sadeh, A., & Appareddy, V. (1995). Normal sleep in neonates and children. In R. Ferber & M. Kryger (Eds.), *Principles and practice of sleep medicine in the child* (pp. 7–18). Philadelphia, PA: W. B. Saunders.

Archbold, K. H. (2011). Pediatric sleep disorders. In N. S. Redeker & G. P. McEnany (Eds.), *Sleep disorders and sleep promotion in nursing practice* (pp. 219–232). New York, NY: Springer.

Ardestani, S., Inserra, P., Solkoff, D., & Watson, R. R. (1999). The role of cytokines and chemokines on tumor progression: A review. *Cancer Detection and Prevention, 23*(3), 215–225.

Association of Sleep Disorders Centers and the Association for Psychophysiological Study of Sleep. (1979). *Diagnostic classification of sleep and arousal disorders* (1st ed.). *Sleep, 2*(1), 1–154.

Atwood, C. W., Jr., Strollo, P. J., Jr., & Givelber, R. (2011). Medical therapy for obstructive sleep apnea. In M. H. Kryger, T. Roth, & W. C. Dement (Eds.), *Principles and practice of sleep medicine* (5th ed., pp. 1219–1232). Philadelphia, PA: Saunders.

Aurora, R. N., Zak, R. S., Maganti, R. K., Auerbach, S. H., Casey, K. R., Chowdhuri, S., ... (2010). Standards of practice committee American Academy of Sleep Medicine. Best practice guide for the treatment of REM sleep behavior disorder (RBD). *Journal of Clinical Sleep Medicine, 15*(6), 85–95.

Barnabei, V. M., Grady, D., Stovall, D. W., Cauley, J. A., Lin, F., Stuenkel, C. A., ... Pickar, J. H. (2002). Menopausal symptoms in older women and the effects of treatment with hormone therapy. *Obstetrics and Gynecology, 100*(6), 1209–1218.

Barnes, P. M., Bloom, B., & Nahin, R. L. (2008). Complementary and alternative medicine use among adults and children: United States, 2007. *National Health Statistics Report, 10*(12), 1–23.

Bastian, C. H., Vallieres, A., & Morin, C. M. (2001). Validation of the Insomnia Severity Index as an outcome measure for insomnia research. *Sleep Medicine, 2*(4), 297–307.

Beijers, R., Jansen, J., Riksen-Walraven, M., & deWeerth, C. (2011). Attachment and infant waking: A longitudinal study from birth through the first year of life. *Journal of Developmental and Behavioral Pediatrics, 32*(7), 1–9.

Benca, R. (2005). Mood disorders. In M. H. Kryger, T. Roth, & W. C. Dement (Eds.), *Principles and practice of sleep medicine* (pp. 1311–1326). Philadelphia, PA: Elsevier/Saunders.

Benson, K. L., & Zarcone, V. P. (2005). Schizophrenia. In M. H. Kryger, T. Roth, & W. C. Dement (Eds.), *Principles and practice of sleep medicine* (pp. 1327–1336). Philadelphia, PA: Elsevier/Saunders.

Berry, R. B. (2012). *Fundamentals of sleep medicine*. Philadelphia, PA: Elsevier/Saunders.

Blake, J. (2010). Development of an online sleep diary for physician and patient use. *Knowledge Management and E-Learning: An International Journal, 2*(2). Retrieved from http://www.kmel-journal.org/ojs/index.php/online-publication/article/viewPDFInterstitial/63/47

Bliwise, D. L. (2005). Normal aging. In M. H. Kryger, T. Roth, & W. C. Dement (Eds.), *Principles and practice of sleep medicine* (pp. 24–38). Philadelphia, PA: Elsevier Saunders.

Bloomfield, E. R., & Shatkin, J. P. (2009). Parasomnias and movement disorders in children and adolescents. *Child and Adolescent Psychiatric Clinics of North America, 18*(4), 947–965.

Boeve, B. F., Silber, M. H., Saper, C. B., Ferman, T. J., Dickson, D. W., Parisi, J. E., ... Braak, H. (2007). Pathophysiology of REM sleep behavior disorder and relevance to neurodegenerative disease. *Brain, 130*(Pt. 11), 2770–2788.

Bootzin, R. R. (2005). Preface. In M. L. Perlis, C. Jungquist, M.T. Smith, and D. Posner. *Cognitive behavioral treatment of insomnia: A session-by-session guide.* New York, NY: Springer Publishing.

Bootzin, R. R., & Perlis, M. L. (2011). Stimulus control therapy. In M. L. Perlis, M. Aloia, & B. Kuhn (Eds.), *Behavioral treatments for sleep disorders: A comprehensive primer of behavioral sleep medicine interventions* (pp. 21–30). Boston, MA: Elsevier

Bootzin, R. R., Epstein, D., & Ward, J. M. (1991). Stimulus control instructions. In P. Hauri (Ed.), *Case studies in insomnia* (pp. 19–28). New York, NY: Plenum.

Borbély, A. A. (1982). A two process model of sleep regulation. *Human Neurobiology, 1*(3), 195–204.

Borelli, F., & Ernst, E. (2010). Alternative and complementary therapies for the menopause. *Maturitas, 66*(4), 333–343.

Brenes, G. A., Miller, M. E., Stanley, M. A., Williamson, J. D., Knudson, M., & McCall, W. V. (2009). Insomnia in older adults with generalized anxiety disorder. *American Journal of Geriatric Psychiatry, 17*(6), 465–472.

Brown, C. D., Higgins, M., Donato, K. A., Rohde, F. C., Garrison, R., Obarzanek, E.,...Horan, M. (2000). Body mass index and the prevalence of hypertension and dyslipidemia. *Obesity Research, 8*(9), 605–619.

Brown, G., Cardinali, D., & Pandi-Perumal, S. R. (2010). Melantonin and mental illness. In S. R. Pandi-Perumal & M. Kramer (Eds.), *Sleep and mental illness* (pp. 199–229). New York, NY: Cambridge University Press.

Buchanan, P., & Grunstein, R. (2011). Positive airway pressure treatment for obstructive sleep apnea-hypopnea syndrome. In M. H. Kryger, T. Roth, & W. C. Dement (Eds.), *Principles and practice of sleep medicine* (5th ed., pp.1233–1249). Philadelphia, PA: Saunders.

Burgess, H. J. (2011). Using bright light and melatonin to adjust to night work. In M. L. Perlis, M. Aloia, & B. Kuhn (Eds.), *Behavioral treatments for sleep disorders: A comprehensive primer of behavioral sleep medicine interventions* (pp.159–166). Boston, MA: Elsevier.

Buysse, D. J., & Perlis, M. L. (1996).The evaluation and treatment of insomnia. *Journal of Practical Psychiatry and Behavioral Health,* March, 80–93.

Buysse, D. J., Reynolds, C. F. III, Monk, T. H., Berman, S. R., & Kupfer, D. J. (1989).The Pittsburgh sleep quality index: A new instrument for psychiatric practice and research, *Psychiatry Research, 28*(2), 193–213.

Byars, K. (2011). Scheduled awakenings: A behavioral protocol for treating sleep walking and sleep terrors in children. In M. L. Perlis, M. Aloia, & B. Kuhn (Eds.), *Behavioral treatments for sleep disorders: A comprehensive primer of behavioral sleep medicine interventions* (pp. 325–332). Boston, MA: Elsevier.

Cao, M. T., Guilleminault, C., & Kushida, C. A. (2011). Clinical features and evaluation of obstructive sleep apnea and upper airway resistance syndrome. In M. H. Kryger, T. Roth, & W. C. Dement (Eds.), *Principles and practice of sleep medicine* (5th ed., pp. 1206–1218). Philadelphia, PA: Saunders.

Carskadon, M. A., & Dement, W. C. (1982). The multiple sleep latency test: What does it measure? *Sleep, 5*(Suppl. 2), 67–72.

Carskadon, M. A., & Dement, W. C. (2000). Normal human sleep: An overview. In M. H. Kryger, T. Roth, & W. C. Dement (Eds.), *Principles and practice of sleep medicine* (3rd ed., pp. 15–25). Philadelphia, PA: Saunders.

Carskadon, M. A., & Dement, W. C. (2005). Normal human sleep: An overview. In M. H. Kryger, T. Roth, & W. C. Dement (Eds.), *Principles and practice of sleep medicine* (pp. 13–23). Philadelphia, PA: Elsevier/Saunders.

Carskadon, M. A., Dement, W. C., Mitler, M. M., Roth, T., Westbrook, P. R., & Keenan, S. (1986). Guidelines for the multiple sleep latency test (MSLT): A standard measure of sleepiness, *Sleep, 9*(4), 519–524.

Catterall, J. R., Calverley, P. M., MacNee, W., Warren, P. M., Shapiro, C. M., Douglas, N. J., & Flenley, D. C. (1985). Mechanism of transient nocturnal hypoxemia in hypoxic chronic bronchitis and emphysema. *Journal of Applied Physiology, 59*(6), 1698–1703.

Chabas, D., Taheri, S., Renier, C., & Mignot, E. (2003). The genetics of narcolepsy. *Annual Review of Genomics in Human Genetics, 4*, 459–483.

Chen, K. M., Chen, M. H., Chao, H. C., Hung, H. M., Lin, H. S., & Li, C. H. (2009). Sleep quality, depression state, and health status of older adults after silver yoga exercises: Cluster randomized trial. *International Journal of Nursing Studies, 46*(2), 154–163.

Chervin, R. D., Archbold, K. H., Dillon, J. E., Panahi, P., Pituch, K. J., Dahl, R. E., & Guilleminault, C. (2002). Inattention, hyperactivity, and symptoms of sleep-disordered breathing. *Pediatrics, 109*(3), 449–456.

Chervin, R. D., Hedger, K., Dillon, J. E., & Pituch, K. J. (2000). Pediatric sleep questionnaire (PSQ): Validity and reliability of scales for sleep-disordered breathing, snoring, sleepiness, and behavioral problems. *Sleep Medicine, 1*(1), 21–32.

Chesson, A., Jr., Hartse, K., Anderson, W. M., Davila, D., Johnson, S., Littner, M.,...Rafecas, J. (2000). Practice parameters for the evaluation of chronic insomnia. An American Academy of Sleep Medicine Report. Standards of Practice Committee of the American Academy of Sleep Medicine. *Sleep, 23*(2), 237–241.

Chesson, A. L., Jr., Wise, M., Davila, D., Johnson, S., Littner, M., Anderson, W. M.,...Rafecas, J. (1999). Practice parameters for the treatment of restless legs syndrome and periodic limb movement disorder. An American Academy of Sleep Medicine Report, Standards of Practice Committee of the American Academy of Sleep Medicine. *Sleep, 22*(7), 961–968.

Chou, T. C., Scammell, T. E., Gooley, J. J., Gaus, S. E., Saper, C. B., & Lu, J. (2003). Critical role of dorsomedial hypothalamic nucleus in a wide range of behavior circadian rhythms. *The Journal of Neuroscience, 23*(33), 10691–10702.

Chung, F., & Elsaid, H. (2009). Screening for obstructive sleep apnea before surgery: Why is it important? *Current Opinions in Anesthesiology, 22*(3), 405–411.

Chung, F., Yegneswaran, B., Liao, P., Chung, S. A., Vairavanathan, S., Islam, S.,...Shapiro, C. M. (2008). STOP Questionnaire: A tool to screen patients for obstructive sleep apnea. *Anesthesiology, 108*(5), 812–821.

Conroy, D. A., Arnett, J. T., & Brower, K. J. (2010). Sleep and substance use and abuse. In S. R. Pandi-Perumal & M. Cramer (Eds.), *Sleep in mental illness* (pp. 283–288). New York, NY: Cambridge University Press.

Crabtree, V. M., & Williams, N. A. (2009). Normal sleep in children and adolescents. *Child and Adolescent Psychiatric Clinics of North America, 18*(4), 799–811.

Crystal, S., Sambamoorghi, U., Walkup, J. T., & Akincingial, A. (2003). Diagnosis and treatment of depression in the elderly Medicare population: Predictors, disparities, and trends. *Journal of the American Geriatrics Society, 51*(12), 1718–1728.

Cueller, N. G., & Ratcliffe, S. J. (2009). Does valerian improve sleepiness and symptom severity in people with restless legs syndrome? *Alternative Therapies in Health and Medicine, 15*(2), 22–28.

Cueller, N. G., & Ratcliffe, S. J. (2008). A comparison of glycemic control, sleep, fatigue, and depression in type 2 diabetes with and without restless legs syndrome. *Journal of Clinical Sleep Medicine, 4*(10), 50–56.

Cueller, N. G., & Redeker, N. S. (2011). Sleep-related movement disorders and parasomnias. In N. S. Redeker & G. P. McEnany (Eds.), *Sleep disorders and sleep promotion in nursing practice* (pp. 121–140). New York, NY: Springer.

Cueller, N. G., Strumpf, N. E., & Ratcliffe, S. J. (2007). Symptoms of restless legs syndrome in older adults: Outcomes on sleep quality, sleepiness, fatigue, depression, and quality of life. *Journal of the American Geriatrics Society, 55*(9), 1387–1392.

Dart, R. A., Gregoire, J. R., Gutterman, D. D., & Woolf, S. H. (2003). The association of hypertension and secondary cardiovascular disease with sleep-disordered breathing. *Chest, 123*(1), 244–260.

Davis, K. L., Stewart, D. G., Friedman, J. I., Buchsbaum, M., Harvey, P. D., Hof, P. R.,...Haroutunian, V. (2003). White matter changes in schizophrenia: Evidence for myelin-related dysfunction. *Archives of General Psychiatry, 60*(5), 443–456.

Dement, W. C. (2011). History of sleep physiology and medicine. In M. H. Kryger, T. Roth, & W. C. Dement (Eds.), *Principles and practice of sleep medicine* (5th ed., pp. 3–15). Philadelphia, PA: Saunders.

Di Fiore, T. (2005). Use of sleep studies in the neonatal intensive care unit. *Neonatal Network, 24*(1), 23–30.

Douglas, N. J. (2011). Sleep in patients with asthma and chronic obstructive pulmonary disease. In M. H. Kryger, T. Roth, & W. C. Dement (Eds.), *Principles and practice of sleep medicine* (5th ed., pp. 1294–1307). Philadelphia, PA: Saunders.

Driscoll, H. C., Serody, L., Patrick, S., Maurer, J., Bensasi, S., Houck, P. R.,...Reynolds, C. F. (2008). Sleeping well, aging well: A descriptive and cross-sectional study of sleep in "successful agers" 75 and older. *American Journal of Geriatric Psychiatry, 16*(1), 74–82.

Dunlop, R. J., & Campbell, C. W. (2000). Cytokines and advanced cancer. *Journal of Pain and Symptom Management, 20*(3), 214–232.

Edinger, J. D., & Carney, C. E. (2008). *Overcoming insomnia: A cognitive-behavioral therapy approach workbook (treatments that work)*. Oxford, UK: Oxford University Press.

Edwards, N., Blyton, D. M., Hennessy, A., & Sullivan, C. E. (2005). Severity of sleep-disordered breathing improves following parturition. *Sleep, 28*(6), 737–741.

Ellen, R. L. B., Marshall, S. C., Palayew, M., Molnar, F. J., Wilson, K. G., & Man-Son-Hing, M. (2006). Systematic review of motor vehicle crash risk in persons with sleep apnea. *Journal of Clinical Sleep Medicine, 2*(2), 193–200.

Endeshaw, Y. (2006). Clinical characteristics of obstructive sleep apnea in community-dwelling older adults. *Journal of the American Geriatric Society, 54*(11), 1740–1744.

Engel, J. K. (2006). *Pediatric assessment* (5th ed.). St. Louis, MO: Mosby.

Epstein, D. R., & Bootzin, R. R. (2002). Insomnia. *Nursing Clinics of North America, 37*(4), 611–631.

Epstein, L. J., Kristo, D., Strollo, P. J., Jr., Friedman, N., Malhotra, A., Patil, S. P.,...Weinstein, M. D. (2009). Clinical guideline for the evaluation, management, and long-term care of obstructive sleep apnea in adults. *Journal of Clinical Sleep Medicine, 5*(3), 263–276.

Espie, C. A. (2011). Paradoxical intention therapy (61–70).

Espie, C. A., MacMahon, K. M. A., Kelly, H. L., Broomfeild, N. M., Douglas, N. J., Engleman, H. M.,...Wilson, P. (2007). Randomized clinical effectiveness trial of a nurse-administered small-group cognitive behavioral therapy for persistent insomnia in general practice. *Sleep, 30*(5), 574–584.

Faraco, J., & Mignot, E. (2011). Genetics of sleep and sleep disorders in humans. In M. H. Kryger, T. Roth, & W. C. Dement (Eds.), *Principles and practice of sleep medicine* (5th ed., pp. 184–198). Philadelphia, PA: Saunders.

Feinberg, I., & Guazzelli, M. (1999). Schizophrenia: A disorder of the corollary discharge systems that integrate the motor systems of thought with the sensory systems of consciousness. *British Journal of Psychiatry, 174*, 196–204.

Floyd, J. A., Medler, S. M., Aer, J. W., & Janisse, J. J. (2000). Age-related changes in initiation and maintenance of sleep: A meta-analysis. *Research in Nursing and Health, 23*(2), 106–117.

Foley, D. J., Vitiello, M. V., Bliwise, D. L., Ancoli-Israel, S., Monjan, A. A., & Walsh, J. K. (2007). Frequent napping is associated with excessive daytime sleepiness, depression, pain and nocturia in older adults: Findings from the National Sleep Foundation 'Sleep in America Survey'. *American Journal of Geriatric Psychiatry, 15*(4), 344–350.

Freedman, R. R. (2005). Hot flashes: Behavioral treatments, mechanisms, and relation to sleep. *American Journal of Medicine, 118*(Suppl. 12B), 124–130.

Freedman, R. R., & Roehrs, T. A. (2006). Effects of REM sleep and ambient temperature on hot flash-induced sleep disturbance. *Menopause, 13*(4), 576–583.

Friedman, M., Tanyeri, H., La Rosa, M., Landsberg, R., Vaidyanathan, K., Pieri, S., & Caldarelli, D. (1999). Clinical predictors of obstructive sleep apnea. *Laryngoscope, 109*(12), 1901–1907.

Fuller, P. M., Gooley, J. J., & Saper, C. B. (2006). Neurobiology of the sleep-wake cycle: Sleep architecture, circadian regulation, and regulatory feedback. *Journal of Biological Rhythms, 21*(6), 482–493.

Galland, B. C., Taylor, B. J., Elder, D. E., & Herbison, P. (2011). Normal sleep pattern in infants and children: A systematic review of observational studies. *Sleep Medicine Reviews*, 1–10. doi:10.1016/j.smrv.2011.06.001

Garcia-Borreguero, D., Allen, R. P., Kohnen, R., Högl, B., Trenkwalder, C., Oertel, W.,...Earley, C. J. (2007). Diagnostic standards for dopaminergic augmentation of restless legs syndrome: Report from World Association of Sleep Medicine-International Restless Legs Syndrome Study Group consensus conference at the Max Planck Institute. *Sleep Medicine, 8*(5), 520–530.

Gillian, J. C., & Ancoli-Israel, S. (2005). The impact of age on sleep and sleep disorders. In G. Salzman (Ed.), *Clinical geriatric psychopharmacology* (pp. 483–512). Philadelphia, PA: Lippincott Williams & Wilkins.

Goff, D. C., & Coyle, J. T. (2001). The emerging role of glutamate in the pathyophysiology and treatment of schizophrenia. *American Journal of Psychiatry, 158*(9), 1367–1377.

Gold, M. A., & Dahl, R. E. (2011). Using motivational interviewing to facilitate healthier sleep-related behaviors in adolescents. In M. L. Perlis, M. Aloia, & B. Kuhn (Eds.), *Behavioral treatments for sleep disorders: A comprehensive primer of behavioral sleep medicine interventions* (pp. 367–381). Boston, MA: Elsevier.

Goldfarb, I. G., Petersen, R. B., Tabaton, M., Brown, P., LeBlanc, A. C., Montagna, P.,...Pendelbury, W. W. (1992). Fatal familial insomnia and familial Creutzfeldt-Jakob disease: Disease phenotype determined by DNA polymorphism. *Science, 258*(2053), 806–808.

Goodlin-Jones, B. L., Burnham, M. M., Gaylor, E. E., & Anders, T. F. (2001). Night waking, sleep-wake organization, and self-soothing in the first year of life. *Journal of Developmental and Behavioral Pediatrics, 22*(4), 226–233.

Gottlieb, D. J., O'Conner, G. T., & Wilk, J. B. (2007). Genome-wide association of sleep and circadian phenotypes. *BMC Medical Genetics, 8*(Suppl. 1), S9.

Gozal, D. (1998). Sleep-disordered breathing and school performance in children. *Pediatrics, 102*(3), 616–620.

Grigg-Damberger, M., Gozal, D., Marcus, C. L., Quan, S. F., Rosen, C. L., Chervin, R. D.,...Iber, C. (2007). The visual scoring of sleep and arousal in infant and children. *Journal of Clinical Sleep Medicine, 15*(3), 201–240.

Guilleminault, C., & Cao, M.T. (2011). Narcolepsy: Diagnosis and treatment. In M. H. Kryger, T. Roth, & W. C. Dement (Eds.), *Principles and practice of sleep medicine* (5th ed., pp. 957–968). Philadelphia, PA: Saunders.

Guilleminault, C., Lirisoglu, C., & Ohayon, M. M. (2004). C-reactive protein and sleep-disordered breathing. *Sleep, 27*(8), 1507–1511.

Guilleminault, C., & Pelayo, R. (2000). Narcolepsy in children: A practical guide to its diagnosis, treatment and follow-up. *Paediatric Drugs,* (2). 1–9.

Guilleminault, C., Querra-Salva, M., Chowdhuri, S., & Poyares, D. (2000). Normal pregnancy, daytime sleeping, snoring, and blood pressure. *Sleep Medicine, 1*(4), 289–297.

Guttuso, T., Kurlan, R., McDermott, M. P., & Kieburtz, K. (2003). Gabapentin's effects on hot flashes in postmenopausal women: A randomized controlled trial. *Obstetrics and Gynecology, 101*(2), 337–345.

Hagenauer, M. H., Perryman, J. I., Lee, T. M., & Carskadon, M. A. (2009). Adolescent changes in the homeostatic and circadian regulation of sleep. *Developmental Neuroscience, 31*(4), 276–284.

Halbower, A. Cv., & Marcus, C. L. (2003). Sleep disorders in children. *Current Opinion in Pulmonary Medicine, 9*(6), 471–476.

Haniffa, M., Lasserson, T. J., & Smith, I. (2004). Interventions to improve compliance with continuous positive airway pressure for obstructive sleep apnoea. *Cochrane Database of Systematic Reviews,* (4). Art. no.: CD003531.

Hanley, P. J., Gabor, J. Y., Chan, C., & Pierratos, A. (2003). Daytime sleepiness in patients with CRF: Impact of nocturnal hemodialysis. *American Journal of Kidney Disorders, 41*(2), 403–410.

Harrison, P. J., & Own, M. J. (2003). Genes for schizophrenia? Recent findings and their pathophysiological implications. *Lancet, 361,* 417–419.

Hastings, M., O'Neill, J. S., & Maywood, E. S. (2007). Circadian clocks: Regulators of endocrine and metabolic rhythms. *Journal of Endocrinology, 195*(2), 187–198.

Hauck, Y. L., Hall, W. A., Dhaliwal, S. S., Bennett, E., & Wells, G. (2011). The effectiveness of an early parenting intervention for mothers with infants with sleep and settling concerns: A prospective non-equivalent before-after design. *Journal of Clinical Nursing,* 1–11. doi:10.1111/j.13652702.2011.03734.x

Hauri, P. J. (1991). Sleep hygiene, relaxation therapy, and cognitive interventions. In P. J. Hauri (Ed.), *Case studies in insomnia* (pp. 65–84). New York, NY: Plenum.

Hedman, C., Pohjasvaara, T., Tolonen, U., Suhonen-Malm, A. S., & Myllyla, V. V. (2002). Effects of pregnancy on mother's sleep. *Sleep Medicine, 3*(1), 37–42.

Hening, W. A., Allen, R. P., Earley, C. J., Picchietti, D. L., & Silber, M. H. (2004). A review by the Restless Legs Syndrome Task Force of the Standards of Practice Committee of the American Academy of Sleep Medicine. An update on the dopaminegic treatment of restless legs syndrome and periodic limb movement disorder. *Sleep, 27*(3), 560–583.

Hoban, T. F. (2010). Sleep disorders in children. *Annals of the New York Academy of Sciences, 1184,* 1–14.

Hoddes, E., Zarcone, V. P., Smythe, H., Phillips, R., & Dement, W. C. (1973). Quantification of sleepiness: A new approach. *Psychophysiology, 10*(4), 431–436.

Hollander, L. F., Freeman, F. W., Sammel, M. D., Berlin, J. A., Grisso, J. A., & Battistinni, M. (2001). Sleep quality, estradiol levels, and behavioral factors in late reproductive age women. *Obstetrics and Gynecology, 98*(3), 391–397.

Hoque, R., & Chesson, A. L., Jr. (2010). Pharmacologically induced/exacerbated restless legs syndrome, periodic limb movements of sleep, and REM behavior disorder/REM sleep without atonia: Literature review, qualitative scoring, and comparative analysis. *Journal of Clinical Sleep Medicine, 6*(1), 79–83.

Horne, J. A., & Ostberg, O. (1976). A self-assessment questionnaire to determine morningness-eveningness in human circadian rhythms. *International Journal of Chronobiology, 4*(2), 97–110.

Howard, B., & Wong, J. (2001). Sleep disorders. *Pediatric Reviews, 22*(10), 327–341.

Iber, C., Ancoli-Israel, S., Chesson, A., & Quan, S. F. (2007). *The AASM manual for the scoring of sleep and associated events: Rules, terminology, and technical specifications* (1st ed.). Westchester, IL: American Academy of Sleep Medicine.

International Restless Legs Syndrome Study Group (IRLSSG). (2003). Validation of the International Restless Legs Syndrome Study Group rating scale for restless legs syndrome. *Sleep Medicine, 4*(2), 121–132.

Jeste, D.V., Alexopoulos, G. S., Bartels, S. J., Cummings, J. L., Gallo, J. J., Gottlieb, G. L.,...Lebowitz, B. D. (1999). Consensus statement on the upcoming crisis in geriatric mental health: Research agenda for the next two decades. *Archives of General Psychiatry, 56*(9), 848–853.

Jetnalani, A. N. (2011). Psychopharmacology. In K. Cheng & K. M. Myers (Eds.), *Child and adolescent psychiatry: The essentials* (2nd ed., pp.455–491). Philadelphia, PA: Lippincott Williams & Wilkins.

Johns, M. W. (1991). A new method for measuring daytime sleepiness: The Epworth Sleepiness Scale. *Sleep, 14*(6), 540–545.

Johns, M. W. (1992). Reliability and factor analysis of the Epworth Sleepiness Scale. *Sleep, 15*(4), 376–381.

Johns, M.W. (1993). Daytime sleepiness, snoring, and obstructive sleep apnea. The Epworth Sleepiness Scale. *Chest, 103*(1), 30–36.

Johns, M.W. (1994). Sleepiness in different situations measured by the Epworth Sleepiness Scale. *Sleep, 17*, 703–710.

Jones, C. R., Campbell, S. S., Zone, S. E., Cooper, F., DeSano, A., Murphy, P. J.,... Ptáček, L. J. (1999). Familial advanced sleep-phase syndrome: A short period circadian rhythm variant in humans. *Nature Medicine, 5*(9), 1062–1065.

Kadotani, H., Kadotani, T., Young, T., Peppard, P. E., Finn, L., Colrain, I. M.,... Mignot, E. (2001). Association between apolipoprotein E epsilon 4 and sleep-disordered breathing in adults. *Journal of the American Medical Association, 285*(22), 2888–2890.

Kazenwadel, J., Pollmacher, T., Trenkwalder, C., Oertel, W. H., Kohnen, R., Künzel, M., & Krüger, H. P. (1995). New actigraphic assessment method for periodic leg movements (PLM). *Sleep, 18*(8), 689–697.

Kemlink, D., Pretl, M., Sonka, K., & Nevsimalova, S. (2008). A comparison of polysomnographic and actigraphic evaluation of periodic limb movements in sleep. *Neurology Research, 30*(3), 234–239.

Khalsa, S. B. (2004). Treatment of chronic insomnia with yoga: A preliminary study with sleep-wake diaries. *Applied Psychophysiology and Biofeedback, 29*(4), 269–278.

Knutson, K. L., & Lauderdale, D. S. (2009). Sociodemographic and behavioral predictors of bed time and wake time among U.S. adolescents aged 15–17 years. *The Journal of Pediatrics, 154*(3), 426–430.

Koch, B. C., Hagen, E. C., Nagtegaal, J. E., Boringa, J. B. S., Kerkhof, G. A., & Ter Wee, P. M. (2009). Effects of nocturnal hemodialysis on melatonin rhythm and sleep-wake behavior: An uncontrolled trial. *American Journal of Kidney Disease, 53*(4), 658–664.

Kodak, T., & Piazza, C. C. (2011). Bedtime fading with response cost for children with multiple sleep problems. In M. L. Perlis, M. Aloia, & B. Kuhn (Eds.), *Behavioral treatments for sleep disorders: A comprehensive primer of behavioral sleep medicine interventions* (pp. 285–292). Boston, MA: Elsevier.

Krishnan, V., & Nestler, E. J. (2008). The molecular neurobiology of expression. *Nature, 455*(7215), 894–902.

Krystal, A. D. (2011). Pharmacologic treatment: Other medications. In M. H. Kryger, T. Roth, & W. C. Dement (Eds.), *Principles and practice of sleep medicine* (5th ed., pp. 916–930). Philadelphia, PA: Saunders.

Kushida, C. A., Efron, B., & Guilleminault, C. (1997). A predictive morphometric model for the obstructive sleep apnea syndrome. *Annals of Internal Medicine, 127*(8, Pt. 1), 581–587.

Lacks, P., & Rotert, M. (1986). Knowledge and practice of sleep hygiene techniques in insomniacs and good sleepers. *Behavioral Research and Therapy, 24*(3), 365–368.

Landolt, H. P., & Dijk, D-J. (2011). Genetic basis of sleep in healthy humans. In M. H. Kryger, T. Roth, & W. C. Dement (Eds.), *Principles and practice of sleep medicine* (5th ed., pp. 175–183). Philadelphia, PA: Saunders.

Lawler, S. P., & Cameron, L. D. (2006). A randomized, controlled trial of massage therapy as a treatment for migraine. *Annals of Behavioral Medicine, 32*(1), 50–59.

Lee, W., Hagubadi, S., Kryger, M. H., & Moklesi, B. (2008). Epidemiology of obstructive sleep apnea: A population-based perspective. *Expert Review in Respiratory Medicine, 2*(3), 349–364.

Lentz, M. J., Landis, C. A., Rothermel, J., & Shaver, J. L. (1999). Effects of selective slow wave sleep disruption on musculoskeletal pain and fatigue in middle aged women. *Journal of Rheumatology, 26*(7), 1586–1592.

Lewith, G. T., Godfrey, A. D., & Prescott, P. (2005). A single-blinded, randomized pilot study evaluating the aroma of lavandula augustifolia as a treatment for mild insomnia. *Journal of Alternative and Complementary Medicine, 11*(4), 631–637.

Libbus, K., Baker, J., Osgood, J., Phillips, T., & Valentine, D. (1995). Persistent fatigue in well women. *Women and Health, 23*(1), 57–72.

Lichstein, K. L., Riedel, B. W., Wilson, N. M., Lester, K. W., & Aguillard, R. N. (2001). Relaxation and sleep compression for late-life insomnia: A placebo-controlled trial. *Journal of Consulting and Clinical Psychology, 69*(2), 227–229.

Lichstein, K. L., Taylor, D. J., McCrae, C. S., & Thomas, S. J. (2011). Relaxation for insomnia. In M. L. Perlis, M. Aloia, & B. Kuhn (Eds.), *Behavioral treatments for sleep disorders: A comprehensive primer of behavioral sleep medicine interventions* (pp. 45–54). Boston, MA: Elsevier.

Lichstein, K. L., Thomas, S. J., & McCurry, S. M. (2011). Sleep compression. In M. L. Perlis, M. Aloia, & B. Kuhn (Eds.), *Behavioral treatments for sleep disorders: A comprehensive primer of behavioral sleep medicine interventions* (pp. 55–60). Boston, MA: Elsevier.

Lin, C. M., Davidson, T. M., & Ancoli-Israel, S. (2008). Gender differences in obstructive sleep apnea and treatment implications. *Sleep Medicine Reviews, 12*(6), 481–496.

Lu, J., Sherman, D., Devor, M., & Saper, C. B. (2006). A putative flip-flop switch for control of REM sleep. *Nature, 441*(7093), 589–594.

Lucille Packard Children's Hospital at Standford. (2011). *Infant Sleep.* Retrieved from www.lpch.org/DiseaseHealthInfo/Health Library/growth/infhab.html

Lyon, P., Cohen, M., & Quintner, J. (2011). An evolutionary stress-response hypothesis for chronic widespread pain (fibromyalgia syndrome). *Pain Medicine, 12*(8), 1167–1178.

Maccario, M., Ruggles, K. M., & Meriwether, M. W. (1987). Post-traumatic narcolepsy. *Military Medicine, 152*(7), 370–371.

Mahowald, M. W., & Schenck, C. H. (2011). REM sleep parasomnias. In M. H. Kryger, T. Roth, & W. C. Dement (Eds.), *Principles and practice of sleep medicine* (5th ed., pp. 175–183). Philadelphia, PA: Saunders.

Majde, J. A., & Krueger, J. M. (2005). Links between the innate immune system and sleep. *Journal of Allergy and Clinical Immunology, 116*(6), 1188–1198.

Mallampati, S. R., Gatt, S. P., Gugino, L. D., Desai, S. P., Waraksa, B., Freiberger, D., & Liu, P. L. (1985). A clinical sign to predict difficult tracheal intubation: A prospective study. *Canadian Anesthesia Society Journal, 32*(4), 429–434.

Malow, B. A. (2011). Approach to the patient with disordered sleep. In M. H. Kryer, T. Roth, and W. C. Dement (Eds.), *Principles and practice of sleep medicine* (5th ed., pp. 641–646). St. Louis, MO: Elsevier.

Manconi, M., Govoni, V., DeVito, A., Economou, N. T., Cesnik, E., Mollica, G., & Granieri, E. (2004). Pregnancy as a risk factor for restless legs syndrome. *Sleep Medicine, 5*(3), 305–308.

Markhov, D., & Goldman, M. (2006). Normal sleep and circadian rhythms: Neurobiologic mechanisms underlying sleep and wakefulness. *Psychiatric Clinics of North America, 29*(4), 841–853, Abstract No. vii.

McGinty, D., & Szymusiak, R. (2003). Hypothalamic regulation of sleep and arousal. *Frontiers in Bioscience, 1*(8s), 1074–1083.

McGinty, D., & Szymusiak, R. (2011). Sleep mechanisms and phylogeny. In M. H. Kryer, T. Roth, & W. C. Dement (Eds.). *Principles and practice of sleep medicine* (5th ed., pp.76–91). St. Louis, MO: Elsevier.

Michaud, M., Paquet, J., Lavigne, G., Desautels, A., & Montplaisir, J. (2002). Sleep laboratory diagnosis of restless legs syndrome. *European Neurology, 48*(2), 108–113.

Mindell, J. A., Emslie, G., Blumer, J., Genel, M., Glaze, D., Ivanenko, A.,…Banas, B. (2006). Pharmacologic management of insomnia in children and adolescents: Consensus statement. *Pediatrics, 117*(6), E1223–E1232.

Mindell, J. A., Kuhn, B., Lewin, D. S., Meltzer, L. J., & Sadeh, A. (2006). Behavioral treatment of bedtime problems and night waking in infants and young children. An American Academy of Sleep Medicine review. *Sleep, 29*(10), 1263–1276.

Mindell, J. A., Meltzer, L. J., Carskadon, M. A., & Chervin, R. D. (2009). Developmental aspects of sleep hygiene: Findings from the 2004 National Sleep Foundation Sleep in America poll. *Sleep Medicine, 10*(7), 771–779.

Mindell, J. A., Sadeh, A., Kohyama, J., & How, T. H. (2009). Parental behaviors and sleep outcomes in infants and toddlers: A cross-cultural comparison. *Sleep Medicine, 11*(4), 393–399.

Mindell, J. A., Sadeh, A., Wiegand, B., How, T. H., & Goh, D. Y. (2010). Cross-cultural differences in infant and toddler sleep. *Sleep Medicine, 11*(3), 274–280.

Minoguchi, K., Yokoe, T., Tazaki, T., Minoguchi, H., Tanaka, A., Oda, N.,…Adachi, M. (2005). Increased carotid intima-media thickness and serum inflammatory markers in obstructive sleep apnea. *American Journal of Respiratory and Critical Care Medicine, 172*(5), 625–630.

Monk, T. H., Reynolds, C. F., III, Kupfer, D. J., Buysse, D. J., Coble, P. A., Hayes, A. J.,…Ritenour, A. M. (1994). The Pittsburgh sleep diary. *Journal of Sleep Research, 3*(2), 111–120.

Montgomery-Downs, H. E., & Gozal, D. (2006). Sleep habits and risk factors for sleep-disordered breathing in infants and young toddlers in Louisville, KY. *Sleep Medicine, 7*(3), 211–219.

Montplasir, J., Allen, R. P., Walters, A., & Ferini-Strambi, L. (2011). Restless legs syndrome and periodic limb movements during sleep. In M. H. Kryger, T. Roth, & W. C. Dement (Eds.), *Principles and practice of sleep medicine* (5th ed., pp. 1026–1037). Philadelphia, PA: Saunders.

Moore, M., Kirchner, H. L., Drotar, D., Johnson, N., Rosen, C., Ancoli-Israel, S., & Redline, S. (2009). Relationships among sleepiness, sleep time, and psychological functioning in adolescents. *Journal of Pediatric Psychology, 34*(10), 1175–1183.

Morgenthaler, T., Alessi, C., Friedman, L., Owens, J., Kapur, V., Boehlecke, B.,…Swick, T. J. (2007). Practice parameters for the use of sp-actigraphy in the assessment of sleep and sleep disorders: An update for 2007. *Sleep, 30*(4), 519–529.

Morgenthaler, T. I., Kapur, V. K., Brown, T., Swick, T. J., Alessi, C., Aurora, R. N.,…Zak, R. (2007). Standards of Practice Committee of the American Academy of Sleep Medicine. Practice parameters for the treatment of narcolepsy and other hypersomnias of central origin. *Sleep, 30*(12), 1705–1711.

Morgenthaler, T. I., Kramer, M., Alessi, C., Friedman, L., Boehlecke, B., Brown, T.,…Swick, T. (2006). Practice parameters for the psychological and behavioral treatment of insomnia: An update. *Sleep, 29*(11), 1415–1419.

Morgenthaler, T. I., Lee-Chiong, T., Alessi, C., Friedman, L., Aurora, R. N., Boehlecke, B.,…Zak, R. (2007). Practice parameters for the clinical evaluation and treatment of circadian rhythm sleep disorders. An American Academy of Sleep Medicine report. *Sleep, 30*(11), 1445–1459.

Morin, C. M. (2011). Psychological and behavioral treatments for insomnia I: Approaches and efficacy. In M. H. Kryger, T. Roth, & W. C. Dement (Eds.), *Principles and practice of sleep medicine* (5th ed., pp. 866–883). Philadelphia. PA: Saunders.

National Center for Complementary and Alternative Medicine (NCCAM), National Institutes of Health (NIH). (2007). *Acupuncture*. NCCAM Publication No. D404. Retrieved from http://nccam.nih.gov/health/acupuncture/introduction.htm

National Center for Complementary and Alternative Medicine (NCCAM), National Institutes of Health (NIH). (2011a). *Massage therapy*. Retrieved from http://nccam.nih.gov/health/massage

National Center for Complementary and Alternative Medicine (NCCAM), National Institutes of Health (NIH). (2011b). *Mindfulness-based stress reduction*. Retrieved from. http://nccam.nih.gov/health/acupuncture/introduction.htm

National Center for Complementary and Alternative Medicine (NCCAM), National Institutes of Health (NIH). (2011c). *Tai chi*. Retrieved from http://nccam.nih.gov/health/taichi/introduction.htm

National Center for Complementary and Alternative Medicine (NCCAM), National Institutes of Health (NIH). (2011d). *Yoga for health*. Retrieved from http://nccam.nih.gov/health/yoga/introduction.htm

National Heart, Lung, and Blood Institute. (2005). *Your guide to healthy sleep*(p. 62). Retrieved from www.nhlbi.nih.gov/health/public/sleep/healthy_sleep.pdf

National Sleep Foundation. (2005). *2005 Sleep in America polls*. Retrieved from www.sleepfoundation.org/article/sleep-america-polls/2005-adult-sleep-habits-and-styles

National Sleep Foundation. (2008). *Sleep diary*. Retrieved from http://science-education.nih.gov/supplements/nih3/sleep/guide/nih_sleep_masters.pdf

Netzer, N. C., Stoohs, R. A., Netzer, C. M., Clark, K., & Strohl, K. P. (1999). Using the Berlin Questionnaire to identify patients at risk for the sleep apnea syndrome. *Annals of Internal Medicine, 131*(7), 485–491.

Newman, A. B., Foster, G., Givelber, R., Nieto, F. J., Redline, S., & Young, T. B. (2005). Progression and regression of sleep-disordered breathing with changes in weight: The Sleep Heart Health Study. *Archives of Internal Medicine, 165*(20), 2408–2413.

O'Brian, L., Hendrix, N., Felt, B., Hoban, T., Ruzicka, D., & Chervin, R. (2007). Aggressive behavior, bullying, and sleep-disordered breathing in schoolchildren. *Sleep, 30*(Suppl.), A100–A101.

Ohayon, M. M., Carskadon, M. A., Guilleminault, C., & Vitiello, M. V. (2004). Meta-analysis of quantitative sleep parameters from childhood to old age in healthy individuals: Developing normative sleep values across the lifespan. *Sleep, 27*(7), 1255–1273.

Ong, J. C., & Manber, R. (2011). Mindfulness-based therapy for insomnia. In M. L. Perlis, M. Aloia, & B. Kuhn (Eds.), *Behavioral treatments for sleep disorders: A comprehensive primer of behavioral sleep medicine interventions* (pp. 133–142). Boston, MA: Elsevier.

Opp, M. R. (2005). Cytokines and sleep. *Sleep Medicine Reviews, 9*(5), 355–364.

Owens, J. A., Belon, K., & Moss, P. (2010). Impact of delaying school start time on adolescent sleep, mood, and behavior. *Archives of Pediatric and Adolescent Medicine, 164*(7), 608–614.

Owens, J. A., & Dalzell, V. (2005). Use of the 'BEARS' sleep screening tool in a pediatric residents' continuity clinic: A pilot study. *Sleep Medicine, 6*(1), 63–69.

Owens, J. A., Spirito, A., & McGuinn, M. (2000). The children's sleep habits questionnaire (CSHQ): Psychometric properties of a survey instrument for school-aged children. *Sleep, 23*(8), 1043–1051.

Owens, J. A., Spirito, A., & McGuinn, M. (2010). Use of pharmacotherapy for insomnia in child psychiatry practice: A national survey. *Sleep Medicine, 11*(7), 692–700.

Parker, K. P., Bliwise, D. L., & Rye, D. B. (2000). Hemodialysis disrupts basic sleep regulatory mechanisms: building hypotheses. *Nursing Research, 49*(6), 327–332.

Partonen, T., & Spence, D. W. (2010). Sleep in seasonal affective disorder. In S. R. Pandi-Perumal & M. Cramer (Eds.), *Sleep in mental illness* (pp. 283–288). New York, NY: Cambridge University Press.

Peppard, P. E., Young, T. B., Palta, M., Dempsey, J., & Skatrud, J. (2000). Longitudinal study of moderate weight change and sleep disordered breathing. *Journal of the American Medical Association, 284*, 3105–3131.

Perlis, M. L., Aloia, M., & Kuhn, B. (Eds.). (2011). *Behavioral treatments for sleep disorders: A comprehensive primer of behavioral sleep medicine interventions*. Boston, MA: Elsevier.

Perlis, M. L., & Gehrman, P. R. (2011). Cognitive restructuring: Cognitive therapy for catastrophic sleep beliefs. In M. L. Perlis, M. Aloia, & B. Kuhn (Eds.), *Behavioral treatments for sleep disorders: A comprehensive primer of behavioral sleep medicine interventions* (pp. 119–126). Boston, MA: Elsevier.

Perlis, M. L., Jungquist, C., Smith, M. T., & Posner, D. (2005). *Cognitive behavioral treatment of insomnia: A session-by-session guide*. New York, NY: Springer.

Petit, D., Montplaisir, J., & Boeve, B. F. (2005). Alzheimer's disease and other dementias. In M. H. Kryger, T. Roth, & W. C. Dement (Eds.), *Principles and practice of sleep medicine* (pp. 853–862). Philadelphia, PA: Elsevier/Saunders.

Phillips, B. A., & Kryger, M. H. (2011). Management of obstructive sleep apnea-hypopnea syndrome. In M. H. Kryger, T. Roth, & W. C. Dement (Eds.), *Principles and practice of sleep medicine* (5th ed., pp. 1278–1293). Philadelphia, PA: Saunders.

Poblano, A., Marquez, A., & Hernandez, G. (2006). Apnea in infants. *Indian Journal of Pediatrics, 73*, 1085–1088.

Polo-Kantola, P., Erkkola, R., & Irjala, K. (1999). Climacteric symptoms and sleep quality. *Obstetrics and Gynecology, 94*(2), 219–224.

Posner, D., & Gehrman, P. (2011). Sleep hygiene. In M. L. Perlis, M. Aloia, & B. Kuhn (Eds.), *Behavioral treatments for sleep disorders: A comprehensive primer of behavioral sleep medicine interventions* (pp. 31–44). Boston, MA: Elsevier.

Postuma, R. B., Gagnon, J., F., Vendette, M., Fantini, M. L., Massicotte-Marquez, J., & Montplaisir, J. (2009). Quantifying the risk of neurodegenerative disease in idiopathic REM sleep behavior disorder. *Neurology, 72*(15), 1296–1300.

Punjabi, N. M., & Beamer, B. A. (2009). Alterations in glucose disposal in sleep-disordered breathing. *American Journal of Respiratory and Critical Care Medicine, 179*(3), 235–240.

Raherison, C., Abouelfath, A., Le Gros, V., Taytard, A., & Molimard, M. (2006). Underdiagnosis of nocturnal symptoms in asthma in general practice. *Journal of Asthma, 43*(3), 199–202.

Ramsawh, H., Stein, M. B., & Mellman, T. A. (2011). Anxiety disorders. In M. H. Kryger, T. Roth, & W. C. Dement (Eds.), *Principles and practice of sleep medicine* (5th ed., pp. 1473–1487). Philadelphia, PA: Saunders.

Randler, C. (2008). Differences in sleep and circadian preference between Eastern and Western German adolescents. *Chronobiology International, 25*(4), 565–575.

Redeker, N. S. (2011). Developmental aspects of sleep. In N. S. Redeker & G. P. McEnany (Eds.), *Sleep disorders and sleep promotion in nursing practice* (pp. 19–32). New York, NY: Springer.

Reid, K. J., Martinovich, Z., Finkel, S., Statsinger, J., Golden, R., Harter, K., & Zee, P. C. (2006). Sleep: A marker of physical and mental health in the elderly. *American Journal of Geriatric Psychiatry, 14*(10), 860–866.

Reid, K. J., & Zee, P. C. (2011). Circadian disorders of the sleep-wake cycle. In M. H. Kryger, T. Roth, & W. C. Dement (Eds.), *Principles and practice of sleep medicine* (5th ed., pp. 470–482). Philadelphia, PA: Saunders.

Richards, K. C. (1998). Effect of a back massage and relaxation intervention on sleep in critically ill patients. *American Journal of Critical Care, 7*(4), 288–299.

Rieman, D., & Perlis, M. L. (2009). The treatments of chronic insomnia: A review of benzodiazepine receptor agonists and psychological and behavioral therapies. *Sleep Medicine Reviews, 13*(3), 205–214.

Rijsman, R., Neven, A. K., Graffelman, W., Kemp, B., & de Weerd, A. (2004). Epidemiology of restless legs in the Netherlands. *European Journal of Neurology, 11*(9), 607–611.

Roehrs, T., & Roth, T. (2011). Medication and substance abuse. In M. H. Kryger, T. Roth, & W. C. Dement (Eds.), *Principles and practice of sleep medicine* (5th ed., pp. 1512–1522). Philadelphia, PA: Saunders.

Rogers, A. E. (2011). Scheduled sleep periods as an adjuvant treatment for narcolepsy. In M. L. Perlis, M. Aloia, & B. Kuhn (Eds.), *Behavioral treatments for sleep disorders: A comprehensive primer of behavioral sleep medicine interventions* (pp. 237–240). Boston, MA: Elsevier.

Rose, K. M., & Bourguignon, C. M. (2011). Complementary and alternative sleep medicine. In N. S. Redeker & G. P. McEnany (Eds.), *Sleep disorders and sleep promotion in nursing practice* (pp. 233–242). New York, NY: Springer.

Roth, T., Zammit, G., Kushida, C., Doohramji, K., Mathias, S. D., Wong, J. M., & Buysee, D. J. (2002). A new questionnaire to detect sleep disorders. *Sleep Medicine, 3*(2), 99–108.

Rowat, A. M., Wardlaw, J. M., & Dennis, M. S. (2007). Abnormal breathing patterns in stroke: Relationship with location of acute stroke lesion and prior cerebrovascular disease. *Journal of Neurological and Neurosurgical Psychiatry, 78*(3), 277–279.

Russo, P. M., Bruni, O., Lucidi, F., Ferri, R., & Violani, C. (2007). Sleep habits and circadian preference in Italian children and adolescents. *Journal of Sleep Research, 16*(2), 163–169.

Sack, R. L., Auckley, D., Auger, R. R., Carskadon, M. A., Wright, K. P., Jr., Vitiello, M. V., & Zhdanova, I. V. (2007a). Circadian rhythm sleep disorders: Part I, basic principles, shift work and jet lag disorders. An American Academy of Sleep Medicine review. *Sleep, 30*(11), 1460–1483.

Sack, R. L., Auckley, D., Auger, R. R., Carskadon, M. A., Wright, K. P., Jr., Vitiello, M. V., & Zhdanova, I. V. (2007b). Circadian rhythm sleep disorders: Part II, advanced sleep phase disorder, delayed sleep phase disorder, free-running disorder, and irregular sleep-wake rhythm. An American Academy of Sleep Medicine review. *Sleep, 30*(11), 1484–1501.

Sadock, B. J., & Sadock, V. A. (2003). *Synopsis of psychiatry: Behavior sciences/clinical psychiatry* (9th ed.). Philadephia, PA: Lippincott Williams & Wilkins.

Sateia, M. J., Doghramji, K., Hauri, P. J., & Morin, C. M. (2000). Evaluation of chronic insomnia. An American Academy of Sleep Medicine report. *Sleep, 23*(2), 243–308.

Scheer, F. A. J. L., & Shea, S. A. (2009). Fundamentals of the circadian system. In C. J. Amlaner & P. M. Fuller (Eds.), *Basics of sleep guide* (2nd ed., chap. 18A, pp. 199–221). Westchester, IL: Sleep Research Society.

Schutte-Rodin, S., Broch, L., Buysse, D., Dorsey, C., & Sateia, M. (2008). Clinical guideline for the evaluation and management of chronic insomnia in adults. *Journal of Clinical Sleep Medicine, 4*(5), 487–504.

Shneerson, J. M., & Simonds, A. K. (2002). Noninvasive ventilation for chest wall and neuromuscular disorders. *The European Respiratory Journal: Official Journal of the European Society of Respiratory Physiology, 20*(2), 480–487.

Siddiqui, S., Kavanagh, D., Traynor, J., Mak, M., Deighan, C., & Geddes, C. (2005). Risk factors for restless legs syndrome in dialysis patients. *Nephron Clinical Practice, 101*(3), C155-C160.

Silvestri, R., & Bromfield, E. (2004). Recurrent nightmares and disorders of arousal in temporal lobe epilepsy. *Brain Research Bulletin, 63*(5), 369–376.

Slifer, K. J. (2011). Promoting positive airway pressure adherence in children using escape extinction within a multi-component behavior therapy approach. In M. L. Perlis, M. Aloia, & B. Kuhn (Eds.), *Behavioral treatments for sleep disorders: A comprehensive primer of behavioral sleep medicine interventions* (pp. 351–366). Boston, MA: Elsevier.

Smith, I., Nadig, V., & Lasserson, T. J. (2009). Educational, supportive, and behavioural interventions to improve usage of continuous positive airway pressure machines for adults with obstructive sleep apnoea. *Cochrane Database of Systematic Reviews*, (2), Art. no.: CD007736.

Smith, M., Fogg, L., & Eastman, C. (2009). Practical interventions to promote circadian adaptation to permanent night shift work: Study 4. *Biological Rhythms, 24*(2), 161–172.

Smith, M. T., Perlis, M. L., Park, A., Smith, M. S., Pennington, J., Giles, D. E., & Buysse, D. J. (2002). Comparative meta-analysis of pharmacotherapy and behavior therapy for persistent insomnia. *The American Journal of Psychiatry, 159*(1), 5–11.

Snyder, D. M., Goodlin-Jones, B. L., Pionk, M. J., & Stein, M. T. (2010). Inconsolable night-time awakening: Beyond night terrors. *Journal of Developmental and Behavioral Pediatrics, 31*(3), S7–S10.

Soden, K., Vincent, K., Craske, S., Lucas, C., & Ashley, S. (2004). A randomized controlled trial of aromatherapy massage in a hospice setting. *Palliative Medicine, 18*(2), 87–92.

Spielman, A. J., Saskin, P., & Thorpy, M. J. (1987). Treatment of chronic insomnia by restriction of time in bed. *Sleep, 10*(1), 45–56.

Spielman, A. J., Yang, C-M., & Glovinsky, P. B. (2011). Sleep restriction therapy. In M. L. Perlis, M. Aloia, & B. Kuhn (Eds.), *Behavioral treatments for sleep disorders: A comprehensive primer of behavioral sleep medicine interventions*. Boston, MA: Elsevier.

Stahl, S. M. (2009). Fibromyalgia—pathways and neurotransmitters. *Human Psychopharmacology, 24*(Suppl. 1), S11–S17.

Stearns, V., Beebe, K. L., Iyengar, M., & Dube, E. (2003). Paroxetine controlled release in the treatment of menopausal hot flashes: A randomized controlled trial. *Journal of the American Medical Association, 289*(21), 2827–2834.

Stefansson, H., Rye, D. B., Hicks, A., Petursson, H., Ingason, A., Thorgeirss, T. E., . . . Stefansson, K. (2007). A genetic risk factor for periodic limb movements in sleep. *New England Journal of Medicine, 357*(7), 639–647.

Stein, M. B., & Mellman, T. A. (2005). Anxiety disorders. In M. H. Kryger, T. Roth, & W. C. Dement (Eds.), *Principles and practice of sleep medicine* (pp. 418–434). Philadelphia, PA: Elsevier/Saunders.

Substance Abuse and Mental Health Services Administration (SAMHSA). (2007). *An Action Plan for Behavioral Health Workforce Development*. Retrieved from http://www.samhsa.gov/Workforce/Annapolis/WorkforceActionPlan.pdf

Super, E., & Johnson, K. P. (2011). Pediatric sleep problems. In K. Cheng & K. M. Myers (Eds.), *Child and adolescent psychiatry: The essentials* (2nd ed.). Philadelphia, PA: Wolters Kluwer/Lippincott Williams & Wilkins.

Tarokh, L., & Carskadon, M. A. (2010). Developmental changes in human sleep EEG during early adolescence. *Sleep*, 33(6), 801–809.

Thomas, K. A., & Burr, R. I. (2006). Melatonin level and pattern in postpartum versus pregnant nulliparous women. *Journal of Obstetric, Gynecologic, and Neonatal Nursing, 35*(5), 608–615.

Touchette, E., Petit, D., Paquet, J., Bolvin, M., Japel, C., Tremblay, R. E., & Montplaisir, J. Y. (2005). Factors associated with fragmented sleep at night across early childhood. *Archives of Pediatric and Adolescent Medicine, 159*(3), 242–249.

Trenkwalder, C., & Arnulf, I. (2011). Parkinsonism. In M. H. Kryger, T. Roth, & W. C. Dement (Eds.), *Principles and practice of sleep medicine* (5th ed., pp. 980–992). Philadelphia, PA: Saunders.

Tyron, W. W. (1991). *Activity measurement in psychology and medicine*. New York, NY: Plenum.

Vaughn, B. V., & D'Cruz, O'N. F. (2011). Cardinal manifestations of sleep disorders. In M. H. Kryger, T. Roth, & W. C. Dement (Eds.), *Principles and practice of sleep medicine* (5th ed., pp. 647–657). Philadelphia, PA: Saunders.

Vaz Fragoso, C. A., & Gill, T. M. (2007). Sleep complaints in community-living older persons: A multi-factorial geriatric syndrome. *Journal of the American Geriatrics Society, 55*(11), 1853–1866.

Vgontzas, A. N., Bixler, E. O., & Chrousos, G. P. (2003). Metabolic disturbances in obesity versus sleep apnea: The importance of visceral obesity and insulin resistance. *Journal of Internal Medicine, 254*(1), 32–44.

Vitiello, M. V. (2006). Sleep and normal aging. *Sleep Medicine Clinics, 1*(2), 171–176.

Vitiello, M. V., Moe, K. E., & Prinz, P. N. (2002). Sleep complaints cosegregate with illness in older adults: Clinical research informed by and informing epidemiological studies of sleep. *Journal of Psychosomatic Research, 53*(1), 555–559.

Walsh, J. K., & Roth, T. (2011). Pharmacologic treatment of insomnia: Benzodiazepine receptor agonists. In M. H. Kryger, T.

Roth, & W. C. Dement (Eds.), *Principles and practice of sleep medicine* (5th ed., pp. 905–915). Philadelphia, PA: Saunders.

Ward, T. M., Gay, C., Anders, T. F., Alkon, A., & Lee, K. A. (2008). Sleep and napping patterns in 3-to 5-year old children attending full-day childcare centers. *Journal of Pediatric Psychology, 33*(6), 666–672.

Wellman, A., & White, D. P. (2011). Central sleep apnea and periodic breathing. In M. H. Kryger, T. Roth, & W. C. Dement (Eds.), *Principles and practice of sleep medicine* (5th ed., pp. 1140–1152). Philadelphia, PA: Saunders.

Winbush, N. Y., Gross, C. R., & Kreitzer, M. J. (2007). The effects of mindfulness-based stress reduction on sleep disturbance: A systematic review. *Explore: The Journal of Science and Healing, 3*(6), 585–591.

Winkelmann, J., Schormair, B., Lichtner, P., Ripke, S., Xiong, L., Jalilzadeh, S.,...Meitinger, T. (2007). Genome-wide association study of restless legs syndrome identifies common variants in three genomic regions. *National Genetics, 39*(8), 1000–1006.

Wolfson, A. R., Crowley, S. J., Anwer, U., & Bassett, J. L. (2003). Changes in sleep patterns and depressive symptoms in first-time mothers: Last trimester to 1-year postpartum. *Behavioral Sleep Medicine, 1*(1), 54–67.

Wolfson, A. R., Spaulding, N. L., Dandrow, C., & Baroni, E. M. (2007). Middle school start times: The importance of a good night's sleep for young adolescents. *Behavioral Sleep Medicine, 5*(3), 194–209.

Wood, P. B., Glabus, M. F., Simpson, R., & Patterson, J. C., II. (2009). Changes in gray matter density in fibromyalgia: Correlation with dopamine metabolism. *Journal of Pain, 10*(6), 609–618.

Woodward, S., & Freedman, R. R. (1994). The thermoregulatory effects of menopausal hot flashes on sleep. *Sleep, 17* (6), 497–501.

World Health Organization. (1992). *International classification of diseases, 10th revision (ICD-10)*. Geneva, Switzerland: Author.

Wu, Y. H., Fischer, D. F., Kalsbeek, A., Garidou-Boof, M-L., der Vliet, J. V., Heijningen, C. V.,...Swaab, D. F. (2006). Pineal clock gene oscillation is disturbed in Alzheimer's disease, due to disconnection from the "master clock." *FASEB Journal, 20*(11), 1874–1876.

Wu, Y. H., & Swaab, D. F. (2005). The human pineal gland and melatonin in aging and Alzheimer's disease. *Journal of Pineal Research, 38*(3), 145–152.

Yeung, W., Chung, K., Leung, Y., Zhang, S., & Saw, A. C. K. (2009). Traditional needle acupuncture treatment for insomnia: A systematic review of randomized controlled trials. *Sleep Medicine, 10*(7), 694–704.

Young, T., Finn, L., Austin, D., & Peterson, A. (2003). Menopausal status and sleep-disordered breathing in the Wisconsin Sleep Cohort Study. *American Journal of Respiratory and Critical Care Medicine, 167*(9), 1181–1185.

Young, T., Peppard, P. E., & Gottlieb, D. J. (2002). Epidemiology of obstructive sleep apnea. *American Journal of Respiratory and Critical Care Medicine, 165*(9), 1217–1239.

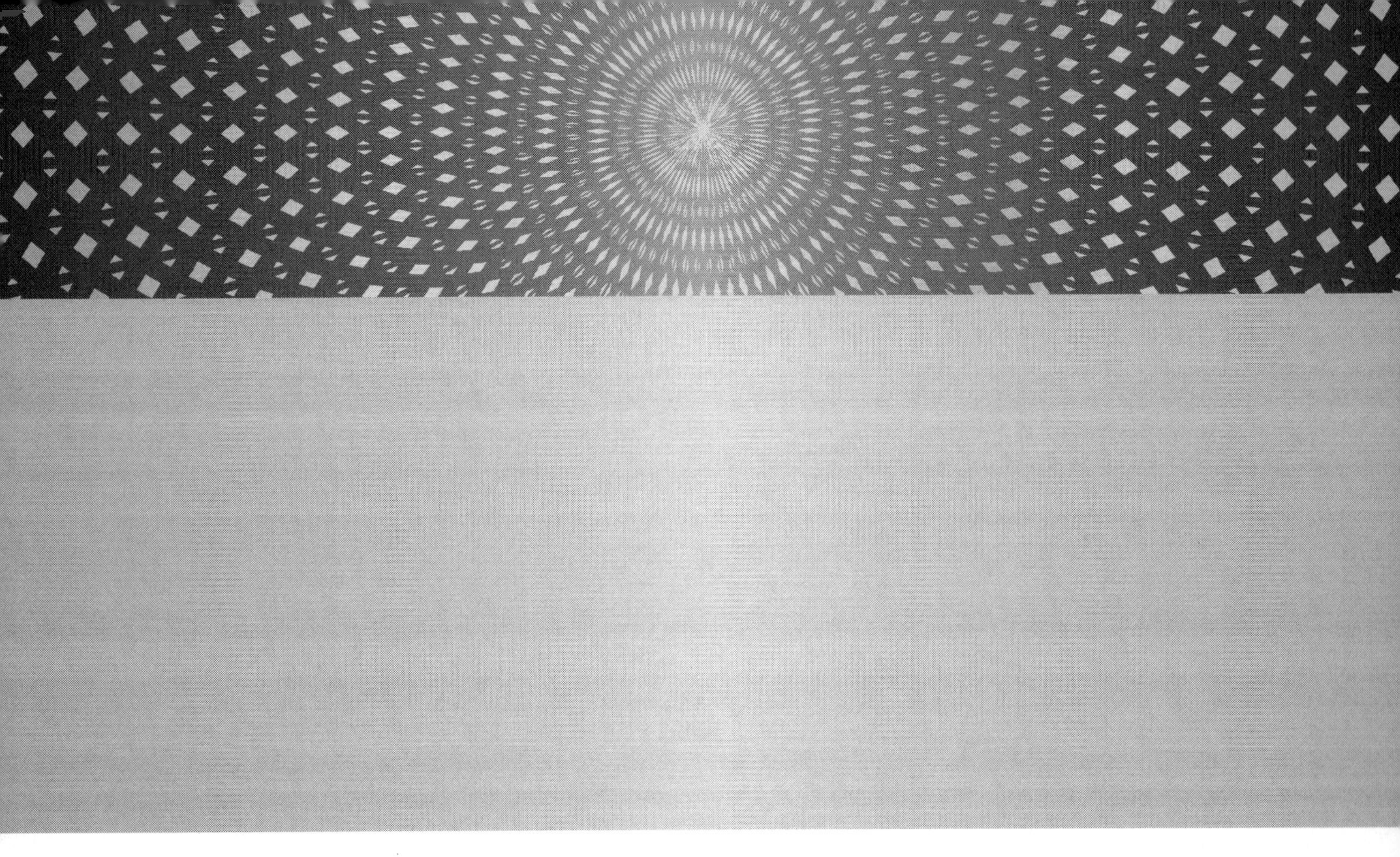

CHAPTER CONTENTS

Food is part of everyone's life, and it is needed for survival. While the appetite center is under the control of the hypothalamus, culture, environment, and emotions play a major role in our attitudes regarding food. When anxiety and stress occur in one's life, food may be used in a dysfunctional manner, resulting in serious eating disorders (EDs) that may be life threatening (Cyr, 2008).

There are numerous biological theories related to hunger and satiation. One theory of hunger is the stomach contraction theory, which postulates that when hungry, our stomach responds by contracting. Washburn (Hara, 1997) attempted to prove this theory by swallowing a balloon and then inflating it. Once the balloon was fully inflated, he felt no hunger. But this theory failed to explain why individuals who had their stomach removed continued to feel hungry (Hara, 1997).

Other theories maintain that glucose and insulin levels remain fairly constant under normal conditions. Insulin levels increase, however, when we feel hungry. In other words, hunger levels increase when the blood glucose levels are low (Heller & Heller, 1991). Bash (Franken, 1994) studied transfusing blood from a fully satiated dog to a starving dog. On completion of the transfusion, the starving dog's stomach ceased to contract, supporting the glucose theory.

The heat-production theory studied the relationship between environmental temperature and hunger. This theory suggests that when environmental temperatures drop, we become hungry, and when temperatures rise,

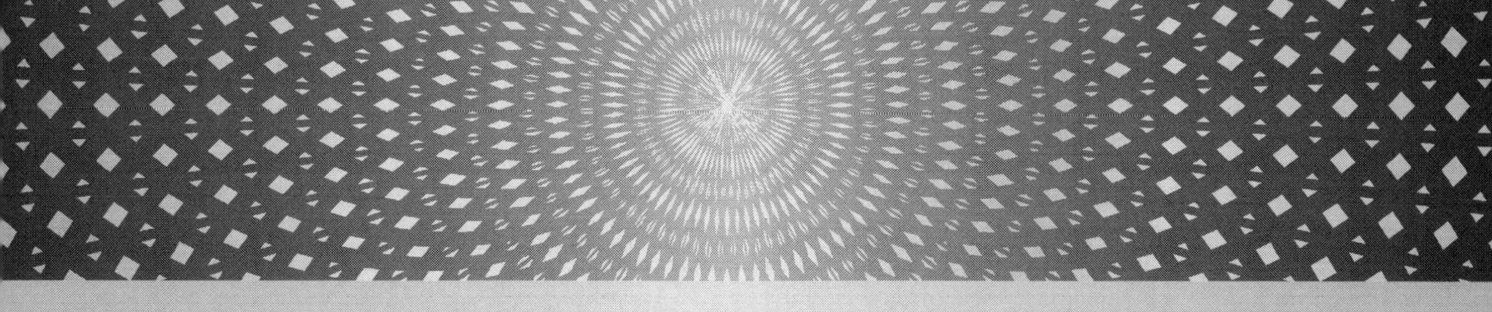

CHAPTER 12

Integrative Management of Disordered Eating

Deborah B. Fahs, Robert Krause, and Kathleen R. Tusaie

hunger decreases. People generally eat more in the winter and less in the summer months, supporting this theory of hunger (Hara, 1997).

But hunger is not based on biology alone (Hara, 1997). Environmental triggers for eating include taste and texture of food as well as the temperature, the type of food, social interactions with others, and stress (Halmi, 2000). Hunger and eating can be a result of learned and cognitive affects. For example, at 8 a.m. we feel hungry because the clock tells us it is breakfast time.

Smells have an influence on our sense of hunger. A freshly cooked, hot pizza stimulates hunger, but smell, taste, and texture of food is also a culturally learned behavior (Hara, 1997).

Color impacts on hunger and eating behaviors as well. When we feel hungry, we may bite into a bright, succulent orange section or a crisp red apple. We would not want to eat a blue orange or apple because, in general, nature does not produce blue foods. In fact, blue has been known to be an appetite suppressant (Hara, 1997).

Hunger and satiety are not one and the same. Satiety functions on two levels: the brain and the gastrointestinal (GI) tract. There are two locations in the hypothalamus that control hunger and eating, which are the lateral hypothalamus telling us when to begin eating and the ventromedial nuclei telling us to stop eating when we feel satiated. Feeling satiated is also a mechanism of the GI tract, which controls short-term eating (Hara, 1997).

Eating is greatly influenced by social media. We see food in magazines and watch television shows on food preparation. We see people socializing over food in restaurants and at parties. We count calories and we worry about not getting enough food or about eating too much food (Cyr, 2008).

Eating is complex in nature and can lead to obesity or disorders such as bulimia nervosa (BN) or anorexia nervosa (AN) (Hara, 1997; Halmi, 2000). Obesity is defined as "exceeding the average weight for one's height, bone structure, age, and sex by a given percentage, above 25%" (Hara, 1997, p. 2). But why are some people obese and others are not? Does the difference lie in different hunger and satiety mechanisms? Studies on twins showed that when raised apart from each other, they still weigh about the same. Similarly, weights of adopted children are comparable to their biological rather than adopted parents (Hara, 1997).

The "set point theory" maintains that our weight is predetermined and our body strives to maintain that level of weight set by the hypothalamus. This theory states that dieting is ineffective as the fewer calories one takes in, the more the body attempts to maintain that "set point," or predetermined weight (Franken, 1994). More simply, this describes obesity in terms of the "set point" being too high as a result of damage to the ventromedial hypothalamus (Hara, 1997).

Another theory views hunger from a cognitive perspective. This theory states that hunger and satiety are biologically determined by hunger boundaries and the space between the two are cognitively established. People determine how much they think they should eat and if set too low than what is biologically recognized, the body reacts by inducing hunger (Hara, 1997).

But what mechanisms trigger EDs? Some classify EDs as psychosomatic in nature, believing that there is a symbiotic relationship between the mind and the body that is manifested in a configuration of symptoms. These individuals feel their body is problematic, thus initiate particular behaviors to solve the problem. They view their bodies as barriers to emotional growth; thus emotional conflict begins to develop (Krantz, 1999). Many of these patients have been traumatized in some manner, which forms an undermining and uncontrolled relationship between the conscious being and the body (Attias & Goodwin, 1999).

Obesity and EDs such as BN and AN are generally considered very separate and unrelated problems, especially as they relate to etiology. However, the unhealthy behaviors associated with BN and AN such as vomiting, laxative use, fasting, and so on, are thought to be brought on by a negative experience of the body: the common thread to obesity and other EDs (Riva, 2011).

A 4-year longitudinal study on teenage girls studied emotional and behavioral risk factors for the onset of obesity. This study demonstrated that those girls who used maladaptive compensatory behaviors for weight loss were at risk for obesity 4 years later. It was concluded that adolescents who practice unhealthy weight loss behaviors are at risk for not only obesity but also for BN and AN. Prevention and treatment interventions should concentrate on the causes of all three eating behaviors (Riva, 2011).

It is well recognized that EDs are familial in nature. Many patients with EDs have been known to suffer from childhood separation anxiety. They see their bodies as "transitional objects" (Sadock & Sadock, 2007, p. 736). In real terms, this may translate into indecisiveness relative to food. Eating may symbolize a longing to connect with the caretaker and purging or vomiting may signify an avenue to separate from the caregiver. Low levels of nurturance from the caregivers have been associated with BN (Sadock & Sadock, 2007).

Mothering skills and attachment issues may play a role in the development of EDs. An unstable parent-infant relationship may lead to dysfunctional eating patterns. The lack of parental affection is replaced by food consumption, therefore, the person associates food with emotional communication (American Psychiatric Association [APA], 2006).

Anxiety disorders are common antecedents in EDs. Anxious individuals, feeling fearful in certain situations, transfer the attention from the situation into themselves and become exceedingly self-focused. The "allocentric lock theory," which describes the person as being locked into an "observer view" with a negative perceived image of one's body, is proposed as the precursor to both obesity and EDs. In other words, people view their bodies on the basis of appearance instead of performance (Riva, 2011).

These people view themselves from an external perspective. For example, the adolescent girl is emotionally stimulated by a thin model while watching television. Subsequently, she begins to focus on her own body but in a negative view, "I am not thin like the beautiful model." She compares her external features to that of the model, "My body looks fat in that mirror." Lastly, the individual develops an "allocentric" view of herself, "I look horrible in that mirror" (Riva, 2011). These individuals develop a hatred of their body even after considerable weight loss and the person continues on a torrid quest to improve her body at all costs (Riva, 2011). Compounding the problem is that many cultures link a thin body with happiness, success, and social likeability. Obesity is related to laziness, lack of willpower, and poor self-control (Riva, 2011).

Other studies have focused on the influential theory of liking as opposed to wanting food. Liking is referred to as the enjoyment of eating a given food and wanting refers to appetite motivation. Research has shown that these two entities espouse different neural relationships. Theory dictates that liking and wanting are conflicting components (Berridge, 2008).

Research has demonstrated that there are neurobiological and behavioral links between substance dependence and overindulgence of highly processed foods. This led to a theory that food addiction may be a commonality to both obesity and EDs (Gearhardt, Yokum, Orr, Stice, Corbin, & Brownell, 2011). This chapter will discuss the integrated management of BN, AN, and obesity across the life span.

DEFINITION OF BULIMIA NERVOSA

According to the *DSM-IV-TR* Diagnostic Criteria (APA, 2000a), BN is characterized by eating much larger amounts of food, within a 2-hour time frame, than the average person would eat in that same period of time. This is coupled with a lack of control over the eating event and is followed by recurrent compensatory behaviors such as vomiting, laxative, diuretic, enema use, or excessive exercise, all in an attempt to manage weight. The binge eating and compensatory behaviors occur at least two times a week for a period of 3 months (APA, 2000a).

There are two types of BN. The purging type involves the misuse of laxatives or diuretics along with the self-induced vomiting. The nonpurging type entails the compensatory behaviors such as fasting or excessive exercise; however, the individual does not employ the use of laxatives, diuretics, enemas, or self-induced vomiting (APA, 2000a). Bulimics possess a morbid fear of becoming fat and base their self-image on body size and shape (Sadock & Sadock, 2007). Approximately half of the patients with BN have experienced a short or protracted prior episode of AN (Sadock & Sadock, 2007). However, binging and purging does not occur during episodes of AN (APA, 2000a).

EPIDEMIOLOGY

EDs are surprisingly common and potentially life threatening conditions with high morbidity and mortality. Obesity is a global pandemic with more than one billion adults overweight (body mass index [BMI]>25kg/m2) and 300 million obese (BMI>30kg/m2). In the United States, 65% of adults are overweight, 32.3% are obese, and children's rates of obesity are continuing to grow. Furthermore, between 1980 and 2004, the prevalence of obesity doubled in adults and tripled in children (Fiegal, Carroll, Ogden, & Curtin, 2010; Ogden, Carroll, Curtin, Lamb, & Flegal, 2010).

BN is more common than AN (Sadock & Sadock, 2007). BN has been known to affect approximately 1.1% to 4.2% of women across a lifetime span (Franco, 2010). While the prevalence among males is approximately one tenth that of females (Sadock & Sadock, 2007), it is on the rise in men and women of all backgrounds and is becoming increasingly prevalent in most continents (Hudson, Pope, & Kessler, 2007; Lazzaro-Smith, 2008; Watters, 2010).

One in five women will engage in some form of disordered eating during her lifetime (Renfrew Center Foundation for Eating Disorders, 2003) with the mean onset between 18 to 21 years of age (Williams, Goodie, & Motsinger, 2008). The great majority of patients with BN are unmarried, college educated, and in their mid-20s (Rushing, Jones, & Carney, 2003).

It has been found that children as young as five already have knowledge about weight control and dieting. They understand that vomiting results in weight loss (Franco, 2010). In females with extreme dieting, prevalence rates climbed to 18 times more likely to develop an eating disorder within 6 months than those females who did not engage in dieting or who engaged in less severe dieting behaviors (Pratt & Woolfenden, 2009). But many individuals do not even recognize that they have disordered eating (Johnson, Spitzer, & Williams, 2001).

ETIOLOGY OF BN

BIOLOGICAL FACTORS

Studies conducted on dieting women and men showed differences in serotonin and circulating tryptophan (the precursor necessary to synthesize serotonin) levels. Serotonin levels were significantly lower in the dieting women than in the men. This study suggests that women may have a biological predisposition for the development of EDs. Because serotonin supports satiety, it stands to reason that decreased levels of serotonin metabolism are found in individuals suffering from BN (Halmi, 2000).

People with BN may have lower levels of activity in the sympathetic nervous system. Abnormalities in dopamine (DA) levels are associated with BN in that aberrant dopaminergic pathways can cause a decreased feeling of satisfaction after eating, resulting in binge and purge EDs. Cerebrospinal fluid (CSF) B-endorphin levels are found to be decreased in women with BN correlating with a higher level of depression (Halmi, 2000). These endorphin levels become elevated in some individuals after vomiting, resulting in a feeling of well-being (Sadock & Sadock, 2007).

Biological factors that set the stage for BN include females who are genetically heavier than others but at the same time internalize the notion of appearing thin. Women who have engaged in numerous dieting behaviors with little to no success are also in danger of purging behaviors as their basal metabolic rates have decreased (Robert-McComb, 2001).

SOCIAL AND PSYCHOLOGICAL FACTORS OF BN

Risk factors for the development of BN include: overweight parents, a history of childhood obesity, disparaging comments made by family members regarding the child's weight or body shape, early onset of menarche, familial history of psychiatric illness, disconnected relationships between the parent and the child, and high parental expectations placed on the child (Pratt & Woolfenden, 2009). Patients with BN have been known to possess a low self-concept, lack social support from family members, have an increased apprehension regarding body weight and shape, and demonstrate poor coping skills (Ghaderi & Pure, 2003). Other predisposing familial precursors are parental overprotectiveness, poor conflict resolution, and enmeshment (Robert-McComb, 2001). The individual may begin to exhibit feelings of perfectionism accompanied by a negative self-esteem (Pratt & Woolfenden, 2009).

Onset of EDs tend to develop in the adolescent girls as body fat begins to develop, thus, body dissatisfaction increases (Kalodner & Delucia-Waack, 2003). Societal influences play a major role in the development of BN since thinness is associated with femininity and physical attractiveness. Females idolize thin actresses and models. Young girls appear to be more concerned with their appearance than boys and connect popularity and attractiveness with being thin (Robert-McComb, 2001). Additionally, adolescent girls see dependence as a desirable trait in a society that really values independence. When these two views cause conflict, confusion and inadequacy result, culminating in a loss of control. Girls may find that dieting can generate a means to reestablish self-control (Robert-McComb, 2001).

BN is correlated with depression, anxiety, and relationship difficulties (Kalodner & Delucia-Waack, 2003). These individuals are known to seek societal approval but are not able to understand or affirm their own personal needs. They tend to have poor coping skills, avoid conflict, and feel high levels of stress (Robert-McComb, 2001). Patients with BN are found to demonstrate more anger but also tend to be more outgoing than individuals suffering from AN (Sadock & Sadock, 2007).

There are comorbidities associated with BN. There may be an associated depression and one third to half of all individuals with BN also have personality disorders (APA, 2006). Individuals with BN may demonstrate compulsive and impulsive behaviors as well as an unstable affect (Harrop & Marlatt, 2009). Substance abuse and attempts at shoplifting are linked with BN (Sadock & Sadock, 2007) as well as increased suicide and mortality rates (Crow et al., 2009).

Personality traits that may increase the risk for developing BN include "impulsivity, stress reactivity, novelty seeking, affective dysregulation, interpersonal sensitivity, and low self-esteem" (Harrop & Marlatt, 2009, p. 395). These individuals are known to be high achievers (Sadock & Sadock, 2007). They may have troubled relationships with peers (Saukko, 2000).

Depression, irritability, anxiety, or stress can ignite BN. Unlike their anorexic counterparts, patients with BN may be more difficult to detect, as they appear with normal body weight (Franco, 2010). These patients tend to be egocentric, thus, tend to seek help more willingly than patients with AN (Sadock & Sadock, 2007). It has been estimated, however, that between 50% and 90% of adults with BN may not obtain treatment for their disorder (Mond, Hay, Rodgers, & Owen, 2007).

ASSESSMENT

Early detection and treatment of EDs are crucial to improved outcomes (National Collaborating Centre for Mental Health, 2004). Although primary care providers are in a unique position to uncover EDs, many cases go undetected despite the existence of associated medical problems. Researchers have found that only 1 in 10 cases of BN are identified by health professionals (Whitehouse, Cooper, & Vize, 1992; Walsh & Garner, 1997; Johnson et al., 2001).

The majority of patients with BN do not have obvious signs on physical examination. Possible findings in patients with advanced BN include: emaciated appearance, pallor, and sunken cheeks. Nails and hair can become brittle. Subconjunctival hemorrhage, dental decay, and loss of tooth enamel can occur from vomiting. The person may present with low energy, fatigue, and vertigo. They may complain of bloating, heartburn, or sore throat (Williams et al., 2008). The abdomen may become tender to palpation. Arrhythmias, palpitations, and murmurs might be audible on cardiac exam. Bulimics may complain of shortness of breath, chest pain, headaches, joint pain, and irregular menses (Allen & Dalton, 2011).

Patient may engage in self-induced vomiting by placing a finger down the throat causing calluses on the dorsum of the hand (Russell's sign), although some patients are able to vomit without this action. The self-induced vomiting serves two purposes: minimizing the bloated feeling and subsequent abdominal pain associated with eating large amounts of food and avoiding weight gain. Individuals generally feel depressed (Sadock & Sadock, 2007) and ashamed (Franco, 2010) after the purging episode. Health care professionals should be cognizant that patients may present in loose clothing in order to hide the weight loss (Forbush, Heatherton, & Keel, 2007).

Hypocalcemia and diminished deep tendon reflexes (DTRs) might occur (American Academy of Pediatrics, Committee on Adolescence, 2003) along with fluid and electrolyte disturbances. Metabolic alkalosis or acidosis may occur from excessive vomiting or frequent stooling secondary to laxative use. Other serious signs of BN are esophageal tears with subsequent bleeding and gastric rupture (Mehler, 2011).

Although the majority of complications will resolve once healthy eating habits and weight are restored (Williams et al., 2008), the lack of treatment for BN can result in death with the mortality rate estimated at 5%. (Dichter, Cohen, & Connolly, 2002). Due to co-morbid physical and emotional conditions, BN is one of the most complex and difficult psychiatric disorders to treat (Crow et al., 2009).

SCREENING INSTRUMENTS

EDs should be screened for in the primary care setting as studies have shown that persons suffering from EDs use primary health services with frequency (Simon, Schmidt, & Pilling, 2005). Many primary care providers, however, are inadequate in identifying these patients as they do not link emotional and psychological factors with individuals suffering from BN (Flahavan, 2006).

The lack of identifying individuals suffering from BN may be due, in part, to time constraints in provision of care. Interestingly, physicians rate themselves as competent or very competent in diagnosing EDs but 84% did not screen for them (Flahavan, 2006). Health providers must be particularly attuned to signs and symptoms of BN as it is seldom that an individual will disclose this disorder (Becker et al., 1999). A screening tool that is both accurate in establishing the diagnosis and time efficient is ideal (Striegel-Moore, Perrin, DeBar, Wilson, Rossell, & Kraemer, 2010).

There are many tools developed to detect and measure EDs yet there is no one accepted tool (Striegel-Moore et al., 2010). The first step to identifying BN should be the clinical interview (Franco, 2010) and it is recommended that, if possible, all screening tools be accompanied by a detailed assessment conducted by a health professional (Chakraborty & Basu, 2010).

The Eating Disorder Examination (EDE) interview is the most widely used and accepted tool for diagnosing EDs (Fairburn & Cooper, 1993). It is an investigator-based interview in which the participants answer questions that are rated without further probing. It is important that the participant understands the purpose of the interview and that the interviewer and participant establish a good rapport before beginning the examination. Questions focus on the preceding 28 days but some questions may include events that have occurred within the past 3 months. This instrument and rating scale can be found in Fairburn (2008).

The Eating Disorder Examination Questionnaire (EDE-Q) is a 35-item, self-report version of the EDE used when an interview is not feasible or possible (APA, 2006). It is gaining increasing interest for measuring ED symptoms and eliminates the time factor associated with the interview process (Fairburn & Beglin, 1994). It may provide more detailed information than other screening tools (Allen, Fursland, Watson, & Byrne, 2011). It can be found at: Appendix in Fairburn (2008). Information about the tool can also be found at www.psychiatry.ox.ac.uk/research units/credo

The Patient Health Questionnaire (PHQ) is a tool for screening mental disorders in general but has also been used to screen for binge EDs. It should only be used, however, in combination with follow-up questions (Striegel-Moore et al., 2010). Use is only made available in accordance with the Terms of Use at www.pfizer.com

The Yale-Brown-Cornell Eating Disorder Scale (YBC-ED) can be administered by the provider and takes approximately 10 to 40 minutes to complete (Chakraborty & Basu, 2010). It is a 65-item symptom checklist with 19 additional questions addressing rituals and preoccupations related to eating. This screening tool requires a trained administrator (APA, 2006). It can be retrieved at: www.ncbi.nlm.nih.gov/pubmed/7897615

The Diagnostic Survey for Eating Disorders (DSED) is a 12-section survey. The survey includes patient demographics, weight history, body image, dieting history, binge eating, purging behaviors, exercise, sexual functioning, menstruation patterns, medical and psychiatric history, life adjustment, and family history (APA, 2006). It can be found in Garner and Garfinkel (1985).

The Sick, Control, One Stone (14ob/6.5 kg), Fat, Food (SCOFF) questionnaire is a five-item screening tool that can lead to the diagnosis of BN. The patient answers a yes or no to areas addressing self-induced vomiting, loss of control over eating, considerable weight loss, body image, preoccupation with eating, and obsessive concern with body shape. Although simple to use, this tool may pose time difficulties in the busy practice setting (Morgan, Reid, & Lacey, 1999). It can be retrieved from: http://psychcentral.com/eatingquiz.htm

The National Institute for Health and Clinical Excellence (NICE) survey entails one or two questions, for example, "Do you think you have an eating problem?" and "Do you worry excessively about your weight?" (National Collaborating Centre for Mental Health, 2004). This questionnaire may be of more practical use in the primary care setting (Flahavan, 2006). Information pertaining to this can be found at www.nice.org.uk/CG009NICEguideline.

The Readiness and Motivation Interview (RMI) is a tool used to evaluate the patient's motivation or readiness to accept change (Geller & Drab, 1999). This tool is based upon the transtheoretical model of change in which individuals can be grouped into one of five readiness stages. The first stage is precontemplation where the patient is either not aware or not willing to make a change in his or her life. Contemplation is the second stage, where the patient begins to consider change. The third stage is preparation or contemplating a change in the near future. Taking action is the fourth stage, in which the patient actively attempts to make changes in his or her behavior, and the fifth stage involves maintenance behaviors to avoid setbacks (Prochaska, 1979; Prochaska, DiClemente, & Norcross, 1992). This information can be found in Geller and Drab (1999).

Other self-report screening instruments are the Bulimia Test Revised (BULIT-R), a 36-item questionnaire designed to evaluate eating behaviors and attitudes about BN (APA, 2006). An example of the questionnaire can be found in Robert-McComb (2001). Note that the BULIT-R may not be copied. Copies must be obtained from Mark H. Thelan, PhD, Department of Psychology, 210 McAlester Hall, University of Missouri, Columbia, MO, 65211, with permission.

The Eating Attitudes Test (EAT) is a brief 26-item self-report that screens for symptoms and concerns related to BN (APA, 2006). It can be viewed at www.santarosanutrition.com/files/Download/EAT26Test120105.pdf

The Eating Disorders Inventory-3 (EDI-3), which has been revised, is a standardized measurement of psychological traits and symptoms assessing attitudes and behaviors related to eating, weight, and shape. It operates on 11 subscales presented in a six-point, forced-choice format assessing attitudes concerning eating, weight, and shape. Eight additional items assess general psychological traits (APA, 2006). Information about the instrument as well as the revisions can be found in: Garner (1991). It can also be found in: Garner (2004), *Eating* Disorder *Inventory-3: Professional Manual.*

The Questionnaire on Eating and Weight Patterns–Revised (QEWP-R) measures the nature and the number of binge eating episodes (APA, 2006). Information about this questionnaire can be obtained from: Spitzer, Uanovski, and Marcus (1993), *The Questionnaire on Eating and Weight Patterns–Revised (QEWP-R).*

CONCORDANCE

It is vital that the PMH-APRN be acutely aware that BN is a particular area of psychiatric nursing that must be dealt with very carefully. Establishing and maintaining a therapeutic relationship is central to managing this disorder (Treasure et al., 1995). The PMH-APRN must identify signs and symptoms early on so that a diagnosis can be reached in a timely manner. Further, the PMH-APRN should be able to identify risk factors associated with BN (Patching & Lawler, 2009).

Critical to the PMH-APRN-patient interaction is an attempt to build a relationship based on trust and mutual respect. This serves as the foundation for the therapeutic relationship, especially in light of the chronicity of the disorder. The PMH-APRN must learn to adapt her approach throughout the course of the relationship. Patients may be reluctant to disclose specifics and may withhold vital information due to feelings of shame (APA, 2006).

It is important to acknowledge the patient's anxieties and to recognize that asking them to gain weight may compound these anxieties. Initially, the PMH-APRN should foster the relationship by validating the patient's feelings and demonstrating an understanding of emotions underlying the BN. It is also important to communicate that treatment takes time and that a rapid change is unrealistic (APA, 2006).

Individuals with BN are reluctant to disclose eating and body concerns not only to health professionals, but across all intimate relationships. Self-disclosure difficulties related to eating and weight, and impact on dissatisfaction with body image may result in depression (Evans & Wertheim, 2001). Patients may be hesitant to disclose to the PMH-APRN for fear of negative reactions such as rejection, feelings of burdening the PMH-APRN, creating an undesirable impression of one's self, showing vulnerability, shame, and regret for not disclosing sooner. These negative outcomes, however, may in time, result in a positive patient-therapist outcome (Faber, 2006).

Helping the patient understand that a team approach is most effective in developing a plan of care is paramount. The team involves the psychiatric professional, the primary health provider, dieticians, dentists, and in the case of children and adolescents, teachers (APA, 2006).

It is important to recognize the experience of living with an ED from the patient's standpoint rather than exclusively from a medical model perspective (Patching & Lawler, 2009). Beginning therapy using the scientific model may not be in the best interests of the patient as it may not provide an in-depth understanding of the patient's lived experience. Thus, interventional therapy will likely be established by the health care professional without shared decision by the patient. Recovery should be a decision made by the individual and the pace of recovery must also be the individual's choice (Patching & Lawler, 2009).

Self-determination and self-help groups can be significant contributors toward recovery in individuals with BN. Recovering, however, will only transpire when the individual is "ready to gain a strong sense of self devoid of their condition" (Patching & Lawler, 2009, p. 20). The PMH-APRN must understand the patient's social and cultural circumstances before treatment regimes can be addressed (Patching & Lawler, 2009).

Therapeutic interventions should begin by facilitating the individual's sense of self-worth rather than focusing on nutritional components and body image. The PMH-APRN must possess an awareness of social and behavioral factors leading to the ED and convey a compassionate and supportive attitude toward the patient. The patient must be ready to address the BN in order to make the choice to work toward recovery. Interventions must initially focus on the feelings of the individual rather than on establishing a cure (Patching & Lawler, 2009).

The PMH-APRN must understand that there is a maladaptive relationship between the person's mind and body (Lazzaro-Smith, 2008). The individual feels that her life is structured and controlled and that being thin makes her feel special and worthwhile (Williams et al., 2008). She feels both estranged and fearful of her body and, therefore, disconnects her mind from her body. Patients intellectualize this maladaptive behavior, but underlying it is the feeling of body hatred, shame, and dissociation (Lazzaro-Smith, 2008).

The patient becomes disconnected with her own emotions and eats to avoid dealing with these emotions. She subsequently judges herself when she does feel emotion. Excessive anxiety and difficulty formulating relationships with others results in overeating and purging (Lazzaro-Smith, 2008). It is therefore crucial that a collaborative approach between the patient and the PMH-APRN be established. The PMH-APRN should ask questions in a nonconfrontational manner in order to engage with the patient in the treatment process (Williams et al., 2008).

Once the diagnosis is made, it is important that the PMH-APRN assess the patient's readiness to change her perceptions so that the patient's maladaptive coping mechanisms can begin to recede. This may take some time and therapy must proceed according to the patient's needs. The patient must develop a "safety zone" both within her or his own body as well as basic self-regulation skills. The change process can completely engulf the patient and may backfire if the patient is not ready to begin the process of self-awareness. Rather than managing to let go of her pain, she may become increasingly fearful (Lazzaro-Smith, 2008).

The PMH-APRN must help the patient deal with any unresolved trauma and build foundational skills before healing can occur (Lazzaro-Smith, 2008). If the patient appears unmotivated to change, the PMH-APRN should communicate her concerns but acknowledge that she will be available if the patient decides to change. If there are life-threatening medical complications, however, the PMH-APRN must intervene by initiating inpatient hospitalization, preferably in a unit specializing in EDs (APA, 2006).

EXPECTED OUTCOMES

Specific goals suggested by the APA (2006) are to encourage the patient with BN to:

- Decrease or eliminate the binge eating and purging
- Address and resolve medical complications associated with BN
- Motivate oneself to participate in the plan of care
- Develop an understanding of her or his own health and eating habits
- Change maladaptive thoughts and feelings toward eating
- Seek help and treatment for underlying psychiatric conditions
- Allow for family support and counseling when necessary
- Be aware of the potential for relapse and seek help when necessary

Healing from EDs involves not only cessation of symptoms but insight into a healthy merging of the body and the self. Patients should have an awareness of who they are and what they feel. They should feel empowered to make other choices in their lives. Lazzaro-Smith (2008) describes healthy outcomes for patients with EDs:

- Understanding that exercise in moderation is healthy
- Understanding the body's need for nourishment
- Having the ability to enjoy food
- Feeling a sense of vitality
- Developing a sense of self-identity beyond the ED
- Being able to accept and not judge oneself
- Realizing individuals have a choice
- Engaging rather than avoiding others
- Establishing new priorities in one's life
- Allowing oneself to have feelings and desires
- Feeling less fearful of one's emotions
- Understanding that relaxation should be pleasurable

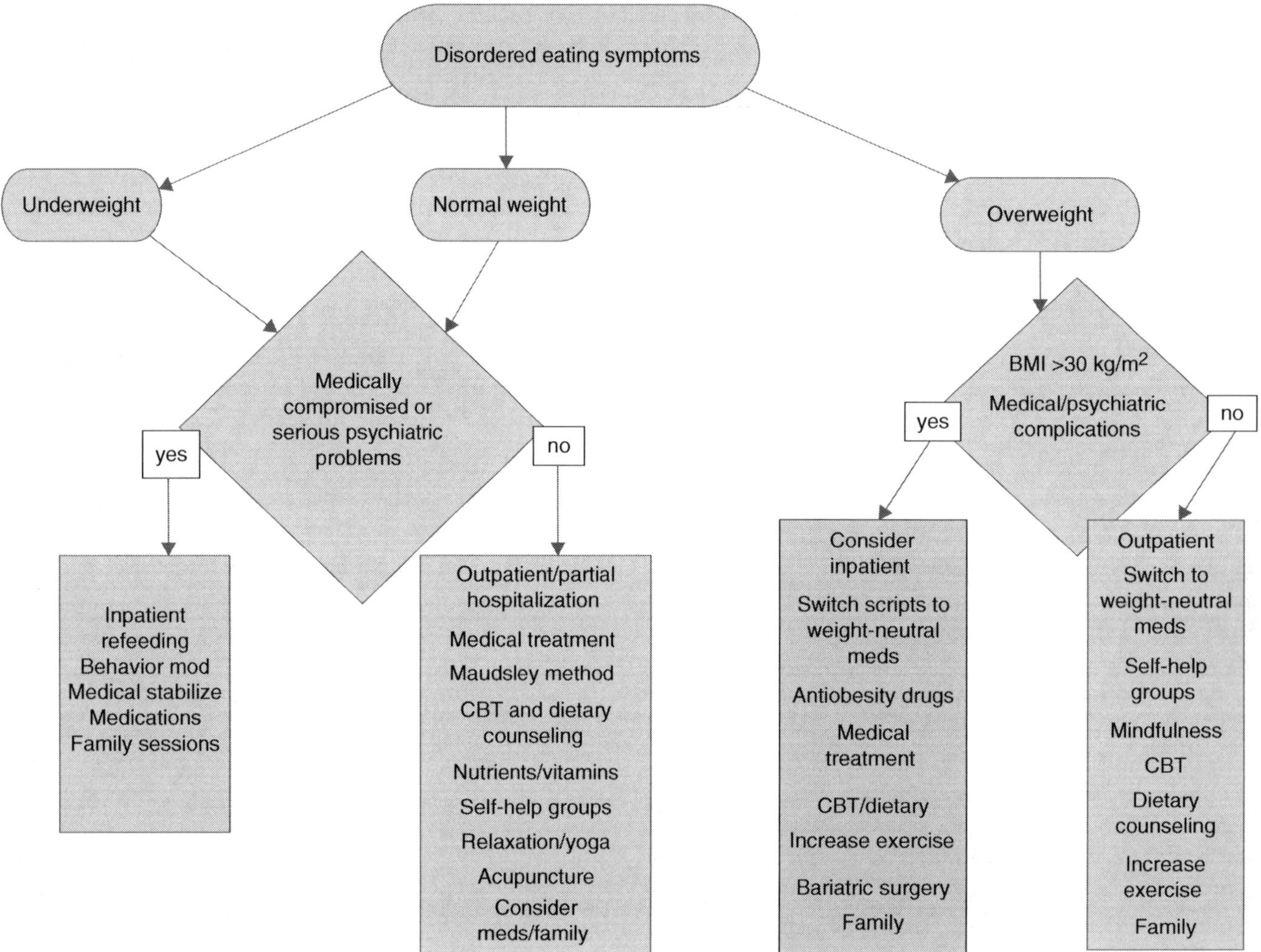

Figure 12-1 Decision Tree for Use of Pharmacologic and Non-pharmacologic Treatment of Disordered Eating

Strong communication skills are central to health and wellness. Robert-McComb (2001) outlines healing outcomes for EDs, which are the ability to:

- Self-disclose to the health professional and others without feeling hostile or competitive
- Creatively problem solve and resolve conflicts
- Learn to healthfully express feelings

TREATMENT INITIATION/ACUTE FOLLOW-UP

Once the diagnosis is made, a baseline medical and psychiatric assessment should be performed (see Figure 12-1). This should be repeated at least weekly once treatment is initiated. Prior to beginning treatment, it is important to understand the patient's psychological and cognitive development, age, family circumstances, as well as psychodynamic issues and any comorbidities. It is preferable that the patient's family cooperate in his or her care (APA, 2006).

Although most patients with BN can be treated in outpatient settings, those who present with life-threatening complications such as emaciation, severe electrolyte imbalance, dehydration, cardiac or GI complications, or a drop to 75% of ideal body weight do require hospitalization (APA, 2006). These cases may require management with nasogastric feedings, daily weights, checking vital signs, measuring intake and output, as well as frequent monitoring to identify fluid volume overload related to overfeeding (Franco, 2010). Harmful psychiatric behaviors such as suicidal ideation or impulsive/compulsive self-harm behaviors must be dealt with in an urgent manner (Williams et al., 2008).

Inpatient treatment is aimed at normalizing the eating patterns and educating the bulimic to consume adequate food to maintain his or her body weight. This entails establishing regular eating times, serving food on trays to teach bulimics portion size, providing a 30-minute time interval to complete the meal that is preselected by the dietician, observing the patient during mealtime, and locking bathroom doors for 1 hour after meals to prevent vomiting (Vitale, Lotito, & Maglie, 2009).

Group sessions to encourage patients' thoughts and feelings regarding eating are scheduled directly after meals since this is a particularly stressful time for patients. In addition, group therapy is scheduled throughout the day with the intent of improving communications skills and developing healthier coping mechanisms. Additional topics such as nutritional counseling and the medical consequences of eating disorders must also be addressed (Vitale et al., 2009).

The majority of individuals can be treated in outpatient settings or partial hospitalization programs specializing in EDs. The treatment setting should be discussed jointly with the patient. These programs vary in intensity but it is recommended that they be structured to 5 days/week for 8 hours/day (APA, 2006).

The initial and most intensive outpatient treatment is Partial Hospitalization. Although similar to inpatient care, the patient is allowed to leave the facility in the evening and return the following day. This allows the patient to separate from the staff and experience some degree of familiarity in their lives. Time at home allows patients to reflect on troublesome areas of their lives as well as more positive ones. Patients are encouraged to discuss these experiences with staff. The treatment plan is similar to inpatient hospitalization (Vitale et al., 2009).

The next level of care is Intensive Outpatient. Most of these programs consist of at least three meetings weekly for 3 hours each. Meetings are generally held in the evening so that patients can attend work or school. The patient should have a physical exam and a dental checkup prior to admission (Vitale et al., 2009).

Individuals with less severe BN are considered for individual or group therapy. These sessions are scheduled one to three times weekly and should include a treatment team that consists of a counselor or therapist, dietician, medical practitioner, and family members (if appropriate) (Vitale et al., 2009).

Prior to treatment, a family history should be obtained as well as a history of substance abuse, obesity, family interactions, exercise, and feelings about the individual's appearance. It is important that the PMH-APRN identify family stressors but not cast blame upon the family as there is no evidence that proves families are the cause of EDs (APA, 2006). Collaboration and communication between various levels of service is necessary in order to facilitate effective intervention (Flahavan, 2006).

It is important to use a nonjudgmental approach to patients with BN. The first step in assessment and treatment is to start a conversation about the patient's eating patterns. Questions such as, "Would it be okay if we discussed your eating habits?" and "I'm concerned about your eating" or "May we discuss how you typically eat?" are appropriate (Williams et al., 2008, p. 193).

The next step is to assess the patient's motivation to change their eating habits. Helpful questions include "On a scale of 1 to 10, how important is it for you to change your eating?," "What might make it more important?," and "How would your life be different if you didn't need to spend so much time thinking about your eating?" (Williams et al., 2008, p. 193).

Next, the PMH-APRN should attempt to determine the precursors and consequences of disordered eating. Examples of questions are, "When are you most likely to binge?" and "How do you feel before you binge? After you binge? Before you purge? After you purge? What happens after you purge?" (Williams et al., 2008).

The last two steps involve developing substitutes for binging and changing negative thinking (APA, 2006). Items to consider are, "When you feel an urge to binge, what could you do instead of binging?" "Consider activities that you could do in the situation when you are most likely to binge." Other questions might include "Who determines how you think about yourself?" or "What can you control?" (Williams et al., 2008, p. 193).

There are a multitude of therapies designed to treat patients with BN which are listed in Table 12-1 Therapies Used to Treat Bulimia Nervosa. Cognitive Behavioral Therapy (CBT) has been found to be the single most effective intervention for BN. It is associated with a more rapid response than other forms of therapy but is more successful in conjunction with other psychodynamic interventions (APA, 2006).

This therapy addresses the dieting/binge eating/ extreme weight control issues by attempting to normalize eating patterns. This is accomplished by exploring individual thoughts and feelings about food and body image. CBT encourages patients to change their original thoughts related to disordered eating toward healthier alternative behaviors (Hay, Bacaltchuk, Stefano, & Kashyap, 2009). Although effective in the treatment of BN, most individuals do not receive such evidence-based treatment. Reasons cited are that treatment appears to be aimed at comorbid mental health problems or medical complications associated with the ED or at weight problems rather than for the BN itself (Mond, Hay, Rodgers, & Owen, 2007).

TABLE 12-1: THERAPIES USED TO TREAT BULIMIA NERVOSA

TYPE OF THERAPY	DESCRIPTION
Cognitive-Analytic Therapy (CAT)	Combination of cognitive & psychotherapy Focuses on interpersonal & transference issues
Cognitive Orientation Therapy	Helps patient focus on meaning of behavior Therapist explores themes with patient & the belief around the theme Therapy should NOT be focused solely around BN Therapist should NOT attempt to convince patient that his or her belief is unusual
Exposure and Response Prevention Therapy	Food is given along with psychological prevention to avoid weight control behaviors Therapy continues until behaviors associated with BN are reduced
Hypnobehavioral Therapy	Combines psychological behavioral technique with hypnosis to modify behaviors associated with BN
Dialectical Behavioral Therapy (DBT)	Defines emotional dysregulation as central problem with BN Patient simultaneously views vomiting with relief & disgust Premise is that binging & purging are used to control or change traumatic emotional states Therapy based on emotional regulation skills & authenticating patient's self-worth
Self-Help Groups	Considered modified cognitive behavioral therapy Booklet mailed to patient who manages on his or her own No support from health professional Patient instructed to maintain food diary & increase food intake awareness
Unguided Self-Help	Booklet provided to patient with support from either professional or nonprofessional who may or may not have expertise in BN Also available are online self-help programs
12-Step Program	Used for adjunctive treatment or follow-up care Allows patients to work through relationship difficulties that may be associated with BN Provides patient with "reality check" when needed Group members support one another Allows patient to escape isolation that may be associated with BN
Family Therapy	Many patients view this as crucial to their recovery Particularly to be considered with adolescents or children Most effective in younger patients with early onset symptoms Not shown to be effective in adults with chronic BN
Nutritional Therapy	Key to managing BN Goals focused on reestablishing healthy eating habits Expectation is to gain 2–3 pounds/week Supplement diet with vitamins, minerals, & stool softeners (never laxatives) May be advantageous for therapist to share a meal with patient to view eating habits
Alternative Therapies	Relaxation & breathing techniques Bright light therapy Transcranial magnetic stimulation Yoga Accupuncture

Source: Griffiths & Cahnnon-Little (1993); Bachar et al. (1999); Williams (2003); APA (2006); Sadock & Sadock (2007); Lazzaro-Smith (2008); Hay et al. (2009); McIver et al. (2009); Wisniewski et al. (2009); Franco (2010); Allen & Dalton (2011).

Historically, psychodynamic therapy has been used most often in treating EDs. This approach describes pathology of the self as it relates to BN. Because the patient cannot depend on others to satisfy their need for self-esteem, they turn to food as an alternative to meet those needs. Successful therapy is aimed at the patient relying on humans for need fulfillment beginning with the therapist. This involves three stages of treatment. Stage 1 explores the interpersonal meaning of the BN, which identifies one or more interpersonal, problematic areas. Stage 2 focuses on supporting the patient through change resulting in cessation of BN. The third stage is aimed at helping the patient find ways to cope with future interpersonal problems. Eating habits and body attitudes are never attended to during psychodynamic therapy (Hay et al., 2009). For those patients who are unresponsive to psychodynamic therapy, a small number do respond to fluoxetine, or family or group psychotherapy (APA, 2006).

Another form of therapy is Psychodynamic/ Psychoanalytic Therapy. Clinical data indicate that this approach, either in individual or group format, is helpful once the binging and purging symptoms improve. This therapy focuses on developmental issues, identity formation, body image, self-esteem issues, sexual conflict, family problems, coping patterns, and problem solving (APA, 2006).

Cognitive-Analytic Therapy (CAT) combines cognitive and psychodynamic therapy (Hay et al., 2009). It focuses on interpersonal and transference issues (Chakraborty & Basu, 2010). While used to treat BN, this therapy is most often used for patients with AN (Hay et al., 2009).

Cognitive Orientation Therapy helps the patient focus on the meaning of his or her behavior, using themes exploring why the patient avoids certain emotions and then systematically alters this belief around a theme. The therapist should not focus the therapy solely around the eating disorder but around each individual theme. At no time should the therapist attempt to convince the patient that his or her belief is unusual or strange (Bachar, Latzer, Kreitler, & Berry, 1999).

Exposure and Response Prevention Therapy was first developed as a treatment for obsessive-compulsive disorder, and in the 1980s was modified as a form of therapy for individuals with BN. The patient is given food along with a psychological prevention approach in avoiding weight control behaviors associated with BN until those behaviors have diminished (Carter, Bulik, McIntosh, & Cue, 2002). This therapy, however, has not gained widespread acceptance for its use (Hay et al., 2009). The hypnobehavioral psychotherapy approach also uses psychological behavioral techniques but combines this with hypnosis to modify behaviors associated with BN (Griffiths & Cahnnon-Little, 1993).

One of the most recent and promising therapies for BN has been dialectical behavioral therapy (DBT). The premise of this therapy defines emotional dysregulation as the central problem in BN with binging and purging behaviors used to control or change traumatic emotional states. The dialectical approach views the patient's emotional state as oppositional in nature, meaning the patient simultaneously views vomiting with both relief and disgust (Hay et al., 2009). The therapy assists the patient in visualizing both sides of the behavior, that is, the vomiting is detestable but at the same time, the patient is gaining some positive reinforcement. This explains why the patient wishes to stop the vomiting but cannot resist. Therapy is based on emotional regulation skills authenticating the patient's self-worth (Hay et al., 2009).

Self-help groups, considered a modified form of CBT, is another approach in the treatment of BN. Typically, an instruction booklet is mailed to the person who manages on his or her own with no support from health care professionals (Williams, 2003). The individual is instructed to maintain a food diary and to increase awareness as to her food intake and any feelings or issues surrounding food. The manual helps formulate both a diagnosis and more effective problem-solving methods (Allen & Dalton, 2011).

A variant to self-help groups involves unguided self-help in which a booklet is provided along with support from either a professional or nonprofessional who may not have expertise in the area of BN (Williams, 2003). Predictors of positive outcomes include individuals who are self-directed at the outset of treatment (Franco, 2010). Recently, online self-help programs have been made available (APA, 2006).

Support groups and/or 12-step programs may be valuable as adjunctive treatment or for follow-up care but there are few data supporting short- or long-term effects (Yager et al. 2006). Therapists feel group therapy is important as it provides a forum for patients to work through relationship difficulties that may be associated with BN. Group members learn to support each other and receive reality checks when needed. These group encounters often help the individual escape the isolation often associated with ED (Levine & Mishna, 2007). Others concur that 12-step programs should not be recommended as the sole approach for individuals with BN as it does not address nutrition or behavioral deficits (APA, 2000b).

In the case of dysfunctional family dynamics, family therapy or marital counseling may be helpful (Franco, 2010). Family therapy has been found to be equivalent to time-limited psychodynamic psychotherapy in decreasing symptoms associated with BN. It should be considered in most cases, in particular when treating children and adolescent patients still living with their parents (APA, 2006). Some patients feel that their ED is based upon dysfunctional family dynamics rather than an individual problem (Lazzaro-Smith, 2008) and view it as a crucial element to their recovery (Chakraborty & Basu, 2010). This type of therapy was most effective in younger patients with early onset of symptoms. It was not shown to be effective in adults with chronic BN (Chakraborty & Basu, 2010).

Alternative approaches to treating BN are relaxation and breathing techniques, which can be used in conjunction with traditional therapeutic approaches (Lazzaro-Smith, 2008). Bright light therapy has been shown to decrease binge frequency. Other studies have recognized the effects of transcranial magnetic stimulation (APA, 2006). Yoga may be an important adjunctive treatment for ED (McIver, O'Halloran, & McGartland, 2009). Acupuncture has also been used to treat BN (Faris et al., 2007).

Nutritional rehabilitation is a key component in managing BN. Goals are focused on reestablishing the patient's nutritional condition and restoring healthy eating habits. The patient is expected to gain 2 to 3 pounds per week and should ingest anywhere from 1,000–1,600 kcal/day. Any concurrent medical complications and comorbidities must be attended to (APA, 2006). See Table 12-3 for complications associated with BN.

The diet should be supplemented with vitamins, minerals, and stool softeners if constipated. Laxatives should never be used unless medically indicated (Franco, 2010). It may be advantageous to share a meal with the patient so that the PMH-APRN can observe the patient's eating patterns (i.e., cutting, separating food, mashing). This way the PMH-APRN can assess any difficulties the patient may have in eating certain foods (APA, 2006).

Foods that appeal to people with BN are those high in calories, sweet, soft, and smooth in texture, such as cupcakes or sweet buns (Sadock & Sadock, 2007). The food is ingested in secrecy and is eaten quickly (Franco, 2010). Individuals with BN may regard some foods as "safe" and others as "forbidden." They may consume large portions of fruits and vegetables with the identical caloric count as a candy bar but do not view this as binge eating since fruits and vegetables are healthy, or "safe," foods. The bulimic may feel bored and depressed prior to binging, followed by that same depression and a lack of self-control following binge eating (Rushing et al., 2003).

Typically, bulimics will eat normally around friends and family but binge in privacy. Some individuals schedule their daily routines around binging and purging episodes. Since binging can become expensive, some steal food from grocery stores (Rushing et al., 2003).

Mental health literacy (MHL) refers to "knowledge and beliefs about mental disorders that aid their recognition, management, or prevention" (Jorm et al., 1997, p. 182). Low MHL among persons suffering from mental disorders is the reason they may not seek treatment (Jorm et al., 1997; Andrews, Sanderson, Slade, & Issakidis, 2000). One study (Mond, Myers, Crosby, Hay, & Mitchell, 2009) found that two thirds of individuals recognized they had an ED, but less than 40% had sought treatment from a health care professional. Only 1 in 10 had sought treatment from a mental health professional (Mond et al., 2009), even though 80% had reported symptoms of anxiety or depression to a health care provider.

Many individuals with BN prefer lifestyle modifications such as the use of vitamins or minerals and are leery of the use of prescription medication. While some sufferers feel that their disorder would be difficult to treat, others feel that their behavior is normal and desirable (Mond et al., 2008). Therefore, there must be efforts made to improve MHL in individuals with BN. Primary care provider (PCPs) and other health care providers must be cognizant of the individual's belief system and how this might impact their seeking of and adherence to treatment (Mond et al., 2008).

One of the goals of recovery for individuals suffering from BN is normalizing eating; however, there are many barriers toward achieving this goal. One roadblock is that the BN becomes the individual's sense of identity. They believe the BN provides them with a sense of control, allowing them to better cope with the demands of life. It is also provides an avenue for circumventing difficult experiences (Cockell, Geller, & Linden, 2002). Because of these factors, individuals with BN are neither motivated nor anxious to alter their eating patterns (Geller, Cockell, & Drab, 2001). Disagreements between patients and health care providers are common and habitual relapses and dropout rates in treatments are problematic in patients with BN (Pike, 1998).

Although cognitive behavioral therapy and interpersonal therapy are efficacious treatment approaches, other studies have examined the impact on the extent of patient involvement in the treatment plan and its results on clinical outcomes (Agras, Walsh, Fairburn, Wilson, & Kraemer, 2000). Traditional approaches to therapy include the establishment of a bond and a partnership with the patient (Horvath & Greenberg, 1989). More recent modalities accentuate client motivation, honesty, and confidence in the provider's competence (Agnew-Davies, Stiles, Hardy, Barkham, & Shapiro, 1998).

Motivational approaches that originated in the area of substance abuse treatment operate by promoting patients' autonomy and accountability for their health (Miller & Rollnick, 2002). There is a difference between the motivational and direct treatment approach in that the patient must be ready to address and accept treatment. Additionally, the health care provider must address any client ambivalence. Safety issues such as establishing appropriate nutritional intake are major themes among both the direct and motivational approach to therapy (Miller & Rollnick, 2002).

The motivational approach does not assume to understand the patient's experience in dealing with BN nor their feelings about healing. The purpose of motivational therapy is not to label the client as resistant but instead, aims to determine when the client is ready to begin therapy. Additionally, motivational therapy allows for a dynamic and collaborative relationship between the patient and provider rather than holding the provider solely responsible for the treatment plan (Miller & Rollnick, 2002).

Motivational therapy is accomplished by showing interest and concern in the patient's experience and by facilitating frank dialogue as to the meaning behind the ED. This approach differs from traditional approaches in that the emphasis is on patient readiness and feelings about recovery rather than established protocols addressing weight gain and nutritional wellness (Miller & Rollnick, 2002).

Central to the treatment of BN are issues related to patient disclosure. The inability to self-disclose results in isolation and repressed feelings that may result in mental illness (Jourard, 1971). Disclosure depends not only on the type of information to be revealed and the surroundings in which the disclosure will occur, but also to whom that information will be disclosed (Rogers, Griffin, Wykle, & Fitzpatrick, 2009). Because disclosing to a professional enhances patient healing, it is considered a fundamental element of therapy (Faber & Hall, 2002). The ability to self-disclose gauges an individual's mental health in attaining self-actualization. It decreases levels of anxiety and allows for personal growth (Jourard, 1971).

MAINTENANCE

It is important that the PMH-APRN provide ongoing support and follow-up for the patient with BN (Flahavan, 2006). Duration of follow-up care appeared to have the greatest influence on recovery. Unfortunately, 25 years of research shows that BN still shows an unsatisfactory outcome in many patients and more refined interventions may be central to favorable outcomes (Steinhausen & Weber, 2009).

The overall short-term success rates for individuals with BN who undergo psychosocial treatment and/or medication therapy is reported to be 50% to 70%. Relapse rates of 30% to 85% have been reported anywhere from 6 months to 6 years post-treatment follow-up. Despite available treatment modalities, mortality rates continue to be high (Chakraborty & Basu, 2010).

BN is shown to have higher rates of partial and full recovery when compared to patients with AN. Patients undergoing treatment tend to have much better outcomes than those who go untreated. Despite various modalities used to treat BN, psychotherapy tends to be turbulent and lengthy in nature (Sadock & Sadock, 2007).

The course of BN may become chronic, lasting for more than a decade. The care of the chronically ill bulimic patient can be challenging, and treatment must be altered as necessary to meet the needs of the patient. Progress alternating with relapses may occur only in minute intervals. Communication among health care professionals involved in the treatment plan is vital among this subgroup of patients, and more frequent outpatient services may be necessary, especially to prevent hospitalization (APA, 2006).

It is necessary to continually reassess the patient's use of alcohol and other substance use throughout the recovery period, as in general these patients have difficulty with impulse control (APA, 2006). The PMH-APRN should assess for symptoms of major depression and anxiety as a high percentage of patients with ED report a lifetime history of both illnesses. Additionally, the PMH-APRN must assess for concurrent personality disorders, particularly impulsive, affective, and narcissistic traits, as well as borderline personality disorders (APA, 2006).

PHARMACOTHERAPY OF BN

Research supports the use of medication in the treatment of BN (Allen & Dalton, 2011). There are a range of medications used to treat BN, but the key priorities according to the 2004 NICE guidelines are the combination of psychological treatments such as CBT and medication. Pharmacological treatment, however, is associated with high noncompliance rates and relapse (Becker, 2003). Table 12-2 provides a list of medications used for treating BN.

The NICE guidelines consider Selective Serotonin Reuptake Inhibitor (SSRIs), particularly fluoxetine, the drug of choice in the treatment of BN in terms of side effect profile and symptom alleviation (Flament, Bissada, & Spettigue, 2011). The APA (2006) recommends antidepressants such as fluoxetine or sertraline but does not recommend tricyclic antidepressants (TCAs) or monoamine oxidase inhibitors (MAOIs) as first-line treatment.

TABLE 12-2: MEDICATIONS USED TO TREAT BULIMIA NERVOSA

TYPE OF EATING DISORDER	MEDICATION	CLASSIFICATION	INDICATIONS FOR USE	DOSE	ADVERSE REACTIONS
Bulimia Nervosa	Fluoxetine	SSRI	Considered 1st-line treatment for Bulimia Nervosa	60 mg QD	Somnolence, nervousness, headache, suicidal behavior, constipation, sexual dysfunction, vomiting, tremor, increased appetite, weight loss, diaphoresis, vertigo, asthemia
	Sertraline	SSRI	Sertraline has also been shown effective in treatment of Bulimia Nervosa	50–200 mg QD	Headache, suicidal behavior, agitation, palpitations, chest pain, sexual dysfunction, myalgias, dry mouth, vomiting, increased appetite

Source: APA (2006); Yager (2006); Flament et al. (2011); Spartto & Woods (2005).

The most studied SSRI in the treatment of BN has been fluoxetine. This is the only medication approved by the U.S. Food and Drug Administration (FDA) for the treatment of BN (Williams et al., 2008). While many studies have shown reduction in binging, vomiting frequency, and an improvement in depression and eating habits, other studies have yielded mixed results, that is, no efficacious results relative to placebo. Other studies have shown an improvement in preventing relapse or worsening eating behaviors while on fluoxetine but it appeared to have no effect on self-image or eating attitudes. The dose shown to be most effective in reducing symptoms was 60 mg/d (Flament et al., 2011).

Sertraline has also been shown to be efficacious in decreasing bulimic symptoms (Milano et al., 2004). Both fluoxetine and sertraline have been useful in treating symptoms of depression, anxiety, and obsessive-compulsive behaviors that may accompany BN. SSRIs should be taken for a minimum of 9 to 12 months (APA, 2006).

Tricycylic antidepressants in a random controlled trial (RCT) showed a mean reduction in the frequency of BN (47%–91%) symptoms, which was significantly superior to placebo. Desipramine and amitriplyline were the most promising with imipramine being less effective (Flament et al., 2011). The dose should be similar to that of treating depression (APA, 2006). The disadvantage of TCAs, however, is the side effect profile, which may be both unpleasant and fatal in an overdose. Because of this, TCAs are not considered front-line treatment for BN in adults (APA, 2006) and should never be used for children or adolescents (Flament et al., 2011).

Phenelzine, isocarboxazid, and brofaromine have been used in the treatment of BN. While initially these medications showed a reduction in symptoms (up to 35%), all initial responders relapsed within a 6-month period, and by the fourth year, 20% of the responders had experienced severe hypertensive episodes, with one resulting in death. Isocarboxazid appeared to have the most significant reduction in symptoms with no adverse side effects. Phenelzine showed promising results as well. Although brofaromine, which is a reversible MAOI, is effective, it is not commercially available in the United States. These medications, due to their side effect profiles and drug interactions are not considered first-line treatment for BN, nor are they FDA approved for the treatment of BN (APA, 2006).

Lithium showed significant improvement in depressed bulimic individuals. Phenytoin and carbamazepine also showed efficacious results. Topiramate was found to be well tolerated and showed improvement in symptoms of BN (Flament et al., 2011). While effective for binge reduction, its utility is limited for patients with BN as it causes weight loss (APA, 2006).

Norepinephrine dopamine reuptake inhibitor (NDRI) bupropion was found to be effective compared to placebo but has been linked with seizure activity; therefore, it is not indicated in treatment of BN (Horne et al., 1988). Trazadone was effective in the treatment of BN but was associated with drowsiness and dizziness (Hudson, Pope, Keck, & McElroy, 1989).

Phenytoin has been used to treat BN but in recent studies has not shown to be efficacious. Weight gain is a known side effect. Valproate and carbamazepine increase appetite; therefore, neither has been useful in the treatment of binge eating. Topiramate has shown a significant decrease in binge-eating episodes but also causes weight loss. Methylphenidate has been shown to be helpful for patients with BN and concurrent attention deficit hyperactivity disorder (ADHD; APA, 2006) but is known to cause weight loss (Spartto & Woods, 2005).

Although some progress has been made in the treatment of BN, there is still considerable information to be learned. Medication therapy should address not only dietary restraint or binge eating but "maladaptive weight and shape-related cognitions" (Flament et al., 2011). Adding antidepressants to behavioral weight control or other therapies does not appear to produce significant results in binge suppression as compared to using medication alone. Medications, however, may be used to treat comorbid conditions such as depression and anxiety (APA, 2006).

MANAGING SIDE EFFECTS

Several medications may need to be trialed to identify the medication with the most optimal response and the least number of side effects. If the patient is nonresponsive to medication, the PMH-APRN must ascertain whether the patient is taking the medication shortly before vomiting. It may be helpful to assess serum levels of mediations to determine if the effective drug levels have been achieved; although correlations have yet to be identified (APA, 2006). The PMH-APRN must evaluate the psychodynamic factors between the patient and PMH-APRN, as this may add to nonadherence in treatment and treatment resistance.

The PMH-APRN should advise the patient to take fluoxetine in the afternoon since it may cause nervousness and insomnia. The medication may cause vertigo or drowsiness so the patient should be cautioned against driving or operating machinery until the effects of the drug are known. With both fluoxetine and sertraline, the patient should watch for mood changes and suicidal tendencies. The patient should avoid alcohol and should avoid discontinuing the drug abruptly (Nursing, 2007).

Side effects of fluoxetine include insomnia, nausea, constipation, asthenia, decrease in libidio and an inability to reach orgasm. Although 60 mg of fluoxidine is the recommended dose in the treatment of BN, titrating downward helps to manage these effects. Stool softeners, not laxatives, are recommended to manage constipation associated with SSRIs (APA, 2006).

Common side effects for TCAs are sedation, constipation, dry mouth, and weight gain. These medications should be used with caution in the patient who is at risk for suicide as the medication is both toxic and potentially lethal when overdosed (APA, 2006). Because they cause sedation, the patient should be advised to take the medication at bedtime. The patient should not drive or engage in activities that require them to be alert until central nervous system (CNS) side effects are known. Advising the patient to chew hard candy or gum may relieve the dry mouth associated with TCAs. The patient should be told to use sunscreen to avoid photosensitive reactions. The patient should stop the drug only under the direction of the health provider (Nursing, 2007).

MAOIs should be avoided in treating BN due to its risk of spontaneous hypotensive crisis (APA, 2006).

Lithium carbonate should be used with caution in patients who may have a rapid shift in fluid volume as the medication levels may change dramatically. Lithium and valproic acid cause unwanted weight gain, which limits its use in treating patients with BN (APA, 2006). If prescribed, the patient should take the medication with food to avoid GI upset. They should be aware of symptoms associated with toxicity such as vomiting, diarrhea, tremors, muscle weakness, and decreased coordination. The patient should carry a medical identification band so that others are aware the patient is taking this medication (Nursing, 2007).

Topiramate can cause adverse effects such as word-finding difficulties and paresthesias. These side effects can be managed by slow, upward titrating of the dose. Weight loss is common with this medication, and therefore may be unacceptable in the treatment of BN. No data are reported for the use of these medications in children and adolescents with BN (APA, 2006).

Although methylphenidate can be used to treat BN, it has many side effects, including weight loss, so it must be used with caution (Nursing, 2007). Patients should be monitored for abuse of this medication (APA, 2006).

PROGNOSIS

Approximately 70% of individuals with BN will not show evidence of the disorder within 10 years of follow-up after

TABLE 12-3: COMPLICATIONS ASSOCIATED WITH BULIMIA NERVOSA

SYSTEM	COMPLICATION	MANIFESTATION & CAUSE
Gastrointestinal	Cheilosis	A form of stomatitis; pale maceration at angle of mouth
	Pharyngeal pain	Chronic irritation from vomiting
	Dental caries, erosion, & periodontal disease	Vomiting gastric contents
	Gingivitis	Vomiting gastric contents
	Sialadenosis or noninflammatory hypertrophy of salivary glands	Peripheral autonomic neuropathy for disordered metabolism and secretion
	Enlarged parotid glands	Unclear; thought to be pancreatic enzymes expelled into mouth or result of eating high carbohydrate foods consumed over a short time period; or chronic vomiting
	Esophagitis	Frequent contact with gastric contents
	Hematemesis	Mallory-Weiss tears of gastroesophageal junction
	GERD	Relaxed lower gastroesophageal sphincter due to repeated vomiting over many months
	Mallory-Weiss tears	Gastroesophageal bleeding resulting from frequent vomiting & erosion
	Barrett's esophagus	Reported in BN but unknown if increased prevalence with BN; periodic endoscopies to screen
	Boerhaave's syndrome (esophageal rupture)	Rare but may follow self-induced emesis; patient complains of chest pain and painful swallowing
	Melanosis Coli	Dark tone of the colonic mucosa
	Diarrhea	Misuse of laxatives
	Cathartic Colon	Loss of peristalsis due to long-term laxative use
	Constipation	Prolonged use of laxatives
	Rectal prolapse	Prolonged use of laxatives & constipation
Skin	Russell's sign	Abrasions & calluses on dorsum of hands & knuckles associated with inserting fingers & hands down the throat to induce vomiting
	Dehydration	Misuse of diuretics
	Dry skin and brittle hair and nails	Improper nutritional status associated with vomiting & diuretic use
Eyes	Subconjunctival Hemorrhage	Excessive and pronounced vomiting
	Sunken Eyes	Dehydration with vomiting & diuretic use
Cardiac (Williams, 2003)	Arrhythmias	Prolonged QT intervals or T-wave abnormalities associated with hypokalemia
	Hypotension	Fluid volume deficit
	Hypertension	Diet pill toxicity
	Low Cardiac Output	Hypovolemia
	Cardiomyopathy	Potassium disturbances
	Impaired left ventricular function	Abuse of ipecac to induce vomiting

(Continued)

TABLE 12-3: COMPLICATIONS ASSOCIATED WITH BULIMIA NERVOSA (*Continued*)

SYSTEM	COMPLICATION	MANIFESTATION & CAUSE
Endocrine (Williams et al., 2008; Rushing et al., 2003)	Menstrual Disturbances/ Amenorrhea or Oligomenorrhea—common in active bulimia but does not affect future ability to conceive in those who recover	Decrease in gonadotropin-releasing hormone and/or hormonal mechanism of leptin
	Hypoglycemia	Inadequate food intake
	Osteopenia	Poor calcium intake
Neurologic (Williams et al., 2008)	Cognitive impairment	Long-term nutritional deficits
	Peripheral neuropathy	Vitamin deficiency
	Seizures	Frequent purging
Pulmonary (Williams et al., 2008)	Aspiration pneumonia	Vomiting
	Pneumomediastinum	Vomiting
	Pneumothorax or rib fractures	Forceful vomiting
Laboratory Abnormalities (Mehler, 2011)	↑ fractionated amylase (↑ salivary amylase over pancreatic amylase)(mehler)	↑ salivary (not pancreatic) activity
	Hypokalemia (Rushing)	Purging, laxative, diuretics
	Hypochloremia	Purging episodes
	Hyperphophatemia	Purging episodes
	Metabolic alkalosis ↓ serum pH	Purging episodes
	Metabolic acidosis ↑ serum pH	Laxative abuse
	↑ Serum bicarbonate level	Vomiting & diuretic use
	↑ Serum sodium	Laxative use
	↓ Serum sodium	Purging or diuretic use
	Pseudo-Bartter Syndrome, which is hypokalemia, hypocholremia, metabolic alkalosis, hyperaldosteronism, hyperplasia of the juxtaglomerular apparatus; lack of intrinsic pathology & resolves once offending behavior has discontinued	Deficient chloride channels seen with chronic laxative & diuretic abuse & vomiting
	↑ Blood Urea Nitrogen	Fluid Volume Deficit

receiving treatment (Berkman, Lohr, & Bulik, 2007); recovery rates are varied (estimated between 24%–76%) depending on the criteria and definitions used to describe it (D'Abundo & Chally, 2004). Standardized mortality ratios are not significantly different when matched with the expected rate in age and sex (Berkman et al., 2007).

Medically, recovery rates are measured by maintenance of weight, return of menses, and less obsession with body shape and weight. But women may measure their recovery by different parameters. They describe recovery as feeling in control of their lives and a better sense of self (D'Abundo & Chally, 2004).

ANOREXIA NERVOSA

AN is often described as a refusal to maintain a healthy body weight combined with obsessive fears of gaining weight. With a 5.6% rate of death per decade of illness, AN has the highest rate of death of any psychiatric disorder (Sullivan, 1995; Attia & Walsh, 2009). AN is 10 times more prevalent in females than males and begins most often in adolescence (Woodside et al., 2001). AN affects approximately 0.5% to 1% of the female population in the United States. AN is likely under-diagnosed and under-treated due to a failure of persons with the disorder to seek treatment and a failure of treaters to properly refer for viable treatment protocols and ultimately a lack of reliable methods of intervention (Attia & Walsh, 2009).

ASSESSMENT

There are numerous tools that are available for clinicians and clients and their families to use in diagnosing AN and other EDs. This section will outline some of the available assessment tools and questionnaires that are available for use.

The Eating Attitudes Test (EAT) is one of the more widely used standardized measuring tools of signs and symptoms that are characteristic of EDs. The EAT was updated to the current 26-item version, the EAT-26. The EAT-26 can be either self-administered or administered by clinicians (Garner, Olmsted, Bohr, & Garfinkel, 1982). There is another variation of the test that is available for use with children, known as the Children's Eating Attitude Test or ChEAT (Maloney, Mcquire, & Daniels, 1988).

The Anorectic Behavior Observation Scale (ABOS) is an assessment tool that is given to the patient's family members who then rate the patient's behaviors and attitudes about eating (Uehara et al., 2002). The Yale-Brown-Cornell Eating Disorder Scale views each patient's illness as possessing unique characteristics and rates the severity of the illness (Mazure, Halmi, Sunday, Romano, & Einhorn, 2008). The SCOFF is used in the primary care setting. It is a short, easy-to-use tool that is sensitive but may produce false positives (Morgan et al., 1999).

The Eating Disorder Examination (EDE) is an assessment tool used by investigators and researchers to identify individuals with EDs with a high degree of reliability (Fairburn & Cooper, 1993). Another tool used for research is the Body Shape Questionnaire. This assessment tool examines the body image of women with EDs. It has been validated as a tool in multiple languages (Waren et al., 2008).

ETIOLOGY

Biological, psychological, and sociological factors are associated with underlying causes of AN. This is complicated by the likely factor that with no single likely etiology AN is likely both the product of complex bio-psycho and social factors and in turn co-creates factors that may be taken subsequently as causal.

BIOLOGICAL FACTORS OF AN

Caloric restriction, voluntarily or involuntarily, appears to be a factor in the onset of AN. (Attia & Walsh, 2009; Dean, Bilsky, & Negus 2009). There appears to be evidence of endogenous opiate production during caloric restriction. Dean et al. continue, "The devotion to dieting and weight loss continues to the exclusion of virtually all other interests, much like an alcoholic or heronin-dependent person becomes preoccupied with the acquisition and use of the addictive substance. Like the addicted, the anorexic patients use denial as a major defense, and frequently refuse hospitalization and treatment until overpowered by physical disease or pressure from the family or an employer" (p. 144). There would be a clear evolutionarily selective benefit for production of endogenous opioids during periods of starvation. Through much of the history of humanity, as in the animal kingdom, there have been periods of food abundance and periods of scarcity. Organisms that develop the ability to tolerate the significant discomfort and pain associated with severe caloric restriction would confer a selection and survival benefit. Thus the ability to produce endogenous opiates during periods of extreme caloric restriction might allow an organism to continue to hunt or gather for longer periods of time before succumbing to starvation.

Jensen and Mejihede (2000), proceeding from the hypothesis that AN is a psychotic issue, state, "One of the diagnostic criteria for aorexia nervosa is body image disturbance that is characterised by feeling and judging oneself to be fat and by claiming to "see" oneself as fat despite being underweight. The bizarre body self-image in AN can be regarded as a psychotic way of thinking" (p. 87). They describe the successful use of olanzapine to restore normal body weight as well as addressing the underlying psychotic body image issue. Evidence has shown that olanzapine appears to interfere with satiation, leading to weight gain due to increased fat deposition. This weight gain is often marked with comorbidities, including the negative effects on glucose and lipoprotein metabolism. In another study of 18 AN subjects treated with olanzapine, subjects reported significant reduction in anxiety, difficulty eating, and core disordered eating symptoms (Malin et al., 2003). This was not a controlled study and thus limited in the scope of the conclusion.

We may see the restriction in caloric intake resulting in increased endogenous opiates and the addict-like avoidance of treatment as well as the "psychotic"-like self-image issues as resulting from the common source of intense brain reward provided when the person with AN has the opiate response and is threatened with losing the intense pleasure and satiation given by this response. The resulting body dysmorphia, rather than being a strictly psychotic process, is as other writers have suggested, the intense self-justifying denial that accompanies processes more similar to substance abuse.

GENETICS

A number of researchers have found evidence to suggest that there is an inherited predisposition toward AN. Estimates have ranged from 50% to as high as 86% (Wade, Bulik, Neale, & Kendler, 2000; Kortegaard, Hoerder, Joergensen, Gillberg, & Kyvik, 2001).

DISTINGUISHING BETWEEN CAUSES AND EFFECTS OF AN

AN has both biological factors and can lead to serious other pathological conditions. Among the causes appear to be obstetric and perinatal factors. Perinatal factors have been implicated in increased risk of developing AN, including maternal anemia, diabetes mellitis, and preclampsia, among others. Multiple factors increase the likelihood of developing AN (Favaro & Tenconi, 2006). Further effects of dieting and starvation on brain development suggest changes that exist after recovery (Frank, Bailer, Henry, Wagner, & Kaye, 2004).

Effects. Potentially life-threatening complications that accompany signs of severe starvation include peripheral cyanosis, hypothermia, bradycardia, dizziness, electrocardiograph (ECG) abnormalities including sinus bradycardia, prolonged interval, and increased vagal tone. GI symptoms include constipation, oesophageal varices, hepatic stenosis, abnormal gastric motility, and pancreatitis. Refeeding syndrome can include fluid and electrolyte disorders, especially hypophoshatemia, neurological, pulmonary, cardiac, neuromuscular, and haematological complications. Common endocrine problems are growth retardation, osteoporosis, and hypogonadism. Premenopausal osteoporisis has been an overlooked consequence of AN. Impaired linear growth and short stature are possible complications in adolescents resulting from neuroendocrine control of growth hormone (GH) and closely linked to nutritional status.

SOCIOLOGICAL AND PSYCHOLOGICAL FACTORS

Periods of weight loss appear to correlate with the onset of AN. Societal norms such as a beauty ideal for women that involves unhealthy low weight and body fat or other sub-cultural groups emphasis on reducing weight may contribute toward specific groups of girls and boys being at risk for AN. These, among others, may include modeling, and ballet, and for boys, wrestling, where "making weight" may include intense periods of fasting.

Psychoanalytic approaches attempt to make sense of the meaning of the food restriction. What symbolic role does it serve for the patient? They locate the etiology of the illness in the intrapsychic conflict or failure to develop adequately. For example, Farrell (1995) examines this as a function of disturbances in the mother-daughter relationship. In Farrell's words, "I think more than the symptom has to change; it is not just about wanting to get a person to eat, or to stop binging, but to understand what it means for them in the intricate and complex interactions of their internal world" (p. 3).

In a similar vein, the feminist view of the underlying cause of AN and EDs lies not so much in the biology of the person suffering from AN but in society and culture. As Wolf (1991) writes, Western society has "a cultural fixation on female thinness..." but this fixation "is not an obsession about female beauty but an obsession about female obedience" (p. 187). For Wolf and other feminists, the beauty ideal of thinness operates to serve the interests of patriarchal culture by keeping women focused on "their plate" and not on issues beyond it. Like other aspects of the cultural ideal of beauty, thinness is a quest that becomes preoccupying, demanding a significant amount of investment in time and money on special diets and products. While initially control of caloric intake is an act of defiance through control over what will enter the body when perhaps other things are out of control, it ultimately results in a loss of power as it becomes a consuming preoccupation that results in a weak and sexless body (Eastland, n.d.).

EXPECTED OUTCOMES

Although AN is an illness with a significant incidence of negative outcomes, treatment can be very effective. It is important to note that no treatment has been clearly identified as offering definitive positive outcomes for AN and that there is a significant relapse rate approaching 50% (Attia & Walsh, 2009). A limitation in adequate treatment is recognition and diagnosis of the condition. Treatment is initiated after the patient presents either to a primary care provider or directly to a psychiatric provider. Patients may have significant cognitive and emotional investment in obtaining body weight or morphology that is damaging to their overall health and well-being. Thus the primary goal of treatment is regaining normal weight and improvement in identified cognitive distortions. In order to do this, the patient's condition may require, in severe cases, a period of hospital of acute stabilization (Lock, Le Grange, Agras, & Christopher, 2000).

Referral to a structural behavioral program should be made if patients have insufficient weight gain through less intensive treatment approaches. The criteria are often given as less than 75% of ideal body weight, or for adult patients, a BMI of less than 16.5, or for children or adolescents who do not gain the expected amount of weight, or due to serious medical or psychiatric complications such as cardiovascular abnormalities or suicidal ideation (Lock et al., 2000).

Though partial hospital or intensive outpatient programs or the least restrictive program needed to achieve desired results are preferable, sometimes the medical condition of a patient necessitates hospitalization. Medical concerns must be addressed first, and assessment of vital signs, complete blood count (CBC), lytes, blood urea nitrogen (BUN), Creat, liver function, thyroid function, ECG are indicated. The next priority is given to providing patients with adequate calories to regain weight. The standard recommendations are as follows: 3,500 kcal over maintenance requirements needed for every pound gained; 1,800 kcal per day to start and then when medically stable, every 2 to 7 days diet increased by 400 Kcal/day. Every 48 to 72 hours until 380 kcal/day is reached, most in the form of solid food. The patient should be weighed 3 times a week and expected to gain .75 lbs over previous weight. During the acute phase refeeding while the patient is inpatient, they should begin with 1,500 kcal/day, increase slowly to 3,500 kcal/day divided into several meals a day with a very low weight goal to gain 1 to 2 lbs/week.

SPECIAL CONSIDERATIONS

An important condition to be aware of when reintroducing food to a person who has had significant weight loss is refeeding syndrome (Attia &Walsh, 2009). Refeeding syndrome is a rare but potentially life-threatening condition characterized by shifts in fluid electrolytes and minerals, potentially leading to hypophosphatemia, hypomagnesemia, hypokalemia, glucose intolerance, fluid overload, and thiamine deficiency. These pathophysiologic

TABLE 12-4: MEDICATIONS USED TO TREAT ANOREXIA NERVOSA

MEDICATION	CLASSIFICATION	INDICATION	DOSE	ADVERSE REACTIONS
Olanzapine	Atypical antipsychotic	First-line agent for psychotic disorders, recommended due to its specific properties increasing appetite and decreasing anxiety	5 mg doses have been studied in AN Effective dosing range from 2.5–20 mg/day Comes in oral disintegrating tablets and Intramuscular (IM) if oral not tolerated	Potential for neuroleptic malingant syndome, and metabolic syndrome, including alteration of lipids and glucose and weight gain (though this is a desired effect in AN)
	SSRI	Used in AN but evidence is lacking for efficacy		
Estrogen	Hormone	Not found to be effective (Teng, 2011)		
Zync	Essential nutrient	essential nutrient (Shay & Mangian, 2000)	15–20 mg/day United States Department of Agriculture (USDA)	Large doses can weaken the immune system

conditions can result in congestive heart failure (CHF), arrythmias, skeletal muscle weakness, respiratory failure, metabolic acidosis, ataxia, seizures, encephalopathy, and possibly death (Lock et al., 2000).

The Maudsley Method of family therapy usually lasts 1 year and involves between 15 and 20 sessions. There are three phases of the treatment, including weight restoration, returning control over eating to the patient, and establishing a healthy identity. In the first phase, the therapist helps the patient focus on the physiological, cognitive, and emotional effects of malnutrition associated with AN. During this phase, restoring the adolescent's weight is a priority. The patient learns to externalize the illness psychologically during this phase. During the second phase, the patient gradually takes control over his or her own eating again. The final phase begins when the patient is able to maintain his or her weight above 95% of ideal weight on his or her own and no longer engages in self-starvation. Treatment focuses on the psychological impact AN has had on the patient's identity and the formation of a healthy identity. This method of therapy is evidence-based and requires that the parents take part in the adolescent's treatment. Therapists who perform this modality are often specially trained and receive certification in family-based treatment (Grange, 2005).

OBESITY

The increase in obesity is problematic because obesity is associated with chronic illnesses such as diabetes, hyperlipidemia, coronary disease, and stroke. Chronic obesity is also associated with higher rates of health care problems and costs than either smoking or alcohol abuse (Sturm, 2002) and lower overall quality of life. Obesity will be discussed as it relates to psychiatric problems in this chapter.

RELATIONSHIP BETWEEN PSYCHIATRIC DISORDERS AND OBESITY

There is a bidirectional relationship between obesity and certain mental disorders such as binge eating, anxiety, schizophrenia, and mood disorders. Evidence suggests that those with serious mental illness (SMI) have about twice the rate of obesity than the overall U.S. population (Daumit et al., 2003; Fiegal et al., 2010).

Many clinical studies demonstrate high rates of obesity in individuals with schizophrenia and mood disorders, but they often include individuals taking medications that cause weight gain. The Clinical Antipsychotic Trials of Intervention Effectiveness (CATIE) reported

TABLE 12-5: THERAPIES USED TO TREAT ANOREXIA NERVOSA

THERAPY	DESCRIPTION
Behavior Modification (in patient)	Uses rewards and reinforcements to help patients obtain normal weight and eating habits Provides food Directly supervises refeeding
NG Tube (in patient)	Refeeding with nasal gastric tube where appropriate due to medical status, provides needed calories & necessary nutrition to maintain medical stability
Interpersonal Therapy	
Dietary	
Cognitive Behavioral Therapy (CBT)	
Family Therapy	Behavioral conditioning within the context of structured family therapy
Maudsley Method	See detailed description in Wallis, Rhodes, KOhn, & Madden, 2007.
Yoga	Decreases anxiety & helps form healthy relationship between body & mind

Source: Liebman, Minuchin, & Baker (1974); Palazzoli (1978); Lock et al. (2000); Grange (2005); Attia & Walsh (2009); Carei, Fyfe-Johnson, Breuner, & Brown (2010).

that adults taking antipsychotics were more likely than controls to have metabolic syndrome (McEvoy, Meyer, & Goff, 2005). This side effect is discussed in more detail in Chapter 5 on psychotropic drugs and Chapter 10 on management of psychotic symptoms. However, when studying drug-naive individuals with early onset schizophrenia, higher levels of intra-abdominal obesity were identified than in normal controls (Petry, Barry, Pietrzak, & Wagner, 2008; Saarni, Saarni, & Fogelholm, 2009). So in addition to side effects of psychotropic medications, there are additional explanations for this obesity in individuals with SMI.

Brain abnormalities related to the disease itself, poverty, environment, and lifestyle factors all contribute to obesity. Brain changes in schizophrenia include multiple abnormalities in structure and function. For example, smaller temporal lobes are partially responsible for poorer decision and choices, and other cortical changes interfere with cause and effect reasoning. So, the lifestyle choices and eating behaviors of some individuals with schizophrenia may be traced to neurobiological pathology and not only choices or motivation for change.

When examining the relationship between depression and obesity, individuals who were depressed had a significantly higher risk for obesity than nondepressed individuals (Blaine, 2008). Furthermore, stress and anxiety have long been associated with overeating. But stress may actually lead to decreased eating in some individuals. Stressful threats relating to physical discomfort often result in decreased eating, while those threats related to ego such as work tasks, increased eating. For obese individuals or those on a restrictive diet, stress especially related to interpersonal issues may increase eating because the individual is distracted from his or her restrictive efforts. This variable relationship between stress and eating was also found in childhood when eating habits are developed (Roemmich, Wright, & Epstein, 2002). The exact mechanisms for these connections are unclear but these descriptive findings validate the strong relationship between obesity and several psychiatric disorders.

ETIOLOGY

The multitude of etiological explanations for obesity represent the multidimensional nature of this disorder. The origins may go back as far as conception. The search for causes basically explore inheritable, biological factors and environmental influences. Because the great increase in obesity has occurred in less than a generation, this shift is not correlated with a change in biological function related to evolution. And findings from twin studies are controversial with some reporting 30% to 70% of obesity related to heritability, while others have found a stronger link to the adiposity of the parent, whether biological or adopted (Devlin, Yanoski, & Wilson, 2000). So, biological and heritability factors contribute to but are not clearly causative for obesity.

Further neurobiological research has identified the origins and maintenance of obesity related to gene products such as leptin and its receptor, agouti signaling protein, and carboxypeptidase E. Leptin has been identified as a mediator in the development of diabetes in obese individuals who are leptin-deficient Friedman, J. & Haloos, J. (1998). However, there is no one gene identified as causative in obesity. Other biological pathways are also being explored.

Another possible biological explanation is to identify overstimulation of the hypothalamic-pituitary-adrenal axis and sympathetic nervous system. This overstimulation leads to a range of symptoms. Most notable for obesity is the production of glucocorticoids that stimulate hepatic gluconeogenesis. This inhibits insulin actions on the muscles and adipose tissue to promote visceral adiposity and the metabolic syndrome (Bjorntorp, 2001).

In addition to biological hypotheses, psychological explanations center on coping with stressors and trauma. EDs are seen as powerful coping mechanisms that help an individual to manage parts of his or her life experience that seem too much to bear. Although the behavior is harmful, the individual perceives it as immediately supportive and feels threatened without it. Weight gain becomes shameful in our culture of thinness and often the overeating masks dissociative states that complicate treatment. When trauma occurs, coping ability and affect regulation is further compromised.

A variation of this psychological explanation is the problem of handling the sensation of desire. In the absence of secure attachments, a baby or child may develop difficulty managing all forms of desire. When a baby's physical and attachment needs are not met, safety is threatened and any sensations experienced such as hunger may be experienced with much distress. The body sensations themselves become a source of fear. Negative internal states in response to sensing desires may include shame, guilt, sadness, and anger. This is an offshoot of attachment theory (Bowlby, 1982).

Yet another psychological explanation focusing upon interpersonal forces is the meaning of food associated with love in many families. Providing food and eating food prepared by a relative represents caring and love.

This association may contribute to children being encouraged to overeat to please others, and this overeating then becomes a habit. This explanation is based in Sullivan's Interpersonal Theory (Sullivan, 1953) as well as Bowen's Family System Theory (Bowlby, 1982).

Placing obesity within the addiction framework is another approach to understand the dynamics of obesity. Natural rewards such as food, drugs, and sex activate reward centers in the brain and produce elevated levels of DA. Similar patterns of neural activation are identified in addictive-like eating behavior and substance abuse. There is elevated activation in reward circuitry in response to food cues and reduced activation of inhibitory regions in response to food intake (Gearhardt et al., 2011).

Causative explanations also include behavioral factors such as sedentary lifestyles and intake of micronutrient-poor foods such as french fries and soda. In other words, too many calories are consumed relative to activity level. Furthermore, studies of the SMI report activity level lower than the general population (Brown, Birtwistle, Roe, & Thompson, 1999; McCreadie, 2003). This decrease in activity level is tied to increased use of technology, decreasing leisure time activities, and the overall ease of acquiring food today compared to our Stone Age ancestors (Sacks, Bray, & Carey, 2009).

Cultural influences can also be recognized by the difference in rates of obesity. The prevalence of significant obesity (BMI over 30) in the U.S. population is 29% for Caucasians, 34% for Hispanics, and 40% for African Americans. Fully 78% of African American females are overweight or obese. Furthermore, social class also contributes. The likelihood of being overweight in the poorest 25% of the population is twice that of people in the highest quarter of economic class. There are many reasons for this association.

People living in poverty find it hard to be physically active and often lack access to quality supermarkets. Leisure time is rare and concerns with neighborhood safety keep both children and adults indoors. Poor individuals are less likely to work for companies with fitness facilities, and there is no discretionary income to join health clubs or to have personal trainers. Poor schools have worse facilities and fewer organized sports, and safety issues prevent children from walking or biking to school. Furthermore, if one does not own a car, a trip to a supermarket might require several transfers on a bus and then the task of carrying groceries on the return trip. Rarely can obesity be reduced to one cause, function, or meaning. There are neurobiological, cultural, developmental, familial environmental, and psychological factors all contributing, but the relative degree of influence for each in the development and maintenance of obesity remains debatable. The treatment approach will be based upon the client's beliefs as well as the theoretical framework of the PMH-APRN and latest evidence of effectiveness.

CONCORDANCE

Engaging the client who is obese may be complicated because many are ambivalent about treatment because aspects of the treatment (dietary control) may not be positively valued. Furthermore, there is shame and secrecy associated with overeating and binge eating, and there may also have been adverse experiences in past treatment. In fact, negative opinions by health care providers about obese individuals were reported in the September 2003 issue of *Obesity* and *American Medical News.* It was also reported in June 2011 that ob-gyn physicians in some parts of the United States were refusing to treat patients over 200 pounds. This is a form of discrimination and may have a strong influence on clients' decisions to seek treatment.

To facilitate engagement, it is important to convey acceptance and knowledge about EDs, encourage active involvement of the client in the assessment and case formulation, and instill hope for overcoming the eating problem (Vitousek, Watson, & Wilson, 1998).

Furthermore, providing education about psychological and physical factors contributing to disordered eating provides an alternate way of thinking about their behavior in place of shame and self-blame. Normalizing the overeating as a coping style helps relax shame and defensiveness and creates a sense of safety in the treatment setting. This environment then assists with relationship building and developing agreement about the plan of treatment to pursue.

Clients' motivation to change can be assessed and motivational interviewing techniques used to facilitate behavioral change. Refer to Chapter 4 for an overview of motivational interviewing. It is important to complete a physical and behavioral/emotional assessment before starting treatment. The following issues require attention before beginning treatment of obesity: compromised physical health, suicide risk, clinical depression, psychosis, persistent substance abuse, major life crisis, and inability to attend treatment due to work or other constraints (Grillo & Mitchell, 2010). Following the jointly developed approach to these issues, a plan for the eating problem can be revisited. The behavioral/emotional assessment should also include a discussion about self-image. Assumptions should not be made about the experience of being obese and opportunities to express positive as well as negative aspects need to be provided. Thus, a holistic plan can be developed.

Possible questions to assess the client's perceptions include:

1. What does it mean to you to be overweight? Why are some people overweight and others not?
2. What is the relationship between health and weight? What is the relationship between your weight and your health?
3. Have you tried to lose weight? Describe. What have been barriers to weight loss?
4. Compared to your friends and family, are you the same size, larger, smaller?
5. Has anyone ever told you should lose weight?
6. How has your weight influenced your activities and your life?

ASSESSMENT

It is difficult to hide obesity. The most common assessment tool is the BMI (BMI). This is calculated from the height and weight of an individual (BMI = kg/m2). It is essential to weigh and measure height, not merely take the client's word for this. Overweight is BMI>25kg/m2 and obese is BMI>30 kg/m2. For more information about assessing obesity and calculators for adults and children see this Centers for Disease Control and Prevention website: www.cdc.gov/healthyweight/assessing/bmi/adult_bmi/index.html#Other%20Ways

Of course, once obesity is established as being physically present, there needs to be further assessment to determine lifestyle patterns (exercise, smoking, caloric intake) as well as the presence of psychiatric disorders and physical problems such as hypertension, cardiovascular disease, or diabetes. Furthermore, several chronic illnesses are also associated with obesity and should be identified and treated first. These include hyperthyroidism, Cushing's Syndrome, and polycystic ovary syndrome (NIH, 2006).

It is important to explore relationships between medications and weight changes. See Chapter 5 for common side effects of psychotropic drugs as well as those drugs that are usually weight neutral. Questionnaires may be completed before the first interview. A standard questionnaire to identify psychiatric problems is usually used. The Dissociative Experience Scale (DES; Bernstein & Putnam, 1986) to identify degree of dissociation is useful for planning and can be downloaded at this site: http://discussingdissociation.wordpress.com/dissociative-experiences-scale-des/

Questionnaires specific to eating problems often used include the EDE-Q (Fairburn & Beglin, 1994) and the Clinical Impairment Scale (CIA; Bohn & Fairburn, 2008). The CIA identifies the impact of the symptoms on clients' functioning. Both questionnaires focus on the past 28 days, are short, and can be downloaded at the following website: www.psychiatry.ox.ac.uk/credo

EXPECTED OUTCOMES

Expected outcomes of treatment include the following:

- Development of a trusting relationship
- Enhanced body awareness and mindfulness
- Development of additional coping strategies
- Enhanced self-understanding and acceptance
- Weight loss. Even a modest loss of weight (<10%) significantly improves blood pressure, cholesterol levels, and glycemic control (Miller et al., 2002).
- Maintenance of lifestyle modifications

TREATMENT INITIATION AND ACUTE FOLLOW-UP

Treatment includes psychotherapy, behavioral approaches as well as pharmacological, and as a last resort bariatric surgery. Following the assessment and case formulation, a shift to weight-neutral medication is first if the client is taking psychiatric medications known to cause weight gain. If weight loss does not proceed, then begin more extensive treatment approaches. First, it is vital to assist the client in developing skills (other than overeating) to self-soothe or to overcome hyperarousal by practicing mindfulness techniques and/or describing thoughts, feelings, and inner sensations in five senses. This may take several sessions and lead to increased engagement in therapy, and more safety because there is less triggering of uncomfortable feelings and increased self-efficacy. With increased motivation and decreased overstimulation of the limbic system, there is more potential for change and dealing with underlying traumas (Ogden, Minton, & Pain, 2006). Levine describes many somatic techniques in *Waking the Tiger: Healing Trauma* (Levine, 1997). PMH-APRNs who are certified in the use of Eye Movement Desensitization Reprogramming (EMDR) often use this approach to maximize safety (Shapiro, 2009). The neurobiological basis for this approach is described in theory of neuroception by Porges (2004). As the client learns grounding and centering techniques, the ambivalence for change begins to shift.

Following the withdrawal of overeating as a source of soothing, if additional/alternative coping skills are not developed, there is a risk of the development of other addictive behaviors for self-soothing and avoidance of withdrawal

TABLE 12-6: MEDICATIONS USED TO TREAT OBESITY

NAME	ACTION	COMMON SIDE EFFECTS
FDA Approved		
Sibutramine	SNRI similar to stimulant	Cardiac complications (Banned in Europe.)
Orlistat	Blocks lipase activity	Hepatoxic (OTC lower dose available as ALI) Fecal soiling
Phentermine	Similar to amphetamines	Addictive, depression, anxiety, insomnia
Off-Label Use		
Glucophage	Antidiabetic agent	GI distress, lactic acidosis
Topiramate	Anticonvulsant	Cognitive deficit (memory, concentration impairment) Nausea, dizziness, metabolic acidosis
Bupropion	Dopamine & norepinephrine Reuptake inhibitor	Nervousness, seizure, insomnia
Over the Counter		
Ephedra-containing supplements		Hypertension, increased cardiac input, sudden death
In Clinical Trials		
Contrave	Bupoprion & Naltrexone (an opioid antagonist)	TBD
Lorcaserin	Selective serotonin 2C agonist	TBD

Source: Adapted from Hendricks, Rothman, & Greenway (2009); Mitchell & Grillo (2010).

symptoms. This may include substance abuse, gambling, promiscuity, shopping, or other addictions. This idea of cross-addiction is supported by reports showing low striatal DA levels in obese individuals, as well as a greater striatal response to the presentation of palatable foods (Stice, Yokum, Blum, & Bohon, 2010; Wang, Volkow, Thanos, & Fowler, 2004). Furthermore, post-weight loss addictions have been reported to be a predictor of weight regain after bariatric surgery (Odom et al., 2010).

Using cognitive behavioral therapy approaches has been identified as a clear leading treatment for obesity in several systematic reviews (Grillo & Mitchell, 2010). There are manuals with specific steps to guide this approach such as Integrative Cognitive Affective Therapy (ICAT) for binge eating, which emphasizes motivational enhancement and regulation of emotional responses; dialectical behavioral therapy, which can be adapted for EDs, and CBT-E which modifies cognitive-behavioral techniques (Grillo & Mitchell, 2010). This CBT-E approach involves education about EDs, establishing real-time monitoring of eating and connected thoughts, feelings, and events and the establishment of regular eating routines while involving significant others in this planning. Next, analysis of over-valuation of body shape and weight and finally, teaching problem solving is the final step in this approach.

Decreasing caloric intake and increasing exercise is also recommended. Offering information about nutritional choices and strategies for gradually increasing exercise is available at this website: www.cdc.gov or www.ahrq.gov

Individual or group sessions weekly or bimonthly for at least 3 months have been associated with sustained weight loss. Referrals to community supports are also helpful. Overeaters Annonymous is based upon the addiction model and has meetings in person as well as telephone meetings. See their website: www.oa.org/

Weight Watchers is based upon increased exercise, decreased caloric intake combined with mindfulness about eating, and group support. It is available in most communities as well as online. See website: www.weightwatchers.com/templates/marketing/Landing_1col_nonav.aspx?PageId=1163821

PHARMACOLOGICAL INTERVENTIONS

For individuals with BMI >30 kg/m2, use pharmacology. This may involve FDA-approved medications, off-label, or over-the-counter medications. Anti-obesity medications attempt to regulate appetite. Many endogenous mediators regulate appetite and metabolism. These mediators include gut, pancreatic, and adipose neuropeptides, which are targeted with the goal of amplifying or blocking anorexigenic and lipolytic signaling. Anti-obesity drugs have been characterized by dilemmas such as safety, efficacy, abuse, and adverse effects (Kim, Jieru, Valentino, Colon-Gonzalez, & Waldman, 2011). It is most effective to also include lifestyle changes and some form of counseling or therapy.

BARIATRIC SURGERY

For individuals with BMI >40kg/m2 with medical complications, bariatric surgery is considered. Surgery produces the most rapid weight loss (approximately 61% of excess weight), but is not without risks (Maggard et al., 2005). Earlier techniques such as jejunoileal bypass are no longer available due to unacceptable side effects and significant mortality. Procedures available now include Roux-en-Y gastric bypass, adjustable banding, gastric stapling, and gastroplasty, which cause nutrient malabsorption and/or gastric restriction. In an attempt to eliminate the surgical risks, clinical trials are under way for transoral gastroplasty, in which the stomach is stapled or sutured to reduce its capacity via oral insertion of flexible devices (Cote & Edmundowicz, 2009).

However, a BMI >40 poses a five-fold risk of depression and approximately half of the applicants for bariatric surgery are depressed. Binge eating has been reported to be present in 25% of applicants compared to 2% of the general population and applicants also often report abnormal patterns of dieting and strict restrictions on foods (Kalarchian, Marcus, & Levine, 2007). Therefore, presurgical psychiatric evaluation is an important aspect of preparation. Additional criteria for surgery include ages 16 to 65, failure of long-term nonsurgical weight loss attempts, motivated and well-informed about postsurgical issues, commitment to lifestyle changes, and absence of psychosis or severe untreated depression (Schneider & Mun, 2005).

Following bariatric surgery, there are other eating problems. Nausea and vomiting due to overeating, eating too fast, and not chewing well occurs in the majority of people. There may be self-induced vomiting to relieve a sensation of food being stuck in the upper digestive tract. Protein malnutrition or vitamin deficiency may develop. Multivitamins reduce the risk but do not eliminate deficiencies and symptoms such as hair loss, and skin problems may develop. Another group of symptoms labeled "dumping syndrome" are related to malabsorption and include lightheadedness, sweating, flushing, palpitations, cramps, and diarrhea. Dietary changes to avoid high sugar and carbohydrates often relieve these symptoms.

Although surgical intervention provides rapid weight loss initially, maintenance of long-term loss is less than ideal. Laparascopic adjustable gastric banding offers poor outcomes in severely overweight individuals. In a recent study, 82 individuals were followed for 12 years after surgery. Although most expressed satisfaction with the procedure, mean body mass decreased to 33.79 from 41.57, but the proportion having diabetes or sleep apnea increased and nearly half had the band removed (Himpens et al., 2011).

MAINTENANCE/TERMINATION

Unfortunately, individuals who have been involved in lifestyle modification generally lose weight, but regain about 35% of their lost weight in the first year following treatment and over 50% return to baseline weight in 5 years (Sarwer, von Sydow Green, Vetter, & Wadden, 2009). Statistics on the effectiveness of adding psychotherapy are in the initial phases, but are hopeful. In spite of partial lapses, individuals seem to be able to apply their new coping skills before a full relapse occurs. The continued use of supportive community groups and self-help programs are also helpful.

Many individuals experience improved satisfaction with their body image issues after significant weight loss. However, the majority of individuals who have had bariatric surgery undergo body-contouring surgery to correct loose skin in the abdomen, breasts, and other areas.

To minimize relapse, the PMH-APRN should discuss this possibility with clients and identify possible triggers for activating the eating problems and early warning signs. Then a plan of action should be considered and include how to shift the problematic eating and how to cope with the trigger. Generally, if the problematic eating persists for 3 weeks, it is best to seek professional help (Grillo & Mitchell, 2010).

It is a challenge to balance the use of specific manualized programs with the flexibility of individualized therapy based on the client's progress. However, once the treatment goals have been met, sessions should be terminated. This allows the individual to resolve some of the aspects of the eating disorder rather than seeing improvement as a result of ongoing therapy. Of course, there are reasons for longer-term treatment. These include development or reoccurrence of a psychiatric problem, which would then result in a shift in the overall treatment plan. Another reason to continue treatment of the eating disorder is if there is considerable disruption of functioning and health. The number of sessions and follow-up checks require concordance between the PMH-APRN and the client.

Of course, the ideal approach to the obesity problem is primary prevention. Beginning healthy lifestyles and eating patterns in childhood and also considering this side effect when prescribing psychotropic medications are examples of obesity prevention.

SPECIAL CONSIDERATIONS

Although EDs have a higher prevalence rate in Western culture, rates of ED appear to be increasing globally (James, 2008). People in some Asian and Middle Eastern countries have developed a decrease in activity level and an increase in access to high fat and high calorie foods. This has led to an increase in obesity at a much faster rate than seen in the United States. Pressure to lose weight and remain thin has crossed Western borders affecting diverse ethnic populations. PMH-APRNs should inquire about weight and shape concerns among minority and non-Western individuals, especially those who are transitioning to Western societies (APA, 2006).

Competitive athletes are at special risk for EDs. Cultural attitudes toward thinness, performance anxiety, and critical self-image may increase this risk. Parents and coaches encourage weight loss in the athlete, as a lean body is synonymous with a competitive edge. Girls as young as 5 years old who participate in sports show a greater obsession with weight than those who do not (APA, 2006).

It is well known that there is a familial tendency in families with EDs. The PMH-APRN must carefully assess the patient's mothering skills and attachment styles to minimize the risk of the development of BN in the offspring (APA, 2006).

Patient education on the nature, course, and treatment of BN is vital to patients. When possible, family members should be included in the treatment plan as well as in meal planning, limit setting, and support groups (Williams et al., 2008).

PMH-APRNs should have a greater awareness of BN among patients and screen for ED, particularly in light of the secretive nature of these disorders. Screening tools should be used for this purpose (Dichter et al., 2002).

PEDIATRIC POINTERS

Most EDs occur in adolescence and the early 20s. Children as young as 7-years of age have been affected but in general, BN is rarely seen in children under 12 years old. These children generally have comorbidities such as obsessive behaviors and depression (APA, 2006). The PMH-APRN should be aware that children presenting with physical symptoms such as nausea, abdominal pain, feeling full, or difficulty swallowing may be suffering from BN. There may be weight loss that is severe and rapid. Parents may report the child shows avoidance behavior toward food or anxiety related to meals (APA, 2006).

There are a number of comorbidities that must be recognized in children suffering from BN. BN may emerge between the ages of 14 to 18; the same age substance abuse rates begin to occur (Harrop & Marlatt, 2009). The combination of BN and substance abuse can be a challenge to manage; therefore, it is the PMH-APRN's role to develop strategies aimed at prevention. Obsessive-compulsive disorders, phobias, and generalized anxiety disorder that occur in childhood may place children in jeopardy for the development of BN. This necessitates early identification for those children at risk (Kaye et al., 2004)

Children as young as six years old may begin to perceive the idea of thinness and its relationship to society and cultural ideals. Because this is a critical developmental period, it is crucial to begin prevention efforts during the early childhood years (Robert-McComb,

(*Continued*)

PEDIATRIC POINTERS (*Continued*)

2001). Additionally, prevention programs focused on sexual, emotional, and physical abuse are imperative in that many women who seek treatment for EDs have personal history of abuse or sexual assault (Robert-McComb, 2001).

The PMH-APRN must assess the child's level of stress and the impact it may have on the child. Life events such as domestic violence; death of a family member, friend, or pet; birth of a sibling or illness of a relative; exposure to illicit drugs; and poverty may trigger disordered eating (Robert-McComb, 2001).

It is important that the PMH-APRN involve the parents in the assessment and treatment plan of children and when appropriate, the school and any other health professionals who have worked with the child. Because the child, and the parents for that matter, may not reveal valuable information, it is important to build a trusting relationship so the child feels comfortable divulging such information. It is important to understand that the assessment phase for pediatric patients may take hours to complete (APA, 2006).

It is recommended that the model used in treating children is the interdisciplinary team approach. This team may include the pediatrician; a specialist in adolescent medicine for teens; a nutritionist; teachers and guidance counselors, school coaches, and the psychiatric professional. It is important that the care be tailored to the developmental stage of the child. The team should have open lines of communication and every member must have a clear understanding of each other's responsibilities (APA, 2006).

Observing the family interaction, in particular their interaction around eating, is central to understanding the family dynamics. Family members experience anguish in understanding and interacting with their children, therefore, the PMH-APRN must listen empathically (APA, 2006).

Since BN is common among adolescent females, primary prevention is crucial. Education is central to prevention and should be disseminated in classrooms, church groups, athletic programs, dormitories, student health services, and other extracurricular locations (APA, 2006).

It is not uncommon that the psychiatric professional be contacted by school administrators to manage students with serious disordered eating. Students should remain in school if possible unless they become severely ill. It may be necessary to "make student attendance contingent on participation in a suitable treatment program" (APA, 2006). When the patient is severely ill but still attending school, clinicians must closely monitor weight, vital signs, and laboratory values. Since BN is characterized as a psychiatric disability, policy and procedures must be maintained under the Americans With Disabilities Act (APA, 2006).

Compulsive exercise is one manifestation of patients with BN; therefore, it is necessary to monitor the level and amount of exercise in children and adolescents. Female athletes involved in ballet and gymnastics are especially at risk. Male bodybuilders are at risk as well and may be using anabolic steroids (APA, 2006).

The "40 Developmental Assets" of Healthy Communities lists building blocks toward healthy development in children and young people. The goal is to help children grow into healthy and responsible adults. The developmental categories include: support, empowerment, boundaries and expectations, constructive use of time, commitment to learning, positive values, social competencies, and positive identity formation (Robert-McComb, 2001). Furthermore, the promotion of healthy environments and recommended actions to prevent childhood obesity are reported by the Institute of Medicine's 2011 report, *Early Childhood Obesity Prevention Policies,* available at www.iom.edu. The main recommendations include growth monitoring, increased physical activity, healthy eating, limiting screen time (computers and television), and ensuring adequate sleep time.

(*Continued*)

PEDIATRIC POINTERS (*Continued*)

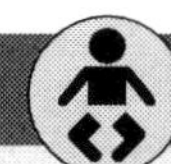

Researchers are applying concepts of mindfulness to eating in the school setting (Burke, 2010). See www.dukehealth.org/health_library/advice_from_doctors/your_childs_health/mindfulness_and_health_in_children for more information.

New technology is being tested for use in EDs. These approaches include the use of Internet-based self-help programs and the use of personal digital assistants to teach CBT in real time and used as needed as well as to provide social support (Jones et al., 2008). However, these approaches are only beginning to be evaluated for effectiveness and are not yet clinically available.

When working with children who are overweight, it is important to also include parents to maximize effective parenting skills as well as to recognize the child's anxiety. Furthermore, parents have long been held responsible for undernourishment and failure to thrive under child abuse and neglect framework. Some states now have legal precedent for considering overnourishment and severe obesity as child abuse. Therefore, severe obesity in children resulting in severe weight-related health problems may be part of mandated reporting (Murtagh, 2007).

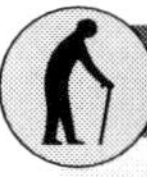

AGING ALERTS

Although EDs are common in middle and late life, many go unnoticed. As the baby boomer population ages, EDs will become more of a clinical issue (Zerbe, 2003). This is attributed to body image concerns and the fact that EDs are becoming more widespread (APA, 2006). When they do occur, however, there is significant morbidity and mortality (Zerbe, 2003). A marital crisis, death of a loved one, or divorce may trigger BN. The fear of aging also has an impact in the development of BN in the older adult (APA, 2006).

The ability to recognize these disorders in the older population may be difficult to distinguish from other psychiatric and medical conditions (Zerbe, 2003). BN should be considered in the differential diagnosis for any older adult with unexplained weight loss (Lapid et al., 2010).

The older adult generally presents with a greater severity of disordered eating but has fewer body image difficulties. They tend to deny their symptoms (Cumella & Kally, 2008). Comorbid conditions exist in many older patients, most commonly major depression (Lapid et al., 2010). Other comorbidies include bipolar disorder, suicide attempts, and sexual abuse histories (Cumella & Kally, 2008).

Distinguishing depression from EDs may be challenging to the health professional in that both may present with weight loss, memory impairment, concentration problems, and body image preoccupation (although this is rare in depression). Other symptoms that point to EDs in middle and late life are the use of over-the-counter, prescribed, or illicit substances to produce weight loss; overexercising; difficulties making life transitions; inability to mourn major losses in life; fear of aging; feeling in competition with younger generations, and setting unrealistic goals for oneself (Zerbe, 2003).

The PMH-APRN must rule out physical causes of weight loss or vomiting prior to making the diagnosis. She must distinguish whether it is a true BN or if the elderly person is angry about aging and losing his or her independence (Zerbe, 2003).

Patients suspected of BN should be given a complete physical examination to rule out physiological causes such as malignancy,

(*Continued*)

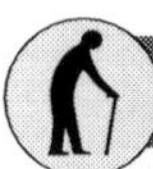

AGING ALERTS (*Continued*)

diabetes mellitis, substance abuse, or infection. It may be necessary to involve a nutritionist in the plan of care. The PMH-APRN must also be alert for comorbid mediation conditions such as osteopenia and osteoporosis (APA, 2006).

It is crucial to understand how the individual is coping with natural life transitions and, in particular, one's own mortality. Although there is a knowledge gap pertaining to diagnosis and treatment of ED in the older adult, additional research will most likely occur with the aging baby boomer generation (Zerbe, 2003).

Older adults are more likely than younger adults to experience functional limitations associated with chronic illnesses, which create a stress-pain-depression cycle leading to activity limitations and lifestyle patterns that contribute to obesity. Consequences of obesity in the elderly include respiratory problems (mechanical impairment combined with changes in lung structure resulting from aging), arthritis and osteoarthritis (strain on joints), skin conditions (itching, redness, breakdown, rashes), atherosclerotic cardiovascular disease, diabetes, cancer, and gallbladder disease (Newman, 2009).

Appropriate nutritional counseling is important to ensure daily nutritional requirements are met during caloric reduction. Loss of fat-free body mass in older adults is associated with significant morbidity and mortality.

In general, stretching, aerobic, and strengthening exercises are recommended. The Silver Sneakers program is offered by several insurance companies and pays for membership at a health club for older adults.

RESOURCES FOR PATIENTS/FAMILIES

BOOKS

50 Ways to Soothe Yourself Without Food (2009) by S. Albers

The Taming of the Chew: A Holistic Approach to Stop Compulsive Eating (1998) by D. Lamothe

ORGANIZATIONS

American Anorexia Bulimia Association
www.aabainc.org
212-575-6200

Center for the Study of Anorexia and Bulimia
www.csabnyc.org
212-595-3449

National Association of Anorexia Nervosa and Associated Disorders, Inc
www.anad.org
630-577-1330

National Eating Disorders Association (NEDA)
www.nationaleatingdisorders.org
800-931-2237

National Institute of Mental Health
www.nimh.nih.gov/health/topics/eating-disorders/index.shtml

SUPPORT GROUPS AND TREATMENT

Internet Mental Health, Anorexia Nervosa
www.mentalhealth.com/dis/p20-et01.html

Online support groups for post-bariatric surgery as well as obesity: www.dailystrength.org

Psychcentral: Eating Disorders Support Group
Psychcentral.com/?Cat=&Board=eating

Remuda Ranch
The Hospital for Eating Disorders
www.remudaranch.com
Wickenburg, Arizona
1-800-445-1900

The Renfrew Center
www.renfrewcenter.com
1-800-RENFREW

Support groups for eating disorders—State by state
www.edreferral.com/support_groups_for_eating-disorders.htm

REFERENCES

Agnew-Davies, R. K., Stiles, W. B., Hardy, G. E., Barkham, M., & Shapiro, D. A. (1998). Alliance structure assessed by the Agnew Relationship Measure (ARM). *British Journal of Clinical Psychology, 37*, 155–172.

Agras, W. S., Walsh, B. T., Fairburn, C. G., Wilson, G. T., & Kraemer, H. C. (2000). A multicenter comparison of cognitive-behavioral therapy and interpersonal psychotherapy for bulimia nervosa. *Archives of General Psychiatry, 55*, 459–466.

Albers, S. (2009). 50 ways to soothe yourself without food. Oakland, CA: Harbinger Publications

Allen, K. L., Fursland, A., Watson, H., & Byrne, S. M. (2011). Eating disorder diagnoses in general practice settings: Comparison with structured clinical interview and self-report questionnaires. *Journal of Mental Health, 20*(3), 270–280.

Allen, S., & Dalton, W. T. (2011). Treatment of eating disorders in primary care: A systematic review. *Journal of Health Psychology, 16*, 1165–1176. doi: 10.1177/1359105311402244

Amercian Academy of Pediatrics, Committee on Adolescence. (2003). Identifying and treating eating disorders. *Pediatrics, 111*(1), 204–211.

American Psychiatric Association. (2000a). *Diagnostic and statistical manual of mental disorders* (4th ed., text rev.). Washington, DC: Author.

American Psychiatric Association. (2000b). *Practice guidelines for the treatment of individuals with eating disorders* (2nd ed.). Washington, DC: Author.

American Psychiatric Association. (2006). *Practice guidelines for the treatment of patients with eating disorders* (3rd ed.). Washington, DC: Author. Retrieved from www.appi.org/CustomerService/Pages/Permissions.aspx

Andrews, G., Sanderson, K., Slade, T., & Issakidis, C. (2000). Why does the burden of disease persist? Relating the burden of anxiety and depression to effectiveness of treatment. *Bulletin of the World Health Organization, 78*, 446–454.

Attia, E., & Walsh, T. (2009). Behavioral management for anorexia nervosa. *New England Journal of Medicine, 360*, 500–506.

Attias, R., & Goodwin, J. (1999). A place to begin: Images of the body in transformation. In J. Goodwin & R. Attias (Eds.), *Splintered reflections: Images of the body in trauma*. New York, NY: Basic Books.

Bachar, E., Latzer, Y., Kreitler, S., & Berry, E. M. (1999). Empirical comparison of two psychological therapies. *Journal of Psychotherapy Practice and Research, 8*(2), 115–128.

Becker, A. E. (2003). Outpatient management of eating disorders in adults. *Current Women's Health Reports, 3*(3), 221–229.

Becker, A.E., Grinspoon, S.K., Klibanski, A., & Herzog, D.B. (1999). Eating Disorders. *The New England Journal of Medicine, 340*, 1092–1098.

Berkman, N. D., Lohr, K. N., & Bulik, C. M. (2007). Outcomes of eating disorders: A systematic review of the literature. *International Journal of Eating Disorders, 40*(4), 293–309.

Bernstein, E., & Putnam, F. (1986). Development, reliability, and validity of a dissociation scale. *Journal of Nervous and Mental Disorders, 174*, 727–735.

Berridge, K. C. (2008). 'Liking' and 'wanting' food rewards: Brain substrates and roles in eating disorders. *Physiology and Behavior, 97*(14), 537–550.

Bjorntorp, P. (2001). Do stress reactions cause abdominal obesity and comorbidities? *Obesity Review, 2*, 73–86.

Blaine, B. (2008). Does depression cause obesity? A metaanalysis of longitudinal studies of depression and weight control. *Journal of Health Psychology, 13*, 1190–1197.

Bohn, K., & Fairburn, C. G. (2008). Clinical Impairment Assessment Questionnaire. In CG Fairburn (Ed,), *Cognitive behavior therapy and eating disorders* (pp. 315-318). New York,NY: Guilford Press.

Bowen, M. (1978). Family therapy in clinical practice. New York: Jason Arason.

Bowlby, J. (1982). *Attachment and loss*. New York, NY: Basic Books.

Brown, S., Birtwistle, J., Roe, L., & Thompson, C. (1999). The unhealthy lifestyle of people with schizophrenia. *Psychological Medicine, 29*(3), 697–701.

Burke, C. (2010). Mindfulness-based approaches with children and adolescents: A preliminary review of current research in an emergent field. *Journal of Child and Family Studies, 19*(2), 133–144.

Carei, T., Fyfe-Johnson, A., Breuner, C., & Brown, M. (2010). Randomized controlled clinical trial of yoga in the treatment of eating disorders. *Journal of Adolescent Health, 46*(4), 346–351.

Carter, F. A., Bulik, C. M., McIntosh, V. V., & Cue, J. P. (2002). Cue reactivity as a predictor of outcome with bulimia nervosa. *International Journal of Eating Disorders, 31*, 240–250.

Chakraborty, K., & Basu, D. (2010). Mangement of anorexia and bulimia nervosa: An evidence-based review. *Indian Journal of Psychiatry, 52*(2), 174–186.

Cockell, S. J., Geller, J., & Linden, W. (2002). Measuring shifts from precontemplation to contemplation in anorexia nervosa: The development of a decisional balance scale for anorexia nervosa. *European Eating Disorders Review, 10*, 359–375.

Cote, G., & Edmundowicz, S. (2009). Emerging technology: Endoluminal treatment of obesity. *Gastrointestinal Endoscopy, 70*(5), 991–999.

Crow, S. J., Peterson, C. B., Swanson, S. A., Raymond, N. C., Specker, S., Eckert, E. D., & Mitchell, J. E. (2009). Increased mortality in bulimia nervosa and other eating disorders. *American Journal of Psychiatry, 166*(12), 1342–1346.

Cumella, E. J., & Kally, Z. (2008). Comparison of middle-age and young women inpatients with eating disorders. *Eating and Weight Disorders, 13*(4), 183–190.

Cyr, N. R. (2008). Considerations for patients who have eating disorders. *AORN Journal, 88*(5), 807–815.

D'Abundo, M., & Chally, P. (2004). Stuggling with recovery: Participant perspectives on battling an eating disorder. *Qualitative Health Research, 14*, 1094–1096.

Daumit, G., Clark, J. M., Steinwachs, D., Graham, C., Lehman, A., & Ford, D. (2003). Prevalence and correlates of obesity in a community sample of individuals with severe and persistent mental illness. *Journal of Nervous and Mental Disorders, 191*(12), 799–805.

Dean, R., Bilsky, E., & Negus, S. (2009). *Opiate receptors and antagonists: From bench to clinic*. New York, NY: Humana Press, 411.

Devlin, M., Yanovski, S., & Wilson, G. (2000). Obesity: What mental health professionals need to know. *American Journal of Psychiatry, 157*, 854–866.

Dichter, J. R., Cohen, J., & Connolly, P. M. (2002). Bulimia nervosa: Knowledge, awareness, and skill levels among advanced practice PMH-APRNs. *Journal of the American Academy of PMH-APRN Practitioners, 14*(6), 269–275.

Eastland, T. (n.d.). *Eating disorders a feminist issue*. Retrieved from www.vanderbilt.edu/AnS/psychology/health_psychology/feminist.htm

Evans, L., & Wertheim, E. H. (2001). *An examination of willingness to self-disclose in women with bulimic symptoms considering the contest of disclosure and negative affect levels. Wiley Periodicals.* Melbourne, Victoria: La Troube Unversity, 344–348.

Faber, B. (2006). *Self–disclosure in psychotherapy.* New York, NY: Guilford.

Faber, B., & Hall, D. (2002). Disclosure to therapists: What is and what is not discussed in therapy. *Journal of Clinical Psychology, 58*, 359–370.

Fairburn, C. G. (2008). *Cognitive behavior therapy and eating disorders.* New York, NY: Guilford.

Fairburn, C. G., & Beglin, S. J. (1994). Assessment of eating disorders: Interview or self-report questionnaire? *International Journal of Eating Disorders, 16*, 363–370.

Fairburn, C., & Cooper, Z. (1993). The eating disorder examination. In C. Fairburn & G. Wilson (Eds.), *Binge eating: Nature, assessment and treatment* (12th ed., pp. 317–360). New York, NY: Guilford.

Fairburn, C., & Cooper, Z. (1993). The eating disorder examination. In C. Fairburn & G. Wilson (Eds.), *Binge eating: Nature, assessment and treatment* (12th ed., pp. 317–360). New York, NY: Guilford.

Faris, P. L., Hofbauer, R. D., Daughters, R., VandenLangenberg, E., Iversen, L., Goodale, R. L.,...Hartman, B. K. (2007). De-stabilization of the positive vago-vagal reflex in bulimia nervosa. *Journal of Physiological Behavior, 94*(1), 136–153. doi: 10.1016/j.physbeh.2007.11.036

Farrell, E. (1995). *Lost for words: The psychoanalysis of anorexia and bulimia.* New York, NY: Other Press, LLC.

Favaro, A., & Tenconi, E. (2006). Perinatal factors and the risk of developing anorexia nervosa and bulimia nervosa. *Archives of General Psychiatry, 63*, 82–88.

Fiegal, K., Carroll, M., Ogden, C., & Curtin, L. (2010). Prevalence and trends in obesity among U.S. adults, 1999–2008. *Journal of the American Medical Association, 303*(3), 235–241.

Flahavan, C. (2006). Detection, assessment, and management of eating disorders: How involved are GPs? *Irish Journal of Psychiatric Medicine, 23*(2), 96–99.

Flament, M. F., Bissada, H., & Spettigue, W. (2011). Evidence-based pharmacology of eating disorders. *International Journal of Neuropsychopharmacology, 15*(2), 1–19. doi: 10.1017/SI461145711000381

Forbush, K., Heatherton, T. F., & Keel, P. K. (2007). Relationships between perfectionism and specific disordered eating behaviors. *International Journal of Eating Disorders, 40*(1), 37–41.

Franco, K. N. (2010). *Eating disorders. Disease management project Cleveland Clinic Center for Continuing Education.* Retrieved from http://www.clevelandclinicmeded.com/medicalpubs/disease managment/psychiatry-psych

Frank, G., Bailer, U., Henry, S., Wagner, A., & Kaye, W. (2004). Neuroimaging studies in eating disorders. *Central Nervous System, 9*, 539–548.

Franken, R. E. (1994). *Human motivation* (3rd ed.). Pacific Grove, CA: Brooks/Cole.

Garner, D., Olmsted, M., Bohr, Y., & Garfinkel, P. (1982). The eating attitudes test: Psychometric features and clinical correlates. *Psychological Medicine, 12*, 871–878.

Garner, D. M. (1991). *Eating disorder inventory-2. Professional manual.* Odessa, FL: Psychological Assessment Reources.

Garner, D. M. (2004). *Eating disorder inventory-3. Professional manual.* Lutz, FL: Psychological Assessment Resources.

Garner, D. M., & Garfinkel, P. E. (1985). *Handbook of psychotherapy for anorexia nervosa and bulimia.* New York, NY: Guilford.

Gearhardt, A. N., Yokum, S., Orr, P. T., Stice, E., Corbin, W. R., & Brownell, D. (2011). Neural correlates of food addiction. *Archives of General Psychiatry, 68*(8), 808–816. Retrieved from www.archgenpsychiatry.com

Geller, J., Cockell, S. J., & Drab, D. L. (2001). Assessing readiness for change in the eating disorders: The psychometric properties of the readiness and motivation interview. *Psychological Assessment, 13*, 180–198.

Geller, J., & Drab, D. L. (1999). The readiness and motivation interview: A symptom specific measure of readiness for change in the eating disorders. *European Eating Disorders Review, 7*, 259–278.

Ghaderi, A., & Pure, S. B. (2003). Pure and guided self-help for full and sub-threshold bulimia nervosa and binge eating disorder. *British Journal of Clinical Psychology, 42*(3), 257–269.

Grange, D. (2005). The Maudsley family-based treatment for adolescent anorexia nervosa. *World Psychiatry, 4*(3), 142–146. Retrieved from http://www.ncbi.nlm.nih.gov/pubmed/16633532

Griffiths, R. A., & Cahnnon-Little, L. (1993). The hypnotizability of patients with bulimia nervosa and partial syndromes participating in controlled treatment outcome study. *Contemporary Hypnosis, 10*, 81–87.

Grillo, C., & Mitchel, J. (2010). *The treatment of eating disorders*: A clinical handbook. New York, NY: Guilford Press.

Halmi, K. (2000). *Basic biological overview of eating disorders. Back to Psychopharmacology: The fourth generation of progress.* Retrieved from http://www.acnp.org/g4/GN401000155/CH151.html

Hara, T. (1997). *Hunger and eating.* Northridge, CA: California State University. Retrieved from http://www.csun.edu/-vcpsyh/students/hunger.htm

Harrop, E. N., & Marlatt, G. A. (2009). The comorbitidy of substance use disorders and eating disorders in women: Prevalence, etiology, and treatment. *Additive Behaviors.* doi: 10.1016/j.addbeh.2009.12.016

Hay, P. P. J., Bacaltchuk, J., Stefano, S., & Kashyap, P. (2009). *Psychological treatments for bulimia nervosa and binging (Review).* Retrieved from http://www.thecochranelibrary.com

Heller, R. F., & Heller, R. F. (1991). *The carbohydrate addict's diet.* New York, NY: Penguin.

Hendricks, E., Rothman, R. & Greenway, F. (2009). How Physician Specialists use drugs to treat obesity. *Obesity, 17*(9), 1730-1735.

Himpens, J., Cadiere, G., Bazi, M., Vouche, M., Cadiere, B., & Dapri, G. (2011). Long-term outcomes of laparascopid adjustable gastric banding. *Archives of Surgery, 146*(7), 902–907.

Horne, R. L., Ferguson, J. M., Pope, H. G., Hudson, J. I., Lineberry, C. G., Ascher, J., & Cato, A. (1988). Treatment of bulimia with bupropion: A multicenter controlled trial. *Journal of Clinical Psychiatry, 49,* 262–266.

Horvath, A. O., & Greenberg, L. S. (1989). Development of validation of the working alliance inventory. *Journal of Counseling Psychology, 36,* 223–233.

Hudson, J. I., Pope, H. G., Keck, P. E., & McElroy, S. L. (1989). Treatment of bulimia nervosa with trazadone: Short-term response and long-term follow up. *Clinical Neuropharmacology, 12,* 538–546.

Hudson, J. I., Pope, Jr., H. G., & Kessler, R. C. (2007). The prevalence and correlates of eating disorders in the national comorbidity survey replication. *Biological Psychiatry, 61*(3), 348–358. doi: 10:1016/jbiopsych.2006.03.040

James, W. (2008). The epidemiology of obesity: The size of the problem. *Journal of Internal Medicine, 263*(4), 336–352.

Jensen, V., & Mejhede, A. (2000). Anorexia nervosa: Treatment with Olanzapine. *The British Journal of Psychiatry, 177,* 87.

Johnson, J. G., Spitzer, R. L., & Williams, B. W. (2001). Health problems, impairment, and illnesses associated with bulimia nervosa and binge eating disorder among primary care and obstetric gynaecology patients. *Psychological Medicine, 31,* 1455–1466.

Jones, M., Luce, K. H., Osborne, M., Taylor, K., Cunning, D., Doyle, A., . . . Wilfley, D. E. (2008). Randomized controlled trial of an internet-facilitated intervention for reducing binge eating and overweight in adolescents. *Pediatrics, 121,* 453–462.

Jorm, A. F., Korten, A. E., Jacomb, P. A., Christensen, H., Rodgers, B., & Pollitt, P. (1997). Mental health literacy: A survey of the public's ability to recognize mental disorders and their beliefs about the effectiveness of treatment. *Medical Journal of Australia, 6,* 182–186.

Jourard, S. (1971). Self-disclosure: An experimental anaylsis of the transparent self. New York, NY: Wiley InterScience.

Kalarchian, M., Marcus, M., & Levine, M. (2007). Psychiatric disorders among bariatric surgery candidates. *American Journal of Psychiatry, 164,* 328–334.

Kalodner, C. R., & DeLucia-Waack, J. L. (2003). Theory and research on eating disorders and disturbances in women: Suggestions for practice. In M. Kopala & Keitel (Eds.), *Handbook of counseling women* (pp. 506–532). Thousand Oaks, CA: Sage Publications.

Kaye, W. H., Bulik, C. M., Thornton, L., Barbarich, N., Masters, K., & the Price Foundation Collaborative Group. (2004). Comorbidity of anxiety disorders with anorexia and bulimia nervosa. *The American Journal of Psychiatry, 161,* 2215–2221.

Kim, G., Jieru, L., Valentino, M., Colon-Gonzalez, F., & Waldman, S. (2011). Regulation of appetite to treat obesity. *Expert Reviews of Clinical Pharmacology, 4*(2), 243–259.

Klump, K., Miller, K., Keel, P., McGue, M., & Lacono, W. (2001). Genetic and environmental influences on anorexia nervosa syndromes in a population-based twin sample. *Psychological Medicine, 31*(4), 737–740.

Kortegaard, L., Hoerder, K., Joergensen, J., Gillberg, C., & Kyvik, K. (2001). A preliminary population-based twin study of self-reported eating disorder. *Psychological Medicine, 31*(2), 361–365.

Krantz, A. M. (1999, fall/winter). Growing into her body: Dance/movement therapy for women with eating disorders. *American Journal of Dance Therapy, 21*(2), 81–103.

Lamothe, D. (1998). *The taming of the chew: A holistic approach to stop compulsive eating.* New York and London: Penguin.

Lapid, M. I., Prom, M. C., Burton, M. C., McAlpine, D. E., Sutor, B., & Rummans, T. A. (2010). Eating disorders in the elderly. *Int Psychogeriatrics, 4,* 523–536.

Lazzaro-Smith, M. (2008). Healing eating disorders with body-centered therapies. *Sage Living Psychotherapy-Healing from Eating Disorders, 7*(2), 1–15.

Levine, D., & Mishna, G. (2007). A self psychological and relational approach to group therapy for university students with bulimia. *International Journal of Group Psychotherapy, 57*(2), 167–185. doi: 10.152/ijgp.2007.57.2.167

Liebman, R., Minuchin, S., & Baker, L. (1974). An integrated treatment program for anorexia nervosa. *American Journal of Psychiatry, 131*(4), 432–436.

Lippincott Williams & Wilkins. (2012). *Nursing drug handbook.* Philadelphia, PA: Author.

Lock, J., Le Grange, D., Agras, S., & Christopher, D. (2000). *Treatment manual for anorexia nervosa: A family-based approach.* New York, NY: Guilford.

Maggard, M., Shugarman, L., Suttorp, M., Maglione, M., Sugarmen, H., & Livingston, E. (2005). Meta-analysis: Surgical treatment of obesity. *Annals of Internal Medicine, 142,* 547–559.

Malin, A., Gaskil, J., McConah, C., Frank, G., Lavia, M., Scholar, L., & Kaye, W. (2003). Olanzapine treatment of anorexia nervosa: A retrospective study. Wiley InterScience. Retrieved from http://eatingdisorders.ucsd.edu/research/imaging/PDFs/2003/malina2003olanzapine.pdf

Maloney, M., Mcquire, J., & Daniels, S. (1988). Reliability testing of a children's version of the eating attitude test. *Journal of the American Academy of Child and Adolescent Psychiatry,* 27, 541–543.

Mazure, C., Halmi, K., Sunday, S., Romano, S., & Einhorn, A. (2008). The Yale-Brown-Cornell Eating Disorder Scale: Development, use, reliability, and validity. *International Journal of Eating Disorders, 41*(3), 265–272.

McCreadie, R. (2003). Diet, smoking, and cardiovascular risk in people with schizophrenia: Descriptive study. *British Journal of Psychiatry, 183,* 534–539.

McEvoy, J., Meyer, J., & Goff, D. (2005). Prevalence of metabolic syndrome in patients with schizophrenia: Baseline results from the Clinical Antipsychotic Trials of Intervention Effectiveness and comparison with NHANES III. *Schizophrenia Research, 80,* 19–35.

McIver, S., O'Halloran, P., & McGartland, M. (2009). Yoga as a treatment for binge eating disorder: A preliminary study. *Complement Therapies in Medicine, 17*(4), 196–202.

Mehler, P. S. (2011). Medical complications of bulimia nervosa and their treatments. *International Journal of Eating Disorders, 44*(2), 95–104. doi: 10.1002/eat.20825

Milano, W., Petrella, C., Sabatino, C., Capasso, A. (2004). Treatment of bulimia nervosa with sertraline: A randomized controlled trial. *Advances in Therapy,* 21, 232–237.

Miller, E., Erlinger, T., Young, D., Megan, J., Charleston, J., Rhodes, D., . . . Lawrence, A. (2002). Results of the diet, exercise, and weight loss intervention trial (DEW-IT). *Hypertension, 40*(5), 612–618.

Miller, W., & Rollnick, S. (2002). *Motivational interviewing: Preparing people for change.* New York, NY: Guilford.

Mond, J. M., Hay, P., Rodgers, B., & Owen, C. (2007). Health service utilization for eating disorders: Findings from a community-based study. *International Journal of Eating Disorders, 40,* 399–408.

Mond, J. M., Hay, P., Rodgers, B., & Owen, C. (2008). Mental health literacy and eating disorders: What do women with bulimic eating disorders think and know about bulimia nervosa and its treatment? *Journal of Mental Health, 17*(6), 565–575.

Mond, J. M., Myers, T. C., Crosby, R. D., Hay, P. J., & Mitchell, J. E. (2009). Bulimic eating disorders in primary care: Hidden morbidity still? *Journal for Clinical Psychology in Medical Settings, 17,* 56–63. doi: 10.1007/s10880-009-9180-9

Morgan, J., Reid, F., & Lacey, J. (1999). The SCOFF questionnaire: Assessment of a new screening tool for eating disorders. *British Medical Journal, 319*(7223), 1467–1468.

Murtagh, L. (2007). Judicial intervention for morbidly obese children. *Journal of Law and Medical Ethics, 35*(3), 497–499.

National Collaborating Centre for Mental Health. (2004). Core interventions in the treatment and management of anorexia nervosa, bulimia nervosa, and related eating disorders. *National Clinical Practice Guidelines No. 9,* Leicester and London: British Psychological Society and Gaskell. Retrieved from http://www.nice.orguk/pdf/cg009niceguidance.pdf

Newman, A. (2009). Obesity in older adults. *The Online Journal of Issues in Nursing, 14*(1), manuscript 3.

National Institutes of Health. NIH Publication No. 01–3680. (2006). *Understanding adult obesity*. Retrieved from http://win.niddk.gov/publications/understanding.htm

Odom, J., Zalesin, K., Washington, T., Miller, W., Hakmeh, B., Zaremba, D. L.,... McCullough, P. A. (2010). Behavioral predictors of weight regain after bariatric surgery. *Obesity Surgery, 20*(3), 349–356.

Ogden, C., Carroll, M., Curtin, L., Lamb, M., & Flegal, K. (2010). Prevalence and trends of high body mass index in US children and adolescents, 2007–2008. *Journal of the American Medical Association, 303*(3), 242–249.

Ogden, C., Minton, K., & Pain, C. (2006). *Trauma and the body: A sensorimotor approach to psychotherapy.* New York and London: Norton.

Palazzoli, M. (1978). *Self-starvation: From individual to family therapy in the treatment of anorexia nervosa.* Northvale, NJ: J. Aronson.

Patching, J., & Lawler, J. (2009). Understanding women's experiences of developing an eating disorder and recovering: A life-history approach. *Nursing Inquiry, 16*(1), 10–21.

Petry, N., Barry, D., Pietrzak, R., & Wagner, J. (2008). Overweight and obesity associated with psychiatric disorders: Results from National Epidemiologic Survey of Alcohol and Related Conditions. *Psychosomatic Medicine, 70,* 288–297.

Pike, K. (1998). Long-term course of anorexia nervosa: Response, relapse, remission, and recovery. *Clinical Psychology Review, 18,* 447–475.

Porges, S. (2004). Neuroception: A subconscious system for detecting threats and safety. *Zero to Three, 32,* 19–24.

Pratt, B. M., & Woolfenden, S. (2009). *Interventions for preventing eating disorders in children and adolescents.* Retrieved from http://www.thecochranelibrary.com

Prochaska, J. O. (1979). *Systems of psychotherapy: A transtheoretical analysis.* Homewood, IL: Dorsey.

Prochaska, J. O., DiClemente, C. C., & Norcross, J. C. (1992). In search of how people change. *American Psychologist, 47,* 1102–1114.

Renfrew Center Foundation for Eating Disorders. (2003). *Eating disorders 101 guide: A summary of issues, statistics, and resources.* Retrieved from http://www.renfrew.org

Riva, G. (2011). The key to unlocking the virtual body: Virtual reality in the treatment of obesity and eating disorders. *Journal of Diabetes Science and Technology, 5*(2), 283–292.

Robert-McComb, J. J. (2001). *Eating disorders in women and children: Prevention, stress management, and treatment.* Boca Raton, FL: CRC.

Roemmich, J., Wright, S., & Epstein, L. (2002). Dietary restraint and stress induced snacking. *Obesity Research, 10,* 1120–1126.

Rogers, V. L., Griffin, M. Q., Wykle, M. L., & Fitzpatrick, J. J. (2009). Internet versus face-to-face therapy: Emotional self-disclosure issues for young adults. *Issues in Mental Health Nursing, 30,* 596–602.

Rushing, J. M., Jones, L. E., & Carney, C. P. (2003). Bulimia nervosa: A primary care review. *Primary Care Companion Journal of Clinical Psychiatry, 5*(5), 217–226.

Saarni, S., Saarni, S. E., & Fogelholm, M. (2009). Body composition in psychotic disorders. *Psychological Medicine, 39,* 801–810.

Sacks, F., Bray, G., & Carey, V. (2009). Comparison of weight-loss diets with different compositions of fat, protein, and carbohydrates. *New England Journal of Medicine, 360,* 859–873.

Sadock, B. J., & Sadock, V. A. (2007). Kaplan and Sadock's synopsis of psychiatry: Behavioral sciences/clinical psychiatry (10th ed.). *Bulimia nervosa and eating disorder not otherwise specified.* Retrieved from mk:@MSITStore:C:/DOCUME-/Home/LOCALS-1Temp/jZip/jZipD213/jZip12196/KS

Sarwer, D., von Sydow Green, A., Vetter, M., & Wadden, T. (2009). Behavior therapy for obesity: Where are we now? *Current Opinion on Endocrinology, 16*(5), 347–352.

Saukko, P. (2000). Between voice and discourse: Quilting interviews on anorexia. *Qualitative Inquiry, 6,* 299–317.

Schneider, B., & Mun, E. (2005). Surgical management of morbid obesity. *Diabetes Care, 28,* 475–480.

Shapiro, R. (Ed.). (2009). *EMDR solutions II for depression, eating disorders, and more.* New York and London: Norton.

Shay, N., & Mangian, H. (2000). Neurobiology of zinc-influenced eating behavior. *Journal of Nutrition, 130*(5), 1493S– 1499S.

Simon, J., Schmidt, U., & Pilling, S. (2005). The health service use and cost of eating disorders. *Psychological Medicine, 35,* 1543–1551.

Spitzer, R. L., Uanovski, S. Z., & Marcus, M. D. (1993). *The questionnaire on eating and weight patterns-revised (QEWP-R).* New York, NY: New York State Psychiatric Institute.

Spratto, G. R., & Woods, A. L. (2005). *PDR Nurse's Drug Handbook.* Clifton Park, NY: Thomson Delmar Learning.

Steinhausen, H. C., & Weber, W. (2009). The outcome of bulimia nervosa: Findings from one-quarter century of research. *American Journal of Psychiatry, 166*(12), 1331–1341.

Stice, E., Yokum, S., Blum, K., & Bohon, C. (2010). Weight gain is associated with reduced response to palatable foods. *Journal of Neuroscience, 30*(39), 13105–13109.

Striegel-Moore, R. H., Perrin, N., DeBar, L., Wilson, G. T., Rossell, F., & Kraemer, H. C. (2010). Screening for binge eating disorders using the patient health questionnaire in a community sample. *International Journal of Eating Disorders, 43*(4), 337–343. doi: 10.1002/eat.20694

Sturm, R. (2002). The effects of obesity, smoking, and drinking on medical problems and costs. *Health Affairs, 21*(2), 245–253.

Sullivan, H. (1953). *The interpersonal theory of psychiatry*. New York, NY: Norton.

Sullivan, P. (1995). Mortality in anorexia nervosa. *American Journal of Psychiatry, 152*, 1073–1074.

Teng, K. (2011) Premenopausal osteoporosis, an overlooked consequence of anorexia nervosa. *The Cleveland Clinic Journal of Medicine, 78*(1), 50–58. Retrieved from http://ccjm.org/content/78/1/50.full/ doi:10.3949/ccjm.78a.10023.

Treasure, J., Todd, G., Brolly, M., Tiller, J., Nehmed, A., Denman, F. (1995). A pilot study of a randomized trial of cognitive analytical therapy vs educational behavioral therapy for adult anorexia nervosa. *Behavioral Research and Therapy, 33*:363–367.

Uehara, T., Takeuchi, K., Ohmori, I., Kawashima, Y., Goto, M., Mikuni, M., & Vandereycken, W. (2002). Factor-analytic study of the anorectic behavior observation scale in Japan: Comparison with the original Belgian study. *Psychiatry Research, 111*, 241–246.

Vitale, E., Lotito, L., & Maglie, R. B. (2009). A psychoneuroendocrino-immune approach in the nursing treatment of anorexia and bulimia nervosa. *Immunopharmacology and Immunotoxicology, 3*(1), 39–50.

Vitousek, K., Watson, S., & Wilson, G. (1998). Enhancing motivation for change in treatment resistant eating disorders. *Clinical Psychology Review, 1*, 391–420.

Wade, T., Bulik, C., Neale, M., & Kendler, K. (2000). Anorexia nervosa and major depression: Shared genetic and environmental risk factors. *American Journal of Psychiatry*, 157(3), 469–471.

Walsh, B., & Garner, D. M. (1997). Diagnostic issues. In D. M. Garner & P. Garfinkel (Eds.), *Handbook of treatment for eating disorders*. New York, NY: Guilford.

Wang, G., Volkow, N., Thanos, P., & Fowler, J. (2004). Similarities between obesity and drug addiction as assessed by neurofunctional imaging: A concept review. *Journal of Addictive Disorders, 23*(3), 39–53.

Waren, C., Cepeda-Benito, A., Gleaves, D., Moreno, S., Rodriguez, S., Fernandez, M.,... Pearson, C. (2008). English and Spanish versions of the body shape questionnaire: Measurement equivalence across ethnicity and clinical status. *International Journal of Eating Disorders, 41*(3), 265–272.

Watters, E. (2010, January 10, 2010, p. mm40 of NY edition). The Americanization of mental illness. *The New York Times*. Retrieved from http://www.nytimes.com

Whitehouse, A. M., Cooper, P. J., Vize, C. V., Hill, C., & Vogel, L. (1992). Prevalence of eating disorders in three Cambridge general practices: Hidden and conspicuous morbidity. *The British Journal of General Practice, 42*(355), 57–60.

Williams, C. (2003). New technologies in self-help: Another effective way to get better? *European Eating Disorders Review, 11*, 170–182.

Williams, P. M., Goodie, J., & Motsinger, C. D. (2008). Treating eating disorders in primary care. *American Family Physician, 77*(2), 187–195.

Wisniewski, L., Warren, M., Heiden, M. (2009). Dialectical behavioural therapy in the treatment of eating disorders. In Wisniewski (Ed). *Interventions for body image and eating disorders* (pp. 234–250). East Hawthorn, Victoria Australia: IP Communications.

Wolf, N. (1991). *The beauty myth*. New York, NY: William Morrow.

Woodside, B., Garfinkel, P., Lin, E., Goering, P., Kaplan, A., Goldbloom, D., & Kennedy, S. (2001). Comparisons of men with full or partial eating disorders, men without eating disorders, and women with eating disorders in the community. *American Journal of Psychiatry, 158*, 570–574.

Yager, J., Devlin, M. J., Halmi, K. A., Herzog, D. G., Mitchell, J. E., Powers, P., Zerbe, K. (2006). *Practice guidelines for the treatment of patients with eating disorders (third edition)*. American Psychiatric Association.

Zerbe, K. J. (2003). Eating disorders in middle and late life: A neglected problem. *Primary Psychiatry, 10*(6), 76–78.

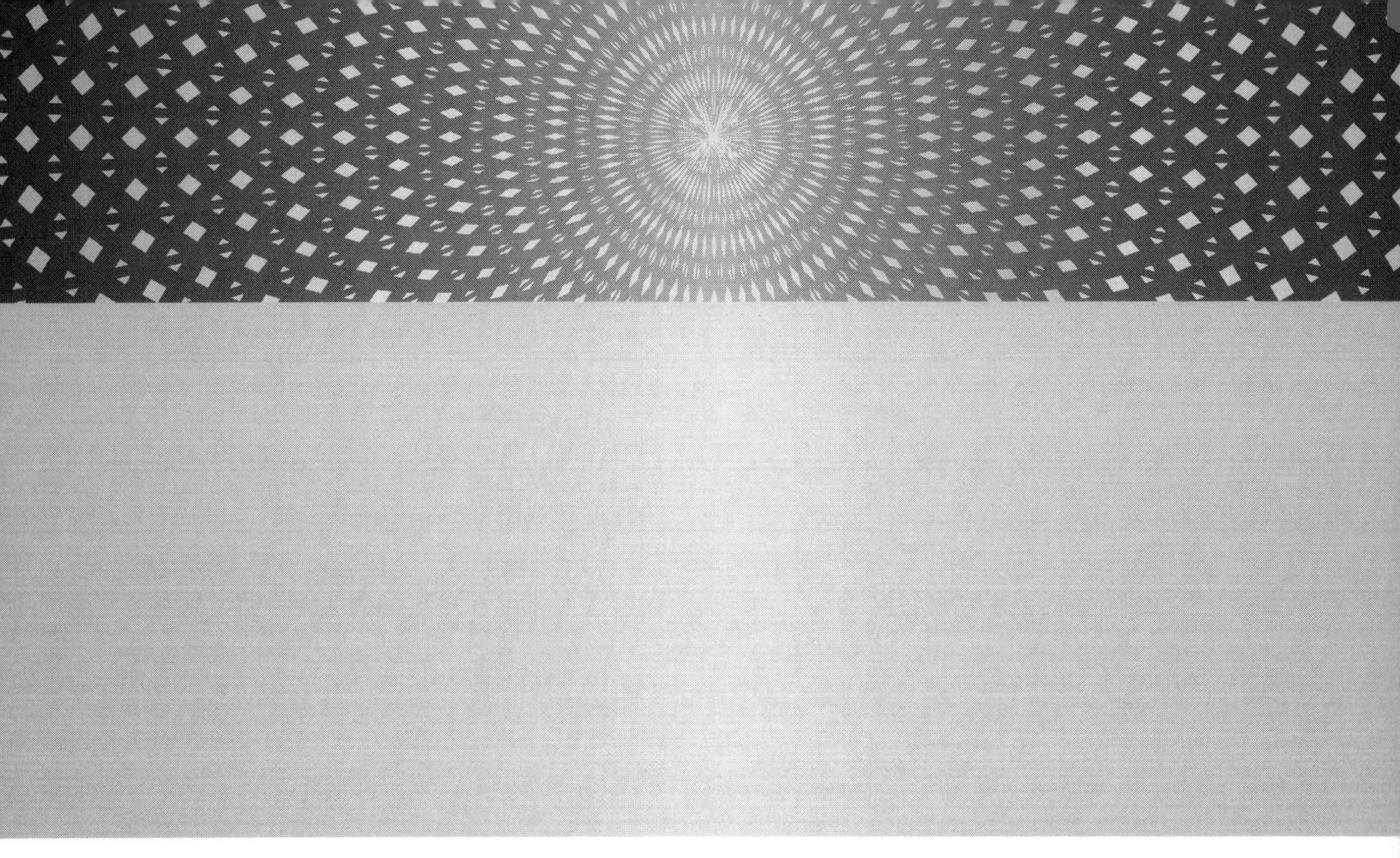

CHAPTER CONTENTS

Cognitive disorders are characterized by a significant decline in the ability to think and reason and often impairments in short-term memory. They are the most prevalent psychiatric disorders of late life, as the aging brain is sensitive and vulnerable to drugs, disease, and environmental factors. As cognitive disorders include both acute onset (delirium) and gradual onset (dementia), they may overlap or be difficult to diagnose. Variance in classification and nomenclature between the American Psychiatric Association (APA), *Diagnostic and Statistical Manual* (*DSM-IV*), and the National Institute for Neurological Disorders and Stroke (NINDS) adds to the challenge of determining specific incidence and prevalence of the various disorders. But we know these conditions are likely to increase.

In 2011, the leading edge of the "baby boom" generation born after World War II officially entered their later adult years by becoming age 65 at the rate of 10,000 per day. This increase will continue for the next 17 years until the last child born in 1964 turns 65 (Cohn & Taylor, 2010). Currently 39 million Americans are over the age of 65 (Administration on Aging, 2008). By the year 2030 the elderly population is expected to more than double. The accelerated rate of growth among the most vulnerable of the elderly, those over age 85, is expected to grow from 5.7 million to 19 million by 2050. As advanced age is the greatest risk factor for the development of a cognitive disorder, the incidence and prevalence of these impairments also are expected to increase. These demographics

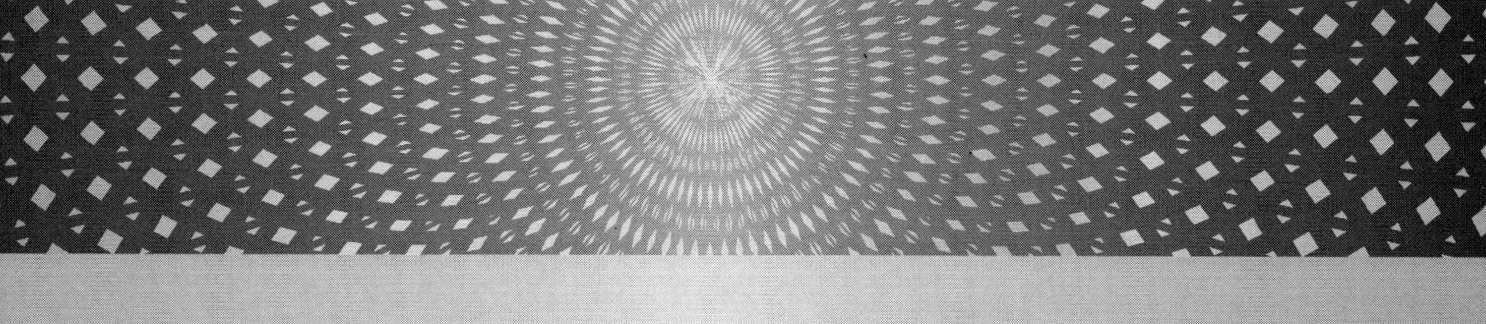

CHAPTER 13
Integrative Management of Disordered Cognition

Anita Thompson Heisterman

will have profound effects on the health care system, and advanced practice psychiatric nurses (PMH-APRNs) in both acute and primary care are very likely to become more involved in the assessment and treatment of persons presenting with cognitive concerns.

Although older adults are most at risk for developing a cognitive disorder, the young are not spared as head injury is a significant risk factor for the development of cognitive impairment both immediately following the injury but also appearing later in life with symptoms of memory loss and often progressing to dementia. There is recognition that athletes who have had repeated head injuries can develop dementia in later life. Veterans returning from combat missions in Iraq (Operation Iraqi Freedom) or Afghanistan (Operation Enduring Freedom) are increasingly diagnosed with Traumatic Brain Injury (TBI) from blast injuries. Barnes et al. (2011) describe it as the "signature wound" of those conflicts. Though initial symptoms may be subtle, significant cognitive impairments may develop as the condition progresses over time.

CLASSIFICATION OF COGNITIVE DISORDERS

Cognitive disorders are broadly classified by the APA into one of three categories: (a) delirium, dementia, amnestic and other cognitive disorders; (b) mental disorders resulting from a general medical condition; and (c) substance-related disorders (APA, 2000). While the cognitive changes associated with the dementias are permanent, those associated with delirium may be reversible, depending on the responsible causal factors. When the cause of delirium is eliminated or subsides, the cognitive deficits usually resolve within a few days or sometimes weeks. Dementia, in contrast, results from primary brain pathology that usually is irreversible, chronic, progressive, and less amenable to treatment.

Although cognitive disorders may vary in etiology, and symptom presentation, the assessment and management of dementia, from mild cognitive impairment (MCI) to progressive chronic disorders, are similar. Delirium, as an acute cognitive disorder and possible medical emergency, requires a more immediate assessment, and management may involve hospitalization. Dementia will be used as the prototype for assessment and management of chronic cognitive disorders, including MCI, TBI, and amnestic disorders. Etiology and symptom presentation of the most common forms of dementias will be presented later in the chapter.

GENERAL PRINCIPLES FOR ASSESSMENT OF OLDER ADULTS

Detection of cognitive impairments particularly in older adults can be a challenge for the most skilled clinician. Clients may not report symptoms and may endure debilitating symptoms and functional decline because they fear the loss of independence or are embarrassed to report symptoms. Conditions that may contribute to cognitive impairments such as depression, alcoholism, and poor nutrition are commonly not reported, and nonspecific presentations such as fatigue, apathy, and poor concentration are typical. Even when reported, a cognitive change could signal depression, dementia of the Alzheimer's type (Alzheimer's disease [AD]), an underlying urinary track infection (UTI), or a myriad of other physical illnesses. As the PMH-APRN is well aware, dementia, delirium, and depression are not mutually exclusive conditions and all three conditions can be present in the same individual at any given time. In fact, 50% of persons with Alzheimer's disease will experience depression at some time in the course of the illness.

Though specific assessment parameters will be discussed with both delirium and dementia, an initial comprehensive biopsychosocial assessment is critical to detect and treat cognitive disorders. Aspects of a comprehensive assessment include physical, mental, functional, and social components, along with review of medications. Such thorough initial assessment will make it possible for the PMH-APRN to gather data that can later help the clinician discern changes from baseline functioning. Likewise, each episode of care, though more focused, should include psychosocial as well as physical assessment. Follow-up after each episode of care to review the goals of treatment, evaluate progress towards remission of target symptoms, and prevent harm through careful assessment of medication use is good practice. Assessment tools used during initial evaluation and in subsequent visits to aid in the detection of changes in cognition, mood, and functional status are particularly helpful and will be described further in the chapter.

Older adults use 33% of all prescription and 40% of all the over-the-counter medications consumed in the United States and are at increased risk for cognitive impairments (Roose, Pollock, & Devanand, 2004). Many drugs affect the central nervous system, and normal age-associated changes in protein and fat distribution, diminished renal function, and hepatic disease can affect pharmacokinetics, making clearance of drugs from the body unpredictable. Assessment of medication can be accomplished by using the "brown bag method." This involves asking the patient and family to bring all prescription and nonprescription medication to the appointment. The PMH-APRN can then review and eliminate unneeded medications, teach the patient about side effects and precautions, and possibly prevent an episode of delirium.

Additional considerations in assessment of the older adult are to establish communication, include the family (unless contraindicated) as an integral part of assessment, and gather information about family and social functioning. Family members are often reliable informants, contributing crucial information for assessment, bringing practical expertise and knowledge in caring for the individual, and providing critical social support. A cultural assessment to discern health beliefs and practices that may be relevant to patient care is another important component of a comprehensive assessment. A multidimensional assessment includes formal resources and support systems, such as Meals on Wheels or the informal support of the neighbor who brings in the mail and talks about the news. The presence of these support systems frequently makes the difference between the patient remaining at home and being institutionalized. The empathic PMH-APRN will adapt communication strategies based on the client's presentation. Allowing more time to gather information for the initial assessment or collecting it over two sessions can preserve patient energy and facilitate communication.

DELIRIUM

Delirium is characterized by a rapid onset of cognitive disturbance and altered consciousness induced by any process, disorder, or agent that disrupts the integrity of the central nervous system and impairs its functioning at a cellular level. The three hallmark diagnostic features of delirium are disordered cognition, impaired ability to maintain or shift attention, and disturbance of consciousness. Although these are vital components of the diagnostic criteria for delirium in the *DSM-IV-TR* (APA, 2000), additional features of delirium may include a disrupted sleep–wake cycle, and an abnormality of psychomotor behavior, either hyperactive or hypoactive. Hypoactive forms where the client presents as apathetic rather than agitated are often missed.

While delirium is the most common psychiatric syndrome found in general medical settings, it is associated with significant mortality and morbidity both during and post hospitalization (Balas et al., 2007; McAvay et al., 2006). The PMH-APRN will encounter patients who present with delirium requiring hospitalization as well as those returning home from acute care with incomplete remission of delirium. Clients who have preexisting cognitive impairments limiting capacity for self-care are at risk for delirium due to poor management of food and fluid intake, medications, and emerging illness. The APRN will increasingly be involved in treating and managing episodes of delirium resulting from urinary and upper respiratory infections (URIs), dehydration, and medication-related mishaps.

ASSESSMENT OF DELIRIUM

Clinical practice guidelines for delirium include diagnosis, assessment of clinical status, management, and intervention (APA, 2004). Delirium is a medical emergency and prompt diagnosis and treatment of the underlying cause is imperative. The goal of the PMH-APRN is to identify clients who are vulnerable to the development of delirium, recognize early signs of delirium, determine the etiology, and rapidly institute measures to correct underlying causes. In addition to early diagnosis and prompt medical treatment, therapeutic goals include managing the acute confusion to prevent injury or further cognitive decline, and education of the family or caregiver regarding the importance of prompt medical evaluation of any change in behavior.

A thorough history aids in the diagnosis of delirium. Obtain information about the onset, duration, and course of the episode from a reliable informant who knows the client well, can describe changes from his normal baseline status, and can report any precipitating biopsychosocial stressors. Ask about the hallmark symptoms of delirium: inability to focus attention, fluctuating consciousness, and disorganized thinking. Review all medications, dosages, changes in schedule, new or discontinued drugs, and use of over-the-counter drugs and botanicals. Particularly look for psychoactive drugs such as sedative-hypnotics, antidepressants, opioids, and anticholinergics. Review medical conditions including presence of pain. Ask about psychosocial factors such as loss of a family member, friend, or caregiver; a change in residence; or a recent change in the patient's behavior or mood indicating depression.

A thorough but targeted physical health assessment is crucial to determine the etiology of delirium. Laboratory evaluation should be based on presenting symptoms and directed to the common conditions that underlie delirium. These must always include a complete blood count, urinalysis, electrolytes, blood urea nitrogen, creatinine, glucose, thyroid function tests, and B12 and folate, along with a chest X-ray if there is evidence of upper respiratory infection (URI), and an electrocardiogram if there is evidence of heart disease. Additional laboratory analyses might be warranted based on physical findings or history including those assessing for syphilis (Veneral Disease Research Laboratory test [VDRL], Rapid Plasma Reagin [RPR]), or heavy metal screening (lead, mercury, arsenic). Diagnostic scans such as CT or MRI may be ordered especially for patients who have sustained recent head trauma, present with first episode of delirium, or are younger with atypical presentations. These can aid in detection of a subdural hematoma, hydrocephalus, cerebral vasculitis, or tumor.

SCREENING INSTRUMENTS FOR DELIRIUM

In the primary care setting, observation along with a brief history can determine the diagnosis, if not the etiology of the episode of delirium, but assessment tools may enhance detection. Two of these are the Delirium Observation Screening Scale or DOS, a 25-item instrument based on the *DSM-IV-TR* criteria for delirium (Schuurmans, Shortridge-Baggett, & Duursma, 2003), and the more widely used Confusion Assessment Method (CAM), a combination nine-item standardized instrument to assist clinicians with no psychiatric training in the recognition and detection of delirium, along with a four-item diagnostic algorithm (Inouye et al., 2000; Woodford & George, 2007). The CAM was developed in 1990 and was based on criteria from the older *DSM-III-R*. It has endured as a valid instrument to assist the clinician in attending to the hallmark features of delirium: acute onset, fluctuating course, inattention, altered level of consciousness, and cognitive disorganization. Although it has high reliability and validity for detection of delirium in inpatient settings, the CAM has not been validated for use in outpatient settings (Wei, Fearing, Sternberg, & Inouye, 2008). However, it enjoys widespread clinical use because of its ease of application and utility in both acute and long-term care environments. Exhibit 13-1 depicts the features of the CAM based on symptoms of delirium that could be used by the clinician to guide the interview with the client's caregiver.

SHARED DECISION MAKING/ACHIEVING CONCORDANCE

Many episodes of delirium will require hospitalization, but if the underlying cause of the delirium can be promptly and easily reversed, outpatient management is preferred, since hospitalization is itself a risk factor for development of delirium. Of prime consideration is the extent to which family or friends are available to assist and constantly observe the patient at home.

OUTCOMES

Outcomes will include resolution of the underlying cause of the delirium, ensuring safety of the patient and caregiver, resolution of perceptual distortions,

EXHIBIT 13-1: CONFUSION ASSESSMENT METHOD (CAM) QUESTIONNAIRE

OBSERVATIONS BY INTERVIEWER

Interviewer: Immediately after completing the interview, please answer the following questions based on what you observed during the interview, Modified Mini-Cog Test, and Digit Span Test.

ACUTE ONSET

1. a. Is there evidence of an acute change in mental status from the patient's baseline?

Yes - 1
No - 2
Uncertain - 8

b. (IF YES) Please describe change and source of information:

____

____

INATTENTION

2. a. Did the patient have difficulty focusing attention, for example being easily distractible, or having difficulty keeping track of what was being said?

Not present at any time during interview - 1
Present at some time during interview, but in mild form - 2
Present at some time during interview, in marked form - 3
Uncertain - 8

b. (IF PRESENT) Did this behavior fluctuate during the interview, that is, tend to come and go or increase and decrease in severity?

Yes - 1
No - 2
Uncertain - 8
Not applicable (NA) - 9

c. (IF PRESENT) Please describe this behavior:

____

____

____

DISORGANIZED THINKING

3. a. Was the patient's thinking disorganized or incoherent, such as rambling or irrelevant conversation, unclear or illogical flow of ideas, or unpredictable switching from subject to subject?

Not present at any time during interview - 1
Present at some time during interview, but in mild form - 2
Present at some time during interview, in marked form - 3
Uncertain - 8

b. (IF PRESENT) Did this behavior fluctuate during the interview, that is, tend to come and go or increase and decrease in severity?

Yes - 1
No - 2
Uncertain - 8
NA - 9

c. (IF PRESENT) Please describe this behavior:

____

____

____

(Continued)

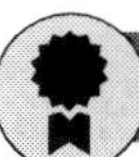

EXHIBIT 13-1: CONFUSION ASSESSMENT METHOD (CAM) QUESTIONNAIRE (*Continued*)

ALTERED LEVEL OF CONSCIOUSNESS

4. a. Overall, how would you rate this patient's level of consciousness?

GO TO Q5 ← Alert (Normal) - 1
Vigilant (Hyperalert, overly sensitive to environmental stimuli, startled very easily) - 2
Lethargic (Drowsy, easily aroused) - 3
Stupor (Difficult to arouse) - 4
Coma (Unarousable) - 5
Uncertain - 8

b. (IF OTHER THAN ALERT) Did this behavior fluctuate during the interview, that is, tend to come and go or increase and decrease in severity?

Yes - 1
No - 2
Uncertain - 8
NA - 9

c. (IF OTHER THAN ALERT) Please describe this behavior:

____
____
____

DISORIENTATION

5. a. Was the patient disoriented at any time during the interview, such as thinking he/she was somewhere other than the hospital, using the wrong bed, or misjudging the time of day?

Not present at any time during interview - 1
Present at some time during interview, but in mild form - 2
Present at some time during interview, in marked form - 3
Uncertain - 8

b. (IF PRESENT) Did this behavior fluctuate during the interview, that is, tend to come and go or increase and decrease in severity?

Yes - 1
No - 2
Uncertain - 8
NA - 9

c. (IF PRESENT) Please describe this behavior:

____
____
____

MEMORY IMPAIRMENT

6. a. Did the patient demonstrate any memory problems during the interview, such as inability to remember events in the hospital or difficulty remembering instructions?

Not present at any time during interview - 1
Present at some time during interview, but in mild form - 2
Present at some time during interview, in marked form - 3
Uncertain - 8

b. (IF PRESENT) Did this behavior fluctuate during the interview, that is, tend to come and go or increase and decrease in severity?

Yes - 1
No - 2
Uncertain - 8
NA - 9

(*Continued*)

EXHIBIT 13-1: CONFUSION ASSESSMENT METHOD (CAM) QUESTIONNAIRE (*Continued*)

c. (IF PRESENT) Please describe this behavior:

____

____

____

PERCEPTUAL DISTURBANCES

7. a. Did the patient have any evidence of perceptual disturbances, for example, hallucinations, illusions, or misinterpretations (such as thinking something was moving when it was not)?

   Not present at any time during interview - 1
   Present at some time during interview, but in mild form - 2
   Present at some time during interview, in marked form - 3
   Uncertain - 8

   b. (IF PRESENT) Did this behavior fluctuate during the interview, that is, tend to come and go or increase and decrease in severity?

   Yes - 1
   No - 2
   Uncertain - 8
   NA - 9

   c. (IF PRESENT) Please describe these perceptual changes:

____

____

____

PSYCHOMOTOR AGITATION

8. a. (Part 1) At any time during the interview, did the patient have an unusually increased level of motor activity, such as restlessness, picking at bedclothes, tapping fingers, or making frequent sudden changes of position?

   Not present at any time during interview - 1
   Present at some time during interview, but in mild form - 2
   Present at some time during interview, in marked form - 3
   Uncertain - 8

   b. (IF PRESENT) Did this behavior fluctuate during the interview, that is, tend to come and go or increase and decrease in severity?

   Yes - 1
   No - 2
   Uncertain - 8
   NA - 9

   c. (IF PRESENT) Please describe this behavior:

____

____

____

PSYCHOMOTOR RETARDATION

8. a. (Part 2) At any time during the interview, did the patient have an unusually decreased level of motor activity, such as sluggishness, staring into space, staying in one position for a long time, or moving very slowly?

   Not present at any time during interview - 1
   Present at some time during interview, but in mild form - 2
   Present at some time during interview, in marked form - 3
   Uncertain - 8

(Continued)

EXHIBIT 13-1: CONFUSION ASSESSMENT METHOD (CAM) QUESTIONNAIRE (*Continued*)

b. (IF PRESENT) Did this behavior fluctuate during the interview, that is, tend to come and go or increase and decrease in severity?

Yes - 1
No - 2
Uncertain - 8
NA - 9

c. (IF PRESENT) Please describe this behavior:

____
____
____

ALTERED SLEEP–WAKE CYCLE

9. a. Did the patient have evidence of disturbance of the sleep–wake cycle, such as excessive daytime sleepiness with insomnia at night?

Yes - 1
No - 2
Uncertain - 8

b. (IF YES) Please describe the disturbance:

____
____

Source: From Inouye, S. K. (2003). *The Confusion Assessment Method (CAM): Training Manual and Coding Guide*. New Haven, CT: Yale University School of Medicine. Used with permission.

elimination of patient anxiety, and restoration of the client to his previous level of cognitive and functional capacity.

TREATMENT OF DELIRIUM

PHARMACOLOGIC INTERVENTIONS

Medications should be minimized, used as a last resort, and triggered only by target symptoms such as severely agitated behavior, hallucinations, or paranoia severe enough to cause the client distress. If the client is having such symptoms, he should be treated in the hospital. Therefore it would be very unlikely that the PMH-APRN in primary care will be prescribing or administering medication for agitated behaviors associated with delirium. Response to medication should be tracked using clinical observation. Expert consensus guidelines recommend tapering the use of antipsychotics over a week once the delirium has been stabilized (Alexopoulos, Streim, Carpenter, & Docherty, 2004). The PMH-APRN may be involved in tapering medication as the patients is discharged from the hospital with delirium not completely resolved.

SUPPORTIVE INTERVENTIONS

Although delirium may not be managed in the primary care setting, the primary care PMH-APRN can consult with the treatment team to ensure that they are aware of the patient's baseline functioning. The PMH-APRN in the acute care setting may be the pivotal clinician ensuring the hospitalized patient receives appropriate supportive measures that prevent risk for injury, iatrogenic illness due to medication administration, further disability, and decline associated with immobility and use of restraints, and sensory deprivation or overload. Supportive measures focus on avoiding risk and increasing protective factors for the resolution of delirium. These include, but are not limited to, (a) close observation, (b) involvement of the family in care, (c) management of the environment to ensure adequate and appropriate levels of stimulation, (d) frequent reorientation of the patient to the environment with explanation for all procedures, (e) ensuring adequate hydration and nutrition by offering fluids regularly, (f) establishment and implementation of a toileting schedule, (g) mobilization of the patient to maintain conditioning, (h) utilization of comfort measures to decrease pain, and (i) client and family education regarding the transient and reversible nature of delirium to allay anxiety.

PREVENTION

Prevention of episodes of delirium is the best intervention. The PMH-APRN can practice primary, secondary, and tertiary prevention by (a) identifying and eliminating some of the risk factors associated with delirium by minimizing drug regimens and recommending influenza vaccines, (b) prompt recognition and treatment of conditions that may cause delirium, and (c) teaching caregivers of persons with cognitive impairment how to recognize acute changes in behavior as delirium and the importance of seeking prompt care to avoid further decline in functional status.

MILD COGNITIVE IMPAIRMENT

It is recognized that there are normal cognitive changes associated with aging. Speed of processing and retrieval and reaction time become slower with advancing age but the impairments do not affect function and generally are not progressive. Not all age-related cognitive slowing is benign, however, and some symptoms may represent the preclinical stages of dementia, leading to a diagnosis of MCI (Geldmacher, 2007). Core clinical criteria to refine the diagnosis of MCI are in development (Albert et al., 2011) and will further assist in early diagnosis and detection.

MCI is defined as problems with memory or language severe enough to be noticeable to others or to be detected on cognitive tests, but not severe enough to interfere with activities of daily living (ADLs). Scores between 26 and 30 on the Mini Mental Status Exam (MM) and less than 26 on the more sensitive Montreal Cognitive Assessment (MoCA) are indicative of MCI (American Geriatrics Society, 2011a). If memory loss is the predominant feature, this is amnestic MCI. The prevalence of MCI is estimated at 10% to 20% for those over age 65. MCI may remain the diagnosis for many years or may progress to dementia. Fifteen percent of this group will develop dementia within 1 year and half within 4 years (Alzheimer's Association, 2011).

DEMENTIA

The term *dementia* is from the Latin *de mens* meaning "out of the mind" and has often been used to describe the presence of a psychiatric, rather than a cognitive disorder. Simply defined, dementia is a clinical state characterized by loss of memory and other cognitive abilities severe enough to impair normal function (Geldmacher, 2007).

Although there are several different types of dementia, all forms affect memory and cognition. Unlike delirium, consciousness is usually not affected until later stages. Dementias are sometimes classified as primary or cortical types, of which Alzheimer's disease is the prototype, and subcortical, of which vascular dementia (VD) is the prototype. Further classification of dementias due to infections, toxins, structural abnormalities, and other, possibly reversible causes has been proposed, and nomenclature of the major dementias may, and often does, differ. The landscape is changing as developments in imaging, biomarkers, and recognition of new subtypes of cognitive impairment emerge from research and clinical practice. A new category, *neurocognitive disorders*, has been proposed for the *DSM-5* to replace the *DSM-IV* categories of delirium, dementia, amnestic, and other cognitive disorders. For now, the last published APA nomenclature for Alzheimer's and VD will be used, frontotemporal dementia (FTD) as a broader category will replace Picks Disease, and a more current nomenclature of TBI will replace post head trauma dementia. Lewy Body dementia (LBD) as a specific entity will be described. The rarer forms of dementia will be briefly noted primarily in how they may present and differ.

Dementia is a syndrome characterized by progressive and global cognitive decline resulting from one or many of several biological etiologies. The United States National Institute of Neurological Disorders (NINDS, 2007) reported prevalence rates of dementia at between 4 and 6.8 million people. AD, is thought to be responsible for between 50% and 75% of all dementias, followed by VD (15–25%), and LBD (10%) (Alzheimer's Association, 2011). The incidence and prevalence of AD directly correlates with increased age, since every 5 years after age 65 the rate of AD doubles. AD is present in one of eight, or 13% of people aged 65 years and older, and the incidence rises to nearly one of every two people aged 85 and older (Alzheimer's Association, 2011). Currently 5.4 million Americans have AD, but it is projected that by midcentury the number of people with this illness will reach as many as 16 million.

ETIOLOGY

As there are multiple etiologies of dementia, there are many associated risk factors. The causes are difficult to differentiate because they are imprecise, can sometimes be confirmed only upon postmortem examination, and can overlap, as in AD and VD. The risk factors for dementia include age, family history, genetics, cerebral vascular disease, head trauma, and the presence of MCI (Alzheimer's Association, 2011). Persons with lower levels of education and lower socioeconomic status have higher rates of dementia. Extension of education may be protective due to developing more cognitive reserve (Hall et al., 2009). The many risk factors associated with lower economic status may account for higher levels of dementia in this population.

ALZHEIMER'S DEMENTIA

AD is the most prevalent of the dementias. It is a degenerative progressive neuropsychiatric disorder resulting in global impairment of cognition, emotions, and behavior leading to physical and functional decline and death. The precise etiology of AD is unknown and most likely multifactoral, a combination of genetic vulnerability and exposure to environmental and psychosocial stressors. The role of various biopsychosocial factors such as genetics, inflammation, oxidative stress, vascular changes, metabolic factors, beta-amyloid and tau proteins, lifestyles and education levels, hormones, and growth factors are being investigated.

The hallmark pathological features of AD are the presence of neurofibrillary tangles and beta amyloid plaques in the brain on postmortem examination, and the definitive diagnosis of AD is based on their presence. The disease process of AD results in neuronal death and the disruption of neurotransmission, especially that of the neurotransmitter acetylcholine (ACh), which is critically important to memory and cognition. Acetylcholinesterase inhibitors have demonstrated their efficacy in slowing the process of Alzheimer's disease (Craig & Birks, 2006; Loy & Schneider, 2006), and neuronal destruction with concomitant disruption of ACh transmission is thought to be a cause of cognitive impairment in AD.

AD may be transmitted genetically, as evidenced by the certain development of AD in adult clients with Down's syndrome (resulting from a defect in chromosome 21. See Figure 13-1 for an illustration of this pathology in Alzheimer's Disease), and those with familial AD who have genetic mutations on chromosomes 1, 14, and 21. People who carry the apolipoprotein E (apoE) gene found on chromosome 19 also carry higher risk for the disorder. Other chromosomes are being investigated to determine if they have a role in the formation of the beta amyloid plaques.

Damage to cells from oxygen free radicals (oxidative stress) may cause neuron dysfunction resulting in production of tangles and plaques and cell death. Inflammatory processes and high cholesterol levels have been investigated as a cause of AD. An immunologic defect also has been implicated as a cause of AD because of abnormally high antibody titers found in some patients (Alzheimer's Association, 2011).

Psychosocial and environmental factors such as exposure to environmental toxins, diet, lifestyle, and psychological stress have been implicated. More highly educated individuals and those with higher incomes have lower rates of AD. Education and participating in intellectually stimulating activities are thought to reduce risk. Industrialized countries seem to have higher rates of AD than do developing countries; however, this may partially be due to a longer life span in which to develop the illness.

VASCULAR DEMENTIA

VD results from multiple infarcts in the cortex and the white matter of the brain following brain hemorrhage or ischemia. It tends to appear comorbidly with AD rather than as a discrete entity (Vishwanathan, Rocca, & Tzourio, 2009). Although its incidence is thought to be considerably less than AD, it may be the most common dementia in men and in those older than 85 years of age. Risk factors for VD parallel those for cerebrovascular accident and include hypertension, smoking, hyperlipidemia, atrial fibrillation, and diabetes. The course of VD has a more abrupt onset and stepwise pattern of progression when compared to the progressive and gradual cognitive decline of AD.

The specific symptomatology seen with this dementia depends on the sectors of the brain affected and the extent to which they are damaged. Frequently, there is accompanying neurologic evidence of cerebrovascular disease, such as paresis or paralysis of a limb or headaches. Diagnostic testing (MRI and CT scan) often verify vascular brain disease in people with this particular dementia. On physical examination the patient may have carotid bruits, fundoscopic abnormalities, or enlarged heart chambers and focal neurologic signs (NIND, 2007).

DEMENTIA WITH LEWY BODIES

LBD is a type of dementia that is quite distinct and more prevalent than once thought. The exact incidence of LBD is unknown but is estimated at 10% of all dementias. Because LBD is characterized by earlier and more prominent visual hallucinations, parkinsonian features, behavior disturbances, and parasomnias, the psychiatric PMH-APRN may be one of the first clinicians to diagnosis and treat clients with this form of dementia. When antipsychotic drugs are used to treat the hallucinations, these clients often have significant adverse effects and worsening of agitated behaviors (NIND, 2007).

Lewy Bodies are the defining lesions found in the substantia nigra of persons with Parkinson's disease. These lesions are found in the limbic and cortical areas of the

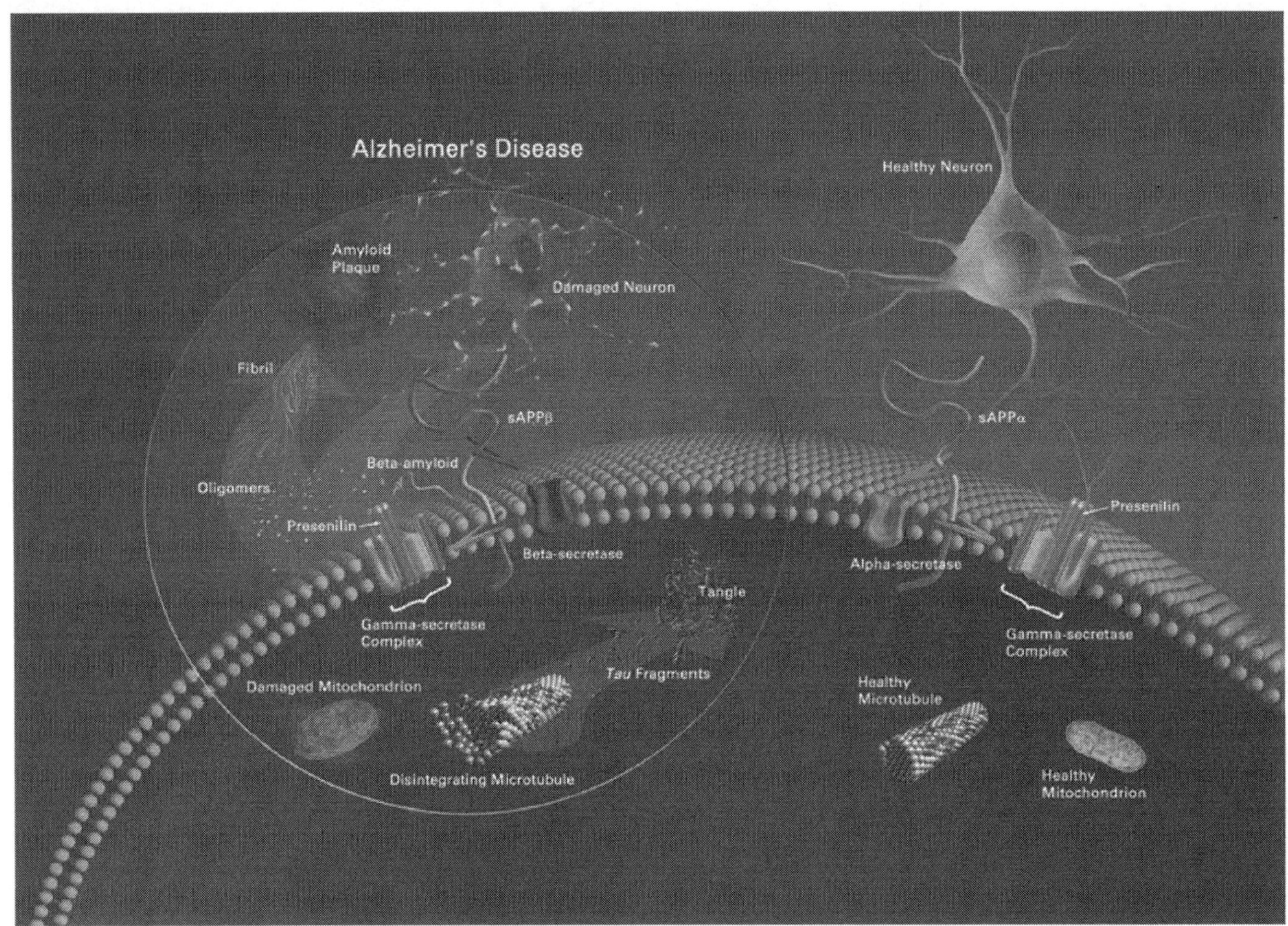

Figure 13-1 X Pathology of Alzheimer's Disease

Source: Used courtesy of the National Institute of Aging, National Institutes of Health website: www.nia.nih.gov

brain in a subgroup of individuals with late onset dementia. The presence of Lewy inclusion bodies in the cerebral cortex on autopsy confirms the diagnosis. Because of some clinical similarity, LBD can be mistaken for AD.

DEMENTIA IN PARKINSON'S DISEASE

Parkinson's disease is a neurodegenerative illness characterized by a decreasing number of neurons in the substantia nigra, resulting in a depletion of the neurotransmitter, dopamine. This disease affects 1 million Americans and, though its predominate clinical picture is that of motor disturbance, the cognitive decline of dementia is estimated between 20% to more than 30% of affected clients (NIND, 2006). The client exhibits resting tremor, slowness, and rigidity along with postural instability. The gait disturbance and cognitive deficits accompanying this disease vary, although the course is insidious and progressive. The dementia of Parkinson's disease does not impair the client's language capabilities, as do many of the other dementias, but it does not spare the client's memory retrieval and executive functioning.

Though patients with Parkinson's disease may receive specialty care for the illness though a neurologist, they are likely to be seen in primary care for other conditions. Because treatment with dopamine precursors and agonists to enhance movement may cause side effects appearing as hallucinations and delusions, the psychiatric PMH-APRN may be involved in the care of persons with this illness.

FRONTOTEMPORAL DEMENTIA

FTD, of which Pick's Disease is a subtype, accounts for about 5% of the progressive dementias. Onset occurs between ages 40 and 60 years, and men are more likely to be affected. Those with a first-degree relative with Pick's disease are at greater risk for development of the disease. (NIND, 2007). Although the cause is unknown, abnormal function of tau protein is associated with the illness (NIND, 2007). In the beginning stages, the victims of this disorder have less disorientation and memory loss than those with Alzheimer's disease, and more personality changes, including loss of social constraints, resulting in frequent behavioral problems. Therefore, the psychiatric PMH-APRN may be consulted at onset of the illness. A second type presents with aphasia rather than behavioral symptoms.

OTHER FORMS OF DEMENTIA

Huntington's disease is a hereditary disorder caused by a faulty gene for a protein (huntingtin). As it is an autosomal dominant trait, children of affected parents have a 50% chance of inheriting the trait-carrying gene. Men and women are equally affected with inevitable manifestation of the disease in persons with the trait in their thirties or forties. As the course from onset to death is approximately 15 years (NINDS, 2007), it is not a dementia associated with older adults.

Dementia due to HIV/AIDS was initially associated with a younger population though advances in treatment have enabled persons with the illness to live longer. In untreated HIV AIDS, the detection of dementia is confounded by infections, tumors, and adverse reactions to drugs. The clinician should be alert for mild cognitive decline or neurological symptoms such as headaches, vision changes, and neuropathies that might signal central nervous system involvement in the patient with AIDS. Symptoms may alternate between memory loss and confusion and mental clarity and can stabilize for months before resuming downward progression.

Dementia due to TBI may present in younger populations as a result of accidents and combat, but is also a risk for older adults as a result of falls. Barnes et al. (2011), in a review of medical records of nearly 300,000 veterans age 55 and over, found those who had had a previous TBI were more than twice as likely to develop dementia. Symptoms of TBI can be mild, moderate, or severe, depending on the extent of the injury. Mild and subtle symptoms include physical symptoms such as headache, dizziness, and blurred vision and neuropsychiatric symptoms such as difficulty with memory, attention, concentration, mood, and sleep. Although mild symptoms may appear to resolve, they can progress over years to measurable MCI and dementia. Language and communication problems along with emotional and behavioral problems are typical with TBI (NIND, 2011).

Creutzfeldt-Jakob disease is a rare disease caused by a protein called a prion body that affects multiple neurological systems. As it has a worldwide incidence of about one new case per 1 million people per year (NINDS, 2007), the PMH-APRN is unlikely to encounter a patient with this form of dementia. However, as the initial symptoms are more suggestive of psychiatric, rather than cognitive disorder, it is possible the psychiatric PMH-APRN would be the first clinician consulted in those rare situations.

AMNESTIC DISORDERS

Amnestic disorders are characterized by short-term memory loss and decline in social and occupational functioning. Although differing etiologies are responsible for amnestic disorders, Korsakoff's syndrome, one of the substance-induced persisting amnestic disorders, is most prevalent. A client with this disorder has great difficulty with recent, or episodic memory, and therefore has difficulty learning new information. Because of the inability to recall recent events, the individual fills in memory gaps with fabricated or imagined data and stories can become quite fantastic. Wernicke's syndrome describes the physical symptoms of ataxia, confusion, and paralysis of some of the motor muscles of the eye, while Korsakoff's results from lack of treatment at this stage. Both syndromes, Wernicke's and Korsakoff's, are caused by the client's chronic alcohol use, resulting in poor nutritional intake and resulting thiamine deficiency that interferes with production of glucose in the brain. This syndrome usually is found in the 40- to 70-year-old client with a history of steady and progressive alcohol intake (Kopelman, Thomson, Guerrini, & Marshall, 2009).

CLINICAL SIGNS AND COURSE OF DEMENTIA

For the remainder of the chapter, AD will be used as a prototype for all the dementias, because it is the most common, and except where noted earlier, the dementias have similar illness trajectories, outcomes, and approaches to treatment. The decline in intellectual ability and cognitive functional capacity seen in AD occurs over a 2- to 10-year period. Subtle changes in recent memory and personality occur early and may go unrecognized by all but the individual. As this prodromal phase ends, memory impairment becomes more severe and deficits in visuospatial and executive function appear. Difficulty finding words (aphasia) and performing tasks (apraxia) worsen. Eventually the client experiences agnosia, the failure to recognize objects and people.

Staging of the symptoms of AD into early, intermediate, and severe dementia with characteristic clusters of symptoms assists in the description of the course of decline and guides the clinician to areas of assessment during the history. Staging also informs choice of interventions and assists clients and families to know where they are in the process of the illness, a question they frequently ask. The three broad categories of early, moderate, and severe have been further refined using one of several dementia rating and staging scales described with screening instruments. Though the diagnosis of dementia is based on both cognitive and functional capacity, the landscape continues to change, as MCI is now included as a first stage by some and biomarkers that can identify preclinical disease have been identified but are not yet ready for use in clinical practice.

Amnestic MCI described previously is probably the prodromal stage of dementia. At this stage the client may temporarily forget where he placed an item, may forget names, and may find the word he was about to utter, slipping away. The line between benign age-related slowing of cognitive processing and retrieval of information and MCI can be quite blurred.

EARLY STAGE

Early dementia is characterized by impaired short-term memory and inability to learn new material. Individuals may forget where they put something and repeat the same questions. Word finding becomes difficult and the client may attempt to compensate by describing the item when the name cannot be located. Complex tasks once easy for the patient such as balancing a checkbook or cooking a meal become impossible. Changes in affect, behavior, and judgment are typical. Social skills are initially preserved but irritability and defensiveness may occur if the memory impairment is noted and addressed. Compensation for deficits can occur in the early stage unless there is change of routine, such as a trip to a relative. Many families describe the long-awaited vacation becoming a nightmare when the older adult becomes agitated due to being in an unfamiliar environment. Apraxia, disorders of skilled movement, become evident at this stage. Ideomotor apraxia is the difficulty of translating an idea into the corresponding action, resulting in impairments in managing routine tasks, and creating safety risks.

INTERMEDIATE STAGE

In this stage the patient's ability to learn new material and perform ADL's declines as the patient develops agnosia, or failure to recognize items, which may lead to misperception of the environment and further risk of injury. Significant agitation due to paranoid ideation, wandering, hoarding, and inappropriate sexual behavior often begin in this stage. Reporting on a variety of studies, Tampi et al. (2011, Part I) found that between 33% and 80% of persons with dementia exhibit some type of behavior disturbance during the course of the illness. Behavior and affect may worsen over the course of the day, with more impairment toward evening.

LATE STAGE

In later stages, the individual will require total ADL assistance, will be unable to recognize even close family members, and will eventually develop dysphasia. The risk for dehydration and malnutrition is high along with infection; a typical causes of death in those affected.

SHARED DECISION MAKING/ACHIEVING CONCORDANCE

Clinical practice guidelines for AD stress the importance of early recognition and treatment to preserve function and help the patient and family plan for the future. The importance of early recognition and treatment of all types of dementia cannot be overstated. Recognition of those conditions that are reversible can restore cognition in some, and early diagnosis of AD can assist the patient and family to secure resources, receive treatment, and preserve function as long as possible.

Due to cognitive impairment, communication strategies for conveying diagnostic and treatment information may need to be modified. The PMH-APRN should start with the premise that the client can understand, particularly in the earlier stages of the disease process. Simple, clear information, use of visual aids, and allowing ample time to discuss options and ask questions will enhance communication and the therapeutic alliance. Discussion of the benefits as well as the limitations and side effects of medications will assist the client and family in making informed decisions regarding treatment options. It is particularly important to create an emotionally supportive milieu and focus on interventions that can improve quality of life and preserve function despite the inevitable trajectory of the illness.

Clients are often very anxious, may be suspicious, and are concerned about loss of independence. Difficult discussions about driving safety, accepting more assistance with ADLs, and planning for the time when transition to assisted living or skilled care may need to occur are very sensitive and complicated. Allaying anxiety and focusing on strengths, while acknowledging the realities of the illness, are essential. Although caregivers may, and often do, need time apart from the client to fully discuss their concerns, the PMH-APRN should always include the client in discussions that occur in the clinic setting, address remarks to the client, and provide contact information for the caregiver to enable opportunities to provide information and discuss concerns that would be too painful or disruptive to discuss in the presence of the client. The ideal is to ask both client and caregiver if the caregiver can provide their view of the situation during the clinic visit. Modeling how to initiate and discuss concerns openly together can assist families in coping with painful topics.

In middle to later stages of dementia, it is important to continue efforts to communicate directly with the client through attentive listening, providing reassuring verbal and nonverbal cues, and observing nonverbal behaviors of the client that signal comfort or distress.

The recognition of caregiver burden and the importance of establishmenting a supportive treatment alliance with caregivers cannot be overstated. Much research supports the psychological and physical impact on caregivers for a person with dementia (Andren & Elmstahl, 2008; Campbell, 2009; Gaugler et al., 2010; Wright et al., 2010). Management of dementia begins with enlistment of caregivers as integral members of the treatment team. The PMH-APRN provides emotional support and guidance to caregivers and works closely with them in monitoring and evaluating both psychosocial and pharmacological interventions. Most families struggle valiantly to assist the patient with lost abilities. They have learned what interventions are most effective, and, instead of offering advice, the PMH-APRN can listen to their concerns and learn what resources they need to continue the difficult work of caregiving. Information regarding the illness, the expected course, treatment, and intervention options, along with community resources and referrals to the Alzheimer's Association (see website listing), and other support services should be offered. Information about respite care and long-term care options can be provided as well as guidance on legal issues such as durable power of attorney and guardianship. These issues can be initiated with the patient and family with sensitivity as to their readiness to discuss these topics. As noted, availability of the clinician to offer caregiver support outside the clinic hours can both secure the alliance and prevent or delay caregiver distress and institutionalization of the patient. A structured telephone support intervention has been demonstrated to lower burden scores and improve coping of dementia caregivers (Tremont, Davis, Bishop, & Fortinsky, 2011).

Although the client is the primary focus of assessment and intervention, family-centered care is critical to quality treatment outcomes. Accordingly, assessment of caregivers and interventions to support them are crucial. The PMH-APRN needs to assess caregivers for depression and anxiety as well as the identified client. In addition to screening instruments noted in Chapters 8 (affective disorders) and 9 (anxiety disorders), there are a myriad of caregiver self-assessment instruments measuring burden, quality of life, and needs (Deeken, Taylor, Mangan, Yabroff, & Ingham, 2003). Although used primarily in research settings rather than clinical practice, a simple, easy-to-use instrument could be given to caregivers to elicit information regarding concerns, burden, and stress level prior to the clinic appointment. The Zarit Burden Interview (ZBI), a popular caregiver self-report questionnaire, is the most widely used instrument for measurement of caregiver burden. It originated as a 29-item questionnaire (Zarit, Reever, & Bach-Peterson, 1980). The revised version contains 22 items. Each item on the interview is a statement that the caregiver is asked to endorse using a 5-point scale. Response options range from 0 (Never) to 4 (Nearly Always). The use of the ZBI for educational and clinical purposes without cost requires permission, which can be obtained at www.mapitrust.org. There is a substantial fee for commercial use.

Caregiver support and education groups are likely to be helpful to caregivers and should be recommended. The use of psychoeducational approaches that require active participation from caregivers has been demonstrated to be most effective in enhancing family coping. Other interventions such as individual supportive psychotherapy, cognitive behavioral therapy, respite care, day care, and others have shown small but meaningful effects on reducing caregiver burden and depressive symptoms but have been more difficult to evaluate due to lack of research and more variation in how they are measured (Pinquart & Sorensen, 2006). The Alzheimer's Association is one of the best resources for providing psychoeducational interventions, along with a vast array of other services, for caregivers of persons with any type of cognitive impairment.

ASSESSMENT

Determining the presence of cognitive disorders and designing appropriate treatment for persons with dementia is a complex and stepwise process. Various groups, both nationally and internationally, have developed clinical practice guidelines for the treatment of Alzheimer's disease. The guidelines assist the clinician from assessment and diagnosis to working with clients and families at the last stages of the disease (Albert et al., 2011; Alexopoulos, Jeste, & Chung, 2005; American Geriatrics Society, 2011; Jack et al., 2011; McCullough, 2009; Sperling et al., 2011a). The history taking should ideally include a family member or other person in addition to the identified patient, who may, because of the illness, not be a reliable informant. Family caregiver questionnaires have been demonstrated to be an efficient and reliable way of screening for dementia in primary care (Monnot, Brosey, & Ross, 2005). When taking the history, the clinician needs to ask questions designed to assess the major symptoms of AD, including memory (the ability to learn and retain new information); cognition (handling complex tasks, reasoning ability, orientation, and language); and behavior. Given the importance of assessing functional status, specific questions regarding ADL's and instrumental activities of daily living (IADL) should be included as well. In determining the presence of dementia, a comprehensive history, physical examination, and diagnostic laboratory tests are necessary. The physical examination should include a neurological examination and a mental status exam with a formal assessment of cognition and memory. To determine treatment approaches and facilitate shared decision making, the clinician needs to determine the health status and capability of the likely caregiver along with the safety of the patient's home environment.

Knowledge of the diagnostic criteria for dementia will guide PMH-APRN assessment of the client. *DSM-IV-TR* criteria for Dementia of the Alzheimer's Type includes the presence of gradual and insidious cognitive decline and impairment in social and occupational functioning from a previous higher level. The cognitive decline may include aphasia, apraxia, and/or agnosia in addition to decline in memory and executive functioning (planning, organizing, and sequencing).

HISTORY

The history needs to be conducted with a reliable informant if possible, as the client may not be able to provide accurate information regarding his history or current functioning. Often the diagnosis of dementia can be made on the basis of a comprehensive history alone. All patients with memory complaints should have a careful targeted history, not just those with suspected dementia. The use of diagnostic criteria from *DSM-IV-TR* and assessment parameters from the Clinical Practice Guidelines can be used to assess and document symptoms related to the disorder and to ask about onset, duration, and progression for each. Assessment may be made more challenging if the client has been resistant to coming for "a checkup" and the visit was initiated by a concerned family member. Active listening, allowing more time and privacy, and arranging a subsequent visit to collect further data are useful strategies.

PHYSICAL

Physical assessment of the older patient with suspected dementia often requires very good communication skills and the ability to establish therapeutic rapport. The client may attempt to hide symptoms, fearing that detection of the cognitive disorder may result in loss of independence or embarrassment. In the early stages the patient preserves social skills and is frequently able to appear intact. He may make up responses on the MM rather than appear impaired. A careful physical examination, including neurological assessment, may reveal reversible causes of dementia, detect impending delirium, differentiate VD, and aid in early detection of primary progressive dementia. Components of the physical examination are found in Exhibit 13-2.

Based on the history and physical obtained, the clinician may obtain diagnostic tests to rule out reversible causes of dementia and differentiate between dementias. Diagnostic tests to assess for delirium and conditions causing cognitive impairment are found in Exhibit 13-3. Basic diagnostics for patients being evaluated for dementia include those noted as baseline and those noted as additional (B12 and folate, serology, and CT or MRI scan). If indicated, some patients may require a more comprehensive neuropsychiatric evaluation, Positron emission tomographt (PET) or single photon emission computed tomography (SPECT) scan.

MENTAL STATUS EXAMINATION

The mental status examination is best presented as part of the physical examination and after rapport has been established to maximize patient comfort and allay anxiety. Components of the MSE include mood and affect,

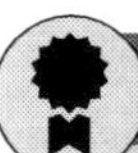

EXHIBIT 13-2: GUIDE TO THE HISTORY AND PHYSICAL EXAMINATION

HISTORY

Does the client have difficulty learning and retaining new information? Does she lose things, forget appointments, and have difficulty remembering a recent conversation? Was this abrupt? Is it getting better or worse? How long has this been present?

Does the client have difficulty managing complex tasks? Is he able to balance the checkbook, organize bills, and plan a simple garden?

Does the client have difficulty reasoning? Can she manage a minor crisis at home or work such as a change in routine or a heavier workload?

Is the client having difficulty with spatial organization and orientation? Does he seem distractible? Is he having difficulty organizing things at home or driving? Often caregivers report that they realized there was a problem when their family member was unable to remember how to drive home.

Is the client having difficulty with language? Does she substitute words, try to identify items with a description, or avoid conversations?

Is the client exhibiting a change in behavior? Is the client less responsive, more irritable or misinterpreting visual stimuli? Is the patient depressed, anxious, or paranoid?

Obtain medical history, including psychiatric illness, head injury, and systemic or neurologic illness, as these are risk factors for dementia.

Assess current medications, including use of botanicals, over the counter (OTC).

Ask about use of alcohol, tobacco, and other substances as well as exposure to toxins.

Obtain a family medical history, including presence of AD and VD, and early onset dementias.

Assess instrumental activities of daily living by using the FAQ or other screening tool.

Ask about recent changes, losses, and other stressors.

Obtain psychosocial history from family as well as cultural information.

Assess the caregiver for caregiver stress. Instruments have been used in research, but some tools may be adaptable for clinical use.

Assess for elder abuse and neglect using the SAFE Questions or other screening tool. S—Ask about stress and safety; A—Ask about physical, psychological, sexual, financial, abuse or neglect; F. Ask about family and friends; E—Ask about an emergency plan.

PHYSICAL

Obtain vital signs (VS) with orthostatic blood pressure (B/P) to assess falls risk, nutritional status, and medication effects.

Weigh client to assess nutrition, establish baseline, collect data related to diagnosis.

Assess hearing and vision.

Conduct complete physical with emphasis on cardiovascular, neurological, and respiratory status.

Genitourinary exam, unless critical, can be delayed to a subsequent visit.

Conduct cardiovascular exam. Listen for carotid bruits.

Assess gait, balance, and mobility. Signs suggestive of Parkinson's should be noted.

Assess cranial nerves, motor nerves, and sensory system and reflexes. Focal neurological signs such as weakness, sensory loss, Babinski's sign, exaggerated reflexes, and visual field defects are diagnostic for VD.

Assess cognition using the MM. The MM should be presented as part of the physical examination of the patient to allay anxiety. The family may need to be reminded not to prompt or help.

Screen for signs of abuse and neglect. Particularly look for signs of dehydration, multiple skin lesions in various stages of evolution, bruises and welts on the trunk, rectal or vaginal bleeding, pressure sores, infestations traumatic alopecia, poor hygiene, wrist or ankle lesions, occult fracture, pain or gait disturbance. Look for behavioral signs such as depression and anxiety.

Obtain diagnostic evaluations noted in text Exhibit 13-3. Assess need for CT or MRI.

EXHIBIT 13-3: LABORATORY TESTS TO DETECT CAUSE FOR DELIRIUM

Renal failure (*blood urea nitrogen [BUN], Creatinine, Albumin*)
Diabetes (*Serum Glucose*)
Malnutrition (*B12, Folate*)
Hepatic dysfunction (*Liver Enzymes, Aspartate ammotransferase test [AST], Bilirubin*)
Thyroid dysfunction (*thyrois stimulating hormone [TSH], T3, T4*)
Infection (*Sedimentation Rate, Urinalysis, white blood count [WBC]*)
Cardiac status (*electrocardiogram [EKG], troponin level*)
Electrolytes (*NA+, K+, Ca2+, Cl-, Mg+*)
Drug and alcohol screen

speech, perception, judgment and insight, and cognition and memory. In clients with disordered cognition, the MSE is often primarily, but not exclusively, focused on the components of cognition including attention, memory, language and speech, visuospatial skills, and executive functioning.

Mood and Affect

It is critically important to assess mood and affect as depression is prevalent particularly in early stages of dementia and frequently older adults with undiagnosed depression report problems with memory and concentration. Treatment of depression leads to improved functional capacity in clients with dementia and resolution of memory impairments in those who suffer from depression. As older adults have the highest rates of completed suicides, the PMH-APRN must always assess suicide risk. In later stages of dementia it is sometimes difficult to distinguish depressed affect from apathy associated with the disease progression. Therefore, asking about mood, observing affect, and asking the family about behavior are important at each appointment. The Geriatric Depression Scale (GDS), a 30-item questionnaire developed by Brink et al. (1982), the shorter 15-item version (Sheikh & Yesavage, 1986), and other the screening instruments described in Chapter 8 for detection of depression are valuable clinical tools to both detect depression and track treatment response. Assessment of mood and affect can also assist with differential diagnosis, as the person with a rarer form of dementia may present with a euphoric or labile affect and an expansive or irritable mood.

Perceptual Distortions

Perceptual distortions, including delusions and hallucinations, are a common feature of most forms of dementia and, in some cases such as Lewy Body dementia, benign hallucinations are a prominent feature. Tampi et al. (2011, Part I) in a review of multiple studies found hallucinations, paranoia, accusatory behavior, and delusions in 45% of patients less than one month after formal diagnosis. Usually these are symptoms occurring in the moderate stage of dementia but suspiciousness can appear earlier. A median of over 36% of clients had delusions and 23% had hallucinations at some point during the course of the illness (Tampi et al., 2011, Part I). These rates were even greater in long-term care settings. The psychotic cluster of symptoms may lead to behavioral symptoms such as agitation and aggression, wandering, and screaming. Although these difficult symptoms and behaviors may have prompted the initial visit and are likely to prompt phone calls to the PMH-APRN once the relationship is established, the family may find it difficult to discuss them in the initial clinical interview in the presence of the patient. Accordingly, a symptom checklist the caregiver can complete or a separate interview time facilitates assessment and intervention.

Judgment and Insight

Judgment and insight are usually assessed in the context of the cognitive evaluation along with the client's history, general presentation, and demeanor. The MSE standard question, "What would you do if you found a stamped addressed envelope on the ground?" can reveal errors in judgment. However, at this point in a comprehensive assessment the PMH-APRN most likely has a sense of the client's judgment ability through the process of the clinical interview. Clients with cognitive impairment may report having no idea why they are coming to the appointment, may insist they are able to perform all ADLs without assistance, and may be irritated with the family for expressing concern. In early stages of the illness, the client may believe he is competent to continue to drive or perform other activities that are no longer safe.

Cognition and Memory

A rapid cognitive screening examination for detection of Alzheimer's disease in primary care settings developed by

Geldmacher (2003) suggests the clinician open the interview by asking a question to assess abstract thinking such as: "Tell me what you enjoy doing in your spare time." If the response is abstract and well formed, no further formal assessment is indicated. If it is vague, without detail or not concrete, further evaluation is warranted.

The assessment of memory is complex as there are four subtypes of memory: episodic (related to personal experiences such as what one ate for breakfast), semantic (related to facts such as who is the President of the country), procedural (such as remembering how to drive), and working (the capacity to briefly retain information such as dialing a phone number) (Woodford & George, 2007). Simple diagnostic tools are very useful for the assessment of cognition in each of these domains. Geldmacher (2003) suggests rapid cognitive screening of learning can be assessed by asking the client to repeat and remember three words. Working memory or calculation is assessed by asking him to state how much money he would have by adding a penny, a nickel, a dime, and a quarter. Semantic memory as well as language comprehension can be evaluated by naming the parts of clothing (e.g., lapel, collar, sleeve) as the examiner points to them. Finally, some aspects of procedural memory, ideomotor praxis, and temporoparietal function can be evaluated by asking the client to demonstrate opening a door with a key, slicing bread, using his left hand to point to the examiners' left hand, and giving a two-stage command such as "Before pointing to the ceiling, point to the door." The clock draw test is described later and is used to assess both visuospatial and executive functions. If the patient does not do well on two or more of these measures, Geldmacher suggests further evaluation with a standardized measure of cognition such as the MM, diagnostic lab work, a neurological examination, or imaging. Referral for more sophisticated neuropsychological testing may be indicated to inform the diagnosis and differentiate the type of cognitive impairment.

DIAGNOSTIC TOOLS

Cognitive Screening Tools

Screening tools that assess cognition, mental status, and memory can assist the PMH-APRN in diagnosis as well as monitoring effectiveness of interventions. There are a multitude of assessment tools available but those most used in primary care include the Short, Portable Mental Status Questionnaire (SPMSQ) (Pfeiffer, 1982), the Folstein MM (Folstein, Folstein, & Hugh, 1975), the Clock Draw Test (CDT) (Shulman, Shedletsky, & Silver, 1986), the MiniCog (Borson, Scanlan, Watanabe, Tu, & Lessing, 2006), and the MoCA (Nasreddine et al., 2005).

The MM has been the most familiar screening measurement worldwide and remains the standard for the assessment of memory. It has excellent reliability and validity and is widely used in primary care practice for detecting and tracking progressive cognitive impairment. Scores below 23 were initially recommended for sensitivity and specificity for dementia but in highly educated community populations, scores between 24 and 27 should trigger further evaluation. The tool now has age- and education-related cutoffs. One limitation is the "ceiling effect." Scores of 30 do not mean the person has no cognitive impairment, and scores of 0 do not mean an absence of cognition (Woodford & George, 2007). A second version, the MM-2, has just been published. It avoids the ceiling effect, is more sensitive to MCI, and is available in short, standard, and expanded formats. All versions of the MM are copyrighted and require permission to use. Information as to how to purchase the instrument and who may administer it can be obtained at www.parinc.com.

The SPMSQ was developed for use in primary care. It is a 10-item screening tool asking the client the date, month, and year, the day of the week, the name of the place, the client's phone number, his age, and date of birth, the name of the current president, the president before the current, and the client's mother's maiden name, and then count backward from 20 by 3s. One point is given for each incorrect answer. A score of less than 2 indicates normal mental functioning; 3–4 errors, MCI; 5–7 errors, moderate cognitive impairment; and more than 8, severe cognitive impairment. One less error is allowed if the client has post secondary education and one more if he has less than an eighth grade education (Pfeiffer, 1975). Permission to use the SPMSQ in service and research programs can be obtained by emailing Dr. Pfeiffer at epfeiffer@health.usf.edu.

Since neither the MM nor the SPMSQ assesses abstract thinking and frontal executive function, the PMH-APRN can add the Clock Draw Test (CDT) (Shulman et al., 1986) to cover these dimensions of assessment or use another screening instrument that includes the CDT, such as the Mini Cog or the MoCA. For the CDT the client is asked to draw a clock, put the numbers on it, and place the hands at 20 after 8, or 10 after 11. This simple assessment tool tests executive functioning, visuospatial skills, and general organization. Like the MM, it is sensitive to changes over time. There are multiple manners in which this tool can be scored, but the simplest is a three-point system allotting one point for the drawing, one for the numbers in the correct position, and one for the time depicted correctly. The CDT alone can be used in clinical practice without permission.

The Mini Cog adds a three-word recall test to the CDT and is a good brief instrument for use in primary care. The client is given 3 minutes to draw the clock. If the client is unable to remember any of the three words after performing the CDT or draws the clock incorrectly, cognition is impaired. As this measure is not scored, it has value only in detecting the presence or absence of cognitive impairment but not for rating severity or monitoring progression of the disease (Woodford & George, 2009). If cognition is impaired, the MMSE should be administered. The Mini Cog is licensed for print distribution by Dr. Borson only for use as a clinical aide. Permission can be obtained by contacting Dr. Borson at soob@u.washington.edu. The instrument and it's use can also be accessed through the Hartford Institute for Geriatric Nursing at www.hartfordign.org

Another brief assessment measure is to ask the client to name as many animals as possible in a 1 minute span of time and each answer is scored one point. Scores below 12 are abnormal and correlate well with scores below 23 on the MM. This measure assists in the assessment of verbal fluency and semantic memory, but a more comprehensive screening should be prompted by a score below 12. The naming test is not copyrighted and can be used in clinical practice.

The MoCA developed by Nasreddine et al. (2005) was designed as a brief screening tool to detect MCI and assess attention and concentration, executive functions, memory, language, visuospatial skills, abstract thinking calculations, and orientation. Visuospatial domains are assessed by asking the client to follow a numbered and lettered trail sequence and copy a cube. The clock draw test is used for executive function. Recognition is tested by asking the client to name three animals pictured. Memory is assessed by repeating a list of five words twice and asking the client to repeat them and then to recall them after 5 minutes. Repetition of five numbers forward and three backward, tapping at each A in a list of letters, and counting backward from 100 by sevens five times (serial sevens), tests for attention. Language is assessed by repeating two sentences and naming the maximum number of words beginning with the letter F. Asking the similarity between an orange and a banana, train and bicycle, and watch and ruler assesses the ability to think abstractly. Finally, orientation is assessed by asking the date, month, year, day, place, and city. The total score is 30 and scores below 26 indicate the presence of cognitive impairment and a need for further assessment if a diagnosis of dementia has not yet been made. This 10-minute screening instrument is both comprehensive and reliable and can be used in clinical practice without permission, if administered free of charge. The MoCA is better than the original MM at screening for MCI, and is therefore a valuable measure to aid in early detection of cognitive impairments. The MoCA can be accessed at www.mocatest.org and can be used for clinical and educational purposes but may not be used for commercial or research purposes without permission.

Functional Assessment Screening Tools

The patient's ability to complete simple tasks and instrumental activities of daily living can be assessed using the *Functional Assessment Questionnaire* (FAQ) (Pfeiffer, 1982). The FAQ is a 10-point list of functional activities completed by the informant rather than the patient. The lower the score, the more impaired the client.

Physical ADL can be assessed using the Physical Self-Maintenance Scale (PSMS) developed by Lawton and Brody (1969) or the Katz Index of Independence in Activities of Daily Living (Katz ADL). These rank physical ADLs, including ability to bathe, dress, toilet, transfer, and feed oneself, along, with continence. The PSMS asks the caregiver to rank patient ability to perform toileting, feeding, dressing, grooming, physical ambulation, and bathing on a 1 to 5 scale, with 1 being independent and 5 totally dependent on others for care. The higher the score, the more impaired the client. Both can be accessed for educational purposes through the Hartford Institute for Geriatric Nursing at www.hartfordign.org. There are some hybrid tools that combine functional and instrumental assessment, but perhaps most useful to clinical practice are dementia rating scales that help identify and assign stage of illness or degree of severity based on function.

Dementia Rating/Staging Tools

Determining the stage and severity of dementia is important in clinical practice to assist the PMH-APRN in determining interventions, both pharmacologic and nonpharmacologic, in tracking progression of the disease, and in assisting and educating patients and caregivers. For example, selection of pharmacological agents is approved for different levels of disease severity and use of cholinesterase inhibitors is not recommended once dementia is severe, as ACh is no longer being produced in sufficient quantity to warrant this intervention. Instruments to quantify stage and severity of dementia are valuable measures in diagnosis and management of patients with dementia.

The four most commonly used instruments to rate and stage dementia are the Functional Assessment Staging Scale (FAST) (Reisberg, 1988); the Global Deterioration Scale (Reisberg, Ferris, DeLeon, & Crook, 1982); the Clinical Dementia Rating Scale (CDR) (Morris, 1997); and the Blessed Dementia Rating Scale (BDRS) (Blessed, Tomlinson, & Roth, 1968). A further instrument copyrighted and used in specialty practice by neuropsychologists trained in its use is the Dementia Rating Scale or DRS-2 (Mattis, 2004).

The FAST is a seven-stage scale based on client function and correlating in earlier stages to MM scores. Stage 1 is presence of no deficits, and stage 2 is possible MCI with subjective functional deficit, and MM scores of 28 to 29. Stage 3 is MCI with objective functional decline and MM scores of 24–28. Stage 4 is mild dementia with deficits in IADLs, such as paying bills and cooking, and MM scores of 19 to 20, and stage 5 is moderate dementia with client needing assistance with clothing selection and an MM score of 15. Stage 6, moderately severe dementia, is divided into five substages that descend from needing help dressing to bathing to toileting to urinary then fecal incontinence, and MM scores descend from 9 to 1. Stage 7, severe dementia, is similarly staged into six substages that descend from only speaking a few words to inability to walk or sit up. For further information and permission for usage, contact Barry Reisberg, M.D., at barry.reisberg@nyumc.org

The BDRS is a 22-item scale that assesses instrumental and physical ADLs, along with behavior. It is completed by a reliable informant, rather than the client. Questions 1 through 8 pertain to IADLs; questions 9 through 11 addressing eating, dressing, and continence have higher point values, and questions 12 through 22 are related to behaviors associated with dementia. A higher score up to 27 indicates more severity.

The CDR is a rating of six domains: memory, orientation, judgment and problem solving, community affairs, home and hobbies, and personal care. Each domain is rated on a five-point scale: 0 for no impairment; 0.5 for questionable impairment; 1, mild impairment; 2, moderate; and 3, severe impairment. Personal care is scored on a four-point scale without the 0.5 rating and the algorithm for scoring has memory weighted more heavily. The instrument has both global and sum of box scores with the later being more easily calculated and more sensitive to changes over time (O'Bryan et al., 2008). The CDR has been well validated as a reliable instrument for staging dementia in both clinical and research settings, can be applied in primary care settings in about 15 minutes and has been translated into 14 languages (Olde Rikkert et al., 2011). The Washington University Alzheimer's Disease Research Center holds the copyright for the CDR, and it is available for clinical use and non profit research without permission. Users of the instrument should be trained in its use, and this can be done online.

DIFFERENTIAL DIAGNOSIS

As previously noted, categories of dementia are not mutually exclusive and mixed dementias are common, challenging the most capable clinician. Detecting causes of cognitive decline such as that associated with major depressive disorder and delirium is the most critical component of assessment for the PMH-APRN. Depression that initially presents with difficulty concentrating or poor memory may be misdiagnosed as dementia. When depression is suspected, further evaluation should occur, including the use of a screening tool for depression such as the Geriatric Depression Scale (Yesavage; see Chapter 8). Delirium can be differentiated from dementia and depression by acute onset, the coexistence of another medical condition, memory disturbance of short duration, and rapid decline in functioning, along with the hallmark symptoms of impaired cognition, fluctuating consciousness, and inability to shift or maintain attention. Instead of delirium, this condition may be diagnosed as acute confusional state or dementia due to a general medical condition if there is evidence from the history, physical examination, or laboratory tests that the disturbance is due to a medical condition other than Alzheimer's disease or VD. Guidelines for differentiating delirium, depression, and dementia and for differentiating types of dementia are found in Table 13-1.

EXPECTED OUTCOMES

Due to the chronic progressive debilitating nature of dementia, overall treatment and management are aimed at improving the quality of life of patient and caregiver by:

- Preventing or slowing further cognitive and functional decline
- Preserving function, stable mood, and adaptive behaviors
- Controlling symptoms and providing comfort
- Preserving dignity and quality of life
- Preventing accident and injury, and promoting safety
- Promoting healthy behavior, and preventing illness in both client and caregiver
- Supporting caregivers

TABLE 13-1: DIFFERENTIAL DIAGNOSIS OF COMMON CONDITIONS PRESENTING WITH COGNITIVE IMPAIRMENTS

DISORDER	ONSET/PROGRESSION	SYMPTOMS
Delirium	Rapid (hours to days)/fluctuating	Fluctuating level of consciousness, disorientation
Dementia, Alzheimer's type	Insidious onset/ gradual progression	Global cognitive impairment with memory deficits
Dementia, Vascular type	May be rapid, immediately following vascular incident such as cerebrovascular accident (CVA), or transient ischemic attack (TIA) Stepwise progression	Stepwise deterioration in cognition and memory coincident with vascular events
Dementia Lewy Body type	Insidious onset/fluctuating progression	Parkinson features with gait disturbance. Visual hallucinations, rapid eye movement sleep (REM) sleep disturbance. Sensitivity to neuroleptics
Dementia Frontotemporal type	Insidious onset/ gradual progression	Early personality change. Problems with executive function. May be speech impairments. Grasp and pout reflexes
Depression	Usually gradual. Differentiates from bereavement, which has sudden onset.	Sleep disturbance, appetite changes, weight loss or gain, anhedonia, sadness, feeling of worthlessness, guilt, somatic focus, hopelessness, helplessness
Sleep disorders	Variable depending on the cause	Difficulty initiating and maintaining sleep, daytime sleepiness, disruption in daytime function
Substance abuse	Generally gradual	Substance use out of control, affecting the ability to function. Unexplained falls, episodes of confusion, and withdrawal symptoms

Specific interventions to achieve these goals are extensive and fall into two broad categories: treatment of the cognitive disorder, and treatment of behavioral and psychological symptoms with both psychopharmacological and nonpharmacological measures. Refer to Table 13-2, Medications Commonly Used for Treatment of Cognitive Disorders, and Exhibit 13-4, Nonpharmacologic Interventions for the Treatment of Cognitive Impairments.

Some general treatment principles from the American Geriatrics Society Guide to Dementia Diagnosis and Treatment (2011b) include:

- Identify and treat comorbid conditions to prevent further disability.
- Promote cognitive health through activities such as exercise, cognitive stimulation, stress reduction, and emotionally supportive milieus.
- Identify, treat, and monitor target symptoms.
- Assess and manage mood and behaviors.
- Avoid anticholinergic and limit psychotropic medications.
- Monitor the environment for safety and advise and intervene to avoid the hazards of wandering and risks of driving.
- Provide support and resources, including referrals, for clients and caregivers for access to financial, legal, and educational information.

TREATMENT

INITIATING TREATMENT TO PRESERVE COGNITIVE AND FUNCTIONAL STATUS

The clinician must initially determine the cause of symptoms and institute measures to treat comorbid medical conditions that may exacerbate cognitive impairment and lead to further functional decline in the client with dementia. Alert the family that a sudden change in behavior or mental status in a loved one with dementia may signal a medical condition and requires immediate evaluation to

TABLE 13-2: MEDICATIONS COMMONLY USED FOR TREATMENT OF COGNITIVE DISORDERS

CLASSIFICATION	MEDICATION	DOSAGE	SIDE EFFECTS
Cholinesterase Inhibitor (CI) Selective Acetylcholinesterase Inhibitor (ACI) Cognitive Enhancer	Donepezil (Aricept)	5–10 mg daily Use 5 mg starting dose for minimum of one month; then increase to 10 mg maintenance dose. 23 mg once daily is a different formulation and is approved to be used only in moderate to severe stages of dementia.	GI: Nausea, diarrhea Vomiting, loss of appetite, weight loss Excessive salivation and rhinorrhea Insomnia, nightmares Dizziness, hypotension Syncopal episodes Muscle cramps Fatigue
Cholinesterase Inhibitor (CI) Selective Acetylcholinesterase Inhibitor(ACI) Cognitive Enhancer	Galantamine (Razadyne) (Razadyne ER)	Usual dosage range 16–24 mg per day Immediate release: start with 8 mg twice daily (4 mg for older adults). Increase after each 4 weeks for a maximum dosage of 16 mg twice daily. Extended release: start with 8 mg daily each morning. Increase to maximum of 24 mg daily.	GI: Nausea, diarrhea Vomiting, loss of appetite, weight loss Headache Dizziness, hypotension Rare syncope Fatigue, depression
Cholinesterase Inhibitor (CI) Acetylcholinesterase Inhibitor(ACI) and butyrylcholinesterase inhibitor Cognitive Enhancer	Rivastigmine (Exelon)	Oral dosage: 6–12 mg in divided dosages. Start with 1.5 mg twice a day. Transdermal dosage: start with 4.6 mg/24 hr. patch for 4 weeks; then increase to 9.5 mg/24 hours.	GI: Nausea, diarrhea Vomiting, loss of appetite, weight loss, increased gastric acid secretion Headache, dizziness Fatigue, sweating Rare syncope
N-methyl-D-aspartate (NMDA) receptor antagonist NMDA is subtype of glutamate receptor antagonist Cognitive Enhancer	Memantine (Namenda)	Titration pack Initial 5 mg per day, increasing by 5 mg each week for a total dosage of 10 mg twice a day. 10 mg twice daily	Dizziness Headache Constipation

avoid further decline. See Figure 13-2 for direction for treatment initiation.

Initiation of treatment for dementia requires consideration of the stage of the illness and the degree of functional capacity. A stage-based approach can assist decision making regarding treatment interventions. Active management through all the stages significantly improves quality of life, helps preserve function, and enhances coordination of care and use of resources (Grossberg et al., 2010). An individualized multimodal and multidisciplinary treatment plan based on symptoms and capacity based on input from the client and family can be developed with input from the client and family. The PMH-APRN must be vigilant and forthcoming about expected symptoms at each stage of impairment and proactive regarding treatment options. Although hearing the diagnosis can be devastating, the PMH-APRN can share the findings in an empathic manner, allowing time for processing, and focusing on preservation of strength and function, rather than disability. Offering pharmacological and psychosocial interventions with demonstrated efficacy at the correct point in the disease progression, along with a caring presence, and contact information for questions and concerns can promote a strong partnership in managing the illness. Treatment interventions are planned in concordance with the family, and plans to obtain further neurological or neuropsychiatric evaluations used to determine the diagnosis, need to be discussed at this meeting. The PMH-APRN may need to refer the patient to a specialist

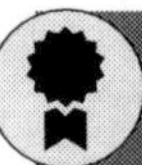

EXHIBIT 13.4: NONPHARMACOLOGICAL INTERVENTIONS FOR THE TREATMENT OF COGNITIVE IMPAIRMENTS

Psychotherapy
Cognitive behavioral therapy
Cognitive retraining
Psychoeducation
Psychotherapy
Reality orientation
Reminiscence therapy
Skills training
Support groups
Supportive psychotherapy

Somatic
Bright light therapy

Complementary/Alternative Interventions
Aromatherapy
Behavioral interventions
Computer-assisted (cognitive enhancing games)
Environmental modifications
Exercise
Herbals and dietary supplements
Massage-therapeutic touch
Nutrition
Relaxation breathing
Meditation
Music
Tai Chi
Visualization
Yoga

such as neurologist, geriatrician, or psychiatrist if the diagnosis is complex or unclear, if cognitive impairment occurs before age 60, or if specialty care for the management of the illness is indicated.

On the initial diagnostic visit the PMH-APRN will identify the presence and severity of symptoms and prepare the patient and family for subsequent visits that will occur 2–3 times a year or as needed to monitor cognitive and behavioral symptoms over the course of the illness. On each visit, assessment of safety concerns is crucial. Such issues as the patient's risk for wandering, agitation resulting in harm to himself or his caregiver, falls, self-harm accidents or suicidal ideation, and the adequacy of the support system should be addressed. The PMH-APRN assists the family to ensure appropriate levels of supervision for ADLs based on the stage of functional and cognitive decline, and plans with the family to address and eliminate safety risks associated with falls, wandering, and environmental hazards. It is often the clinician's role to raise the difficult issue of driving cessation and to plan with the patient and family how and when to relinquish driving. Involving the patient in this decision gives him more control and allows time to plan for transportation alternatives.

INITIATING TREATMENT TO MANAGE BEHAVIORAL OR MOOD DISTURBANCES

Psychosocial management begins with the establishment of an alliance with the patient and family. The PMH-APRN provides emotional support and guidance to patients and caregivers and enlists family as integral members of the team in monitoring and evaluating interventions. Most families struggle heroically to assist the patient with lost abilities. They have learned what interventions are most effective but may require additional guidance on how to manage behavioral disturbances and psychotic symptoms that may emerge. The role of the PMH-APRN is to elicit concerns and help caregivers find the resources required to continue the difficult work of caregiving or to process their feelings when the caregiving demands outstrip their resources and the patient requires long-term care. Referrals to the Alzheimer's Association (www.alz.org) and other support services should be offered. Information about respite care, long-term care options, and guidance on legal and financial planning is welcomed. In the early stages it is important to involve the patient in planning health care and transfer of assets as he makes his wishes known while he still has the capacity to make decisions. The PMH-APRN should refer the patient and family to social services for resource information and access to legal expertise for decisions regarding durable power of attorney and guardianship.

NONPHARMACOLOGICAL INTERVENTIONS

Through the progression of the illness but particularly in MCI and the early and middle stages of dementia, expert consensus guidelines (Alexopoulos et al., 2007) recommend the client be encouraged to stay cognitively, socially, and physically active, and emotionally engaged, and to follow a heart-healthy diet along with management of cardiac risk factors.

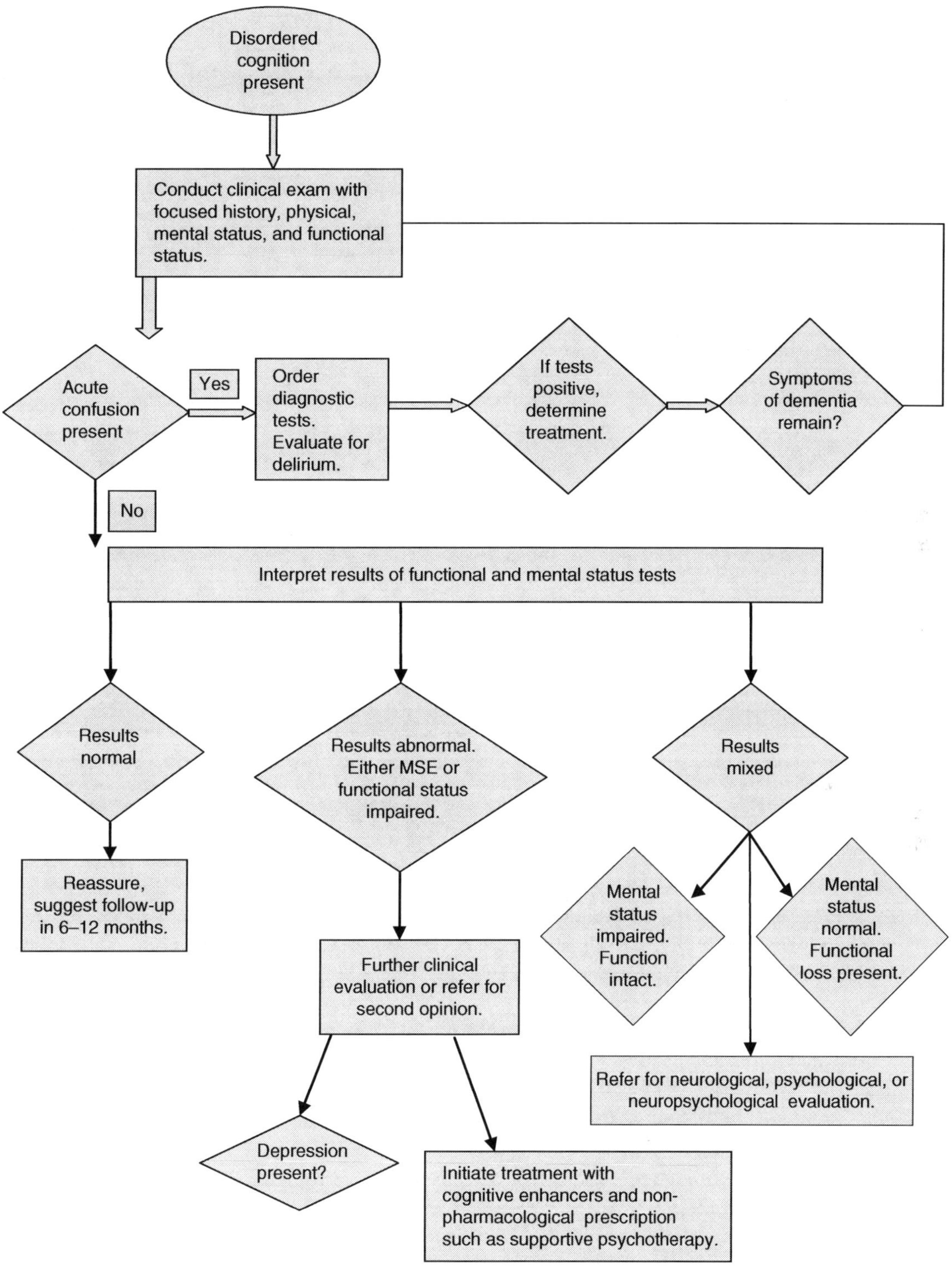

Figure 13-2 Treatment Initiation Decision Tree

Source: Inouye, S., van Dyck, C., Alessi, C., Balkin, S., Siegal, A., & Horowitz, R. (1990). Clarifying Confusion: The Confusion Assessment Method. *Annals of Internal Medicine, 113*(12), 941–948.

Cognition-oriented treatments including reality orientation, cognitive retraining, and skills training have been associated with slight cognitive gains (Bottiroli, Cavallini, & Vecchi, 2008; Gross & Rebok, 2011; Hall et al., 2009; Valenzuela & Sachdev, 2009). Stimulation-oriented treatments include activities that have been shown to improve mood, cognition, and function, such as music, crafts, and games (Gerdner, 2007). Occupational therapy programs focusing on activity and socialization and day treatment programs have demonstrated benefits to cognitive function.

In the early stages of dementia the patient and caregiver can employ strategies such as using an appointment book or personal data assistant (PDA) establishing a routine, keeping activities manageable, and engaging in stimulating, enjoyable, and stress-free activity to help preserve function. Stimulating memory, cueing, and reinforcement of attempts to fully engage in ADL performance are helpful. Some psychological treatments associated with short-term improvements in memory include cognitive behavioral approaches, reminiscence therapy, and supportive psychotherapy. There is little evidence to support validation therapy, simulated presence therapy, and sensory integration (Neal & Briggs, 2004).

Physical activity has been associated with improvements in cognition and function and should be recommended for all patients with MCI or dementia (Abbott et al., 2004; Larson et al., 2006; McDougal, Becker, Acee et al., 2010; McDougal, Becker, Pituch et al., 2010).

Difficult behaviors such as wandering and agitation, screaming, and acute confusion at sundown often emerge in the moderate stages of dementia. Symptoms of psychosis such as delusions and hallucinations are typical of this stage as well. Behavior-oriented treatments that focus on recognition of triggers for problem behaviors and modification of the environment to eliminate them are helpful, as is caregiver education and support, activity programs, music, and light therapy (Alexopoulos, Jeste, & Chung, 2005; Essential Evidence Plus, 2007). At this stage of the illness, comprehension is often better than expression, so attempts to maintain communication should be encouraged although the caregiver may become frustrated with repetitive questions and accusations based on delusions. Suggestions to caregivers might include avoiding changes in routine, ensuring the client has daily activity and physical exercise, using distraction, and avoiding arguments. The use of adult day care and respite for caregivers is helpful for both patient and family. Safety measures such as disconnecting the stove, locks on doors, and Safe Return bracelets need to be in place by this stage, and provision for constant supervision is required.

Caregivers are very creative at recognition and modification of environmental factors but may need added support and education to be most effective. Supportive psychotherapy and support and education groups are likely to be helpful to caregivers and should be recommended. Hain (2011) reported on a study by Gitlin, Winter, Dennis, Hodgson, & Hauck (2010) that found a home-based intervention reduced dependence, increased engagement of patients, and improved caregiver well-being and confidence. It is at this moderate stage of illness with the emergence of behavioral symptoms that client needs often begin to outstrip caregiver resources, financial, physical, and emotional. Transition to long-term care often begins at this point in the illness trajectory.

In the final, severe stage of dementia, the client is totally dependent on others and requires nursing care. If the client is still at home, the family can be guided to provide nursing care, including establishment of a toileting schedule, provision of soft foods to avoid aspiration, and safety measures. Usually the client will be in a nursing home or transitioning to one at this stage. A referral to Hospice may enable the family to continue to provide care at home. Frequently caregivers need support to assist with feelings related to the decision to transition the client to nursing home care.

COMPLEMENTARY AND ALTERNATIVE INTERVENTIONS FOR PATIENTS AND CAREGIVERS

The presence of a progressive neurodegenerative illness requires enormous adjustments for both patient and caregiver from diagnosis to final stages. Naturally, most people will experience stress as they struggle to cope with new realities. Complementary and alternative interventions can offer stress relief and the prospect of improved ability to cope and better quality of life for caregivers and lessening of catastrophic reactions for patients. Interventions such as mediation, yoga, relaxation breathing, progressive relaxation, tai chi, and others have demonstrated promise for symptom relief in persons with disordered cognition. But none have been proven to specifically improve cognition. Some herbal and dietary supplements may be helpful and the placebo effect cannot be underestimated. However, there is also great potential for fraud as claims about the effectiveness of various modalities are based on little scientific evidence and patients and families seek any new treatment that offers the promise of improvement. Additionally, many supplements have side effects that may be harmful alone or in combination with other medications the patient may be taking.

According to the National Center for Complementary and Alternative Medicine (NCCAM, 2011), there are currently four broad major classifications of CAM, including natural products, mind-body interventions, manipulative and body-based methods, and an undefined category named "others." Some practices fall into more than one category. Natural products include the use of herbal and other supplements. Mind-body interventions include relaxation therapy, meditation, biofeedback, hypnosis, and imagery. Manipulative and body-based methods include chiropractic, acupuncture, and massage therapy. Other modalities include movement therapies such as tai chi, Feldenkrais, Alexander techniques, and Pilates; the manipulation of energy fields including the use of magnet therapy, light therapy, and healing touch; and the use of traditional healers and spiritually based practices such as chanting and prayer.

A number of herbals, supplements, and dietary foods including ginkgo biloba, coenzyme Q10, vitamin B supplements, omega-3 fatty acids, and others have been promoted as memory enhancers and excellent and current reviews are available on the Alzheimer's Association website at www.alz.org. Some foods such as blueberries, deep water fish, and tumeric are thought to have antioxidant properties that support health and preserve cognition. Following a heart-healthy diet is recommended since what is cardioprotective, is neuroprotective. However, few supplements, once the damage has occurred, have been found to improve cognition. Although initially demonstrating promise, ginkgo biloba, touted as a cognitive enhancer, has been studied in two well-controlled investigations and was found not to either improve cognition or prevent decline in normal subjects and those with MCI (Birks & Grimley-Evans, 2004; DeKosky et al., 2008; Snitz et al., 2009). Patients need to be informed about the anticoagulant effects of ginkgo and to be cautioned to observe for bleeding if used with other anticoagulants. Of all the supplements, dietary foods, and herbals, only omega-3 fatty acids have been demonstrated to have a positive effect on cognition, most likely because of their antioxidant properties and effects on heart, blood vessels, and nerve membranes. Patients and families will bring questions about various products, including medicinal foods, advertised for memory loss, and the PMH-APRN needs to be aware of the most current research and refer clients to reliable sources of information such as the Alzheimer's Association and the Center for Complementary and Alternative Medicine.

Stress and resulting sympathetic release of cortisol is known to reduce cognition and further compromise functioning. Though there is no strong evidence that mind-body modalities such as relaxation therapy, relaxation breathing, and meditation improve cognitive scores in persons with dementia, they might be protective and have been demonstrated to reduce stress in clients and improve coping and self efficacy in caregivers (Innes, Selfe, Brown, Rose, & Thompson-Heisterman, 2012; Sierpina, Sierpina, Loera, & Grumbles, 2005). Similarly, yoga and tai chi have not been found to improve cognition, but have been very effective in reducing stress and agitated behaviors and improving strength, balance, and general well-being. Although massage therapy is classified as a manual alternative therapy, rather than a mind-body therapy, its use in relaxation and reduction of agitated behaviors in one review was effective in half the investigations of its use (Sierpina et al., 2005).

Other modalities such as movement and exercise (Abbott et al., 2004; Larson et al., 2006; McDougal, Becker, Acee et al., 2010; McDougal, Becker, Pituch et al., 2010); bright light (Burns, Allen, Tomenson, Duignan, & Burn, 2009); and music (Gerdner, 2007); have been effective in managing agitated behaviors and improving sleep. Multisensory environments known as Snoezelen rooms that incorporate music, aromatherapy, appealing nature sounds, and visual images of sunrises or starry skies have been found to diminish agitation and wandering. Reminiscence groups and story telling have anecdotal reports of efficacy but no strong evidence base (Sierpina et al., 2005). One manner of stress reduction is to help the client and caregiver change their perception of the stressor. Helping them find meaning in the illness and the caregiving can enhance coping. Incorporation of culturally appropriate and individualized spiritual practices can be very supportive.

In summary, a review of complementary and integrative approaches to dementia demonstrates the need for holistic care, support of caregivers, the importance of social and behavioral interventions, and the limited role of medications and botanicals (Sierpina et al., 2005). In fact, most of the care of persons with impaired cognition involves some type of CAM, as traditional treatment is limited. PMH-APRN's not only need to incorporate CAM into the care of persons with disordered cognition, but need to learn from clients and caregivers what measures have been most helpful to them, and protect them from unscrupulous marketers of products that have no efficacy.

PHARMACOLOGICAL INTERVENTIONS

Pharmacological Interventions for Cognitive and Functional Losses

Consensus treatment guidelines recommend use of a cholinesterase inhibitor for patients in early-stage dementia, and some authors suggest use of these medications for amnestic MCI as well. The recommendations are based on the proven efficacy of the drugs in slowing the cognitive decline and functional impairments associated with dementia. The neuropathologic changes characteristic of AD lead to deficits in the enzyme that synthesizes ACh. Loss of cholinergic neurons and loss of ACh, which has an important role in learning and memory, led to the cholinergic hypothesis to account for the symptom pattern of memory loss in patients with AD (Geldmacher, 2007). Thus, cholinesterase inhibitors were developed to counteract the effects of decreased ACh by preventing the destruction of ACh by the enzyme, acetylcholinesterase.

The three cholinersterase inhibitors (ChEIs) are Donepezil (Aricept), Rivastigmine (Exelon), and Galantamine (Reminyl or Razadyne). Geldmacher (2007) in a review of the evidence from randomized, double-blind, placebo-controlled trials found all were equally effective in slowing cognitive decline and in delaying transition to nursing home placement.... Earlier published evidence suggests both Donepezil (Birks & Harvey, 2004) and Rivastigmine (Grimley-Evans, Iakovidou, & Tsolake, 2004) may be effective in treating cognitive symptoms. Donepezil (Aricept) can be given once a day beginning at 5 mg and titrated to 10 mg daily. Donepezil is now available in 23 mg daily formulation, and is only approved for use only in moderate to severe stages of dementia. Rivastigmine (Exelon) is available in both an oral dosing that must be given twice a day (see Table 13-2), and a transdermal formulation if the patient is unable to tolerate the typical nausea, vomiting, and diarrhea associated with the cholinergic effects of the oral formulation. The transdermal formulation is started at 4.6 mg/24 hours for a month, and then, if well tolerated, titrated to the terminal dose of 9.5 mg/24 hours. Galantamine (Reminyl or Razadye) is the third possible choice and is available in a sustained release formulation that allows once-daily dosing. The initial dose is 8 mg daily and it can be titrated up to 16 mg, then the maintenance dosage of 24 mg daily. The ChEI agents are depicted in Table 13-2.

The gastrointestinal (GI) side effects of the ChEI agents can be significant when first initiated and occur because of the effect on the cholinergic receptors in the GI tract. To mitigate the side effects, dosing should begin at the lowest point for one month, then be titrated up. The medications should be taken after eating. Ginger ale can help alleviate nausea and over-the-counter preparations such as immodium can stop diarrhea.

As the progression of dementia is slowed by an average of two years but is not stopped by the use of ChEI agents, memantine (Namenda) was developed and approved by the Food and Drug Administration (FDA) as an agent for moderate to severe dementia. Therefore, it is used as a second-line agent to be added to ChEI agents when there is clinical and measurable change in cognition or functional status. Memantine is a N-Methyl-D-Aspartate glutamate receptor antagonist, which is thought to counteract the effect of excessive glutamate levels in the cortex of AD patients, that may contribute to memory deficits (Geldmacher, 2007). It has shown some benefits for patients with mild cognitive loss due to VD but has not been studied as a first-line treatment for AD. The client should receive serial follow-up with clinical interviews and use of cognitive and functional measures to determine stage of illness and when to initiate Memantine.

Memantine is initiated with a titration pack. The initial dose is 5 mg daily for 1 week, then 5 mg twice a day for week 2, 10 mg in the morning and 5 mg in the evening week 3, and then 10 mg twice a day. Side effects are generally mild but may include dizziness, constipation, and headache. Some clients become too energized on the medication. The lowest effective therapeutic dose is 10 mg daily and if side effects are not tolerated, reduction of dosage is indicated. Lower dosing is also indicated if there is renal impairment.

In summary, decisions to initiate and continue cognitive enhancement drugs should be based on an individualized assessment with evaluation of risks and benefits and on the choice of the agent profile, including tolerability of adverse effects, cost, and ease of use (Quaseem et al., 2008). Though these drugs have demonstrated clinically significant results, if quality of life is poor or the client is in later stages of dementia, or slowing of cognitive decline is no longer a goal, there is no reason to initiate or continue use. The adverse GI effects of the cholinesterase inhibitors and the expense of memantine may outweigh any benefit of use.

Pharmacological Treatment of Mood, Psychosis, and Behavioral Symptoms

Depression is very prevalent in persons with disordered cognition arising most likely from both the psychosocial and biological effects of the chronic debilitating illness. Persons with MCI or dementia are likely to exhibit depression in the early to early-middle stages of the illness. An increase in irritability rather than clear dysphoria may indicate presence of depression. Differentiation of depression from apathy can be challenging but usually the person with apathy does not report poor mood.

Symptoms and treatment of depression were well described in Chapter 8, and the drugs of choice for treatment are the same, the Selective serotonin reuptake inhibitors (SSRIs) or Serotonin-norephranephrine reuptake inhibitor (SNRIs). For specific information, please refer to Chaper 8. Citalopram (Celexa) is commonly used for patients with dementia due to its lower potential for side effects, and Duloxetine (Cymbalta) is the agent of choice for the patient who has neuropathic pain and depression. Treatment of depression will improve functional status and quality of life even if it has no direct effect on cognition, though it often has an effect in the short term.

As previously noted, psychosis and agitation are common in dementia, particularly in the intermediate stages. Medications should be avoided and nonpharmacological interventions, as previously described, used before considering medication. The PMH-APRN should perform a careful assessment of behavior to detect occult pain, depression, sleep deprivation, or delirium. Treatment of all causes should be initiated for possible resolution before using psychotropic drugs.

If symptoms remain, assess and modify the environment and provide safety, and institute nonpharmacological measures. For example, provision of a daily routine with exercise alternating with rest, along with an emotionally calming and supportive interpersonal milieu may alleviate anxiety and eliminate agitated behaviors. If there are no other choices, identify target symptoms and institute drug therapy very cautiously. Second-generation antipsychotics, particularly quetiapine (Seroquel), risperidone (Risperdal), and olanzapine (Zyprexa), have been used to manage hallucinations and agitation in persons with cognitive impairment. All now have an FDA black box warning for use in elderly persons with dementia due to association with death from cardiac events. In addition to physical risks, recent investigations by Vigen et al. (2011) demonstrated the use of atypical antipsychotics as being associated with worsening cognition in persons with Alzheimer's disease.

If there is no alternative, all agents should be started at the lowest possible dosage and monitored carefully with frequent contact with the clinician. Prior to initiating treatment, the family must be given full information about the risks and benefits and must give consent, and this conversation should be documented.

Tampi et al. (2011, Part II) recommend the following guidelines. First, define the symptomatology and obtain informed consent. If the patient has hypomanic or manic symptoms, initiate a mood stabilizer such as carbamazepine or divalproex first, then add an atypical antipsychotic if needed. If there are psychotic symptoms, use an atypical antipsychotic in monotherapy. If there is agitation or aggression. choose an SSRI or mood stabilizer or trazodone. Trazodone is the treatment of choice for sleep disturbances. An SSRI is usually the treatment of choice for anxiety, a mood stabilizer for physical aggression or severe agitation, and trazodone for limited agitation associated with sun downing and for treatment of sleep disturbance. Benzodiazepines such as lorazepam (Ativan) can be used for short-term management of anxiety and agitation but must be used with caution due to the potential for falls, worsening of cognition, and further disinhibition.

All of these agents have been described in previous chapters on affective and psychotic disorders. Therefore dosing and side effects and cautions for use will not be repeated here, other than a note regarding the importance of obtaining baseline liver function and complete blood count (CBC) testing prior to initiation of treatment with mood-stabilizing drugs.

The importance of careful monitoring, frequent follow-up, and determination of efficacy of the psychotropic drugs cannot be overstated. All should be tapered, if possible, after a 3 to 4 month asymptomatic period.

ACUTE FOLLOW-UP AND MAINTENANCE TREATMENT

Following initiation of any medication, the practitioner should contact the client within first month or sooner as needed and have the client return in 3 months. Management of behavioral symptoms, acute confusion, physical illness, or sleep disturbances may require a more urgent visit.

Maintenance treatment for disordered cognition requires serial follow-up depending on treatment options. If treatment with cognitive enhancers has been maximized and the patient is on both a cholinesterase inhibitor and memantine and is stable, annual visits are indicated and there is no need to conduct further neuropsychological testing, as the treatment options will not change.

If the client has a diagnosis of MCI, full evaluation that ideally would include a referral for neuropsychological assessment each year is indicated to detect changes in scores and initiate treatment early to slow further cognitive decline. Bedside testing and brief cognitive assessment measures of cognition for persons of high education levels who have MCI are usually not sensitive enough to detect changes.

For any client with disordered cognition, if there are declines in memory, mood, or function, or if the family is in need of support and guidance, visits should be scheduled every 6 months and they should be instructed to schedule them earlier as needed.

PEDIATRIC POINTERS

A discussion of cognitive disorders in children such as Autism Spectrum disorders, developmental disorders, and others is beyond the scope of this chapter and should be managed in specialty care. The reader is referred to Chapter 14 for further information. However, any etiology such as trauma, tumors, infections, drugs and toxins, metabolic disturbance, and stress that affects adults can also cause disordered cognition in children.

What affects one member of a family, such as caring for an adult with disordered cognition, affects all members of the family. Families caring for both adult parents and children may be particularly stressed and have difficulty meeting the needs of each. It is helpful to families to offer anticipatory guidance regarding how they may feel caring for the client as he becomes increasingly dependent. Children may exhibit distress through behaviors such as withdrawal, anger, and poor performance at school. The PMH-APRN can offer education, support, and family counseling along with referral to support and community groups. The family can be encouraged to build in time together for respite and relaxation. Children and adolescents can be included in caregiving and can assist the client to stay socially, cognitively, emotionally, and physically engaged through activities such as sharing photos, reminiscing, making a memory book, baking cookies, dancing, listening to music, and taking walks together with the client. The PMH-APRN can encourage all family members to express their feelings of grief and frustration openly.

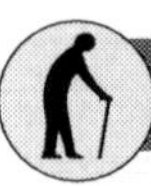

AGING ALERTS

As age is the greatest risk factor for development of a cognitive disorder, but is not a normal feature of aging, screening of memory should be part of an annual wellness visit for all persons over age 65 to establish a baseline, promote cognitive health, and provide early detection and treatment of cognitive disorders. Although affective disorders are also not a normal feature of aging, similarly, screening for mood disorders should be part of annual wellness visits for elders to promote healthy aging, establish a baseline to detect changes, and treat depression if present. Particularly in older adults, mental health and physical health are closely intertwined. Psychiatric illness, such as depression, may present as memory loss with difficulty concentrating and attending, and forms of dementia may initially appear with behavioral symptoms suggesting psychiatric illness.

Detection of depression in older adults is critical, as older adults, particularly those diagnosed with a chronic illness and those with a new diagnosis of dementia, are at increased risk for suicide (Seyfried, Kales, Ignatio, Conwell, & Valenstein, 2011). Although those over age 65 accounted for only 13% of the national population until 2011, the ratio of attempts

(Continued)

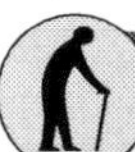

AGING ALERTS (*Continued*)

to completed suicides was 100–200:1 in the young and 4:1 in the elderly. Though those over 65 in 2007 had a suicide rate of 16 per 100,000, the risk of suicide accrues with age and is gender related. White men over the age of 75 have a rate of 36 per 100,000 deaths (CDC, 2011). Elderly white men with a chronic illness, pain, access to firearms, a history of substance abuse, no kin or social support, and no faith in community are at greatest risk for suicide. These statistics may be conservative estimates of suicide prevalence, as passive or accidental suicides are not reported, nor are assisted suicides.

Suicide is tragic and often preventable. A landmark report by the National Study for Suicide Prevention (2003) found 20% of elderly persons who committed suicide had visited a physician within 24 hours of their act, 41% within a week, and 75% within the month prior to suicide. PMH-APRNs have significant opportunities to prevent potential suicide through careful and thorough assessment and treatment of depression. Along with a complete clinical interview, the Geriatric Depression Scale or the Hamilton Depression Scale described in Chapter 8 are particularly well suited for screening for depression in older adults.

CONCLUSION

As the prevalence of disorders of cognition continues to rise dramatically, the need for PMH-APRNs, across care settings will continue to rise as well. PMH-APRNs by virtue of grounding in biopsychosocial frameworks of assessment and treatment and interdisciplinary models of practice, are the ideal practitioners to provide care to clients with cognitive disorders, their families, and their caregivers.

RESOURCES

FOR CLIENTS

Alzheimer's Association: www.alz.org; http://alzheimer's.org
The Alzheimer's Association website provides up-to-date information about the disease with links to related websites and local and regional support groups that are found throughout the country in large and small communities. Family members can find the support group closest to them (1) by calling the Alzheimer's Association chapters, which usually are listed in the phone book; (2) by calling the Alzheimer's Association for a chapter referral (1-800-272-3900, fax 312-335-1110); (3) by accessing their website at www.alz.org; or (4) by calling their Area Agency on Aging or the Eldercare Locator (1-800-667-1116). Families also may receive the Alzheimer's Association Newsletter to keep abreast of developments in research, legislation, and techniques of care.

Alzheimer's Disease Education and Referral Center: adear@alzheimers.org
The Alzheimer's Disease Education and Referral Center (Box 8250, Silver Spring, MD, 20907-8250, 1-800-438-4380, fax 301-495-3334, e-mail adear@alzheimers.org) is a service of the National Institute on Aging, which is a national resource for information on all aspects of Alzheimer's disease for both professionals and families. This center also provides referrals to national and state resources.

National Institutes of Health, National Institute on Aging: www/nia.nih.gov
This is the website for the National Institutes of Health, National Institute on Aging, providing comprehensive information related to all aspects of aging and many links to related websites. It is a useful site for professionals and the public.

National Institute of Neurological Disorders of the National Institutes of Health: www.nind.nih.gov
The National Institute of Neurological Disorders of the National Institutes of Health website provides comprehensive information on a number of neurological disorders and links to support groups, resource information and clinical trials.

U.S. government's official web portal: www.usa.gov/Citizen/Topics/Health/caregivers.shtml
This website provides links to a wealth of resources for caregivers including eldercare locator, veterans services, Medicaid, and Medicare information and more. It is an ideal site to start a search for more specific resources.

Family Caregiver Alliance: www.caregiver.org
This is the website for the Family Caregiver Alliance offering support, education, and resource information for caregivers.

Association for Frontotemporal Degeneration: www.theaftd.org
The Association for Frontotemporal Degeneration website provides clinical information, support for caregivers, a variety of resources on management of the symptoms of the illness, and information regarding how to locate current clinical trials.

FOR THE PROFESSIONAL PMH-APRN

Hartford Institute for Geriatric Nursing: www.hartfordign.org
The Hartford Institute for Geriatric Nursing provides extensive resources for nurses caring for older adults including a myriad of assessment tools and education as to how to administer them. The site contains many of the instruments described in the chapter and permissions have been obtained for use in education and clinical practice to improve the care of older adults. The site contains www.ConsultGeri.org, the clinical website of the Hartford Institute for Geriatric Nursing, New York. Improving Care for Healthsystem Elders program and links to the www.nursingcenter.com/AJNolderadults site and the Try This series, with free videos demonstrating assessment of cognition. continuing education unit (CEU) credit can be obtained if purchased.

University of Iowa, Hartford Center for Geriatric Nursing Excellence: www.nursing.uiowa.edu/hartford/
The University of Iowa, Hartford Center for Geriatric Nursing Excellence has developed many evidence-based practice guidelines and interventions for older adults with cognitive, affective, and behavioral impairments. Guidelines can be ordered through this website.

REFERENCES

Abbott, R. D., White, R., Ross, G. W., Masaki, K. H., Curb, J. D., & Petrovich, H. (2004). Walking and dementia in physically capable elderly men. *JAMA, 292*(12), 14471453.

Administration on Aging. (2008). A profile of older Americans, 2010. USDHHS. Retrieved from www.aoa.gov

Albert, M. S., DeKosky, S. T., Dickson, D., Dubois, B., Feldman, H. H., Fox, N. C.,...Phelps, C. H. (2011). The diagnosis of mild cognitive impairment due to Alzheimer's disease: Recommendations from the National Institute on Aging and Alzheimer's Association workgroup. *Alzheimer's & Dementia.* The Alzheimer's Association.

Alexopoulos, G. S., Jeste, D. V., & Chung, H. (2005). The expert consensus guideline series: Treatment of dementia and its behavioral disturbances. *Postgraduate Medicine Special Report.*

Alexopoulos, G. S., Streim, J., Carpenter, D., & Docherty, J. P. (2004). Expert consensus panel for using antipsychotic drugs in older patients: Using antipsychotic agents in older patients. *Journal of Clinical Psychiatry, 65*(Suppl. 2:5), 99–104.

Alzheimer's Association. (2011). 2011 Alzheimer's Disease Facts and Figures. *Alzheimer's & Dementia* Vol. 7, Issue 2, 208–244.

American Geriatrics Society. (2011a). A guide to dementia diagnosis and treatment. Retrieved from www.americangeriatrics.org.

American Geriatrics Society. (2011b). Guide to the management of psychotic disorders and neuropsychiatric symptoms of dementia in older adults. Retrieved from www.americangeriatrics.org.

American Psychiatric Association. (2000). *Diagnostic and statistical manual of mental disorders* (4th ed.). Washington, DC: Author.

Andren, S., & Elmstahl, S. (2008). The relationship between caregiver burden, caregivers' perceived health and their sense of coherence in caring for elders with dementia. *Journal of Clinical Nursing, 17*(6), 790–799.

Balas, M. C., Deutschman, C. S., Sullivan-Marx, E. M., Strumpf, N. E., Alston, R. P., & Richmond, T. S. (2007). Delirium in older patients in surgical intensive care units. *Journal of Nursing Scholarship, 39*(2), 147–154.

Barnes, D., Krueger, K., Byers, A., diaz-Arrastia, R., & Yaffe, K. (2011) Traumatic brain injury and risk of dementia in older veterans. *Alzheimer's and Dementia, 7*(4), 2–117.

Birks, J. S., & Grimley-Evans, J. (2004). Ginkgo biloba for cognitive impairment and dementia. (Cochrane Review). In *The Cochrane Library* Issue 2, 2004. Chichester, United Kingdom: John Wiley & Sons.

Blessed, G., Tomlinson, B. E., & Roth, M. (1968). The association between quantitative measures of dementia and of senile change in the cerebral grey matter of elderly subjects. *British Journal of Psychiatry, 114*(512), 797–811.

Borson, S., Scanlan, J. M., Watanabe, J., Tu, S., & Lessing, M. (2006). Improving identification of cognitive impairment in primary care. *International Journal of Geriatric Psychiatry, 21*(4), 349–355.

Bottiroli, S., Cavallini, E., & Vecchi, T. (2008). Long term effects of memory training in the elderly: A longitudinal study. *Archives of Gerontology and Geriatrics, 47*(2), 277–299.

Brink, T. A., Yesavage, J. A., Lum, O., Heersema, P., Adey, M., & Rose, T. L. (1982). Screening tests for geriatric depression. *Clinical Gerontologist, 1*, 37–44.

Burns, A., Allen, H., Tomenson, B., Duignan, D., & Burn, J. (2009). Bright light therapy for agitation in dementia: A randomized controlled study. *International Geriatrics, 21*(4), 711–721.

Campbell, J. (2009). A model of consequences of dementia caregivers' stress process: Influence on the behavioral symptoms of dementia and caregivers' behavior-related reactions. *Research and Theory for Nursing Practice, 23*(3), 181–202.

Centers for Disease Control (CDC). (2011). Retrieved from http://www.cde.gov

Cohn, D'V., & Taylor, P. (2010). Baby boomers approach age 65-glumly. *Pew Research Center Publications.*

Craig, D., & Birks, J. (2006). Galantamine for vascular cognitive impairment. *Cochrane Database of Systematic Review,* (1), CD004746.

Deeken, J. F., Taylor, K. L., Mangan, P., Yabroff, K. R., & Ingham, J. M. (2003). Care for caregivers: A review of self-report instruments developed to measure the burden, needs and quality of life of informal caregivers. *Journal of Pain and Symptom Management, 26*(4), 922–953.

DeKosky, S. T., Williamson, J. D., Fitzpatrick, A. L., Kronmal, R. A., Ives, D. G., Saxton, J. A., ... Furberg, C. D. (2008). Ginkgo biloba for prevention of dementia: A randomized controlled trial. *Journal of the American Medical Association, 300*(19), 27–30.

Essential Evidence Plus. (2007). *Duodecim Medical Publications Ltd.* Retrieved from www.essentialevidenceplus.com

Folstein, M. E., Folstein, S. E., & McHugh, P. R. (1975). Mini-Mental State: A practical method for grading the cognitive state of patients for the clinician. *Journal of Psychiatric Research, 12*(3), 189F–195F.

Gaugler, J. E., Wall, M. M., Kane, R. L., Menk, J. S., Sarsour, K., Johnson, J. A.,...Newcomer, R. (2010). The effects of incident and persistent behavioral problems on change in caregiver burden and nursing home admission of person with dementia. *Medical Care, 48*(10), 875–883.

Geldmacher, D. (2003). Contemporary diagnosis and management of Alzheimer's dementia. *Handbooks in Health Care Company*. Newtown, PA.

Geldmacher, D. (2007). Treatment guidelines for Alzheimer's Disease: Redefining perceptions in primary care. *Primary Care Companion to Journal of Clinical Psychiatry, 9*(2), 113–129.

Gerdner, L. (2007). Individualized music for elders with dementia. *University of Iowa Gerontological Nursing Interventions Research Center, Research Translation Dissemination Core,* Iowa City, IA.

Gitlin, L. N., Winter, L., Dennis, M. P., Hodgson, N., & Hauck, W. W. (2010). A biobehavioural home-based intervention and the well-being of patients with dementia and their caregivers: the COPE randomized trial. *JAMA, 304,* 983–991.

Gross, A. L., & Rebok, G. W. (2011). Memory training and strategy use in older adults: Results from the ACTIVE study. *Psychology and Aging, 26*(3), 503–517.

Grossberg, G. T., Christernsen, D. D., Grffith, P. A., Kerwin, D. R., Hust, G., & Hall, E. G. (2010). The art of sharing the diagnosis and management of Alzheimer's disease with patients and caregivers. Recommendations of an expert consensus panel. *Journal of Clinical Psychiatry (Primary Care Companion), 12*(1), e1–e9.

Hain, D. J. (2011). Home-based bio-behavioral intervention reduces dependence, increased engagement of patients with dementia in the short term and improved care giver well-being and confidence. *Evidence Based Nursing, 14,* 39–40.

Hall, C. B., Lipton, R. B., Sliwinski, M., Katz, M. J., Derby, C. B., & Verghese, J. (2009). Cognitive activities delay onset of memory decline in persons who develop dementia. *Neurology, 73,* 356–361.

Innes, K., Kit-Selfe, T., Brown, C., Rose, K., & Tompson-Heisterman, A. (2012). The effects of meditation on perceived stress and related indices of psychological status and sympathetic activation in persons with Alzheimer's Disease and their caregivers: A pilot study. *Evidence-Based Complementary and Alternative Medicine.*

Inouye, S., vanDyke, C., Allessi, C., Balkin, S., Siegal, A., & Horowitz, R. (1990). Clarifying confusion: The Confusion Assessment Method. *Annals of Internal Medicine* 113(12), 941–948.

Inouye, S., vanDyke, C. H., Allessi, C., Balkin, S., Siegal, A. P., & Horowitz, R. I. (2000). Confusion Assessment Method. In American Psychiatric Association. *Handbook of Psychiatric Measures* (pp. 398, 399). Washington, DC, American Psychiatric Association.

Jack, C. R., Albert, M. S., Knopman, D. S., McKhann, G. M., Sperling, R. A., Carrillo, M. C.,...& Phelps, C. H. (2011). Introduction to the recommendations from the National Institute on Aging and the Alzheimer's Association workgroup o the diagnostic guidelines for Alzheimer's disease. *Alzheimer's & Dementia.* The Alzheimer's Association.

Kopelman, M. D., Thomson, A. D., Guerrini, I., & Marshall, E. J. (2009). The Korsakoff Syndrome: Clinical aspects, psychology and treatment. *Oxford Journals, 44*(2), 148–154.

Larson, E. B., Wang, L., Bowen, J. D., McCormick, W. C., Teri, L., Crane, P., & Kukull, W. (2006). Exercise is associated with reduced risk for incident dementia among persons 65 years of age and older. *Annuals of Internal Medicine, 144*(2), 73–81.

Lawton, M. P., & Brody, E. M. (1969). Assessment of older people self maintaining and instrumental activities of daily living. *The Gerontologist, 9,* 179–186.

Loy, C., & Schneider, L. (2006). Galantamine for Alzheimer's disease and mild cognitive impairment. *Cochrane Database of Systematic Reviews,* (1), CD001747.

Mattis, S. (2004). Dementia Rating Scale-2. *Psychological Assessment Resources.* Retrieved from www.parinc.com

McAvay, G., Van Ness, P. H., Bogardus, S. T., Zhang, Y., Leslie, D. L., Leo-Summers, L. S., & Inouye, S. K. (2006). Older adults discharged from the hospital with delirium: 1-year outcomes. *Journal American Geriatrics Society, 54*(8), 1245–1250.

McDougal, G. J., Becker, H., Acee, T. W., Vaughan, P. W., Pituch, K., & Delville, C. (2010). Health training intervention for community dwelling elderly in the Senior WISE study. *Archives of Psychiatric Nursing, 24*(2), 125–136.

McDougal, G. J., Becker, H., Pituch, K., Acee, T. W., Vaughan, P. W., & Delville, C. L. (2010). The SeniorWISE study:

Improving everyday memory in older adults. *Archives of Psychiatric Nursing, 24*(5), 291–306.

Monnot, M., Brosey, M., & Ross, E. (2005). Screening for dementia: Family caregiver questionnaires reliably predict dementia. *Journal American Board Family Practitioners, 18*, 240–256.

Morris, J. C. (1997). Clinical dementia rating scale: A reliable and valid diagnostic and staging measure for dementia of the Alzheimer Type. *International Psychogeriatrics, 9*(1), 173–176.

Nasreddine, Z. S., Phillips, N. A., Bedirian, V., Charbonneau, S., Whitehead, V., Collin,... Chertkow, H. (2005). The Montreal Cognitive Assessment, MoCA: A brief screening tool for mild cognitive impairment. *Journal of the American Geriatrics Society, 53*(4), 695–699.

National Center for Complementary and Alternative Medicine (NCCAM). Retrieved from www.nccam.nih.gov

National Institute of Neurological Disorders. (2006). *Parkinson's disease: Hope through research.* NIH Publication No. 06-139

National Institute of Neurological Disorders. (2007). *The dementias: Hope through research.* Retrieved from *www.ninds.nih.gov*

National Institute of Neurological Disorders. (2011). *Traumatic brain injury: Hope through research.* Retrieved from www.ninds.nih.gov

National Strategy for Suicide Prevention. (2003). At a glance-Suicide among the elderly. United States Department of Health and Human Services.

Neal, M., & Briggs, M. (2004). Validation therapy for dementia. (Cochrane Review). In *The Cochrane Library*. Chichester, United Kingdom: John Wiley & Sons.

O' Bryant, S. E., Waring, S. C., Cullum, C. M., Hall, J., Lacritz, L., Massman, P. J.,... Doody, R. (2008). Staging dementia using Clinical Dementia Rating Scale Sum of Boxes Scores. *Archives of Neurology, 65*, 8.

Olde Rikkert, M. G. M., Tona, K. D, Janssen, L., Burns, A., Lobo, A., Robert, P.,... Waldemar, G. (2011). Validity, reliability and feasibility of clinical staging scales in dementia: A systematic review. *American Journal of Alzheimer's Disease and Other Dementias, 26*(5), 357–385.

Pfeiffer, E. (1975). A short, portable mental status questionnaire for the assessment of organic brain deficit in elderly patients. *Journal of the American Geriatrics Society, 23*(10), 433–441.

Pfeiffer, R. I., Kurosaki, T. T., Harrah, C. H., Chance, J. M., & Filos, S. (1982). Measurement of functional activities of older adults in the community. *Journal of Gerontology, 37*, 323–329.

Pinquart, M., & Sorensen, S. (2006). Helping caregivers of persons with dementia: which interventions work and how large are their effects? *International Psychogeriatrics, 18*(4), 577–595.

Qaseem, A., Snow, V., Cross, T., Forciea, A., Hopkins, R., Shekelle, P.,... Owens, J. (2008). Current pharmacologic treatment of dementia: A clinical practice guideline form the American College of Physicians and the American Academy of Family Physicians. *Annuals of Internal Medicine, 148*, 340–378.

Reisberg, B. (1988). Functional assessment staging (FAST) of Alzheimer's Disease. *Psychopharmacology Bulletin, 24*, 653–659.

Reisberg, B., Ferris, S. H., deLeon, M. J., & Crook, T. (1982). The Global Deterioration Scale for assessment of primary degenerative dementia. *American Journal of Psychiatry, 139*, 1136, 1139.

Schuurmans, M. J., Shortridge-Baggett, L. M., & Duursma, S. A. (2003). The Delirium Observation Screening Scale: A screening instrument for delirium. *Research and Theory for Nursing Practice, 17*(1), 31–50.

Seyfried, L. S., Kales, H. C., Ignatio, R. V., Conwell, Y., & Valenstein, M. (2011). Predictors of suicide in patients with dementia. *Alzheimer's and Dementia: The Journal of the Alzheimer's Association, 7*(6), 567–573.

Sheikh, J. I., & Yesavage, J. A. (1986). Geriatric depression scale (GDS): Recent evidence and development of a shorter version. *Clinical Gerontology, 5*, 165–173.

Shulman, K. I., Shedletsky, R., & Silver, I. R. (1986). The challenge of time: Clock drawing and cognitive function in the elderly. *International Journal of Geriatric Psychiatry, 1*, 135–140.

Sierpina, V. S., Sierpina, M., Loera, J. A., & Grumbles, L. (2005). Complementary and integrative approaches to dementia. *Southern Medical Journal, 98*(6), 636–645.

Snitz, B. E., O'Meara, E. S., Carlson, M. C., Arnold, A. M., Ives, D. G., Rapp, S. R.,... DeKosky. (2009). Ginkgo biloba for preventing cognitive decline in older adults: A randomized trial. *Journal of the American Medial Association, 23:302*(24), 2663–2670.

Sperling, R. A., Aisen, P. S., Beckett, L. A., Bennett, D. A., Craft, S., Fagan, A. M.,... Phelps, C. H. (2011). Toward defining the preclinical stages of Alzheimer's disease: recommendations from the National Institute on Aging and the Alzheimer's Association workgroup. *Alzheimer's & Dementia*. Alzheimer's Association in press.

Tampi, R. R., Williamson, D., Muralee, S., Mittal, V., McEnerney, N., Thomas, J., & Cash, M. (2011). Behavioral and psychological symptoms of dementia: Part I-epidemiology, neurobiology, heritability and evaluation. *Clinical Geriatrics, 19*(5), 41–46.

Tampi, R. R., Williamson, D., Muralee, S., Mittal, V., McEnerney, N., Thomas, J., & Cash, M. (2011). Behavioral and psychological symptoms of dementia: Part II-treatment. *Clinical Geriatrics, 19*(6), 31–40.

Tremont, G., Davis, J. D., Bishop, D. S., & Fortinsky, R. H. (2011). Telephone delivered psychosocial intervention reduces burden in dementia caregivers. *American Journal of Alzheimer's and Other Dementias, 26*, 36–43.

Valenzuela, M., & Sachdev, P. (2009). Can cognitive exercise prevent the onset of dementia: systematic review of randomized clinical trials with longitudinal follow-up. *American Journal of Geriatric psychiatry, 17*(3), 179–187.

Vigen, C. L. P., Mack, W. J., Keefe, R. S. E., Sano, M., Sultzer, D., Stroup, T. S., Dagerman, K. S., Hsiao, J. K., Lebowitz, B.

D., Lyketsos, C. G., Tariot, P. N., Zheng, L., Schneider, L. S. (2011). Cognitive effects of atypical antipsychotic medications in patients with Alzheimer's Disease: Outcomes from the CATIE-AD. *American Journal of Psychiatry, 168*(8), 831–839.

Vishwanathan, A., Rocca, W. A., & Tzourio, C. (2009). Vascular risk factors and dementia: How to move forward? *Neurology, 72*(4), 368–374.

Wei, L. A., Fearing, M. A., Sternberg, E. J., & Inouye, S. K. (2008). The Confusion Assessment Method: A systematic review of current usage. *Journal of the American Geriatric Society,* 56(12), 2358–2359.

Woodford, H. J., & George, J. (2007). Cognitive assessment in the elderly: A review of clinical methods. *Oxford Journal of Medicine, 1*, 469–484.

Wright, M. J., Battista, M. A., Pate, D. S., Hierholzer, R., Magelof, J., & Howsepian, A. A. (2010). Domain-specific associations between burden and mood state in dementia caregivers. *Clinical Gerotologist, 33*, 3237–3247.

Zarit, S. H., Reever, K. E., & Bach-Peterson, J. (1980). Relatives of the impaired elderly: Correlates of feelings of burden. *Gerontologist,* 20, 649–655.

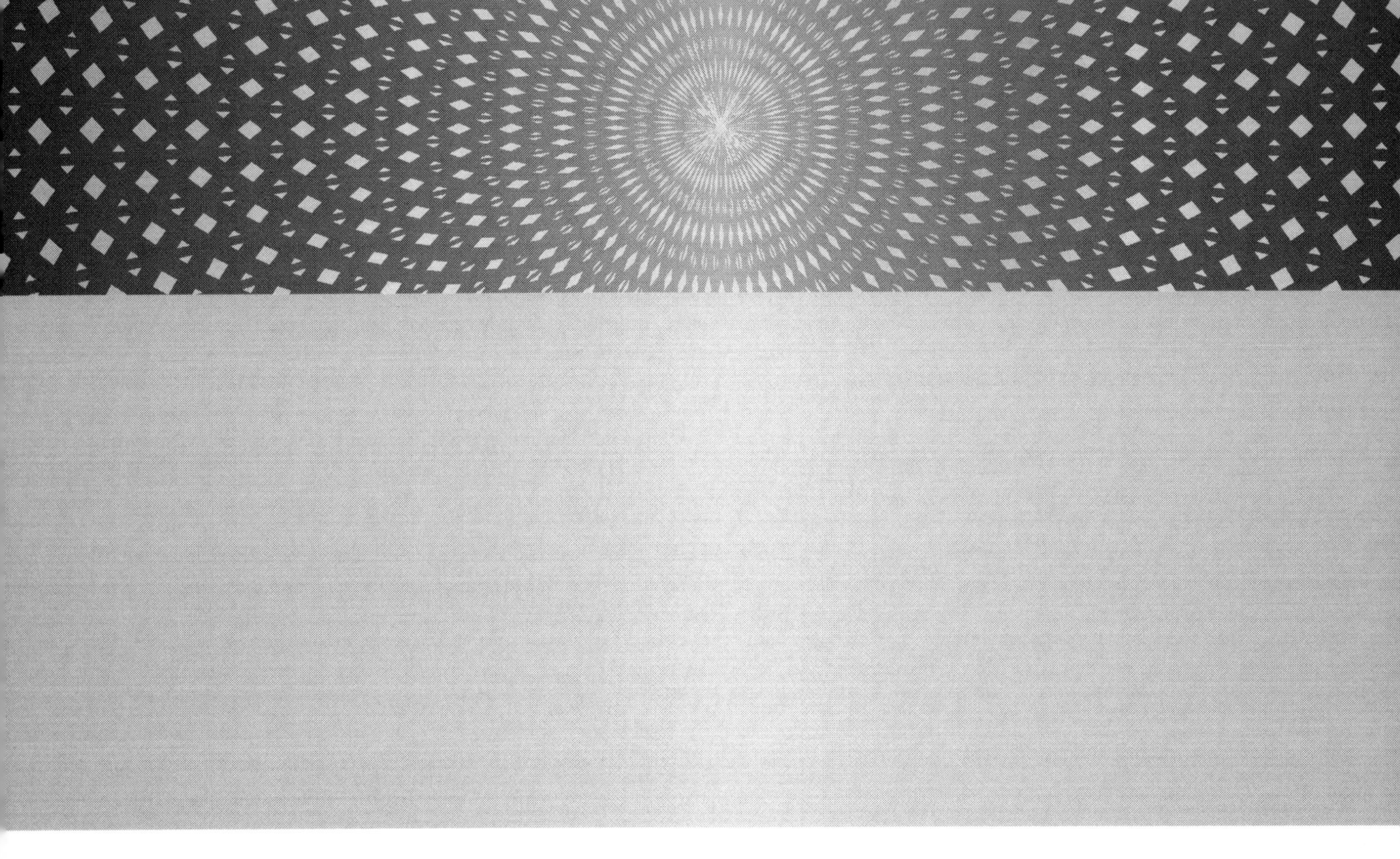

CHAPTER CONTENTS

Attention Deficit Hyperactivity Disorders (ADHD) and Autism Spectrum Disorders (ASD) are chronic neurological disorders originating in childhood. Recent research suggests that over 30% of children with ASD also meet criteria for ADHD. Furthermore, another 20% of children with ASD demonstrate subthreshold levels of ADHD symptoms (Matson & Nebal-Schwalm, 2007; Yerys et al., 2009). This comorbidity is important because the presence of ADHD symptoms influence cognition, autistic traits, and adaptive behavior. Although both disorders initially present in a similar social and biological manner, they are different disorders. It is important not to overlook either diagnosis in facilitating the most effective treatment. Only by understanding both disorders can the highest level of functioning be reached for the child as well as their family. This chapter includes information on both ADHD and ASD.

OVERVIEW OF ATTENTION DEFICIT DISORDER/ ATTENTION DEFICIT/HYPERACTIVITY DISORDER

Features of Attention Deficit Disorder (ADD) or ADHD were first identified in children in the 19th century (Greydanus, Pratt, & Patel, 2007). According to Greydanus et al. (2007), Heinrich Hoffman was a German physician and medical writer/illustrator who, in 1854, wrote about a young child, Fidgety Phillip, who had traits of what is now called ADHD. Other terms for ADHD

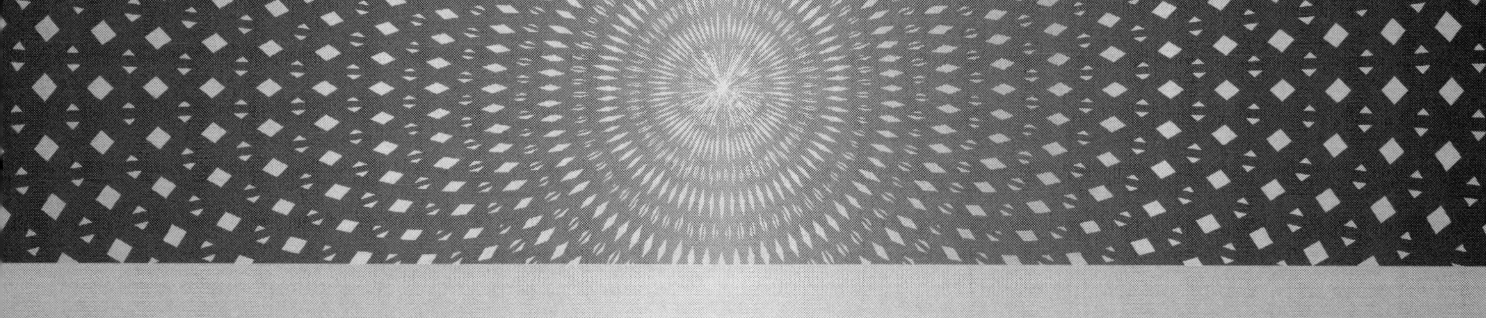

CHAPTER 14

Integrative Management of Disordered Attention

Lisa Barry and Marianne Tarraza

in the 20th century included the hyperkinetic syndrome and hyperactive reaction of childhood (Greydanus et al., 2007). Greydanus et al. (2007), point out that ADHD was described over a century ago as a disorder of children in which there was unruly behavior and hyperactivity, noted mainly in boys. Between 1916 and 1927, attention dysfunction and conduct disorder-like behavior were noted in children diagnosed with encephalitis lethargica (Von Economo's disease) and the pathophysiology was considered to be encephalitis with subsequent brain damage (Greydanus et al., 2007). According to Greydanus et al. (2007), there was also a group of children identified with these same symptoms without overt encephalitis and eventually they were diagnosed with minimum brain damage or dysfunction.

ADHD is one of the most common neuropsychiatric conditions of childhood and its effect on childhood development may be far-reaching (Buitelaar & Medori, 2010). The prevalence of ADHD is characterized by symptoms of inattention, hyperactivity, and impulsivity with childhood onset that often persists into adolescence and adulthood. ADHD is a neurobehavioral disorder with abnormalities in the noradrenergic, serotonergic, and dopaminergic neurotransmitter systems (Greydanus et al., 2007). According to the National Comorbidity Survey, the worldwide prevalence of ADHD in children is 8% to 12% and is estimated to be 4% in adults in the United States (Faraone & Mick, 2010). Although formerly recognized as a typical disorder in childhood, the notion of ADHD in adults was officially

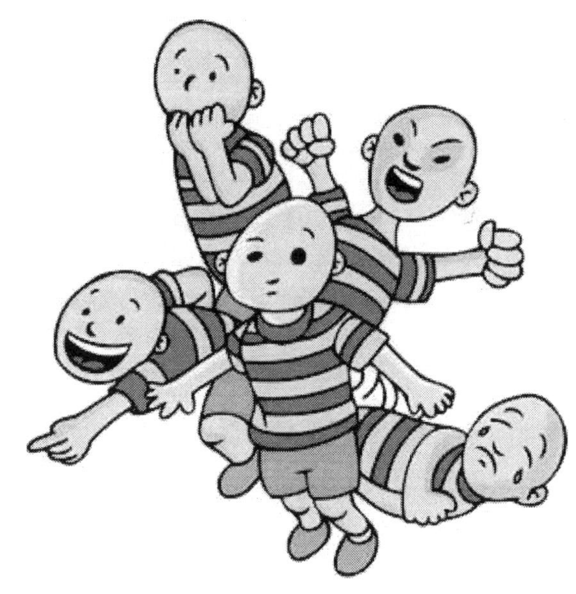

adopted more than 25 years ago when diagnostic criteria first appeared in the third edition of the *Diagnostic and Statistical Manual of Mental Disorders* (*DSM-III*) in 1980 (Dodson, 2005 as cited in Peterson, McDonagh, & Fu, 2008). However, adult ADHD is not a separate phenomenon and requires symptoms before the age of 7 as one of the criteria. The ADHD criterion was not updated in the *DSM-IV-TR*. The growth of psychiatric literature over the past few years has sparked an interest regarding the need to reevaluate ADHD criteria with the advent of the *DSM-5* targeted for May of 2013. According to Kieling,

C., Kieling, R.R., Rohde, L.A., Frick, P.J., Moffitt, T., Nigg, J.T., Tannock, R., & Castellanos, F.X. (2010), as prospective and retrospective data indicate that only half of adults who are assessed for ADHD symptoms report their presence by age 7, an extension of the age at onset criterion is both prudent and necessary and provides support for a recommendation that the presence of symptoms be required by age 12. The International Classification of Diseases is the enumeration of specific conditions and groups of conditions determined by an internationally representative expert committee that advises the World Health Organization (WHO) and is the preferred system used in the United Kingdom and most European countries. The International Classification of Diseases (ICD)-6 published in 1949 was the first to contain a section on mental disorders. In the early 1960s numerous proposals to improve the classification of mental disorders resulted from the extensive consultation process organized by the WHO to draft the Eighth Revision of the International Classification of Diseases (ICD-8) (WHO, 1993). The *DSM-IV-TR* and the ICD-10 are the current diagnostic classification systems utilized to establish diagnostic criteria.

Children with ADHD have deficits compared to other children of the same age in attending to and completing tasks such as schoolwork, impulse control, and activity-level modulation (Pelham, Famianto, & Massetti, 2005). They also have a host of impairments in multiple domains of functioning, including adult relationships (e.g., noncompliance with adult requests), school functioning (e.g., classroom disruption, poor achievement), and peer and sibling relationships (e.g., annoying, intrusive, overbearing, and aggressive behaviors) which continue into adolescence and adulthood even though core symptoms may improve with age (Pelham et al., 2005). Often times a child with ADHD will be described as being "lazy." Adolescents with ADHD are more likely than controls to drop out of school and to experience social problems in school, as well as conduct disorder (CD) symptoms, and early onset of substance use (Modesto-Lowe, Danforth, & Brooks, 2008). Similarly, adults with ADHD are more likely than controls to be unskilled workers, develop substance use disorders, and have psychopathology and antisocial behavior (Modesto-Lowe et al., 2008). Regardless of the developmental stage, ADHD can severely impact daily functioning and relationships without proper management.

Although there are many theories, no single etiology for ADHD has been substantiated (Rader, McCauley, & Callen, 2009). Rader et al. (2009) identify risk factors that affect a child's brain development and behavior and may lead to ADHD as genetic factors, behavioral disorders, medical conditions that affect brain development, and various environmental influences on the developing brain (e.g., toxins such as lead and alcohol; nutritional deficiencies). Greydanus et al. (2007) indicate that areas of the brain involved in attentional dysfunction include the cortex (prefrontal and parietal), brain stem (reticular formation), thalamus, basal ganglia, cingulate gyrus, and limbic structures (amygdala-hippocampus). Current research in ADHD is looking at identifying different types of attentional dysfunction based on these areas of the brain and this process of brain mapping will allow more specific anti-ADHD medications in the future (Greydanus et al., 2007). Genetic factors account for 80% of the etiology of ADHD and family, twin, and adoption studies support the theory that ADHD is a highly heritable disorder, with the majority of patients having a first- or second-degree relative with a history of ADHD or learning disorder (Millichap, 2008). Millichap (2008) reveals that learning disability is reported in 70% of patients and among their relatives and is frequently associated with ADHD as an interrelated, overlapping problem. Little is known about the causes of ADHD in girls because the incidence is relatively infrequent and gender differences factor into the prevalence of ADHD (Millichap, 2008).

ADHD shows high heterogeneity and comorbidity with other psychiatric disorders in children, adolescents, and adults (Schmidt & Petermann, 2009). Comorbidities that may be present in children and adolescents with ADHD are Oppositional Defiant Disorder (ODD), CD, mood disorders, childhood anxiety disorders, cognitive performance and learning disabilities, tic disorders, and substance use disorders (Ebert, Loosen, Nurcombe, & Leckman, 2008). Barkley and Newcorn (2009) identify adult comorbidities as anxiety disorders (47%), mood disorders (38%), impulse control (20%), and substance use disorders (SUD, 15%). Comorbidities may differ in frequency between adults and children with ADHD, as adults are more likely than children to have one or more anxiety disorders, SUD, personality disorders, or social phobias, and children are more likely to have comorbid ODD and separation anxiety (Barkley & Newcorn, 2009). Recognizing comorbidities and identifying differential diagnoses is crucial for the appropriate management of ADHD, since a diagnosed mood or anxiety disorder should be treated prior to treating ADHD.

AUTISM SPECTRUM

Autism Spectrum (ASD) disorder currently encompass three *DSM-IV* diagnoses: Autistic disorder, Asperger's disorder, pervasive developmental disorder not otherwise specified (PDD-NOS), and two disorders that are closely associated, these being Rett's disorder (Rett's Syndrome), and childhood disintegrative disorder (CDD). CDD is a neurodevelopment disorder that is characterized by distinct and pervasive impairment in multiple developmental areas primarily in the realm of social skills, communication, and behavior (American Psychological Association, 2000).

The common characteristics of these diagnoses include a variety of symptoms that are differentiated diagnostically and encompass a wide range of outcomes and impairment. Subsequently, the inclusion of the symptoms within a chapter on attention disorders is purposeful since there is often either a comorbid attention deficit diagnosis, or there are inherent attention delays which respond to medications for ADHD, or the primary presenting symptom may be consistent with attention deficits.

The development of the clarity of the diagnosis has evolved and continues to be refined. The term *Autism Spectrum* is a synonym that is widely accepted by parents and experts. In both the *DSM II* and *I* the symptoms that are now consistent with autism spectrum were considered within the diagnosis of schizophrenia. Previously, ASD was primarily considered a developmental disorder, however more recently it is associated with a higher incidence of medical disorders including seizures, sleep disturbances, gastrointestinal (GI) symptoms, metabolic issues, hormonal imbalances, infection, and allergies (Bauman, 2006).

Autism was first identified in 1942 by Leo Kanner from John Hopkins in his paper/lecture where he described a syndrome of "Autistic Aloneness," while Hans Asperger in 1938 coined the term Aspergers as a similar disorder that is separated by degrees of intellect (Matson, Nebel-Schalm, & Matson, 2006). Since that time there has been much debate about the clarification of the diagnosis, integration of biomedical and behavioral analysis, and cohesive scales that are clinically relevant.

The evolving fund of knowledge that surrounds the differentiation of these diagnoses lends itself to the agreement that the foundation of treatment consistent with best outcomes is that of early diagnosis and intervention. Historically, Aspergers has not been clarified until late adolescent years or later, while there is an increasing body of evidence that supports a diagnosis of PDD or autism as early as age 2. The use of rating scales in combination with clinical observations and *DSM* criteria are the tools that are used to consider the accuracy of the diagnosis. The disorder is a lifelong chronic disorder with variations in functional capacity that can be managed with a multitude of treatment recommendations.

ETIOLOGY

The etiology of ADHD involves complex interactions of neuroanatomical and neurochemical systems based on twin and adoption family genetic studies, DA transport gene studies, neuroimaging studies, and neurotransmitter data (Sadock & Sadock, 2007). In Sadock and Sadock (2007), contributory factors for ADHD include prenatal toxic exposures, prematurity, and prenatal mechanical insult to the fetal nervous system. There is no scientific evidence indicating that food additives, colorings, preservatives, and sugar are causative factors of ADHD, although they continue to be proposed as possible causes of hyperactive behavior (Sadock & Sadock, 2007).

ADHD AND THE BRAIN

Numerous studies suggest impaired frontal lobe functioning in people suffering from ADHD, which is evident in studies of metabolic functioning such as Single Photon Emission Computer Tomography (SPECT) and PET (Positron Emission Tomography) scans (Preston, O'Neal, & Talaga, 2005). Studies using PET scans have found lower cerebral blood flow and metabolic rates in the frontal lobe areas of children with ADHD than in controls (Sadock & Sadock, 2007). Pet scans have also shown that adolescent females with ADHD have globally lower glucose metabolism than both normal control females and males with the disorder (Sadock & Sadock, 2007). Zametkin et al. (1990) studied hyperactivity in adults by using PET of the brain with use of a technique involving a radioactive tracer that permits the measurement of regional glucose metabolism. A pilot study found evidence suggestive of depressed global cerebral glucose metabolism and possible frontal hypometabolism in the brains of hyperactive adults (Zametkin et al., 1990). According to Zametkin et al. (1990) the patients in their study had not been treated with stimulants, had no history of substance abuse, and were hyperactive themselves as children. In regards to gender, the global glucose metabolism was 1.9% higher in the brains of women with hyperactivity than in those of men with hyperactivity, but 12.7% lower in the hyperactive women versus the normal women (Zametkin et al., 1990). This supports the findings in Sadock and Sadock (2007) regarding the PET scan results that showed adolescent females with ADHD have globally lower glucose metabolism than both normal control females and males with the disorder.

There also have been significant advances in neuroimaging research in the last decade, prompting the use of electrophysiological studies which have identified abnormalities in the frontal cortex and basal ganglia associated with deficits of inhibitory and attentional control (Ryan & McDougall, 2009). The frontal cortex is the part of the brain where executive functioning such as problem solving, planning, reasoning, and attention occur. It functions in close association with other brain regions that consist of cerebral systems specifically designed for individual mental tasks (Buchsbaum, 2004). The frontal cortex participates with other brain regions in aspects of learning and memory, and attention and motivation, in part through its central role in working memory (Buchsbaum, 2004). It surrounds the limbic system and is also associated with aggression and impulse control. The vast majority of volumetric studies found prefrontal volume and cortical thickness reductions in children and adults with ADHD (Cherkasova & Hechtman, 2009, Figure 14-1). Although executive function deficits in ADHD are now well-supported and there is considerable neuroimaging evidence of frontalstriatal abnormalities, there is now a growing recognition in the field that pathophysiology of ADHD may not be limited to deficits in executive function and the frontalstriatal circuitry (Cherkasova & Hechtman, 2009). Cherkasova and Hechtman (2009) report that individuals with ADHD may suffer from a more general deficit, including impairments in attentional functions (e.g., alerting and orienting), regulation of arousal, and reward processing, and there is now accumulating evidence of structural and functional abnormalities in nonfrontostriatal brain regions, white matter tracts, and connectivity among brain regions.

The occiput is at the bottom, and the left side of the image represents the right side of the brain. The two subjects were selected as representative of the hyperactive and control groups. The left images indicate areas of relatively high glucose metabolism, whereas the right images indicate areas of lower glucose metabolism. (The purple halo is an artifact.) Comparison of the brain of an ADHD child and a non-ADHD child (PET scan), Zametkin et al. (1990), is shown in Figure 14-1.

The basal ganglia contain a cluster of structures (caudate, putamen, globus pallidius) located in the center of the brain that coordinate messages between multiple other brain areas (WebMD, 2009). These structures have an inhibitory function and take cues from the senses and integrate them into movements. Therefore, if the basal ganglia functions improperly, it decreases inhibition, resulting in the hyperactivity seen in ADHD.

Although the cerebellum has been traditionally thought of as a structure involved primarily in motor control, recent evidence has implicated it in numerous cognitive and affective functions and demonstrated cerebellar-cortical connections with regions involved in higher order cognitive operations, including those of the cerebellum with the prefrontal cortex (Cherkasova & Hechtman, 2009). Cherkasova and Hechtman (2009) identify temporal information processing, motor sequencing and planning, working memory, shifting of attention, implicit learning, emotional regulation, and executive functions as a wide range of cerebellar functions that have attracted the attention of ADHD researchers. There is a paucity of research on cerebellar function, despite strong and consistent evidence of cerebellar volume reductions in ADHD and recent incorporations of cerebellum into models of pathophysiology of ADHD (Cherkasova & Hechtman, 2009). The two fMRI studies referenced in Cherkasova and Hechtman (2009) provide evidence of functional abnormalities of the cerebellum in ADHD and of responsivity of cerebellar activity to stimulant medication, suggesting that cerebellar dysfunction may underlie the impaired ability of individuals with ADHD to predict event occurrence, which could in part explain poor behavioral adjustment in the contexts of expectancy violations.

The temporal and parietal areas are also of emerging interest in ADHD research, the latter of which is relevant to attentional functioning. In Cherkasova and Hechtman (2009), the temporal lobe is of interest due to its role in auditory processing of linguistic information, of which impairment has been reported with ADHD. The amygdala and hippocampus are temporal subcortical structures that are involved with processing reward information, the latter of which was mentioned earlier in

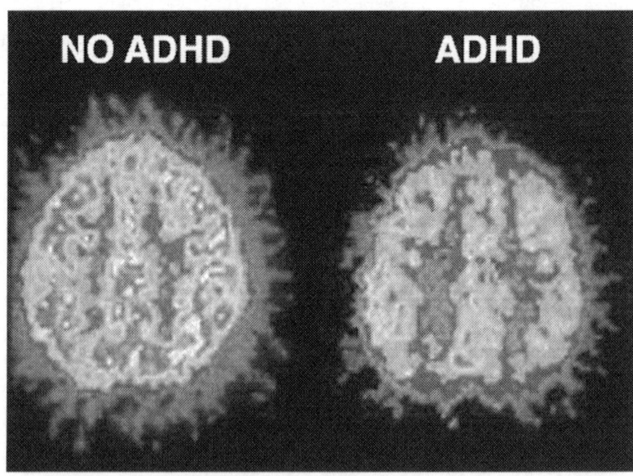

Figure 14-1 Representative Transverse Images (Left, Normal Control; Right, Patient With Attention-Deficit Disorder with Hyperactivity) through Plane A, Approximately 94 mm Above the Canthomeatal Line

this chapter as a function that has gained growing recognition, and there may be additional structures involved with ADHD beyond executive functioning (Cherkasova & Hechtman, 2009). The limbic system, which consists of the amygdala, hippocampus, and other brain structures, is responsible for emotional expression and behavior, both of which are important components of ADHD. The Reticular Activating System (RAS) is part of the brainstem reticular formation that plays a central role in bodily and behavioral alertness (Stedman's Medical Dictionary for the Health Profession and Nursing, 2005). According to the article "The Subcortical Areas Involved in ADHD," the RAS is a stimuli filter which helps to maintain self-control and allows the mind to attend, both of which are major deficits in individuals who have ADHD. The mechanism of action in the RAS that causes ADHD symptomatology remains unclear.

ADHD AND THE ROLE OF NEUROTRANSMITTERS

DA and noradrenaline (NA) (norepinephrine) are two neurotransmitters that are essential to prefrontal cortex function, and small changes in these neurotransmitters can have marked effects (Kaplan & Newcorn, 2011). NA is often believed to strengthen attention to stimuli via enhanced network connections sometimes referred to as increasing signal, and DA is involved in attention to stimuli but also seems to weaken unnecessary connections or decrease noise (Kaplan & Newcorn, 2011). DA influences behaviors such as risk taking and impulsivity, whereas norepinephrine modulates attention, arousal, and mood (Rader et al., 2009). Volkow et al. (2009) point out that evidence from brain imaging studies have shown that brain DA neurotransmission is disrupted in ADHD and these deficits may underlie core symptoms of inattention and impulsivity.

Rader et al. (2009) reports that current research suggests that rather than acting specifically on DA, stimulants create a calming effect by increasing serotonin levels. Nikolas et al. in Stannard Gromisch (2010), note that DA and norepinephrine are associated with the reward processing but the emotional dysregulation seen in ADHD is associated with impulse control and aggression related to serotonergic activity. Reward deficits in ADHD are characterized by a failure to delay gratification, impaired response to partial schedules of reinforcement, and preference for small immediate rewards over larger delayed rewards (Volkow et al., 2009). The serotonin transporter gene linked to ADHD is 5HTTLPR (Gromisch, 2010). The researchers found that two variants of 5HTTLPR, the "short" and "long" allelic variants, have been linked to ADHD and comorbid disorders such as conduct disorder and mood problems and that these 5HTTLPR alleles result in either low or high serotonin transporter activity (Gromisch, 2010).

Sadock and Sadock (2007) discuss how animal studies have shown that the locus ceruleus, consisting of mainly noradrenergic neurons, plays a role in attention. The locus ceruleus (LC), according to Berridge and Waterhouse (2003), serves at least two general behavior functions: (1) The LC contributes to the induction and maintenance of forebrain neuronal and behavioral activity states appropriate for the acquisition of sensory information (e.g., waking), and (2) Within the waking state, norepinephrine LC enhances and/or modulates the collection and processing of salient sensory information via actions on sensory, memory, and attentional and motor processes, the latter of which can be both short term and long term in nature and can occur within perceptual, attentional, and memory systems. Based on these observations, it is posited that dysregulation of the LC-noradrenergic system may result in deficits in a variety of cognitive and affective processes that are, in turn, associated with numerous cognitive and affective disorders such as ADHD, narcolepsy, and stress-related disorders (Berridge & Waterhouse, 2003). It is important to consider Berridge and Waterhouse's (2003) specification that whether or not deficiencies in noradrenergic neurotransmission contribute to the etiology of these disorders, actions of noradrenergic systems likely contribute to the efficacy of a variety of medications used in the treatment of these conditions. This will become apparent later in this chapter when we address medication management for the treatment of ADHD.

ADHD AND GENETICS

There is strong and consistent evidence from family, twin, and adoption studies from all over the world that ADHD symptoms are transmitted in families and influenced by genetic factors (Ryan & McDougall, 2009). Ryan and McDougall state that research shows, if a parent has ADHD, there is a greater than 50% chance that at least one of their children will also have the disorder. Although the mechanism for inheritance remains unknown, Plomin and Bergeman (1991), Faraone et al. (2001), Voeller (2004), and Salmon (2005), as cited in Ryan and McDougall (2009), report that the high population prevalence of ADHD (5% to 10%) and modest risk to first degree relatives (about 15% to 20%) suggest that the process of transmission is complex and likely to be mediated by environmental factors and gender.

Hawkins et al. (1998), Farrington (2007), and Thapar et al. (2007), as cited in Ryan and McDougall (2009), reveal that further studies have highlighted a strong heritable component with hyperactivity and impulsivity and chronic antisocial behavior persisting into adulthood.

Genetic studies have identified a few genes with polymorphisms associated with ADHD, with the most replicated being two DA genes (e.g., dopamine D4 receptor [DRD4] and dopamine transporter [DAT1] genes), and environmental studies have identified important nongenetic risk factors (e.g., maternal smoking during pregnancy and lead levels) (Volkow et al., 2009). The gene encoding the DA transfer, DAT1, was the initial gene candidate studied and is the principal target for methylphenidate and other psychostimulant medications used to treat individuals with ADHD (Volkow et al., 1998; Seeman & Madras, 1998 as cited in Kirley et al., 2002). The gene encoding the DA D4 receptor, DRD4, has also attracted interest as a candidate gene, and studies by Benjamin et al. (1996) and Ebstein et al. (1996), as cited in Kirley et al. (2002), suggest an association between this gene and the personality trait of novelty seeking, a behavior also seen in ADHD. The DA D4 receptor mediates the postsynaptic action of DA (Kirley et al., 2002). Daly et al. (1999), as cited in Kirley et al. (2002), reported an association between the DA receptor gene 148 bp DRD5 allele and ADHD, using a family-based study design. Other researchers have found significant evidence of association regarding this polymorphism and Payton et al. (2001), as cited in Kirley et al. (2002), also found a trend of association between the 148 bp DRD5 allele and ADHD children.

A study conducted by Volkow et al. (2009) using PET to measure DA synaptic markers (transporters and D2/D3 receptors) included 53 nonmedicated adults with ADHD and 44 healthy controls between 2001 and 2009 at Brookhaven National Laboratory in Long Island, NY. Findings suggest that there is a disruption in the mesoaccumbens DA pathway in ADHD, and PET imaging revealed a lower D2/D3 receptor and DAT (DA presynaptic marker) availabilities in those with ADHD than in the control group (Volkow et al., 2009). According to Volkow et al. (2009), the results of the PET imaging were documented in two key brain regions for reward and motivation (accumbens and midbrain) and also corroborated disruption of synaptic DA markers in caudate in adults with ADHD, providing preliminary evidence that the hypothalamus may also be affected.

Genetic studies suggest that the genetic architecture of ADHD is complex and the handful of genome-wide scans that have been conducted thus far show divergent findings and are, therefore, inconclusive (Faraone & Mick, 2010). Although candidate gene studies of ADHD have produced substantial evidence implicating several genes in the etiology of the disorder, these associations are small and consistent with the idea that the genetic vulnerability to ADHD is mediated by many genes of small effect, which will require studies that provide enough statistical power for detection of these genes (Faraone & Mick, 2010). Faraone and Mick (2010) reported no statistically significant association with acetylcholine receptors, glutamate receptors, and brain-derived neurotropic factors (BDNF) and ADHD, although 20 SNPs (single nucleotide polymorphisms) in the BDNF gene were tagged in the IMAGE project. The influence of specific receptor genes warrants further research to be conducted regarding the neurochemistry of ADHD.

Single nucleotide polymorphisms or SNP (pronounced "snip") are worth mentioning in this chapter since they are the newest medical advance related to genetics and will be a useful tool in a nurse practitioners evidence-based practice. There has been a recent flurry of SNP discovery and detection due to recent advances in technology, coupled with the unique ability of these genetic variations to facilitate gene identification. According to the article, "SNPs: Variations on a Theme," 2007), a SNP is a small genetic change, or variation, that can occur within a person's DNA sequence. There are millions of SNPs available in the human body ("SNPs: Variations on a Theme," 2007) and the genetic code is specified by four nucleotide "letters" A (adenine), C (cytosine), T (thymine), and G (guanine). SNP variation occurs when a single nucleotide, such as an A, replaces one of the other three nucleotide letters—C, G, or T ("SNPs: Variations on a Theme"). The article reports that it will only be a matter of time before physicians can screen patients for susceptibility to a disease by analyzing their DNA for specific SNP profiles. Studying the genetics of drug responses could be instrumental in the creation of "personalized medicine," the ability to target a drug to those individuals most likely to benefit. SNPs are not responsible for a disease state but instead serve as excellent biological markers for pinpointing a disease on the human genome map ("SNPs: Variations on a Theme").

ADHD AND ENVIRONMENT

Biederman et al. (2002b), as cited in Ryan and McDougall (2009), found that adverse psychosocial factors contributed to the risk of ADHD and its associated morbidity and dysfunction, after controlling for confounding factors such as parental mental health and gender. Individual differences in genetic risk factors are likely to alter the sensitivity of a child or young person to environmental risks which may explain why some children seem more vulnerable than others to psychosocial stressors (Caspi et al., 2002 as cited in Ryan & McDougall, 2009). Modesto-Lowe et al. (2008) reported that studies focusing on the interactions between mothers and their sons indicated high levels of child-rearing stressors induced by the child's ADHD symptoms. These parents typically displayed high levels of overreactivity, a tendency to be more critical of their children, and were less rewarding and less responsive to their children than parents of children without ADHD (Modesto-Lowe et al., 2008). Modesto-Lowe et al. (2008), explain than the degree of parental dysfunction appears to correlate with the presence and severity of ADHD-related disruptive disorders such as ODD and CD. Ebert et al. (2008) report that ADHD and ODD/CD have been found to co-occur in 30% to 50% of cases in both epidemiologic and clinical samples. Research studies show that parents of children with ADHD are found to have lower self-confidence and less warmth and involvement with their children and use physical discipline significantly more than the parents of control children do (Modesto-Lowe et al., 2008).

Stressful psychic events, disruption of family equilibrium, and other anxiety-inducing factors contribute to the initiation or perpetuation of ADHD and include predisposing factors such as the child's temperament, genetic-familial factors, and the demands of society to adhere to a routinized way of behaving and performing (Sadock & Sadock, 2007). Overall, Modesto-Lowe et al. (2008), reveal that available cross-national data replicate the U.S. findings and indicate that parents of children with ADHD experience higher levels of parental stress, resulting in adverse effects on parental functioning. It is pointed out by Modesto-Lowe et al. (2008), that some of the studies referenced may have included heterogeneous samples of children, including both children with ADHD and those with comorbid disruptive disorders.

In addition to considering the challenges of being a child with ADHD, providers must also consider how the challenges of parenting are exacerbated when raising a child with ADHD regardless of or in addition to the presence of comorbidities. These parental challenges affirm the need for provision of supports and resources for parents and primary caretakers caring for or raising children with ADD or ADHD with comorbidities, the latter of which is often present in children and adults. Most researchers and clinicians currently concede that genetics, biological, environmental, and psychosocial factors all play a crucial role in the assessment, management, treatment, and prognosis of ADHD in children, adolescents, and adults.

ASSESSMENT

Barkley and Newcorn (2009) report that although ADHD is a developmental disorder, up to 85% of children with ADHD are at risk for having the disorder as adults. The *DSM-IV-TR* (American Psychiatric Association [APA], 2000) is a diagnostic tool used for collaboration with insurance companies and other providers as a common language, but the true assessment process commands a holistic, biopsychosocial approach individualized to the needs of each individual child, adolescent, and adult. The goal of assessment is to differentiate between those children with behavioral symptoms of ADHD that are persistent versus symptoms that are occasionally exhibited or occur because of some external cause (Smith, 2007). According to Pelham et al. (2005), the main focus of assessment in ADHD should be impairment and adaptive skills. Barkley and Newcorn (2009) recommend the following for assessment of adults with ADHD:

1. Obtain patient's self-report on current functioning using the *DSM-IV-TR* criteria as well as functioning before the age of 16.
2. Obtain corroboration of symptoms and evidence of impairment in several major life activities.
3. Obtain evidence of a chronic course of illness without periods of remission.
4. Define impairment relative to the average person.
5. Explain impairment that developed after 16 years of age.
6. Use rating scales for adult ADHD.
7. Rule out a low IQ, learning disabilities, and other co-occurring disorders (comorbid disorders are common in ADHD and can make accurate diagnosis difficult).

For children and adolescents, the above assessment recommendations could be adopted with the following considerations:

1. Obtain child, adolescent, and parent reports on current functioning using the *DSM-IV-TR*.
2. Obtain corroboration of symptoms and evidence of impairment in activities in school, home, and with peers.
3. Obtain evidence of a chronic course of illness without periods of remission (this often helps distinguish anxiety and mania from ADHD symptoms as there is usually remission with these comorbid disorders).

4. Define impairment relative to the average child, taking into consideration the hormonal influences of adolescence.
5. Nonapplicable for children and adolescents.
6. Use rating scales for child and adolescent ADHD.
7. Rule out a low IQ, learning disabilities, and other co-occurring disorders (comorbid disorders are also common in children and adolescents with ADHD and can make accurate diagnosis difficult).
8. Consideration of high IQ in children and adults is also valuable as oftentimes adults can't recall having difficulty with ADHD symptoms before the age of 7 because they had above average intelligence and adapted well throughout elementary and middle school.

A comprehensive initial psychiatric evaluation is essential for each individual, regardless if the only chief complaint being presented is ADD/ADHD. Information gathered during this process, in addition to conducting a mental status exam, will be useful in identifying differential diagnoses. It is important to address or rule out substance use issues during the assessment process if a diagnosis of ADHD is made and stimulants are being considered. Rader et al. (2009) point out that hyperactivity and impulsivity seem particularly common in younger children and by adolescence the hyperactivity associated with ADHD wanes and the consequences of childhood ADHD become evident, including the development of coexisting problems, which will be addressed later in this chapter. The predominantly inattentive type has several characteristics such as easy distractibility, forgetfulness, daydreaming, disorganization, poor concentration, losing or misplacing things, and difficulty completing tasks (e.g., classroom or homework assignments) (Rader et al., 2009). The majority of adults seem to present with the inattentive type of ADHD and usually describe difficulties managing the household or performing in a work setting. Other symptoms experienced by adults are chronic lateness, marital difficulties, clumsiness/laziness, poor listening skills, angry outbursts, difficulty prioritizing and starting tasks, reckless driving/traffic accidents, and restlessness/inability to relax. With the exclusion of marital difficulties and reckless driving, the symptoms listed are also experienced by many children and adolescents with ADHD. Many adults also report that family, peers, and colleagues have remarked on their symptomatology.

Screening tools specific for children and adults are also useful during the assessment process and should be documented in the initial evaluation. There are a plethora of rating scales for assessing ADHD in children and adults. The scales presented in this chapter are the most commonly utilized scales. Rosier et al. (2006) state that most scales are of two types: self-rated (SR), and observer rated (OR). The majority of the rating scales are designed to assess the 18 diagnostic criteria of the *DSM-IV* (Rosier et al., 2006). Rader et al. (2009) report that scales used in the assessment of childhood ADHD may be used in the evaluation of ADHD but are not recommended in the diagnosis of the condition. Diagnostic tests such as lead levels, thyroid hormone levels, neuroimaging, and electroencephalography are also not needed to establish the diagnosis of ADHD but they may be warranted based on specific history and physical examination findings (Rader et al., 2009). The input of parents/caregivers and teachers is a crucial part of the assessment process to determine a child's symptoms in various settings. According to Rader et al. (2009), the American Academy of Pediatrics (AAP) devised the following questions to be used as an initial screening test:

1. How is your child doing in school?
2. Are there any problems with learning that you or the teachers have noticed?
3. Is your child happy in school?
4. Are you concerned with any behavioral problems in school, at home, or when your child is playing with friends?
5. Is your child having problems completing classwork or homework?

Rating scales for the assessment of childhood ADHD (Rader et al., 2009) include:

BROADBAND ASSESSMENTS

- Behavior Assessment System for children
- Child Behavior Checklist/Teacher Report Form
- Conners Rating Scales (long form)

NARROWBAND ASSESSMENTS

- ADHD Rating Scale
- Behavior Assessment System for Children—Monitor for ADHD
- Childhood Attention Problems Scale
- Comprehensive Teacher's Rating Scale
- Conners Rating Scales (short form)
- Disruptive Behavior Rating Scale
- Vanderbilt Assessment Scale

ASSESSMENT OF MEDICATION ADVERSE EFFECT

- Side Effects Rating Scale

Rating scales for the assessment of adult ADHD (Rosier et al., 2006):

- Conners Adult ADHD Rating Scales (CAARS-SR and CAARS-OR)
- Current Symptoms Scale (CSS-SR and CSS-OR), Adult Self Report Scale (ASRS), and the ASRS Screener
- ADHD Rating Scale-IV (ADHD-RS-IV)
- Brown ADD Rating Scale (Brown ADD-RS)
- ADHD-SR and ADHD-OR

The following descriptions of the adult rating scales are cited in the Rosier et al. (2006) article. The Conners Adult ADHD Rating Scale (CAARS-OR and CAARS-SR) include self–report and observer–report scales which both have a long, a short, and a screening version. The CAARS measures emotional lability and problems with self-concept in addition to the calculation of *DSM-IV* oriented inattention, impulsivity, and hyperactivity scores. The Current Symptoms Scales (CSS-OR and CSS-SR) in comparison to the CAARS, focus exclusively on the *DSM-IV* defined psychopathology, and both scales use the 18 *DSM-IV* items. A specific feature of the two CSS scales is the opportunity to rate ADHD-interfered functional deficits and the symptoms of ODD.

The Adult Self-Report Scale (ASRS) and the ASRS Screener are official instruments of the WHO and contain 18 *DSM-IV* items. The screener has four inattention items and two hyperactivity items which highly correlate with the full scale ASRS and are available in different languages. The screener is widely used by professionals in assessing adult ADHD. The ADHD Rating Scale (ADHD-RS-IV) was originally designed for children and adolescents but has been used in studies with adults, particularly in pharmacological trials. This scale is also available in Spanish.

The Brown ADD Rating Scale (Brown ADD-RS) was developed before the *DSM-IV* concept was published. The primary focus is on inattention versus hyperactivity and impulsivity. Other symptom domains are assessed such as organizing work, managing affective interference, sustaining energy and effort, and working memory. The ADHD-SR and the ADHD-OR were originally designed for the use in German-speaking countries and the principles of construction of the ADHD-SR are similar to those of the ASRS. In the case of the ADHD-OR, the selection and graduation of the 18 *DSM-IV* items was done using the ADHD-RS as a model. Both scales contain the 18 *DSM-IV* items of inattention, hyperactivity, and impulsivity.

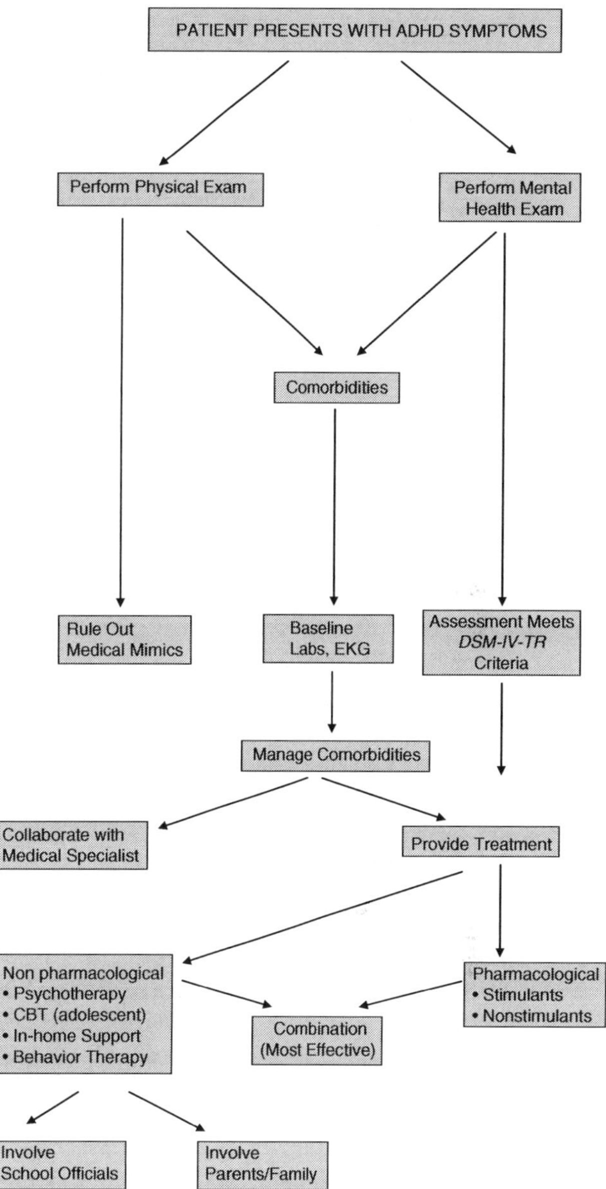

Figure 14-2 Decision Tree: Child/Adolescent With ADHD

DECISION TREE

Figure 14-2 depicts a decision tree for managing children and adolescents with ADHD and Figure 14-3 shows one for managing adults with ADHD. A biopsychosocial approach is crucial in the assessment process when diagnosing ADHD in children, adolescents, and adults. A mental health and physical exam are important components of a thorough evaluation. It is recommended that a physical exam be performed by the appropriate provider such as a pediatrician or primary care physician (PCP) to rule out or manage medical comorbidities and/or medical mimics before a diagnosis of ADHD is made or before stimulants are prescribed.

Nonpharmacological approaches complement medication management and a multidisciplinary approach

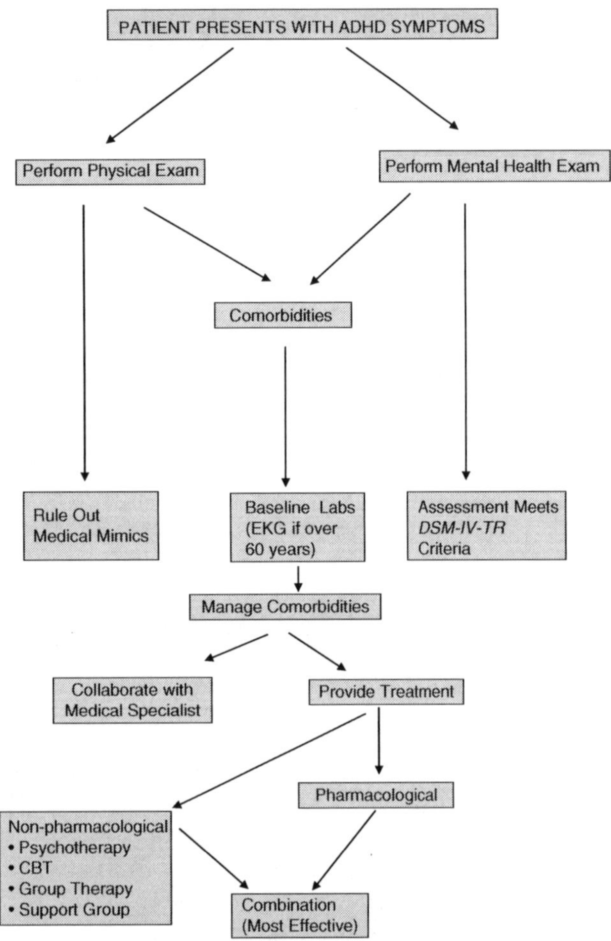

Figure 14-3 Decision Tree: Adult With ADHD

can be beneficial for all ages. Children and adolescents may have multiple venues in which collaboration is essential for a thorough assessment of symptoms observed by adults, that is, parents, school officials, and coaches. Adults often receive feedback from family, friends, and coworkers regarding ADHD symptomatology.

DIAGNOSIS

According to Smith (2007), the diagnosis of ADHD is based on certain behavioral criteria, as no biological markers currently exist to identify this condition. Conner (2002), as cited in Smith (2007), revealed a few key points that increase the likelihood of an ADHD diagnosis:

1. When children's symptoms develop very early and when their symptoms are much more severe than what is expected for their developmental level.
2. When children's symptoms are apparent in contexts other than the home environment, such as in the school or community.
3. When children's symptoms continue past the duration of an environmental stressor (e.g., parental divorce, trauma).

Although school age children with ADHD have been diagnosed and effectively treated, limited knowledge is available on the diagnosis and treatment of preschool children (Arons et al., 2002, as cited in Smith, 2007). Connor (2002), as cited in Smith (2007), reports that experts are increasingly diagnosing preschool children with ADHD and treating them for this disorder, despite this lack of knowledge and understanding. Conner (2002), as cited in Smith (2007), continues by stating that the core symptoms of ADHD (i.e., inattention, impulsivity, and hyperactivity) are common behaviors for many children in the preschool years which creates a challenge in diagnosing this disorder. Consequently, a diagnosis is not possible using a single test Cantwell, 1996, (as cited in Smith 2007) and Blackman, 1999 (as cited in Smith 2007) suggests that ADHD assessment should incorporate standardized rating scales, direct observations of behavior, structured interviews and direct measures of attention, hyperactivity and impulsivity. Schaughency and Rothlind (1991), as cited in Smith (2007), have identified the following as among the most important sequence of questions that have been suggested by numerous authors to assist in the assessment and diagnosis of ADHD:

1. Does the child meet *DSM-IV* criteria?
2. Are there alternative explanations for the symptoms?
3. Are the symptoms developmentally inappropriate?
4. Do the symptoms impair the child's functioning?

The revised and the original Conners' Parent and Teacher Rating Scale (CRS; Connors, 1997), as cited in Smith (2007), was referenced by 19 articles and was the most popular rating scale used in research studies for the assessment of ADHD in preschool children (it is used for ages 3–17).

It is questionable whether the *DSM-IV* criteria are adequate to characterize adult ADHD since no validation study in adults has ever been performed (Rosier et al., 2006). According to Rosier et al. (2006) the set of 18 *DSM-IV* symptoms characterizing the different ADHD types was originally developed for use in child psychiatry and Wender (1995), Murphy and Barkley (1996), and McGough and Barkley (2004), as cited in Rosier et al. (2006), state that some of the *DSM-IV* symptoms are clearly inappropriate such as "runs and climbs excessively" or "has difficulty playing quietly." The subjective experiences of the child are not part of the diagnostic criteria but play a substantial role in psychopathology for adults, the latter of who have an increased ability and accuracy of self-recognition of symptomatology. Although the subjective experiences of children are not part of the diagnostic criteria, it is beneficial to include them in the assessment and diagnostic process, in an age appropriate manner, to exercise good practice. As mentioned previously, the *DSM-IVTR* (American Psychiatric Association, 2000) criteria for adults with ADHD is being reviewed for the *DSM-5*.

PSYCHIATRIC COMORBIDITIES

Comorbidity or co-occurring refers to the presence of one or more disorders occurring simultaneously with the primary disorder. Overall, up to 44% of people classified with ADHD have at least one other psychiatric disorder, 32% have two others, and 11% have at least three other disorders (Barkley, 1999 as cited in Decker, McIntosh, Kelly, Nicholls, & Dean, 2001). Ebert et al. (2008) identify comorbid conditions in children and adolescents as oppositional.

Oppositional Defiance Disorder (ODD), Conduct Disorder (CD), anxiety disorders, cognitive performance and learning disabilities, Tic Disorders and Substance-Use Disorders. ODD is characterized by a pattern of negativistic, hostile, and defiant behavior, and CD is a more severe and less common disorder of habitual rule breaking defined by a pattern of aggression, destruction, lying, stealing, or truancy (Ebert et al., 2008).

ADHD and ODD/CD have been found to co-occur in 30% to 50% of cases in both epidemiologic and clinical samples and while CD is a strong predictor of substance abuse, ODD without CD is not (Ebert et al., 2008). Mood Disorders can also co-occur in children with ADHD and Ebert et al. (2008) report that in epidemiologic studies and several controlled, prospective studies, higher rates of depression were found in ADHD children. Children with comorbid mania at either baseline or follow-up assessment had other correlates expected in mania, including additional psychopathology, psychiatric hospitalizations, and severely impaired psychosocial functioning as well as a greater family history of mood disorders. According to Ebert et al. (2008), ADHD children with comorbid anxiety disorders had increased psychiatric treatment, and more impaired psychosocial functioning as well as a greater family history of anxiety disorders.

Children with ADHD perform more poorly than controls on standard measures of intelligence and achievement (Ebert et al., 2008). Decker et al. (2001) relate that historically there has been an overlap between ADHD and learning disabilities (LDs). Barkley (1996), as cited in Decker et al. (2001), estimates that between 19% and 26% of individuals with ADHD also meet criteria for at least one type of LD. Lambert and Sandoval (1980), as cited in Decker et al. (2001) estimated about 30% to 40% of children classified with LD also met ADHD criteria. Problems with attention often influence behavior in multiple settings, including the classroom, and make learning more difficult for both memory encoding and retrieval (Decker et al., 2001). Children with ADHD also have higher rates of Tic Disorders according to Ebert et al. (2008), that may contribute additional dysfunction due to distractions and social impairments directly attributable to the movements or vocalizations themselves. Juveniles with ADHD are at risk for cigarette smoking and substance abuse during adolescence, according to combined data from retrospective accounts of adults and prospective observations of youth (Ebert et al., 2008). ASD, including Asperger's Disorder, will be discussed in a separate section at the end of this chapter.

Sleep disorders can also coexist with ADHD and can modify prognosis and treatment responses (Corkum et al., 2010). According to Meltzer and Mindell (2006), as cited in Corkum et al. (2006), ADHD has one of the highest rates of sleep problems of all child mental health disorders. Corkum et al. (2011) report that depending on the operational definition of sleep problems used, the prevalence estimates of sleep problems based on parent reportings have varied widely, but have been consistently high (i.e., 50% to 80%). The most common sleep problems reported by parents of children with ADHD are difficulties initiating or maintaining sleep, both of which typically shorten sleep duration and can cause problems for the family and child (Corkum et al., 2011). Corkum et al. (2011) point out that although sleep problems are common in children with ADHD these are often overlooked and rarely included in research examining the comorbidity of ADHD, as evidenced by the exclusion of sleep disorders in the Multimodal Treatment of Children with Attention Deficit Hyperactivity Disorder (MTA) study, which is the largest treatment trial of ADHD. Melatonin is a common sleep aid used to treat sleep disorders in children in addition to sleep hygiene and behavioral strategies.

There are only a few studies addressing the issue of ADHD with comorbid Eating Disorders, most of which utilized different methodologies and had small samples limiting the generalizability of the results (Nazar et al., 2008). According to Nazar et al. (2008), available studies suggest that adult women with ADHD have a higher risk of developing an Eating Disorder.

Comorbidities in adults with ADHD include substance abuse, affective disorders, antisocial and borderline personality disorders (Schmidt & Petermann, 2009). Barkley and Newcorn (2009) point out that many adults with ADHD also have co-occurring psychiatric disorders, including anxiety (47%), mood (38%), impulse control (20%), and SUD (15%). Barkley and Newcorn (2009) report that symptoms of ADHD can be concealed by more robust symptoms of co-occurring conditions and conversely, comorbid anxiety and learning disorders can be obscured by more obvious ADHD symptoms. The following is a description of each comorbid disorder as described by Schmidt and Petermann (2009).

In prospective studies a strong association was found between the consumption of substances, behavior disorders in childhood, and a negative social environment. Individuals who use stimulating substances report a better "drive" and ability to concentrate which has consequences for the diagnostic process. Clarification is necessary to decipher if the symptoms can be regarded as reactions to the substance abuse rather than as ADHD specific symptoms.

Many individuals show extreme reactions to frustrating events due to emotional instability and emotional reactivity with depressive disorders. Some studies regard ADHD as a risk factor for developing a bipolar affective disorder and in one study, a comorbidity of ADHD and major depression was found in 15% of the cases, while 7.6% of the sample met the diagnostic criteria for a dysthymic disorder and 10.4% of a bipolar affective disorder. ADHD and bipolar affective disorder are clearly distinguishable.

An overall increased level of arousal as well as the tendency to hyperfocus can facilitate the development of an anxiety disorder. A caveat is that the tendency to hyperfocus can also be a symptom of ADHD in children and adults. Biederman (2005) as cited in Schmidt and Petermann (2009), reported a life time prevalence rate of comorbid anxiety disorders in 50% of the patients affected by ADHD in adulthood. According to Kathleen Nadeau PhD, people with ADHD have a disregulated attention system versus a short attention span due to their ability to hyperfocus (Kolberg & Nadeau, 2002). Nadeau points out that examples of hyperfocusing might be a child playing a video game to the exclusion of playing with friends and an adult who is shopping or surfing the web for hours versus going to a movie (Kolberg & Nadeau, 2002). The risk of developing an antisocial personality disorder is elevated in the presence of oppositional behavior and the development of a conduct disorder. These symptoms are often exhibited in the form of aggressive traffic behavior, delinquency, and as substance and alcohol abuse. The domain of delinquency in particular plays a significant role, with different studies highlighting the relation of ADHD, comorbid antisocial personality disorder, and delinquent behavior. A study of 129 inmates compared to a control group conducted by Rosier et al. (2004), as cited in Schmidt and Petermann (2009), reported a 45% prevalence rate of ADHD according to the *DSM-IV* criteria. The prevalence rates in numerous other international studies on the interrelation of ADHD and delinquency are lower.

The biggest diagnostic challenge is the comorbidity of ADHD and borderline personality disorder. A study conducted by Fossati et al. (2002), as cited in Schmidt and Petermann (2009), involving 42 patients with borderline personality disorder, revealed that 59.5% reported ADHD symptoms in childhood. Another study also reported a clear link between ADHD and borderline personality disorder.

In summary, preschool age seems to be an important developmental stage in which ADHD symptoms can first be assessed and the transition into adulthood can be regarded as a crucial developmental transition point. The assumption that ADHD is a disorder that only occurs in childhood has dominated clinical psychology for many years due to the high comorbidity with other disorders.

MEDICAL COMORBIDITIES

Ruling out medical comorbidities and medical mimics are a crucial component of the initial assessment process. Medical comorbidities seen in children and adolescents with ADHD are obesity, thyroid disorders, seizures, impaired vision or hearing, learning, speech and language disorders, and mild mental retardation. Obesity, fibromyalgia, hypertension, thyroid disorders, seizures, and nicotine dependence are comorbidities seen in adults with ADHD. The acronym THINCMED is a useful mnemonic utilized by practitioners to rule out medical mimics for children, adolescents and adults with ADHD. The following are medical conditions that can mimic psychiatric symptoms: **T**umors, **H**ormones, **I**nfectious diseases, **N**utrition, **C**entral nervous system, **M**iscellaneous, **E**lectrolyte abnormalities, and **D**rugs (Hedaya, 1996). A more detailed discussion of common medical comorbidities which co-occur with psychiatric syndromes will be presented in Chapter 19.

ACHIEVING CONCORDANCE

Shared decision making begins with the establishment of a positive, therapeutic relationship in which the individual and/or family feels validated and understood. The placebo effect is usually associated with medication trials in a research setting, however, a placebo effect may develop for the client during the initial evaluation with the instillation of hope through the development of a therapeutic relationship. Employing active listening skills in a nonjudgmental manner will allow the client to develop a sense of trust that the nurse practitioner is an ally operating in their best interest. The Institute of Medicine of the National Academies has emphasized the importance of client-centered care that is grounded in respect and sensitivity to client preferences, needs, and values and that recognizes clients and families as equal partners with mental health or other human service professionals (Bussing & Lall, 2010). Bussing and Lall (2010) eloquently state that in a clear departure from paternalistic power structures still common in much of medicine, these concepts emphasize equal partnerships between clinicians and clients or families.

Consideration and validation of negative experiences the client or family may have had is a crucial component of the initial meeting. Many adults with ADHD have endured their symptoms of ADHD without support or treatment. The nurse practitioner's willingness to be empathic and his/her ability to exude sensitivity related to the client's lost time is crucial in establishing trust and understanding. Clients must have a safe environment to articulate their story and recognize their active role in choosing their course of treatment. Recognition that clients are the experts on their bodies, together with the nurse practitioner's medication knowledge, allows a team approach to be implemented. In the case of children, parents, teachers, and other adults who have observed the child's behavior in various settings are a valuable resource since they witness behaviors that may not be apparent on the initial evaluation. Parents often report feeling unheard by providers, resulting in valid anger, frustration, and mistrust in the medical field.

The Psychiatric Mental Health Advanced Practice Nurse (PMH-APRN) must learn strategies to manage their countertransference (projection of their own unresolved conflicts related to information the client is presenting) and gain an understanding of their own beliefs regarding ADHD. Weekly clinical supervision or monthly peer supervision is highly recommended in order for the nurse practitioner to manage his/her own feelings and conflicts. The supervision process is an opportunity to process feelings and conflicts and receive feedback from an objective colleague. This process will aid the nurse practitioner in maintaining healthy boundaries in the therapeutic relationship.

EXPECTED OUTCOMES

There are additional elements for the PMH-APRN to consider regarding expectations, when working with individuals with ADHD across the life span. Although ongoing evaluation of evidence-based conventional and nonconventional treatments for ADHD is essential for best clinical practice, the development of basic goals, in collaboration with the individual, can be a driving force in the treatment process.

- Establishment of a therapeutic relationship of trust and nonjudgmental acceptance
- Safe environment that fosters honesty and provides validation
- Alleviation of ADHD symptomatology
- Grief related to years of impaired functioning without treatment
- Biopsychosocial, holistic approach
- Increased knowledge for management of ADHD
- Acquisition of strategies for maintenance and relapse prevention
- Age appropriate shared decision making for empowerment
- Utilization of resources and supports
- Ongoing evaluation of treatment success
- Implementation of new treatments when necessary
- Improved overall level of functioning

TREATMENT INITIATION

Treatment initiation is the next step now that the diagnosis of ADHD has been established. As Waite (2007) so precisely states, the goal of treatment is to improve the individual's quality of life; therefore, patients and NPs should work collaboratively to develop a treatment plan. Although the subjective experiences of children are not part of the diagnostic criteria, it is beneficial to include them in the assessment and diagnostic process, in an age appropriate manner, to exercise good practice. As mentioned previously, the *DSM-IV-TR* (American Psychiatric Association, 2000) criteria for adults with ADHD is being reviewed for the *DSM-5*.

Although pharmacological treatment is considered as the first line treatment for ADHD, it is important to consider nonpharmacological treatments such as psychosocial interventions for children and adults. As with other mental health disorders, medication is only one component of treatment and there is evidence that a combination of nonpharmacological and pharmacological treatments are the most effective. It is essential that mental health professionals familiarize themselves with emerging research findings about widely used complementary and alternative medicine (CAM) treatments of ADHD in order to provide individuals with accurate information on efficacy, safety, and appropriate use (Lake, 2010). No nonpharmacological treatments have been empirically proven to treat adult ADHD, although research suggests possible benefits with Cognitive Behavioral Therapy (CBT) (Safren et al., 2005 as cited in Waite, 2007). It is an asset to have a plethora of treatment options available since the needs of each individual treated for ADHD are diverse. Some parents are ambivalent about starting their children on stimulants and are more likely to consider CAM therapies. This parental concern is valid and verifies the importance of the nurse practitioner's need to examine their own values and belief about alternative medicine, as mentioned in the concordance section of this chapter, in the treatment of ADHD.

NONPHARMACOLOGICAL TREATMENTS

Cheng and Jetmalani (2009) report that although the majority of children with ADHD are treated by their primary care pediatricians, most children, especially those with comorbidities, display symptoms in multiple environments and require multimodal treatment (academic, family, individual, and medical interventions). The pediatrician may become the focal point for facilitating collaborations between a team of professionals to provide comprehensive treatment (Cheng & Jetmalani, 2009). These professionals may include teachers, child psychologists and psychiatrists, psychiatric and family nurse practitioners, clinical counselors and social workers, occupational therapists, and sleep specialists. Bussing and Lall (2010) state that the one missing ingredient in suboptimal ADHD treatment may be insufficient partnering between families and treatment providers. The number of successful treatment outcomes has not increased, despite our increased understanding of ADHD and its evidence-based treatments (Bussing & Lall, 2010).

Bussing and Lall (2010) have provided strategies for effective parenting, such as partnered treatment plan development and implementation and monitoring. These strategies involve increasing a families knowledge regarding research-based efficacy concepts, the latter of which is provided in the NAMI publication "Choosing the Right Treatment: What Family Members Need to Know About Evidenced-Base Practices" (Bussing & Lall, 2010). This strategy engages families and professionals in a team approach with the common goal of improving quality of life for patient and family. In regards to implementation and monitoring, it is crucial to consider what outcomes matter to the family in addition to what the provider views as most important (again we revisit the importance of the nurse practitioner's awareness of their own beliefs and values and ability to maintain openness).

BEHAVIOR-MODIFICATION

Behavior modification techniques may include daily report cards targeting problem behavior with positive reinforcement for school-age children and these approaches can be taught to parents and school personnel to reinforce appropriate behavior and minimize interactions that injure the child's self-esteem (Zametkin & Ernst, 1999). Other strategies are employed through behavioral modification systems such as a token economy, star charts, response costs, and positive reinforcement (Ryan & McDougall, 2009).

According to Antshel and Barkley (2008), Behavioral Parent Training (BPT) techniques generally consist of training parents in general operant conditioning techniques, such as contingent application of reinforcement or punishment after appropriate/inappropriate behaviors. The BPT programs seem effective for children who have disruptive behaviors whether or not they have co-occurring ADHD, although most of the studies on BPT are of short duration and do not assess maintenance of treatment effects (Antshel & Barkley, 2008). Antshel and Barkley (2008) point out that teachers often receive explicit training in classroom behavioral management during their training and education which speaks to why more research has occurred on the application of behavior management methods in the classroom than with parent training.

Behavior therapy has been shown to be effective in supporting children and young people to develop social skills and improve academic performance (Ryan & McDougall, 2009). The key to success is consistency with implementation of strategies, structure, and maintenance.

COGNITIVE BEHAVIORAL THERAPY

CBT is not demonstrated as efficacious in children who have ADHD but there are reasons to be optimistic that CBT may be more efficacious in adolescents who have

ADHD (Anthshel & Barkley, 2008). Anthshel, Faraone, and Kunwar (2008) also concede that CBT may be efficacious in reducing functional impairments in adults. Safren and colleagues, as cited in Anthshel et al. (2008), developed a supplemental CBT Program for adults with ADHD who were receiving medication, and initial results from a small-scale study of this manualized therapy have shown significant benefits beyond those achieved by medication alone. Ramsay and Rostain, as cited in Anthshel et al. (2008), also created a CBT Program for adults with ADHD which was an open study of 43 adults with ADHD who were treated for 6 months with a combination of pharmacotherapy and CBT. The combined treatment approach, according to Anthshel et al. (2008), was effective across both symptom and functional parameters. As Barkley, Biederman, and others' longitudinal samples continue to age, we will know more about the continuation of ADHD in middle and late adulthood (Anthshel et al., 2008).

CBT combines cognitive interventions with behavioral therapy and the aim of CBT is to interrupt the cognition cycle and link thoughts, feelings and behavior to improve overall day to day functioning (Ryan & McDougall, 2009). According to Ryan and McDougall, CBT builds on the principles of behavior therapy as outlined by aiming to enhance skills of self-control achieved through enabling children and young people to develop skills of reflection, self-regulation, positive self-reinforcement, and self-evaluation.

INDIVIDUAL, FAMILY, AND GROUP THERAPY

Play therapy could be valuable when treating children with ADHD considering environment factors may influence behavioral issues. Individual therapy for adolescents and adults can assist with gaining understanding in an articulate manner of how ADHD symptomatology can affect their quality of life. Adults who were not diagnosed or treated in their youth may embark in a grieving process regarding a lost opportunity to have experienced improved functioning and academic performance.

Parents and siblings of the child with ADHD, or in the case of adults, their partners, children, and colleagues are directly affected by the behaviors of the individual with ADHD. There is a lack of robust studies to evaluate the effectiveness of family therapy for ADHD, according to Ryan and McDougall (2009), although family interventions are widely used. Like many other psychological interventions, group therapy has a paucity of literature reviewing the effectiveness of these interventions (Ryan & McDougall, 2009). Ryan and McDougall point out that group interventions are cost-effective in terms of time and resources and they can provide opportunities for peer support, role modeling, and interpersonal skills-building; however, a caveat is that group interventions can also be intimidating and perpetuate difficulties associated with socialization for young people who are shy and lack confidence.

COMPLEMENTARY AND ALTERNATIVE THERAPIES

The frequency of CAM therapies in children who have ADHD ranges between 12% and 64% with the lower estimates likely the result of a narrow definition of CAM (Weber & Newmark, 2007). According to Weber and Newmark (2007), the treatments for ADHD include nutritional interventions, biofeedback, herbal and natural products, vitamins and minerals, homeopathy, massage and yoga, the beneficial impact of playing in green spaces, and the detriment of neurotoxicants.

NUTRITIONAL INTERVENTIONS

The verdict is controversial as to whether or not nutritional supplements are effective in treating ADHD. According to Ballard, Hall, and Kaufmann (2010), a randomized controlled trial (RCT) of 63 children, ages 6 to 12 years, with ADHD were randomly assigned supplementation with the most abundant polyunsaturated fatty acids (PUFA), docosahexanoic (DHA), or placebo for 4 months, found no significant differences in ADHD symptoms after the first 2 months. Written tests, objective attention evaluation by computer, and standardized objective measures such as the Conner's Rating Scales were used to measure outcomes (Ballard et al., 2010). A deficiency of these fatty acids was thought to contribute to a range of developmental disorders, including ADHD, since they are essential for brain development and function (Ballard et al., 2010). According to Weber and Newmark (2007), children are at a particular risk for low concentrations of these omega-3 fatty acids because of the recommendation that children not consume fish on a frequent basis due to its high mercury content.

ELECTROENCEPHALOGRAPHIC BIOFEEDBACK

Electroencephalographic (EEG) biofeedback is a growing area of research for ADHD and is based on the finding that children who have ADHD demonstrate abnormal quantitative EEG results in a pattern of underactivity in the majority of cases, or hyperarousal in some patients

(Weber & Newmark, 2007). Weber and Newmark (2007) conclude that future studies need to be conducted to randomize participants to treatment allocation with a placebo form of EEG biofeedback as the control.

HERBAL AND NATURAL HEALTH PRODUCTS

Ginsengs and ginkgo are believed to have nontropic effects to improve memory and facilitate learning and although the study found improvement in ADHD symptoms over the 4 week intervention, efficacy could not be determined because no comparison group was studied (Weber & Newmark, 2007).

VITAMINS AND MINERALS

There is research that indicates low levels of zinc in children with ADHD. Zinc reduced symptoms of hyperactivity, impulsivity, and socialization difficulties in children and adolescents with ADHD but did not improve symptoms of inattention. To prevent toxicity it is important to monitor liver enzymes and serum or cell membrane levels if using vitamins and minerals higher than the recommended dosage (Weber & Newmark, 2007).

HOMEOPATHY

According to Weber and Newmark (2007), homeopathy is based on the belief that "like treats like" and that the energetics of a small amount of substance can have healing effects on individuals. Findings led investigators to conclude that the effectiveness of homeopathy may be the result of the nonspecific effects of the interaction with the homeopath and not the actual remedy given, which indicates a need for further research to explore this possibility (Weber & Newmark, 2007).

MASSAGE AND YOGA

Although a limited sample size, Weber and Newmark (2007) revealed that the investigators reported improvement in ADHD symptoms in the yoga group on some of the measures of the Conner's Parent Rating Scale. According to Weber and Newmark (2007), the adolescents with ADHD in the massage group were rated by their teachers to have decreased symptoms of hyperactivity, anxiety, and inattention but the difference was not statistically better than the improvement seen in the relaxation group.

PLAYING IN GREEN SPACES

The environment contains a variety of chemicals and toxins, many of which are linked to neurodevelopmental disorders and the symptoms of the toxic effects of mercury and lead are similar to the symptoms of ADHD (Weber & Newmark, 2007). Weber and Newmark (2007) point out that many parents have always believed that a connection to nature is beneficial to children.

PHARMACOLOGICAL TREATMENTS

Between 1980 and 2007, there was almost an eight-fold increase of ADHD prevalence in the United States compared with rates of 40 years ago. Before 1970 the diagnosis of ADHD was relatively rare for schoolchildren and almost nonexistent for adolescents and adults (Connor, 2011). Safer and colleagues, as cited in Connor (2011), estimated the prevalence of ADHD in American schoolchildren as 1% in the 1970s, 3% to 5% in the 1980s, 4% to 5% in the mid to late 1990s and in 2007, using data from the National Survey of Children's Health. Visor and colleagues, as cited in Connor (2011), reported that 7.8% of youths aged 4 to 17 years had a diagnosis of ADHD and 4.3% reported current use of medication for the disorder.

As was discussed earlier in the chapter, DA and NA are two neurotransmitters that are essential to prefrontal cortex (PFC) function, and small changes in these neurotransmitters can have marked effects (Kaplan & Newcorn, 2011). In 1937, according to Kaplan and Newcorn (2011), Charles Bradley published a paper describing a "spectacular" improvement in the school performance of behaviorally disordered children who were treated with dl-amphetamine (benzedrine). This marked the beginning of modern child psychopharmacology and documented that amphetamines (AMP) were a potentially effective treatment for the condition that subsequently became known as ADHD. Methylphenidate (MPH) (Ritalin) followed in the 1950s with reports by Knovel and colleagues and others, as cited in Kaplan and Newcorn (2011). Stimulants are amongst the most well-researched psychotropics and their high degree of efficacy has been demonstrated in multiple randomized controlled studies in which they were shown to improve the core ADHD symptoms of hyperactivity, impulsivity, and inattention, in addition to academic productivity or task completion, family interactions, aggression, school disruption, peer interactions, and antisocial behaviors. Stimulants may even decrease the risk for subsequent comorbid psychiatric disorders and academic failure (Kaplan & Newcorn, 2011).

OVERDIAGNOSING AND OVERPRESCRIBING

According to Connor (2011), controversy and public debate over the diagnosis and medication treatment of ADHD continue to exist despite it being the most extensively studied pediatric mental health disorder. The increase in stimulant prescribing for pediatric ADHD was only part of a shift to an emphasis on medication interventions for the treatment of children with early-onset and complex behavioral and mental health disorders (Connor, 2011). Stimulant use among adults has also increased over the past few years with more young and older adults being diagnosed with ADHD. According to Connor (2011), comprehensive provider ADHD evaluation practices are essential for accomplishing evidence-based stimulant prescribing and for reducing unwanted variation in stimulant prescribing rates.

Constant monitoring of signs of stimulant abuse such as running out early or losing prescriptions may be a sign that a patient is abusing or selling his/her medication. Adderall and Ritalin are the stimulants of choice that can be snorted and result in a high. Because Vyvanse is a prodrug there is less abuse potential and it is a preferred stimulant in college-aged youth living on college campuses. It is important to document education regarding stimulant use and a signed consent form stating a patient will not abuse or sell their medication. Fortunately stimulants don't require tapering if a potential for substance abuse is suspected. It is a challenge to assess whether or not a patient is reporting ADHD symptoms to obtain stimulant use. Although patients who are untreated with ADHD exhibit unsafe driving, the patient who is abusing stimulants is also considered to be unsafe due to significant impairment that ensues from overuse of stimulants. *Diversion* is the practice by which legitimate stimulant prescriptions for ADHD are diverted for reasons other than treating ADHD (Connor, 2011).

STIMULANTS

Kaplan and Newcorn (2011) report that several preparations of AMP and MPH are available in the United States, in both generic and branded formulations. In the past few years, ADHD changed from a condition that manifests only during school hours to one that can potentially impair the patient's functioning in all settings throughout the day, and so came the dawn of longer-acting extended release preparations (i.e., Extended Release (ER), Long Acting (LA), Sustained Release (SR), Extended Release (XR). A list of pharmacological agents to treat ADHD are listed in Table 14-1. Longer acting stimulants are only dosed once a day versus twice or more with the short acting preparations, the latter causing a challenge for adherence in children and adults (Kaplan & Newcorn, 2011). Vyvanse is a prodrug (a prodrug must undergo chemical conversion by metabolic processes before becoming an active pharmacological agent), and has a different delivery system in the body as compared to other stimulants. It does not convert to dextroamphetamine until lisdexamphetamine (Vyvanse) reaches the gastrointestinal tract. Therefore it may take 1 to 1½ hours to take effect. It is delivered in the body similar to a slow intravenous drip for duration of effectiveness lasting 12 to 14 hours. A caveat is to always consider that rates of metabolism may vary between individuals. It is delivered similar to a slow intravenous drip throughout the day versus a quick release of half the dose within hours a part.

Stimulants are contraindicated in patients who have cardiac defect diseases, unstable or moderate to severe hypertension, symptomatic cardiovascular disease, advanced arteriosclerosis, known hyperpsensitivity or idiosyncrasy to sympathomimetic amines, tics/Tourette Syndrome, hyperthyroidism, glaucoma, increased anxiety, a history of substance abuse, and during or within 14 days after the administration of monoamine oxidase inhibitors (MAOI) (Kaplan & Newcorn, 2011).

RESPONSE

Kaplan and Newcorn (2011) report that in children and adolescents, AMP and MPH are equally efficacious at the group level when dosed comparably, with a response rate of 65% to 75%. The overall stimulant response rate increases to as much as 85% if the two classes of medications are tried, with an observable response in 30 to 90 minutes. Overall, immediate release (IR) methylphenidate is the most well-studied drug for treatment of ADHD in adults (Peterson et al., 2008). Peterson et al. (2008) point out that, with regard to efficacy, the chances of clinically significant improvement were 2.7 to 3.3 times greater in trials of primarily immediate release (IR) methylphenidate than in trials with longer-acting forms of buproprion or longer-acting stimulants.

NONSTIMULANTS

When children, adolescents, and adults cannot tolerate side effects or fail to respond to stimulants, a nonstimulant is

TABLE 14-1: PHARMACOLOGICAL TREATMENTS FOR ADHD

MEDICATIONS	USUAL DOSAGE	MAX DOSAGE	CONSIDERATIONS
METHYLPHENIDATES			
Short Acting Ritalin	**Children** 2 mg/kg/day	60 mg/day	6 years and older
	Adults 20–30 mg/day	40–60 mg/day	
Focalin (Dexmethylphenidate)	2.5–10 mg bid	10 mg bid	2.5 mg bid in 4 hour intervals. Adjust in weekly intervals by 2.5–5 mg/day
Intermediate Acting			
Ritalin SR	20–30 mg/day bid	60 mg/day	Older SR
Long Acting			
Concerta	18 mg/day qam	72 mg/day	Newer SR
Focalin XR	**Children** 2.5–10 mg/day/ qam	20 mg qam	Same titration as IR but qam
	Adults 10 mg/day/qam	20 mg/day	Adjust weekly intervals by 10 mg/day
Ritalin LA	20 mg/day	60 mg/day	Adjust weekly 10mg increments
AMPHETAMINES			
Short Acting			
Dexedrine	**Children** 5–10 mg/day/ qam/bid	40 mg/day	6 and older increase 5 mg/week
	Adult 5–40 mg/day	40 mg/day	Divided
Intermediate Acting			
Adderall	**Children** 5 mg/qam/bid	40 mg/day	6 and older increase 5 mg/week
	Adult 10 mg/day	40 mg/day	12 and older increase by 5 mg/week
Long Acting			
Adderall XR	10 mg/day/qam	30 mg/day	Increase 5–10 mg/week
Dexedrine Spansules	5–40 mg/day/qam	40 mg/day	
Vyvanse	30 mg/day	70 mg/day	Increase 10–20 mg/weekly
Non-stimulants			
Strattera (Atomoxetine)	**Children** 0.5 mg/kg/day	1.4 mg/kg/day	70 kg or less. After 7 days increase to 1.2 mg/kg/day qam or divided
	Adults 40 mg/day	100 mg/day	Over 70 kg After 7 days increase to 80mg/day qam or divided after 2–4 weeks increase to 100 mg
Tenex (Guanfacine)	1 mg/qhs	2 mg/day	After 3–4 weeks increase to 2 mg/day. Monitor BP
Intuniv (Guanfacine Extended Release)	1 mg/qhs	4 mg/day	Increase by 1mg/week. Monitor BP
Wellbutrin (buproprion)	225–450 mg	150 mg/tid	Divided
Buproprion SR	200–450 mg	200 mg/bid	Divided
Buproprion XL	150–450 mg	450 mg/qam	Once qam. May cause anxiety

LA = long acting; BP = blood pressure.

considered for treating ADHD. Parents who are ambivalent about giving their child stimulants may be more apt to consider a nonstimulant. Adolescents or adults with a history of or potential for substance abuse may be a candidate for nonstimulant treatment. Strattera (Atomoxetine), a selective NA transport blocker indicated for the treatment of ADHD, is approved for children over 6 years of age and has been effective in children and adults (Ryan & McDougall, 2009). Strattera has a tendency to worsen motor tics.

According to Ryan and McDougall (2009), the effectiveness of Atomoxetine for children is currently being reviewed as part of the Cochrane Collaboration.

Intuniv (Tenex) is a centrally acting alpha 2A agonist and antihypertensive used in the treatment of ADHD. It is also indicated for the treatment of ODD, CD, PDD, and Tourette's Syndrome and motor tics, all of which can co-occur with ADHD. Although the mechanism of Guanfacine extended release (GXR) action in ADHD in unknown, the drug is a selective a-2A receptor agonist thought to directly engage postsynaptic the postsynapticly in the prefrontal cortex (PFC), an area of the brain believed to play a major role in attentional and organizational functions that preclinical research has linked to ADHD (Sallee, 2010). According to Sallee (2010), Guanfacine was originally developed as an IR agent and its extended release (GXR) form became available for use in November of 2009.

Wellbutrin (bupropion) is a norepinephrine DA reuptake inhibitor and antidepressant. It is also used in the treatment of smoking cessation and ADHD. It is not as effective as first line stimulants in many cases. Wellbutrin increases DA neurotransmission in the PFC. It may lower the seizure threshold and is contraindicated in bulimia.

ACUTE FOLLOW UP/MAINTENANCE

Best practice guidelines suggest a return visit in 2 weeks, following the initial evaluation after starting on medications. Two-week follow-up visits are also indicated if medications are being tapered, titrated or with the addition of a new medication. As the patient becomes stable on a dosage of medication, consecutive 1-, 2-, and 3-month visits are appropriate. A patient taking stimulants should have follow-up visits at no longer than 3-month intervals. Review side effects, efficacy, and monitor for an underlying mood disorder at each consecutive visit.

Children and adolescents may take "drug holidays" from stimulant usage. The advantage of stimulants is that they don't require tapering or cause discontinuation syndrome. Patients will often choose not to take their stimulants on the weekends or vacations. This is an individual preference with consideration for the severity of their symptomatology. Elicit feedback from support people and all disciplines involved in the treatment of children and adolescents. Repeat rating scales during follow-up visits to determine efficacy.

MANAGING SIDE EFFECTS

The following is a side effect profile according to Kaplan and Newcorn (2011): The most common side effects of stimulants are insomnia and anorexia. Other common side effects are headache, weight loss, new onset tics and irritability, with less frequent side effects being nausea, abdominal pain, palpitations, dizziness, drowsiness, and changes in pulse. Allergic reactions, fever, arthralgia, psychosis, depression, and sudden death (specifically in preexisting cardiac conditions) are rare side effects of stimulants.

Insomnia can be managed by Melatonin (regular or CR). Clonidine and Trazodone can be used to promote sleep in children and adults, although Clonidine is used more in children as it also helps reduce aggressive behaviors in children. Other sleep aids such as Lunesta and Ambien can be used for adults and should be taken ½ to 1 hour before bedtime. Taking the stimulant before noontime may also help to promote sleep. Good sleep hygiene is important for children, adolescents, and adults. Examples include: no food before bedtime, engage in calming activities before bedtime, establish an earlier bedtime, and avoid daytime naps. A pattern of going to bed and rising at the same time also helps to reestablish a good sleep pattern.

Anorexia is common with the use of stimulants. Most patients will report a decreased appetite but report that they continue to eat nutritiously. Vyvanse may be taken with or without food. Taking amphetamines with food may delay peak actions for 2 to 3 hours. If nausea and vomiting occur, switching to another agent or nonstimulant may be effective.

ADDITIONAL CONSIDERATIONS

1. Do not administer Guanfacine extended release with high fat meals because this increases exposure.
2. Gastrointestinal acidifying agents such as ascorbic and fruit juices and urinary acidifying agents lower amphetamine plasma levels and therefore may

also lower therapeutic efficacy of amphetamines. Therefore, routinely ask about vitamin use during initial evaluation such as vitamin C and multivitamins which contain vitamin C. Suggest they take vitamin C at nighttime (Stahl, 2011).

3. Proton Pump Inhibitors such as Prilosec and Nexium can interfere with the absorption of Adderall and Adderall XR by increasing amphetamine plasma levels and potentiate amphetamines actions. Vyvanse is a better choice in this case.
4. Start low and go slow when prescribing, to decrease side effects.
5. It is important to create an accurate diagnosis of ADHD as there are statistics that indicate people with ADHD have more driving accidents due to difficulty focusing.
6. With short acting Ritalin and Dexadrine there may be a rebound effect when the drug is wearing off, resulting in much worse ADHD symptoms versus a return to usual symptoms.
7. Parents are often diagnosed with ADHD when their children are diagnosed, as they can relate to their child's symptomatology which unfolds during the initial assessment with the use of rating scales and obtaining a family history.
8. Educate adolescents and adults regarding the fact that stimulants mask the effects of alcohol and consequently they may be unable to judge their true level of intoxication.
9. Some patients report that extended release stimulants such as Adderall XR lose efficacy in the late afternoon and may require supplementation with an immediate release agent such as Adderall IR. As mentioned earlier in this chapter, some patients, due to their individual metabolism, can tolerate taking an extended release stimulant twice a day with effectiveness and without any effect on sleep pattern. This is important to assess at each visit, in addition to appetite.

CULTURAL CONSIDERATIONS

Although the prevalence of ADHD is similar across cultures, cultural differences can be a major factor in determining whether ADHD symptoms are seen by individuals as problematic, and if they are, whether a person seeks care and remains adherent to treatment (Goldman et al., 1998, as cited in Buitelaar, Kan, & Asherson, 2011). Livingston

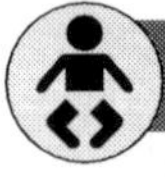

PEDIATRIC POINTERS

1. Take blood pressure and pulse before starting stimulants since they increase blood pressure and heart rate. Monitor vital signs 1 to 3 months after initial treatment and 6 to 12 months at regular follow-up visits, when stable on dosage. A heart condition does not exempt children and adolescents from being treated with stimulants, but careful monitoring will be necessary throughout treatment by a pediatrician or ideally a pediatric cardiologist.
2. Baseline and periodic monitoring of height and weight is crucial in children due to stimulant-induced growth suppression. Recommendations for periodic monitoring of height and weight were included in treatment guidelines and drug product labeling instructions (Vitiello, 2008). The average preschooler treated with stimulants requires short-acting agents due to low weight.
3. Take a baseline electrocardiogram (EKG) prior to starting stimulants for children with preexisting heart conditions or to rule out congenital heart disease or arrhythmias that could predispose a child to sudden cardiac arrest. Repeat an EKG later if the child is younger than age 12 since some cardiac abnormalities are not present until adolescence.
4. A nutritional diet and exercise regime are an important part of the treatment plan in conjunction with medication management.
5. Check interactions with other psychiatric and medical medications the child may be taking.
6. Collaborate with PCP and other providers regarding medical conditions and medication adjustments in order to establish continuity of care.

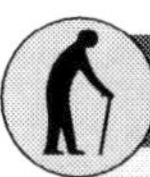

AGING ALERTS

1. Take a baseline electrocardiogram (EKG) for adults over the age of 50 to rule out cardiac abnormalities. Consult with a cardiologist as needed to discuss stimulant use in adults with various heart conditions.
2. Take a baseline blood pressure and pulse before starting stimulants, monitor 1 to 3 months after initiation of treatment and 6 to 12 months at regular follow-up visits when stable on dosage.
3. Check interactions with other psychiatric and medical medications since many older adults are on multiple medications. Collaborate with primary care provider and other specialists regarding medical conditions and adjustments made to medication regime (i.e., blood pressure).
4. Routinely ask if antihypertensive medications have been adjusted by their PCP and document changes in the medical record. *Caveat*: Be cautious when considering antihypertensives such as Clonidine or Intuniv in the treatment of ADHD in older adults who are already taking antihypertensive agents.

(1999), as cited in Buitelaar et al. (2011) points out that attitudes and beliefs about illness, choice of care, access to care, degree of trust toward majority institutions and authority figures, and religious beliefs and tolerance for certain behaviors, in addition to cultural differences in familial, educational, and social expectations can affect whether people seek treatment.

Cultural sensitivity is an essential quality that contributes to the establishment of an atherapeutic relationship between the individual and/or family and nurse practitioner. The nurse practitioner must gain knowledge of diverse cultural practices and examine their own cultural attitudes and beliefs, which could be detrimental to establishing and maintaining a therapeutic alliance.

AUTISM SPECTRUM DISORDER

PREVALENCE

In 2009, Maine Children's Services formed an Evidence Based Advisory committee that was charged with designing a guideline for evaluating the strength of evidence regarding specific treatment approaches (Maine Children's Services Autism Advisory Committee Report). This project was initiated after the identification of the rapid growth of ASD in the state of Maine and throughout the United States. For example, in Maine the number of identified ASD children grew from 594 children receiving special services in 2000 to 2,231 in 2008, an increase of more than 200% (Maine Children's Services Autism Advisory Committee Report, 2009). In the United States the cost over the lifetime of an individual with ASD is approx $3.2 million with a $35 billion annual national cost (Ganz, 2007). It is important to recognize that the increased number of diagnosed cases is not correlated with an increased incidence but rather a refinement of the diagnostic symptoms/features and a greater understanding of the diagnostic indicators. This knowledge helps to identify what types of lifetime support may be needed for functional improvement and a greater understanding of what specific types of needs correlate with what treatments are considered best practice. From the perspective of fiscal responsibility, patient safety, allocation of resources, and accountable care, these factors all coincide to support the use of reviewed evidence based framework in which to approach treatment.

The increased number of diagnosed cases that receive services is staggering. However it also lends itself to the consideration of a population of now adults who perhaps have been misdiagnosed or have spent a lifetime separated from societal norms without adequate support. Societal costs that are associated with either misdiagnosed or undiagnosed individuals are difficult to quantify but must be in the forefront of public health policy decision making. The cost of undiagnosed or untreated individuals, both adults and children, can be more staggering than the increase utilization of services.

ETIOLOGY/RISK FACTORS

While there is no single causative factor for ASD there is a general consensus that it is an abnormality in brain structure and function (Autism Society.org). The causative factors are multimodal including genetics, infectious, neurological, metabolic, immunologic, and environmental.

Brain scans show differences in the shape and structure of the brain in children with autism versus neuro-typical children. In many families there appears to be a pattern of autism or related disabilities, however, with research focused on identification of a specific gene this has not yet been determined (National Institute of Mental Health [NIMH] Parents guide). Rather it appears that it is a combination of a genetic predisposition that is "turned on" by environmental factors similarly to oncogenes. In addition, ASD occurs more frequently with certain medical conditions such as Fragile X syndrome, tuberous sclerosis, congenital rubella, and untreated phenylketonuria (PKU). Environmental toxins such as heavy metals may also play a role in the trigger of the genetic material (NIMH Parents guide). There is a higher incidence of seizures in ASD with an estimate of one out of every four (Eunice Kennedy Shriver National Institute of Child Health and Human Development, 2003). It is difficult to determine if the presence or absence of seizures is related to the disorder, lack of sleep, or an independent diagnosis particularly since there is evidence of abnormality of brain structure and function. Fragile X syndrome is a genetic disorder that causes symptoms similar to ASD and relates to approximately one in three children who meet the criteria for both disorders (Zafeirou, Ververi, & Vargiami, 2007; Eunice Kennedy Shriver National Institute of Child Health and Human Development). Since Fragile X syndrome is caused by a mutation on a single gene there is a range of genetic influence with one in 25 children diagnosed with ASD also having the gene that causes Fragile X. Tuberous sclerosis occurs in one out of four people with ASD (Smalley, 1998; Zafeirou et al., 2007). Tuberous sclerosis is a rare genetic disorder that causes tumor growth in organs, including the brain, that are nonmalignant. When located in the brain there are neurological effects including seizures, mental retardation, epilepsy, and so on.

Nutritional variations and the degree of influence are subject to debate. There is evidence that children have an increase in GI disturbances such as lactose intolerance, food allergies, reflux, diarrhea, or constipation, but this may not be a direct correlation to the disorder (NIMH Parents guide).

SYMPTOMS

The symptoms of ASD are at times difficult to associate with one another given the scope of spheres of influence in which they occur. In general the patient presents with symptoms in three domains, social, communication, and behavior. There is a description of patterns rather than a cadre of symptoms that fit a particular mold. The clinician should be skilled in identification of the developmental norms in all of these domains so that along with the caregiver the recognition of a pattern of developmental differences can be diagnostically determined so that early intervention can be considered.

In most cases, parents or guardians are the first to notice at times odd or peculiar behaviors that may seem pertinent only to them. In the past decade, pediatric providers have increasingly paid more attention to the concerns of parents, whereas previously these subtleties were often dismissed. Early symptoms that can be seen in infants are related to interacting with parents. For example, infants may seem preoccupied and make little eye contact or not coo and babble with their parents (NIMH). In other cases there is almost a "ceasing" of interaction that is noticed after age 2 or 3 when the child falls silent, withdrawn, or indifferent to their surroundings, actually regressing (Wiggins, Rice, & Baio, 2009).

As the child enters school these behaviors can be more noticeable and contribute to the challenges of social impairment, which in itself is a domain of developmental delay. A child on the playground may demonstrate oddities that become flags and result in teasing from their peers. Some children may live in a fantasy world and play out that fantasy in school, becoming a target of separation from their peers.

Along with oddities in behavior, a primary area of separation from norms is in the domain of social impairment. The scope of the degree in which this affects the prognosis can vary depending on the available resources in the community. *DSM-IV-TR* summarizes social impairment in four areas: absence or minimal eye contact, failure to respond to people and the surrounding environment, minimal sharing of toys or experiences even when pleasurable, and unusual responses when others are in distress (American Psychiatric Association, 2000). These behaviors can be a source of frustration for people in the child's environment and can contribute to a multitude of reactions from parents, caregivers, peers, and teachers. The seemingly "apathetic" child creates few friendships and is often alone but little is known about the internal process of what that may actually feel like to the child. Treatment is geared toward an attempt to create behavioral programs to teach social skills when there is little understanding regarding what is the true experience of the child. Repetitive and stereotypical behaviors can vary from unusual to extreme (American Psychiatric Association, 2000). Behaviors can be extremely pattern specific and reflective of obsessive-compulsive symptoms in regard to repetition of patterns. They may demonstrate what may seem to be obsessional thoughts when they hyper-focus on a particular item of interest. They can demonstrate "persistent intense preoccupation" (Wiggins et al., 2009). They may become overly interested in objects, numbers, or science topics. This does not mean that every child who is overly interested in a particular subject is at risk for ASD. The significance must impair their function and be in conjunction with a multitude of symptoms rather than a single area.

Since social cues encompass a wide range of manners, the classroom and the playground are in a sense the laboratory for research development. Often these children misinterpret those around them and do not respond in a socially normative way. They may seem to be "black and white" or "serious" and not demonstrate the ability to shift from reality to what may be a light-hearted joke. Facial expressions, movements, tone of voice, intolerance to other's opinions, and inability to predict other's actions are areas that for a child of normal development are innate whereas an ASD child does not respond in a normative way. Again, these children develop few friendships and relationships, which is associated with the hallmark identification of the disorder. Inability to comprehend and navigate nonverbal communication, read other people's body language, and identify with another's feelings may be misinterpreted as several other psychiatric disorders.

Communication discrepancies are also a prominent area of delay. The AAP developmental milestones define growth points where the child's development is expected to reach certain targets (AAP). Recognition of the divergence of communication may hearken to the infancy stage when there may be an absence of cooing or the disruption of that interaction as the child grows and becomes more seemingly withdrawn. Communication or lack thereof can be demonstrated in behaviors that are seemingly nonrelated. The inability to express needs can result in aggressiveness from many perspectives. Screaming, grabbing, and, at times, seemingly "out of control" behavior may be misinterpreted both diagnostically and developmentally when in fact these behaviors are related to a frustration with not being able to express a need through communicative measures. Asperger's children may have a fund of exceedingly high language development but may also demonstrate communication variance in the way they detail and ramble about a particular interest. There also may be elements to their language that are understood by their caregivers only and not accepted by peers or in a social environment. The term "echolalia" can be associated with communication difficulties with ASD children (repeating words or phrases that they hear), which can be associated with prodromal psychotic disorders. Communication can be summarized as an area that is less subjective than social and behavioral inconsistencies in these children, making any communication delay an area of immediate assessment.

Since the constellation of these symptoms is along a continuum, these children are at risk for aggressive behavior, anxiety, and depression, which may be the presenting symptoms that are identified. In addition, because of the levels of potential hyper-focus and seemingly lack of focus they are often either misdiagnosed with ADHD or they have a comorbid diagnosis. Treatment is dependent on the level of functional impairment. Fortunately, the education of pediatric providers, teachers, and parents has focused early intervention as associated with improved outcomes, which can have an effect on the prevention of other psychiatric disorders. As recent as the late 1990s these children could get through school without accurate or comprehensive diagnosis only to present with depression as a young adult where the primary disorder is in the realm of ASD.

TREATMENT

There has been controversy surrounding treatment for ASD. From dietary treatment to nonapproved medications and a variety of therapeutic interventions, parents and caregivers have been bombarded with ideas that have not always been associated with improvement or good outcomes. This speaks to the heightened awareness and passion about the long-term effects of the disorder on autonomy, family, and society. This is not to say that the modalities of treatment both conventional and nonconventional are not intended for the betterment of the individuals who are affected. However, given the degree of variability of supported evidence that has demonstrated consistent improvement, the Maine Autism Advisory Group set out to evaluate the research specifically for Autism Spectrum. The focus was on providing a guideline that has demonstrated efficacy (Maine Children's Services Autism Advisory Committee Report, 2009).

DECISION TREE

Figure 14-4 summarizes the decision tree for managing patients with ASD. Patients typically present with signs and symptoms of four domains. These can occur alone or in combination. They include social, communication, language, and behavior. A careful mental health and physical exam may or may not reveal if the patient has ASD. If

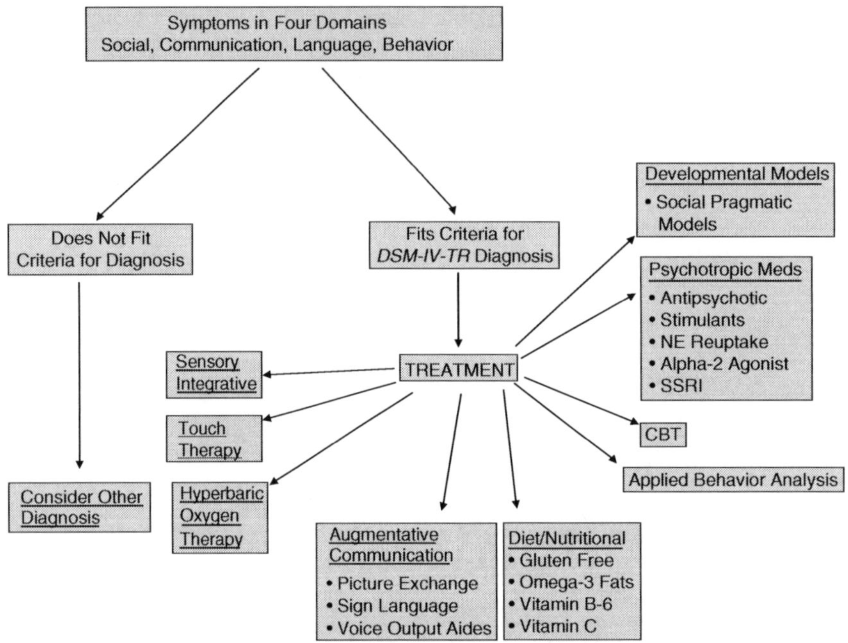

Figure 14-4 Autism Spectrum Disorder

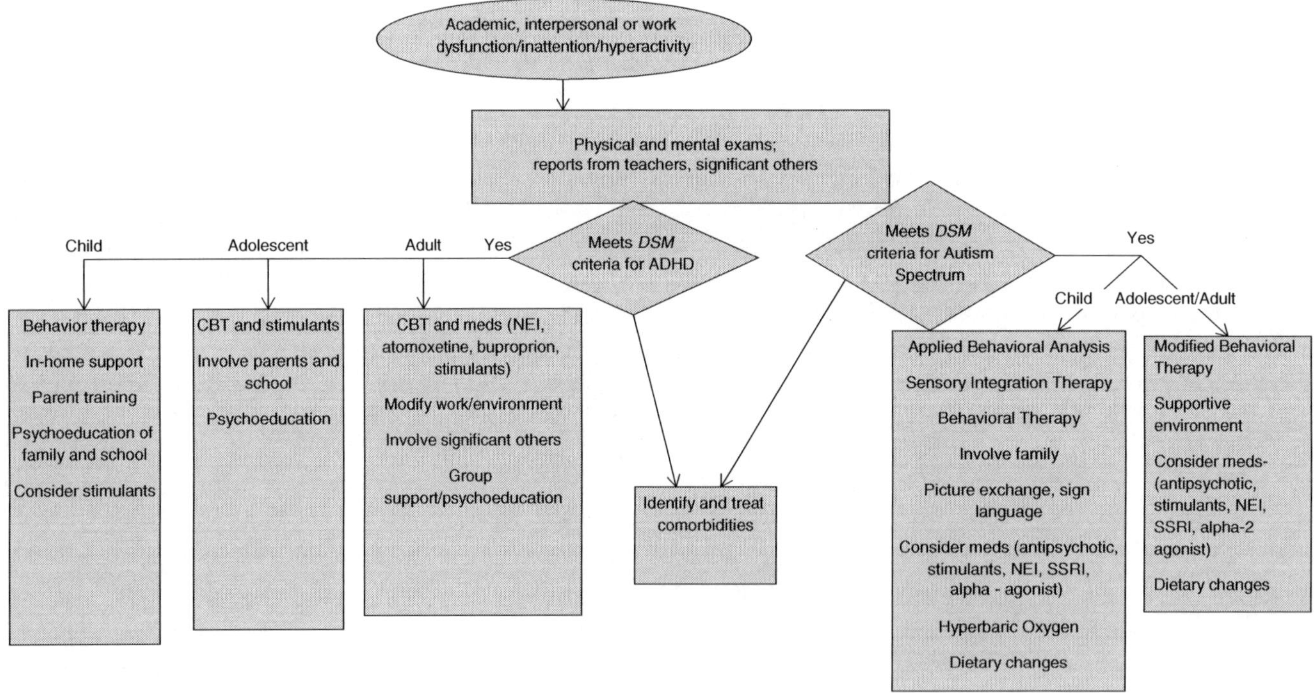

Figure 14-5 Initiating Treatment for Symptoms of Disordered Attention

patients are suspected and meet *DSM-IV-TR* criteria, consideration should be given to a multimodality approach to therapy. Applied Behavioral Analysis is the most effective treatment for demonstrating improved outcomes in several domains for target symptoms. The management also includes psychotropic medications (antipsychotics serotonin-specific reuptake inhibitor [SSRI], NE reuptakes, and stimulants). Diet and nutrition has been used with mixed results. CBT should also be considered. Other experimental approaches include hyperbaric oxygen therapy, developmental models, and social therapy. Augmentive communication has been used in certain cases with effect. Often patients require multimodality therapy in an effort to find the best combination.

SPECIAL POPULATIONS

While there is no one medication or treatment that is recommended for ASD, the management is focused on symptoms and developmental growth. A significant amount of information is available on the NIMH parents' guide for educational resources for parents and caregivers of patients with ASD. Careful preparation of children's stages of growth into adolescents and adults will require ongoing support and education. These are areas for development of support service projects that will serve to address the unique needs of these individuals as they enter adulthood. All ASD patients should be monitored for comorbid psychiatric diagnosis and medical disorders. Despite a growing body of evidence and diagnostic refined techniques there is little known regarding the treatment of the aging adult with ASD. This is a gap in the research and as the generation of newly diagnosed ASD children/young adults enter the older adult phase there needs to be further inquiry on the supports/treatment into older adulthood.

The assessment of the individual who presents with symptoms consistent with disordered attention requires a careful review that is initiated by some form of recognition of a social, academic or professionally functional impairment. Figure 14-5 depicts the multifaceted approach that the APRN should take when considering differential diagnosis and determining treatment recommendations. The complexities of the potential diagnosis (if any) are aided by the collaboration with supportive parties who are able to provide external information so that the clinician can perform a detailed comprehensive assessment. The diagnostic intricacies of individuals whose lives are impacted by attention difficulty requires skill and knowledge and are key to the initiation of treatment recommendations.

RESOURCES

BOOKS

Adventures in Fast Forward Life: Life, Love, and Work for the ADD Adult (1996) by K. G. Nadeau

Asperger's Syndrome: A Guide for Parents and Professionals (1998) by T. Attwood

Help4ADD@High School (1998) by K. G. Nadeau

Delivered from Distraction: Getting the Most Out of Life With Attention Deficit Disorder (2005) by E. M. Hallowell and J. Ratey

Freaks, Geeks, and Asperger Syndrome; A User Guide to Adolescence (2002) by L. Jackson

ADD-Friendly Ways to Organize Your Life (2002) by J. Kolberg and K. G. Nadeau

ADD in the Workplace: Choices, Changes and Challenges (1997) by K. G. Nadeau

Learning to Slow Down and Pay Attention: A Book for Kids About ADHD (2004) by K. Nadeau, C. Beyl (Illustrator), and E. B. Dixon

School Strategies for ADD Teens (1999) by K. G. Nadeau

Survival Guide for College Students With ADD or LD (2006) by K. G. Nadeau

Ten Things That Every Child With Autism Wish You Knew (2005) by E. Notbohm

Autism's False Prophets: Bad Science, Risky Medicine and the Search for a Cure (2008) by P. A. Offit

Children With Autism: A Parents Guide (2nd ed, 2000) by M. Powers

Autistics' Guide to Dating: A Book by Autistics, for Autistics and Those Who Love Them or Who Are in Love With Them (2008) by E. M. Ramey and J. J. Ramey

Driven to Distraction: Recognizing and Coping With Attention Deficit Disorder (ADD) From Childhood to Adulthood (1994) by E.M Hallowell and J. Ratey

WEBSITES

ADHD &You: www.adhdandyou.com/?utm_source=adhdsupport&utm_medium=vanity&utm_campaign=adhdsupport2012

Attention Deficit Disorder Association: www.add.org

CDC (Center for Disease Control), nnbddd (National Center on Birth Defects and Developmental Disabilities CDC.gov/ncbddd/adhd

National Institute of Mental Health: www.nimh.nih.gov

National Resource Center on ADHD: A program of CHADD (Children and Adults with ADHD): http://help4adhd.org; 1-800-233-4050

NICHD-Eunice Kennedy Shriver National Institute of Child Health and Human Development. Available at http://www.nichd.nih.gov/

WebMD: www.webmd.com

REFERENCES

American Psychiatric Association. (2000). *Diagnostic and statistical manual of mental disorders* (4th ed. TR, pp. 65–67). Washington, DC: Author.

Anthshel, K. M., & Barkley, R. (2008). Psychosocial interventions in attention deficit hyperactivity disorder. *Child and Adolescent Psychiatric Clinics of North America, 17*, 421–437.

Anthshel, K., Faraone, S. V., & Kunwar, A. (2008). ADHD in adults: How to recognize and treat. *Psychiatric Times, 48*(12). Retrieved from www.psychiatrictimes.com

Attwood, T. (1998). *Asperger's syndrome: A guide for parents and professionals*. London: Jessica Kingsley.

Autism Society. Retrieved from http://www.autism-society.org/about-autism/symptons

Ballard, W., Hall, M. N., & Kaufmann, L. (2010). Do dietary interventions improve ADHD symptoms in children? *Journal of Family Practice, 59*(4), 234–235.

Barkley, R., & Newcorn, J. H. (2009). Assessing adults with ADHD and comorbidities. *Prime Care Companion, Journal of Clinical Psychiatry, 11*(1), 25.

Bauman, M. L. (2006). Beyond behaviors-biomedical diagnoses in autism spectrum disorders. *Autism Adovate, 45*(5), 27–29.

Berridge, C. W., & Waterhouse, B. D. (2003). The locus coeruleus-noradrenergic system: Modulation of behavioral state and state dependent cognitive processes. *Brain Research Reviews, 42*, 33–84.

Buchsbaum, M. S. (2004). Frontal cortex function. *American Journal of Psychiatry, 161*(12), 2178.

Buitelaar, J., & Medori, R. (2010). Treating attention-deficit/hyperactivity disorder beyond symptom control alone in children and adolescents: A review of the potential benefit of long-acting stimulants. *European Child Adolescent Psychiatry, 19*, 325–340.

Buitelaar, J. K., Kan, C. C., & Asherson, P. (2011). *ADHD in adults: Characterization, diagnosis and treatment.* New York, NY: Cambridge University Press.

Bussing, R., & Lall, A. (2010). Keys to success in ADHD treatment. Strategies for effective partnering with families. *Psychiatric Times, 27*(10). Retrieved from www.psychiatrictimes.com

Cheng, K., & Jetmalani, A. (2009). It takes a village to treat ADHD: Community and clinica l collaborations. *Psychiatric Times, 8*(10). Retrieved from www.psychiatrictimes.com

Cherkasova, M. V., & Hechtman, L. (2009). Neuroimaging in attention-deficit hyperactivity disorder: Beyond the frontal-striatal circuitry. *The Canadian Journal of Psychiatry, 54*(10), 651–664.

Connor, D. F. (2011). Problems of overdiagnosing and overprescribing in ADHD. *Psychiatric Times, 28*(8). Retrieved from www.psychiatrictimes.com

Corkum, P., Davidson, T., & MacPherson, M. (2011). A framework for the assessment and treatment of sleep problems in children with attention deficit hyperactivity disorder. *Pediatric Clinics of North America, 58*, 667–683.

Decker, S. L., McIntosh, D. E., Kelly, A. M., Nichols, S. K., & Dean, R. S. (2001). Comorbidity among individuals classified with attention disorders. *International Journal of Neuroscience, 110*, 43–54.

Ebert, M. H., Loosen, P. T., Nurcombe, B., & Leckman, J. F. (2008). *Current diagnosis and treatment psychiatry* (2nd ed.). New York, NY: Mcgraw Hill.

Eunice Kennedy Shriver National Institute of Child Health and Human Development. (2003). *NIH, PHS, DHHS Families and Fragile X Syndrome* (NIH-96-3402). Washington, DC: U.S. Government Printing Office.

Faraone, S., & Mick, E. (2010). Molecular genetics of attention deficit hyperactvity disorder. *Psychiatric Clinics of North America, 33*, 159–180.

Ganz, M. L. (2007). The lifetime distribution of the societal costs of autism. *Archives of Pediatrics & Adolescent Medicine, 161*(4), 343–349.

Greydanus, D. E., Pratt, H. D., & Patel, P. R. (2007). Attention-deficit hyperactivity disorder across the lifespan: The child, adolescent and adult. *Disease-a-Month, 53*, 70–131.

Gromisch, E. S. (2010). Neurotransmitters involved in ADHD. *Psych Central*. Retrieved from http: //psycentral.com

Hallowell, E. M., & Ratey, J. (1994). *Driven to Distraction: Recognizing and Coping With Attention Deficit Disorder (ADD) From Childhood to Adulthood*. New York: Pantheon Books.

Hallowell, E. M., & Ratey, J. (2006). *Delivered from distraction: Getting the most out of life with attention deficit disorder.* New York: Ballantine Books.

Hedaya, R. J. (1996). *Understanding biological psychiatry* (1st ed., pp. 189–200). New York, NY: W. W. Norton & Company.

Jackson, L. (2002). *Freaks, geeks, and Asperger syndrome: A user guide to adolescence*. London: Jessica Kingsley.

Kaplan, G., & Newcorn, J. H. (2011). Pharmacotherapy for child and adolescent attention deficit hyperactivity disorder. *Pediatric Clinics of North America, 58*, 99–120.

Kieling, C., Kieling, R. R., Rohde, L. A., Frieh, P., Moffitt, T., Nigg, J. T., . . . Castellanos, F. X. (2010). The age at onset of attention deficit hyperactivity disorder. *American Journal of Psychiatry, 167*(1), 14–16.

Kirley, A., Hawi, Z., Phil, M., Daly, G., McCarron, M., Mullins, C., . . . Gill, M. (2002). Dopaminergic system genes in ADHD: Toward a biological hypothesis. *Neuropsychopharmacology, 27*(4), 607–619.

Kolberg, J., & Nadeau, K. (2002). *ADD-friendly ways to organize your life*. New York, NY: Routledge.

Lake, J. (2010). Integrative management of ADHD: What the evidence suggests. *Psychiatric Times, 27*(7). Retrieved from www.psychiatrictimes.com

Matson, J. L., Benavidez, D. A., Compton, L. S., Paclawskyj, T., & Baglio, C. (1996). Behavioral treatment of autistic persons: A review of research from 1980 to present. *Research in Developmental Disabilities, 17*, 433–465.

Matson, J. L., Nebel-Schalm, M., & Matson, M. L. (2006). A review of the methodological issues in the differential diagnosis of autism spectrum disorders in children. *Research in Autism Spectrum Disorders, 1*, 38–54. doi: 10.1016/j.rasd.2006.07.004

Matson, J., & Nebel-Schwalm, M. (2007). Comorbid psychopathology with autism spectrum disorder: An overview. *Research in Developmental Disabilities, 28*, 342–352.

Millichap, J. G. (2008). Etiologic classifications of attention-deficit/hyperactivity disorder. *Pediatrics, 121*(2), 358–365.

Modesto-Lowe, V., Danforth, J. S., & Brooks, D. (2008). ADHD: Does parenting style matter? *Clinical Pediatrics, 47*(9), 865–872.

Nadeau, K. G. (1996). *Adventures in fast forward life: Life. love, and work for the ADD adult*. Florence, KY: Brunner/Mazel.

Nadeau. K. G. (1997). *ADD in the workplace: Choices, changes, and challenges*. Florence, KY: Brunner/Mazel.

Nadeau, K. G. (1998). Help4AAA@high school. Bethesda, MD: Advantage Books.

Nadeau, K. G. (1999). *School strategis for ADD teens*. Bethesda, MD: Advantage Books.

Nadeau, K. G. (2004). *Learning to slow down and pay attention: A book for kids about ADHD*. Washington, DC: American Psychological Press.

Nadeau, K. G. (2006) *Survival guide for college students with ADD or LD*. (2006) Washington, DC: Magination Press.

National Institute of Mental Health. (2002). "A Parent's Guide to Autism Spectrum Disorder." NIMH Â·. N.p., n.d. Web. 03 July 2012. <http://www.nimh.nih.gov/health/publications/a-parents-guide-to-autism-spectrum-disorder/index.shtml>.

Nazar, B. P., Pinni, C. M. d. S., Coutinho, G., Segenreich, D., Duchesne, M., Appolinario, J. C., & Mattos, P. (2008). Review of literature of attention-deficit/hyperactivity disorder with comorbid eating disorder. *Revista Brasileira de Psiquiatria, 30*(34), 384–389.

Notbohm, E. ((2005). *The things that every child with autism wish you knew*. London: Jessica Kingsley.

Offit, P. A. (2008). *Autism's false prophets: Bad science, risky medicine, and the search for a cure*. New York: Columbia University Press

Pelham Jr., W. E., Fabiano, G. H., & Masseti, G. M. (2005). Evidence-based assessment of attention deficit hyperactivity disorder in children and adolescents. *Journal of Clinical Child and Adolescent Psychology, 34*(3), 449–476.

Peterson, K., McDonagh, M. S., & Fu, R. (2008). Comparative benefits and harms of competing medications for adults with attention-deficit hyperactivity disorder: A systematic review and indirect comparison meta-analysis. *Psychopharmacology, 197*(1), 1–11.

Powers, M. *Children with autism: A parent's guide*. Bethesda, MD: Woodbine House.

Preston, J. D., O'Neal, J. H., & Talago, M. C. (2005). *Handbook of clinical psychopharmacology for therapists* (4th ed.). Oakland, CA: New Harbinger Publication.

Rader, R., McCauley, L., & Callen, E. (2009). Current strategies in the diagnosis and treatment of childhood attention-deficit/hyperactivity disorder. *American Family Physician, 79*(8), 657–665.

Ramey, E. M., & Ramey, J. J. (2008). *Autistic's guide to dating: a book for autistics and those who love them or who are in in love with them*. London: Jessica Kingsley.

Rosier, M., Retz, W., Thomas, J., Schneider, M., Stieglitz R. D., & Falkai, P. (2006). Psychopathological rating scales for diagnostic use in adults with attention deficit hyperactivity disorder. *European Archives of Psychiatry and Clinical Neuroscience, 256*(1), 1/3–1/11.

Ryan, N., & McDougall, T. (2009). *Nursing children and young people with ADHD*. New York, NY: Routledge.

Sadock, B. J., & Sadock, V. A. (2007). *Synopsis of psychiatry behavioral science/clinical psychology* (10th ed.). Philadelphia, PA: Wolters, Kluwer/Lippincott, Williams & Wilkins.

Sallee, F. R. (2010). Guanfacine extended release for ADHD. *Current Psychiatry, 9*(1), 49–60.

Schmidt, S., & Petermann, F. (2009). Developmental psychology: Attention deficit hyperactivity disorder. *BMC Psychiatry, 9*, 58, Retrieved from www.biomedcentral.com

Smalley, S. L. (1998). Autism and tuberous sclerosis. *Journal of Autism and Developmental Disorders, 28*(5), 407–414.

Smith, K. G. (2007). Systematic review of measures used to diagnose attention-deficit/hyperactivity disorder in research on preschool children. *Topics in Early Childhood Special Education, 27*(3), 164–173.

SNP's: Variations on a theme. (2007). Retrieved from www.ncbi.nlm.nih.govl

Stahl, S. M. (2011). *The prescriber's guide. Stahl's essential psychopharmacology* (4th ed.). New York, NY: Cambridge University.

State of Maine. (2009). *Interventions for autistic spectrum disorder. Report of the Maine Children's Services Advisory Committee Report*. Retrieved from www.main.gov/dhhs/ocfs/cbhs/ebpac/asd-report2009.pdf

Stedman's Medical Dictionary for the Health Profession and Nursing (5th ed.). (2005). Baltimore, MD: Lippincott, Williams & Wilkins.

The subcortical areas involved in ADHD. Retrieved from www.macalester.edu/psychology

Vitiello, B. (2008). Understanding the risk of using medication for attention deficit hyperactivity disorder with respect to physical growth and cardiovascular function. *Child and Adolescent Psychiatry Clinics of North America, 17*, 459–474.

Volkow, N. D., Wang, G. J., Kollins, S. H., Wigal, T. L., Newcorn, J. H., Telang, F., Fowler, J. S., Zhu, W., Logan, J., Ma, Y., Pradhan, K., Wong, C., & Swanson, J. (2009). *Evaluating dopamine reward pathway in ADHD: clinical implications*. JAMA, 302 (10), 1084-1091.

Waite, R. (2007). Women and attention deficit disorders: A great burden overlooked. *Journal of the American Academy of Nurse Practitioners, 19*(30), 116–125.

Weber, W., & Newmark, S. (2007). Complementary and alternative medical therapies for attention-deficit/hyperactivity disorder and autism. *Pediatric Clinics of North America, 54*, 983–1006.

WebMD. (2009). *Brain and nervous system health center*. Retrieved from www.webmd.com/brain/picture-of-the-brain

WHO. (1993). *ICD-10 classification mental & behavioral disorders. Diagnostic criteria for research*. Retrieved from www.who.int/classification/icd

Wiggins, L. D., Rice, C. E., & Baio, J. (2009). Developmental regression in children with an autism spectrum disorder identified by a population-based surveillance system. *Autism, 13*(4), 357–374.

Yerys, B., Wallace, G., Sokoloff, J., Shook, D., James, J., & Kenworthy, L. (2009). Attention deficit hyperactive disorder symptoms modify cognitive and behavioral responses in children with autism spectrum disorder. *Autism Research, 2*(6), 322–333.

Zafeirou, D. I., Ververi, A., & Vargiami, E. (2007). Childhood autism and associated comorbidities. *Brain and Development, 29*(5), 257–272.

Zametkin, A. J., & Ernst, M. (1999). Problems in the management of attention-deficit/hyperactivity disorder. *The New England Journal of Medicine, 340*(1), 40–46.

Zametkin, A. J., Nordahl, T. E., Gross, M., King, A. X., Semple, W. E., Rumsey, J., . . . Cohen, M. R. (1990). Cerebral glucose metabolism in adults with hyperactivity of childhood onset. *The New England Journal of Medicine, 323*(20), 1361–1366.

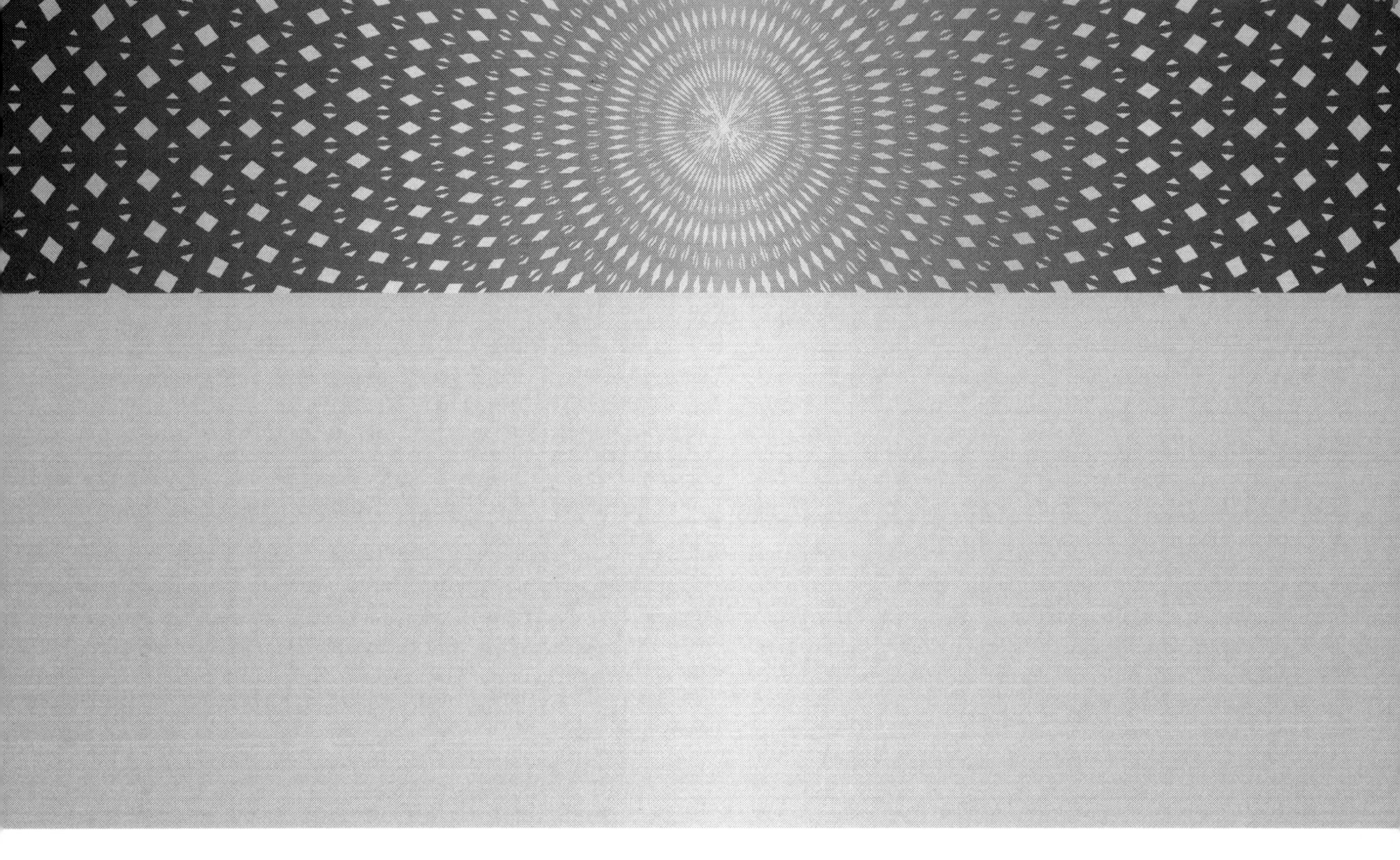

CHAPTER CONTENTS

OVERVIEW

Working with individuals who are self-injuring or contemplating suicide is complicated and difficult. This chapter will provide information to assist with methodical and sound clinical approaches in the assessment and treatment of individuals who are considering or actually self-injuring. Experiencing an individual who is self-injuring is a reality for most Psychiatrice Mental Health Advance Pracice Nurses (PMH-APRNs) and the literature providing evidence-based approaches to treatment is increasing.

AWARENESS OF OWN REACTIONS

By exploring one's own reactions and gaining an increased awareness of effective approaches, working with individuals who are self-injuring will become less daunting.

DEFINITIONS

Understanding the continuum of self-injurious behavior (SIB) begins with definitions of terms used in the literature as well as clinical practice. "Suicidal behavior is a broad term that includes death by suicide and intentional, nonfatal, self-injurious acts committed with or without intent to die" (Linehan et al., 2006b). Nonsuicidal self-injurious behavior (NSSIB) is the infliction of deliberate

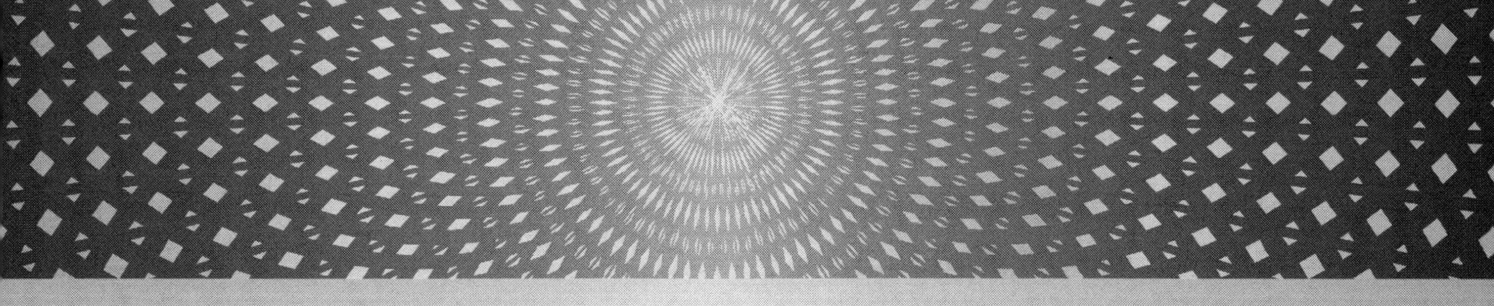

CHAPTER 15

Integrated Management of Self-Directed Injury

Ann M. Mitchell, Irene Kane, Kirstyn M. Kameg, Ereka R. Spino, and Bona Hong

bodily damage, usually by cutting oneself, without the intention to die (Nock, 2009; Brausch & Gutierrez, 2010; Gutierrez et al., 2001). Differentiating NSSIB from the plethora of terms (see Exhibit 15-1) used throughout the literature to describe suicide-related behaviors is critical because risk and other factors such as depressive symptoms, suicidal ideation, self-esteem, and support are not the same (Hankin & Abela, 2011; Jacobson & Gould, 2007; Muehlenkamp, 2006). In addition, suicidal behavior is often associated with mental disorders such as depression, substance dependence, and schizophrenia. More specifically, borderline personality disorder is only one of two *DSM-IV-TR* diagnoses in which suicidal behavior is a decisive factor (Linehan et al., 2006a, b).

NSSIB has been associated with many psychiatric diagnoses; however, there are incidences where no concomitant disorder is present (Nock, Joiner, Gordon, Lloyd-Richardson, & Prinstein, 2006). NSSIB does not involve explicit suicidal intent (SI) to end one's life as does suicidal behaviors; nonetheless, a higher risk for suicide attempts has been reported in individuals with a NSSIB history (Jacobson & Gould, 2007). Because the Centers for Disease Control and Prevention (2010) report that suicide is the third leading cause of death among 15- to 24-year-olds (accounting for about 12% of deaths annually); and is the 11th leading cause of death for all ages, a comprehensive understanding of NSSIB and its relation to suicidal behaviors including: Theoretical underpinnings, functions, risk factors, and approaches to care is required for AP-PMHNs to accurately implement an evidence-based nursing process. As Jacobson and Gould (2007) point out, the intent behind the act, its function, and epidemiology are important in prevention and treatment.

EPIDEMIOLOGY

"Worldwide, almost a million people die by suicide each year. Intentional, nonfatal, self-inflicted injuries, including both suicide attempts and acts without SI, also have a very high prevalence" (Comtois & Linehan, 2006, p. 161). NSSIB is most typically associated with a higher and growing incidence (13% to 23%) among adolescents (Ross & Heath, 2002; Nock, 2009; Hankin & Abela, 2011); with a 7.5% rate recently reported for onset in younger adolescence (Hilt et al., 2008). A small prevalence rate (1% to 4%) for adults is reported for NSSIB. Several studies noted a greater prevalence of NSSIB in females, whereas other studies found equivalent rates leading to inconclusive gender data (Jacobson & Gould, 2007). The prevailing data indicate no difference related to ethnicity or socioeconomic class (Nock et al., 2006; Yates, Tracy, & Luthar, 2008). Engaging in NSSIB varied per study, age group, and evidence of impairment, with one study suggesting a decrease in NSSI over time (Jacobson & Gould, 2007).

Significant steps must be taken within psychiatry, clinical psychology, and psychiatric nursing to aid in the

EXHIBIT 15-1: KEY TERMS

Nonsuicidal self-injurious behavior (NSSIB): deliberate, self-inflicted damage to body tissue without suicidal intent (SI) and for purposes not socially sanctioned (Nock et al., 2006; Ross, Heath, & Toste, 2009)

Self-injurious behavior (SIB): broad group of deliberate and direct self-harming behaviors (Nock et al., 2006)

Para-suicide: nonlethal, intentional self-harm (McGlothlin, 2008)

Suicide attempt: unsuccessful SIB with intent to die (APA Practice Guidelines, 2006)

Suicidal gesture: planned suicide attempt for the purpose of influencing others (Varcarolis, 2003)

Suicidal ideation: self-destructive thoughts (Varcarolis, 2003)

SI: subjective self-destructive expectations and desires to die (McGlothlin, 2008)

Suicide threat: verbal or nonverbal actions which communicate a suicidal or planned suicidal act (McGlothlin, 2008)

Suicide: purposeful, self-destructive ending of one's life (Varcarolis, 2003)

field of suicide prevention. Unfortunately, there is no data to suggest a program or specific treatment that offers a decrease in the rate of suicidal acts, which remains a central problem (Comtois & Linehan, 2006). That is, existing treatments need to be evaluated for use as a standard of care and for distinguishing NSSIB and SIB; and additionally, new treatments need to be developed and disseminated.

DIFFERENTIATING SUICIDE ATTEMPTS FROM SIB

It is important to differentiate NSSIB from suicide attempts with SI. Many studies have shown that suicidal behavior occurs at higher rates among adolescents, females, those who have mental and/or alcohol or substance use disorders, those who have a family history of mental disorders, and those who have a history of violence or victimization (Nock et al., 2008).

THE CASE APPROACH TO ASSESS NSSIB/SIB

Shea's Case Approach can readily be used as the first step of the nursing process to assess the client who presents with SIBs. Wilkinson (2012) observes that "assessment is more than writing information on an assessment form." The Case Approach encourages an exploration process that matches the critical thinking process. Wilkinson notes it is required to accurately assess a client's behavior while applying a myriad of theories, establishing a therapeutic alliance, and interpreting data. Interestingly, Shea's Case Approach prompted with the pneumonic from The American Association of Suicidology (AAS) serves to capture the evidence-based distinctions observed by researchers (Hankin & Abela, 2011; Jacobson & Gould, 2007; Muehlenkamp, 2004, 2005, 2006; Nock, 2006, 2009; Rosen, 1988; Ross & Heath, 2002; Shea, 1998, 2007; Shneidman, 1985; Walsh & Rosen, 1988; Wilkinson, 2011). (See Table 15-1).

ASSESSMENT

The formal structure required in a psychiatric interview (Wilkinson, 2012) can easily be fulfilled using the Case Approach incorporating "Behavioral Incidents" and "Gentle Assumptions" (Shea, 1998, 2007), which capture evidence-based observations and multiple theoretical frameworks. The Case Approach also goes hand-in-hand with the use of good communication techniques advocated for critical thinking during the assessment by the nurse (Wilkinson, 2012). The AAS recommends an easily remembered pneumonic to assess for the warning signs of acute risk for suicide (see Exhibit 15-2). This pneumonic can provide the clinician with a ready reference for "Behavioral Incidents" and "Gentle Assumptions" exploration throughout the 4-step Case Approach process.

Shea (1998) and Shea (2007) recommend using the 4-step Case Approach which organizes the clinician's multitude of assessment questions into time contiguous categories: past, recent, presenting, and immediate events. The fundamental components of suicidal assessment

TABLE 15-1: DIFFERENTIATING SIB AND NSSIB

ASSESSMENT FOCUS	SUICIDE ATTEMPT (SIB)	SELF-INJURY (NSSIB)
Attitude toward life and death	Repulsed by life Motivation to end a life as a solution to difficulties (terminating consciousness) (Jacobson & Gould, 2007; Muehlenkamp, 2004, 2006; Nock et al., 2006; Shea, 1998, 2007)	Less repulsed by life Morbid and dysfunctional coping strategy with motivation to live (attracted to life) (Jacobson & Gould, 2007; Muehlenkamp, 2004, 2006; Nock et al., 2006; Shea, 1998, 2007)
Suicidal ideation	Yes (Muehlenkamp, 2004, 2006)	None or low during self-injury (Muehlenkamp, 2004, 2006)
Level of physical damage and potential lethality	Serious physical damage, lethal means of self-harm (Jacobson & Gould, 2007; Shneidman, 1985; Shea, 1998, 2007)	Little physical damage, nonlethal means of self-harm (Muehlenkamp, 2004, 2006; Nock et al., 2006; Walsh & Rosen, 1988)
Presence of chronic, repetitive pattern of self-injurious acts	Rarely a chronic repetition, some repeated overdoses (Jacobson & Gould, 2007; Muehlenkamp, 2004, 2006; Shea, 1998, 2007; Shneidman, 1985)	Frequently a chronic, high-rate pattern: often cutting, self-hitting (Jacobson & Gould, 2007; Muehlenkamp, 2004, 2006; Nock et al., 2006; Shea, 1998, 2007; Walsh & Rosen, 1988)
Level of psychological pain	Unendurable, persistent (Nock et al., 2006; Shneidman, 1985)	Uncomfortable, intermittent (Nock et al., 2006; Walsh & Rosen, 1988)
Association with pain analgesia during self-injury	Increased pain, increased methods, increased suicide attempts (Nock et al., 2006; Shneidman, 1985)	Lower number of NSSI episodes, use of fewer NSSI methods (Nock et al., 2006; Walsh & Rosen, 1988)
Presence of constriction of cognition	Extreme constriction; suicide seen as the only way out; tunnel vision; seeking a final solution (Jacobson & Gould, 2007; Nock et al., 2006; Shneidman, 1985)	Little or no constriction; choices and options remain available; seeking a temporary solution (Jacobson & Gould, 2007; Nock et al., 2006; Walsh & Rosen, 1988)
Decrease in discomfort following the act	Not immediate; treatment required for improvement (Jacobson & Gould, 2007; Nock et al., 2006; Shneidman, 1985)	Rapid improvement and return to usual cognition and affect; successful "alteration of consciousness;" reinforced by calming effect (Jacobson & Gould, 2007; Nock et al., 2006; Shea, 1998, 2007; Walsh & Rosen, 1988)
Risk factors	Previous SIB/NSSIB and suicide attempt, family dysfunction, pain analgesia (Nock et al., 2006; Wilkinson, 2011)	Previous NSSIB, symptoms of depression and anxiety, borderline personality disorder most common—but not limited to (Nock et al., 2006; Wilkinson, 2011)
Gender	More female attempts than male (Muehlenkamp, 2004, 2006; Nock, 2009)	No conclusive gender differences (Jacobson & Gould, 2007; Muehlenkamp, 2004, 2006; Nock et al., 2006)

NSIB = nonsuicidal self-injurious behavior; SIB = self-injurious behavior.

emphasized throughout Shea's Case Approach include the use of the validity techniques of behavioral incidents, gentle assumptions, symptom amplification, denial of the specific, and normalization.

Step 1 is the "exploration of presenting events," which Shea (1998) describes as "exploring how close the client came to completing suicide" and how the client feels about being alive. Questions for Step 1 involve understanding the seriousness of the "Behavioral Incident," the attempt, including why it did not work, method and planning, level of stress and hopelessness, involvement of alcohol or drugs, and interpersonal factors. However, the method with the Case Approach is critical and asks the client to describe the event from beginning to end versus

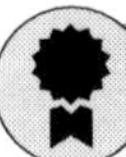

EXHIBIT 15-2: IS PATH WARM

IS PATH WARM?
I Ideations
S Substance Abuse

P Purposelessness
A Anxiety
T Trapped
H Hopelessness

W Withdrawal
A Anger
R Recklessness
M Mood Change

Retrieved July 5, 2011 from www.suicidology.org/web/guest/stats-and-tools/warning-signs. *Reprinted with permission from the American Association of Suicidology (AAS), a membership organization for all those involved in suicide prevention and intervention, or touched by suicide. AAS is a leader in the advancement of scientific and programmatic efforts in suicide prevention through research, education and training, the development of standards and resources, and survivor support services. For more information, visit www.suicidology.org.*

memorizing a list of questions to impose upon the client. As the client's narrative unfolds, the clinician uses "Gentle Assumptions," softened questions or statements, and "Behavioral Incidents," specific facts or detailed questions and statements carefully applied using "Shame Attenuation," if indicated, to help the client tell their story without fear or shame (Shea, 1998). Normalization, knowing that others may have experienced similar symptoms or feelings, may be employed to assist the client who denies or hesitates to admit to a symptom out of embarrassment, anxiety, or fear of care outcome if shared (Shea, 1998, 2007).

Step 2 continues with getting an overview of the client's history of attempts (past 6 to 8 weeks) to obtain greater understanding of the suicidal risk versus NSSIB. Shea (1998, 2007) notes there is no "cookbook" approach for the clinician, but suggests strategically applying and alternating straightforward "Behavioral Incidents" exploration with "Gentle Assumptions" to determine lethality frequency, duration, and intensity.

The completion of a recent history assessment leads to Step 3, which is judiciously spending time examining the most serious past suicide attempts or gestures to determine "triage decisions for client safety" (Shea, 1998). Safety is critical as clients may be inclined to downplay or distort their negative behaviors. It is important to employ what Shea (2007) describes as "Symptom Amplification" to ascertain behavioral incident downplay; and, "Denial of the Specific" to ascertain methods of SI by direct inquiry. An example of a symptom amplification question is, "How many suicide attempts have you made since the time you described that you first felt down," whereas asking the client, "Have you thought about overdosing?" compels the patient to deny a specific method.

Finally, Step 4 centers on current suicidal ideation to assess client safety needs. In addition to the accumulating interview information gathered throughout Steps 1–3, Shea (1998) and Shea (2007) stress the need to obtain corroborative reports from significant others to evaluate information as well as available support. If the 4-step assessment process results in a high lethality assessment, then the clinician should consider immediate safety contracting with the client (see Exhibit 15-3). As can be readily ascertained, the "IS PATH WARM" pneumonic offers a complementary assessment guide for use with the Case Approach to assist with the interview process if desired.

RELATIONSHIP-BUILDING DURING ASSESSMENT

Clinical interviewing even with modeling the Case Approach as an evidence-based guide is a complex process that requires ongoing skill-building through practice, role-play, and supervision to carefully assess the suicidal client. Shea and Barney (2007a, 2007b) introduced the concept of "facilics," from Latin "grace of movement," which is the study of how interviewers structure an interview, the topics chosen, and how topics are explored within the constraints of the interview setting. The purpose of "facilics" is to increase awareness of interviewing skills to ultimately improve interview effectiveness by building a strong relationship with the client. Interview content (the topics explored during the assessment) is crucial to a comprehensive, prespecified database. The "process" of the interview, which facilitates the nurse interviewer-client relationship, is equally if not more important to a productive assessment. For practice, identify the validity techniques for assessment employed in the "process" examples below.

Enhancing engagement, addressing resistance and anger, and exploring psychodynamic processes or defense mechanisms are identified by Shea and Barney (2007a, 2007b) as examples of classic "process" regions requiring interviewer attention. Enhancing engagement with the client involves nondirective or active listening and comprises

EXHIBIT 15-3: CRISIS PLAN

A crisis plan or no-suicide or no-harm contract may be established with a client in an attempt to help the client remain safe from self-harm for a specific period of time. Together, the PMH-APRN and client develop a plan with at least three strategies to use when suicidal thoughts occur. This may involve calling a friend for general discussion as a distraction, activities such as walking/exercising or listening to favorite music, and finally, agreement by the client to get in touch with their chosen or assigned clinician if they are in an outpatient setting, to go to an emergency room; or if they are in an inpatient setting, to seek out their inpatient nurse when self-injurious feelings are uncontrollable (Yufit & Lester, 2005; McMyler & Pryjmachuk, 2008). Although there is no solid evidence that those who contract for safety are less likely to commit suicide (Shea, 1998; McMyler & Pryjmachuk, 2008), a recent study done on client's perceptions of no-suicide contracts found that clients reported positive attitudes toward written no-suicide agreements irrespective of age, gender, presence or absence of an Axis II diagnosis, or ratings of overall treatment helpfulness (Davis, Williams, & Hays, 2002). Multiple attempters may doubt the usefulness of this technique (Davis, Williams, & Hays, 2002); and, additional research suggests that no-suicide or no-harm agreements are not an effective NSSIB/SIB deterrent (Kroll, 2000; Farrow & O'Brien, 2003). The 4-step Case Approach process for suicide risk assessment may best protect the client.

the process region of "free facilitation" to advance the interview Case Approach steps. For example:

Client: I'm just so nervous all the time.... I'm not sure what's wrong.

Nurse: Tell me more about this feeling and what's happening...

Client: All of a sudden I just feel very anxious and my heart is racing and I feel like I'm not me...that's when I start scratching at my arm...

Nurse: And...

Client: When I start scratching, I get me back...

Nurse: Get me back?...

Strengthening the engagement process using an effective listening process with this client provides important content information that facilitates development of a comprehensive assessment toward completion of the Case Approach and accurate diagnosis related to self-injury.

A second process region is "transforming resistance" (Shea and Barney, 2007a, 2007b, p. 30). When the client actively opposes the engagement attempts of the nurse interviewer with anger or nonresponses, the objective is to transform the resistance to enable assessment continuation of the Case Approach. For example:

Client: Just because I scratch myself, I'm not crazy...stop.... I want to leave.... I'm going.

Nurse: Let's just pause a minute before you get up...you're concerned about being crazy...

Client: I'm not...but I'm here.... I don't belong here.

Nurse: We're here to talk about that nervousness that you just described. If we talk a bit more, we will work together so that you have other options when that nervous feeling takes over...you can help me understand better what happens...

Client: *Quiet, thinking*. ...Okay...for a little longer, but I'm not crazy.

Transforming resistance allows the client to ventilate feelings without fear of shame, redirect the anger, and move forward toward active participation in their plan of care with a more precise assessment of self-injury contributing factors.

The psychodynamic region is the focus of interviewer attention to the client's intellect and interpretive ability, self-concept and defense mechanisms with insight into issues and ability to reflect, and willingness to participate in recommended therapy (Shea & Barney, 2007a, 2007b). For example:

Client: My parents had strict rules...no drinking ...just a little party time. Good grades are expected. Sometimes I feel as if I can't be that good...maybe I don't want to be...

Nurse: How do you think the strict rules have impacted the behaviors you were sharing a few minutes ago?

Client: I guess...maybe.... I don't know.... I get so nervous thinking about what I have to do. Then

I feel so bad and not myself, so I start scratching at me...then I just want to go out and forget about it all. Yet I know I still want to be somebody....I get so confused and I don't want to hurt my parents...they're strict....I still love them, but I wish sometimes they would just go away....I don't mean I don't want them...I mean...let me be...

Nurse: You want your parents to give you more space to do some of your planning...

Client: Yes, I guess. Maybe I can do what I think will work...make my own rules...try my way...

Nurse: So you find that maybe your parents' making all the rules doesn't give you the chance to try some on your own?

Self-reflection, ego strength, and ability to interpret feelings without fear of shame or guilt shed light on the process and give valid insights into this client's ability to participate in therapy recommendations that will focus on behavioral alternatives to self-injury. Importantly, employing "Shame Attenuation" (Barney & Shea, 2007) in this example of self-reflection is a technique that increases obtaining reliable information concurrently with strengthening the nurse-client relationship (www.cmellc.com/psychcongress/syllabus/data/425-Shea-Happiness-Hand-Outs.pdf).

Transitions, which Shea and Barney (2007a, 2007b) label as gates in the "facilic" movement, are used by interviewers throughout the content and process of the interview. Transitions or gates can be spontaneous and natural, unfolding without effort (e.g., Tell me more...; How do you mean?...), and may take the client back (referred gate) to previous information (e.g., Earlier you mentioned...), providing graceful, unforced forward movement through topic transitions throughout the interview. These transitions enhance engagement and relationship building with clients.

Conversely, "phantom" (forced) transitions (e.g., What were your parents like in their teen years?...) or "implied" (mildly connected transitions) (e.g., Tell me what it was like for you in your earlier school years...) prevent the forward process of the interview with ill-timed comments such as a query into historical data and should be generally avoided. Recognition and conscious use of transitions is considered a powerful tool to be willfully used to enable the interview process.

Sequential use of the Case Approach steps coalesced with content, process, and transition awareness strengthens the relationship-building process toward a comprehensive self-directed suicidal injury assessment. Besides self-awareness and utilization of an interviewing method like the 4-step Case Approach and the IS PATH WARM complementary assessment pneumonic described earlier, there are also a number of important assessment tools or questionnaires that may be utilized for prompts and all-inclusive information compilation during this important process. The Inventory of Statements about Self-injury (ISAS) is a measure designed to comprehensively assess the functions of nonsuicidal self-injury (NSSI). The ISAS assesses 13 functions of NSSI, as well as the frequency of 12 NSSI behaviors (Klonsky & Glenn, 2009).

There are also a number of assessment tools (Claes et al., 2005) that assess for SIBs or suicidal ideations and behaviors which are readily available for use by the clinician (see Exhibit 15-4). It contains a list of some of these assessment tools and where to find them.

Suicide risk assessment is a systematic process in which the nurse uses the assessment data to formulate a clinical judgment, which serves as the foundation for appropriate treatment and management (Simon, 2008). Assessment data identifies risk factors and protective factors, which are combined with a specific "now" suicide inquiry to determine level of risk as low, medium, or high (see Figure 15-1).

The American Psychiatric Association's (APA) Practice Guidelines for the Treatment of Psychiatric Disorders Compendium (2006) identified empirically-based suicide risk factors which are factors that increase the risk for suicide (see Table 15-2).

These risk factors are subsequently evaluated along with protective factors which decrease the risk for suicide (see Table 15-3).

Using the Case Approach to assess these factors along with the specific inquiry regarding suicidal ideation and suicidal plans, allows the nurse interviewer to classify the client as low, moderate, or high lethality risk (see Table 15-4).

Multiple theoretical frameworks encompassing social, psychodynamic, genetic, cognitive, and diagnostic factors have been proffered to explain how NSSIB evolves and is discerned from SIB (Ross & Heath, 2003; Muehlenkamp, 2005; Walsh, 2005; Jacobson & Gould, 2007; Bureau et al., 2010). Research has shown that although often times these two scenarios coincide with one another, care and treatment needs to be tailored to individual needs.

Integrating therapeutic assessment models provides the clinician with a broad-based opportunity to individualize an evidence-based approach to guide the comprehensive assessment and management of the client's specific NSSIB/SIB behavior. However, interviewing techniques that will elicit suicidal behaviors and intent

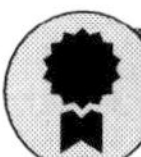

EXHIBIT 15-4: ASSESSMENT INSTRUMENTS

Chronic Self-Destructiveness Scale (CSDS) by Kelly, K., Byrne, D., Przybyla, D. P.J., Eberly, C., Eberly B., Greendlinger, V., & Gorsky, J. (1985). Chronic self-destructiveness: Conceptualization, measurement, and initial validation of the construct. *Motivation and Emotion, 9*(2), 135–151.

Self-Harm Behavior Survey by Favazza, R. A. (1986). *Self-Harm Behavior Survey*. Columbia, MI: Author.

Favazza, R. A., & Conterio, K. (1988). The plight of chronic self-mutilators. *Community Mental Health Journal, 24*(1), 22–30.

Self-Injury Survey by Simpson, E., Zlotnick, C., Begin, A., Costello, E., & Pearlstein, T. (1994). *Self-Injury Survey*. Providence, RI: Author.

Self-Injurious Behavior Questionnaire (SIB-Q) by Schroeder, R. S., Rojahn, J., & Reese, M. R. (1997). Brief Report: Reliability and validity of instruments for asessing psychotropic medication effects on self-injurious behavior in mental retardation. *Journal of Autism and Developmental Disorders, 27*(1), 89–102.

Self-Injury Questionnaire (SIQ) by Vanderlinden, J., & Vandereycken, W. (1997). *Trauma, dissociation, and impulse dyscontrol in eating disorders*. Philadelphia, PA: Routledge.

Timed Self-Injurious Behavior Scale by Brasic, R. J., Barnett, Y. J., Ahn, C. S., Nadrich, H. R., Will, V. M., & Clair, A. (1997). Clinical assessment of self-injurious behavior. *Psychological Reports*, 80(1), 155–160.

Deliberate Self-Harm Inventory (DSHI) by Gratz, L. K. (2001). Measurement of deliberate self-harm: preliminary data on the deliberate self-harm inventory. *Journal of Psychopathology and Behavioral Assessment, 23*(4), 253–263.

Adolescent Risk Inventory by Lescano, M. C., Hadley, S. W., Beausoleil, I. N., Brown, K. L., D'eramo, D., & Zimskind, A. (2007). A brief screening measure of adolescent risk behavior. *Child Psychiatry and Human Development, 37*(4), 325–326.

Self-Harm Inventory by Sansone, R. A., & Sansone, L. A. (2010). Measuring self-harm behavior with the self-harm inventory. *Psychiatry, 7*(4), 16–20.

Sansone, R. A., Wiederman, M. W., & Sansone, L. A. (1998). The self-harm inventory (SHI): Development of a scale for identifying self-destructive behaviors and borderline personality disorder. *Journal of Clinical Psychology, 54*(7), 973–983.

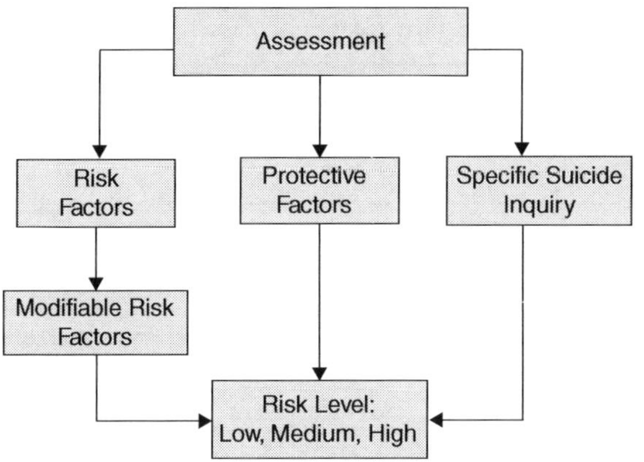

Figure 15-1 Level of Risk

Source: Adapted from Jacobs, D. (2003) and used with permission from Suicide Assessment Presentation to the University of Michigan Depression Center Colloquium Series. Retrieved September 2011 from *www.stopasuicide.org/downloads/sites/docs/SuicideAssessment_slides.ppt.*

also require practical interviewing strategies for accurate assessment and ensuing treatment decisions vested in the theoretical models.

INTEGRATION

Nock (2009) conceptualizes an integrated model that collates theoretical frameworks into one unified model to explain the development and maintenance of NSSI behaviors that also applies to understanding SIB (see Figure 15-2). Why an individual would choose SIB is elucidated through an understanding of how epidemiology, function, and intent lead to NSSIB and potentially SIB. Nock's model postulates how factors such as child abuse or family dysfunction influence an individual's intrapersonal and interpersonal factors leading to engaging in NSSIB or SIB behaviors as a way to regulate routine life experiences.

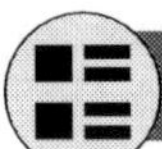

TABLE 15-2: RISK FACTORS

Demographic	Male; widowed, divorced, single; increases with age; white
Psychosocial	Lack of social support; unemployment; drop in socioeconomic status; *firearm access*, loss
Psychiatric	*Psychiatric diagnosis*; comorbidity
Physical Illness	Malignant neoplasms; HIV/AIDS; peptic ulcer disease; hemodialysis; systemic lupus erthematosis; pain syndromes; functional impairment; diseases of nervous system
Psychological Dimensions	*Hopelessness; psychic pain/anxiety; psychological turmoil; decreased self-esteem; fragile narcissism, and perfectionism*
Behavioral Dimensions	*Impulsivity; aggression; severe anxiety; panic attacks; agitation; intoxication*; prior suicide attempt; global insomnia
Cognitive Dimensions	*Thought constriction; polarized thinking*
Childhood Trauma	Sexual/physical abuse; neglect; parental loss
Genetic and Familial	Family history of suicide; mental illness, or abuse

Italics = Modifiable.

Source: Used with permission from Jacobs, D. (2003) Suicide Assessment Presentation to the University of Michigan Depression Center Colloquium Series. Retrieved September 2011 from *www.stopasuicide.org/downloads/sites/docs/SuicideAssessment_slides.ppt*.

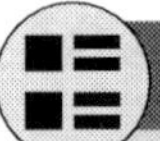

TABLE 15-3: PROTECTIVE FACTORS

PROTECTIVE FACTOR	DESCRIPTION AND EFFECT ON SUICIDE RISK
Stable social support system	One's social support system may offer acceptance, support and company to distract from feelings of self-worthlessness
Availability and ability to use adaptive coping skills	Individual coping and problem-solving abilities enable finding other, less self-destructive ways to deal with feelings in order to alleviate the desperation and despair felt with depression and suicidal ideation
Actively participating in one's treatment	Availability of resources and being involved actively in one's treatment may enable coming forward to discuss uncomfortable or unwanted feelings with the treatment team
Sense of hopefulness	Allows ability to see the "light at the end of the tunnel" and helps to alleviate the impulse toward self harm
Spiritual inclinations	Strong cultural identity and spiritual beliefs or being afraid of suicide or death may help prevent acting on impulsive ideas
Pregnancy or having children under the age of eighteen in the home	Family cohesion and adults modeling healthy adjustment may promote a sense of being needed thereby alleviating self-harm

Source: Adapted from White, J. (2006/2007). Suicide risk and protective factors for youth, *Crosscurrents, 10*(2), 10.

CONCORDANCE

It is important for the PMH-APRN to understand that simply asking about suicide will not necessarily mean that accurate or complete information will be obtained. Cultural, social, or religious beliefs about suicide may restrict a person's willingness to talk about the possibility of suicide during the assessment, as well as the likelihood of acting on suicidal impulses. Therefore, incorporating the influence of these beliefs within a professional summary is indicated to ensure a "concordant" picture is painted for an individual so comprehensive care may be planned.

TABLE 15-4: LETHALITY RISK

LEVEL OF RISK	DIRECT	INDIRECT
High Lethality	Suicide (e.g., overdose, hanging, jumping from a height, use of a gun)	Situational Risk Taking (e.g., getting into a car with strangers, walking alone in a dangerous area)
	Single Episode	Single Episode
	Suicide Repeaters	High-Risk Stunts (e.g., walking on a high-pitched roof or in high-speed traffic)
Medium Lethality		Late-Phase Anorexia
	Multiple Episodes	Multiple Episodes
	Atypical or Major Self-Injury (e.g., mutilation of the face, eyes, genitals, breasts, or damage involving multiple sutures, self-enucleation, autocastration)	Acute Drunkenness Sexual Risk Taking (e.g., having sex with strangers, unprotected anal intercourse)
Low Lethality		
	Single Episode	Single Episode
	Common Self-Injury (e.g., wrist, arm, and leg cutting, self-burning, self-hitting, excoriation)	Chronic Substance Abuse (alcohol, marijuana, cocaine, inhalant, hallucinogens, ecstasy, IV drug, etc.) Unauthorized Discontinuance or Misuse/Abuse of Prescribed Psychotropic Medications Bulimia Use of Laxatives Obesity
	Multiple Episodes	Multiple Episodes

Source: After Pattison & Kahan (1983), printed with permission from Walsh, B.W. (2006). *Treating Self-Injury: A Practical Guide*. Guilford Press, New York.

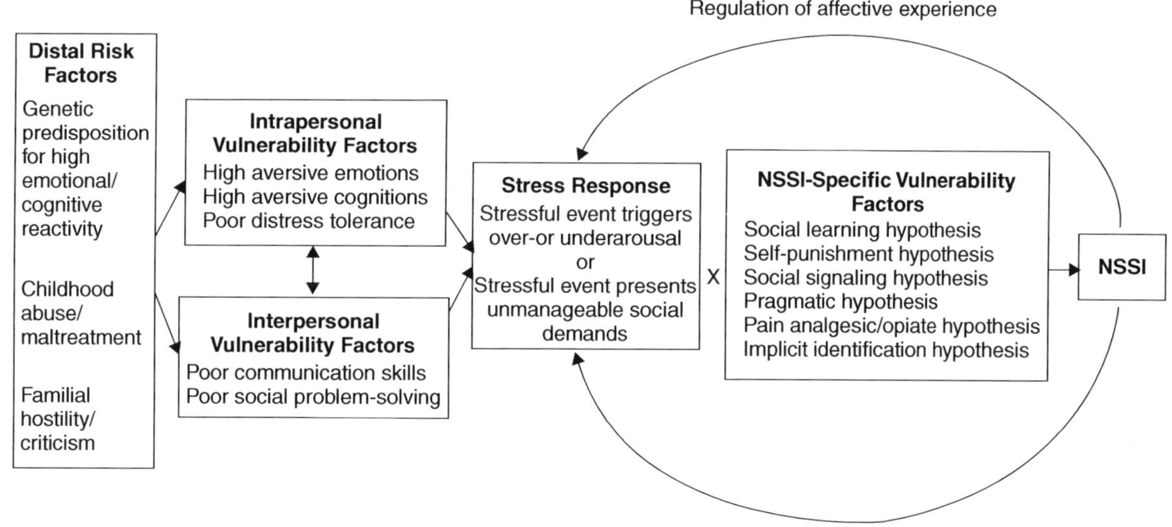

Figure 15-2 Why do People Hurt Themselves?

Source: Printed with permission from Nock, M. (2009). Why do people hurt themselves? *Current Psychological Directions in Science, 18*, 79.

EXPECTED OUTCOMES

A comprehensive Case Approach assessment utilizing Shea's content, process, and transition principles and validity techniques provides evidence-based practice opportunities to form the beginning of a trusting therapeutic relationship leading to an accurate diagnosis. Once the PMH-APRN comprehensively reviews all assessment data and determines diagnostic lethality risk, preparation of a plan of care that includes developing and implementing effective nursing interventions is the task at hand for both short- and long-term risk management (Muehlenkamp, 2004, 2005, 2006; Cutcliffe et. al., 2007; Jacobson & Gould, 2007; Shea, 2007; Shea & Barney, 2007a, 2007b; Nock, 2011; Wilkinson, 2012). Evidence-based planning and practice interventions ensue with ensuring safety and security for the patient first, assisting the patient in gaining insight into self-skills, and deriving patient goals vested in hope as recurrent intervention themes in the sound management of the client at risk for suicide.

If inpatient care is indicated for the at-risk client, the focus is on acute interventions (e.g., observation status, individual therapy, medications, etc.) that facilitate discharge and return to the community. When multidisciplinary assessment and collaborative evaluations indicate that the risk for suicide is eliminated, discharge may be imminent. However, previous research has identified that follow-up care for the suicidal patient is critical, given the risk for suicide (14% for men and 22% for women) following discharge (Muehlenkamp, 2004, 2005, 2006; Cutcliffe, Stevenson, Jackson, & Smith, 2007; Jacobson & Gould, 2007; Shea & Barney, 2007a, 2007b; Nock, 2011; Wilkinson, 2012).

Impending discharge highlights the critical need for not only accurate, empathic-generated inpatient Case Approach assessment of suicide risk prior to discharge, but also, continuation of ongoing suicide risk assessment in the outpatient setting. The brief, short-term treatment initiated on the inpatient unit is the start of the recovery process that must be maintained with qualified long-term clinical intervention (Cutcliffe, Stevenson, Jackson, & Smith, 2007). Reassurance of continuity of care upon discharge to the care of an outpatient clinician ensures an uninterrupted care-planning process (Muehlenkamp, 2004, 2005, 2006; Nock, 2011).

Whether the client receives care as an inpatient or within an outpatient setting, Cutcliffe, Stevenson, Jackson, and Smith (2007) describe a core process composed of three stages where the PMH-APRN sets the stage for interaction interventions with empathic, nonbiased care that guides the suicidal patient toward attaining power over suicidality; and ultimately, emerging with the confidence to live again. Complementing the principles of the Case Approach, creating a warm, interpersonal setting, offering security while exploring insight into suicidal beliefs, and making sense of suicidal thoughts to reset goals and establish a hopeful future are central to the nurse's approach. As the client is developing novel skills to cope with suicidal thoughts, the PMH-APRN uses evidence-based findings to individualize and enhance therapeutic skills specific to the client.

INITIATION OF TREATMENT

The PMH-APRN develops a plan of care that is discussed with the patient, nurse, family, and others to prescribe evidence-based interventions toward desired outcomes based upon information gathered throughout the Case Approach, the IS PATH WARM assessment pneumonic, and according to the Standards of Psychiatric and Mental Health Clinical Nursing Practice, Standard V (Planning) (1998, 2009). The purpose of the plan is to guide interventions, document progress, and achieve desired patient outcomes. For the suicidal patient, this means planning interventions based on the risk factors, protective factors, and suicide inquiry (see Figure 15-3).

A major aspect of prevention and successful treatment needs to be placed on distinguishing between NSSIB and SIB using evidence-based assessment. Multiple theoretical frameworks encompassing social, psychodynamic, genetic, cognitive, and diagnostic factors have been proffered to explain how NSSIB evolves and are discerned from SIB (Ross & Heath 2003; Muehlenkamp, 2005; Walsh, 2005; Jacobson & Gould 2007; Bureau et al., 2010). The practitioner is able to gain insight by establishing a trusting relationship, providing education to the client and family, and focusing on relapse prevention. Therapy allows the client to feel comfort in discussing self-inflicted injury with or without SI. It also gives the practitioner the ability to create a safety plan to help the

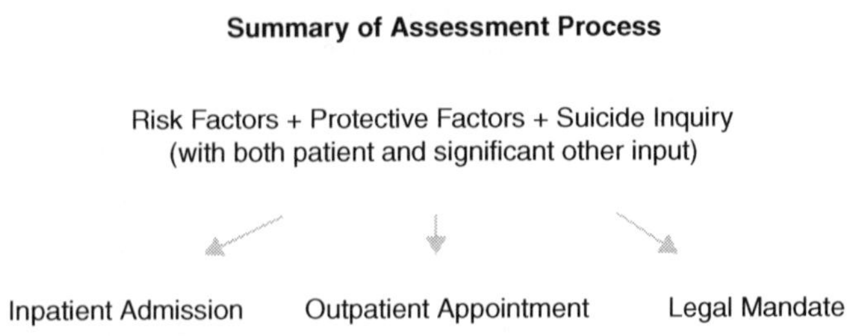

Summary of Assessment Process

Risk Factors + Protective Factors + Suicide Inquiry
(with both patient and significant other input)

Inpatient Admission | Outpatient Appointment | Legal Mandate

Figure 15-3 Assessment Process

client build coping skills while the practitioner provides education on symptoms and on recognizing stressful factors contributing to the behavior. Psychotherapy vested in multiple theoretical frameworks offers treatment options feasible for the practitioner and specific to the client. The choice depends on the individual situation and the status of the client.

COGNITIVE BEHAVIORAL THERAPY

"Most clinicians agree that patients who harm themselves deliberately are among the most complex and therapeutically challenging patients they are confronted with" (Slee, Arensman, Garnefski, & Spinhoven, 2007). The population is stated to be classified as "heterogeneous" due to specific qualities including: number of previous episodes of NSSIB/SIB, motives for NSSIB/SIB, and psychological and psychiatric problems. There is a necessity for psychotherapeutic interventions, which allow clinicians to individually adapt the treatment options to the patient's needs.

Cognitive behavioral therapy (CBT) focuses on "stressors, emotional and behavioral responses, cognitive errors, and developmental factors that contribute to suicidal attempt" (Stewart, Quinn, Plever, & Emmerson, 2009). Research has shown that people who complete suicide have shortfalls in problem-solving and experience depressing, hopeless attitudes when evaluated against the general population (Stewart et al., 2009). As a result, an approach such as CBT may assist the client in thinking more logically and examining their problems with hope and encouragement.

Furthermore, a successful therapeutic treatment should address cognitive, emotional, behavioral, and interpersonal problems associated with NSSIB/SIB. Slee et al. (2007) discuss three different cognitive behavioral therapies and compares the diverse techniques which allow researchers and practitioners to individualize therapy choices. For example, Marsha Linehan, PhD, felt that standard CBT placed an emphasis on aiding patients in altering their thoughts and behaviors, which she found to be unsuccessful due to clients feeling misinterpreted, with many ending up noncompliant with the treatment options (Slee et al., 2007). Taking these limitations into consideration, Linehan created a treatment program called dialectical behavioral therapy (DBT) (Linehan, 2006a, 2006b). This type of therapy combines "general cognitive behavioral techniques with elements from Zen" (Slee et al., 2007). In general, the therapy shares principles related to CBT including: emotional regulation, interpersonal efficiency, distress tolerance, core mindfulness, and self-management skills. Furthermore, Zen principles are added, focusing on promoting a nonjudgmental attitude toward one's own thoughts and emotions, which prevents negative mood behaviors that often lead to the recurrence of NSSIB/SIB. Research has demonstrated positive impacts of DBT such as: "reducing both the number and severity of repeated NSSI episodes, reducing the number of hospital days, and improving general and social functioning, as well as treatment compliance over a 1-year follow-up period" (Slee et al., 2007). On the other hand, little differences were demonstrated between DBT and treatment as usual (TAU) when it came to depression, hopelessness, suicidal ideation, and reasons for living. Given the circumstances and complexity of treating this patient population, the results found are hopeful since some of the elements of DBT can be applied directly, while other aspects can be further researched.

The second elaborated CBT related specifically to NSSIB/SIB was developed by Berk, Henriques, Warman, Brown, and Beck (2004). Its creation branch off Beck's Cognitive Therapy and focuses on repetition with the diverse aspect of brief, 10-session treatments. The interventions used include the following: "a multi-step crisis-plan, a detailed cognitive conceptualization of the irrational negative beliefs associated with self-harm, and the use of coping cards" (Slee et al., 2007). Positive features of this therapy include its short length, which may lead to more compliance with treatment and may be more appropriate for community mental health centers since clients are not present for long periods of time. A great deal of studies have not been conducted pertaining to this treatment's efficacy, but there has been strong evidence stating that during the follow-up period of a year and half, approximately half of the participants were less likely to reengage in NSSIB/SIB, and their depressed and hopeless moods showed some improvement.

Additionally, the third type of CBT, created by Rudd, Joiner, and Rajab (1996), encompasses a broader population of NSSIB/SIB clients. The primary focus of this therapy is that NSSIB/SIB is the main problem rather than an underlying issue. Techniques developed from this therapy comprise: "symptom management, restructuring the patient's belief system, and building skills such as interpersonal assertiveness, distress tolerance, and problem solving" (Slee et al., 2007). An additional emphasis is placed on creating a strong therapeutic alliance which in the end becomes the foundation of well-being and support during a crisis. While this specific therapy lacks controlled clinical trials, CBT centered on cognitive restructuring seems to be successful in treating NSSIB/SIB.

In general, after reviewing these therapies, four key components create a core of the treatment effectiveness. First a therapeutic and trusting relationship needs to be established between the client and the therapist, which will allow for more information to be divulged and in the end result in a beneficial outcome for the client. Enhancing emotional regulation skills is also a component that deals with reducing negative thoughts and developing a mindful attitude. In addition, cognitive restructuring aids in reducing cognitive distortions focused on hopelessness and depression. Last, improving behavioral skills allows the client to become a better problem solver and establishes confidence (Slee et al., 2007). All in all, the primary goal is to motivate practitioners to address and search for the mechanisms listed above while working with NSSIB/SIB clients and to further inspire them to target specific areas individualized for each case to improve and make their work more effective.

DIALECTICAL BEHAVIOR THERAPY

Research on dialectical behavior therapy (DBT) place emphasis on its usefulness in borderline personality disorder clients with or without SI. DBT falls under the cognitive behavioral therapies and it places emphasis on suicidal and dangerous, severe, destabilizing behaviors. Standard treatment addresses five main areas including: (1) increasing behavioral capabilities; (2) improving motivation for skillful behavior; (3) assuring generalization of gains to the natural environment; (4) structuring the treatment environment so that it reinforces functional rather than dysfunctional behaviors; and (5) enhancing therapist capabilities and motivation to treat patients effectively (Linehan et al., 2006a, 2006b; Linehan et al., 1983).

Furthermore, these functions are delivered individually, as group training, by telephone, and in consultation with a team of therapists in order to enhance the overall effectiveness. Several research studies have been performed comparing DBT to nonbehavioral community treatment by experts (CTBE), and results have shown a positive outcome with DBT in treating suicidal clients and clients with borderline personality disorder. More specifically, it has been demonstrated that DBT was more effective in preventing suicidal attempts by half compared to CTBE. Also, DBT decreased emergency room visits and inpatient care for suicidal ideation and was able to keep clients in treatment and decrease noncompliance (Linehan et al., 2006a, 2006b).

MOTIVATIONAL INTERVIEWING

"Motivational interviewing, a client-centered, goal-oriented method for enhancing intrinsic motivation for change by exploring ambivalence may appear to many clinicians as an unlikely treatment for suicidal patients" (Zerler, 2009). On the other hand, research suggests that it is an approach that can be applied efficiently to clinical crises and suicidal clients. Oftentimes, clients who express self-injury with or without SI are categorized as unreliable and have the inability to make positive decisions. In turn, they are hospitalized "for their own good" to decrease anxieties of those who are at stake of taking responsibility (Zerler, 2009). Motivational interviewing focuses on endorsing self-sufficiency, establishing a therapeutic union, and discovering ambivalence (Zerler, 2009). This type of therapy pertains to emphasizing the fact that the choice is in the clients hands, and by recognizing their ability to make proper decisions and deal with their negative feelings versus judging them as helpless and assuming the role of the rescuer, may be more effective. By acting in this manner, the clinician may provide the client with confidence in making life-affirming changes, and research has demonstrated that with motivational interviewing there has been reduced rates of involuntary commitment, inpatient psychiatric hospitalization, and use of emergency services.

MINDFULNESS-BASED COGNITIVE THERAPY

Thought suppression is a technique intended to perform mental control associated with depression, which may in turn increase the frequency of unwanted thoughts (Hepburn, et al., 2009). It is instinct that when negative ideas come to mind to disregard them, which usually works for a short period of time, but later, an increase in the discarded material occurs. Suicidal individuals are particularly at risk for developing depression in the future and research is being conducted using mindfulness-based cognitive therapy (MBCT) and looking at the effects on thought suppression (Hepburn et al, 2009). This population is particularly at high risk to suppress their thoughts which can lead to exacerbation of NSSIB/SIB. "MCTB is a relapse-prevention treatment combining CBT with mindfulness training. Mindfulness can be defined as purposeful, nonjudgmental, and present-moment awareness" (Hepburn et al., 2009). The primary aim of MBCT is to encourage clients to acclimatize ways of managing their thoughts and feelings by acknowledging them, compared to suppressing them. Preliminary evidence suggests that

MBCT for suicidality may decrease innate thought suppression and in turn decrease depression.

FUTURE-ORIENTED GROUP TRAINING THERAPY

General psychiatric treatment requires clinicians to assess suicide risk and once it is addressed, the focus on suicidal thoughts is often set aside. A common attitude among practitioners is that once depression or anxiety symptoms are relieved and treated, then suicidal thoughts will diminish. However, research has shown that it is necessary to detect and place importance on suicidal thinking in order to decrease the return and power of the thoughts (van Beek, Kerkhof, & Beekman, 2009). Future-oriented group training for patients with suicidal thoughts was developed in an attempt to decrease the incidence and intensity of suicidal thinking. Cognitive behavioral techniques serve as the basis with "hopelessness, worrying, and future perspectives taken from the theories of Beck, McLeod, and others, concerning the lack of positive expectations characteristic for many suicidal patients" (van Beek et al., 2009). The main objective is to avoid the social isolation most participants encounter, which inhibits their ability to develop cognitive and problem-solving skills. The interventions in this therapy assist patients in envisioning rational outlooks for the future and in turn by creating this; their hopelessness and negative thinking will likely diminish. This group training is effective for clients with suicidal ideation and works to assist them early in the suicidal process. Further research needs to be conducted pertaining to the specific elements of this therapy that are responsible for the positive alterations, but it has been shown to be simple to incorporate and appropriate to use for an extensive range of comorbid psychiatric disorders. In summary, the goal of future oriented group training is to help clients to make life livable by realistically focusing on what the future might have to offer (van Beek et al., 2009).

PHARMACOLOGIC MANAGEMENT

Although a systematic review of NSSIB-specific treatment strategies suggest that approaches utilizing largely CBT may prove most efficacious in NSSIB treatment (Muehlenkamp, 2006), there may be cases in which medications are warranted. There are currently not any Food and Drug Administration (FDA)-approved medications for the treatment of NSSIB; however, medications may need to be prescribed to treat comorbid conditions and/or some of the symptoms such as impulsivity associated with self-injury. Common comorbidities include mood disorders and anxiety disorders. Castille et al. (2007) examined the diagnostic composition of 105 self-harmers and results revealed that 56.4% were diagnosed with a mood disorder; 30.4% were diagnosed with anxiety disorders; 4.3% were diagnosed with post-traumatic stress disorder; and 4.3% with eating disorders. Other diagnoses commonly associated with self-injury include borderline personality disorder and dissociative disorders.

SIB has been described in the literature as an impulse control problem that may have a biological basis, including dysfunction in serotonergic and/or dopaminergic neurotransmission. It is likely that low serotonin function as well as dopaminergic overstimulation increase both impulsivity and aggressive behavior (Swann, 2003). Selective serotonin reuptake inhibitors (SSRIs) can reduce impulsive and aggressive behavior (Reist, Nakamura, Sagart, Sokolski, & Fujimoto, 2003) and have also been found to be effective for aggressive and self-injury in people with learning disabilities (Branford et al., 1998; Davanzo, Belin, Widawski, & King, 1998). Additionally, there is some evidence that endogenous opioids are thought to be involved in the initiation and maintenance of SIB (Villalba & Harrington, 2000) and administration of the opioid antagonist, naltrexone, can reduce self-injury (Symons, Thompson, & Rodriguez, 2004).

Most of the evidence for the pharmacologic treatment of NSSIB comes from case reports and open label studies. In theory, enhancing serotonergic transmission may assist in reducing impulsivity and irritability, two symptoms frequently reported by self-injurers. Two case reports indicate the successful reduction in SIB in the form of biting with the use of fluoxetine in an 11-year-old boy and citalopram in a 30-year-old man (Velazquez, Ward-Chene, & Loogsian, 2000; Martin & Guth, 2005). According to Fong (2003), SSRIs appear to be an appropriate first-line treatment for NSSIB secondary to their overall safety profile, tolerability, efficacy in treating mood lability, and documented evidence of low serotonergic transmission in patients who self-injure. No particular SSRI has emerged as superior over the others in terms of treating NSSIB. PMH-APRNs should base their initial selection on the overall symptom profile that the patient in presenting with (i.e., patients with predominant complaints of anxiety and feeling activated may benefit from an SSRI that is more sedating, such as citalopram or escitalopram, and patients reporting lethargy and lack of motivation may benefit from a more stimulating SSRI such as fluoxetine).

There have also been case reports of utilizing atypical antipsychotics for the treatment of impulsivity and mood

TABLE 15-5: SELECTED PHARMACOLOGIC TREATMENTS FOR NSSIB

SSRIs	DOSE RANGE	FDA APPROVED CONDITIONS	SIDE EFFECTS	DRUG INTERACTIONS
Fluoxetine (Prozac)	10–80 mg/day	MDD*, OCD*, PMDD, BN, Panic Disorder	**	2 D6 inhibition (can increase blood levels of beta blockers, atomoxetine, and thioridazine) 3A4 inhibition (can increase blood levels of alprazolam, buspirone, trazolam, HMG CoA reductase inhibitors, and pimozide) Can increase tricyclic antidepressant levels
Sertraline (Zoloft)	25–200 mg/day	MDD, PMDD, Panic Disorder, PTSD, Social Phobia, OCD*	**	2 D6 inhibition (can increase blood levels of beta blockers, atomoxetine, and thioridazine) 3A4 inhibition (can increase blood levels of alprazolam, buspirone, trazolam, HMG CoA reductase inhibitors, and pimozide) Can increase tricyclic antidepressant levels
Paroxetine (Paxil)	10–60 mg/day	MDD, OCD, Panic Disorder, Social Phobia, PTSD, GAD, PMDD	**	2 D6 inhibition (can increase blood levels of beta blockers, atomoxetine, and thioridazine) Can increase tricyclic antidepressant levels
Fluvoxamine (Luvox)	50–300 mg/day	OCD*, Social Phobia	**	1A2 inhibition (can increase blood levels of duloxetine, theophylline and clozapine) 3A4 inhibition (can increase blood levels of alprazolam, buspirone, trazolam, HMG CoA reductase inhibitors, and pimozide) Can increase tricyclic antidepressant levels
Citalopram (Celexa)	10–40 mg/day	MDD	**	2 D6 inhibition (can increase blood levels of beta blockers, atomoxetine, and thioridazine) Can increase tricyclic antidepressant levels
Escitalopram (Lexapro)	10–20 mg/day	MDD*, GAD	**	Few known adverse drug reactions
SNRIs				
Venlafaxine (Effexor XR)	37.5–300 mg/day	MDD, GAD, Social Phobia, Panic Disorder	***	Few known adverse drug reactions
Duloxetine (Cymbalta)	20–120 mg/day	MDD, Diabetic Peripheral Neuropathic Pain, Fibromyalgia, GAD	*** Rare cases of hepatotoxicity have been reported	2 D6 inhibition (can increase blood levels of beta blockers, atomoxetine, and thioridazine) Can increase tricyclic antidepressant levels
Desvenlafaxine (Pristiq)	50–100 mg/day	MDD	***	Few known adverse drug reactions

NDRIs				
Bupropion (Wellbutrin SR) (Wellbutrin XL)	SR (150–300 mg/day) XL (150–450 mg/day)	MDD Seasonal Affective Disorder (XL) Nicotine Addiction	Initial anxiety/activation, insomnia, headache, tinnitus, agitation, weight loss; less sexual side effects (often used as an augmentation agent for sexual dysfunction) Contraindicated in patients with a history of seizure disorders	2 D6 inhibition (can increase blood levels of beta blockers, atomoxetine, and thioridazine)
Alpha 2 Antagonist				
Mirtazapine (Remeron)	15–45 mg/day	MDD	Weight gain, sedation, dry mouth, constipation, increased suicidal thinking in youth < 24 years	Few known adverse drug reactions
Mood Stabilizers				
Valproate (Depakote ER)	750–3000 mg per day (dosed to achieve plasma level between 50–100 mg/ml)	Acute mania and mixed episodes Migraine prophylaxis Seizure disorders	Sedation, GI upset, weight gain, ataxia, alopecia, thrombocytopenia, elevated liver function tests	Inhibits metabolism of lamotrigine Aspirin can increase valproate levels Levels can be reduced by carbamazepine, phenytoin, phenobarbital, and rifampin
Lamotrigine (Lamictal)	100–400 mg/day	Maintenance treatment of Bipolar I Seizure disorders	Sedation, dizziness, ataxia, GI upset, headaches, poor corrdination, fatigue Risk of Steven Johnson's syndrome	Valproate increases levels (increases risk of rash) Levels can be reduced by carbamazepine, phenytoin, phenobarbital, rifampin, and oral contraceptives
Topiramate (Topamax)	50–300 mg/day as adjunctive treatment of Bipolar disorder	Seizure disorders Migraine prophylaxis	Sedation, ataxia, appetite loss, weight loss, GI upset, confusion, memory problems	Levels can be reduced by carbamazepine, phenytoin, phenobarbital, and rifampin Can decrease both valproate and phenytoin levels Can increase levels of metformin
Atypical Antipsychotics				
Olanzapine (Zyprexa)	10–20 mg/day	Schizophrenia Bipolar maintenance Acute mania/mixed mania	**** Significant weight gain Significant cardiometabolic risk	May increase effect of antiphypertensive agents Need to lower dose if given with 1A2 inhibitors
Risperidone (Risperdal)	2–8 mg/day	Schizophrenia Acute mania/mixed Autism related irritability in children ages 5–16	**** Higher risk of EPS and risk of elevated prolactin levels	May increase effect of antiphypertensive agents Levels can be increased by duloxetine, fluoxetine, sertraline, citalopram, and paroxetine

(*Continued*)

TABLE 15-5: SELECTED PHARMACOLOGIC TREATMENTS FOR NSSIB (*Continued*)

ATYPICAL ANTIPSYCHOTICS	DOSE RANGE	FDA APPROVED CONDITIONS	SIDE EFFECTS	DRUG INTERACTIONS
Quetiapine (Seroquel) (Seroquel XR)	25–800 mg/day	Schizophrenia Bipolar maintenance Acute mania Bipolar depression (XR)	****	Levels can be increased by duloxetine, fluoxetine, sertraline, fluvoxamine, citalopram, and paroxetine
Ziprasidone (Geodon)	40–200 mg/day	Schizophrenia Acute mania/mixed	**** Less weight gain compared to other atypical Do not use in patients with history of QTc prolongation or if taking other meds known to prolong QTc interval	May increase effect of antiphypertensive agents
Aripirazole (Abilify)	2–30 mg/day	Schizophrenia Acute mania/mixed Bipolar maintenance Depression (adjunct)	**** More activating compared to other atypicals Less weight gain compared to other atypicals	Levels can be increased by fluoxetine, fluvoxamine, citalopram, and ketoconazole

SSRIs = Selective Serotonin Reuptake Inhibitors; SNRIs = Serotonin Norepinephrine Reuptake Inhibitors; NDRIs = Norepeinephrine Dopamine Reuptake Inhibitors; MDD = Major Depressive Disorder; OCD = Obsessive Compulsive Disorder; PMDD = Premenstrual Dysphoric Disorder; BN = Bulimia Nervosa; PTSD = Post Traumatic Stress Disorder; GAD = Generalized Anxiety Disorder; HMG CoA = 3-hydroxy-3-methylglutaryl-coenzyme A, GI = gastrointestinal; EPS = Extrapyramidal Symptoms.

*FDA approved for use in individuals <age 18.

**Common side effects include: initial anxiety, GI upset, headache, sweating, sexual side effects, risk of causing suicidal thinking (risk increased in individuals <24 years of age), risk of inducing hypomania/mania.

***Common side effects include: initial anxiety, GI upset, headache, sweating, sexual side effects, risk of causing suicidal thinking (risk increased in individuals <24 years of age), risk of inducing hypomania/mania, elevation of blood pressure.

Atypical Antipsychotics

****Common side effects include: sedation, weight gain, orthostatic hypotension, extrapyramidal side effects, cardiometabolic risk.

Need to monitor lipids, blood sugar, weight, body mass index (BMI), and vital signs.

Source: Stahl, S. M. (2009). *The Prescriber's Guide: Stahl's Essential Psychopharmacology* (3rd Ed.). Cambridge, UK: Cambridge University Press.

dysregulation that can accompany NSSIB. Although NSSIB can occur across a spectrum of Axis I and Axis II psychiatric disorders, the diagnosis that has been most studied in regards to utilization of psychotropic medications to treat self-injury is borderline personality disorder. Two meta-analyses of medications used in the treatment of borderline personality disorder were recently conducted. Ingenhoven and Duivenvoorder (2011) reviewed 10 studies and pooled the effect size of antipsychotics on impulsive behavioral dyscontrol and found that antipsychotics have limited effectiveness on impulsive and aggressive behaviors in patients with borderline personality disorder. Vita, De Peri, and Sacchetti (2011) also conducted a meta-analysis of several classes of psychotropic agents used in the treatment of borderline personality disorder. Randomized controlled trials demonstrated the highest effect size for anticonvulsants and a lower effect size for both first- and second-generation antipsychotics for the treatment of impulsive-behavioral dysregulation. There was no evidence that antidepressants were efficacious for impulsivity (Vita et al., 2011). Lieb, Vollm, Rucker, Timmer, and Stoffers (2010) conducted a Cochrane systematic review of 27 trials and found the most beneficial effects related to reduction of impulsivity was with topamax, lamotrigine, and depakote and the second-generation antipsychotics, aripirazole and olanzapine.

As noted above, there are no FDA medications approved for NSSIB. When treating patients who engage in self-injury, PMH-APRNs must take into account whether there is an Axis I psychiatric condition that accompanies the self-injury and if so, select a medication that has FDA approval or a strong evidence base to support prescription of that agent. If there is not a diagnosable Axis I condition present, the PMH-APRN should take into account the major symptom clusters that the patient is presenting with as well as the presence of medical comorbidities. All medications are associated with side effects and the risk of drug interactions. PMH-APRNs should have knowledge of the risks associated with the medications and prescribe medication cautiously in this population of patients who often have high levels of impulsivity and mood dysregulation. See Table 15-5 for a list of selected pharmacologic agents that can be utilized for the treatment of NSSIB.

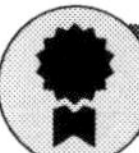

EXHIBIT 15-5: CASE STUDY

Connie is an 18-year-old nursing student who is attending her freshman year at a local university. Her longtime friend, Lisa, attending the same university, noticed scratches on Connie's forearm when they met for a Friday night party. Upon talking to Connie, she learns that Connie has been feeling anxious and unsure if she made the right choice for her major, and feeling that it's too late to change her mind, but states that the availability of beer in the dorm is helping her to cope. Connie tells her that when she scratches her arm like she did last week, the stress "melts away" and she feels a "sense of relief." Lisa tells Connie she is concerned, but Connie tells her not to worry. Uncomfortable with this answer, Lisa says, "Well, I'm just going to talk to my mom because I'm not sure how to help you with this." Connie shrugs and tells her there is really no need to do that because she will be fine and starts out the door for the party. Lisa notes how giddy Connie acts at the party when she drinks more beer than Lisa has ever noticed before. They leave the party together, but upon returning to the dorm Connie just falls into bed into a deep sleep.

Lisa shares her information about Connie the next day with her mother saying she does not know how to help her, but she is worried. Lisa's mother lets her know that the best action would be to call Connie's parents and offers to do so with her.

Upon hearing Lisa's story, Connie's parents immediately plan an impromptu visit to surprise Connie. When her parents meet Connie at their usual restaurant, they casually call attention to the arm scratches, and Connie breaks down in tears. She lets them know how she has been feeling and her parents agree that a visit to their family doctor is their next step. Connie objects saying, "I'm fine—really!," but when her parents insist, she hesitantly agrees. They leave for an emergency office appointment where the nurse practitioner begins the assessment.

TABLE 15-6: CARE PLAN

RISK FACTORS	NURSING ASSESSMENT CASE APPROACH	OUTCOME/EVALUATION
Step 1 Presenting Suicidal Events	Build an empathic, therapeutic relationship using active listening, case approach principles (Muehlenkamp, 2004–2006; Cutcliffe, et. al., 2007; Jacobson & Gould, 2007; Shea, 2007; Shea & Barney, 2007a, b; Nock, 2011; Wilkinson, 2012)	Comprehensive assessment with suicidal risk evaluation and improved patient insight (Muehlenkamp, 2004–2006; Cutcliffe, et. al., 2007; Jacobson & Gould, 2007; Shea, 2007; Shea & Barney, 2007a, b; Nock, 2011; Wilkinson, 2012)
1. Self-inflicted cuts on arm	1. Objective Data, Behavioral Incident, Gentle Assumptions: Tell me about the cuts on your arm…and this happened about the time…this was something you planned or it just happened…and were you thinking about killing yourself when you were cutting (Clarify; Behavioral Incident)…and you mentioned feeling…(Encourage; Gentle Assumptions)	1. Client explores self- injurious behavior with nurse; conveys understanding of level of self-control toward behavioral choice; shares desire to live concurrent with denying suicidal ideation so that client safety is prioritized
2. Anxiety	2. Objective Data, Behavioral Incident, Gentle Assumptions: How has your "nervousness" affected your routines? Tell me about the thoughts you have when you are feeling anxious…(Identify contributing stressors, explore; Behavioral Incident)…do you have ways you use to cope when feeling nervous…your hands are trembling a bit…is this how you would describe being nervous when you are in the dorm? (Open-ended question; Gentle Assumption)	2. Client gains greater understanding and defines how anxiety, and self-injury are connected and related to level of self-control and behavioral choices/alternatives
3. Feeling trapped with elements of hopelessness	3. Objective Data, Behavioral Incident, Gentle Assumptions: The sensation of feeling trapped…define what you mean by trapped…and, what's happening around you when this occurs (Clarify, Explore; Behavioral Incident)…Tell me more about your career thoughts (Establish connection, strengthen positive association; Gentle Assumptions)	3. Client defines issues creating "trapped" feelings contributing to sense of hopelessness; identifies areas for preferred focus
4. Substance use	4. Objective Data, Behavioral Incident, Gentle Assumptions: How much do you drink during a typical week?…Type? And what happens after you drink? (Information gathering, clarify; Behavioral Incident)…How does drinking seem to help you at the time you decide to "join your friends for a six pack?" (Open-ended question; Gentle Assumption)	4. Client shares circumstances surrounding alcohol consumption, thereby participating in self-understanding of contributing factors to decision making action
Step 2 Recent Suicidal Events		
1. Self-inflicted arm cuts "last week"	1. Objective Data, Behavioral Incident, Gentle Assumptions: The cuts you are rubbing on your arm…you said this happened last week…you started to explain what was happening with school and mentioned something about a group you are working on a project with?…walk me through what was going on step-by-step…(Clarify; Behavioral Incident)…it sounds like working with this group is very difficult and makes you feel…(Encourage; Reflect; Empathy; Gentle Assumptions)	1 & 2. Client explores self-injurious behavior and its relation to perceived stressors, (e.g. school, work group). Nurse explores/clarifies recent events facts to determine how close client has come to attempting suicide
2. Substance use	2. Objective Data, Behavioral Incident, Gentle Assumptions: When you shared how much you were drinking at the party…were you thinking about drinking so that you could just sleep…and sleep…simply pass out as you did from the party with Lisa (Information gathering, clarify; Behavioral Incident, Open-ended question; Gentle Assumption)	

(Continued)

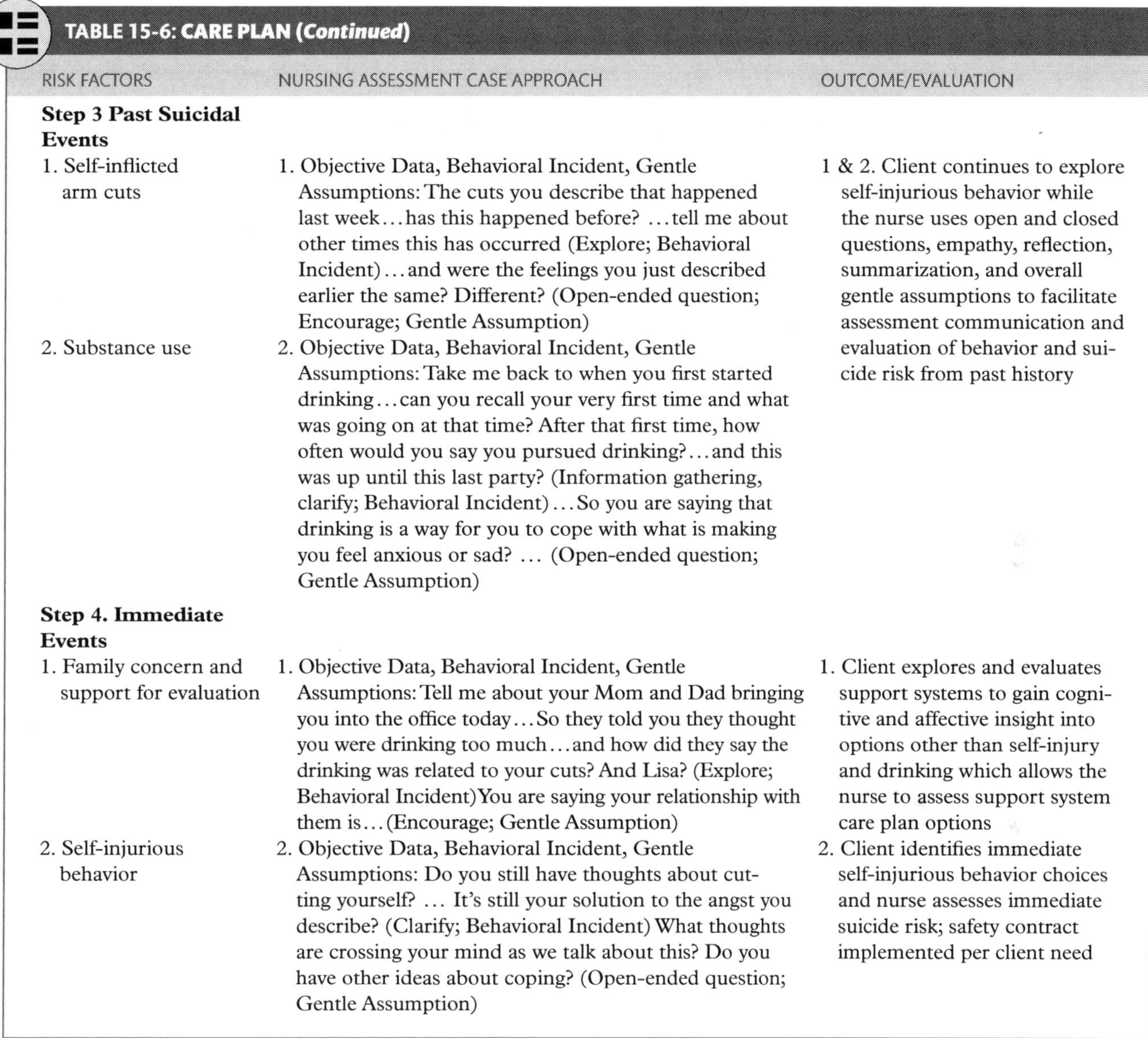

TABLE 15-6: CARE PLAN (*Continued*)

RISK FACTORS	NURSING ASSESSMENT CASE APPROACH	OUTCOME/EVALUATION
Step 3 Past Suicidal Events		
1. Self-inflicted arm cuts	1. Objective Data, Behavioral Incident, Gentle Assumptions: The cuts you describe that happened last week...has this happened before? ...tell me about other times this has occurred (Explore; Behavioral Incident)...and were the feelings you just described earlier the same? Different? (Open-ended question; Encourage; Gentle Assumption)	1 & 2. Client continues to explore self-injurious behavior while the nurse uses open and closed questions, empathy, reflection, summarization, and overall gentle assumptions to facilitate assessment communication and evaluation of behavior and suicide risk from past history
2. Substance use	2. Objective Data, Behavioral Incident, Gentle Assumptions: Take me back to when you first started drinking...can you recall your very first time and what was going on at that time? After that first time, how often would you say you pursued drinking?...and this was up until this last party? (Information gathering, clarify; Behavioral Incident)...So you are saying that drinking is a way for you to cope with what is making you feel anxious or sad? ... (Open-ended question; Gentle Assumption)	
Step 4. Immediate Events		
1. Family concern and support for evaluation	1. Objective Data, Behavioral Incident, Gentle Assumptions: Tell me about your Mom and Dad bringing you into the office today...So they told you they thought you were drinking too much...and how did they say the drinking was related to your cuts? And Lisa? (Explore; Behavioral Incident) You are saying your relationship with them is...(Encourage; Gentle Assumption)	1. Client explores and evaluates support systems to gain cognitive and affective insight into options other than self-injury and drinking which allows the nurse to assess support system care plan options
2. Self-injurious behavior	2. Objective Data, Behavioral Incident, Gentle Assumptions: Do you still have thoughts about cutting yourself? ... It's still your solution to the angst you describe? (Clarify; Behavioral Incident) What thoughts are crossing your mind as we talk about this? Do you have other ideas about coping? (Open-ended question; Gentle Assumption)	2. Client identifies immediate self-injurious behavior choices and nurse assesses immediate suicide risk; safety contract implemented per client need

FOLLOW-UP AND MAINTENANCE

Treatment and prevention is an ongoing process and every contact with these clients is crucial for screening and assessment. At the heart of follow-up and maintenance is a sound care plan coordinated with the client and family vested in the Case Approach. A Case Study and Care Plan example illustrate the steps (see Exhibit 15-5; see Table 15-6).

Self-help strategies are encouraged to give self-confidence to the client, thereby promoting self-care as much as possible. Incorporate families into treatment strategies since they are oftentimes the client's support group and usually are the first to notice any changes in behavior or mood. Most importantly, all health care providers need to be aware of the plan of care and designated referrals. A great number of clients will first be seen at the primary care level, and it is vital for APNs to be aware of the patient with NSSIB/SIB and their ongoing health care status. Collaborative health care, informed by mental health expertise and delivered by APNs in primary health care settings, may provide one way to improve the health outcomes of patients.

SPECIAL CONSIDERATIONS

Trichtillimania and dermatillimania are usually presented when discussing anxiety or impulse control problems, but these behaviors are also examples of self-injury.

Trichtillimania, the inability to resist impulses to pull out one's hair, results in hair loss and distress ranging from insignificant to severe. This behavior may start during childhood or later in life. It is secretive and results in tension reduction or a sense of pleasure. The distress is related to fear of exposure, feeling that something is wrong, and sometimes inability to work. There are often comorbidities of mood disorder, obsessive-compulsive disorder, or other anxiety disorders. Another similar behavior is compulsive skin picking. For more information see www.skinpick.com/.

Treatment includes behavioral techniques as well as psychopharmacology (Franklin & Tolin, 2007). Habit reversal is the most effective approach and involves designing competitive behaviors to inhibit the behavior. Psychopharmacology usually involves the use of SSRIs. There is minimal available evidence for treatment, with most information reported as case studies.

SELECTED INTERNET RESOURCES FOR CLIENTS AND FAMILIES

American Association of Suicidology: www.suicidology.org

American Foundation for Suicide Prevention: www.afsp.org

International Society for the Study of Self Injury: www.isssweb.org

National Institute of Mental Health: www.nimh.nih.gov

PEDIATRIC POINTERS

Mental Health Assessment of Children and Adolescents

The mental health assessment of children is a specialized process taking into consideration where they are developmentally. It needs to be more specific, with fewer open-ended questions and simple phrasing, because children have a narrower vocabulary than adolescents. Artistic and play media like drawing, puppets, and dolls are often used to engage children and evaluate their perceptions, fine motor skills, and intellectual functions (Boyd, 2012). A comprehensive evaluation of children's mental status is performed by using a combination of different means such as a medical history and physical exam, a biopsychosocial history, a mental status examination, and the child's school performance. The clinical interview is the primary assessment tool that, in general, follows the same format as for older children and adults (Boyd, 2012). It's important that the PMH-APRN take into consideration the developmental level of each child in terms of language, cognitive, emotional, and social development. Since parents are generally the primary caregivers, they are significant partners in the child's evaluation and treatment. Other family members may also play a valuable role in the evaluation and treatment processes.

Preschool-aged children have difficulty talking about and describing how they feel in addition to having more concrete thinking. Play is useful for this age of children because it is a way for them to transfer their real life experiences to symbolic and nonliteral representations (Boyd, 2012). Sensorimotor skills, cognitive styles, language, emotional and behavioral responsiveness, coping styles, and problem-solving skills can be observed from play. Children younger than 5 years of age may be assessed in a playroom if one is available, while any rules for play should be explained to ensure safety.

The use of specialized tools for children may also be utilized. Lidz (2003) developed a tool that the PMH-APRN may use to assess preschoolers play. The Devereux Early Childhood Assessment (DECA) instrument is used to measure factors of attachment, initiative, and self-control in children 2 to 5 years of age (Hamrin, Deering, & Scahill, 2008).

School-aged children from 5 to 11 years of age have more verbal skills and can tolerate more periods of direct questioning than preschool-aged children. The PMH-APRN may use competitive board games or cards to establish rapport.

Adolescents have an increased command of language and developmentally have the

(Continued)

PEDIATRIC POINTERS (*Continued*)

capacity for abstract and formal operations thinking (Boyd, 2012; Webb, 2002). They have a more complex social world and in addition, an increased sense of self-consciousness, fear of being shamed, and demands for privacy (Boyd, 2012). For this reason, it is important for the PMH-APRN to communicate with respect, honesty, and genuineness in order to build rapport. Adolescents may also be concerned about confidentiality; therefore, the PMH-APRN needs to be straightforward with them about what will and will not be shared with their parents.

Adapting Dialectical Behavior Therapy for Children

The study by Perepletchikova and colleagues (2011) describes the adaptation of DBT for use with preadolescent children, as well as its feasibility and efficacy for preadolescents with suicidality and/or self-injury. DBT that is used for adults and adolescents was modified according to the developmental level of children in the study, and the ability of the children to understand and utilize the adapted skills was tested. In addition, not only the children but also their caregivers (e.g., parents) were included for training and feedback. Adaptation of DBT skills included materials modified for the children, experiential exercises, in-session practice, role play, and multimedia presentations. Materials were simplified and condensed into large font sizes with cartoons, colors, limited amounts of text per page, and language geared for a second-grade reading level.

The sample for this study was recruited from regular classes from a local school. There were a total of 11 children consisting of 6 girls and 5 boys ranging in age from 8 years to 11 years and 6 months. The majority were Caucasian (73%), while 64% presented clinically significant symptoms of depression, anxiety, or both, and/or endorsed suicidal ideation. Both children and parents completed a variety of questionnaires. Children completed questionnaires to assess their mood and feelings, their coping strategies, and self-control, and a skills training and homework review questionnaire. Parents completed questionnaires including an emotion regulation checklist, a social skills ratings scale, parent version, and a skills training attitude inventory. Group skills training and homework review with the children was conducted twice a week for 6 weeks. Both children and parents showed moderate to high acceptability of the skills training. Changes in children's symptoms over time were also seen. Depressive symptoms, suicidal ideation, and behavioral problems decreased while adaptive coping skills increased. However, in more conservative analyses, only a decrease in depressive symptoms retained significance.

The results of this study demonstrate initial acceptability, feasibility, and efficacy of the adapted DBT skills for children. Children's understanding and utilization of skills, which are important outcomes to consider, were supported by therapists' observations during homework review. Since DBT skills training requires parental reinforcement and involvement in skills practice to enhance children's ability to use these skills, the researchers are in the process of developing a caregiver training component. Limitations include that this study was conducted with a small nonclinical sample, there was no control group, and the duration of the intervention was short. However, the preliminary results do show promise.

Screening for Adolescent Self-Injury

Tusaie, Acierto, Murry, Fitzgerald, and Chiu (2009) did a survey of Ohio Advanced Practice Nurses (APRNs) to assess their screening for adolescent self-injury. Little research has been done to examine the role of APRNs in screening for self-injury, although they play an important role in adolescent health care in both inpatient and outpatient settings. It is imperative that APRNs screen for self-injury because the consequences are far-reaching including physically, socially, and psychologically. Again

(*Continued*)

PEDIATRIC POINTERS (*Continued*)

the relationship between NSSIB and SIB needs to be highlighted. Studies show that many adolescents who self-injure have also made one or more suicide attempts (Skegg, 2005; Gardner, 2008).

Two-hundred fifty surveys were sent out to Ohio APRNs, with a return rate of 40.8% (n=102). Five surveys were excluded from analysis because they responded that they weren't currently practicing or they did not provide information about their practice. Among the APRNs that did respond, 71.1% (n=69) reported observing patients between 11 and 22 years who had evidence of self-injury. However, only 44.3% reported that they actually screened for self-injury. Further, only about 25% of practicing APRNs had formal educational content on assessing for intentional self-injury in their graduate programs (Tusaie et al., 2009).

This study also highlights that APRNs see adolescent patients with evidence of self-harm across specialty areas. Identification of self-harm was also increased by over 20% with purposeful screening. Screening may help to interrupt the repetition of self-harm, increase positive coping skills, and save lives. The other finding from this study was a self-identified knowledge deficit of APRNs, although the majority had an interest in learning more about it (Tusaie et al., 2009).

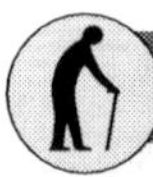

AGING ALERTS

Risk Factors and Prevention of Suicide in Older Adults

Although a large number of suicides occur in adolescents and middle age, "late-life suicide is a cause for great concern and warrants ongoing attention from researchers, health care providers, policy makers, and society at large" (Conwell, Van Orden, & Caine, 2011). Just as across the life span, so too in the geriatric population it is vital to identify risk and protective factors in order to conduct prevention efforts in this age category. Psychiatric illness is one of the most important risk factors. For instance, these authors looked at rates of psychiatric and substance abuse disorders that were present in older people who died by suicide and noted that psychiatric illnesses were present in 71% to 97% of the deaths by suicide (Conwell, Van Orden, & Caine, 2011, p. 454). Further, an elder's overall physical health and functioning will impact various aspects of their lives. Not only does the number of physical illness have an impact on suicide, but the outcomes of these illnesses on functioning, pain, and threats to their independence also play an essential role. Additionally, similar to all suicide risks, social factors have a role in suicide in older adults as well. Stressful life events may trigger reactions and in this population these can include events associated with aging such as: threats to health and function, losses through bereavement, or the break of a relationship with family and/or friends or other sources of support. The promotion of connection at personal, family, and community levels may be a key strategy of suicide prevention in the elderly (Conwell, Van Orden, & Caine, 2011), as well as for others.

REFERENCES

American Psychiatric Association. (2006). *Practice guidelines for the treatment of psychiatric disorders compendium*. Arlington, VA:American Psychiatric Association.

Barney, C., & Shea, S. C. (2007). The art of effectively teaching clinical interviewing skills using role-playing: A primer. *Psychiatric Clinics of North America, 30*, e31–e50.

Berk, M., Henriques, G., Warman, D., Brown, G., & Beck, A. (2004). A cognitive therapy intervention for suicide attempters: An overview of the treatment and case examples. *Cognitive and Behavioral Practice, 11*, 265–277.

Boyd, M. A. (2012). *Psychiatric nursing: Contemporary practice* (5th ed.). Philadelphia, PA: Lippincott Williams & Williams.

Branford, D., Bhaumik, S., & Naik, B. (1998). Selective serotonin reuptake inhibitors for the treatment of perseverative and maladaptive behaviors of people with intellectual disability. *Journal of Intellectual Disability Research, 42*, 301–306.

Brasic, J. R., Barnett, J. Y., Ahn, S. C., Nadrich, R. H., Will, M. V., & Clair, A. (1997). Clinical assessment of self-injurious behavior. *Psychological Reports, 80*(1), 155–160.

Brausch, A. M., & Gutierrez, P. M. (2010). Differences in non-suicidal self-injury and suicide attempts in adolescents. *Journal of Youth and Adolescence, 39*, 233–242.

Bureau, J-F., Martin, J., Freynet, N., Poirier, A. A., Lafontaine, M-F., & Cloutier, P. (2010). Perceived dimensions of parenting and non-suicidal self-injury in young adults. *Journal of Youth and Adolescence, 39*, 484–494.

Castille, K., Prout, M., Marczyk, G., Shmidheiser, M., Yoder, S., & Howlett, B. (2007). The early maladaptive schemas of self-mutilators: Implications for therapy. *Journal of Cognitive Psychotherapy, 21*(1), 58–71.

Centers for Disease Control and Prevention. (2010). *Injury prevention and control: Data and statistics (WISQARS)*. Retrieved from www.cdc.gov/injury/wisqars/index.html

Claes, L., Vandereycken, W., & Vertommen, H. (2005). Clinical assessment of self-injurious behaviors: An overview of rating scales and self-reporting questionnaires. *Advances in Psychology Research, 36*, 183–209.

Comtois, K. A., & Linehan, M. M. (2006). Psychosocial treatments of suicidal behaviors: A practice-friendly review. *Journal of Clinical Psychology, 62*(2), 161–170. doi: 10.1002/jclp.20220

Conwell, Y., Van Orden, K., & Caine, E. (2011). Suicide in older adults. *Psychiatric Clinics of North America, 34*(2), 451–468.

Cutcliffe, J. R., Stevenson, C., Jackson, S., & Smith, P. (2007). Reconnecting the person with humanity. Crisis, 28(2), 207–210.

Davanzo, P. A., Belin, T. R., Widawski, M. H., & King, B. H. (1998). Paroxetine treatment of aggression and self-injury in persons with mental retardation. *American Journal of Mental Retardation, 102*, 427–437.

Davis, S. E., Williams, I. S., & Hays, L. W. (2002). Psychiatric inpatients' perceptions of written no- suicide agreements: An exploratory study. *Suicide and Life-Threatening Behavior, 32*(1), 51–66.

Farrow, T. L., & O'Brien, A. J. (2003). No-suicide contracts and informed consent: An analysis of ethical issues. *Nursing Ethics, 10*(2), 199–207.

Favazza, A. R., & Conterio, K. (1988). The plight of chronic self-mutilators. *Community Mental Health Journal, 24*(1), 22–30.

Favazza, A. R. (1986). *Self-harm behavior survey*. Columbia, MI: Author.

Fong, T. (2003). Self-mutilation: Impulsive traits, high pain threshold suggest new drug therapies. *Current Psychiatry, 2*(2), 15–23.

Franklin, M., & Tolin, D. (2007). *Treatment of Trichotillomania*. New York, NY: Springer-Verlag.

Gardner, F. (2008). Analysis of self-harm. *Community Care, 1725*, 22.

Gratz, K. L. (2001). Measurement of deliberate self-harm: Preliminary data on the deliberate self-harm inventory. *Journal of Psychopathology and Behavioral Assessment, 23*(4), 253–263.

Gutierrez, P. M., Osman, A., Barrios, F. X., & Kopper, B. A. (2001). Development and initial validation of the self-harm behavior questionnaire. *Journal of Personality Assessment, 77*(3), 475–490.

Hamrin, V., Deering, G. C., & Scahill, L. (2008). Mental health assessment of children and adolescents. In M. A. Boyd (Ed.), *Psychiatric nursing: Contemporary practice* (pp. 596–615). Philadelphia, PA: Lippincott Williams & Wilkins.

Hankin, B. L., & Abela, J. R. Z. (2011). Nonsuicidal self-injury in adolescence: Prospective rates and risk factors in a 2½ year longitudinal study. *Psychiatry Research, 186*, 65–70.

Hepburn, S. R., Crane, C., Barnhofer, T., Duggan, D. S., Fennell, M. J., & Williams, M. G. (2009). Mindfullness-based cognitive therapy may reduce thought suppression in previously suicidal participants: Findings from a preliminary study. *British Journal of Clinical Psychology, 48*, 209–215.

Hilt, L. M., Nock, M. K., Lloyd-Richardson, E. E., & Prinstein, M. J. (2008). Longitudinal study of nonsuicidal self-injury among young adolescents: Rates, correlates and preliminary test of an interpersonal model. *The Journal of Early Adolescence, 28*(3), 455–469.

Ingenhoven, T. J. M., & Duivenvoorden, H. J. (2011). Differential effectiveness of antipsychotics in borderline personality disorder. *Journal of Clinical Psychopharmacology, 31*(4), 489–496.

Jacobson, C. M., & Gould, M. (2007). The epidemiology and phenomenology of non-suicidal self-injurious behavior among adolescents: A critical review of the literature. *Archives of Suicide Research, 11*(2), 129–147.

Kelly, K., Byrne, D., Przybyla, D. P. J., Eberly, C., Eberly, B., Greendlinger, V.,...Gorsky, J. (1985). Chronic self-destructiveness: Conceptualization, measurement, and initial validation of the construct. *Motivation and Emotion, 9*(2), 135–151.

Klonsky, E. D., & Glenn, C. R. (2009). Assessing the functions of non-suicidal self-injury: Psychometric properties of the inventory of statements about self-injury (ISAS). *Journal of Psychopathology and Behavioral Assessment, 31*, 215–219.

Kroll, J. Use of no-suicide contracts by psychiatrists in Minnesota. *American Journal of Psychiatry, 157*(10), 1684–1686.

Lescano, C. M., Hadley, W. S., Beausoleil, N. I., Brown, L. K., D'eramo, D., & Zimskind, A. (2007). A brief screening measure of adolescent risk behavior. *Child Psychiatry and Human Development, 37*(4), 325–326.

Lieb, K., Vollm, B., Rucker, G., Timmer, A., & Stoffers, J. M. (2010). Pharmacotherapy for borderline personality disorder: Cochran systematic review of randomized trials. *The British Journal of Psychiatry, 196*, 4–12.

Linehan, M. M., Comtois, K. A., Brown, M. Z., Heard, H. L., & Wagner, A. (2006a). Suicide Attempt Self-Injury Interview (SASII): Development, reliability, and validity of a scale to assess suicide attempts and intentional self-injury. *Psychological Assessment, 18*(3), 303–312.

Linehan, M. M., Comtois, K. A., Murray, A. M., Brown, M. Z., Gallop, R. J., Heard, H. L.,...Tutek, D. A. (2006b). Two-year randomized controlled trial and follow-up of dialectical behavior therapy vs therapy by experts for suicidal behaviors and borderline personality disorder. *Archives of General Psychiatry, 63*, 757–766.

Linehan, M. M., Goodstein, J. L., Nielsen, S. L., & Chiles, J. A. (1983). Reasons for staying alive when you are thinking of killing yourself: The reasons for living inventory. *Journal of Consulting and Clinical Psychology, 51*(2), 276–286.

Martin, P., & Guth, C. (2005). Unusual devastating self-injurious behavior in a patient with a severe learning disability: Treatment with citalopram. *The Psychiatrist, 29*, 108–110.

McGlothlin J. (2008). *Developing clinical skills in suicide assessment, prevention, and treatment*. Alexandria, VA: American Counseling Association.

McMyler, C., & Pryjmachuk, S. (2008). Do "no-suicide" contracts work? *Journal of Psychiatric and Mental Health Nursing, 15*, 512–522.

Muehlenkamp, J. (2005). Self-injurious behavior as a separate clinical syndrome. *American Journal of Orthopsychiatry, 75*(2), 324–333.

Muehlenkamp, J. (2006). Empirically supported treatments and general therapy guidelines for non-suicidal self-injury. *Journal of Mental Health Counseling, 28*(2), 166–185.

Muehlenkamp, J., & Gutierrez, P. (2004). An investigation of differences between self-injurious behavior and suicide attempts in a sample of adolescents. *Suicide and Life-Threatening Behavior, 34*, 12–23.

Nock, M. K. (2009). Why do people hurt themselves? New insights into the nature and functions of self-injury. *Current Directions in Psychological Science, 18*(2), 78–83.

Nock, M. K., Borges, G., Bromet, E. J., Cha, C. B., Kessler, R. C., & Lee, S. (2008). Suicide and suicidal behavior. *Epidemiologic Reviews, 30*, 133–154.

Nock, M. K., Joiner, T. E., Jr., Gordon, K. H., Lloyd-Richardson, E., & Prinstein, M. J. (2006). Non-suicidal self-injury among adolescents: Diagnostic correlates and relation to suicide attempts. *Psychiatry Research, 144*, 65–72.

Perepletchikova, F., Axelrod, R. S., Kaufman, J., Rounsaville, J. B., Douglas-Palumberi, H. & Miller, L. A. (2011). Adapting dialectical behavior therapy for children: Towards a new research agenda for pediatric suicidal and non-suicidal self-injurious behaviors. *Child and Adolescent Mental Health, 16*(2), 116–121.

Reist, C., Nakamura, K., Sagart, E., Sokolski, K. N., & Fujimoto, K. A. (2003). Impulsive aggressive behavior: Open label treatment with citalopram. *Journal of Clinical Psychiatry, 64*(1), 81–85.

Rosen, P. (1988). The kind of cut. *Journal of Emergency Medicine, 6*(6), 543.

Ross, S., & Heath, N. (2002). A study of the frequency of self-mutilation in a community sample of adolescents. *Journal of Youth and Adolescents, 31*(1), 67–77.

Ross, S., Heath, N. L., & Toste, J. R. (2009). Non-suicidal self-injury and eating pathology in high school students. *American Journal of Orthopsychiatry, 79*(1), 83–92.

Rudd, M. D., Joiner, T., & Rajab, M. H. (1996). Relationships among suicide ideators, attempters, and multiple attempters in a young-adult sample. *Journal of Abnormal Psychology, 105*(4), 541–550.

Sansome, A. R., & Sansone, A. L. (2010). Measuring self-harm behavior with the self-harm inventory. *Psychiatry, 7*(4), 16–20.

Sansone, R. A., Wiederman, M. W., & Sansone, L. A. (1998). The self-harm inventory (SHI): Development of a scale for identifying self-destructive behaviors and borderline personality disorder. *Journal of Clinical Psychology, 54*(7), 973–983.

Schroeder, S. R., Rojahn, J., & Reese, R. M. (1997). Brief report: Reliability and validity of instruments for assessing psychotropic medication effects on self-injurious behavior in mental retardation. *Journal of Autism and Developmental Disorders, 27*(1), 89–102.

Shea, S. C. (1998a). *Psychiatric interviewing: The art of understanding–a practical guide for psychiatrists, psychologists, counselors, social workers, nurses, and other mental health professionals* (2nd ed.). Philadelphia, PA: W.B. Saunders.

Shea, S. C. (1998b). The chronological assessment of suicide events: A practical interviewing strategy for the elicitation of suicidal ideation. *The Journal of Clinical Psychiatry, 59*, 8–72.

Shea, S. C. (2007). My favorite tips from the "Clinical Interviewing Tip of the Month" archive. *Psychiatric Clinics of North America, 30*(2), 219–225.

Shea, S. C., & Barney, C. (2007a). Facilic supervision and schematics: The art of training psychiatric residents and other mental health professionals how to structure clinical interviews sensitively. *Psychiatric Clinics of North America, 30*, e51–e96.

Shea, S. C., & Barney, C. (2007b). Macrotraining: A "How-To" primer for using serial role-playing to train complex clinical interviewing tasks such as suicide assessment. *Psychiatric Clinics of North America, 30*(2), e1–e29.

Shneidman, E. S. (1985). Some thoughts on grief and mourning. *Suicide and Life-Threatening Behavior, 15*(1), 51–55.

Simon, R. I. (2008). Naked suicide. *Journal of the American Academy of Psychiatry and the Law, 36*(2), 240–245.

Simpson, E., Zlotnick, C., Begin, A., Costello, E., & Pearlstein, T. (1994). *Self-Injury Survey*. Providence, RI: Authors.

Skegg, K. (2005). Self-harm. *Lancet, 366*, 1471–1483.

Slee, N., Arensman, E., Garnefski, N., & Spinhoven, P. (2007). Cognitive-behavioral therapy for deliberate self-harm. *Crisis, 28*(4), 175–182. doi:10.1027/0227–5910.28.4.175

Stahl, S. M. (2009). *The Prescriber's guide: Stahl's essential psychopharmacology* (3rd ed.). New York, NY: Cambridge University.

Stewart, C. D., Quinn, A., Plever, S., & Emmerson, B. (2009). Comparing cognitive behavior therapy, problem solving therapy, and treatment as usual in a high risk population. *Suicide and Life-Threatening Behavior, 39*(5), 538–547.

Swann, A. C. (2003). Neuroreceptor mechanisms of aggression and its treatment. *Journal of Clinical Psychiatry, 64*(Suppl. 4), 26–35.

Symons, F. J., Thompson, A., & Rodriguez, M. C. (2004). Self-injurious behavior and the efficacy of naltrexone treatment: A quantitative synthesis. *Mental Retardation and Developmental Disabilities Research Reviews, 10*, 193–200.

Tusaie, R. K., Acierto, S., Murray, A., Fitzgerald, K., & Chiu, S. (2009). Screening for adolescent self-injury. *Journal for Nurse Practitioners, 5*(5), 359–364.

van Beek, W., Kerkhof, A., & Beekman, A. (2009). Future oriented group training for suicidal patients: A randomized clinical trial. *BMC Psychiatry, 9*(65).

Vanderlinden, J., & Vandereycken, W. (1997). *Trauma, dissociation, and impulse dyscontrol in eating disorders*. Philadelphia, PA: Routledge.

Varcarolis, E.M. (2003). *Foundations of psychiatric-mental health nursing*. New York, NY: W.B. Saunders.

Velazquez, L., Ward-Chene, L., & Loogsian, S. R. (2000). Fluoxetine in the treatment of self-mutilating behavior. *Journal of the American Academy of Child & Adolescent Psychiatry, 39*, 812–814.

Villalba, R., & Harrington, C. J. (2000). Repetitive self-injurious behavior: Neuropsychiatric perspective and review of pharmacologic treatments. *Seminars in Clinical Neuropsychiatry, 5*, 215–226.

Vita, A., De Peri, L., & Sacchetti, E. (2011). Antipsychotics, antidepressants, anticonvulsants, and placebo on the symptom dimensions of borderline personality disorder: A meta-analysis of randomized controlled and open-label trials. *Journal of Clinical Psychopharmacology, 31*(5), 613–624.

Walsh, B. W. (2006). *Treating self-injury: A practical guide.* New York, NY: Guilford Press.

Walsh, B. W., & Rosen, P. M. (1998). *Self-mutilation: Theory, research and treatment.* New York, NY:Guilford Press.

Webb, L. (2002). Deliberate self-harm in adolescence: A systematic review of psychological and psychosocial factors. *Journal of Advanced Nursing, 38*(3), 235–244.

White, J. (2006/2007). Suicide risk and protective factors for youth. *Crosscurrents, 10*(2), 10.

Wilkinson, J. M. (2012). *Nursing process and critical thinking,* (5th ed.). Saddle River, NJ: Prentice Hall.

Wilkinson, P. O. (2011). Nonsuicidal self-injury: A clear marker for suicide risk. *Journal of the American Academy of Child & Adolescent Psychiatry, 50*(8), 741–743.

Yates, T. M., Tracy, A. J., & Luthar, S. S. (2008). Non-suicidal self-injury among "privileged" youths: Longitudinal and cross-sectional approaches to developmental process. *Journal of Counseling and Clinical Psychology, 76*(1), 52–62.

Yufit, R. I., & Lester, D. (2005). *Assessment, treatment, and prevention of suicidal behavior.* Hoboken, New Jersey:John Wiley & Sons.

Zerler, H. (2009). Motivational interviewing in the assessment and management of suicidality. *Journal of Clinical Psychology: In Session, 65*(11), 1207–1217.

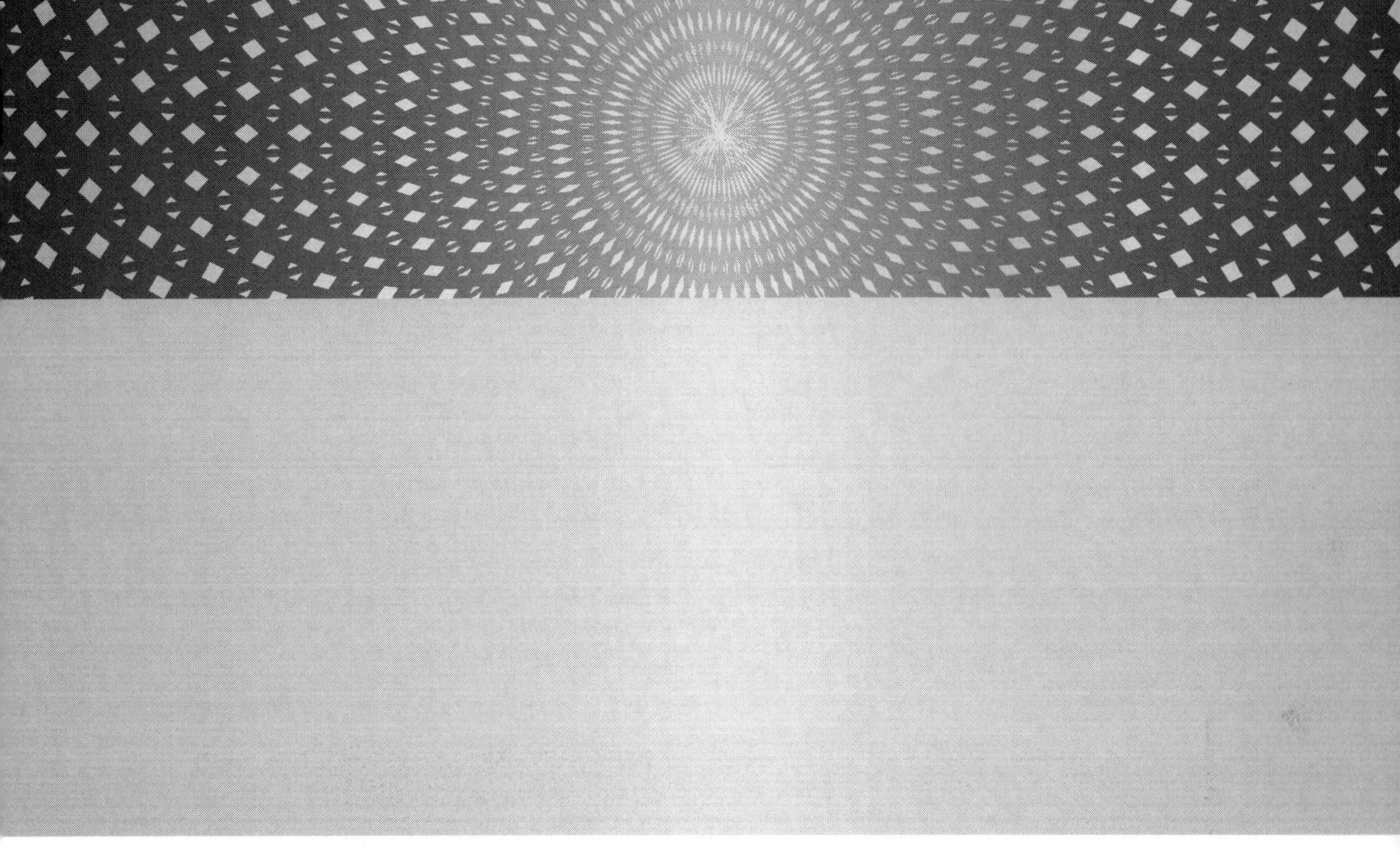

CHAPTER CONTENTS

The World Health Organization (WHO) proclaims violence to be the leading worldwide health problem (WHO, 2002). While some believe that violence is an inevitable part of the human condition, the WHO challenges member nations to participate in the effort to prevent and reduce all types of violence (WHO, 2002) (Table 16-1). Interpersonal violence, the type that U.S. health professionals are most likely to encounter, killed an estimated 520,000 persons worldwide, or 8.8 per 100,000 persons, likely a gross underestimation due to lack of statistics from many countries, and many deaths reported as "accidental" when the true cause was family-inflicted violence (WHO, 2002). The crude death rate due to interpersonal violence per 100,000 persons estimated by a survey of 16 states within the United States was 19.64 in 2008 (CDC, 2011). This chapter will focus upon the other-directed violence that advanced practice nurses (APRN) are likely to encounter in the work-place, and how to identify and treat both the victims and perpetrators of violence, since these are the tasks to which the Psychiatric Mental Health Advanced Practice Nurse (PMH-APRN) is called.

Violence is defined as exertion of physical force so as to injure or abuse; injury by distortion, infringement, or profanity; or destructive, intense, turbulent, or furious force. Specific types of violence include: (1) Assault: slapping, beating, rape, and homicide; threat and/or use of knives, firearms, bombs, or other weapons; (2) Battery: unwanted physical contact or threat to inflict harm such as slapping, biting, kicking, hitting, or spitting;

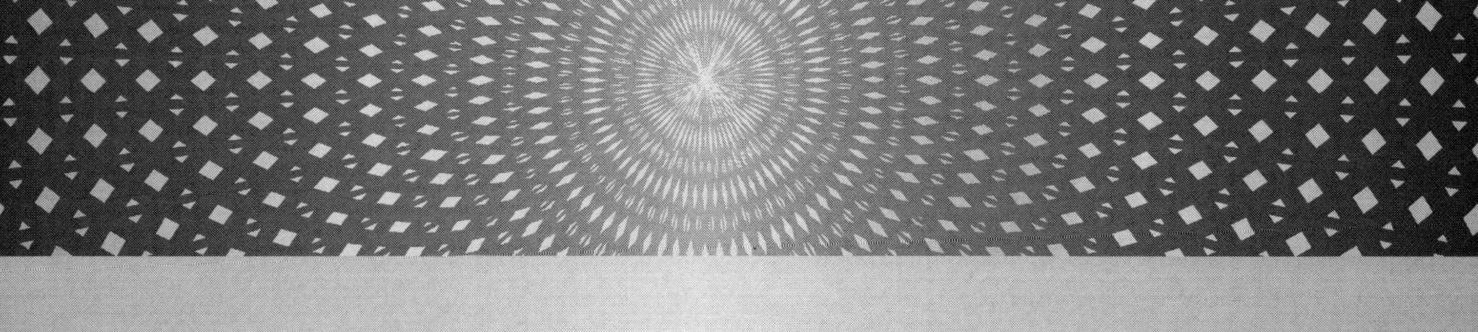

CHAPTER 16

Integrated Management of Other-Directed Violence

Marla McCall

(3) Sexual: rape, fondling, words or conduct of a sexual nature that cause alarm, annoyance, or emotional upset; (4) Verbal: threats that are verbal, written, or communicated via body language (American Psychiatric Nurses Association [APNA] report, 2008; Merriam-Webster, 2011). Recently, the many forms of violence have been the topic of not only lay publications but also of health care and scholarly literature. Other-directed types of violence that PMH-APRNs most frequently encounter include battery, bullying, child abuse, emotional abuse, intimate partner violence (IPV), murder, rape, property destruction, workplace violence, and stalking (see Exhibit 16-1). More rarely the PMH-APRN may encounter survivors of human trafficking, mass violence, or war. Refugee patients may be from areas where rape, of both men and women, and control over birth rate are used systematically as weapons of war; these practices are widespread with numerous historical precedents (Schott, 2011). PMH-APRNs must know how to protect themselves and their coworkers from victimization when violent persons undergo treatment for comorbid psychiatric issues, either voluntarily or by court order. They must also be able to recognize horizontal and vertical violence within the nursing profession, and participate in efforts to curtail its occurrence (Johnson, 2009; Johnson & Rea, 2009). Horizontal violence is violence perpetrated against someone of equal rank, such as nurse to nurse; vertical violence occurs between different ranks, such as from supervisor to employee, or vice versa.

SPECIFIC TYPES OF VIOLENCE—IPV

The WHO found in a 10-nation study that 15% to 54% of women report intimate partner violence (IPV; García-Moreno, Jansen, Ellsberg, & Watts, 2005). IPV is the most prevalent form of violence against women (United Nations [UN], 2006). Furthermore, impunity for violence against women exists in many countries, either explicitly via poor laws, or implicitly as in the United States via poor response of police and other authorities (UN, 2006). The types of violence perpetrated against women included physical abuse, emotional abuse, sexual abuse, and emotional control, and by far the most common abuser was the woman's spouse (García-Moreno et al., 2005). Forty to 45% of women who report IPV also report forced sex (Campbell, 2002; Finkelhor & Yllo, 1985); those same women report that the sex was unprotected, leaving them at higher risk of sexually transmitted diseases (Díaz-Olavarrieta et al., 2009). IPV victims are less effective at negotiating condom use (Swan & O'Connell, 2011). Younger age and lower educational level as well as unmarried marital status are risk factors for female victims; unemployment, substance abuse, and violence toward other men were risk factors for male perpetrators (García-Moreno et al., 2005). Educated women are not exempt, however, as evidenced by a study quote:

> One day he returned home very late. I asked him, "You are so late ... where did you go?" He answered, "I went

EXHIBIT 16-1: STRANGER, ACQUAINTANCE, OR DOMESTIC VIOLENCE

Emotional—control via restriction of freedom, socially isolating, bullying
Verbal—insults, putdowns, character assassination, in person or Internet
Sexual—rape, assault, coercion, sexting, Internet posts, threats
Physical violence—hitting, beating, murder
Stalking—in person, by mail or Internet, frivolous lawsuits
Imprisonment
Child Abuse
Elder Abuse
Terrorism
Hate Crimes
Natural Disaster
Rape in war as a weapon for genocide, natality

Source: Adapted from Simon (2011).

to the red light zone. Do you have any problems with that?" I started shouting at him and he instantly landed a blow on my right eye. I screamed and he grabbed my hair and dragged me from one room to another while constantly kicking and punching me. He did not calm down at that.... He undid his belt and then hit me as much and as long as he wanted. Only those who have been hit with a belt know what it is like.

University-educated woman married to a doctor in Bangladesh (WHO, 2005)

IPV affects 25% to 30% of American women with victims numbering 1.9–3.5 million per year (Tjaden & Thoennes, 2000). Minority immigrant women of Asian descent report an incidence of IPV of 41% to 60% and are also overrepresented in the femicide group, which is defined as IPV leading to death (Asian and Pacific Islander Institute on Domestic Violence, 2011). After intimate partners, children were the largest group of victims in familial murder cases, followed by parents of wives and girlfriends, leading to 226 fatalities in a 6-year period (Dabby, Patel, & Poore, 2010). Multiple studies show that minority women are much less likely to be referred for specialty mental health services to deal with IPV compared with Caucasian women, and are less likely to engage in help-seeking (Rodriguez, Valentine, Son, & Muhammed, 2009).

There is a strong link between patriarchal views and the acceptance of wife battering in many cultures; in countries where men give "bride money" to his wife's family, men are more likely to demand complete control over their wives' lives (Fawole, 2008; Marshall, 2010). This hegemonic view is unfortunately accepted by the women themselves who are often poor, illiterate, and very young when they marry. Among Asian immigrants who resided in the United States an average of 14 years, 25% of respondents both male and female believe that male violence is acceptable for misbehavior of wives such as infidelity, refusing to cook or clean, or nagging (Yoshioka, DiNoia, & Ullah, 2001). These views are common in Bangladesh and other South Asian as well as African cultures (García-Moreno et al., 2005).

Timing of IPV. Individuals are most likely to be victimized when trying to leave an abuser, when they fail to meet any expectation of the abuser, no matter how small, during child custody battles, when a perpetrator abuses substances, or if the victim disagrees with the abuser. As IPV continues, the children are often part of the collateral damage. Infants and children under the age of 3 are more likely to become abused due to their total dependence upon their parents, their high need of care, frequency of crying, and limited ability to modify their needs when dealing with an impaired parent (National Consensus Guidelines [NCG], 2004).

Barriers to Care of IPV. Poverty is the single greatest risk factor for victims due to the inability to escape economically. Barriers to seeking care include language, lack of knowledge regarding resources, stigma associated with both victimization and help seeking, and fear of being labeled as crazy; this is especially true for immigrant Caribbean African women, U.S.-born African Americans, and U.S.-born Latinas (Rodriguez et al., 2009). Limited English language skills are also a severe barrier to receiving good quality care (Rodriguez et al., 2009). Many IPV victims are told by religious communities to keep their IPV a secret (Petersen et al., 2004). Many victims felt self-reliance was virtuous, therefore admitting to need of help with IPV was stigmatizing (Khoury, 2004). Women over 45 reporting long-term abuse in long-term marriages were found very reluctant to divulge abuse for fear of harsh punishment of their spouse, fear of disapproval from adult children, need to preserve the family, and long-standing shame that the abuse was somehow their fault; often their concern for the abuser outweighed their desire to escape abuse (Beaulaurier, Seff, & Newman, 2011).

CHILD ABUSE

When IPV is disclosed, inquiry into parenting styles and methods of child discipline is relevant since child abuse and IPV are often co-occurring (Chan, 2011). PMH-APRNs will encounter both victims and perpetrators of child abuse in the course of their careers, depending upon their service population. For the fiscal year of 2009 in the United States only 8.3% of Child Protective Service (CPS) reports came from medical personnel, a percentage that is likely lower than it should be (Flaherty & Sege, 2005; U.S., Department of Health and Human Services [USDHHS], 2010). While many are legally mandated to report abuse, many persons do not report suspicions of abuse due to ignorance of reporting procedures, fear of recrimination, fear of false accusations, past experience of not feeling as if the report made a difference, and fear that the report might worsen the situation for the child (Flaherty, Sege, Binns, Mattson, & Christoffel, 2000; Yehuda, Altar-Swartz, Ziv, Jedwab, & Benbenishty, 2010).

Signs of physical neglect and abuse include inappropriate or inadequate clothing for weather conditions, poor hygiene, poor physical condition, unexplained injuries, lack of lunch at school, and so on. Victims are likely to present with anxiety disorders or behavioral problems, such as fighting, at school. Bruising of the face and neck and injuries that are not age-appropriate are unusual injuries, and may be signs of abuse. Conduct disorders (CDs) in school-aged children and unexplained physical injuries in younger children should raise the suspicion of child abuse.

Children who are abused suffer vulnerability to lifelong effects including lower educational achievement, earlier onset of mental health problems, physical health problems including immediate injury and long-term chronic illness, poorer peer and social relationships, higher likelihood of substance abuse, earlier sexual activity, and CDs that can lead to juvenile delinquency and adult criminality (NCG, 2004). Therefore early detection of risk factors for child maltreatment and prompt intervention is the goal. However, the most vulnerable children, those under age 4, are least likely to come to the attention of outside agencies and care providers. Thus, PMH-APRNs treating older family members for a variety of mental health problems that are risk factors for child maltreatment are in a unique place to identify at-risk children early, report the abuse, and propose multidisciplinary intervention strategies (Feng, Fetzer, Chen, Yeh, Huang, 2010).

ELDER ABUSE

Estimates of incidence of elder abuse are 4% to 6% of those living at home; however, rates for those living in

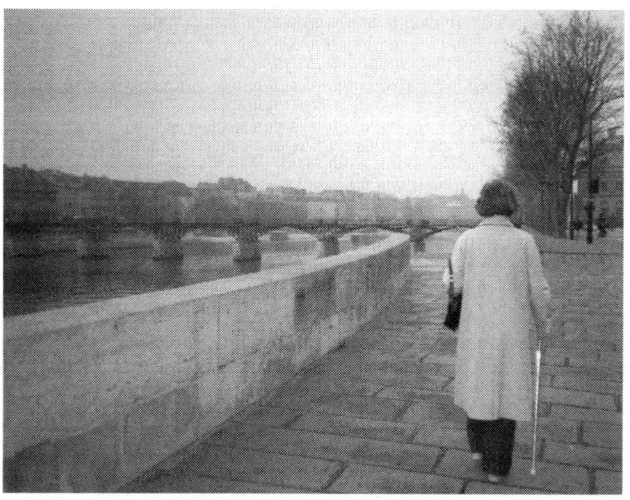

institutions are thought to be much higher (WHO, 2002). Up to 36% of nursing home staff reported witnessing at least one instance of abuse, up to 10% reported having committed at least one act of physical abuse, and 40% reported emotionally abusing an elderly person (Pillemer & Moore, 1990). Elders become victims of abuse with forced labor when their children bring them into the country under sponsorship, then require them to work excruciatingly long hours in businesses such as restaurants. They cannot leave as they are ineligible for social service support while still under sponsorship, and can be threatened with deportation just like victims of human trafficking (Walsh, Olson, Ploeg, Lohfeld, & MacMillan, 2011). Hispanics and African Americans were found in one study to be more likely to become victims of financial abuse, while Asians were more likely to become victims of forced labor (Walsh et al., 2011). Many elders who are abused are immigrants with poor English skills, and most come from cultures where it would be considered shameful to complain (Walsh et al., 2011). Men and women were equally likely to commit elder abuse, but when it occurred between spouses, men were more likely the perpetrators of physical and sexual abuse, and women, the perpetrators of physical neglect or emotional abuse (Walsh et al., 2011). The elderly have a very difficult time leaving abuse, especially if they are medically disabled, or if they are women who have never worked outside the home (Walsh et al., 2011).

RAPE

Estimates of the lifetime prevalence of rape vary from 18% to 30% in the United States, with young Asian Pacific Islander women reporting lifetime prevalence as high as 68% (Asian Pacific Institute on Domestic Violence, 2011;

Garrett, 2011). Previous estimates are that by the age of 18, one in four girls and one in six boys will be sexually assaulted; however rape statistics grossly underestimate the true incidence of sexual assault (*New York Times*, 2011). Fifteen out of 16 assailants never spend a day in jail, two-thirds of assailants are known to the victim, 38% of assailants are acquaintances or friends of the victim, and 44% of victims are under 18 years of age (RAINN, 2011). Sexual assault is one of the leading causes of injuries and death in American women (RAINN, 2011). Sexual assault is one of the most severe traumas with multiple repercussions for both the victim and their family. Negative social reactions from family and friends can worsen recovery and result in more severe post-traumatic stress disorder (PTSD) (Garrett, 2011).

Rape is an underreported crime, with 54% of cases not reported at all (RAINN, 2012). Many victims are discouraged from reporting the crime by law enforcement officials, as well as others, and few cases are adjudicated despite the fact that 50% to 80% of sexual assailants are known to the victim (Avegno, Mills, & Mills, 2007; Garrett, 2011). Knowing the assailant did not reduce the risk of injures in one study conducted in a metropolitan emergency department (ED) (Avegno et al., 2007). Men are even more unlikely to report sexual assault than are women and more frequently report it only if there are physical injuries (Monk-Turner & Light, 2010). Men also delay seeking help for many years after assault (Monk-Turner & Light, 2010).

Workplace sexual assault becomes even more complicated since victims fear for not only their well-being but their livelihood (Garrett, 2011). Complex post-assault issues arise and are often overlooked by medical personnel, due to lack of medical personnel trained in post-sexual assault procedures and lack of available care or difficulties accessing care, as well as difficulty with follow-up of rape victims. Rural women report that rape after leaving a violent relationship is commonplace and often supported by the male peers of the assailant (DeKeseredy & Schwartz, 2008). Reporting abuse is difficult for rural women since the community at large is aware of the abuse, but does not want to become involved, leading to a situation in which the very institutions that are supposed to protect women may perpetuate their abuse (DeKeseredy & Schwartz, 2008). Rural women also report severe issues with confidentiality since many treating professionals know both the assailant and the perpetrator, rural residents may use police scanners to listen to emergency communications, and accessing services can mean the whole community is aware by small things such as parking one's car near service facilities (Annan, 2011).

Date rape is a serious issue on high school and college campuses, with some studies showing that both males, and to a lesser extent females, believe in rape myths, all of which blame the victim. Rape myths include beliefs that the woman owed sex for an expensive date; was to blame for provocative dress; if there was not severe injury, the episode cannot be classified as rape; women cannot be raped by husbands or other intimates; women fantasize about being raped; stranger rape is more prevalent than acquaintance rape; if a woman was drunk, it was her fault (Basow & Minieri, 2011). Attitudes are also culturally dictated. In many countries little legal protection exists for women, and may require their resistance to the point of death in order for an assault to be considered rape, pointing to a worldwide prevalence of a double standard regarding sexual behavior in males versus females (Lee, Kim, & Lim, 2010).

HUMAN TRAFFICKING

While human trafficking is a known phenomenon worldwide, it has become a growing problem in the United States, with the glamorization of sex for hire in popular culture songs and merchandise, that has made buying women and children for sex seem like a socially acceptable activity (Kotrla, 2011). Estimates of current victims of sexual enslavement in the United States are about 200,000 at-risk victims, many of whom begin prostitution as children or adolescents (Busch-Armendariz, Nsonwu, & Cook, 2011). Worldwide, the numbers are much higher. The widespread international traffic of pornography has the largest numbers of consumers in the United States (Hodge, 2008). Internet purchasers of pornographic material may request live acts of violent rape against women in which injuries are "ordered" over the Internet, and then performed and relayed via video conferencing in real time by women who have been entrapped and enslaved by pimps. These women are often lured into entrapping employment agreements via false foreign worker or marriage schemes, child bride websites, or via foreign legal prostitution houses, where the women are recruited by the promise of better working conditions and more money (Hodge, 2008). Women and children from all impoverished nations, and socioeconomic status, as well as U.S. runaway teens, may become victims of these heinous crimes. Juveniles working in prostitution in the United States are estimated to be between 100,000 and 3 million victims (National Juvenile Prostitution Study, 2011). Victims of trafficking need comprehensive services, but their immediate needs are for safe shelter, food, and clothing as well as medical attention. Therapy must be culturally sensitive and can only be undertaken once basic safety needs are met.

BULLYING

Bullying has been defined as intimidation, physical as well as psychological, grounded in tactics to control and socially isolate individuals from others (Arseneault, Bowes, & Shakoor, 2010). This may include verbal harassment, physical assaults, written or Internet-based harassment, or cyberbullying (Kowalski, Limber, & Agaston, 2008). Peer victimization as a child produces feelings of helplessness and low self-worth that translates into later depression and mental health problems. Victims develop a sense of injustice that may lead to participation in violent retaliation, producing even worse outcomes for themselves (Rudolph, Troop-Gordon, Hessel, & Schmidt, 2011). Girls show more internalizing behaviors in the aftermath of bullying, and boys are more likely to show externalizing behaviors. Children who are bullied early and are having problems by the second grade have mental health consequences by fifth grade and more difficult transitions at adolescence than that of nonaffected peers (Rudolph et al., 2011). Bullying predisposes youth who have mental health problems at baseline to become more seriously ill, and is a predictor of suicidal behavior in those individuals who are both bullies and victims (Klomek, Marrocco, Kleinman, Schonfeld, & Gould, 2007).

VIOLENCE TOWARD HEALTH CARE PROFESSIONALS

Violence directed at medical professionals is both underreported and concerning. The Bureau of Labor Statistics data for 2000 shows that 48% of the nonfatal attacks in the workplace took place in health care or social services settings, with nurses, aides, orderlies, and attendants suffering the most nonfatal injuries (Occupational Health and Safety Administration [OSHA], 2000). The Department of Justice reported a 1993–1999 rate of nonfatal assaults on all workers of 12.6 per 1,000 workers. The rate is 16.2 per 1,000 physicians and 21.9 per 1,000 nurses, and is topped by rates of 68.2 per 1,000 mental health professionals and 69 per 1,000 mental health custodial workers (OSHA, 2000). "Work-related violence is the third leading cause of occupational injury fatality in the United States and the second leading cause of death for women at work" (Findorff, McGovern, Wall, & Gerberich as cited by APNA, 2008). The Veterans Administration reported 24,219 incidents of assaultive behavior over a 1-year period; 8,552 of those incidents involved battery or physical assault (Lehmann, McCormick, & Kizer, 1999). Assaults were most frequently on psychiatric units (43.1%), followed by long-term care units (18.5%), and admitting or triage areas (13.4%) (Lehmann et al., 1999).

The PMH-APRNA convened a task force on violence in 2007; they reported that violence against nurses is one of the most difficult problems facing the health care professions and identified horizontal and vertical violence as serious issues in the workplace that can contribute to poor patient care (APNA, 2008; Joint Commission, 2008). Acute agitation is the most common reason persons with a mental disorder receive emergency psychiatric care, or come to the attention of law enforcement or those responsible for emergency psychiatric evaluations. Agitation in the emergency room has many causes including long wait times, substance intoxication and withdrawal, significant illness, mental health crisis, and physical issues. Changes in mental status can be from a variety of physical causes including urinary tract or other infection, hypoxia, hypo- or hyperglycemia, electrolyte disturbances, renal or hepatic failure, thyroid storm, neurological disorders such as stroke and meningitis, and dementia (Mattingly & Small, 2011). Aggressive behavior was the presenting problem in 26% of patients coming to the ED (Dhossche, 1998). Among 112 nursing home patients, 34.8% were referred to psychiatry for agitation and 23.5% for aggressive behavior (Callegari et al., 2006).

TYPES OF VIOLENCE TOWARD HEALTH PROFESSIONALS

PATIENT VIOLENCE TOWARD HEALTH PROFESSIONALS

Violence committed includes verbal abuse (shouting, threatening, and profanity), physical abuse (pushing, hitting, spitting, grabbing, throwing objects, use of weapons), stalking, and defamation (see Exhibit 16-2). Stalking can take the form of physically following a clinician; unwanted or threatening phone calls, voice mails, emails, or text messages; sending of unordered merchandise; gathering personal information about the clinician; driving by their home; or coming to the office when there is no appointment (Simon, 2011, Exhibit 16-2). With smartphone technology, stalkers can use GPS technology to locate the intended victim without their knowledge (Sechrest, 2011). Internet slander of health care professionals occurs when an agitated patient begins making Internet posts with

EXHIBIT 16-2: TYPES OF VIOLENCE AND ABUSE AGAINST MENTAL HEALTH PROVIDERS

Physical
Threats (also Internet), shouting, and profanity
Inappropriate sexual comments
Stalking (also Internet)
False accusations (also Internet)
Frivolous lawsuits
Complaints to licensure boards
Abusive/excessive phone calls, letters (also by third parties)
Vandalism of office, car, personal space, home
Threatening or obscene mail (also Internet)
Trespassing
Loitering in clinic without an appointment
Drive-by and home visits
Displaying knowledge of clinician's personal life; e.g., names of spouse, children

Source: Adapted from Simon (2011).

accusations and other derogatory comments that are difficult to defend against without a large investment of time and money. There are now companies that deal specifically with this last issue due to the seeming proliferation of this type of abuse against many persons.

HORIZONTAL AND VERTICAL VIOLENCE WITHIN NURSING

Horizontal violence refers to peer-to-peer aggression and may take the form of nonverbal innuendo, verbal assaults, withholding information, breaking confidences, or undermining activities at work (Longo, 2007; Thomas & Burk, 2009). Vertical violence refers to similar activities between non-peers, such as between staff and their manager or supervisor. Both psychological and physiological consequences of this type of violence have been reported. Depression, anxiety, PTSD, fatigue, angina, and hypertension as well as increased risk of suicide have been reported by nurses experiencing horizontal and/or vertical violence in the workplace (Hansen, Hogh, & Persson, 2011). These practices have often been referred to as "eating our young" and have been responsible for many difficulties in recruitment and retention of new nurses.

EFFECTS OF VIOLENCE ON SURVIVORS (VICTIMS)

All persons experiencing violence may suffer from injuries, some of them life-altering, as well as somatic complaints such as asthma, arthritis, dizziness, gastrointestinal (GI) disturbances, headaches, and earlier onset of multiple chronic diseases (Scott et al., 2011). Psychiatric symptoms include anxiety, depression, difficulty concentrating, and symptoms of PTSD including hypervigilence, sleep disturbance, appetite disturbance, social withdrawal, difficulty trusting others, fear of future assault, and a greater likelihood of future substance abuse.

Children who are victims of child maltreatment, or who witness violence, often show externalizing behaviors such as aggression and antisocial behaviors, or internalizing behaviors such as depression, anxiety, and withdrawal, as well as executive functioning problems related to anxiety and dissociation (DePrince, Weinsierl, & Combs, 2009). Children experiencing abuse are more likely to suffer from earlier onset of mental health problems, and later in life they are more likely to suffer chronic diseases such as arthritis, chronic pain, and diabetes (Von Korff et al., 2009; Scott et al., 2011). Children who have witnessed community or IPV have higher rates of adolescent substance abuse, depression, anxiety, and antisocial and delinquent behavior (Zinzow et al., 2009). Systematic review of 6,743 refugees from multiple countries showed that they are 20 times more likely to suffer from PTSD than nonrefugee residents of Western countries (Fazel, Wheeler, & Danesh, 2009). Adolescents who have suffered from bullying have become depressed and committed suicide (Klomek, Marrocco, Kleinman, Schonfeld, & Gould, 2007).

SEQUELAE OF IPV

Mental health sequelae of IPV include depression, PTSD, substance abuse, and later poorer functioning (Lee & Haddid, 2009). Physical health problems related to IPV include a higher risk of HIV infection, as well as facial, orthopedic, and other traumatic injuries, anxiety, depression, PTSD, unintended pregnancy, miscarriage, low birth weight babies, multiple abortions, worse overall health, and cardiac, gynecologic, circulatory, musculoskeletal, GI, and neurological complaints (García-Moreno et al., 2005; Sarkar, 2008). Mental health problems of victim mothers lead to poorer parenting, leading to poorer outcomes for their children (Taylor, Guterman, Lee, & Rahoutz, 2009). Among mothers who were reported to child protection agencies for child abuse, 45% had a lifetime prevalence of IPV, and a past-year prevalence of 29% (Hazen, Connelly, Kelleher, Landsverk, & Barth, 2004). Women who are abused while pregnant are more likely to have worse maternal attachment with their infants at 6 months, and are more likely to develop PTSD, as are women who are sexually assaulted by intimate partners (Bogat, DeJonghe, Eye, & Levandosky, 2008).

Multiple studies show that witnessing IPV has later deleterious effects on children and adolescents and is a risk factor for later perpetration of violence (Palazzolo & Roberto, 2010). Adolescents are vulnerable to poor outcomes: Males are more likely to become teenaged fathers; girls are more likely to have unintended and repeat pregnancies, have sex with males who have had multiple partners, and become victims of dating violence (NCG, 2004). Teens who have mothers with a history of both child abuse and IPV are more likely to have conduct problems, problems with peer relationships, substance abuse problems, and mental health problems such as depression and anxiety (Miranda, dela Osla, Granero, & Espeleta, 2009).

Health professional victims of violence may suffer from symptoms of PTSD months after they experience assault (Emergency Nurses Association [ENA], 2010; Richter & Berger, 2006). The numbers of personnel who have been attacked who experience symptoms of anxiety and fear of being assaulted vary widely in studies from as low as 5% to as high as 50% (Coverdale, Louie, & Roberts, 2005). Victims also reported difficulty sleeping, missed days of work, emotional feelings of anger, anxiousness, helplessness, loss of control, and increased irritability, muscular tension, body soreness, and headache (Mahoney, 1991). Two, three, and six months after an assault, 17% of assault victims still met the criteria for PTSD (Richter & Berger, 2006).

OFFICE SAFETY POLICIES

Awareness of the various types of violence is the first step to decreasing or preventing violence. Clinicians living in states where carrying weapons is legal must inform families and patients that they are not to bring weapons to appointments. Office policies wherein new patients are seen at peak times when there are likely to be many others present is common sense. One should never be in the office alone, see an agitated person without family members present, or see a new patient after hours. In the case of psychotic patients, I require a family member to be present at each meeting until it is established that the particular patient has no risk factors for violence. It is a good practice to be very conservative when deciding whether or not it is appropriate at that moment for a patient to be seen in an outpatient setting. While the physical environment is not completely under the control of the PMH-APRN, all clinicians must advocate for safer office settings and require that locked doors and other safeguards such as front office staff, security personnel, and emergency procedures are in place to protect them from a potentially violent patient or family member.

Policies within the workplace to not tolerate any type of vertical or horizontal violence are also important. A clear code of conduct indicating acceptable and disruptive behaviors with reporting and consistent consequences is necessary for a safe environment.

ASSESSMENT

When considering assessment of the potential for violence, there are certain groups of people who are more vulnerable, and certain individuals have characteristics that may indicate a higher likelihood of being violent. Both of these approaches will be discussed.

MIGRANT AND REFUGEE POPULATIONS

By definition, most refugees have suffered adversity, and many classified as migrants left their home of origin due to adverse political or economic situations, often caused by mass violence such as war. A review was performed of the mental health of more than 22,000 migrants and refugees from more than 25 countries in Asia, South and Central America, the Middle East, Africa, Europe, the Pacific, and Caribbean Islands, who left their homelands for new homes in 16 countries in Europe, Iran, Mexico, Argentina, Africa, Southeast Asia, New Zealand, Australia, the United States, and Canada. For refugees, the combined rates of PTSD were 36%, depression 44%, anxiety 40%; for migrants those rates were more similar to overall population estimates (Lindert, Ehrenstein, Priebe, Mielck, et al., 2009). However, these estimates are influenced by differing data collection systems, though the PTSD rates seem to be in keeping with other studies.

EMERGENCY WORKERS ARE AT HIGH RISK

There are numerous reports of both verbal abuse and physical abuse experienced by psychiatric and ED personnel, who frequently encounter violent patients. The Emergency Nurses' Association (ENA, 2010) analyzed four consecutive data rounds collected between May 2009 and February 2010, focusing on violence in the ED as experienced by nurses. Nurses surveyed were approximately 80% staff nurses and about 20% PMH-APRNs. PMH-APRNs are likely to encounter violent patients during intake, admission, or triage duties. Eleven percent of respondents reported victimization with physical violence, and an average of 43.8% reported that they had been victims of verbal abuse. The majority (87.4%) of ED nurses who experienced threats, yelling, name calling, or profanity did not report the event; and 67.4% of those physically abused did not report it (ENA, 2010). Reasons for nurses not reporting abuse included the feeling that abuse was part of their job, the feeling that reporting it would not help matters or would be used as evidence that they were not doing their jobs properly, and the lack of institutional policies regarding such reports (ENA, 2010). Psychiatric patients comprised 44% of the cases of reported physical violence, 57% of the time the patient was under the influence of alcohol, and 48% of the time the patient was under the influence of illicit drugs (ENA, 2010). Seventy-three percent of physically assaultive patients were deemed lucid at the time of the assault by the nurses. Among nurses who did report physical abuse by a patient, 44.9% reported that no action was taken against the perpetrator, 23.4% of perpetrators received a verbal warning, and 11.4% were transferred to psychiatric facilities. Seventy-four percent of nurses who reported physical assault received no response from administration (ENA, 2010). Additionally, witnessing the aftermath of violence by emergency personnel can cause symptoms of PTSD.

PSYCHIATRIC CLINICIANS

Those working in psychiatric inpatient settings are routinely exposed to violence due to the nature of the patient population; the functions of locked inpatient settings to protect the public; the demands of the institutional environment; the inherent limitations of the treatment provided; and staffing patterns wherein there are few registered nurses (RNs) compared to lesser-trained mental health workers, when compared to other nursing specialties. Very violent patients, many of whom have committed violent crimes, are found in state hospitals and, in some localities, in public and private hospital psychiatric units. Several surveys of psychiatric nursing staff on acute units report a 75% to 100% rate of assault over the course of their careers (Caldwell, 1992; Hatch-Maillette, Scalora, Bader, & Bornstein, 2007). Caldwell (1992) reported that 28% of clinical staff and 12% of nonclinical staff were assaulted within the past 6 months. Ninety-four percent of Canadian psychiatric nurses reported at least once assault in their careers and 54% reported more than 10 assaults (Poster, 1996).

> *For psychiatrists, the risk of violence when treating mentally ill patients is more than 4 times greater than the risks facing other physicians. An article from* The Times *of London (Ahuja, 2006) reported that the rate of nonfatal, job-related violent crime among general medical physicians is 16.2 per 1,000. For psychiatrists and mental health professionals, the rate is 68.2 per 1,000. (APNA, 2008)*

For psychiatry staff, assaults often occur during patient containment procedures. During containment procedures, psychiatric staff members were most likely to sustain injuries to extremities, but during random assaults, the injuries were to the head (Erdos & Hughes, 2001). Random assaults are the most frightening, least predictable, and the most difficult to defend against. Among mental health professionals, those in the earliest phases of their careers are mostly likely to become a victim, with 40% to 50% of psychiatric residents experiencing violence during their training (Rueve & Welton, 2008). Personalities of Turkish nurses who were assaulted were assessed: Those who were physically assaulted were less social and less tolerant than others; those who were more help-seeking were more likely to be verbally assaulted (Bilgin, 2009).

Prescribing clinicians should recognize that they often become the focus of patient anger during involuntary detainment as patients quickly realize that these are the persons who can ensure their release with the stroke of a pen (personal communication and personal experience). Flannery reported in a 2004 study of violent Alzheimer's patients that medical residents and experienced nurses were the most likely to be assaulted (Flannery, 2004). Quanbeck and colleagues reported that staff members in state mental institutions most likely to be assaulted were those who had tried to verbally redirect a patient or denied a patient request (Quanbeck et al., 2007).

OTHERS MOST AT RISK FOR VICTIMIZATION

Most at risk of becoming targets of patient violence were persons presently involved in a conflict with the patient at home, at work, or in the neighborhood, followed by persons with a present or past intimate relationship with the patient. Mental health clinicians came next, at close to 10% of the targets, followed by criminal justice personnel, then mass victims, and last, child protection workers (Warren, Mullen, & Ogloff, 2011). WHO reports that 57,000 children were killed as a result of child abuse in 2000, with infants under 1 and children under 4 years of age at greatest risk due to their inability to escape those they depend upon for survival (WHO, 2002). Youth violence is estimated in 2000 to have killed an estimated 199,000 worldwide (WHO, 2002). The elderly are also at risk due to their physical vulnerability, as well as loss of close friends and community contacts that are protective factors. Older men and women experience the same risk for abuse by adult children and relatives, including physical, emotional, and economic abuse, which includes having their monies or properties taken (WHO, 2002). Murder of the elderly can occur when an ill couple makes a pact to end their lives in a murder suicide, or it can be perpetrated upon an unsuspecting elderly spouse (Salari, 2007).

SERIOUSLY MENTALLY ILL ARE ALSO VICTIMS OF VIOLENCE

Seriously mentally ill persons also experience violence as victims in significantly higher numbers than those of the general population, with women at a 13- to 19-fold increased risk for victimization, and men at a 9- to 11-fold increased risk for victimization (Khalifeh & Dean, 2010). Risk factors for women included lack of regular family contact and homelessness, and for men recent substance abuse or lack of an intimate partner increased their risk. For both sexes, earlier onset of psychosis and the presence of a comorbid personality disorder also increased risk of victimization (Khalifeh & Dean, 2010).

Risk factors for becoming a victim of violence are many and include young age; old age; physical disability; living in communities that suffer from street violence and high crime; history of child abuse, sexual abuse, and IPV; substance abuse; mental illness; lesbian, gay, bigendered, transsexual, or questionable orientation (LGBTQ); immigrant or minority status; homelessness; teenaged; and runaway status. The majority of homeless youth experienced multiple trauma in their previous home including neglect, parental substance abuse, and emotional, physical, and/or sexual abuse, with girls more likely than boys to be victims of sexual abuse. Homeless youth were more likely to have tried to commit suicide, and were more likely to have substance abuse and mental health problems as a result of their backgrounds (Ferguson, 2009).

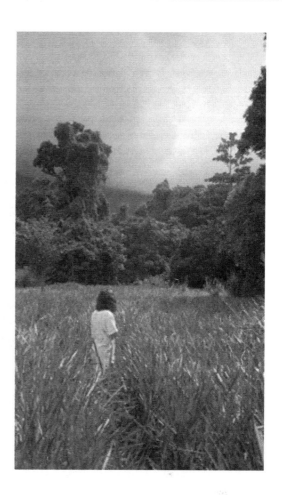

ASSESSMENT OF INDIVIDUAL POTENTIAL FOR VIOLENCE

RULE OUT MEDICAL REASONS FIRST, THEN ASSESS PSYCHIATRIC FACTORS

Urine toxicology screening should be mandatory for patients who present with acute agitation to rule out substances of abuse. Medical reasons such as ingestions, prescription or recreational drug overdose, adverse medication reactions, and head injury should be ruled out. In the elderly, medical problems or prescription drug interactions can often be the cause of agitated delirium. Children presenting violently must be checked for medical problems and ingestions. Mental status factors that predict violence are: threats of violence, active paranoid ideation, persecutory delusions, fear of harm, intoxication with substances, history of violence, history of childhood sexual or physical abuse, and severe agitation (see Table 16-1).

Among those who threaten to kill, in a forensic study of a community-based consultation clinic, assaults were made by 20% of those who uttered the threats in the 12 months following the threat, including homicide and suicide (Warren et al., 2011). Other characteristics predictive of violence in this group of 144 patients included substance abuse, lower educational level, no mental health follow-up, and a history of violence. Over 44% of 613 forensic offenders who threatened violence were convicted of a violent offense in the following 10 years (Warren, Mullen, Thomas, Ogloff, & Burgess, 2007). The most likely perpetrators were substance abusers, younger, mentally disordered, and those without prior convictions; the most likely to commit homicide were those with a diagnosis of schizophrenia (Warren et al., 2008).

TABLE 16-1: PATIENT RISK ASSESSMENT FOR PERPETRATION OF VIOLENCE

AREA TO ASSESS	RISK FACTORS
Mental status examination	Agitation Stated wish to hurt or kill someone Paranoid ideation, command hallucinations, psychosis, thought insertion Feelings of persecution, fear of being harmed, PTSD symptoms Substance abuse
Patient history/ social environment	Childhood sexual or physical abuse, witnessing abuse as a child Previous violent acts Military training Current victimization or recent trauma Severe psychosocial stressors—contentious divorce Cultural background of patriarchal society (risk factor of intimate partner violence only) Unemployment
Patient Personality	Antisocial or borderline personality disorder Narcissism
Medical comorbidity	Organic brain disease Delirium Advanced age and terminal illness in patient or partner

RISK ASSESSMENT QUESTIONNAIRES

INPATIENT

One validated tool for violence prediction used in inpatient settings is the Brøset Violence Checklist (see Exhibit 16-3) that requires nurses to rate six patient behaviors: confusion, irritability, boisterousness, verbal threats, physical threats, and attacks on objects (Abderhalden et al., 2008). Mere assessment of patients for violence potential using a structured tool decreased the incidence of violence (Abderhalden et al., 2008). This effect of assessing violence risk may have caused nursing staff to discuss ways to divert or prevent violence ahead of time (Abderhalden et al., 2008). This tool has favorable reviews from nurses who have implemented it in Norway, Canada, Germany, and the United Kingdom. It is primarily a tool that the nursing staff completes and utilizes while a patient is on an inpatient acute ward to assess daily violence risk (Kennedy, Breslar, Whitaker, & Masterson, 2007). The advantages of the tool are that it assesses behaviors applicable to any patient and takes about five minutes to complete. In a UK trial, seclusions decreased, and this was thought to be due to better anticipation of violence and diversion in the previolence phase by nursing staff (Clark, Brown, & Griffith, 2010).

Another short tool presently under consideration is the V-10 risk assessment (see Exhibit 16-4); it attempts to predict the likelihood of future violence based upon brief clinical and historical information that can be readily obtained and has a high interrater reliability (Bjørkly, Hartvig, Haggen, Brauer, & Mogen, 2009). Questions include previous or current violence, previous or current threats, personality disorder, lack of insight, lack of empathy, suspiciousness, unrealistic planning, previous or current drug abuse, and exposure to future stress (Bjørkly et al., 2009). The tool was found to have validity for predicting future violence and was easy to use, requiring little time to complete in the 3- and 6-month time frames following discharge from acute hospitalization (Hartvig, Roaldset, & Bjørkly, 2011; see Exhibit 16-5).

EXHIBIT 16-3: BRØSET VIOLENCE CHECKLIST

The Brøset Violence Checklist © (BVC)—quick instructions:

Patient/Client data

Score the patient at agreed time on every shift. Absence of behavior gives a score of 0. Presence of behavior gives a score of 1. Maximum score (SUM) is 6. If behavior is normal for a well known client, only an increase in behavior scores 1; e.g., if a well known client normally is confused (has been so for a long time) this will give a score of 0. If an **increase** in confusion is observed this gives a score of 1.

MONDAY / /			
	DAY	EVENING	NIGHT
Confused			
Irritable			
Boisterous			
Verbal threats			
Physical threats			
Atacking objects			
SUM			

TUESDAY / /			
	DAY	EVENING	NIGHT
Confused			
Irritable			
Boisterous			
Verbal threats			
Physical threats			
Atacking objects			
SUM			

WEDNESDAY / /			
	DAY	EVENING	NIGHT
Confused			
Irritable			
Boisterous			
Verbal threats			
Physical threats			
Atacking objects			
SUM			

THURSDAY / /			
	DAY	EVENING	NIGHT
Confused			
Irritable			
Boisterous			
Verbal threats			
Physical threats			
Atacking objects			
SUM			

FRIDAY / /			
	DAY	EVENING	NIGHT
Confused			
Irritable			
Boisterous			
Verbal threats			
Physical threats			
Atacking objects			
SUM			

SATURDAY / /			
	DAY	EVENING	NIGHT
Confused			
Irritable			
Boisterous			
Verbal threats			
Physical threats			
Atacking objects			
SUM			

SUNDAY / /			
	DAY	EVENING	NIGHT
Confused			
Irritable			
Boisterous			
Verbal threats			
Physical threats			
Atacking objects			
SUM			

EXHIBIT 16-4: VIOLENCE RISK SCREENING – 10 (V-RISK-10)

Violence risk screening - 10 (V-RISK-10)

At admission ☐
At discharge ☐
In policlinic ☐

Patient's name:		**Date of birth:**
Female ☐ **Male** ☐		**Patient number:**
Date of admittance:	**Date of discharge:**	**Registration number:**
Signed in by:		**Date:**

Scoring instruction:

The rater collects information about each of the 10 risk factors on the V-RISK-10 checklist. Some examples of important scoring information are described under each item. Put a check in the box to indicate the degree of likelihood that the risk factor applies to the patient in question:

- **No:** Does not apply to this patient
- **Maybe/moderate:** Maybe applies/present to a moderately severe degree
- **Yes:** Definitely applies to a severe degree
- **Do not know:** Too little information to answer

Item	No	Maybe/ moderate	Yes	Do not know
1. Previous and/or current violence *Severe violence refers to physical attack (including with various weapons) towards another individual with intent to inflict severe physical harm.* ***Yes:*** *The individual in question must have committed at least 3 moderately violent aggressive acts or 1 severe violent act. Moderate or less severe aggressive acts such as kicks, blows and shoving that does not cause severe harm to the victim is rated* ***Maybe/moderate.***	☐	☐	☐	☐
2. Previous and /or current threats (verbal/physical) ***Verbal:*** *Statements, yelling and the like, that involve threat of inflicting other individuals physical harm.* ***Physical:*** *Movements and gestures that warn physical attack.*	☐	☐	☐	☐
3. Previous and/or current substance abuse *The patient has a history of abusing alcohol, medication and/or other substances (e.g., amphetamine, heroin, cannabis). Abuse of solvents or glue should be included. To rate* ***Yes****, the patient must have and/or have had extensive abuse/dependence, with reduced occupational or educational functioning, reduced health and/or reduced participation in leisure activities.*	☐	☐	☐	☐
4. Previous and/or current major mental illness ***NB:*** *Whether the patient has or has had a psychotic disorder (e.g., schizophrenia, delusional disorder, psychotic affective disorder). See item 5 to rate personality disorders.*	☐	☐	☐	☐

(Continued)

EXHIBIT 16-4: VIOLENCE RISK SCREENING – 10 (V-RISK-10) (*Continued*)

Item	No	Maybe/ moderate	Yes	Do not know
5. Personality disorder *Of interest here are eccentric (schizoid, paranoid) and impulsive, uninhibited (emotionally unstable, antisocial) types.*	☐	☐	☐	☐
6. Shows lack of insight into illness and/or behavior *This refers to the degree to which the patient lacks insight in his/her mental illness with regard to, for instance, need of medication, social consequences or behaviour related to illness or personality disorder.*	☐	☐	☐	☐
7. Expresses suspicion *The patient expresses suspicion towards other individuals either verbally or nonverbally. The person in question appears to be "on guard" towards the environment.*	☐	☐	☐	☐
8. Shows lack of empathy *The patient appears emotionally cold and without sensitivity towards others' thoughts or emotional situation.*	☐	☐	☐	☐
9. Unrealistic planning *This assesses to which degree the patient him/herself has unrealistic plans for the future (inside or outside the inpatient unit). Is, for instance, the patient him/herself realistic with regard to what he/she can expect of support from family and of professional and social network? It is important to assess whether the patient is cooperative and motivated with regard to following plans.*	☐	☐	☐	☐
10. Future stress-situations *This evaluates the possibility that the patient may be exposed to stress and stressful situations in the future and his/her ability to cope with stress. For example (in and outside inpatient unit): reduced ability to tolerate boundaries, physical proximity to possible victims of violence, substance use, homelessness, spending time in violent environment/association with violent environment, easy access to weapons etc.*	☐	☐	☐	☐

Overall clinical evaluation

Based on clinical judgement, other available information and the checklist:

· How great do you think the violence risk is for this patient? *(Put a check in one of the boxes)*

LOW	MODERATE	HIGH

· Suggestion following overall clinical evaluation: *(Put a check in one of the boxes)*

NO MORE DETAILED VIOLENCE RISK ASSESSMENT	MORE DETAILED VIOLENCE RISK ASSESSMENT

IMPLEMENTATION OF PREVENTIVE MEASURES

Justifications/reasons/arguments should be detailed in patient record and/or discharge summary

Page 2 of 2

OUTPATIENT

The same risk for violence criteria for inpatients holds true for outpatients (see Table 16-1). Information needed to assess propensity for violence may be obtained via the initial psychiatric evaluation or complete patient interview, and by reviewing any patient history files available. Patients requesting an outpatient appointment should be prescreened over the phone asking questions about diagnoses, history, medication adherence issues, reasons for seeking care, current substance abuse, presence of symptoms, and current stressors. Clinicians should be cautious about persons with a history of terminating care with multiple other providers for unclear reasons. If one is fortunate enough to work where records are available electronically, a review of the patient record prior to the first appointment is a must. Asking a patient to sign consents to release their previous records to you prior to the first appointment is reasonable. Patient refusal to do this could be a red flag.

Mental Status Assessment. The mood of the patient as well as presence of psychotic ideation and/or current intoxication with substances must be assessed upon patient arrival. PMH-APRNs must be unafraid to terminate an interview, or refuse to see a patient who is inebriated, very psychotic, or very agitated; the emergency room is the proper referral for such patients. Even patients known to a clinician can decompensate for multiple reasons and a clinician must be alert to signs that a formerly stable patient has become agitated. There are many tragic cases of an experienced clinician suffering injury or death because they failed to heed signs that a patient might be too agitated to be seen in the office, as opposed to in the hospital, and were seen alone in unsecured settings (Simon, 2011). A thorough psychiatric evaluation will contain necessary historical questions about risk factors for later violence; questions regarding gun or other weapon ownership, while considered controversial by some, are required by others. Access to firearms is a reasonable question in mental health, and if presented in a sensitive fashion, it should not be a cause for offense.

Interviewing for Victimization/Perpetration. Women have multiple reasons for not disclosing IPV and for not seeking help for the problem; many felt that when they disclosed the situation they did not receive substantive help, and it was not the help they anticipated (Postmus, Severson, Berry, & Yoo, 2009). Hispanic women living in the United States cited concern for their children as their main reason for staying with an abusing spouse (Kelly, 2009). Latina women living in the United States reported concealing IPV for fear of losing custody of their children, fear that abuse will escalate if they report it, fear of deportation or other legal problems, and fear that they will be unable to provide for their children if they leave an abuser (Kelly, 2009). Men are also victims of IPV but more likely to have participated in mutual IPV themselves; more study of this population is warranted (Hines & Douglas, 2010).

Sensitive questioning using noninflammatory language by an PMH-APRN may cause a victim to be able to report abuse. Asking questions such as, “Has anyone ever pushed you?” “Have you been shouted at or scolded for minor issues?” “Have you been forced to do something you did not want to do?” “Have you had objects thrown at you?” “Has someone destroyed something that belonged to you?” may be less threatening questions than “Have you ever been abused?” (Kelly, 2009). Keep in mind that in many cultures it is considered impolite to talk with outsiders about what is considered a family matter. Victims may be guarded in their responses and worry that affirmative answers would set legal machines in motion. Many victims rationalize that what they are experiencing is not that bad.

Males may be even more ashamed to admit IPV victimization than females. Males who are suffering from PTSD likewise should be questioned about both victimization and perpetration of IPV via gentle questioning about their reasons for symptoms, their anger, mood, whether their family members have been afraid of them, and so on. (Gerlock, Grimesey, Pisciotta, & Harel, 2011). Persons testing positive for immediate risk of imminent harm from an intimate partner with whom they are living should be directed to emergency housing at a friend’s or a local shelter (see Exhibit 16-5).

An excellent resource for health care providers on all aspects of domestic violence is the NCG to Identifying and Responding to Domestic Violence in the Health Care Setting (NCG) found at www.futureswithoutviolence.org/userfiles/file/Consensus.pdf. Appendix E is a detailed assessment tool for uncovering IPV victimization. IPV perpetration in patients with PTSD can be assessed with a tool recently developed especially for veterans that appears generalizable to the other perpetrators (Gerlock et al., 2011).

Child Abuse Victimization/Perpetration. Due to the much higher co-occurrence of child maltreatment with IPV, those who report IPV should be further questioned about child abuse (Chan, 2011). Homes with IPV are more likely to have co-occurring incest (NCG, 2004). Primary care providers are the usual persons who report child abuse, but any child in treatment for internalizing

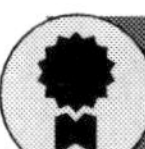

EXHIBIT 16-5: ASSESSMENT FOR IMMEDIATE SAFETY IN IPV–SIGNS A VICTIM MAY NEED EMERGENCY SHELTER

Does your partner

- Embarrass you with put-downs?
- Look at you or act in ways that scare you?
- Control what you do, who you see or talk to, or where you go?
- Stop you from seeing your friends or family members?
- Watch you closely, follow you, or stalk you?
- Take your money or Social Security check, make you ask for money, or refuse to give you money?
- Make all of the decisions?
- Tell you that you're a bad parent or threaten to take away or hurt your children?
- Prevent you from working or attending school?
- Act like the abuse is no big deal, it's your fault, or even deny doing it?
- Destroy your property or threaten to kill your pets?
- Intimidate you with guns, knives, or other weapons?
- Shove you, slap you, choke you, or hit you?
- Force you to try and drop charges?
- Threaten to commit suicide?
- Threaten to kill you?
- Are you in immediate danger?
- Is your partner at the health facility now?
- Do you want to (or have to) go home with your partner?
- Do you have somewhere safe to go?
- Have there been threats or direct abuse of the children?
- Are you afraid your life may be in danger?
- Has the violence gotten worse or is it getting scarier? Is it happening more often?

Source: Adapted from thehotline.org

and externalizing behaviors or executive functioning difficulties should be assessed for the possibility of child maltreatment, since those are the most likely behavioral problems associated with violence in the home (DePrince, Weinzerl, & Combs, 2009). Parents who have deficits in emotion recognition in their children are at risk for perpetrating child abuse (Asla, de Paúl, Pérez-Albéniz, 2011). Traumatized parents may have emotional numbing and therefore have trouble recognizing the needs of their children. Substance abuse, as previously mentioned, is a risk factor for all violence, and is also a risk factor for child maltreatment, maternal attachment difficulties, and worse parenting. Parental aggression and authoritarian parenting styles, as well as harsh overreactive styles, are related to child psychological maltreatment (Rodriquez, 2010). Children of mothers who have suffered both child abuse and IPV are more likely to have severe conduct problems; awareness of this when encountering a child with severe conduct issues can lead to improvement in treatment strategies for both mother and child (Miranda et al., 2009).

There are multiple standardized tools used to assess for risk of child maltreatment; most of these are aimed at evaluation of past child abuse in adults, but some are for those under 18 (Burgermeister, 2007). One newly tested scale, the Child Abuse Risk Assessment Scale, has been used among Chinese parents and is aimed at predicting future child abuse potential (Chan, 2011). The items on this parental self-reporting questionnaire include anger management, violence approval, depressive symptoms, social desirability, stressful conditions, substance abuse, childhood history of witnessed IPV, parental IPV, in-law conflict, and social support. The initial study shows sensitivity and specificity for child abuse; however, it relies on parental self-report, which may or may not be accurate (Chan, 2011).

Interviewing for Elder Abuse. Elderly patients presenting for mental health treatment should be questioned about possible abuse or neglect that can take many forms, including emotional, physical, and financial. There are many subtle factors that contribute to mutual abuse in the elderly with adult child caregivers, so a sensitive interview with the patient alone, as well as with family, may be the best option. Elder abuse is much more complex than a perpetrator-victim model; caring for the elderly involves a complex dynamic because of conflicting needs of the caregiver and the elderly (Phillips, 1986). Inventions that include respite care and improved communication of expectations may be helpful in improving the situation for both the caregivers and the patient (Phillips, 1986). Elder abuse, as with other forms of abuse, is highly underreported. Health care professionals must work at improving their skills at detecting abuse and their comfort with reporting it.

ETIOLOGY: PATIENT POPULATIONS AT RISK FOR PERPETRATING VIOLENCE

GENERAL DIAGNOSTIC CATEGORIES

Disorders most associated with aggression include substance abuse, psychotic disorders, intermittent explosive disorder, cognitive disorders such as delirium and dementia, mood disorders, personality disorders (paranoid, antisocial, borderline, narcissistic), adjustment disorders with disturbance of conduct, CD, and attention deficit disorder (ADHD) (Sadock & Sadock, 2007, pp. 245–246). Smoking by caregivers was shown to be positively correlated with later suicide or self-harm risk in children (Mitrou et al., 2010). While psychotically disordered patients in delusional states are the most feared for violence, it is the comorbid presentation with substance abuse that will most positively predict violent behaviors (Fazel, Gautam, Linsell, Geddes, & Grann, 2009). The dynamic patient factors that may change and thus improve outcomes are substance use, current symptoms of persecutory delusions, command hallucinations, depression, hopelessness, suicidal thoughts, treatment non-adherence, impulsivity, and access to weapons (Anderson & West, 2011). In hospitalized psychiatric patients, male sex, substance abuse, and severity of positive psychotic symptoms (PANSS) were predictors of violence; after admission, however, the most accurate predictive factor was history of violent behavior (Amore et al., 2008). Thus taking a detailed patient history on intake is critical. Static patient factors that increase risk for violence are previous history of violence, age of 25 years or younger, lower intelligence, history of head trauma, history of military service, weapons training, and past diagnosis of major mental illness (Anderson & West, 2011).

DELUSIONAL DISORDERS

Patients who suffer from a specific delusional disorder often labeled "Othello Syndrome" are at very high risk of harming their spouse (Miller, Kummerow, & Mgutshini, 2010). These individuals have a delusional belief that their spouse or significant other is engaged in unfaithful behavior and their uncontrolled irrational jealousy can lead them to violent, if not fatal, acts against their loved one. Psychotic jealousy of this type can be successfully treated with antipsychotic medications. Nonpsychotic jealousy in the case of narcissistic or paranoid personality disorders or obsessive compulsive personality disorders with poor insight can be treated with cognitive behavioral therapy (CBT). Most of these patients will require close follow-up and a lengthy treatment compared with other acutely aggressive patients; the minimum expected duration of CBT is 1 year. During this time patients are taught multiple skills that combine self-awareness, self-soothing, decreasing negative cognitions and false beliefs, improving coping mechanisms, utilization of support systems, and trust building. This disorder may be more frequently encountered in outpatient settings when the target of their delusions seek help, as these perpetrators can be high functioning in other areas of their lives and frequently do not think that they have a problem.

CD AND ANTISOCIAL PERSONALITY DISORDER (APD)

Patients with a previous juvenile diagnosis of CD are at higher risk of aggression (Hodgins, Cree, Alderton, & Mak, 2008). Among persons with a diagnosis of CD before the age of 15, in both men and women, schizophrenia was more prevalent (Odgers et al., 2007). CD diagnosed in childhood is predictive of poor outcomes in adulthood including criminality, poor mental and physical health, domestic violence, and lack of financial autonomy. The outcomes are poorest if CD occurs prior to age 10 and is also co-occurring with a low intelligence quotient (IQ), attention deficit hyperactivity disorder (ADHD), temper outbursts, child abuse, poverty, or a mother with a low IQ (Odgers et al., 2007).

Persons with serious mental illness (SMI) are socialized toward violence by their many experiences of victimization and the need of self-protective action (Swanson et al., 2002). Other predictors of violence are: experience of violence prior to the age of 16, but more so experience of violence after the age of 16; homelessness; poor subjective mental health; witnessing violence; inpatient psychiatric admission in the past year; lower ratings on the Brief Psychiatric Rating Scale; mood disorders; and substance abuse (Swanson et al., 2002). Childhood CD was predictive of aggressive behavior in the Clinical Antipsychotic Trials of Intervention Effectiveness (CATIE) trial that included 1,410 outpatients from across the United States, whereas substance misuse was not (Swanson et al., 2006).

Persons more likely to commit aggressive acts such as emotional abuse and rape tend to be controlling, narcissistic, have low empathy, and low tolerance for frustration. They tend to be impulsive and lack remorse once they have committed a violent act (Garrett, 2011). They may be high functioning in other spheres, and may be considered charming by those who do not know them well.

SUBSTANCE ABUSE, MENTAL ILLNESS, AND ANTISOCIAL PERSONALITY DISORDER

CD, antisocial personality disorder, and SMI in combination have the worst outcomes of increased criminality, increased violent charges, and convictions, in patients with a serious substance abuse dual diagnosis. Additional factors that are predictive of worsened violence are homelessness and a social history of a high number of sexual partners (Mueser et al., 2006). Earlier onset of substance abuse among SMI patients residing in inner cities predicts increased violent antisocial behaviors, as does family substance abuse and increased severity of substance abuse. This suggests that in a person with an SMI, full-blown antisocial personality disorder can develop, in part, as a result of severe substance abuse (Muser et al., 2006).

LOW IQ, HEAD INJURY, CHEMICAL EXPOSURES AS RISK FACTORS FOR VIOLENCE

Intellectual impairment in the form of low IQ is also a risk factor for violence, presumably due to lowered complex reasoning skills. The mean IQ of juveniles committed to Bellevue Hospital for Forensic Psychiatry in New York, after those patients were convicted of committing violent crimes, was significantly lower than that of the general population (Lopez-Leon & Rosner, 2010). Close to half of the subjects that were studied also had a history of head injury, and three had a loss of consciousness (Lopez-Leon & Rosner, 2010). Previous studies of adolescents linked to violent offending found a history of neurological conditions such as traumatic brain injury with loss of consciousness (Williams, Cordan Mewse, Tonks, & Burgess, 2010). Environmental exposures to toxins is linked to violent behaviors; specifically, pre- and postnatal exposure to secondhand smoke, early childhood exposure to lead or arsenic, and later exposure to methyl mercury or polychlorinated biphenyls. Children who are exposed to lead suffer irreversible brain changes that render them much more likely to commit violent offenses as adults (Carpenter & Nevin, 2010).

HISTORY OF TRAUMATIC CHILDHOOD EXPERIENCES

Children who are exposed to abuse, household violence, or adverse experiences are more likely to commit violent acts (Duke, Pettinggell, McMorris, & Borowsky, 2010). Among adolescent inpatient psychiatric patients, those who perpetrated violence were significantly more likely to be childhood victims or witnesses to violence, and were more likely to exhibit symptoms of impulsivity, PTSD, and disassociation than those who did not commit violent acts (Fehon, Grilo, & Lipschitz, 2005). Children of mothers who smoke during pregnancy are more likely to develop CD (Baler, Volkow, Fowler, & Benveniste, 2008; Nigg & Breslau, 2007).

NEUROENDOCRINE, GENETIC, AND HEREDITARY FACTORS

The nature versus nurture debate has been discussed for many years, and there is a large body of evidence that shows neuroendocrine genetic factors influence outcomes. Effects of child abuse in males studied from birth to adulthood are moderated by the gene encoding the enzyme monoamine oxidase A (MAOA), which is responsible for metabolizing norepinephrine (NE), serotonin (5-HT), and dopamine (Capsi et al., 2002). Those with high levels of MAOA expression were much less likely to develop antisocial behavior problems (Capsi et al., 2002).

There is a complex interplay of individual genetic, developmental, and social factors that lead to childhood aggression and antisocial behavior (van Goozen, Fairchild, Snoek, & Harold, 2007). Serotonergic functioning and stress-regulating mechanisms including the hypothalamic-pituitary-adrenal (HPA) axis, hypothalamic-pituitary-gonadal (HPG) axis, and autonomic nervous system are key factors that help to explain both the predisposition toward antisocial behaviors and the persistence or desistance of these behaviors over time (van Goozen et al., 2007).

Two different types of aggression have been identified that apply to both pediatric and adult populations. These are the reactive-hostile-affective-aggression (impulsive), and controlled-proactive-instrumental-predatory (controlled) subtypes, which differ from each other in phenomenological and neurobiological features (Quanbeck et al., 2006; Stanford et al., 2003; Vitiello & Stoff, 1997). Impulsive aggression is linked to reduced serotonergic activity, and shows a high level of biologic arousal; predatory aggressors are more likely to be affectively stable at the time of assault, and their aggression is used for purposes other than harming another (Vitiello & Stoff, 1997).

Abnormalities in the cerebral spinal fluid (CSF) of pretrial violent offenders include low concentrations of 5-hydroxyindoleacetic acid (HIAA), a serotonin metabolite, and high concentrations of homovanillinic acid (HVA) (Soderstrom, Blennow, Manhem, & Forsman, 2001a). In two studies of the CSF of violent aggressive offenders, aggression in psychopathic offenders is linked to serotonergic hypofunctioning and high dopamine turnover, as evidenced by high HVA levels, as well as other CSF protein abnormalities (Soderstrom, Blennow, Manhem, & Forsman, 2001b).

One meta-analysis of data confirmed that genetic factors account for 40% to 50% of population variation in antisocial behavior, but the proportion of genetic influence for aggressive antisocial behavior is greater at 60% to 65% (Tackett, Krueger, Iacono, & McGue, 2005). This may indicate a complex interplay of genes and environment. Adoption studies demonstrate a consistent link between genetics and later criminality (Rutter & Silberg, 2002). Monozygotic twins had a higher concordance rate for criminality than did dizygotic twins. Genetically impaired parents are less likely to provide optimal parenting styles, and genetically predisposed children also evoke negative behavior from the environment that leads them to create, seek out, or elicit negative environmental influences (Rutter & Silberg, 2002). German researchers found a genetic variation among 3,200 outpatients in treatment for personality disorder, ADHD, suicide attempts, and aggression that expressed itself as hypoactivity of the anterior cingulate cortex, which is involved in the processing of emotion and reward in behavioral control (Reif et al., 2009). Emerging research using advanced neuroimaging studies such as MRI/positron emission tomography (PET)/Single-photon emission computed tomography (SPECT) scans demonstrate dysfunction in both the temporal lobes and frontal lobes in persons with violent antisocial psychopathic behavior (Wahlund & Kristiansson, 2009).

Juvenile patients with ADHD, PTSD, and oppositional defiant disorder are more likely to be aggressive. This may be a result of both inherent genetic makeup of individuals and the role of childhood adversity on the serotonin transporter promoter gene (Barzman, Patel, Sonnier, & Strawn, 2010). Children who express higher levels of cortisol and testosterone in some studies have been more aggressive, but there are no clear-cut answers yet to determine if treatment could be tailored to address hormonal issues (Barzman et al., 2010). Attachment difficulties are related to later aggression, and maternal depression is also related to poor mothering; these relationships need more study as well as early intervention to improve infant attachment (Barzman et al., 2010).

EXPECTED OUTCOMES

With all types of violence there are general expectations that interventions will result in the following outcomes:

1. Provision for safety while maintaining self-esteem/dignity.
2. Creation of a cohesive narrative surrounding either the experience of perpetrating violence or surviving the experience of violence.
3. Development of additional coping strategies to facilitate self-control of assaultive or destructive behaviors.
4. Prevention of survivor's emotional/physical reactions from developing into chronic illnesses and disability.

CONCORDANCE IN MANAGEMENT OF INCIDENTS OF VIOLENCE

Patient participation and agreement with treatment is always the primary goal, although this is somewhat more difficult when a patient is acutely agitated. Removal to a less stimulating environment or asking a patient what can be done to help them with the problem that is bothering them are the first lines of actions, after which PRN medication can be offered (see Figure 16-1). Psychiatric patients should be invited to make choices regarding medications and management if at all possible. The goal is patient self-control and self-soothing behavior. If the patient is unable to accept oral medication, or if it is ineffective, voluntary intramuscular (IM) medication can be offered. Only if the previous interventions fail will involuntary medication be given and only then if patient behavior presents a danger to themselves or others.

TREATMENT INITIATION, ACUTE PHASE OF VIOLENCE

Often there is a preattack buildup of anxiety and agitation that can sometimes be caught early and diverted.

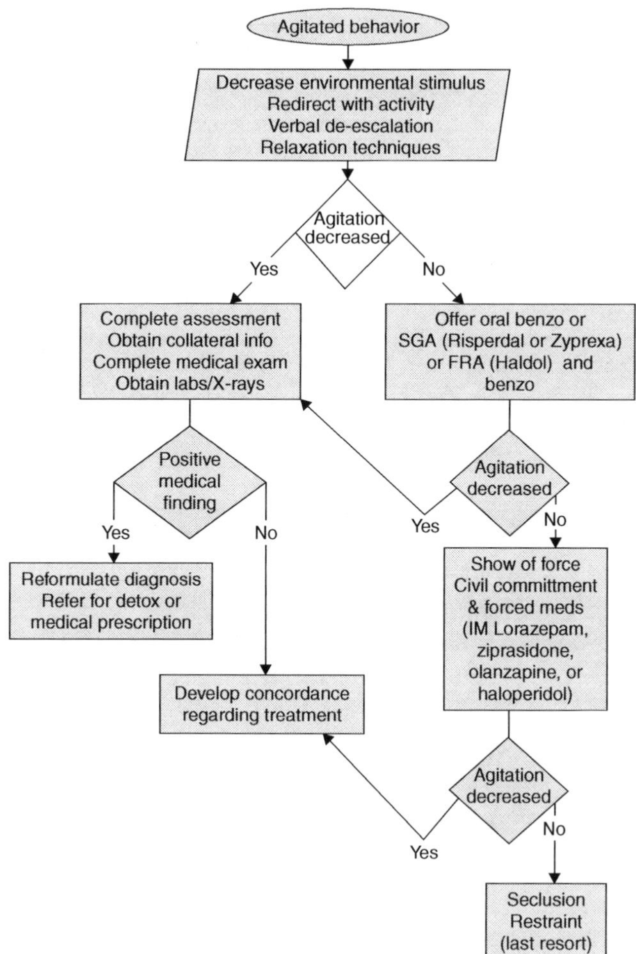

Figure 16-1 Decision Tree for Agitated Behavior

Anticipation of violence is a key point to prevention. Redirection of the potentially violent patient toward productive activity can be a good diversionary tactic that works equally well for all ages. Having quiet rooms or comfort rooms where an agitated patient can go to self-soothe is good practice (Cummings, Granfield, & Caldwell, 2010).

Attacks that are random and unprovoked must be dealt with differently by strategic planning. I have witnessed several cases in which patients with a history of violence suddenly attacked either a staff or peer and began to strike them forcefully and repeatedly. When questioned after such an attack, patients gave reasons such as they felt the victim was talking about them or threatening them, or gave no reason at all, except their perception that the victim was in the way of their goals at that moment. Safety measures when dealing with an acutely delusional or psychotic patient that is not well known to the clinician include: keeping physical distance from the patient; only speaking to a previously unknown patient in the presence of an attendant such as a psychiatric technician or mental health worker; and arranging the room so that quick egress by the clinician or patient is possible. Clinicians should not walk too closely to a patient on the patient unit, and should never turn their back on an unknown patient, or on any patient with a history of violence.

Limited restriction of patient movements on the acute psychiatric unit may be indicated in the case of repeat offenders who lash out unexpectedly at persons not known to them. This entails written orders for denial of patient rights in most states, since patients have the right to be maintained in the least restrictive environment possible. Detailed documentation of the reasons for such restrictions, such as room restrictions and so on, is imperative. Creative milieu management in these incidences can be accomplished by establishing alternate times for a violent patient to eat, exercise, and use the phone, for example, thereby reducing risk of contact with other patients and minimizing the possibility of overstimulation. One way to attempt more concordance with such a patient is to discuss with the patient ways in which they can voluntarily control their movements and aggression. Many patients will voluntarily restrict their own movements about an acute unit, self-isolating to their room when there is too much stimulation in the common areas, such as the day room. Patients can be offered PRN medication and instructed to ask for PRN medication if they feel themselves becoming agitated. Placing such patients with quieter roommates may be helpful, or if at all possible, in rooms by themselves. The same general rules may be used in pediatrics and geriatrics, with considerations in geriatrics for mobility. Minor interventions such as placing an elderly patient closer to the bathroom can greatly reduce their distress.

ACUTE AGITATION

Medication management of violence in psychiatric settings is focused on the management of acute agitation, usually in the emergency room, locked psychiatric unit, or residential psychiatric setting. Typically the techniques of management include oral and IM administration of benzodiazepines, and typical and atypical antipsychotic agents. Patients should be offered the option to take medications orally if they are able, which will help them feel as if they are more in control, and will hopefully improve trust (Mattingly & Small, 2011). Patients should be encouraged to ask for PRN medications if they feel themselves becoming anxious or agitated; patients who appear to be escalating are frequently offered PRN benzodiazepines as a means of averting acute agitation. If patients are unable to make the decision to voluntarily take medications, injections are used as a last resort (Allen, Currier, Carpenter, Ross, & Docherty, 2005).

Benzodiazepines are frequently used as a first-line choice in emergency rooms, especially when the etiology of the agitation is unknown (Allen et al., 2005; Zimbroff, 2008), since alcohol or other drug withdrawal may cause acute agitation. Lorazepam 2 mg IM is frequently used in emergency settings, has favorable tolerability, and has been studied for safety and efficacy (Zimbroff, 2008). One study compared the efficacy of lorazepam 4 mg IM with a combination of haloperidol 10 mg and promethazine 200 mg in an agitated patient; there was a faster onset of sedation with the latter combination (Alexander et al., 2004). Typical antipsychotics have been used for acute agitation for decades, especially haloperidol, usually combined with a benzodiazepine to improve sedation, and often with an anticholinergic agent to reduce the risk of extrapyramidal side effects such as severe dystonia (Callegari et al., 2006; Zimbroff, 2008). Most violent or severely agitated patients medicated emergently receive either of the above combinations or an injectable atypical antipsychotic such as ziprasidone or olanzapine, the two drugs showing similar efficacy in review studies (Callegari et al., 2006). Ziprasidone has recently come into favor due to its rapidity of action in the emergency setting and short half-life of 3–5 hours; however, as with any antipsychotic medication, side effects may occur. In one study, IM ziprasidone was found to be as effective with fewer side effects than IM haloperidol (Brook, Lucey, & Gunn, 2000). Another study found injectable olanzapine highly effective against acute agitation in bipolar mania (Meehan et al., 2001) with longer lasting effects on agitation than either haloperidol or ziprasidone (Callegari et al., 2006).

Among the atypical antipsychotics, oral disintegrating formulations of several atypical antipsychotics including risperidone and olanzapine are fast-acting and highly effective in both reducing agitation and providing sedation that may be considered favorable (Zimbroff, 2008). Both come in oral disintegrating tablets that are difficult to "cheek" or pretend to but not swallow, since they begin dissolving upon contact with moist oral mucosa. A summary of the most common medications used in acute agitation is in Table 16-2 for adults and Table 16-3 for children.

ACUTE FOLLOW-UP: ACUTE DYSTONIA, NMS, ALLERGY

During the acute phase of medication initiation, patients must have vital signs monitored if IM medication has been given, and must be monitored for signs of allergic reaction, or dystonias if typical or atypical antipsychotics have been used; appropriate therapeutic interventions must be made if adverse reactions occur (Baren et al., 2008; Battaglia, 2010; Zeller & Rhodes, 2010).

Acute Dystonia. Acute dystonic reactions require immediate intervention. Patients may display torticollis, locking of the jaw, severe drooling, feeling of tongue thickening, an inability to speak or swallow, oculogyric crisis, or deviation of the eyes in any or all directions. Diphenhydramine 50–100 mg IM should be given immediately for acute dystonic drug reactions. Either diphenhydramine 25–50 mg PO QID or trihexyphenidyl 2 mg PO BID should be continued for 48 to 72 hours to prevent relapse. Both psychotic patients and patients from certain cultures or religions that believe in spiritual possession may mistake severe dystonic reactions for demon possession. I experienced one instance in which a patient with an oculogyric crisis felt that he had become demon possessed, and attempted self-strangulation to rid himself of the demon. Therefore careful monitoring of patients in the hours after a new neuroleptic is started is a safety measure, and patients should be informed of possible severe side effects.

Neuroleptic Malignant Syndrome. Neuroleptic malignant syndrome (NMS) is a life-threatening complication with a 4% to 30% mortality rate. It is characterized by change in mental status, followed by rigidity, hyperthermia, and autonomic dysfunction characterized by labile blood pressure, tachycardia, and profuse diaphoresis (Widjicks, 2010). Dysphagia and mutism may follow, but elevated creatinine kinase (CK) level is the hallmark; levels of more than 1,000 IU/L to as high as 100,000 IU/L have been reported (Widjicks, 2010). Other laboratory abnormalities include leukocytosis in the range of 10,000 to 40,000/mm^3, in which a left shift may be present, electrolyte abnormalities, and mild elevations of alkaline phosphatase, lactate dehydrogenase, and liver transaminases. Myoglobinuric acute renal failure may result from rhabdomyolysis. Low serum iron concentration, mean 5.71 μmol/L, is common (Widjicks, 2010). Risk factors for NMS include rapid increases in dosage of neuroleptics, multiple or large dosage neuroleptics, dehydration, agitation, and previous episodes of NMS (Susman, 2001). The higher the dopamine binding level of the medication, the higher the risk of NMS (Neuhut, 2001). An excellent mnemonic I learned in training for NMS is that it "looks like the flu but can't talk to you." The differential diagnostic marker is elevated CK, which is not present in serotonin syndrome.

NMS is a medical emergency and the patient must be hospitalized at once in intensive care since the need

TABLE 16-2: ADULT MEDICATION DOSES FOR ACUTE AGITATION

MEDICATION	ORAL	INTRAMUSCULAR	INTRAVENOUS
Lorazepam (Ativan®)	1–3 mg	.5–3 mg	1–3 mg
Halperidol (Haldol)	2.5–10 mg (5 mg usual starting dose)	Same as oral	NR
Risperidone (Risperdal®)	1–3 mg	NR	NR
Olanzapine (Zyprexa®)	5–20 mg	2.5–10 mg	Rarely given
Ziprasidone (Geodon®)	NR	10–20 mg	NA

NR = not recommended; NA = not available.

TABLE 16-3: PEDIATRIC MEDICATION DOSES FOR ACUTE AGITATION (AGES 6–18 YEARS OLD)

MEDICATION	ORAL	INTRAMUSCULAR
Lorazepam (Ativan®)[1,2]	.05 mg/kg may repeat	.05 mg/kg may repeat
Hydroxyzine (Atarax) age 6 and older	.6 mg/kg	.5 mg/pound
Halperidol	1–3 mg	1–3 mg, do not exceed .15 mg/kg/day
Risperidone (Risperdal®)	.25–.5 mg/day oral liquid or ODT	NA
Olanzapine (Zyprexa®)	2.5–5 mg/day oral tablet or ODT	5 mg children/10 mg adolescents
Ziprasidone (Geodon®)	Not recommended	5 mg children/10 mg adolescents

Source: Adapted from Sonnier & Barzman (2011).

NR = not recommended, NA = not available, ODT = oral disintegrating tablet.

[1]Safety and efficacy not established in children under 12 years of age (Stahl, 2009)

[2]Safety and efficacy not established in children under 18 years of age (Stahl, 2009)

for airway support is anticipated. Lorazepam 1–2 mg intravenous (IV) or IM is given as a test dose with monitoring of respiratory status (Sadock & Sadock, 2007, p. 995). Drug therapy should be directed at patient symptoms. For hyperthermia, recommended medications are: Bromocriptine 2.5 mg every 8 hours orally or by nasogatric tube (NGT), and amantadine 100 mg BID orally or by NGT. Tylenol is not considered a treatment at this time for hyperthermia in NMS. Dantrolene is given for muscular rigidity with hyperthermia at a dose of 1 mg/kg/day IV every 6 hours to a maximum dose of 10 mg/kg in 24 hours for 8 days, then by mouth (PO) for an additional 7 days (Bottoni, 2002; Sadock & Sadock, 2007 p. 995).

Cooling measures such as cooling blankets and fans may be used. For thromboembolism prevention, antiembolic stockings, chest physiotherapy, range of motion exercises, and frequent turning and repositioning should be instituted. Patients experiencing NMS should have a 14-day washout period after full resolution of symptoms in which no antipsychotic medications are administered. Concomitant lithium administration with neuroleptics should be avoided in patients with a history of NMS, as it is a risk factor for recurrence (Susman & Addonizio, 1988). Often benzodiazepines are given alone during this time period. Rechallenge with antipsychotics must be carefully supervised and should begin with low-potency, low-dose neuroleptics first, with a slow titration (Wijdicks, 2010).

Serotonin syndrome is another acute psychiatric emergency that may occur as a result of either antidepressants or neuroleptics, in combination or alone. While fairly rare, it is a medical emergency due to the symptoms of altered mental status including anxiety, confusion, dysphoria, irritability, and agitation. Autonomic dysfunction includes diaphoresis, labile blood pressure, dilated pupils, hypersalivation, shivering, and tachycardia. Neurological symptoms include myoclonus, hyperreflexia, ataxia, muscular rigidity and tremor, diarrhea, incontinence, and nausea and vomiting (Sadock & Sadock, 2007, p. 1089). For treatment see Chapter 7.

QT Interval Prolongation. Any antipsychotic medication can be implicated in QT prolongation, which may lead to torsades de pointes, a lengthening of the QT interval until fatal ventricular arrhythmia occurs (Glassman & Bigger, 2001). There are no deaths reported to date from torsades de pointes with olanzapine, quetiapine, and risperidone; ziprasidone has a specific warning of QT prolongation but no reported deaths to date. Pimozide, sertindole, haloperidol, and droperidol have had documented cases of torsades de pointes related death; the actual occurrence has been only 10 to 15 cases up until 2001 in over 10,000 person-years of observation (Glassman & Bigger, 2001). Dangerous situations could arise with the mixing of antipsychotics with medications that are themselves likely to cause QT prolongation. While there are many medications that are implicated in QT prolongation, some of the most common ones that might be prescribed to the psychiatric patient population would be tricyclic antidepressants, anti-arrhythmics in Class 1A and Class 3, beta agonists, macrolides, fluoroquinolones, albuterol, azithromycin, bretylium tosylate, and apomorphine. A more complete list of dangerous medication combinations that can cause fatal torsades de pointes is available at www.azcert.org/medical-pros/drug-lists/drug-lists.cfm which is a database and research clearinghouse for this condition.

MAINTENANCE INTERVENTIONS

ANTIEPILEPTIC DRUGS

Huband, Ferriter, Nathan, and Jones (2010) reviewed 14 studies that included 672 patients to determine if antiepileptic drugs helped in managing violence and aggression.

> *Five different antiepileptic drugs were examined. Sodium valproate/divalproex was superior to placebo for outpatient men with recurrent impulsive aggression, for impulsively aggressive adults with cluster B personality disorders, and for youths with conduct disorder, but not for children and adolescents with pervasive developmental disorder. Carbamazepine was superior to placebo in reducing acts of self-directed aggression in women with borderline personality disorder, but not in children with conduct disorder. Oxcarbazepine was superior to placebo for verbal aggression and aggression against objects in adult outpatients. Phenytoin was superior to placebo on the frequency of aggressive acts in male prisoners and in outpatient men including those with personality disorder, but not on the frequency of "behavioral incidents" in delinquent boys. (Huband et al., 2010)*

Topiramate has been used for anger control, but different studies have had various results: One small study claimed effectiveness in a short review time of .8–10 weeks for decreasing anger and aggression at a dose of 50–200 mg a day (Varghese, Rajeev, Norrish, & Khusaiby, 2010). In comorbid antisocial personality disorder and substance use disorders, topiramate had a U-shaped response showing worsening of aggression in low and moderate doses, but only moderately less aggression in high doses of 400 mg, though few patients reached that dosing level due to side effects (Lane et al., 2009). Topiramate is useful for aggression in intellectually disabled adults (Janowsky, Kraus, Barnhill, Elamir, & Davis, 2003). Antidepressants are implicated in worsening of aggression (Mauri et al., 2011). Lithium is well-proven to deter aggression if the aggression is due to agitated mania.

ANTIDEPRESSANTS

Fluoxetine was used in a randomized placebo-controlled study with aggressive alcoholic patients with histories of domestic violence; it is an effective adjunctive intervention to rehabilitation drug therapy, group therapy, self-help groups, and CBT, significantly reducing anger, irritability, and both verbal and physical aggression (George et al., 2011).

GENERAL MEDICATION CONSIDERATIONS

Results of the mentioned studies underline the fact that most psychiatric care providers have their own opinions on which patients will respond to which medication interventions, based upon clinical presentation and the clinician's personal accumulated experience. Unfortunately not much of this knowledge is documented in well-designed, head-to-head, placebo-controlled studies. Commonly used medications are mood stabilizers, both antiepileptic and others; antipsychotics; and in some cases, benzodiazepines or antidepressants, based upon the comorbidities and personality of the patient. When choosing medications, the patient's target symptoms, medical conditions, likelihood of compliance, living situation, access to laboratory studies, cost, convenience, and preferences must be considered. For those afraid of blood draws, or living too far from laboratories to be likely to comply with frequent blood draws, medications that do not require blood level monitoring are obvious first choices. Cost is a factor as well since the cost of medications may range from as little as $4 per month to nearly $1,000 per month. This writer agrees with the authors of the Italian study (Mauri et al., 2006); I rarely use antidepressants unless there is a known depressive element to the patient's history since they can exacerbate agitation and violent tendencies. Female patients of childbearing age should always have a pregnancy test if there is any possibility of pregnancy and be advised to choose a reliable birth control method since most psychotropic medication have some possibility of teratogenesis; a number have known elevated risks for causing birth defects as well as health issues in newborns.

PEDIATRIC CONSIDERATIONS

Atypical antipsychotics, or second generation antipsychotics, have been used for some time in children with disruptive behavior (Findling, 2008), and several acquire Food and Drug Administration (FDA) approval for this use each year. Olanzapine has been effective in adolescent aggression (Janowsky, Barnhill, & Davis, 2003). Valproic acid is frequently used in the pediatric population. Children have a reduced ability to eliminate the drug and are more sensitive to hepatotoxicity, thus must be monitored more closely than adults (Stahl, 2009, pp. 572–573). Lithium and risperidone were found useful in one study for aggression in teens (Ipser & Stein, 2007). Children and adolescents are more at risk of akathisia and dyskinesia than are adults (Barzman et al., 2010). Common pediatric doses are listed in Table 16-3, though there are still not enough randomized controlled trials on the long-term effects of atypical antipsychotics in children.

AGING CONSIDERATIONS

Additional warnings for the elderly include increased incidence of hypotension and possible sudden death in the use of atypical antipsychotics. Most of the typical and atypical antipsychotics are therefore dosed in lower ranges for the elderly due to possible decreased hepatic and renal clearance with resulting increased bioavailability of these drugs. In the case of benzodiazepines, the elderly show increased sensitivity to central nervous effects, therefore doses are often reduced (DiPiro et al., 2005, pp. 106–107).

MANAGING SIDE EFFECTS

Open communication and honest informed consent are keys to both patient satisfaction and the prevention of medication discontinuation without the clinician's agreement. Patients should be advised to inform the clinician of any untoward side effects immediately and receive assurance that their comfort with, and tolerance of, medication is important. Patients should be encouraged that often more than one trial is needed to find the right medication fit.

LABORATORY STUDIES

Many medications require routine laboratory studies to monitor hepatic, renal, and blood cell functioning. Lithium has a narrow therapeutic index so blood trough levels should be checked to determine the therapeutic dose. Patients should be instructed on how to have trough blood levels taken by timing the blood draw ideally around 10 to 12 hours after their last dose. Topiramate is included in pregnancy category D risk, with links to cleft lip and palate in the newborn, risk of metabolic acidosis, and risk of kidney stones; it is also very expensive (FDA, 2011; Stahl, 2009, p. 536). Valproic acid levels must also be monitored with therapeutic levels ranging from 50–125 mcg/ml in stabilized adults, and 40–75 mcg/ml in elderly or medically ill (DiPiro et al., 2005, pp. 1274–1275).

Long-term lithium therapy is implicated in renal failure, as well as thyroid dysfunction; thus regular laboratory studies including renal panel, urinalysis, and monitoring of lithium levels are recommended (Stahl, 2007). In older patients, or in those with a history of cardiac disease, a baseline elctrocardiogram (EKG) may also be ordered if QT prolongation is a concern. Patients must be advised that it may take several weeks to achieve a therapeutic blood level of medication; the range is usually 0.6–1.2 mEq/L in stabilized adults, or 0.4–0.6 mEq/L in elderly or the medically ill. After stabilization, lithium levels should be drawn 1 month later and then at least once a quarter to start, then at 6-month intervals, and at least yearly in the even most stable of patients.

EXTRAPYRAMIDAL SIDE EFFECTS

Akathisia, or the feeling of restlessness, which can become unbearable, is a risk in both antipsychotics and antidepressants. Movement disorders ranging from tremor to Parkinsonian rigidity; severe torticollis and tardive dyskinesia may occur at any time in therapy. With neuroleptics these effects are more likely to occur in the early phase of treatment, with dose increases, or with discontinuation of therapy. Should movement disorders occur with medication discontinuance, a slower tapering off of medications may prove helpful. I experienced a case of a patient who was tapered off of risperidone, but developed a new onset of a rabbit mouth-type movement disorder halfway through the taper. We increased the medication dose slightly, tapered off more slowly with low dose benztropine, and the problem was resolved. Eventually we were able to wean the patient from benztropine as well. Patients should be assessed at every outpatient visit for signs of movement disorders, as often a patient is not initially aware that one is developing. The abnormal involuntary movement scale (AIMS) test is a standard tool used to evaluate movement disorders and is in the public domain.

Pooled data analysis from several studies show East Asians have a significantly greater risk of extrapyramidal symptoms (EPS) with antipsychotics compared with non-East Asians, and significantly worse reactions to haloperidol specifically, therefore lower beginning doses should be used in that population (Omerod, McDowell, Coleman, & Ferner, 2008). β-adrenergic agents are used to treat tremor from EPS.

BLOOD DYSCRASIAS

Rapid and serious neutropenia, sometimes irreversible and potentially fatal, has developed with typical and atypical antipsychotics, valproic acid, clozapine, and carbamazepine. Complete blood counts (CBC with differential) should be monitored at the start of and periodically throughout therapy since neutropenia may develop at any time. Most organizations have policies regarding frequency of laboratory studies, but typically it is before start of treatment, 1 month later, then up to once a month or once a quarter initially, then once every 6 months. Clozapine requires weekly CBCs until stable, every 1 to 2 weeks thereafter, and for at least 6 weeks upon cessation of treatment. The FDA started CARE (Clozaril Administration Registry Enrollment), a national clozapine registry that requires mandatory tracking of patients for the development of neutropenia. The registry is available online at www.clozarilregistry.com. South Asians are more susceptible to agranulocytosis, and black patients have a 77% greater risk of neutropenia than white patients; Askenazi Jews likewise show more changes in total white blood cell counts on clozapine, but no difference in rates of neutropenia and agranulocytosis (Omerod et al., 2008).

ANTICONVULSANT HYPERSENSITIVITY SYNDROME

Life-threatening hypersensitivity reactions may occur with antiepileptic mood stabilizers that also occur due to other causes. The mildest form is usually called erythema multiforme (rash without mucousal involvement); the more severe form, Steven-Johnson's Syndrome, has 10% to 30% body involvement; and the most severe form, toxic epidermal necrolysis, has 30% or more of body involvement (FDA, 2007; Foster, 2011). While all conditions can be caused by drugs and infectious agents, fully half of the cases are idiopathic in nature (Foster, 2011). South Asian Indians and Asians possessing human leukocyte antigen (HLA) allele HLA-B*1502 have an unusually high incidence of developing these serious side effects when exposed to carbamazepine (Hung et al., 2006). Persons from these ethnic groups should be screened for this prior to starting therapy, or other therapies should be considered first line. There are reports of the syndrome developing with the addition of a second antiepileptic for mood control (Chang, Shiah, Yeh, Wang, & Chang, 2006; Mansur, Yaşar, & Göktay, 2008). Though this hypersensitivity reaction does occur in persons of European ancestry, it is rare at 1 to 6 per 10,000 new users (Mockenhaupt, 2006). The mean onset of these reactions is 20 to 30 days, but can occur at any time. Triggering events are an increase of dose, addition of another anticonvulsant, and the possible buildup of toxic arene oxide metabolites over time (Mansur et al., 2008).

The full syndrome begins as an innocuous fever and flu-like symptoms, followed by a maculopapular rash that can progress to a pustular or bulbous rash, and then to systemic organ involvement. Stop the offending medication immediately, administer diphenhydramine 25–50 mg b.i.d., and if other than a very minor rash, add prednisone 10 mg b.i.d. Outpatients should be checked daily; if symptoms are other than very minor, they must be admitted to the hospital for closer observation, laboratory studies, and supportive care (Chang et al., 2006). For patients with a concomitant seizure disorder, benzodiazepines are a safe alternative while deciding on further therapy. The offending medication must be placed on the patient's allergy list. While some have proposed later rechallenge with the same medication, this is not a practice that I would undertake. I have seen multiple cases of mild pustular rash, confined to a small body area, that did remit with medication cessation and antihistamine administration. Patients should be advised to seek immediate medical attention should a rash develop; primary care providers should be enlisted to help with patient management at that point.

SIADH, HYPONATREMIA, ACIDOSIS

Oxcarbazepine is implicated in causing syndrome of inappropriate secretion of antidiuretic hormone

(SIADH) or an SIADH-like mechanism causing excessive retention of free water (Wade, Dang, Nelson, & Wasserberger, 2008). Elderly patients may develop significant hyponatremia (Asconape, 2002). Topiramate is implicated in a dose-dependent acidosis that may become dangerous in patients with renal failure; the drug also increases the risk of acute angle closure glaucoma (which may present as a painful red eye), and kidney stones (Wade et al., 2008). In children, oligohydrosis (decreased sweating) and hyperthermia have been reported (Cerminara, Seri, Bombardieri, Pinci, & Curatolo, 2006); these side effects may also occur in adults.

WEIGHT GAIN, HYPERGLYCEMIA, METABOLIC SYNDROME, CARDIAC EVENTS

All patients taking a typical or atypical antipsychotic must have their weight, fasting blood sugar, and waist circumference measured at the start of therapy and periodically thereafter. Most organizations have policies regarding frequency of these measurements, but quarterly is usually advised. Patients should be instructed to alert the clinician if they gain weight, since weight gain and development of metabolic syndrome are risks in long-term antipsychotic therapy. Those who are already overweight should avoid the medications most notorious for weight gain (olanzapine and risperidone); it would be wise to try second-generation antipsychotics aripiprazole or ziprasidone, which are less likely to cause weight gain (Stahl, 2009, pp. 47, 260, 536, 591); alternately they may try mood stabilizers topiramate or lamotrigine, neither of which is known for weight gain.

African American patients are more likely to show excessive weight gain than Caucasian patients, and East Asians show more elevated prolactin levels than Caucasians (Omerod et al., 2008). Non-white race is associated with a greater incidence of diabetes 10 years after treatment initiation with atypical antipsychotics, and non-whites gained weight faster in trials that contained olanzapine (Omerod, McDowell, Coleman, & Ferner, 2008). African American, Hispanic, and black race were associated with increased cardiac events in one study; Hispanic race was also associated with more adverse reactions to antidepressants (Omerod, McDowell, Coleman, & Ferner, 2008).

Patients must be counseled about diet and exercise and referred to nutrition experts if necessary. Group diet and weight-loss groups are effective interventions. A change of medication may be indicated if a patient has excessive or rapid weight gain.

ELEVATED PROLACTIN LEVEL, HYPOTHYROIDISM, RENAL PROBLEMS, SEXUAL DYSFUNCTION

Any antipsychotic can cause elevation in prolactin levels, but risperidone and amisulpride are particularly implicated. This occurs disproportionately in women of child bearing age, adolescents, and children. Elevated prolactin levels cause a shift in the hypothalamic-pituitary axis, and the end result for women is a decrease in circulating estrogen, for men a decrease in testosterone. Women may experience amenorrhea, and both may have sexual dysfunction. While D2 blockade in mesolimbic and mesocortical brain areas causes the therapeutic effects of antipsychotics, D2 blockade in the striatum causes Parkinsonism, and D2 blockade in the lactotroph cells removes the main inhibitory influence on prolactin secretion (Haddad & Wieck, 2004). Symptoms of prolactinemia include gynecomastia, galactorrhea, infertility, menstrual irregularity, sexual dysfunction, acne, and hirsutism in women due to low estrogen levels and androgen excess; one small study noted a greater risk of development of breast cancer in women with antipsychotic-induced hyperprolactinemia (Haddad & Wieck, 2004). Patients who develop prolactinemia should have a dose decrease, switch to a prolactin-sparing antipsychotic, and if female, start an oral contraceptive containing estrogen and be closely monitored (Haddad & Wieck, 2004).

Up to 30% of patients on long-term lithium therapy develop an elevated thyroid stimulating hormone (TSH) and between 5% and 30% develop goiter. Lithium-induced nephrogenic diabetes inspidus may occur, so careful thyroid monitoring is a must. Serious side effects such as neurotoxicity, severe tremor, delirium, and EPS have occurred, and have been reported in elderly patients receiving lithium with traditional antipsychotics (DiPiro et al., 2005, p. 1278). Many patients also suffer from headache, fatigue, and confusion with lithium therapy, so those complaints must be taken seriously, and if they do not abate, the drug must be withdrawn. Tremor may be treated with a β-adrenergic antagonist medication such as propranolol 20–120 mg a day (DiPiro et al., 2005, p. 1278).

Sexual side effects are one of the most common fears and complaints of patients on any psychotropic, and they must be dealt with on an individual basis, with switch of medications and careful evaluation of other causes, hormonal or other medical.

MOVEMENT DISORDERS

EPS may occur with both typical and atypical antipsychotics, and are frequently cited by patients as reasons for discontinuing medications.

Lifestyle modifications (in the case of weight gain), dose reductions (in the case of mild change in laboratory values), or cessation of medication (in the case of serious side effects) must be undertaken. Working closely with the patient's primary care provider to designate who is following the patient for ordering of necessary laboratory tests, monitoring patient's body mass index (BMI), weight, and vital signs is a good practice. Patients should be advised at the outset to take precautions against pregnancy as none of these medications are considered safe in pregnancy, and some may alter the effectiveness of oral contraceptives. Females who require medications and wish to become pregnant, or inadvertently become pregnant, should be referred to a high-risk antenatal program where medication risks and benefits as well as mood states can be closely monitored by an interdisciplinary team. Patients should be informed in advance that several trials of different medications may be necessary to find the right treatment for them, based upon their individual responses to medications and side effect sensitivity. Pediatric and elderly considerations are similar to those for adults in that greater sensitivity to medications is likely, and dose adjustments downward are recommended; there are a few exceptions in which children metabolize the drugs more quickly than adults, and therefore may need higher doses per kg of weight.

DIETARY MEASURES, CAFFEINE, SUGAR, VITAMINS, AND SUPPLEMENTS

CAFFEINE

Caffeine is a widely used and abused substance in our society. At least one in five adults consumes caffeine in quantities sufficient to cause adverse symptoms (DiPiro et al., 2005, p. 1202). Caffeine is present in coffee, leaf tea, and chocolate, as well as in many energy drinks and athletic performance products. Some of the so-called healthy products marketed at gyms and convenience stores contain high levels of caffeine or other stimulants such as guarana, sometimes mixed with alcohol. Many psychiatric facilities maintain a no-caffeine policy to protect patients from its potent psychoactive properties, which produce agitation and psychiatric destabilization in susceptible patients. Patients who have achieved stability have visited family and consumed caffeine, only to return to us in an aggressive decompensated state, independent of other factors. We advise patients with mood regulation issues to avoid caffeine or stimulants in any form. Caffeine is presently contained in many commercial foods including oatmeal, children's drinks, potato chips, and in a wide variety of packaged beverages, and is being marketed to very young children. Many parents are not aware of the large quantities of caffeine that are marketed to and consumed by their children. It is the most widely abused legal stimulant (Temple, 2009). Adolescents who drank five or more carbonated beverages per week were 30% more like to carry a weapon and to report being violent with a peer (Solnick & Hemenway, 2011).

MICRONUTRIENTS AND SUPPLEMENTS

Leading experts in violence and psychiatry are advocating more research into the role of micronutrients and mental health (Gardner, Kaplan, Rucklidge, Jonsson, & Humble, 2009; Lakhan & Viera, 2008). Vitamin deficiencies, especially B12, are linked to violent behavior, and other vitamins and micronutrients are now being studied in placebo-controlled trials with violent inmates (Gesch, 2009). Omega-3 fatty acids have known mood modulating effects due to their cell signaling and signal transduction; proposed research in using n-3 and n-6 poly unsaturated fatty acids (PUFAs) in violent prison populations is underway (Bhat, 2009; Gesch, 2009). Systematic review of the effects of n-3 fatty acids have shown improvement in depression in the elderly; intake of eicosapentaenoic acid (EPA) and docosahexaenoic acid (DHA) have improved DHA and EPA in plasma phospholipids and increased EPA in red blood cells, which is thought to improve irritability in children with ADHD (Riediger, Othman, Suh, & Moghadasian, 2009). Larger randomized controlled trials are needed in this area.

REFINED FOODS AND SUGAR

Much has been written about irritability and the effects of sugar, diets high in refined foods, food colors, preservatives, and additives. There are no perfect randomized controlled studies that can categorically recommend one diet over another. However, many in psychiatry are recommending a whole foods diet that is high in omega-3 fatty acids, low in sugar and artificial ingredients, and sufficient in protein. For those interested in nutritional studies, there are several excellent websites and books on the subject. Dr. Andrew Weil, with the Arizona Center for Integrative Medicine (http://integrativemedicine.arizona.edu/) is considered an expert in this area. Mediterranean diets are helpful for mood stability and neurotransmitter function (Maize, 2007). Beneficial characteristics of the Mediterranean diet are that it has a low glycemic index, is high in omega-3 fatty acids, and is high in vitamins B6, B12, folate, vitamin D, magnesium, chromium, and zinc. For those who cannot or do not eat fish, a beginning recommended dose of omega-3 fatty acid supplementation is 1,000 mg per day of EPA and 300–500 mg DHA (Low Dog, 2010). Anti-inflammatory foods and those containing protective phytochemicals, such as green tea, spices such as turmeric and ginger, and any antioxidant-rich food, are beneficial (Maize, 2007).

EXERCISE, STRESS MANAGEMENT, EASTERN HEALING

Benefits of vigorous exercise are well documented, and all persons with or without mental health problems benefit from both aerobic and meditative exercises, such as yoga, Qigong, Tai Chi, dancing, running, breathing, and energy work (Chiasson, 2007). Therapeutic modalities from Eastern cultures such as acupuncture, reiki, and shakra work have been used for trauma and aggression reduction as well as to improve cognitive functioning and focus. Child abuse victims who were taught rhythmic exercise for just a few minutes a day improved in cognitive functioning measures in a small pilot study (Goldshtrom, Korman, Goldshtrom, & Bendavid, 2011). These modalities improve overall well-being, reduce stress, and create a sensation of happiness and centering. See Chapter 6 for more information.

ENVIRONMENTAL, CULTURAL, AND MILIEU MANAGEMENT

Planning of the physical environment to prevent patient violence is important. Virtanen and colleagues reported a 16% increase in assaults when inpatient wards were overcrowded (Virtanen et al., 2011). A clean and clutter-free environment that lacks dangerous, heavy, or easily thrown objects is optimal. Clinicians should use strategies to divert the attention of potentially violent patients toward soothing or distracting activities to reduce the risk of patient escalation. Often on inpatient wards, roommates must be shifted in order to avoid toxic combinations of patients. Empathic communication, accurate information, and complete orientation to unit policies can help to deflect patient dissatisfaction and anger. Calming colors (blues, greens, and pastels), homey furnishings, and comfort measures can assist patients in feeling less anxious and more open to therapeutic intervention.

Establishing a culture where nonviolent de-escalation is the modus operandi is essential to provide a therapeutic patient environment that does not retraumatize patients with unnecessary seclusions and restraints. Comfort rooms, where a patient may have quiet, private space to regain self-control, have been used as nonviolent methods to reduce seclusion and restraint use (Cummings et al., 2010). Staff members who adopt a mindset that they are wardens of patients, as opposed to helpers, start a naturally adversarial dynamic in motion. Nonviolent communication that offers patients opportunities to gain self-control is the optimal goal. To that end, the Substance Abuse and Mental Health Services Administration (SAMSHA) has developed a 15-page document called "Roadmap to Seclusion and Restraint Free Mental Health Services" that outlines the philosophy and training materials needed (SAMSHA, 2005). In this document specifics are given on how to train staff and what materials are needed. The training takes 21 to 24 hours and can be accomplished with minimal extra cost and materials. In 2011, SAMSHA published a comprehensive 38-page document that identifies the scope of the problem of seclusion and restraints, and details methods of institutional culture change via staff training and institutional grant initiatives (Huang, 2011). Updates may be found via SAMSHA newsletters (www.samhsa.gov/).

Staff must be able to understand that anger and release of tension are commonly expressed emotions by acutely ill patients on locked inpatient units. Some facilities allow for patients to yell in their rooms, or go to a quiet room voluntarily to scream if needed. Punching bags (bean bags) for patients to express anger are rarely seen these days. Many believe that the use of punching as an anger outlet excites patients and teaches them that physical violence is acceptable. Most often anger management groups, recreational therapy, brief cognitive therapies, and physical exercise are used.

LONGER TERM CBTs AND GROUP INTERVENTIONS

PEDIATRIC CONSIDERATIONS

Children who are raised by mentally ill or violent parents fare much worse in their mental health and social functioning. However, the Star-D Child study, a longitudinal multicenter study of children of depressed mothers, documented that psychiatric symptoms in children significantly improved when their mothers' depression improved. Thus, when attempting to treat a child therapeutically, it is important that parental treatment is also addressed (Pilowsky et al., 2008). School-based prosocial behavioral programs aimed at all children are helpful for children who have been childhood witnesses of IPV or child abuse; however, individual and play therapy are indicated in most cases, depending on age and other mental health comorbidities. Multi-systemic treatment involving all spheres of a child's life is the treatment of choice for adolescents with antisocial behaviors (Curtis, Ronan, Heiblum, & Crellin, 2009). Some schools have implemented early elementary education aimed at reducing violence and improving pro-social behavior that can be effective in assisting both children with trauma backgrounds and those without those backgrounds.

CBT AND DBT

Dialectical behavioral and CBT have been successfully implemented with Canadian incarcerated violent youth, with some reduction in violent behaviors (Quinn & Shera, 2009). Therapies directed at children with PTSD targeting their trauma have been shown to improve executive functioning (DePrince et al., 2009). Structured functional family therapy is effective for reducing recidivism in violent youth on probation, when compared with probation only (Sexton & Turner, 2010). Mindfulness-based stress reduction techniques have been used with urban youth to decrease hostility (Sibinga et al., 2011). Multisystemic treatment, engaging the child or adolescent in the home, at school, and in the community has shown long-term effectiveness with violent juvenile offenders (Curtis et al., 2009). Parenting classes improve short-term outcomes for oppositional defiant disorder and CD in children and adolescents, but may not be predictive of success without continued intervention (Drugli, 2009).

PEDIATRIC CLINICAL CASE STUDY

While working at a locked juvenile acute psychiatric center years ago I encountered a child who was severely sexually and emotionally abused and neglected from the age of 18 months. She attracted the attention of authorities by attempting to stab her brother and burn down her apartment, where she was largely held prisoner by her father and uncle, and molested after her mother was sent to prison. Upon arrival to our unit she was 6 years old but was one of the most violently dangerous patients, attacking and injuring multiple staff persons. She had never been to school, did not know what a fruit or vegetable was, and did not know how to use eating utensils. Within 1 year at our facility, without the use of potentially harmful psychotropics, she was reading at grade level, her violent outbursts were reduced to nearly none, and she was able to be discharged to a reparenting group home, where the children were treated for severe attachment disorders. Our children's program was a behaviorally based program that used a reward and privileges system, as well as consistent individualized nursing care plans focusing on specific recovery goals for each patient. As each goal was achieved, the next level of goals was formulated. Step-by-step improvement in behavioral self-regulation was the aim of the program, along with improved affective functioning.

CBTs FOR PERPETRATORS

CBT for the treatment of aggressive adults who were violent under the influence of drugs or alcohol or in a reactive mood episode has shown some promise. The same can be said for treatment of traumatized individuals who have symptoms of PTSD. In these individuals, therapeutic interventions that address their trauma should reduce externalizing behaviors and improve emotional self-regulation. Individual and diagnosis-based group therapies have been beneficial in these populations using standard CBT techniques and anger management classes.

Service for Treatment and Abatement of Interpersonal Risk (STAIR) has been continuously operated in New York to treat seriously mentally ill state hospital patients with a history of recidivism. They have shown improved outcomes, with less cognitive impairment and less impulsivity for persons who completed the 6-month 72-session program that teaches skills, values, and attitudes necessary for successful living in the community (Yates et al., 2005).

These therapeutic approaches help patients to identify their personal triggers, develop coping mechanisms, learn to self-soothe, learn to elicit help in a nonaggressive fashion, learn to reduce anxiety and stress, and develop healthy lifestyles. Comparing social activity with CBT in psychotic patients with a history of violence in a randomized controlled trial, those who were treated with CBT had improved cognition and reduced anger (Haddock, Barrowclousgh, Shaw, Dunn, Novaco, & Tarrier, 2009). Anger management classes are a helpful group cognitive behavioral intervention for those whose aggression is impulsive. SAMSHA has a detailed guide to anger management classes that can be downloaded from their website (Reilly & Shopshire, 2002).

GROUP MOBILIZATION AND SOCIAL ATTITUDE TRANSFORMATION

Utilizing the theoretical framework of Pablo Friere in "Pedagogy of the Oppressed," male Hispanic men were engaged in facilitated discussion aimed at encouraging self-reflection and behavior change, in a migrant underserved community in which sexual and IPV were problematic (Friere, 1970; Nelson, Lewy, Ricardo, Dovydaitis, Hunter, & Kugel, 2010). Theoretically derived from the work of Frieire, Bandura, and Pajares, the latter of which encourages the notion of a self-system involving self-reflection and planning for alternative strategizing, men were engaged in a discussion that reframed violence as a problem that affects both men and women. The project had two phases. The first collected data on knowledge, attitudes, beliefs, and behaviors of Hispanic farm-working males on sexual violence and IPV. Next, an educational/discussion curriculum was developed and conducted on three sites to educate the same workers on those subjects. The project was called *Hombres Unidos Contra La Violencia Familiar* (Men United Against Family Violence) and included five basic concepts: "(1) Men are naturally loving, sensitive, and nurturing human beings; (2) Violence and acceptance of violence are learned and can be unlearned; (3) Men can and want to help stop violence against women; (4) Men must provide support for each other in order to change the social acceptance of violence; (5) We can only change ourselves; we cannot change anyone else" (Nelson, Lewy, Ricardo, Dovydaitis, Hunter, Kugel, 2010, p. 301). The male participants in the program received a certificate of completion, which was valuable to them as many had never been to school before. They began to mentor other men and discourage them from violent acts, even friends they had in Mexico with whom they were in contact with by phone. The program is continuing and has now spread to a second state, Arizona (Nelson et al., 2010). This is a brilliant example of a culturally sensitive intervention that has the possibility of changing negative cultural influences while bringing about individual positive change.

Schools and colleges are becoming more aware of violence as a campus issue and have initiated studies as well as interventions to change attitudes about violence, especially bullying and rape, with several successes. College and military service personnel programs aimed at changing college students' and active duty military troops' beliefs about rape showed attitude shifts in males, as well as prosocial behaviors such as males intervening in situations prior to a rape occurring (Currier & Carlson, 2009; Foubert, Godin, & Tatum, 2009). Elementary school programs can improve prosocial behavior and reduce the later incidence of violence perpetration (Beets, 2009).

COGNITIVE THERAPY AND ANTISOCIAL PERSONALITY DISORDER

Thus far, cognitive behavioral treatment of violent adults with antisocial personality disorder has not been promising; thus these individuals' prognosis is poor (Gibbon et al., 2010). For CBT to be effective, the patient and clinician must agree on the goals of treatment. In my experience in working with patients with antisocial personality disorder, the primary problem is their very limited insight into their need to change, and little desire to change, therefore they do not readily engage in available treatment options with sincerity. Options may unfortunately be limited to offering medications to reduce emotional reactivity and violent tendencies.

THERAPY INTERVENTIONS FOR PARENTS

Substance-abusing mothers who had irritable infants improved their mothering behaviors with a residential intervention aimed at improving their parenting skills. Pregnant low-income mothers with a history of IPV improved depression with a brief interpersonal therapy intervention aimed at improving their self-efficacy (Zlotnick, Capezza, & Parker, 2010). Mothers who were substance abusers and their toddlers were recruited from outpatient substance abuse treatment. They were randomized into two groups: One group received parent education, and the other group received 12 specialized individual therapy sessions using a mother and toddlers model (Suchman, DeCoste, Castiglioni, & McMahon, 2010). The mothers' therapy was aimed at improving maternal attachment in women who were likely victims of abuse themselves. High parenting stress in substance-abusing mothers is associated with parental aggression, neglect, and low parental functioning. Improving mothers' abilities to "mentalize" or understand their own and their children's emotional experience has the potential to improve maternal empathy and recognition that a child's behavior and affective state are related. Over the course of this 12-week pilot intervention, in the 47 mothers who completed the program, the therapy group showed higher levels of reflective function and lower levels of risk for child maltreatment than the parent education group (Suchman et al., 2010). The therapy group was also more likely to have stopped abusing substances (Suchman et al., 2010). Maternal response to children greatly affects their mental health trajectories; interventions aimed at improving the quality of the maternal-child interaction and parental support will greatly improve a child's recovery in the wake of trauma (Gerwitz, DeGarmo, & Medhanie, 2011).

THERAPEUTIC INTERVENTIONS FOR CHILDREN AND ADOLESCENTS

Multisystemic treatment shows improved outcomes for children and adolescents where school, home, parenting classes and engagement, and community interventions are combined. Children and parents in these programs learn coping mechanisms, which are reinforced in all spheres. The approach seems to have a moderate effect size but there is a problem with high dropout rates (Conner et al., 2006). Children with obsessive compulsive disorder (OCD)/CD and externalizing behaviors have improved behavioral outcomes when their parents are engaged in parent education groups (Drugli, Larsson, Fossum, & Merch, 2010). Children who have experienced IPV have been taught deontic reasoning, or what one may and should do in a given circumstance—an approach that shows hope for improving their skills in relationship negotiation and in decreasing trauma-associated dissociation (DePrince, Chu, & Combs, 2008). Children who are victims of familial trauma experience deficits in executive functioning; school interventions aimed at improving attention in executive functioning could prove helpful for all children's school performance and behavior, since it is difficult to determine which children are victims (DePrince et al., 2009).

COMPLEMENTARY/ALTERNATIVE THERAPIES

Mindfulness-based interventions including meditation, yoga, qi gong, and deep breathing have proven effective for reducing agitation, anger, and violence. Mindfulness has its origins in Buddhist meditation, but has been adapted without religious intent for use in therapy. Mindfulness encourages an awareness of one's emotions, body sensations, and feelings in the present, and encourages acceptance of those feelings without judgment or actions, for example, "Just because I feel mad I do not have to hit." Acceptance and commitment theory helps to ameliorate negative effects of trauma and to improve survivors' resiliency. This method seeks to decrease ruminative thinking, depression, anger, avoidance, and disassociation, and improve commitment to positive values (Lang et al., 2012). Cambodian refugees have utilized Buddhist monks, the practice of meditation, Buddhist teachings, and holy water to reduce anger and improve emotional regulation (Nickerson, 2011). Women who were court-ordered to treatment for alcohol abuse issues and aggression toward an adult household member showed improvement with Mindfulness-Based Modification Therapy (MMT), which targets learning to recognize negative arousal and develop methods to see that there are many options for each situation that presents itself (Wupperman et al., 2011).

TREATMENT FOR PTSD

Persons suffering from trauma will present for treatment during multiple time points in their recovery, with acute stress disorder immediately after an event, or months to years later after prolonged suffering. It is important to assess patient needs from their point of view and refer them to the most skilled care providers, depending on their needs. The PMH-APRN must recognize their own comfort or discomfort with the patient problem, and treat or refer them appropriately. Trauma-specific programs if available can be helpful, but in the least, patients may be referred for eye-movement desensitization processing (EMDR) (see Chapter 9), trauma-focused therapy groups, and individual therapy (NIMH fact sheet; Ponniah & Hollan, 2009; Veterans Administration Guidelines for PTSD, 2010).

Most practitioners agree that specialty training is required to treat severe trauma. There are professional organizations offering specialty certification and training in EMDR (www.emdr.com), as well as advanced training in trauma-focused CBT. Severe trauma victims are best treated in settings where multidisciplinary team support is possible; they can be very needy and can become too challenging for the solo practitioner. Practitioners dealing with severe trauma should have professional support themselves to prevent burnout, and for collaboration. I had the excellent experience of multidisciplinary trauma treatment at Sierra Tucson, where I served as a nurse practitioner intern. On the post-sexual trauma and mood disorder dual diagnosis track, I was able to witness group work, family work, drama therapy, and adjunctive therapies such as equine therapy, life-mapping, and body therapies. While all of these modalities are not available to most, many can benefit from combining community resources to construct a personalized program of recovery, and often the PMH-APRN is the one to orchestrate this.

Trauma-focused CBT strives [for clarity] to improve patients' awareness of their biologic response to traumatic stimuli, gain control over hyperarousal, learn not to descend into helplessness or dissociation, and begin to reframe their experiences with themselves as a victor (Levine, 1997).

THERAPEUTIC MILIEU TREATMENT FOR THE DEVELOPMENTALLY DELAYED VIOLENT PERSON

Priorities (Yuba City, California) is a residential program for developmentally delayed mentally ill adults where I served as the clinical coordinator; the program is behaviorally based and community-milieu oriented. Patients there either failed other placements due to violence, are attempting a step-down from a more restrictive locked facility, have been arrested for minor violent crimes, or are young adults who have aged out of high-level locked juvenile facilities. Nearly all of the patients have been in custodial care in the past, and many are accustomed to high doses of antipsychotic medications as well as limited, if any, contact with the outside community, sometimes for years. Housing is a converted locked 16-bed unit that has been furnished to provide a family-like setting where patients eat communally, play, do recreational activities and sports, attend groups (about 35–40 groups per week), exercise, go on community outings, and live dormitory style. The goals for each patient vary, but in general they are to reduce or eliminate violent acting out, improve independent living skills, work on health improvement and preventive health skills, improve the ability to be out in the community with or without supervision, and improve affective functioning. In just over 18 months in operation at press date, some patients have had success with reduced psychotropic medications, improved physical health (weight loss, exercise, health habits), and are close to reintegration into the community; others have failed and have gone on to more restrictive levels of care (personal observation).

The keys to behavioral change in this program are peer support and CBT specifically targeted at improving communication skills, frustration tolerance, and coping mechanisms. Patients are encouraged to assume responsibility for their feelings and to see themselves as having potential control over their response to frustration. The program involves the use of exercise and healthy lifestyles, and the avoidance of overstimulation, negative peer influences, and substances that can exacerbate anxiety such as methylxanthines.

TRAINING OF PSYCHIATRIC PERSONNEL IN VIOLENCE MANAGEMENT

Most emergency personnel (Gates, Ross, & McQueen, 2006), psychiatric residents (Anderson & West, 2011), and APNs have historically received little formal training during the course of graduate studies in the management of aggression and violence. One study found only one-third of psychiatric residents had received training in how to deal with violent patients, despite the fact that clinicians with less experience are the ones most likely to become victims (Swartz & Park, 1999). Interviews of psychiatric residents and nurses who were assaulted revealed that assaults are underreported and not processed adequately, due to poor training of residents in institutional rules and guidelines for reporting violence, as well as very limited training in assessment for potential violence (Antonius et al., 2010; ENA, 2010; Gates et al., 2006). Residents and nurses felt that they were partly to blame for the violence, that the experience of violence is inherent to the psychiatric profession, and that reporting incidents would reflect negatively upon their performance evaluations; they also simply did not know the institutional policies regarding the reporting of patient violence (Antonius et al., 2010; ENA 2010). The majority of nurses who did report patient violence were underwhelmed with the result, since little, if anything, was done to reprimand or sanction the perpetrators of violence, with few even receiving a verbal warning (ENA, 2010).

The average psychiatric resident surveyed by Antonius and colleagues received 4.7 hours of training in violence management, mostly didactic lectures (Antonius et al., 2010). The American Psychological Association (APA) task force report recommended that this training be increased to a minimum of 10 hours with more training on simulations of patient violence, anticipation of patient violence, and how to escape violence once it has begun, as well as self-defense training (Schwartz & Park, 1999).

In the summer of 2011, I conducted an informal survey of PMH-APRN colleagues holding at least a Master of Science in nursing, from any specialty training program; though most were psychiatric nurse practitioners, a few family nurse practitioners responded. Only 2 of 30 responding remembered any training in their graduate program on how to deal with violent patients. Those who remembered any training stated that it consisted of a few didactic hours of reading on how to recognize a potentially aggressive patient as well as verbal de-escalation techniques. Two colleagues had more than 1 or 2 hours of training, and one had several hours of hands-on clinical training when a violence-threatening family appeared fortuitously in the outpatient PMH-APRN intern's clinic placement. One PMH-APRN remembered 6 to 8 hours of didactic training on the subject, which included CPS reporting and domestic violence. None reported remembering specifics about their training other than environmental control such as how to place oneself in an interview room safely.

BASIC ELEMENTS OF VIOLENCE PREVENTION TRAINING

KNOW THE PHYSICAL ENVIRONMENT AND INSTITUTIONAL POLICIES

Violence prevention training programs for staff and clinicians from all disciplines should include a few components. All workers must be apprised of institutional policies and physical safeguards to prevent violence in each clinical setting to which they are assigned. These safeguards may include panic buttons, barriers, safe unit areas, office furnishings, and placement of furniture to allow quick egress. Placing oneself and the patient so that either may leave the room without passing the other is a good policy. Decorating offices and interview rooms with a minimum of objects that might be used as weapons, and with calming colors such as pink, is helpful. Use shatter-proof barriers in triage or check-in areas and have lockers outside of patient care areas so that contraband such as weapons cannot be brought into the clinical area. Clinicians should be versed in how to summon help, be given permission to refuse to interview a patient they do not feel is safe enough to interview, and be completely familiar with the procedural chain of command in their assigned work area.

APRNs must receive training in the acute management of violence: (1) assessing patient for potential violence; (2) establishing a therapeutic alliance; (3) engaging of family and collateral support systems; (4) verbally de-escalating; (5) self-defense; (6) protecting personal information, as a precaution; (7) managing medication, including emergency rapid tranquilization as well as long-term medication; and (8) seclusion and restraints ("Here's how to prevent assaults on staff," 2001). Some states allow PMH-APRNs to order seclusion and restraints for emergency use; others do not.

Therapeutic training to minimize violence includes training of staff on therapeutic communication, motivational interviewing, maintaining good professional boundaries, transference and countertransference in psychiatric patients, and treatment planning skills. All persons working in health care should take personal precautions so that patient access to personal information is minimized, reducing the potential for a violent patient to target a professional both at work and outside of work. Many psychiatric professionals have unlisted home addresses and telephone numbers, and try to keep as much personal information as possible out of the public domain. Assuring that institutions have safe parking areas, away from places where violent patients could see a clinician entering or exiting their car, is also good advice, though sadly rarely available. Using available security personnel such as a parking lot escort is a common-sense measure.

CRITICAL INCIDENT STRESS MANAGEMENT

Critical incident stress management is a technique used by first responders, emergency personnel, and psychiatry since the late 1980s. This technique encompasses training of staff and first responders before a critical event, leadership during an event, processing the event with those involved, and caring for others after the event. Critical incident stress debriefing (CISD) is a technique wherein persons involved in an incident meet as soon as possible to discuss what happened, process their feelings, offer each other support, and reintegrate back to their usual work (Everly & Boyle, 1999). The originators of this technique continue to claim broad applications and effectiveness (Everly & Boyle, 1999). CISD is considered effective in both improving handling of crisis events and in reducing emergency and other health care workers' symptoms of PTSD (Evans, 1993; Freehill, 1992; Neely & Spitzer, 1997; Wee, Mills, & Koehler, 1999), including mental health nurses (Antai-Otong, 2001). Miller suggested that only a brief form of this method should be used, and only for emergency personnel (Miller, 1999). For certain persons emotional debriefing may actually do harm; thus brief educational debriefing might be a safer alternative (Sijbrandi, Olff, Reitsma, Carlier, & Gersons, 2006). More recent review studies debated the effectiveness of critical incident stress management (CISM), either staunchly defending it as a best practice (Regel, 2007; Wagner, 2005), or calling for the re-evaluation of which groups benefit from this intervention (Jacobs, Horne-Moyer, & Jones, 2004; Mitchell, Sakraida, & Kameg, 2003). Despite the controversy, the technique is still widely employed all over the world and has been in continuous use by many agencies for several decades. Everly and Mitchell (2000), considered the founders of the method, wrote a thorough review of the issues surrounding this controversy and delineated the types of intervention indicated for which groups. They continue to be involved with the International Critical Incident Stress Foundation, of which they are founding members (www.icisf.org).

LEGAL ISSUES

LEGAL RESPONSIBILITIES

When a patient is uttering specific threats to kill or injure others, one has a legal obligation to warn the intended victims, per the mandate resulting from the infamous 1976 Tarasoff case, in which a young woman was murdered by her ex-boyfriend, whose threats were known by the University of California (Herbert & Young, 2002). Recently courts have not held clinicians liable for being unable to foresee potential victims, and therefore their duty to warn is limited (Walcott, Cerundolo, & Beck, 2001). PMH-APRNs are mandated reporters for adult or child abuse. The responsible agencies must be contacted if a child or a vulnerable adult is at imminent risk of harm due to the actions or intended actions of another person. All clinicians must keep abreast of the legal responsibilities in the state where they practice, and ignorance regarding procedures does not absolve them of responsibility (Cooper, Selwood, & Livingston, 2010; Yehuda et al., 2010). When dealing with difficult cases an interdisciplinary team can offer help and support in this process (Feng et al., 2010).

WHEN LEGAL ACTION RATHER THAN FURTHER TREATMENT MUST BE PURSUED

There is no formulaic consensus among clinicians on when a health care provider who is a victim of patient violence should resort to legal action. Each case must be individually evaluated. Decisions must consider the global circumstances of the assault, the individual circumstances, injury sustained, and the likelihood of repeated offense. Ho, Ralston, McCullough, and Coverdale (2009) give insightful reasons to seek criminal prosecution of a violent hospitalized patient. I have encountered very violent patients, recently discharged from either state hospitals or prison, who are nonresponsive to medications, able to inflict great bodily harm, lacking insight, and lacking remorse or empathy. Such patients must, for safety's sake, be moved to criminal incarceration settings, as they are less likely to benefit from usual psychiatric treatment than they are to inflict harm to other patients and staff present in the psychiatric milieu (Ho et al., 2009). Patients who are repetitive perpetrators, who have received usual psychiatric treatment options without adequate response, must also be dealt with by the criminal prosecution.

PROVIDING CULTURALLY COMPETENT CARE

The PMH-APRN must work to develop the skills necessary to provide culturally competent care to an ever-changing demographic in which people from disparate reaches of the world seek relocation in the countries where PMH-APRNs practice. By the year 2050, non-Hispanic Caucasians will be outnumbered by minority residents in the United States (U.S. Census Bureau, 2011). Sensitivity to cultural practices and respect for different views of health, and expectations for care, will require constant education and learning.

SUMMARY COMMENTS

Violence is an ever-present issue in mental health. The ability to predict which patients are at high risk for violence, protect those at risk for victimization, and deal with the aftermath for victims of violence are essential advanced practice nursing skills. Thoughtful planning of the environment of care, as well as the utilization of every therapeutic tool available, including medications, therapy, holistic modalities, social supports, interdisciplinary teams, and sometimes law enforcement, will help to keep both the caregivers and patients in a safe treatment environment. There is a current shortage of clinicians trained to provide comprehensive psychiatric care. Retaining these clinicians by preventing injury and premature retirement from the psychiatric professions is important. Broader issues of culture and society impact this profession, and the current trends of downsizing of public institutional safety nets may create a situation wherein we will see more and more frustrated, untreated, and potentially violent patients and their victims in the future.

Research is needed on pharmacological and biologic interventions as well as sociologic research to further define risk factors and ameliorating factors for violence. Funding must be directed toward the prevention of child abuse and neglect, and the improvement of mental health care of children and mothers. More research in the area of childhood victimization of boys and men is also needed, since a larger proportion of those seen and incarcerated for violence are men. Resources must also be directed at the psychiatric treatment of perpetrators of child abuse so that those who are able to be rehabilitated can receive services. More funding is also needed in the area of substance abuse prevention and treatment, since substance abuse is highly linked to violent behavior. PMH-APRNs are in a unique position to further their skills in interdisciplinary collaboration to develop and test new interventions aimed at health promotion and violence reduction via early identification and intervention.

PEDIATRIC POINTERS

The interests of children cannot be placed on the back burner; the way in which a society treats and cares for the needs of children impacts their mental health for the rest of their life span. Early intervention for children of all ages, but particularly those in the prenatal, postnatal, infant, and preschool periods, must be prioritized if we are to reduce the psychiatric morbidity of the populace at large. The cycle of violence cannot be broken unless we attend to the treatment of substance-abusing parents, IPV, community violence, and poor access to basic health care. Early childhood well-child visits are one of the few opportunities where an at-risk child and professionals who can help may meet.

Health care for all children would ensure that children at least have this small chance of detection of risk situations in their lives. Public health programs must be more aggressive and comprehensive in providing services to at-risk mothers and children. Adolescents from at-risk families are in need of therapeutic interventions at early points in negative trajectories. Schools can impact violence by teaching a culture of nonviolence and providing assessment services for at-risk families. The model of the school-based health clinic should be expanded to include psychiatric care. Childhood and adolescence must once again be recognized as a time of both great vulnerability but also great possibility for change. Children and adolescents who cannot have their needs met at home need able, compassionate adult mentors from other places in the community. Instead of incarcerating youthful minor offenders, we should offer diversion programs where they can receive the psychiatric evaluation, psychoeducation, and school and family interventions that they need.

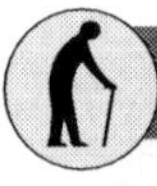

AGING ALERTS

The elderly who are psychiatrically impaired suffer an earlier decline in cognitive and social functioning than their nonpsychiatrically impaired peers (Cooper & Holmes, 1998). Loss of social connections, personal neglect of health due to psychiatric impairment, and the deleterious health effects of long-term psychotropic medications contribute to their declining health status. Role reversals that can occur with aging are profound. Elderly who were once robust, and perhaps even abusive, if mentally ill, become dependent upon those whom they abused. Families may in turn become uncaring due to past abuse, or from the extreme burdens associated with long-term caregiving, which takes a huge toll on the caregiver. Families of the elderly mentally ill perceive greater burden than those who care for elderly with neurological disorders, likely due to perceived stigma and difficulty finding respite. Health and financial tolls on caregivers may also be great. The PMH-APRN can assist families to locate resources that are available. Meanwhile, long-term care of the mentally ill elderly and end-of-life care must be research priorities, as the cost of health care continues to rise. With longer life expectancies, there will likely be a burgeoning population of those who need longer-term and end-of-life custodial care, as more families who are unable to bear the burden seek help from community resources.

With conscientious effort to confront, treat, and prevent the conditions in both individuals and society that are the etiologic conditions for violence, we can hope to better create a less violent society in the future.

RESOURCES FOR GENERAL VIOLENCE PREVENTION

Centers for Disease Control and Prevention: http://www.cdc.gov/ViolencePrevention/index.html
A comprehensive resource covering all types of violence.

CHILD ABUSE

U.S. Department of Health and Human Services Child Abuse Prevention: www.childwelfare.gov/preventing
U.S. Department of Health and Human Services Child Abuse Prevention website has information plus a database of referring and partnering organizations and resources. This site includes state by state statutory information and resources, information about adoption and foster care, organizational training and improvement activities, and comprehensive information about all aspects of child abuse including how it is evaluated judicially, and prioritized in Child Protective Services, plus many links to further reading and education and a search tool.
Assessment tools for detection of child abuse can be obtained from: www.childwelfare.gov/systemwide/assessment/family_assess/sources.cfm

HUMAN TRAFFICKING AND RAPE

Academy for Educational Development: www.humantrafficking.org/content/about_us
Related is the Center for Gender Equality: http://cge.aed.org/AboutUs.cfm
HumanTrafficking.org is a web resource to fight human trafficking, offering information on an international basis: international hotline numbers, advocacy updates, and governmental report links.
Related is Children At Risk: http://childrenatrisk.org

Polaris Project: polaris project.org Hotline: 1-888-3737-888

Mosaic Family Services: www.mosaicServices.org
Based in Dallas, TX, Hotline: 1-214-823-4434
Offers multilingual help and information in Arabic, Bosanski, Burmese, Chinese, Dutch, Spanish, French, Farsi, Gujarati, Hindi, Croatian, Italian, Karen, Kikuyu, Kirundi, Korean, Kurdish, Laotian, Mandarin, Nepali, Russian, Serbian, Somali, Swahili, Thai, Urdu, and Vietnamese; resources; and hotline services. Materials in foreign languages, refugee resettlement and case management services, HIV early intervention program, and multicultural youth substance abuse prevention.

GAY, LESBIAN, AND BIGENDER

Advocates for Youth: www.advocatesforyouth.org/glbtq.htm
A website dedicated to people interested in advocating for LGBTQ youth.

The Trevor Project: www.thetrevorproject.org. 866-4-U-TREVOR (866-488-7386).
The Trevor Project operates the only nationwide, around-the-clock crisis and suicide prevention helpline for LGBTQ youth. The Gay and Lesbian National Hotline 1-888-THE-GLNH provides phone and e-mail peer counseling, as well as information about local resources for GLBTQ teens across the United States. At GLBT National Youth Talkline 1-800-246-PRIDE (7743) Youth, volunteers provide young GLBTQ people (up to age 25) with peer counseling, information, and referrals to local resources. Available Monday–Saturday, 9:30 p.m. to midnight (EST).

Youth Pride, Inc.: www.youthprideri.org/Resources/RecommendedLinks/tabid/188/Default.aspx

DOMESTIC VIOLENCE

The Hotline: www.thehotline.org
National Information and referral source with a quick escape button while browsing to avoid detection by a perpetrator.

Love is Respect: www.loveisrespect.org
Includes information about first-dating violence for teens, information about sexting and texting abuse, as well as a hotline for teens, 24/7 live chat, and campus safety tips.

National Resource Center on Domestic Violence: www.nrcdv.org
Includes a toolkit for runaway and homeless youth.

National Resource Center on Violence Against women: www.vawnet.org/domestic-violence/intervention.php?page=2

SAFE-Stop Abuse for Everyone: www.safe4all.org/resource-list/index?category=16

State by State and Foreign resources and shelters for victims, online forums, education.

Asian and Pacific Islander Institute on Domestic Violence: www.apiidv.org/resources/violence-against-api-women.php
Contains latest research, statistics, information on programs, policy updates, advocacy information, and brochures in multiple Asian languages

RAPE

Men Can Stop Rape: www.mencanstoprape.org

Rape, Abuse, and Incest National Network: http://www.rainn.org

FOR PROFESSIONALS

Rape assessment National Protocol Guide for Medical Forensic Investigation 2004: www.ncjrs.gov/pdffi les1/ovw/206554.pdf

Sexual Assault examiner training: http://taife.com/Courses/2000/2015description.html

U.S. Department of Justice brochure on statutory rape: www.ojp.usdoj.gov/ovc/publications/infores/statutoryrape/trainguide/welcome.html

PTSD

National Center for PTSD: www.ptsd.va.gov
Primarily for veterans and their family members but offers lots of information, a searchable database for scholarly articles, and referrals specific to women and families.

National Institute of Mental Health: www.nimh.nih.gov/health/publications/post-traumatic-stress-disorder-ptsd/index.shtml

Operation We Are Here: www.operationwearehere.com/index.html
Faith-based resources for military families battling PTSD issues.

REFERENCES

Abderhalden, C., Needham, I., Dassen, T., Halfens, R., Haug, H. J., & Fischer, J. E. (2008). Structured risk assessment and violence in acute psychiatric wards: Randomised controlled trial. *British Journal of Psychiatry, 193*(44), 44–50. doi: 10.1192/bjp.bjp.107.045534

Ahuja, 2006, as cited by American Psychiatric Nurses' Association Position Statement on Workplace Violence (2008). Retrieved from http://www.apna.org/files/public/APNA_Workplace_Violence_Position_Paper.pdf

Allen, M. H., Currier, G.W., Carpenter, D., Ross, R.W., Docherty, J. P., & Expert Consensus Panel for Behavioral, E. (2005). The expert consensus guideline series. Treatment of behavioral emergencies 2005. *Journal of psychiatric practice, 11 Suppl 1*, 5–108; quiz 110–102.

Almvik, R., Woods, P., & Rasmussen, K. (2000). The Brøset Violence Checklist (BVC): Sensitivity, specificity and interrater reliability. *Journal of Interpersonal Violence, 15*(12), 1284–1296.

Amore, M., Menchetti, M., Tonti, C., Scalatti, F., Lundgren, E., Esposito, W., & Berardi, D. (2008). Predictors of violent behavior among acute psychiatric patients: Clinical study. *Psychiatry Clinical Neuroscience, 62*(3), 247–255.

Anderson, A., & West, S. G. (2011). Violence against mental health professionals: When the treater becomes the victim. *Innovation in Clinical Neuroscience, 8*(3), 34–39.

Annan, S. L. (2011). "It's not just a job. This is where we live. This is our backyard": The experiences of expert legal and advocate providers with sexually assaulted women in rural areas. *Journal of the American Psychiatric Nurses Association, 17*(2), 139–147. doi: 10.1177/1078390311401024

Antai-Otong, D. (2001). Critical incident stress debriefing: A health promotion model for workplace violence. [Review]. *Perspectives in Psychiatric Care, 37*(4), 125–132.

Antonius, D., Fuchs, L., Herbert, F., Kwon, J., Fried, J. L., Burton, P. R. S.,...Malaspina, D. (2010). Psychiatric assessment of aggressive patients: A violent attack on a resident. [Case Reports Clinical Conference]. *American Journal of Psychiatry, 167*(3), 253–259. doi: 10.1176/appi.ajp.2009.09010063

Arseneault, L., Bowes, L., & Shakoor, S. (2010). Bullying victimization in youths and mental health problems: 'much ado about nothing'?, *Psychological Medicine, 40*(5), 717–729.

Asconape, J. J. (2002). Some common issues in the use of antiepileptic drugs. [Case Reports Review]. *Seminars in Neurology, 22*(1), 27–39. doi: 10.1055/s-2002–33046

Asian and Pacific Islander Institute on Domestic Violence (2011). Statistics on violence against API women, Retrieved from http://www.apiidv.org/resources/violence-against-api-women.php.

Asla, N., de Paúl, J., & Pérez-Albéniz, A. (2011). Emotion recognition in fathers and mothers at high-risk for child physical abuse. *Child Abuse & Neglect, 35*(9), 712–721. doi:10.1016/j.chiabu.2011.05.010

Avegno, J., Mills, T. J., & Mills, L. D. (2009). Sexual Assault Victims in the Emergency Department: Analysis by Demographic and Event Characteristics. *The Journal of Emergency Medicine, 37*(3), 328–334. doi: 10.1016/j.jemermed.2007.10.025

Baler, R. D., Volkow, N. D., Fowler, J. S., & Benveniste, H. (2008). Is fetal brain monoamine oxidase inhibition the missing link between maternal smoking and conduct disorders? *Journal of Psychiatry and Neuroscience, 33*(3), 187–195.

Baren, J. M., Mace, S. E., Hendry, P. L., Dietrich, A. M., Goldman, R. D., & Warden, C. R. (2008). Children's mental health emergencies—part 2 Emergency department evaluation and treatment of children with mental health disorders. *Pediatric Emergency Care, 24*(7), 485–498.

Barzman, D. H., Patel, A., Sonnier, L., & Strawn, J. R. (2010). Neuroendocrine aspects of pediatric aggression: Can hormone measures be clinically useful? *Neuropsychiatric Disease Treatment, 6*, 691–697. doi: 10.2147/ndt.s5832

Basow, S. A., & Minieri, A. (2011). "You owe me": Effects of date cost, who pays, participant gender, and rape myth beliefs on perceptions of rape. *Journal of Interpersonal Violence, 26*(3), 479–497. doi: 10.1177/0886260510363421

Beaulaurier, R. L., Seff, L R., & Newman, F L. (2008). Barriers to help-seeking for older women who experience intimate partner violence: a descriptive model. *J Women Aging, 20*(3–4), 231–248.

Beets, M.W., Flay, B. R., Vuchinich, S., Snyder, F. J., Acock, A., Li, Kin-Kit...Durlak, J. (2009). Use of a Social and Character Development Program to Prevent Substance Use, Violent Behaviors, and Sexual Activity Among Elementary-School Students in Hawaii. *American Journal of Public Health, 99*(8), 1438–1445.

Bhat, R. S. (2009). You are what you eat: of fish, fat and folate in late-life psychiatric disorders. *Current Opinion in Psychiatry, 22*(6), 541–545.

Bilgin, H. (2009). An evaluation of nurses' interpersonal styles and their experiences of violence. *Issues in Mental Health Nursing, 30*, 252–259. doi: 10.1080/01612840802710464

Bjørkly, S., Hartvig, P., Haggen, F. A., Brauer, H., & Mogen, T. A. (2009). Development of a brief screen for violence risk (V-Risk-10) in acute and general psychiatry: An introduction with emphasis on findings from a naturalistic test of interrater reliability. *European Psychiatry, 24*, 388–394.

Bottoni, T. N. (2002). Neuroleptic malignant syndrome: A brief review. *Hospital Physician, 38*(3), 58–63.

Brook, S., Lucey, J.V., & Gunn, K.P. (2000). Intramuscular ziprasidone compared with intramuscular haloperidol in the treatment of acute psychosis. Ziprasidone I.M. Study Group. *The Journal of Clinical Psychiatry, 61*(12), 933–941.

Burgermeister, D. (2007). Childhood adversity: A review of measurement instruments. *Journal of Nursing Measurement, 15*(3), 163–176.

Busch-Armendariz, N. B., Nsonwu, M. B., & Cook, H. L. (2011). Human trafficking victims and their children: Assessing needs, vulnerabilities, strengths, and survivorship. *Journal of Applied Research on Children: Informing Policy for Children at Risk, 2*(1), Article 3. Retrieved from http://digitalcommons.library.tmc.edu/childrenatrisk/vol2/iss1/3

Caldwell, M. F. (1992). Incidence of PTSD among staff victims of patient violence. *Hospital & Community Psychiatry, 43*(8), 838–839.

Callegari, C. M. T., Menchetti, M., Croci, G., Beraldo, S., Costantini, C., & Baranzini, F. (2006). Two years of psychogeriatric consultations in a nursing home: Reasons for referral compared to psychiatrists' assessment. *BMC Health Services Research, 6*(73), doi: 10.1186/1472–6963–6–73

Campbell, J., Jones, A.S., Dienemann, J., Kub, J., Schollenberger, J., O'Campo, P....Wynne, C. (2002). Intimate partner violence and physical health consequences. *Archives of Internal Medicine, 162*(1157–1163).

Carpenter, D. O., & Nevin, R. (2010). Environmental causes of violence. *Physiological Behavior, 99*(2), 260–268. doi: 10.1016/j.physbeh.2009.09.001

Caspi, A., McClay, J.,Moffitt, T. E., Mill, J., Martin, J., Craig, I. W.,...Poulton, R. (2002). Role of genotype in the cycle of violence in maltreated children. *Science 297*(5582), 851–854.

CDC. (2011). National violent death reporting system: Reports violent deaths 2003–2008. Retrieved from http://wisqars.cdc.gov:8080/nvdrs/nvdrsController.jsp

Cerminara, C., Seri, S., Bombardieri, R., Pinci, M., & Curatolo, P. (2006). Hypohidrosis during topiramate treatment: A rare and reversible side effect. *Pediatric Neurology, 34*(5), 392–394. doi:10.1016/j.pediatrneurol.2005.10.004

Chan, K. L. (2011). Co-Occurence of intimate partner violence and child abuse in Hong Kong Chinese families. *Journal of Interpersonal Violence, 26*, 1322–1342. doi: 10.1177/0886260510369136 On 2011

Chan, K. L. (2011). Evaluating the risk of child abuse: The child abuse risk assessment scale (CARAS). *Journal of Interpersonal Violence, 27*(5), 951–973. doi: 10.1177/0886260511423252

Chang, C. C., Shiah, I. S., Yeh, C. B., Wang, T. S., & Chang, H. A. (2006). Lamotrigine-associated anticonvulsant hypersensitivity syndrome in bipolar disorder. *Progress in Neuro-Psychopharmacology and Biological Psychiatry, 30*(4), 741–744. doi: 10.1016/j.pnpbp.2005.11.033

Chiasson, A. M. (2007, January). *Mind-body tools for women.* Paper presented at 6th Annual Women's Mental Health Symposium, University of Arizona, Tucson, AZ.

Clark, D. E., Brown, A. M., & Griffith, P. (2010). The BrØset Violence Checklist: Clinical utility in a secure psychiatric intensive care setting. *Journal of Psychiatric and Mental Health Nursing, 17*(7), 614–620.

Cooper, C., & Holmes, C. (1998). Previous psychiatric history as a risk factor for late-life dementia: A population-based-control study. *Age and Ageing, 27*, 181–188.

Cooper, C., Selwood, A., & Livingston, G. (2009). Knowledge, detection, and reporting of abuse by health and social care professionals: A systematic review. *American Journal of Geriatric Psychiatry, 17*(10), 826–838.

Coverdale, J. H., Louie, A. K., & Roberts, L.W. (2005). Protecting the safety of medical students and residents. [Comment Editorial]. *Academic Psychiatry: The Journal of the American Association of Directors of Psychiatric Residency Training and the Association for Academic Psychiatry, 29*(4), 329–331. doi: 10.1176/appi.ap.29.4.329

Cummings, K. S., Grandfield, S. A., & Coldwell, C. M. (2010). Caring with comfort rooms: Reducing seclusion and restraint use in psychiatric facilities. *Journal of Psychosocial Nursing, 48*(6), 26–30.

Currier, D. M., & Carlson, J. H. (2009). Creating attitudinal change through teaching: how a course on "Women and Violence" changes students' attitudes about violence against women. *Journal of interpersonal violence, 24*(10), 1735–1754. doi: 10.1177/0886260509335239

Curtis, N. M., Ronan, K. R., Heiblum, N., & Crellin, K. (2009). Dissemination and effectiveness of multisystemic treatment in New Zealand: A benchmarking study. *Journal of Family Psychology, 23*(2), 119–129.

Dabby, C., Patel, H., & Poore, G. (2010). *Shattered lives: Homicides, domestic violence and Asian families.* San Francisco: Asian & Pacific Islander Institute on Domestic Violence. Retrieved from http://apiidv.org/files/Homicides.DV.AsianFamilies-APIIDV-2010.pdf

DeJonghe, E. S., Bogat, G. A., Levendosky, A. A., & von Eye, A. (2008). Women survivors of intimate partner violence and post-traumatic stress disorder: prediction and prevention. *J Postgrad Med, 54*(4), 294–300.

DeKeseredy, W. S., & Schwartz, M. D. (2008). Separation/divorce sexual assault in rural Ohio: Survivors' perceptions. *Journal of Prevention& Intervention in the Community, 36*(1–2), 105–119. doi: 10.1080/10852350802022365

DePrince, A. P., Chu, A. T., & Combs, M. D. (2008). Trauma-related predictors of deontic reasoning: A pilot study in a community sample of children. *Child Abuse Neglect, 32*(7), 732–737.

DePrince, A. P., Weinzierl, K. M., & Combs, M. D. (2009). Executive function performance and trauma exposure in a community sample of children. *Child Abuse & Neglect 33*(6), 353–361.

Dhossche, D. M., & Ghani, S. O. (1998). Who brings patients to the psychiatric emergency room? Psychosocial and psychiatric correlates. *General Hospital Psychiatry, 20*(4), 235–240.

Diaz-Olavarrieta, C., Wilson, K.S., Garcia, S.G., Revollo, R., Richmond, K., Paz, F., et al. (2009). The co-occurrence of intimate partner violence and syphilis among pregnant women in Bolivia. *Journal of Women's Health, 18*(12), 2077–2086. doi: 10.1089/jwh.2008.1258

DiPiro, J. T., Talbert, R. L., Yee, G. C., Matzke, G. R., Wells, B. G., & Posey, L. M (Eds.) (2005). *Pharmacotherapy a pathophysiologic approach* (6th ed.). New York, NY: McGraw-Hill.

Drugli, M. B., Larsson, B., Fossum. S., & MØrch, W. T. (2010). Five- to six-year outcome and its prediction for children with ODD/CD treated with parent training. *Journal of Child Psychology and Psychiatry, 51*(5), 559–566. doi: 10.1111/j.1469-7610.2009.02178.

Duke, N. N., Pettingell, S. L., McMorris, B. J., & Borowsky, I. W. (2010). Adolescent violence perpetration: Associations with multiple types of adverse childhood experiences. *Pediatrics, 125*(4), e778–e786. doi: 10.1542/peds.2009–0597

Emergency Nurses Association. (2010). *Emergency Department Violence Surveillance Study*. Des Plaines, IL: Institute for Emergency Nursing Research. Retrieved from http://www.ena.org/IENR/Documents/ENAEVSSReportAugust2010.pdf

Erdos, B. Z. & Hughes, D. H. (2001). Emergency psychiatry: A review of assaults by patients against staff at psychiatric emergency centers. [Review]. *Psychiatric Services, 52*(9), 1175–1177.

Evans, P. (1993). Critical incident stress debriefing. Stress management program succeeds in San Francisco General Hospital's emergency department. *California Hospitals, 7*(6), 20–21.

Everly, G. S., Jr., & Boyle, S. H (1999). Critical incident stress debriefing (CISD): A meta-analysis. [Meta-Analysis]. *International Journal of Emergency Mental Health, 1*(3), 165–168.

Everly, G. S., Jr., & Mitchell, J. T. (2000). The debriefing "controversy" and crisis intervention: A review of lexical and substantive issues. *International Journal of Emergency Mental Health, 2*(4), 211–225.

Fawole, O. I. (2008). Economic violence to women and girls: Is it receiving the necessary attention? *Trauma, Violence & Abuse, 9*, 167–177. doi: 10.1177/1524838008319255

Fazel, S. Gautam, G., Linsell, L., Geddes, J. R., & Grann, M. (2009). Schizophrenia and violence: Systematic review and meta-analysis. *PLoS Medicine, 6*(8), e1000120. doi:10.1371/journal.pmed.1000120

Fazel, M., Wheeler, J, & Danesh, J. Prevalence of serious mental disorder in 7000 refugees resettled in western countries: A systematic review. *The Lancet, 365*(9467), 1309–1314. doi: 10.1016/s0140-6736(05)61027-6

Fehon, D. C., Grilo, C. M,. & Lipschitz, D. S. (2005). A comparison of adolescent inpatients with and without a history of violence perpetration: Impulsivity, PTSD, and violence risk. *Journal Nervous & Mental Disease, 193*(6), 405–411.

Feng, J. Y., Fetzer, S., Chen, Y. W., Yeh, L., & Huang, M. C. (2010). Multidisciplinary collaboration reporting child abuse: A grounded theory study. *International Journal of Nursing Studies, 47*(12), 1483–1490.

Ferguson, K. M. (2009). Exploring family environment characteristics and multiple abuse experiences among homeless youth. *Journal of Interpersonal Violence, 24*(11), 1875–1891.

Findling, R. L. (2008). Atypical antipsychotic treatment of disruptive behavior disorders in children and adolescents. *Journal of Clinical Psychiatry, 69*(Suppl. 4), 9–14.

Finkelhor, D., & Yllo, K. (1985). *License to rape: Sexual abuse of wives*. New York, NY: Rinehart & Winston.

Flaherty, E. G., & Sege, R. (2005). Barriers to physician identification and reporting of child abuse. *Pediatric Annals, 34*(5), 349–356.

Flaherty, E. G., Sege, R., Binns, H. J., Mattson, C. L., & Christoffel, K. K. (2000). Health care providers' experience reporting child abuse in the primary care setting. Pediatric Practice Research Group. *Archives of Pediatric &Adolescent Medicine, 154*(5), 489–493.

Flannery, R. B., Jr. (2004). Characteristics of staff victims of psychiatric patient assaults: Updated review of findings, 1995–2001. [Review]. *American Journal of Alzheimer's Disease and Other Dementias, 19*(1), 35–38.

Foster, C. S. (2011). Steven-Johnson syndrome. *Medscape Reference*. Retrieved from http://emedicine.medscape.com/article/1197450-overview

Foubert, J. D., Godin, E. E., & Tatum, J. L. (2010). In their own words: sophomore college men describe attitude and behavior changes resulting from a rape prevention program 2 years after their participation. *Journal of interpersonal violence, 25*(12), 2237–2257. doi: 10.1177/0886260509354881

Freehill, K. M. (1992). Critical incident stress debriefing in health care. [Review]. *Critical Care Clinics, 8*(3), 491–500.

Friere, P. (1970, 2003). *Pedagogy of the Oppressed*. New York: The Continuum International Publishing Group.

García-Moreno, C., Jansen, H. A., Ellsberg, M., & Watts, L. H. (2005). *WHO multi-country study on women's health and domestic violence against women: Initial results on prevalence, health outcomes and women's responses*. Retrieved from http://www.who.int/gender/violence/who_multicountry_study/en/

Gardner, A., Kaplan, B.J., Rucklidge, J.J., Jonsson, B.H., & Humble, M.B. (2010). Potential of nutrition therapy. *Science, 327*, 268.

Garrett, L. H. (2011). Sexual assault in the workplace. *AAOHN: official journal of the American Occupational Health Nurses Association, 59*(1), 15–22. doi: 10.3928/0891062–20101216–02

Gates, D. M., Ross, C. S., & McQueen, L. (2006). Violence against emergency department workers. [Multicenter Study Research Support, Non-US Gov't Research Support, US Gov't, P.H.S.]. *Journal of Emergency Medicine*, 31(3), 331–337. doi: 10.1016/j.jemermed.2005.12.028

George, D. T., Philips, M. J., Lifshitz, M. Lionetti, T. A., Spero, D. E., Ghassemzedeh, N.,…Rawlings, R. R. (2011). Fluoxetine treatment of alcoholic perpetrators of domestic violence: A 12-week, double-blind, randomized, placebo-controlled intervention study. *Journal of Clinical Psychiatry, 72*(1), 60–65. doi: 10.4088/JCP.09m05256gry

Gerlock, A. A., Grimsey, J. L., Pisciotta, A. K., & Harel, O. (2011). Ask a few more questions. *American Journal of Nursing, 111*(11), 35–39.

Gerwitz, A. H., DeGarmo, D. S., & Medhanie, A. (2011). Effects of mother's parenting practices on child internalizing trajectories following partner violence. *Journal of Family Psychology, 25*(1), 29–38.

Gesch, B. (2009). The theory? Diet causes violence? The lab? Prison. *Science, 325*(Sept. 25), 1614–1616.

Gibbon, S., Duggan, C., Stoffers, J., Huband, N., Vollm, B. A., Ferriter, M., & Lieb, K. (2010). Psychological interventions for antisocial personality disorder. *Cochrane Database of Systematic Reviews, 16*(6), Art. no.: CD007668.

Glassman, A. H. & Bigger, J. T., Jr. (2001). Antipsychotic drugs: Prolonged QTc interval, torsade de pointes, and sudden death. *American Journal of Psychiatry, 158*(11), 1774–1782.

Goldshtrom,Y., Korman, D., Goldshtrom, I., & Bendavid, J. (2011). The effect of rhythmic exercises on cognition and behavior of maltreated children: A pilot study. *Journal of Bodywork and Movement Therapies, 15*(3), 326–334. doi: 10.1016/j.jbmt.2010.06.006

Haddad, P. M., & Wieck, A. (2004). Antipsychotic-induced hyperprolactinaemia: Mechanisms, clinical features and management. *Drugs, 64*(20), 2291–2314.

Haddock, G., Barrowclough, C., Shaw, J. J., Dunn, G., Novac, R. W., & Tarrier, N. (2009). Cognitive-behavioural therapy v. social activity therapy for people with psychosis and a history of violence: Randomised controlled trial. *British Journal of Psychiatry, 194*(2), 152–157. Doi: 10.1192/bjp.bp.107.039859

Hansen, A., Hogh, A., & Persson, R. (2011). Frequency of bullying at work, physiological responses, and mental health. *Journal of Psychosomatic Research, 70*, 19–27.

Hartvig, P., Roaldset, J. O., Moger, T., Ostberg, B., & Bjorkly, S. (2011). The first step in the validation of a new screen for violence risk in acute psychiatry: The inpatient context. *European Psychiatry, 26*(2), 92–99. doi: 10.1016/j.eurpsy.2010.01.003

Hatch-Maillette, M. A., Scalora, M. J., Bader, S. M., & Bornstein, B. H. (2007). A gender-based incidence study of workplace violence in psychiatric and forensic settings. *Violence& Victims, 22*(4), 449–462.

Hazen A. L., Connelly C. D., Kelleher K., Landsverk J., & Barth R. (2004). Intimate partner violence among female caregivers of children reported for child maltreatment. *Child Abuse &Neglect*, 28, 301–319.

Herbert, P. B.Y., K.A. (2002). Tarasoff at twenty-five. *Journal of the American Academy of Psychiatry Law, 30*, 275–281.

Here's how to prevent assaults on staff. (2001). *ED Management: the Monthly Update on Emergency Department Management, 13*(6, Suppl. 1–2), 66–69.

Hines, D. A., & Douglas, E. M. (2010). Intimate terrorism by women toward men: Does it exist? *Journal of Aggressive Conflict & Peace Research, 2*(3), 35–56. doi: 10.5042/jacpr.2010.0335

Ho, J., Ralston, D. C., McCullough, L. B., & Coverdale, J. H. (2009). When should psychiatrists seek criminal prosecution of assaultive psychiatric inpatients? [Review]. *Psychiatric Services, 60*(8), 1113–1117. doi: 10.1176/appi.ps.60.8.1113

Hodge, D. R. (2008). Sexual Trafficking in the United States: A Domestic Problem with Transnational Dimensions. *Social Work, 53*(2), 143–152.

Hodgins, S., Cree, A., Alderton, J., & Mak, T. (2008). From conduct disorder to severe mental illness: Associations with aggressive behaviour, crime and victimization. [Research Support, Non-US Gov't]. *Psychological Medicine, 38*(7), 975–987. doi: 10.1017/S0033291707002164

Huband, N., Ferriter, M., Nathan, R., & Jones, H. (2010). Antiepileptics for aggression and associated impulsivity. (Review). *Cochrane Database of Systematic Reviews*, (2), Art no.: CD003499.

Hung, S. I., Chung, W. W., Jee, S. H., Chen, W. W., Chang, Y. T., Lee, W. R,...Chen, Y. t. (2006). Genetic susceptibility to carbamazepine-induced cutaneous adverse drug reactions. [Comparative Study Research Support, Non-US Gov't]. *Pharmacogenetics and Genomics, 16*(4), 297–306. doi: 10.1097/01.fpc.0000199500.46842.4a

Ipser, J., & Stein, D. J. (2007). Systematic review of pharmacotherapy of disruptive behavior disorders in children and adolescents. *Psychopharmacology, 191*(1), 127–140.

Jacobs, J., Horne-Moyer, H. L., & Jones, R. (2004). The effectiveness of critical incident stress debriefing with primary and secondary trauma victims. *International Journal of Emergency Mental Health, 6*(1), 5–14.

Janowsky, D. S., Barnhill, L. J., & Davis, J. M. (2003). Olanzapine for self-injurious, aggressive, and disruptive behaviors in intellectually disabled adults: A retrospective, open-label, naturalistic trial. *Journal of Clinical Psychiatry, 64*(10), 1258–1265.

Janowsky, D. S., Kraus, J. E., Barnhill, L. J., Elamir, B., & Davis, J. M. (2003). Effects of topiramate on aggressive, self-injurious, and disruptive/destructive behaviors in the intellectually disabled: An open-label retrospective study. *Journal of Clinical Psychopharmacology, 23*(5), 500–504.

Johnson, S. L. (2009). International perspectives on workplace bullying among nurses: A review. *International Nursing Review, 56*(1), 34–40. doi: 10.1111/j.1466–7657.2008.00679.x

Johnson, S., & Rea, R. (2009). Workplace bullying: Concerns for nurse leaders. *Journal of Nursing Administration, 39*, 84–90.

Kelly, U. A. (2009). "I'm a mother first": The influence of mothering in the decision-making processes of battered immigrant Latino women. *Research in Nursing & Health, 32*(3), 286–297. doi: 10.1002/nur.20327

Kennedy, J., Bresler, S., Whitaker, A., & Masterson, B. (2007). Assessing violence risk in psychiatric inpatients: Useful tools. *Psychiatric Times, 24*(8), 1–9.

Khalifeh, H., & Dean, K. (2010). Gender and violence against people with severe mental illness. *International Review of Psychiatry, 22*(5), 535–546.

Klomek, A. B., Marrocco, F., Kleinman, M., Schonfeld, I. S., & Gould, M. S. (2007). Bullying, depression, and suicidality in adolescents. *Journal of the American Academy of Child and Adolescent Psychiatry, 46*(1), 40–49.

Kotrla, K. (2010). Domestic minor sex trafficking in the United States. *Social Work 55*(2), 181–187.

Kowalski, R., Limber, S., & Agatson, P. (2008). *Cyber bullying: Bullying in the digital sage.* Malden, MA: Blackwell.

Lakhan, S. E., &.Vieira, K. F (2008). Nutritional therapies for mental disorders. *Nutrition Journal*, 7(2). doi:10.1186/1475-2891-7-2.

Lane, S. D., Gowin, J. L., Green, C. E., Steinberg, J. L., Moeller, F.G., & Cherek, D. R. (2009). Acute topiramate differentially affects human aggressive responding at low vs. moderate doses in subjects with histories of substance abuse and antisocial behavior. *Pharmacology and Biochemical Behavior, 92*(2), 357–362. doi: 10.1016/j.pbb.2009.01.002

Lang, A. J., Schnurr, P. P., Jain, S., Raman, R., Walser R., Bolton, E. … Benedek. D. (2012). Evaluating transdiagnostic treatment for distress and impairment in veterans: A multi-site randomized controlled trial of acceptance and commitment therapy. *Contemporary Clinical Trials, 33*(1), 116–123. doi:10.1016/j.cct.2011.08.007

Lee, Y. S. & Hadeed, L. (2009). Intimate partner violence among Asian immigrant communities: Health/mental health consequences, help-seeking behaviors, and service utilization. *Trauma Violence & Abuse, 10*(2), 143–170.

Lee, J., Kim, J., & Lim, H. (2010). Rape myth acceptance among Korean college students: The roles of gender, attitudes toward women, and sexual double standard. *Journal of Interpersonal Violence, 25*(7), 1200–1223. doi: 10.1177/0886260509340536

Lehmann, L., McCormick, R., & Kizer, K. (1999). A survey of assaultive behavior in veterans health administration facilities. [Multicenter Study]. *Psychiatric Services, 50*(3), 384–389.

Levine, P. A. (1997). *Waking the Tiger Healing Trauma*, (pp. 193–220). Berkeley: North Atlantic Books.

Levine, J. M. (2003). Elder neglect and abuse: A primer for primary care physicians. *Geriatrics, 58*(10), 37–44.

Lindert, J., Ehrenstein, O.S., Priebe, S., Mielck, A., & Brähler, E. (2009). Depression and anxiety in labor migrants and refugees—A systematic review and meta-analysis. *Social Science & Medicine, 69*(2), 246–257. doi: 10.1016/j.socscimed.2009.04.032

Longo, J. (2007). Horizontal violence among nursing students. *Archives of Psychiatric Nursing, 21,* 177–178.

Lopez-Leon, M., & Rosner, R. (2010). Intellectual quotient of juveniles evaluated in a forensic psychiatry clinic after committing a violent crime. *Journal of Forensic Sciences, 55*(1), 229–231. doi: 10.1111/j.1556–4029.2009.01225.x

Low Dog, T. (2010). The role of nutrition in mental health. *Alternative Therapies, 16*(2), 42–46.

Mahoney, B. S. (1991). The extent, nature and response to victimization of emergency room nurses in Pennsylvania. *Journal of Emergency Nursing, 17*(5) 282–294.

Maize, V. (2007, Jan). What's there to eat? An anti-inflammatory approach to healthy nutrition. Symposium conducted at the 6th Annual Women's Mental Health Program, Tucson, AZ.

Mansur, A. T., Yaşar, Ş. P., & Göktay, F. (2008). Anticonvulsant hypersensitivity syndrome: Clinical and laboratory features. *International Journal of Dermatology, 47*(11), 1184–1189. doi: 10.1111/j.1365–4632.2008.03827.x

Marshall, G. A., & Furr, L. A. (2010). Factors that affect women's attitudes toward domestic violence in Turkey. *Violence and Victims, 25*(2), 265–277.

Mattingly, B. B., & Small, A. D. (2011). Chemical restraint. *Medscape Reference.* Retrieved from http://emedicine.medscape.com/article/109717-overview

Mauri, M. C., Rovera, C., Paletta, S., De Gaspari, I. F., Maffini, M., & Altamura. A. C. (2011). Aggression and psychopharmacological treatments in major psychosis and personality disorders during hospitalisation. *Progress in Neuro-Psychopharmacology & Bioliological Psychiatry, 35*(7), 1631–1635. Retrieved from http://www.sciencedirect.com/science/article/pii/S0278584611001606.

Meehan, K., Zhang, F., David, S., Tohen, M., Janicak, P., Small, J.,…Breier, A. (2001). A double-blind, randomized comparison of the efficacy and safety of intramuscular injections of olanzapine, lorazepam, or placebo in treating acutely agitated patients diagnosed with bipolar mania. *Journal of Clinical Psychopharmacology, 21*(4), 389–397.

Miller, L. (1999). Critical incident stress debriefing: Clinical applications and new directions. [Review]. *International Journal of Emergency Mental Health, 1*(4), 253–265.

Miller, M. A., Kummerow, A. M., & Mgutshini, T. (2010) Othello Syndrome. *Journal of Psychosocial Nursing and Mental Health Services, 48*, 20–27. doi: 10.3928/02793695–201000701–05.

Miranda, J. K., de la Osa, N., Granero, R., & Ezpeleta, L. (2011). Maternal experiences of childhood abuse and intimate partner violence: Psychopathology and functional impairment in clinical children and adolescents. *Child Abuse & Neglect, 35*(9), 700–711. doi: 10.1016/j.chiabu.2011.05.008

Mitchell, A. M., Sakraida, T. J., & Kameg, K. (2003). Critical incident stress debriefing: Implications for best practice. [Review]. *Disaster Management & Response: DMR: An Official Publication of the Emergency Nurses Association, 1*(2), 46–51. doi:10.1016/S1540–2487(03)00008–7

Mitrou, F., Gaude, J., Lawrence, D., Silburn, S., Stanley, R., & Zubrick, S. (2010). Antecedents of hospital admission for deliberate self-harm from a 14-year follow-up study using date-linkage. *BMC Psychiatry,* doi:10.1186/1471–244X-10–82, Retrieved from http://www.biomedcentral.com/1471–244X/10/82

Merriam-Webster Online Dictionary Thesaurus. (2011). Merriam-Webster Retrieved from http://www.merriam-webster.com/

Mockenhaupt, M., Messenheimer, J., Tennis, P., & Schlingmann, J. (2005). Risk of Stevens-Johnson syndrome and toxic epidermal necrolysis in new users of antiepileptics. [Research Support, Non-US Gov't]. *Neurology, 64*(7), 1134–1138. doi: 10.1212/01.WNL.0000156354.20227.F0

Monk-Turner, E., & Light, D. (2010). Male sexual assault and rape: Who seeks counseling? *Sexual Abuse: A Journal of Research and Treatment, 22*(3), 255–265. doi: 10.1177/1079063210366271

Mueser, K., Crocker, A., Frisman, L., Drake, R., Covell, N., & Essock, S. (2006). Conduct disorder and antisocial personality disorder in persons with severe psychiatric and substance use disorders. [Comparative Study Multicenter Study]

Neely, K. W., & Spitzer, W. J. (1997). A model for a statewide critical incident stress (CIS) debriefing program for emergency services personnel. *Prehospital and disaster medicine: the Official Journal of the National Association of EMS Physicians and the World Association for Emergency and Disaster Medicine in Association with the Acute Care Foundation, 12*(2), 114–119.

Nelson, A., Lewy, R., Ricardo, F., Dovydaitis, T., Hunter, A., Mitchell, A., Loe, C., Kugel, C. (2010). Eliciting behavior change in a US sexual violence and intimate partner violence prevention program through utilization of Freire and discussion facilitation. *Health Promot Int, 25*(3), 299–308. doi: 10.1093/heapro/daq024

Neuhut, R., Lindenmayer, J. P., & Silva, R. (2009). Neuroleptic malignant syndrome in children and adolescents on atypical antipsychotic medication: A review. *Journal of Child and Adolescent Psychopharmacology, 19*(4), 415–422.

Nickerson, A., & Hinton, D. E. (2011). Anger regulation in traumatized Cambodian refugees: the perspectives of Buddhist monks. *Culture Medicine & Psychiatry, 35*(3), 396–416. doi: 10.1007/s11013-011-9218-y

Nigg, J. T., & Breslau, N. (2007). Prenatal smoking exposure, low birth weight, and disruptive behavior disorders. *Journal of the American Academy of Child and Adolescent Psychiatry, 46*(3), 362–369. doi:10.1097/01.chi.0000246054.76167.44

Odgers, C. L., Caspi, A., Broadbent, J. M., Dickson, N., Hancox, R. J., Harrington, H. L.,... Moffitt, T. E. (2007). Prediction of differential adult health burden by conduct problem subtypes in males. *Archives of General Psychiatry, 64*, 476–484. Retrieved from http://archpsyc.ama-assn.org/cgi/reprint/64/4/476

Palazzolo, K. E., Roberto, A.J., & Babin, E.A. (2010). The relationship between parents' verbal aggression and young adult children's intimate partner violence victimization and perpetration. *Health Communication, 25*, 357–324. doi: DOI: 10.1080/10410231003775180

Petersen, R., Moracco, K.E., Goldstein, K.M. & Clark, K.A. (2005). Moving Beyond Disclosure: Women's Perspectives on Barriers and Motivators to Seeking Assistance for Intimate Partner Violence. *Women & Health, 40*(3), 63–76. doi: 10.1300/J013v40n03_05

Phillips, L. R. (1986). Caring for the frail elderly at home: Toward a theoretical explanation of the dynamics of poor quality family caregiving. *Advances in Nursing Science, 8*(4), 62–84.

Pillemer, K., & Moore, D. W. (1989). Abuse of patients in nursing homes: findings from a survey of staff. *Gerontologist, 29*(3), 14–20. doi: 10.1093/geront/29.3.314

Pilowsky, D. J., Wickramaratne, P., Talati, A., Tang, M., Hughes, C. W., Garber, J.,...Weissman, M. M. (2008). Children of depressed mothers 1 year after the initiation of maternal treatment: Findings from the STAR*D-Child Study. *American Journal of Psychiatry, 165*(9), 1136–1147. doi: 10.1176/appi.ajp.2008.07081286

Ponniah, K., & Hollon, S. D. (2009). Empirically supported psychological treatments for adult acute stress disorder and posttraumatic stress disorder: A review. *Depression and Anxiety, 26*(12), 1086–1109. doi: 10.1002/da.20635

Poster, E. C. (1996). A multinational study of psychiatric nursing staffs' beliefs and concerns about work safety and patient assault. *Archives of Psychiatric Nursing, 10*(6), 365–373. doi: 10.1016/s0883-9417(96)80050-1

Postmus, J. L., Severson, M., Berry, M., & Yoo, J. A. (2009). Women's experiences of violence and seeking help. *Violence Against Women, 15*(7), 852–868. doi 10.1177/1077801209334445

Quanbeck, C. (2006). Forensic psychiatric aspects of inpatient violence. [Review]. *Psychiatric Clinics of North America, 29*(3), 743–760. doi: 10.1016/j.psc.2006.04.011

Quanbeck, C., McDermott, B., Lam, J., Eisenstark, H., Sokolov, G. & Scott, C. (2007). Categorization of aggressive acts committed by chronically assaultive state hospital patients. *Psychiatric Services, 58*(4), 521–528. doi: 10.1176/appi.ps.58.4.521

Quinn, A., & Shera, W. (2009). Evidence-based practice in group work with incarcerated youth. *International Journal of Law & Psychiatry, 32*(5), 288–293. doi: 10.1016/j.ijlp.2009.06.002

RAINN (Rape Abuse and Incest National Network) (2012). Statistics. Retrieved from raiin.or/statistics

Regel, S. (2007). Post-trauma support in the workplace: the current status and practice of critical incident stress management (CISM) and psychological debriefing (PD) within organizations in the UK. [Review]. *Occupational Medicine, 57*(6), 411–416. doi: 10.1093/occmed/kqm071

Reif, A., Jacob, C., Rujescu, D., Herterich, S., Lang, S., Gutknecht, S.,... Lesch, K-P. (2009). Influence of functional variant of neuronal nitric oxide synthase on impulsive behaviors in humans. *Archives of General Psychiatry, 66*(1), 41–50. doi: 10.1001/archgenpsychiatry.2008.510

Reilly, P., & Shopshire, M. (2002). *Anger Management for Substance Abuse and Mental Health Clients: A Cognitive Behavioral Therapy Manual*. DHHS Pub. No. (SMA) 02-3661. Rockville, MD: Center for Substance Abuse Treatment, Substance Abuse and Mental Health Services Administration, 2002. Retrieved from http://kap.samhsa.gov/products/manuals/pdfs/anger1.pdf

Richter, D., & Berger, K. (2006). Post-traumatic stress disorder following patient assaults among staff members of mental health hospitals: A prospective longitudinal study. [Comparative Study Research Support, Non-US Gov't]. *BMC Psychiatry, 6*(15). doi: 10.1186/1471-244X-6-15

Riediger, N. D., Othman, R. A., Suh, M., & Moghadasian, M. H. (2009). A systemic review of the roles of n-3 fatty acids in health and disease. *Journal of the American Dietetic Association, 109*(4), 668–679.

Rodriguez, C. M. (2010). Parent-child aggression: association with child abuse potential and parenting styles. *Violence and Victims, 25*(6), 728–741.

Rodriguez, M., Valentine, J. M., Son, J. B., & Muhhammad, M. (2009). Intimate partner violence and barriers to mental health care for ethnically diverse populations of women. *Trauma Violence & Abuse, 10*(4), 358–374. doi: 10.1177/1524838009339756

Rudolph, K. D., Troop-Gordon, W., Hessel, E. T., & Schmidt, J. D. (2011). A latent growth curve analysis of early and increasing peer victimization as predictors of mental health across elementary school. *Journal of Clinical Child & Adolescent Psychology, 40*(1), 111–122. doi: 10.1080/15374416.2011.533413

Rueve, M. E., & Welton, R. S. (2008). Violence and mental illness. *Psychiatry, 5*(5), 34–48. Retrieved from http://www.ncbi.nlm.nih.gov/pmc/articles/PMC2686644/pdf/PE_5_5_34.pdf

Rutter, M., & Silberg, J. (2002). Gene-environment interplay in relation to emotional and behavioral disturbance. [Review]. *Annual Review of Psychology*, (53), 463–490. doi: 10.1146/annurev.psych.53.100901.135223

Sadock, B. J., & Sadock V. A. (Eds.). (2007). *Kaplan & Sadock's Synopsis of Psychiatry*. New York, NY: Lippincott, Williams & Wilkins.

Salari, S. (2007). Patterns of intimate partner homicide suicide in later life: strategies for prevention. *Clinical Interventions in Aging, 2*(3), 441–452.

SAMHSA. (2005). *Roadmap to Seclusion and Restraint-Free Mental Health Services*. Retrieved from http://store.samhsa.gov/product/Roadmap-to-Seclusion-and-Restraint-Free-Mental-Health-Services-CD-/SMA06-4055. Retrieved from http://store.samhsa.gov/shin/content/SMA06-4055/SMA06-4055-H.pdf

Schott, R. M. (2011). War rape, natality and genocide. *Journal of Genocide Research, 13*(1–2), 5–21.

Schwartz, T. L., & Park, T. L. (1999). Assaults by patients on psychiatric residents: A survey and training recommendations. [Multicenter Study]. *Psychiatric Services, 50*(3), 381–383.

Scott, K. M., Von Korff, M., Angermeyer, M. C., Benjet, C., Bruffaerts, R., de Girolamo, G.,….Kessler, R. C. (2011). Association of childhood adversities and early-onset mental disorders with adult-onset chronic physical conditions. *Archives of General Psychiatry, 68*(8), 838–844.

Sechrest, D. (2011, Apr.2). *How to keep your smartphone safe from cyber stalkers: Androids, IPhones, and their invisible GPS trails.* [Online forum content Yahoo]. Retrieved from http://www.associatedcontent.com/article/7907031/how_to_keep_your_smartphone_safe_from_pg2.html?cat=59

Sexton, T., & Turner, C. W. (2010). The effectiveness of functional family therapy for youth with behavioral problems in a community practice setting. *Journal of Family Psychology, 24*(3), 339–348. doi: 10.1037/a0019406

Sibinga, E. M., Kerrigan, D., Steward, M. Johnson, K., Magyari, M. S., & Ellen, J. M. (2011). Mindfulness-based stress reduction for urban youth. *Journal of Alternative & Complementary Medicine, 17*(3), 213–218. doi: 10.1089/acm.2009.0605

Sijbrandij, M., Olff, M., Reitsma, J. B., Carlier, I. V., & Gersons, B. P. (2006). Emotional or educational debriefing after psychological trauma: Randomised controlled trial, *British Journal of Psychiatry, 189*, 150–155. doi: 10.1192/bjp.bp.105.021121. Retrieved from http://bjp.rcpsych.org/cgi/content/full/189/2/150

Simon, R. (2011). Patient violence against health care professionals: Safety assessment and management. *Psychiatric Times, 28*(2), 1–8.

Soderstrom, H., Blennow, K., Manhem, A., & Forsman, A. (2001a). CSF studies in violent offenders. I. 5-HIAA as a negative and HVA as a positive predictor of psychopathy. [Research Support, Non-US Gov't]. *Journal of Neural Transmission,* 108(7), 869–878. doi: 10.1007/s007020170037

Soderstrom, H., Blennow, K., Manhem, A., & Forsman, A. (2001b). CSF studies in violent offenders. II. Blood-brain barrier dysfunction without concurrent inflammation or structure degeneration. [Comparative Study Research Support, Non-US Gov't]. *Journal of Neural Transmission, 108*(7), 879–886. doi: 10.1007/s007020170036

Solnick, S. J., & Hemenway, D. (2011). The 'Twinkie Defense': The relationship between carbonated non-diet soft drinks and violence perpetration among Boston high school students. *Injury Prevention*, epub 10/26/11 ahead of print. 10.1136/injuryprev-2011–040117

Sonnier, L., & Barzman, D. H. (2011). Pharmacologic management of acutely agitated pediatric patients. *Pediatric Drugs, 13*(1), 1–10.

Stahl, S. M. (2009). *The prescriber's guide, Stahl's essential psychopharmacology.* (3rd ed.). New York, NY: Cambridge University.

Stanford, M. S., Houston, R. J., Mathias, C. W., Villemarette-Pittman, N. R., Helfritz, L. E., & Conklin, S. M. (2003). Characterizing aggressive behavior. [Research Support, Non-US Gov't]. *Assessment, 10*(2), 183–190. doi: 10.1177/1073191103010002009

Suchman, N. E., DeCoste, C., Castiflioni, N., McMahon, T.J., Rounsaville, B., & Mayes, L. (2010). The Mothers and Toddlers Program, an attachment-based parenting intervention for substance using women: Posttreatment results from a randomized clinical pilot. *Attachment in Human Development, 12*(5), 483–504. doi: 10.1080/14616734.2010.501983.

Susman, V. L. (2001). Clinical management of neuroleptic malignant syndrome. *Psychiatric Quarterly, 72*(4), 325–336.

Susman, V. L., & Addonizio, G. (1988). Recurrence of neuroleptic malignant syndrome. *Journal of Nervous & Mental Disorders, 176*(4), 234–241.

Swan, H., & O'Connell, D. J. (2012). The impact of intimate partner violence on women's condom negotiation efficacy. *Journal of Interpersonal Violence, 27*(4), 775–792. doi: 10.1177/0886260511423240

Swanson, J. W., Swartz, M. S., Essock, S. M., Osher, F. O., Wagner, H. R. Goodman, L. A.,… Meador, K. G. (2002). The social-environmental context of violent behavior in persons treated for severe mental illness. *American Journal of Public Health, 92*(9), 1523–1531. Retrieved from http://ajph.aphapublications.org/cgi/reprint/92/9/1523.

Swanson, J. W., Swartz, M. S., Van Dorn, R. A., Elbogen, E. B., Wagner, H. R., Rosenheck, R. A., & Lieberman, J. A. (2006). A national study of violent behavior in persons with schizophrenia. [Comparative Study Multicenter Study Randomized Controlled Trial Research Support, N.I.H., Extramural Research Support, Non-US Gov't]. *Archives of General Psychiatry, 63*(5), 490–499. doi: 10.1001/archpsyc.63.5.490. Retrieved from http://archpsyc.ama-assn.org/cgi/reprint/63/5/490

Tackett, J., Krueger, R., Iacono, W., & McGue, M. (2005). Symptom-based subfactors of DSM-defined conduct disorder: Evidence for etiologic distinctions. *Journal of Abnormal Psychology, 114*(3), 483–487. doi:10.1037/0021–843X.114.3.483

Taylor, C. A., Guterman, N. B., Lee, S. J., & Rahoutz, P. J. (2009). Intimate partner violence, maternal stress, nativity, and risk for maternal maltreatment of young children. *American Journal of Public Health, 99*(1), 175–183.

Temple, J. L. (2009). Caffeine use in children: What we know, what we have left to learn, and why we should worry. *Neuroscience and Biobehavioral Reviews, 33*, 793–806. doi:10.1016/j.neubiorev.2009.01.001

Thomas, S. P., & Burk, R. (2009). Junior nursing students' experiences of vertical violence during clinical rotations. *Nursing Outlook, 57*, 226–231.

Tjaden, P., & Thoennes, N. (2000a). *Extent, nature, and consequences of intimate partner violence: Findings from the National Violence against Women Survey*. Washington, DC: US Department of Justice.

Tjaden, P., & Thoennes, N. (2000b). *Full report of the prevalence, incidence, and consequences of violence against women: Findings from the National Violence against Women Survey.* Washington, DC: US Department of Justice.

U.S. Census Bureau. (2011). Retrieved from http://www.census.gov/population/www/projections/usinterimproj/

U.S. Department of Health and Human Services, Administration for Children and Families, Administration on Children, Youth and Families, Children's Bureau. (2010). *Child Maltreatment 2009.* Retrieved from http://www.acf.hhs.gov/programs/cb/stats_research/index.htm#can.

van Goozen, S., Fairchild, G., Snoek, H., & Harold, G. T. (2007). The evidence for a neurobiological model of childhood antisocial behavior. [Research Support, Non-US Gov't Review]. *Psychological Bulletin, 133*(1), 149–182. doi: 10.1037/0033–2909.133.1.149

Veterans Administration. (2010). *VA/DoD Clinical Practice Guideline: Management of Post-traumatic Stress.* Washington

D.C.: Department of Veterans Affairs Retrieved from http://www.healthquality.va.gov/PTSD-FULL-2010c.pdf.

Virtanen, M., Vahtera, J., Batty, G. D., Tuisku, K., Pentti, J., Oksanen, T., & Kivimaki, M. (2011). Overcrowding in psychiatric wards and physical assaults on staff: Data-linked longitudinal study. *British Journal of Psychiatry, 198*(2), 149–155. doi: 10.1192/bjp.bp.110.082388

Vitiello, B., & Stoff, D. M. (1997). Subtypes of aggression and their relevance to child psychiatry. [Review]. *Journal of the American Academy of Child and Adolescent Psychiatry, 36*(3), 307–315. doi: 10.1097/00004583–199703000–00008

Von Korff, M., Alonso, J., Ormel, J., Angermeyer, M., Bruffaerts, R., Fleiz, C.,...Uda, H. (2009). Childhood psychosocial stressors and adult onset arthritis: broad spectrum risk factors and allostatic load. *Pain, 143*(1-2), 76–83. doi: 10.1016/j.pain.2009.01.034

Wade, J. F., Dang, C. V., Nelson, L., & Wasserberger, J. (2010). Emergent complications of the newer anticonvulsants. [Review]. *Journal of Emergency Medicine, 38*(2), 231–237. doi: 10.1016/j.jemermed.2008.03.032

Wagner, S. L. (2005). Emergency response service personnel and the critical incident stress debriefing debate. [Review]. *International Journal of Emergency Mental Health, 7*(1), 33–41.

Wahlund, K., & Kristiansson, M. (2009). Aggression, psychopathy and brain imaging - Review and future recommendations. *International Journal of Law & Psychiatry, 32*(4), 266–271. doi: 10.1016/j.ijlp.2009.04.007

Walcott, D. M., Cerundolo, P., & Beck, J. C. (2001). Current analysis of the Tarasoff duty: An evolution towards the limitation of duty to protect. *Behavioral Sciences and the Law, 19*, 325–343. doi: 10.1002/bsl.444

Walsh, C. A., Olson, J. L., Ploeg, J., Lohfeld, L., & MacMillan, H. L. (2011). Elder abuse and oppression: voices of marginalized elders. *Journal of Elder Abuse and Neglect, 23*(1), 17–42. doi: 10.1080/08946566.2011.534705

Warren, L. J, Mullen, P. E., & Ogloff, J. R. (2011). A clinical study of those who utter threats to kill. *Behavioral Sciences and the Law, 29*(2), 141–154. doi: 10.1002/bsl.974

Warren, L., Mullen, P., Thomas, S., Ogloff, J., & Burgess, P. (2008). Threats to kill: A follow-up study. *Psychological Medicine, 38*, 599–605/ doi: 10.1017/S003329170700181X

Wee, D. F., Mills, D. M., & Koehler, G. (1999). The effects of critical incident stress debriefing (CISD) on emergency medical services personnel following the Los Angeles Civil Disturbance. *International Journal of Emergency Mental Health, 1*(1), 33–37.

Widjicks, E. (2010). Neuroleptic malignant syndrome. *Up to Date*. Retrieved from http://www.uptodate.com/contents/neuroleptic-malignant-syndrome

Williams, W. H., Cordan, G., Mewse, A. J., Tonks, J., & Burgess, C. N. (2010). Self-reported traumatic brain injury in male young offenders: A risk factor for re-offending, poor mental health and violence? *Neuropsychological Rehabilitation, 20*(6), 801–812. doi: 10.1080/09602011.2010.519613

Wupperman, P., Marlatt, G. A., Cunningham, A., Bowen, S., Berking, M., Mulvihill-Rivera, N., & Easton, C. (2011). Mindfulness and modification therapy for behavioral dysregulation: Results from a pilot study targeting alcohol use and aggression in women. *Journal of Clinical Psychology*: Advance online publication. doi: 10.1002/jclp.20830

Yates, K., Kunz, M., Czobor, P., Rabinowitz, S., Lindenmayer, J. P., & Volavka, J. (2005). A cognitive, behaviorally based program for patients with persistent mental illness and a history of aggression, crime, or both: Structure and correlates of completers of the program. *Journal of the American Academy of Psychiatry and the Law, 33*(2), 214–222. Retrieved from http://www.jaapl.org/cgi/reprint/33/2/214

Yoshioka, M. R., DiNoia, J., & Ullah, K. (2001). Attitudes toward marital violence: an examination of four asian communities. *Violence Against Women, 7*, 900–926. doi: 10.1177/10778010122182811

Zeller, S. L., & Rhodes, R.W. (2010). Systematic reviews of assessment measures and pharmacologic treatments for agitation. *Clinical Therapeutics, 32*(3), 403–425. doi: 10.1016/j.clinthera.2010.03.006

Zimbroff, D. L. (2008). Pharmacological control of acute agitation: Focus on intramuscular preparations. [Research Support, Non-US Gov't Review]. *CNS Drugs, 22*(3), 199–212.

Zinzow, H. M., Ruggiero, K.J., Hanson, R.., Smith, D.W., Saunders, B.E., & Kilpatrick D.G. (2009). Witnessed community and parental violence in relation to substance use and delinquency in a national sample of adolescents. *Journal of Traumatic Stress, 22*(6), 525–533. doi: doi:10.1002/jts.20469.

Zlotnick, C., Capezza, N., & Parker, D. (2011). An interpersonally based intervention for low-income pregnant women with intimate partner violence: a pilot study. *Archives of Women's Mental Health, 14*(1), 55–65. doi: 10.1007/s00737-010-0195-x

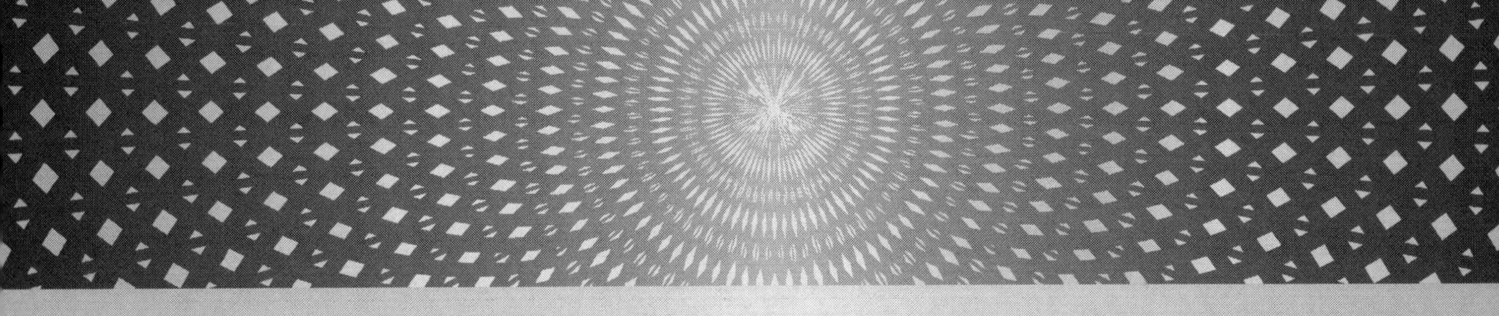

SECTION IV

Special Considerations

CHAPTER CONTENTS

Life is filled with struggle: pain, anxiety, loss, grief, illness, stress, depression; thus, altering mood is often viewed as essential. Alcoholic beverages and nicotine are commonly used to alter mood. Indeed, pharmaceutical companies are built on western medicine's practice to alter mood. Antidepressants, stimulants, anxiolytics, and analgesics all are intended to alter mood. The "problem" seen with mood-altering substances is not the use of alcohol or drugs to alter mood; it is the misuse, dependence on, and the inability to refrain from the use of the drug that is viewed as problematic.

The Substance Abuse & Mental Health Service Administration (SAMHSA) (www.samhsa.gov) and the Centers for Disease Control (cdcinfo@cdc.gov) have complete and comprehensive data available to the public on the incidence of alcohol misuse, illicit drug use, and tobacco use and the relationship of the use of these substances to mental and physical health problems among adults and adolescents. Co-occurring disorder (COD) refers to substance abuse or dependence and a mental disorder. COD is diagnosed when at least one disorder of each type exists independent of the other and is not simply a cluster of symptoms resulting from one disorder. In the late 1970s, practitioners began to recognize that the presence of substance abuse in combination with mental disorders had profound implications for treatment outcomes. This growing awareness led to today's emphasis on recognizing and addressing both disorders and

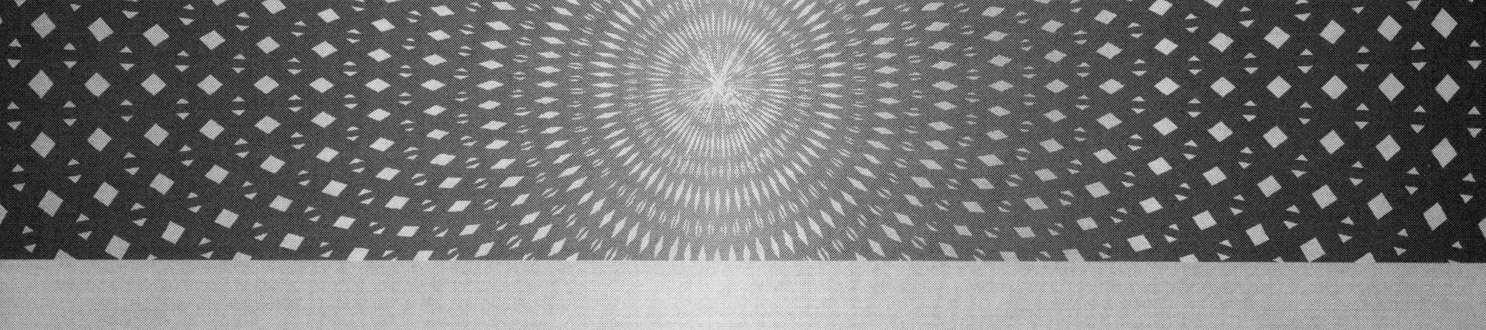

CHAPTER 17

Co-Occurring Substance Misuse and Psychiatric Syndromes

Rita Hanuschock

understanding how they interact with one another. Between 20% and 50% of clients in mental health treatment have a co-occurring substance problem.

The use of substances to alter mood in most cultures is accepted; the misuse or overuse of a substance, in some situations, is accepted. Overindulgence at a bachelor party or one's 21st birthday is acceptable. Overindulgence that is disruptive to the occasion at hand and the inability to refrain from using a substance when such use is clearly a problem are not only unaccepted . . . they carry a societal stigma. Furthermore, due to the disabilities and social costs associated with COD, an accurate understanding of the co-occurrence is vital to prevention and treatment.

DEFINITIONS

Substance misuse is defined as the excessive or otherwise abnormal way of using a substance that departs from medical and/or social norms. It is the use of a substance in a harmful manner other than its intended purpose.

One example is the college freshman who guzzles a fifth of tequila at a party; as she stumbles to the bathroom, she trips, hitting her head hard on the toilet edge. She lies unconscious on the cold tile; if not discovered in time, she will die from an intracranial bleed. Another example is the young mother who took several valium tablets and is found in deep slumber while her newborn cries in the crib.

Dependence is defined as the continued use of a substance, often with development of tolerance and rebound pain or anxiety. More of the substance may be needed for the desired effect, and withdrawal symptoms occur when the drug is stopped. Withdrawal symptoms can occur without cessation of the drug as a result of tolerance.

Opiate analgesics and benzodiazapines are the hallmark drugs that persons can become dependent on. Rebound pain, or pain far exceeding what one started out with, can be seen with dependence on oral narcotics. Likewise, rebound anxiety on large doses of benzodiazepines can occur. Of concern is that tolerance to benzodiazepines can result in seizures even while one is taking the drug.

Examples include the following: A young woman who takes increasing doses of vicodin to control pain due to multiple sclerosis; over time, she finds herself taking 4 times as many pills as she started with, yet her pain is far worse. A woman with Meniere's disease increases her dose of benzodiazepine to control worsening symptoms. She becomes concerned as to the amount she's taking. She phones her prescriber, but before getting to the appointment, she suffers a seizure. These situations exemplify dependence on a substance.

Addictive disorder is an entity in and of itself, not simply "misuse" of a drug or a "physical dependence." Addiction has many overlapping definitions and many common terms such as "Chemical Dependency" and "Substance Abuse Problem." Addiction is often considered a brain disease, as drugs and alcohol exert their mood-altering effects within the brain. Through the examination and study of the nervous system in the context of addiction, science has made strides in understanding its structure and function. Like several other chronic diseases, addiction has no specific known etiology; it has no known cure; if left untreated it can be fatal; it can be treated on a day-to-day basis, enabling a person to stay healthy; sometimes it does not respond to known treatment and a person does fall ill.

DSM-IV definitions divide Addiction into the specific substances differentiating dependence and abuse (American Psychiatric Association, 1994). One definition of Addiction is the *inability to stop* using that which is mood-altering coupled with *negative consequences* because of the use; it is when one cannot stop the use that bad things have happened or are happening. Addiction is not so much about the use of alcohol/drugs but the intrinsic inability to *stop* the use. Persons suffering with addictive disorders are *unable* to stop, even if they "really want to" and even when their life is falling apart.

Like other chronic health problems, addiction is ongoing; there is no cure; if left untreated, it could cause severe illness and be fatal; there is no absolute etiology, although as far back as antiquity it has been seen to run in families supporting a genetic predisposition; it affects not only the person suffering with it but those who love him/her: spouse, parents, family, workplace; it is stigmatized by societies, insurance companies, and health care providers (Coombs, 1997; Davies-Scimeca, 2008). And like most chronic diseases or afflictions, it can be managed. Consider a young man suffering with leukemia; in spite of treatment and temporary remission, it recurs. Insurance readily covers his continued therapy. His family and community rally in support of him. Prayers are offered for him in religious services; fundraisers are held; support overflows.

Now, consider a young man suffering with chronic addiction. In spite of a 30-day treatment program, which was *not* covered by his family's insurance plan, he relapses. His parents do not share this with anyone; there is no fundraiser; he is not eligible for county-funded treatment, as he is insured. If the addiction involves substances that are illegal, he may encounter legal problems and prison time. He may even face felonious charges. He does not enjoy getting high; he is *unable to stop*, even though he desperately wants to. He may be riddled with shame and guilt believing that he has failed; he has no one's sympathy, only their scorn.

These could be two young men from the same community; two different chronic diseases, two very different responses from family, community, and society. Neither young man asked for the disease that afflicts him. Both are desperate for it to "go away." Both may very well die from their diseases. Adding to the suffering of those with addictive disorders and feeding into societal stigma, two of the most common mood-altering substances are legal, generate substantial revenue, and provide abundant jobs: alcoholic beverages and nicotine products.

In most societies and cultures, alcoholic beverages are accepted and held in esteem. The toast to the bride and groom, the expensive bottle of fine wine as a gift, the cold beer at a ball game, the champagne to ring in the New Year—all celebrations where beverage alcohol is joyously consumed. Alcohol, a toxic substance that destroys cells and contributes to organ damage, is celebrated! If one is *unable* to stop the consumption of beverage alcohol when the situation calls for it, they are met with societal disapproval. A groomsman becoming inebriated at a bachelor party is accepted, even expected. It is not at all acceptable for that same groomsman to become inebriated and stumble down the aisle at the wedding ceremony.

Addiction to drugs and/or alcohol is *not* a bad habit. It is *not* a choice that one makes. The exact etiology of addiction is yet to be determined; there clearly is no cure for it. If left untreated it can result in death. Even with treatment, it can recur.

Comprehensive knowledge about addiction is not enough for psychiatric mental health advanced practice registered nurses (PMH-APRNs) to effectively intervene with those suffering from the disorder; understanding and compassion are needed as well.

Clinicians in all practice specialties will encounter substance abuse and addiction as well as COD. This chapter provides education on assessment of persons suffering with chemical dependency, toxic effects of mood-altering substances, the recognition and management of withdrawal symptoms, treatment modalities, and addictive disorders in special populations.

ETIOLOGY OF ADDICTIVE DISORDERS

Does the substance cause the addiction? Perhaps, but if so, why isn't everyone exposed to a substance addicted? Many persons drink alcohol, sometimes heavily; they do not all develop alcoholism. Many persons smoke marijuana in their youth; they do not all continue to use it as they mature. Many persons have snorted cocaine, even injected heroin; they do not all keep using the drug. Everyone who has major surgery is prescribed narcotic medication; some continue and are unable to stop; others stop.

Is it societal, the culture that someone grows up and lives in? Is it learned behavior as one grows up watching parents use mood-altering substances? Is it peer influence? Is it genetic? After all, addictive disorders run in families. Something seems to be "passed on," but is it a gene or something else... something yet to be discovered?

BIOCHEMICAL FACTORS

Dopamine is a neurotransmitter that is essential to our feelings of well-being and joy. When we hear our favorite song, see our favorite person, feel the tingle of love, feel the rush of spontaneous joy... it is dopamine! Research on addiction is focused on dopamine. Nora Volkow, the director of the National Institute of Drug Abuse, and her associates have done extensive research on the Dopamine 2 receptor. Consistently, her research and that of others has shown that persons suffering with addictive disorders have fewer D2 receptors than average (Rosack, 2004; Volkow et al., 1992). Questions remain. Does the person with addictive disorder have fewer D2 receptors at birth? Is the number genetically determined? Is the development of the D2 receptors adversely influenced by something else? Does the substance alter the D2 receptor? Do all persons deficient in D2 receptors develop addiction? Do persons with adequate D2 receptors ever develop addictions?

GENETIC FACTORS

Researchers repeatedly have shown that persons with a family history of alcoholism and/or drug addiction have a greater chance of developing the disorder (Cadoret, Troughton, & Woodworth, 1994; Goodwin, 2003; Leshner, 2003; O'Brien, 2008; Schuckit, 2003).

Understandably, the gene and its multiple alleles responsible for the development of the D2 receptor is the focus of much research (O'Brien, 2008). Additionally, the gene responsible for the development of the opiate mu receptor has also been researched. When an opiate innervates the mu receptor, an increase in dopamine occurs. While no specific gene has been found to cause addiction, researchers are learning a tremendous amount about the human nervous system (Leshner, 2003).

OTHER FACTORS

Neurological, metabolic, and psychosocial causes have all been suspected and researched as being the etiology of the development of the inability to stop the use of a mood-altering substance. Many clinicians and recovering addicts firmly believe that the cause is rooted in a person's spiritual core (S. Strobbe, personal communication, October 10, 2009). The many research studies on the determinants of developing alcohol and drug addiction are vast and extensive. However, in clinical practice, the simple answer to addiction's etiology is that it is caused by multiple and complex biopsychosocial determinants (R. Kump, personal communication, September 20, 2011).

CONCORDANCE

Engaging the individual with a substance use problem in addition to an independent psychiatric problem can be very challenging. Your own beliefs about addictions and abuse require examination to allow for welcoming and competent relationship building. In addition to basic relationship building, the client is usually hesitant and guarded. Therefore, taking information in a matter-of-fact style and not challenging it is vital to this process of engagement. Of course, engagement is necessary before moving on to stabilization, primary treatment, recovery, and relapse prevention. Developing a treatment plan is a process between the PMH-APRN and the person seeking treatment. The path of treatment is dependent on the unique situation presented and the practice situation.

Understanding the individual's current stage of change and matching interventions based on Motivational Interviewing (Rollnick, Miller, & Butler, 2008) is recommended. The stages include the following:

- No problem and/or no interest in change (Precontemplation).
- Might be a problem; might consider change (Contemplation).
- Definitely a problem; getting ready to change (Preparation).
- Actively working on changing, even if slowly (Action).

The spirit of Motivational Interviewing does not include confrontation and lecturing but collaboration, evocation, and honoring autonomy. Collaboration is based upon the realization that the client is ultimately responsible for enacting change and joint decisions are necessary. Evocation brings forth the client's reasons and arguments against change. Remember that ambivalence about change is expected and needs to be processed, not labeled as resistance. Honoring the client's autonomy involves detaching from your own goals and respecting and recognizing the client's goals.

The guiding principles include resisting the righting reflex, understanding, listening, and empowering. Avoid lecturing and educating on the right way. Instead process current ambivalence and together discover and develop what is most appropriate for this client at this time. Understanding and listening to the client's perceptions and appreciating that client's concerns, values, and personal motivations as unique and important is necessary for change to occur. Empowering the client is a process of identifying and exploring the client's strengths and resources available for change. By following the spirit and principles of Motivational Interviewing, PMH-APRNs can assist individuals with COD in planning to change patterns.

EXPECTED OUTCOMES

Although the specific outcomes are individualized following an assessment, there are general expectations related to substance use and psychiatric problems. Short-term outcomes include the following:

- Adhere to plan of treatment for psychiatric syndromes
- Provide safety and medical stabilization
- Engage in and develop therapeutic relationship
- Participate in and complete thorough assessment
- Decrease level of denial
- Verbalize increased understanding of substance abuse/addiction
- Verbalize desire to change
- Identify and make changes in lifestyle to facilitate change

Longer-term outcomes following engagement and stabilization are focused upon recovery and relapse prevention and may include the following:

- Establish a continuing quality of life free from substance abuse/addiction
- Develop awareness of relapse triggers and coping strategies to deal with them
- Develop a meaningful social support system
- Learn and implement expanded positive coping strategies to deal with stress as well as urges to lapse back into chemical use.

EFFECTS OF THE SUBSTANCE AND TOXICITY

This section includes the actions and toxicity of commonly abused substances. This information is important for assessment including triage as well as treatment of individuals with COD.

ETHYL ALCOHOL: C_2H_5OH

This small molecule consisting of two carbon atoms, five hydrogen atoms, and a hydroxyl group is toxic to living cells (Korsten & Lieber, 1992). It is the key ingredient is in all forms of beverage alcohol: beer, wine, whiskey, liquor, sherry. Concentrations are different; the molecule is the same.

Alcohol does not have its own receptor site in the human body, at least not one that is yet known. It does, however, seem to attach to the nerve cell next to the gaba aminobutyric (GABA) and glycine receptors (Welch & Martin, 2003). This close proximal innervention opens chloride channels. Negatively charged chloride ions (Cl^-) rush into the neuron, subsequently relaxing it. It takes positively charged potassium and sodium to create an action potential; with a negative interior, the nerve and the person are relaxed. When alcohol is ingested on a daily basis, the neuron adjusts to this; when alcohol intake is abruptly stopped, the neuron becomes hyperexcited, thus the state of withdrawal.

Alcohol also seems to affect the opiate mu receptor in some individuals, causing an increase in extracellular dopamine in one of the brain's pleasure centers, the nucleus accumbens. This may be responsible for alcohol's ability to create euphoria (O'Brien, 2008).

Alcohol Toxicity. When one receives an injection, the skin is first wiped with an alcohol-saturated swab, to kill germs on the skin's surface. Disinfecting countertops can be effectively done with alcohol. Be it isopropyl or ethyl alcohol, the effect is the same.

C_2H_5OH is a toxic molecule. When it comes into contact with living cells, be they human organ cells or microbes, it reacts chemically by attracting a molecule of water out of the cell. Cells need their water. When this microscopic chemical dance takes place, a cell could die. This dehydrating effect happens with all forms of beverage alcohol to a lesser or greater degree. When human cells dehydrate, irritation first occurs, with subsequent death of the cell.

Imagine dribbling vodka over your hand for a prolonged period of time. First, the skin will redden, then become irritated and excoriated. When one drinks beverage alcohol, the effect is somewhat the same to all tissues bathed in the alcohol. This toxic effect leads to tissue damage, cell death, and scar formation.

Mucosal lining of the mouth, throat, and esophagus can become irritated and friable. Mouth, tongue, and throat cancers can occur, especially when combined with nicotine and the products of nicotine combustion. Irritation of the esophagus makes it friable and vulnerable to the development of varices. Gastic ulceration can occur (Korsten & Lieber, 1992).

Nerve tissue in the brain and periphery can be affected. Peripheral neuropathy from direct contact with alcohol and from alcohol-related vitamin B1 deficiency can lead to pain and the inability to walk. Brain volume shrinks; cerebellar damage can be irreversible, resulting in gait disturbances.

Cognitive functioning declines from the alcohol's direct damage to brain cells. In the presence of alcohol and in the withdrawal state, the body is unable to absorb thiamine (vitamin B1) adequately. As previously mentioned, this contributes to peripheral nerve damage (Victor, 1992).

Within the brain, thiamine deficiency can result in a neurological syndrome termed Wernicke–Korsakoff. Wernicke presents with nystagmus, ataxia, paralysis of ocular muscles, confusion, somnolence, and apathy. Korsakoff presents with profound loss of retentive memory out of proportion to other cognitive impairments in an otherwise alert and responsive person (Victor, 1992). A person with alcohol dependence may present with both or only one of the manifestations. With adequate thiamine supplements over several months, most symptoms improve; the memory loss, however, may be permanent.

Cardiac tissue, when bathed in alcohol, can become scarred and ineffective. Heart failure and compensatory enlargement can occur. At times, a person with alcohol-induced cardiomyopathy may suffer arrhythmias or heart failure so severe that transplant is the only option. Cardiovascular damage from alcohol along with alteration in lipid metabolism contribute to coronary artery disease and hypertension (Woodward, 2003).

The pancreas can be damaged by direct contact with alcohol. When a pancreas cell dies, scar tissue forms. If the scarring is in the pancreatic duct, the enzymes produced for starch digestion do not pass into the stomach. Instead, they stir within pancreatic tissue causing further destruction and severe pain. If alcohol damages the beta cells of the islets of Langerhans, then insulin production declines (Korsten & Lieber, 1992).

Bone marrow is also affected by alcohol. Bone marrow suppression can be seen in laboratory reports (G. B. Collins, personal communication, September 20, 2011). There is a decrease in red and white blood cells with an increase in premature blood cells; platelets are low. The person is at risk for anemia, poor clotting, and infections.

The liver takes the brunt of damage from beverage alcohol. When one drinks alcohol, in any form, it is first absorbed immediately from the stomach into the blood directly to portal circulation. The portal artery delivers the alcohol-infused blood to the liver for metabolizing. On first pass, liver cells metabolize the alcohol molecule into acetylaldehyde. Next, liver cells break the acetylaldehyde into the acetyl molecule that the body uses to make acetylcholine and the aldehyde molecule that the body ultimately disposes. Alcohol causes damage to liver cells in three ways: (1) direct contact by virtue of its chemical nature, (2) natural death due to overworking the cell, and (3) lipid deposits ("fatty liver") that adversely affect the function of hepatic cells.

When liver cells are irritated from constant exposure to alcohol's irritant effect, the result is alcoholic hepatitis. When a liver cell dies, a small scar is formed. Multiple small scars equal one large scar, thus liver cirrhosis occurs.

The hepatic artery is the first tributary of the abdominal aorta. Blood flow through this large artery to a significantly scarred cirrhotic liver is blocked. With no safe passage, the blood backs up into the hepatic artery, then into the abdominal aorta. This pressured system is intensified by a forceful beating heart. The abdominal aorta is intimately adjacent to the esophagus in the mediastinum. Enough pressure can cause seepage through the arterial wall into the esophagus; this esophageal tear is known as a varice. Blood loss into the gastric system can be severe enough to cause death. Varices are surgically repaired by either cauterizing the tear or banding it tightly.

This backup of blood and fluid can cause seepage into the abdominal cavity, creating ascites. Often, the fluid needs to be extracted to prevent infection.

In clinical situations of hepatic failure, one sees ascites, swollen legs, gray discoloration of skin, yellowing of the sclera, and an unpleasant odor.

The liver functions in many ways to keep the human body healthy; cirrhosis compromises these functions. Gluconeogenesis is decreased, contributing to hypoglycemic conditions. Clotting factor production is decreased, leaving the person more susceptible to bleeding, particularly in situations where platelets are low. Protein metabolism is decreased. The cirrhotic liver is unable to adequately remove the ammonia from the protein molecule. Serum ammonia rises with subsequent accumulation in brain tissue. This situation leads to hepatic encephalopathy characterized by somnolence, confusion, coma, and death. Medical treatment to prevent this involves administering oral lactulose, which binds the ammonia and eliminates it through the gastrointestinal (GI) tract.

Persons with cirrhosis to the extent of hepatic failure can be candidates for transplant. Most transplant centers require the person to complete a course of treatment, attend Alcoholics Anonymous (AA) meetings, and maintain abstinence from all alcoholic beverages and mood-altering substances. Following a period of close observation and evidence of sustained sobriety, the person is placed on the transplant list and given a notification beeper. Clinicians have seen situations where the person lives a sober and healthy lifestyle allowing the portion of unscarred liver to heal, recover, and get the work done. They become no longer in need of a transplanted organ; they return the beeper.

It is well known that beverage alcohol is toxic to human cells and causes significant organ damage. Yet it is legal to buy it and drink it. In most cultures, it is a celebrated substance. It is present at weddings, at New Year's Eve celebrations, and definitely at sporting events. It is customary to give fine wine as gifts. The taxes imposed on beverage alcohol are a source of governmental income; yet we know what it is capable of doing simply by its chemical nature.

OPIATES

The opiate narcotics can be categorized into three forms: naturally occurring, semisynthetic, and synthetic. From the many strains of poppy plants, only one provides seeds used for baking and opiates for medication/drugs. The unripened seed pod of the *Papaver somniferum* poppy is expressed to produce opium. From the opium is derived heroin, codeine, and morphine. These are the four naturally occurring opiate agents.

The use of opium can be traced to 4000 B.C. The word *opium* comes from the Greek word for *juice*; morphine is named for the Greek god of dreams (Schuckit, 2003).

Semisynthetic Opiate agents include: hydromorphone (hydrated morphine, Dilaudid), hydrocodone (hydrated codeine, Vicodin), and Buprenorphine (alkaloid derivative of a by-product of opium). A field of these poppies are what Dorothy and her friends walked through as they approached the Emerald City; of course, they fell asleep.

Synthetic opiate agents are made in pharmaceutical laboratories and are many. They include: oxycodone (percodan/Percocet), OxyContin, methadone, fentanyl and sufentanil, meperidine (Demerol), nalbuphin (Nubain), butorphanol (Stadol), tramadol (Ultram), and propoxyphene (Darvon). When taken, they all work at the many opiate receptor sites dispersed throughout the human body. The opiate receptors are composed of amino acids on the cellular membrane.

The body produces intrinsic endorphins, which have affinity for the kappa and delta opiate receptors. All opiate agents taken exogenously have primary affinity for the mu opiate receptor (Borg & Kreek, 2004; Gorelick & Cornish, 2003). It is the mu receptor that research has studied extensively.

When the opiate drugs (agonists) innervate the mu receptor, biochemical changes in the cyclic adenosine monophosphate cascade produce analgesia. These drugs inhibit the release of GABA, which in turn allows greater production of dopamine in the brain's pleasure centers; this results in euphoria (Goodwin, 2003).

Opiate drugs are phenomenal analgesic agents. They are frequently prescribed and rigorously controlled by the Drug Enforcement Agency (DEA) and comparable legislative organizations internationally. Other effects on the body include: somnolence, mood changes, clouded cognitions, decreased respirations, peripheral vasodilatation, histamine release, decreased production of gastric enzymes, decreased production of acetylcholine in the GI tract leading to decreased GI motility, and decreased production of immune cells (Borg & Kreek, 2004).

It is important to know that only the natural and semisynthetic opiate agents will produce positive results for opiates in common urine toxicology drug screens. The synthetic opiates will not. A person may be using oxycodone or another synthetic drug and be opiate-negative on a drug screen. It is also important to know the exact mode of drug urine testing that a laboratory practices. Many laboratories require indications of the specific drugs a clinician is looking for.

Opiate Toxicity. The opiate agents, if taken in large quantities, can lead to respiratory depression and death. As chemicals, they do not share the toxicity that alcohol has on a molecular level. There are certainly side effects, as with any drug. The unpleasant side effects of the opiate drugs are constipation and skin itching. If used in combination with other drugs, their effects are potentiated. If taken frequently, over long periods of time, they have been known to cause renal damage.

The intravenous (IV) use of illicit drugs or misuse of legal drugs brings its own avenue of toxicity; it's not the drug that is toxic, but the myriad problems with IV use. It is difficult to use drugs intravenously outside of clinical settings in a way that is completely sterile. Crushed pills or heroin are put into solution with tap water or often saliva; the drugs are prepared and mixed with fillers that are not sterile or easily dissolved. Needles are shared or rinsed in a common bowl of water. Bacteria, viruses, and particulate matter are introduced into circulation. Problems occur when the microbes lodge in the heart or joints. Endocarditis defines microbial growth within the heart muscle, usually around a valve. Surgical excision and weeks of IV antibiotics are necessary to prevent death. Septic joints often require replacement if surgical clean-out is ineffective. Veins become scarred; skin abcesses can develop; cellulitis and thrombophlebitis can be seen. This is all due to toxic effects of IV drug misuse, not the actual drug that is injected.

It is noteworthy to remember that, as chemical substances are concerned, beverage alcohol is far more toxic to the body than heroin. If a plant is watered daily with a pint of gin, the plant will die. If the plant is sprinkled with heroin mixed with water, most likely it will continue to grow.

SEDATIVES: BENZODIAZEPINES AND BARBITURATES

These medications are prescribed for anxiety, panic, sleep, and sedation in anesthesia (Table 17-1). They are controlled by the Drug Enforcement Agency due to their potential for misuse. As chemicals, they are not directly toxic to human tissue. If taken in large quantities or mixed with beverage alcohol, they will cause significant respiratory depression that could lead to death. Mixing these medications with alcohol is frequently done in suicide attempts.

Benzodiazepines are classified as central nervous system depressants. They are prescribed as antianxiety agents, muscle relaxants, anticonvulsants, and detoxification agents. They all exert their effect at the GABA receptor; GABA is secreted and, as an inhibitory neurotransmitter, opens the channels that permit negatively charged chloride ions to enter the neuron. The neuron relaxes.

The use of these agents is best for brief periods as the situation may warrant. As the central nervous system quickly alters in adaptation to their presence, tolerance develops and more drug is needed for symptom control. With increased tolerance, rebound anxiety occurs that far exceeds the original state; seizure can occur even with high doses, as the body needs more drug to accommodate the need. These drugs differ in potency and half-life.

BARBITURATE DRUGS

The barbiturates were widely prescribed in the 1950s to 1970s for anxiety and sleep. Their use now is limited. Phenobarbitol is commonly prescribed for seizure disorders in humans and animals. It is also a recommended drug to use to manage benzodiazepine, alcohol, and barbiturate withdrawal. Butalbitol is found in the common headache medications Esgic and Fiorinol/Fioricet. Barbiturates are used most frequently in anesthesia induction and include the following:

- Amoobarbital (Amytal)
- Pentobarbital (Nembutal)
- Secobarbital (Seconal)
- Phenobarbital (Luminal)
- Methoexital (Pentothal)
- Butalbital (as contained in Fioricet/Fiorinal/Esgic)

The barbiturates are well known to cause significant respiratory depression and sedation. They are drugs that have been used for successful suicides.

Toxic Effects of Sedatives. These drugs will cause respiratory depression if taken in large quantities; memory deficits can occur and are usually reversible after cessation.

Their primary toxicity is in withdrawal states. When these agents are stopped abruptly, withdrawal symptoms can be severe with high probability of seizure. Highly supervised medical management of withdrawal is recommended.

COCAINE

Cocaine was readily available in common beverages and medicinal products from 1860 through 1914. The first published report of cardiac death from cocaine appeared in 1886. Once the key ingredient in the ever-popular carbonated beverage, it was removed from the recipe in 1903 (Schuckit, 2003).

Cocaine preparations are legally manufactured for ophthalmic, dental, and medical procedures as an anesthetic. The anesthetic effect is due primarily to the blockage of sodium channels along the neuron, minimizing its action potential and the vasoconstrictive properties.

Cocaine is derived from the leaf of the coca plant. Illegal production makes it available in powdered salt forms that can be snorted, rubbed onto mucosa, placed in solution for injection, or mixed with marijuana or tobacco for smoking. The powdered salt can be altered with ether to extract a more potent form of cocaine, freebase, and boiled down to a hard plaster-like substrate crack; these forms are placed in a pipe and smoked (Gorelick & Cornish, 2003).

Cocaine exerts its effects by blocking the reuptake of dopamine and norepinephrine by the presynaptic neuron. It does this very well, causing a flood of these

TABLE 17-1: COMMONLY PRESCRIBED SEDATIVES (SCHUCKIT, 2003)

DRUG	ROUTES	SEDATION	MUSCLE RELAXATION	DEA CLASS
Diazepam (Valium)	po/iv/im	high	high	III
Chlordiazepoxide (Librium)	po	moderate	moderate	III
Lorazepam (Ativan)	po/iv/im	moderate	moderate	III
Alprazolam (Xanax)	po	moderate	mild	
Clonazepam (Klonopin)	po	moderate	mild	

Zolpidem (Ambien) differs in that it has two benzo rings; commonly prescribed for sleep.

Midazolam (Versed) is a benzodiezapine used only in anesthesia; it has specific affinity for receptors in the memory center of the brain, thus providing an amnesic state perioperatively.

Meprobamate (Equanil/Miltown) is a medication that was first introduced in the 1950s as an antidepressant. Currently, if it is prescribed, it is for anxiety.

Carisoprodol (Soma) is a widely prescribed muscle relaxant. Acts as a benzodiazepine in the central nervous system and should be weaned rather than stopped abruptly.

catecholamines throughout the central and peripheral nervous system. In the brain's pleasure centers, this flood is experienced as a euphoric "rush." In the cardiovascular system, it is both inotropic and chronotropic, causing increased heart rate and increased blood pressure

Toxic Effects of Cocaine. Toxicity can occur throughout the body as a result of the catecholamine stimulation and vasoconstriction. When cocaine constricts small arterioles, the bloodflow is shunted into other areas; this, occurring in the presence of forceful cardiac output, can result in hemorrhagic infarcts in brain and cardiac tissue.

Cardiac effects can be seen with arrhythmias, conduction blocks, ischemic infarction, cardiomyopathy, myocardial fibrosis, or myocarditis. Persons will often say they experience chest pain when using cocaine; it is the symptom that often takes them to the emergency room. Sudden cardiac death can occur when the overstimulated heart demands more oxygen, yet the vasoconstricted coronary arteries can't meet the demand.

Mucosal tissue damage from intranasal use can cause septal lesions, ulcers, and sinus cavity wall holes. Not uncommon are meningeal or brain infections and abscesses due to bacterial invasion through sinus wall holes. Secondary damage occurs to olfactory nerve endings and taste buds. GI damage is seen as a direct result of vasoconstriction: ulceration, perforation, GI infarcts, or ischemic colitis. A painful condition seen in neonates exposed to cocaine in utero is necrotizing enterocolitis: the blood vessels to the GI tract of the fetus do not develop in the presence of cocaine; with no perfusion, the GI tract necrotizes.

Lung tissue is compromised when cocaine and its residue become lodged in bronchioles; cocaine deposits can easily be seen on chest imaging. Nervous system toxicity includes acute seizures, stroke, and movement disorders.

Fetal development in the presence of cocaine can cause multiple nervous system abnormalities. Babies will have shrill cries; as they grow, they will have movement disorders and walk on their toes; intelligence is often adversely affected.

Psychiatrically, due to the excess amount of dopamine at the neurosynaptic junction, paranoia, hallucinations, and psychosis occur. Severe paranoia can cause a person to become defensively violent. A person who is cocaine-toxic with severe paranoia may very well attack due to the perception that someone is following them or out to kill them. This is irreversible when the drug is cleared from the system.

AMPHETAMINES

Amphetamines include the following prescription medications:

- Ritalin (methylphenidate)
- Lisdexamfetamine (Vyvanse)
- Dexedrine (dextroamphetamine)
- Adderal (a combination of four amphetamine salts)
- Methamphetamine (Desoxyn)
- Modafinil (Provigil)

Their primary indication is for attention deficit, narcolepsy, and antidepressant augmentation. They exert their effect by increasing dopamine at the neurosynaptic junction but do so somewhat differently than cocaine; they act to cause the nerve to surge more dopamine and norepinephrine into the junction rather than block reuptake.

Toxic Effects. Toxicity results primarily in cardiac and nervous tissue damage due to the catecholamine surge. They do not cause vasoconstriction. They can cause seizure and death if put into solution and injected. If crushed and snorted, they can cause mucosal irritation but to a lesser degree than cocaine.

MARIJUANA

The active ingredient in marijuana is tetrahydrocannabinol or THC. It is a natural occurring plant whose leaves are crushed and then smoked or eaten. Synthetically, it is manufactured as dronabinol (Marinol) for prescription use only. Its indicated medical use is as an antiemetic during chemotherapy, an appetite stimulant in wasting diseases, an adjunct to analgesic medications, and for certain movement disorders. Classified as a hallucinogen, growing, selling, and using natural marijuana is illegal in most countries.

THC binds to phospholipid membranes, particularly in the meninges and myelin and to specific cannabinoid receptors located primarily in the limbic system. The receptors are presumed to be present at birth. Endogenous cannabinoids have been isolated and clearly have a role in appetite and food intake (Welch & Martin, 2003). THC exerts its effects when binding to these sites by causing complex intracellular biochemical changes. The result is changes in sensorial perceptions, increased appetite, psychomotor slowing, delayed reflex response, euphoria, and a decrease in energy and motivation. In cardiac tissue, THC directly stimulates the conduction pathways causing increases in both rate and force.

Toxic Effects of Marijuana. Lung tissue suffers the brunt of toxic effects of marijuana. THC is less of a toxin than the products of combustion inhaled when smoking. Additionally, the chemical products that adhere to the marijuana plant (pesticides, fertilizer) are toxins. Bronchi shrinkage occurs with decompensation of large airway functioning.

Smoking several "blunts" per day (a hollowed-out cigar that is then filled with marijuana), particularly in adolescents and young adults, can lead to irreversible lung damage. Reproductive problems occur from THC, altering pituitary function, sperm formation, and sperm motility. In severe cases, male sterility has resulted. Pesticide residue on marijuana leaves, when inhaled, has been associated with DNA mutation and an increased risk of leukemia in children of the smokers.

Psychiatrically, for persons predisposed to the development of psychotic disorders, marijuana can hasten the onset. Independently, marijuana use can cause paranoia, anhedonia, amotivation, and overall cognitive decline. In instances of heavy, long-term use, cognitive changes are irreversible.

NICOTINE

Nicotine is a phenomenal drug. It can relax as well as stimulate its user. It can calm agitation and sharpen cognition. It can energize one upon awakening from sleep; it can soothe one into a peaceful slumber. It can help one when a laxative is warranted.

When smoking was permitted among patients on psychiatric units, nicotine was used abundantly to help soothe the psyche of anxious and psychotic individuals.

The parasympathetic nervous system has cholinergic receptors that nicotine has a distinct affinity for. No endogenous nicotine has been found; however, the body does make acetylcholine that innervates these receptors. When nicotine innervates the receptors, multiple neurobiochemical cascades occur involving acetylcholine, dopamine, GABA, and norepinephrine. How they all interact to create the many effects of nicotine ingestion is not completely understood. Much of what is written is assumption. Nicotine can be delivered into the body through inhalation (smoking) of cigarettes, cigars, and pipe tobacco; it can be absorbed through mucosa; it can be absorbed through the skin (primarily seen among tobacco workers).

The source of nicotine is the tobacco plant. Tobacco growing and processing and the packaging of the various delivery systems are major industries providing employment and income for many. Nicotine as a drug is legal; as an industry, it provides significant income to governments through taxes applied to it.

Toxic Effects of Nicotine/Tobacco. The toxic effects of nicotine are primarily in the delivery system and thc adjunct toxins used in tobacco growing and processing. The combustion products of smoking are irritating, highly toxic, and clearly carcinogenic. The topical irritation on mucosa of oral tobacco is also toxic and carcinogenic.

Even though smoking is less acceptable than the other legal drugs, it is widely used and very toxic. When human tissue expects delivery of oxygen via the blood but receives more carbon monoxide and other products of combustion, it suffers.

Toxic Changes from Smoking. Cardiovascular changes occur. Smoking alters arterial linings, which leads to platelet aggregation, atherosclerosis, and emboli development; occlusions of femoral arteries can occur, leaving one with neuropathy and loss of muscle tone to the legs; infarcts to brain and heart occur. Lung tissue is affected. Smoking causes multiple pulmonary diseases including cancer, chronic obstructive pulmonary disease (COPD), bronchitis, and asthma. Mucosa are damaged. Smoking and oral tobacco use can cause mouth, tongue, throat, and esophageal cancers.

OTHER PRESCRIPTION MEDICATIONS

Other prescription medications such as gabapentin (Neurontin), pregabalin (Lyrica), lidocaine preparations (injectable), and Desyrel (Trazadone) have been abused. This author has seen and cared for persons who have misused and developed specific addictions to unlikely medications. The incidents were infrequent but noteworthy.

Gabapentin is an antiseizure medication that can be used for anxiety with moderate effectiveness. Pregabalin is a metabolite of gabapentin that is used for neuropathies. In instances of dependence, the patients were admitted for medical management of withdrawal symptoms.

The incident involving injectable lidocaine unfortunately had a negative outcome. The patient was a nurse who was suspected of diverting and using narcotics. No one suspected or found that the diverted drug was injectable lidocaine until death occurred and vials were found in the home.

Desyrel was reported as a misused medication by a patient: "I found myself hoarding the medicine; taking more than prescribed; lying about losing my prescription. It was just like being addicted to Vicodin."

BEHAVIORAL ADDICTIONS

Drugs and chemicals that alter mood do so by altering the intricate and complex biochemical physiology of the human body. Behaviors and situations influence the neurotransmitters that result in mood changes. Emotional changes and the situations that can cause them are due to biochemical changes in neurotransmitter production. Behaviors and situations most known to change mood and seen in addictive situations include sex, gambling, exercise, work, and certain eating behaviors.

NEGATIVE CONSEQUENCES

Substances, drugs, and behaviors that alter mood have their effects and toxicities independent of addiction. If one is unable to stop using a substance or engaging in a certain behavior that alters mood with no negative consequence or potentially negative consequences, then is there any reason to stop using the substance or engaging in the behavior? Addiction as an entity is not about the use of a substance as much as it is about the inability to stop the use when negative consequences occur.

Consuming alcohol is toxic to cells. The more one consumes, the more tissue damage occurs. This is *not* addiction to alcohol. Addiction is when a person suffers a job loss or encounters legal consequences due to alcohol consumption and is *unable* to stop their use.

Addictive disorder is the inability to stop using a substance or engaging in a behavior when coupled with negative consequences. Simply defined, it is when one can't stop and bad things happen. Negative consequences seen in addictive disorders cover the spectrum of simple to extreme.

One can break a toe as one stumbles when intoxicated, and one can cause a fatal accident as one drives while intoxicated. Addiction, even without the influence of the drug, affects a person negatively. It is an affliction that affects the body, mind, and spirit of the person suffering with it. Addiction affects how a person thinks, acts, feels, makes decisions, and relates to others. It is not the drug but the entity that is the addictive disorder.

Denial, repression, minimization, externalization, and rationalization are all things the normal psyche develops and uses to keep the person functioning. Addiction seems to take hold of these normal defense mechanisms and use them for its own propagation.

Humans are vulnerable beings. When the body is cut, it bleeds; when the person loses someone, there is grief; when trauma occurs, there are psychic wounds. Addiction seems to feed on human vulnerability. Childhood trauma does not cause addiction, as many suffer the wounds of trauma without developing addiction. Yet addiction takes advantage of this vulnerability, feeding off of it as though it were fertilizer.

Family members and close coworkers are influenced by the entity of a person's addiction. Their thoughts, feelings, and behaviors are influenced. They will deny, minimize, or rationalize a person's continued using behavior. In some instances, a spouse is more "addicted" than their using partner; it's as though one person in a marriage suffers with severe addiction but their spouse does the drinking/using for them. Family members and even health care workers hope to save the addicted person, to rescue them from the travesties that can happen. Family members often spend thousands of dollars sending their loved one to a treatment center only to be frustrated when relapse occurs.

Like any other chronic disease, addiction can be treated. A person can care for themselves daily with the hope of staying healthy. Addiction is a chronic affliction (disease) that is complex. Health care providers in all specialty areas will encounter those suffering with it. It is critical to know the basics of what to do in caring for the person.

ASSESSMENT

As addiction is a biopsychosocial disease, assessment should include a history and physical exam inclusive of psychiatric and mental status exam (see Exhibit 17-1). When assessing an individual with COD, it is very important to identify periods of abstinence of 30 days or more to understand the nature of mental health symptoms, treatment, and disability as well as readiness for change. Laboratory, imaging, and electrocardiography (EKG) should be done (see Exhibits 17-2 and 17-3). In some cases, examination of cerebrospinal fluid (CSF) is warranted.

EXHIBIT 17-1: OUTLINE FOR BIOPSYCHOSOCIAL ASSESSMENT FOR PERSONS WITH ADDICTIVE DISORDER

- Identifying Information
- Presenting Problem
- Motivation for Seeking Help
- Health Issues
- Surgical History
- Allergies
- Medications Prescribed
- Chemical Dependency History (Alcohol, Opiates, Sedatives, Mjna, Nicotine, OTC)
- Withdrawal Phenomena/Seizures/Overdose/Backouts
- Prior Treatments/Years Sober
- Family History
- Developmental History (Parents, Siblings, Education, Trauma)
- Relationship/Marital History
- Children
- Employment History
- Legal Problems: Past/Current/Pending
- Military History
- Recreational Interests
- Spiritual Beliefs/Practices
- Goals

CONSULTATION AND REFERRAL SOURCES

Depending on the clinical situation and the outcome of the assessment, the PMH-APRN may need to refer a person to a caregiver or facility for further or more appropriate care. It is wise to keep a collection of such persons and facilities to use when the situation mandates such. See Exhibit 17-4 for signs and symptoms requiring immediate medical attention. Also, remember that any statements about self-harm must be taken seriously. Altered mental status, such as during intoxication or withdrawal, places an individual at increased risk for self-harm. Chapter 15, Integrative Management of Self-directed Injury, discusses this issue in more detail.

TOOLS AVAILABLE

There are several psychometric tools available for use in assessing clients for substance use/misuse. A commonly used tool for screening is the CAGE. This is a simple neumonic based on four questions.

Cut down: Have you ever thought of doing so?
Annoyed: Have you become so when others comment on your use?
Guilt: Have you felt this related to using?
Eye opener: Have you used in the morning to get going?

Additional assessment tools include the Addiction Severity Index (ASI), the Alcohol Dependence Scale, the Michigan Alcohol Screening Test (MAST), and the Clinical Institute Withdrawal Assessment for alcohol withdrawal (CIWA).

The ASI is a semistructured interview guide to address seven potential problem areas related to substance abuse. The areas are medical problems, work problems, legal problems, relationship problems, psychiatric problems, uncontrolled use of alcohol, and uncontrolled use of other substances. It is copyrighted and available from Delta Metrics, 1-800-238-2433.

The MAST is not copyrighted and is widely used for screening of alcohol abuse. It is a 25-item questionnaire available on the Internet at several sites. The following site offers several self-tests for substance abuse including the MAST: http://counsellingresource.com/lib/quizzes/drug-testing/alcohol-mast

EXHIBIT 17-2: OUTLINE FOR A COMPLETE HISTORY AND PHYSICAL EXAM FOR PERSONS WITH ADDICTIVE DISORDER

Patient Name: ________________
REFERRAL SOURCE: ________________
PRIMARY CARE PHYSICIAN: ________________
CHIEF COMPLAINT: ________________
BRIEF HISTORY LEADING TO THIS ASSESSMENT: ________________
ATTITUDE AND MOTIVATION: ________________
PAST MEDICAL HISTORY: ________________
MEDICATIONS: ________________
ALLERGIES: ________________
PAST SURGICAL HISTORY: ________________

CHEMICAL DEPENDENCY HISTORY:
(Include amount, frequency, last use)
ALCOHOL: ________________
BENZODIAZAPENES: ________________
OPIATES: ________________
MARIJUANA: ________________
COCAINE: ________________
NICOTINE: ________________
IV USE: ________________
WITHDRAWAL SYMPTOMS: ________________
SEIZURES: ________________
BLACKOUTS: ________________
LEGAL PROBLEMS: ________________
JOB LOSSES: ________________
PRESCRIPTION TAMPERING: ________________
DECEPTION TO OBTAIN: ________________
PRIOR TREATMENTS ________________
PRIOR PERIODS OF SOBRIETY: ________________
PRIOR 12-STEP WORK: ________________
PSYCHIATRIC HISTORY: Hospitalizations; Care; Suicidality
(thoughts past and current; attempts)
____
____

DEVELOPMENTAL/FAMILY HISTORY:
(Born/raised; siblings; education; family history of addictions)
____
____

COMPLETE REVIEW OF SYSTEMS:
Skin: ________________ Rash/tattoos/piercings/abcesses
Hair: ________________
Head: ________________ Hx of head injury/trauma
Endocrine: ________________
Eyes/Vision: ________________
Ears/Hearing: ________________
Nose/Smell: ________________
Mouth/Teeth: ________________
Appetite: ________________
Swallowing: ________________
GI: ________________ GERD/acid reflux
Bowel: ________________ Constipation/diarrhea
Bladder: ________________ Hx of UTI
Heart: ________________ Palpitations/chestpain/SOB
Lungs: ________________ Asthma/COPD/breathing difficulties
Sleep: ________________
Extremities: ________________ Numbness/tingling/joint pain/arthritis
Neuro: ________________ Stroke/dizziness/seizures/tremors
Immune Functions/Hx of STDs ________________
Memory/Cognitions: ________________
Gynecological: ________________ Pregnancies/abortions; menses: regular/last ________________
Men: ________________ Last prostate exam

PHYSICAL EXAM:
Withdrawal Symptoms:
Any observed (tachycardia/tremor/diaphoresis/piloerections/rhinorrhea/hyperreflexia)
____
____

Mental Status:
(It is advised that the mental status exam be written in paragraph form giving the reader enough to have a visual image of the person at time of assessment)
____
____

Skin: ________________
Hair: ________________
Head: ________________
Eyes: ____________ Pupils/sclera/region of margin (ROM)
Ears: ________________
Nose: ________________
Mouth/Dentation: ________________
Neck: ________________ ROM/nodules/thyroid
Heart: ________________ Apical sounds/carotids/capillary refill
Radial and Pedal Pulses: ________________
Lungs: ________________
Extremities: ________________ ROM/lower extremity edema/joints
Neuro: ________________ Reflexes/response to stimuli

PSYCHIATRIC ASSESSMENT:
AXIS I: ________________
AXIS II: ________________
AXIS III: ________________
AXIS IV: ________________
AXIS V: ________________
Plan: ________________

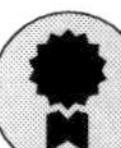

EXHIBIT 17-3: ADJUNCTIVE TESTING

Urine Pharmacology Testing: Most labs test the presence of drugs or metabolites in urine rather than blood; ordering blood toxicology usually demands indication of specific agents to be tested for; serum testing usually takes longer for results

Blood Alcohol Level

Complete Metabolic Panel (CMP)

Complete Blood Count (CBC)

Amylase/Lipase

Magnesium

Thyroid Stimulating Hormone (TSH)

HIV

Hepatitis Panel to look for antibodies to B and C virus

GGT (gamma glutamine transpepsidase: specific for liver cell damage)

HCG (urine) for women of childbearing age

Chest Imaging (for women, wait for results of HCG)

EKG

Imaging if injuries have occurred

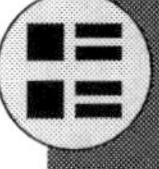

EXHIBIT 17-4: SYMPTOMS AND SIGNS OF WITHDRAWAL OR INTOXICATION THAT MAY REQUIRE IMMEDIATE MEDICAL ATTENTION

- Marked changes in mental status
- Increasing anxiety and panic
- Hallucinations
- Seizures
- Temperature greater than 100.4° F (these patients should also be considered potentially infectious)
- Significant increases and/or decreases in blood pressure or heart rate
- Marked insomnia
- Abdominal pain
- Upper and lower gastrointestinal bleeding
- Changes in responsiveness of pupils
- Heightened deep tendon reflexes and ankle clonus, a reflex beating of the foot when pressed rostrally (i.e., toward the mouth of the patient), indicating profound central nervous system irritability and the potential for seizures

Source: From TIP 45, *Detoxification and Substance Abuse Treatment*, p. 26.

The CIWA is specifically used for alcohol withdrawal assessment and is not copyrighted. It can be found on the University of Washington's Alcohol and Drug Abuse Institute's web page, http://lib.adai.washington.edu/instruments

There are many other self-report tests for abuse available but of course the results are based upon an individual's willingness and readiness to answer honestly. The most effective tool in assessing is trust between the PMH-APRN and the client. Questions such as "What do you use?", "How much and how often?", "What bad things have happened because of your use?", and "What is the reason for wanting to change now?" are most useful.

TREATMENT

The concept of "no wrong door" is recommended by the U.S. Department of Health and Human Services. In other words, an individual requiring treatment for substance abuse/addiction should be seen whether the individual presents at a mental health center, substance abuse center, emergency room, or other setting. To not turn away the person seeking help and to provide seamless services should be the goal. Depending upon the results of the assessment, the individual and PMH-APRN make decisions about the appropriate level of care.

The American Society of Addiction Medicine's Patient Placement Criteria (ASAM PPC-2R) (Center for Substance Abuse Treatment, 2002) envision treatment as a continuum within which there are five levels of care:

- Level 0.5: Early Intervention
- Level I: Outpatient Treatment
- Level II: Intensive Outpatient/Partial Hospitalization Treatment
- Level III: Residential/Inpatient Treatment
- Level IV: Medically Managed Intensive Inpatient services

Another framework to assist with understanding the range of severity and continuum of COD and coordination of level of service is Figure 17-1, the COD conceptual framework (p. 451). This was developed by the National Association of State Mental Health Program Directors and the National Association of State Alcohol and Drug Abuse Directors (Greenberg, 2002). It represents the level of service coordination required, ranging from consultation and collaboration to integration with the higher severity requiring the most intense coordination of services. The entire Substance Abuse & Mental

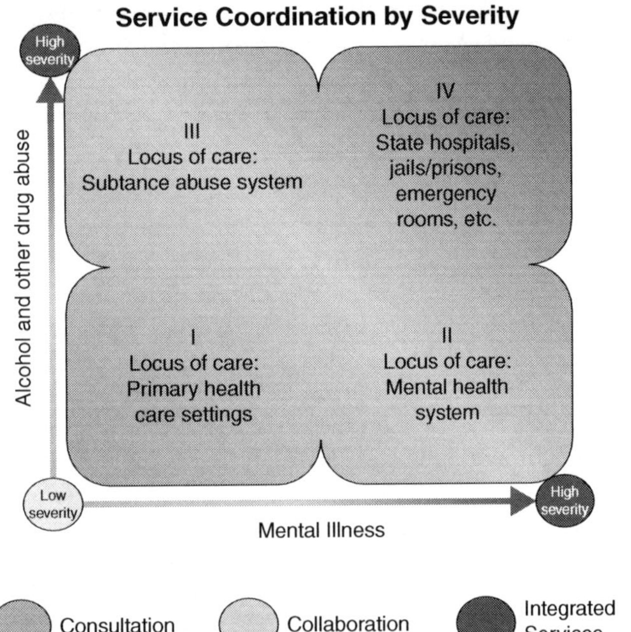

Figure 17-1 COD Conceptual Framework for Service Delivery

Definitions of terms in COD framework:

- **Consultation**: Traditional types of informal relationships among providers, from referrals to requests for exchanging information and keeping each other informed.
- **Collaboration**: Distinguished from consultation on the basis of the formal quality of collaborative agreements, such as memoranda of understanding or service contracts.
- **Integration**: Contributions of professionals in both fields are moved into a single treatment setting and treatment regimen, depending on the needs of the client and the constraints and of the systems.

Health Services Administration *Report to Congress on the Prevention and Treatment of Co-occurring Substance Abuse Disorders and Mental Disorders* (2002), which also contains this figure, can be viewed at www.samhsa.gov/reports/congress2002/execsummary.htm

MANAGEMENT OF PERSONS INTOXICATED WITH ALCOHOL AND SUBSEQUENT WITHDRAWAL

How the PMH-APRN manages a person who is intoxicated or in severe alcohol withdrawal depends upon the clinical setting. The primary goal of treatment is stabilization as well as engagement.

In an office-based practice, if the person is highly intoxicated or in profound withdrawal, calling an ambulance for transport to the appropriate hospital emergency department is the safest and most appropriate intervention. Security personnel or other help may be necessary for assistance until an ambulance arrives.

Alcohol intoxication at levels above 400 mg/dl can cause respiratory depression.

Alcohol withdrawal brings the risk of stroke or seizure. If the office has an alcohol breathalyzer, and the patient can manage using it, it will provide the suspected level of alcohol in the alveolar blood. Notifying the Emergency Room staff and providing a history should be done. In hospital settings, advanced practice nurses are better able to provide direct care and management.

INTOXICATION PRESENT

- Obtain history and order tests as above
- Consider IV fluids: Vitamin-infused saline (Banana Bag with multivitamin [MVI], Thiamine, Folate)
- Thiamine is essential as a neuroprotective intervention
- If IV fluids are not given, administer oral or intramuscular (IM) thiamine (100 mg)
- If blood alcohol levels are greater than 500 mg/dl, admit the person to an intensive care unit (ICU)

WITHDRAWAL PRESENT

Alcohol withdrawal is a nervous system in crisis since it has accommodated to having alcohol in its presence. Four basic steps to simple assessment include:

- Apical Pulse (in withdrawal it will be elevated)
- Blood Pressure (in withdrawal it will be elevated)
- Tremor: Sometimes gross tremor with the entire body shaking; sometimes fine tremor with the tendons in the hand shaking
- Diaphoresis: Sometimes profuse; sometimes palmar sweats

A quick assessment involves

- placing a stethoscope over the heart to obtain a rate
- obtaining a blood pressure, and holding the hand feeling for tremor and diaphoresis

Additional symptoms of withdrawal may include: hyperreflexia, anxiety, and agitation. Be aware that antihypertensive medications may keep the pulse and blood pressure from elevating. Some facilities use specific scale with associated medication protocols for alcohol withdrawal.

MEDICATIONS TO MANAGE ALCOHOL WITHDRAWAL SYMPTOMS

There are medications routinely used to manage alcohol withdrawal symptoms. First and foremost, administer vitamin B1 (thiamine) 100 mg IM/IV or 100 mg po tid for three days, then 100 mg po daily. If withdrawal is severe, continue oral tid dosing or daily IV dosing. Additionally, oral folate 1 mg daily and an MVI are used.

Next, chlordiazepoxide (Libriumis) used orally only for first 24 hours then 25–50 mg po every 4 hours as needed for withdrawal should be administered, then routine dosing based on the amount needed with subsequent taper. Higher doses (75–100 mg) may be given if symptoms increase or worsen. Assessment should be completed every 6 hours documenting pulse, blood pressure, presence of tremor or diaphoresis.

A typical oral taper of Librium is the following:

- 50 mg q. 6 hours × 4 (day 1)
- 40 mg q. 6 hours × 4 (day 2)
- 25 mg q. 6 hours × 4 (day 3)
- 15 mg q. 6 hours × 4 (day 4)
- 10 mg q. 6 hours × 4 (day 5)
- 5 mg q. 6 hours × 2 (day 6)
- A *pro re nata* (PRN) order for librium should be placed in a person's profile to use for worsening withdrawal symptoms (25–50 mg or 10–20 mg every 4 hours).

Librium has a long half-life (30–100 hours). It can be tapered up for worsening withdrawal or down if the person becomes sedate. Symptoms of too much Librium include: ocular nystagmus, ataxia, and slurred speech. It is only effective orally; it is poorly absorbed intramuscularly and cannot be administered intravenously. Librium is metabolized by the liver. In situations where Gamma-glutamyl-transpeptidase (GGT)/alanine aminotransferase (ALT)/aspartate aminotransferase (AST) are severely elevated or in the face of liver cirrhosis, lower doses may be necessary to avoid serum buildup.

Lorazepam (Ativan) is an option in cases of liver impairment as it does not mandate hepatic metabolization, or when an IV agent is indicated. Lorazepam (Ativan) is usually ordered as oral, IV, or IM; usual dose for the first 24 hours: 1–2 mg po/IV every 4 hours as needed, then routine dosing based on total amount needed. Higher doses (4 mg) or greater frequency may be administered if symptoms are severe.

A typical taper (oral) for lorazepam (Ativan) follows:

- 2 mg q. 6 hours (day 1)
- 1.5 mg q 6 hours (day 2)
- 1 mg q 6 hours (day 3)
- 0.5 mg q 6 hours (day 4)
- 0.25 mg tid (day 5)

Ativan has a half-life of 10–20 hours. It is seen as the drug of choice in most medical and ICU settings due to the ability to administer it PO, IV, or IM. IV administration is usually done when a person is in severe withdrawal and hospitalized on medical or ICUs rather than an addictions/detoxification unit or unable to take pills orally. Taper should be slow based on control of symptoms. Some practitioners prefer withdrawal management with oral chlordiazepoxide and IM lorazepam as needed for breakthrough symptoms.

Diazepam (Valium), administered Oral, IV, or IM, is a more sedating benzodiazepine with the unique property to relax muscles. It is long-acting with a half-life of 30–100 hours.

As with the other medications, dosing begins with 5–10 mg q 4 hours as needed for withdrawal symptoms then begin routine dosing based on quantity needed.

Starting dose may vary and as always, to be held if symptoms of oversedation, ocular nystagmus, slurred speech, or ataxia are seen.

A typical diazepam taper may look like this (oral):

- 10 mg q 6 hours × 4 (day 1)
- 7.5 mg q 6 hours × 4 (day 2)
- 5 mg q 6 hours × 4 (day 3)
- 2.5 mg q 6 hours × 4 (day 4)
- 2.5 mg bid × 2 (day 5)

Clonazepam (Klonopin) (oral) is another agent to use for withdrawal, however, it tends to be less anxiolytic than other benzodiazapines. Begin dosing with 1–2 mg every 4 hours for the first 24 hours then determine a routine dose and taper. The half-life is 20–50 hours. Too high a level of benzodiazepine in the blood is characterized by ocular nystagmus, ataxia, and slurred speech; should this occur, hold several doses of the detoxification regimen.

Author's Note: NEVER USE XANAX TO MANAGE ALCOHOL WITHDRAWAL. THE RISK FOR SEIZURE IS GREAT GIVEN THE VERY SHORT HALF-LIFE (8–15 hours).

Phenobarbitol (oral) continues to be used in addictions units or by practitioners familiar with its effects. As a barbiturate, it is sedating and quite effective in managing withdrawal.

Adjunct medications to use in managing a person through alcohol withdrawal include antiemetics, antacids (H2 blockers/Maalox), Inderal for incessant tremor, and antidiarrheal agents.

The medical management of alcohol withdrawal is directed toward prevention of seizure and delirium tremens (DT). Anticonvulsant medications such as phenytoin (Dilantin), carbamazepine (Tegretol), and valproic acid (Depakote) have been shown to have NO effect in preventing alcohol-withdrawal seizures. If a person has an underlying seizure disorder and has been taking an antiseizure medication, it should be continued throughout medical management of withdrawal.

A person who drinks daily in a heavy and steady manner is at risk for seizure and/or DT up to 14 days following cessation of alcohol intake (G. B. Collins, personal communication, September 7, 1985). DT is the most severe manifestation of the alcohol withdrawal syndrome. It presents as a state of profound confusion, delusions, hallucinations, gross body tremors, agitation, insomnia, fever, tachycardia, profuse diaphoresis, restlessness, fumbling movements, and overall overactivation of the autonomic nervous system (Victor, 1992).

Persons experiencing DT should be under constant monitoring with a bedside companion, ideally in an intensive care unit. IV fluids infused with thiamine and folic acid should be given. Benzodiazepines should be used cautiously, avoiding overuse. Lorazepam or diazepam drips or oral chlordiazepoxide are drugs of choice. The goal of drug therapy in managing the person with DT is not the absolute suppression of agitation and tremor, but to blunt them to prevent exhaustion and facilitate the acceptance of fluids and supportive care (Victor, 1992).

Managing a person throughout the duration of DT may find the staff anxious and frustrated. Expert and experienced addictions clinicians should be the caregivers for persons experiencing DT. It is a condition where expert bedside nursing care is the most effective intervention. Family members will be in need of updates, education, and reassurance.

MANAGING PERSONS UNDER THE INFLUENCE OF SEDATIVES (BENZODIAZAPINES, BARBITURATES, MEPROBAMATE, AND CARISOPRODOL) AND WITHDRAWAL

INTOXICATION

The person intoxicated with sedative drugs are somnolent, slow to respond, sluggish, ataxic, and hypo-reflexic. Eyes tend to be glassy with nystagmus. Assessment should include urine pharmacology testing to see if other drugs have been ingested. As these drugs cause significant respiratory depression, emergency care may be in order with hospitalization in an intensive care unit.

WITHDRAWAL

The person experiencing sedative withdrawal presents with profound anxiety, agitation, muscle twitches, hyper-reflexia, and in some cases, muscle rigidity. Severe withdrawal states may present with hallucinations. The ultimate severe sedative withdrawal phenomena on is seizure. Elevation in pulse and blood pressure are not classic symptoms but may be seen.

Ample benzodiazapines should be immediately administered. Chlordiazepoxide, diazepam, or clonazepam are the recommended agents to use. In situations where IV administration is necessary, lorazepam or diazepam may be used.

Dosages should be equivalent to what the person has been using and taper should be slow. The goal of managing sedative withdrawal is seizure prevention.

Gabapentin (Neurontin) may be used as an adjunct medication to assist with decreasing agitation and contribute to seizure prophylaxis. The usual dose is 300 mg PO three to four times daily. When detoxification is complete, gabapentin can be continued for a period of time to reduce latent withdrawal symptoms.

Often, when a person has developed tolerance to sedative agents, withdrawal symptoms and seizure may occur while they are taking large doses. It is not uncommon to see someone who has slowly developed tolerance taking more drug in an effort to control severe rebound anxiety. This occurs primarily with clonazepam but has been observed with lorazepam and diazepam. Converting them to chlordiazepoxide with titration to a stable dose and subsequent slow wean manages withdrawal nicely. Gabapentin and sedating selective serotonin reuptake inhibitor (SSRI) agents are helpful managing latent withdrawal anxiety.

MANAGING PERSONS UNDER THE INFLUENCE OF OPIATES AND OPIATE WITHDRAWAL

How the Advanced Practice Nurse (APN) manages the person who misuses opiates or has dependence on or addiction to opiates depends on the presentation and clinical setting.

IN AN OFFICE-BASED PRACTICE

When a person has become dependent on prescribed opiates and the APN is responsible for managing a taper without hospitalization, a schedule for opiate wean should be carefully designed with weekly clinic visits for monitoring progress. Prescribed opiates should be given weekly. In states that have an automatic reporting system for controlled substances, it should be routinely monitored to determine whether the person is receiving controlled drugs from other prescribers.

When a person identifies misuse and/or addiction, referral to an evaluation with an addiction specialist should be done. Clonidine (Catapres) can be prescribed orally 0.1–0.2 mg four times daily as long as needed for opiate withdrawal symptoms, as long as the person is not constitutionally hypotensive. Other helpful medications: are Baclofen 10–20 mg as needed for muscle aches and neurontin 300 mg every 4 hours as needed for anxiety. Adjunctive medications for nausea and diarrhea should also be prescribed. Prescribed quantities should be only enough to bridge to the appointment with an addiction specialist. If intoxication is evident, an ambulance should be summoned immediately for transport to an emergency department.

INTOXICATION

Opiate intoxication presents with pinpoint pupils, decreased respirations, somnolence, lethargy, and clouded cognitions. A case where a person is unresponsive is an emergency situation and should be treated in an appropriate setting. Narcan 0.4 mg IM or IV can be administered every 15 minutes × 3; narcan will block opiates from innervating the body's opiate receptors.

Over the past 10 years, there has been an epidemic of opiate addiction among young persons 25 years and younger. Primarily, but not exclusively, it is seen in Caucasian young men. Rarely is it seen among young African Americans. The pattern seen is beginning substance misuse with marijuana and alcohol, progressing to prescription narcotics and eventually heroin. The epidemic is most alarming due to the ineffectiveness of traditional treatment modalities. Accidental overdose is common. Many young men are motivated to seek help following the funeral(s) of friend(s) who have accidentally overdosed.

Opiate withdrawal creates profound physical illness and emotional distress. When a person comes for help, they are desperate and fearful of "the sickness" of withdrawal. Usually, this occurs in a hospital emergency department and often following an accidental overdose. Family members are frantic, particularly if overdose is how they discover the drug problem. Creating greater distress is the reality that even though a person may have health insurance, coverage for opiate withdrawal may be denied or severely limited. If care is not delivered or hospitalization denied, a person is at risk for emesis aspiration, dehydration, and accidental overdose.

Opiate withdrawal is easily seen in the distress level of the person. Clinical assessment involves objective observations and subjective reports including the following:

Objective:

- Pupil size (dilated)
  - Piloerections
  - Clammy skin
  - Rhinorrhea (nasal sniffles)
  - Yawning
  - Lacrimation (tearing)
  - Emesis
  - Diarrhea
  - Constant rubbing of leg muscles
  - Restless legs
  - Irritability and agitation
  - Disheveled and distressed appearance
- Pulses tend to be in the nineties; blood pressures tend to be low; respirations tend to be normal.

Ask the person about IV use and examine injection sites for abcesses, phlebitis, and cellulitis.

Auscultate apical pulse listening for murmurs and/or rubs.

Review lab results for abnormalities, particularly elevated white blood cells and the presence of blood-borne pathogens.

Subjective reports from the person includes the following:

- Nausea
- Abdominal cramping
- Body aches
- Flu-like symptoms
- Anxiety
- Cravings to make the "dope sickness" go away
- Restless legs

The person in opiate withdrawal should be treated with sincere compassion. The caregiving team needs to remember that addiction is the *inability* to stop using the substance. Most persons continue using opiates not to "get high" but to avoid the sickness of withdrawal.

MEDICATIONS USED TO MANAGE OPIATE WITHDRAWAL

In hospital settings, assessment for opiate withdrawal and effect of medication should be done minimally every 6 hours. Medications approved and indicated for the treatment of opiate withdrawal include methadone and buprenorphine. In treatment centers for detoxification and addictions treatment, these are the only approved agents unless contraindicated (Stine, Greenwald, & Kosten, 2003).

In hospital settings other than detoxification units, long acting *morphine* or oxycodone (Percodan) can be used to "wean" someone from pain medication (D. W. Streem, October 20, 2010; personal communication, 2010). However, methadone and buprenorphine remain the standards.

Oral methadone in liquid form is the preferable form to use for management of opiate withdrawal. Initial dosing is 2–5 mg every 4 hours as needed for withdrawal symptoms. A recommended first dose should be no greater than 5 mg. If the condition requires more, it will be evident and the prn dosage can be increased. Determine the total dose needed within a 24-hour period to minimize symptoms and keep the person relatively comfortable, and use that as a starting point for routine tapering. If a person receives a total of 16 mg in a 24-hour period with symptoms minimized, a routine dose and taper should follow:

- 4 mg qid for four doses (day 1)
- 3 mg qid for four doses (day 2)
- 2 mg qid for three doses (day 3)
- 1 mg qid for four doses (day 4)
- 0.5 mg qid for four doses (day 5)
- 0.5 mg bid for two doses (day 6)

In cases of severe withdrawal, higher doses may be needed. Forty to 80 mg in divided doses may be necessary. Methadone has a half-life of 24–36 hours. When taken on a routine daily basis for maintenance therapy or chronic pain, it is stored in the liver and released slowly (Pate, Zweben, & Martin, 2003). This is the rationale behind once-daily dosing in methadone maintenance clinics.

It is wise to have a prn order for bedside nurses to use for worsening symptoms.

Additionally, instructions should be given to hold the routine dose for sedation or lethargy. Narcan should be available for immediate use for oversedation or unresponsiveness. Adjunct medications should include an antiemetic and antidiarrheal. Benzodiazapines can be administered for agitation. If emesis and diarrhea do not subside, IV fluids should be given. In situations of abscess due to IV injection, antibiotics may be required; additionally, consultation with infectious disease specialists, dermatology, or general surgery may be required. Baclofen may be helpful to decrease muscle aches 40–60 mg in divided doses/day.

Buprenorphine is a synthetic opiate that in and of itself is both an agonist and antagonist at the mu opiate receptor: 50% of the drug innervates the receptor and 50% of the drug blocks the receptor. This unique property provides a ceiling effect with a very low probability of overdose. It does not seem to produce the eurphoria seen with other opiates. It also has moderate analgesic properties.

In 2003, the Food and Drug Administration (FDA)/DEA approved the sublingual preparation for maintenance dosing for persons with opiate addiction. The regulations mandate that only approved and registered physicians prescribe the drug, keep a log of those they prescribe to, and limit the patient numbers to 100 patients.

The physician must take an approved course, have a DEA number, and register with the DEA for an additional number allowing prescribing privileges for sublingual buprenorphine. These regulations apply only to office-based maintenance therapy with sublingual form. Buprenorphine is a schedule III analgesic; to use for treatment of pain, the prescriber needs only a basic DEA license. PMH-APRNs should follow their State Board formularies if considering prescribing.

Preparations include: injectable Buprenex for IM/IV administration, sublingual tablets, and film with and without added naltrexone. Sublingual buprenorphine comes as Subutex (buprenorphine) (2 mg and 4 mg tabs/filmstrip) and Suboxone (buprenorphine/naltrexone) (2 mg/0.5 mg and 8 mg/2 mg) tabs/filmstrips).

Naltrexone (Suboxone) is added as a safeguard against injectable overdose; the FDA feared the potential for misuse by people crushing, dissolving, and injecting the drug. If this is done, the naltrexone will immediately block the mu receptor.

Sublingually, the naltrexone is benign.

Injectable Buprenex has been used on addiction units for opiate detoxification frequently until the sublingual forms became available. The usual protocol is for a 3–4 day course of treatment for opiate withdrawal as follows:

- 1 ml (0.3 mg) deep IM or slow IV every 6 hours on day 1
- every 8 hours on day 2
- bid on day 3
- once on day 4

Tramadol (Ultram) is a synthetic opiate agent that has mild analgesic properties. It has been known to cause seizures when taken in large quantities. Combined use with SSRI antidepressants has been known to cause serotonin syndrome. It has been misused and is the drug of choice for persons with addictive disorder, therefore it should be used if no other options are available and if the person is not taking an SSRI antidepressant or has a history of seizures. It is suggested for ambulatory use when no other options are available. A typical course to prescribe for management of symptoms on an outpatient basis follows:

- 50 mg po four times (day 1)
- 50 mg po three times (day 2)
- 50 mg po twice (day 3)
- 25 mg po twice (day 4)
- 25 mg po once daily (days 5 and 6)
- Provide a prescription for #12 50 mg tablets along with specific instructions.

Baclofen (Lioresal) is a common muscle relaxant that has been shown to provide effective relief from the muscle cramping resulting from opiate withdrawal. It is not a controlled substance and can be prescribed to help bridge the gap between initial assessment and evaluation by an addictions specialist. Effective doses are 10 mg 4x/day to 20 mg 3x/day. It should be tapered down if a person takes it for more than several weeks.

Clonidine (Catapres) is a fast-acting, short-acting antihypertensive that activates the alpha 2 adrenergic receptors, which in turn quiets the neurological response of opiate withdrawal symptoms. It seems to dull the symptoms of opiate withdrawal and take the edge off. It has long been used for opiate withdrawal symptoms in a variety of clinical settings. It is not a controlled drug. It can be prescribed along with tramadol for ambulatory use. Preparations include oral tablets and patches for 7-day transdermal infusion. Patches are far more expensive than tablets.

Dosing for Catapres tablets:

- Day 1: 0.1 mg every 4 hours as needed for symptom control
- Day 2: 0.1–0.2 mg every 4 hours as needed/tolerated
- Maintain a total daily dose no greater than 1.2 mg/day (divided doses) for several days then begin a slow wean to avoid rebound hypertension

Patches of 1–0.2 mg are applied to skin every 7 days. Caution the person about hypotension and related dizziness. Referral to evaluation with an addiction specialist and a return to a clinic appointment should always be recommended.

MANAGEMENT OF PERSONS WITH STIMULANT INTOXICATION AND WITHDRAWAL

INTOXICATION WITH STIMULANTS

With minimal ingestion, stimulant drugs will produce alertness, sharpened cognitions, decreased appetite with increased energy, pleasurable feelings, and insomnia. As cocaine and prescribed stimulant drugs create a flood of dopamine at the neuroreceptor junction, symptoms of intoxication include agitation, restlessness, inability to sleep, purities and skin picking, hallucinations (visual, auditory, and tactile), impaired cognitions and judgment, hypervigilance, and paranoia. In some instances, stimulant intoxication, particularly with cocaine, will produce symptoms indistinguishable from paranoid schizophrenia.

Severe symptoms should be managed with safety as the primary goal—safety for the person and for others. Emergency hospitalization on a locked psychiatric unit may be necessary. Antipsychotic medication should be administered orally (if possible) or intramuscularly to manage both psychotic symptoms and agitation: haldoperidol (Haldol) 5–10 mg PO or IM along with 50 mg diphenhydramine (Benadryl) PO or 25 mg IM. Benzodiazepines may also be administered to help calm the person. Lorazepam (Ativan) 1–2 mg PO or IM or diazepam (Valium) 5–10 mg PO or IM is used. Diphenhydramine may be administered along with any acutely given antipsychotic medication to prevent dystonia and ocular gyro crisis.

A stimulant overdose, particularly when ingested intravenously, can be fatal. A thorough history and physical exam may not be feasible in some instances.

Emergency care with subsequent Intensive Care admission may be in order. Emergency departments are well-versed in the care of critical cocaine overdoses. Sadly enough, many of these emergencies involve children who are paid to deliver the drug from dealer to client. They are taught to swallow the supply if law enforcement approaches; seizure and death can occur if immediate emergency care is not delivered.

STIMULANT WITHDRAWAL

The person withdrawing from chronic stimulant use experiences depression, somnolence, fatigue, irritability, and anxiety. Intense cravings and vivid using dreams are typical with cocaine withdrawal. In instances where the drug is intranasally ingested, rhinorrhea presents with constant sniffling. Assessment should include examination of the nasal cavities and oral mucosa for lesions. Also, if intravenously ingested, injection sites should be examined for signs of abscess or cellulitis. Testing should include EKG, chest imaging particularly for inhaled misuse, and serum for blood-borne pathogens.

Often, the person in stimulant withdrawal responds well to care that is supportive, understanding, and compassionate. A quiet hospital room where they are allowed to sleep, and a person available to sit with them as they fight cravings can make a profound influence in their healing. Benzodiazepines to help with anxiety may be used; antipsychotics may help with lingering agitation or suspiciousness.

In instances where a person is dependent on or misusing prescribed amphetamines, a taper of the amphetamine administered in divided low doses may be considered. This author has managed Adderall or Ritalin weans over several days with good results. Some clinicians will use a medication combo of imipramine (Tofranil) 25 mg tid along with propranolol (Inderal) 20 mg tid over several days to provide a bit of dopamine at the neuroreceptor site. However, there is no medication regime that is recommended for use in managing stimulant withdrawal. The management of such depends largely on the experience of the clinician and the specific symptoms presented.

MANAGING PERSONS WITH MARIJUANA INTOXICATION AND WITHDRAWAL

INTOXICATION

Marijuana intoxication is commonly known as "being stoned" and presents with euphoria, giddiness, sleepiness, enhanced sensory perceptions, hunger, dry mouth, red sclera, glazed eyes, decreased attention span, decreased reaction time, and due to its effects on cardiac muscle, tachycardia. Severe states of intoxication may present with hallucinations, paranoia, confusion, disorientation, loss of insight, panic, and sometimes aggression.

Management of intoxication is primarily palliative. Safety of the person and environment is the first consideration. Supportive care in a secure environment with frequent contact to assess and reassure is needed. EKG and chest imaging should be obtained, particularly if cardiac and/or pulmonary problems preexist. In severe states, antipsychotic medications will help to decrease anxiety, agitation, and accompanying psychotic symptoms.

WITHDRAWAL

As the THC molecule adheres tightly to lipid tissue throughout the body, its release is gradual with a "self-detox" phenomenon. Symptoms of intoxication may linger for several weeks but usually resolve in several days. Administration of prescribed Marinol is not recommended for withdrawal symptoms. Anxiety, restlessness, cravings, and insomnia often occur which can be managed with neuronti or hydroxyzine. Vivid using dreams are common. Frequent contact, with reassurance and encouragement, are all beneficial in managing withdrawal.

MANAGING NICOTINE WITHDRAWAL

Nicotine, be it in the form of cigarettes or oral tobacco, presents with a most severe withdrawal. The symptoms include agitation, irritability, headache, cravings, constipation, increased appetite, and decreased attention span (Schuckit, 2003).

Medically, nicotine preparations can be administered in the form of transdermal patches (21 mg, 14 mg, 7 mg), gum (2 mg, 4 mg), and lozenges. They can be used in combination; the doses can be decreased slowly over time. The use of nicotine replacement for sustained cessation of smoking or tobacco use is successful when a person is highly motivated. The person should be advised not to chew the gum, rather chew once then place between tongue and cheek to enable the nicotine to be absorbed mucosally.

Varenicline (Chantix) is a medication that blocks nicotine at receptors in the brain's pleasure center. It has significant side effects including nausea, vomiting, constipation, flatulence, appetite fluctuations, insomnia, nightmares, headache, heartburn, and unpleasant lingering taste. Severe side effects reported include the following:

- Swelling/edema of face, throat, tongue, lips, eyes, neck, hands, feet, legs
- Hoarse voice
- Difficulty swallowing
- Difficulty breathing
- Blistering skin
- Chest pain
- Slowed speech
- Suicidal thoughts

Persons highly motivated to stop using nicotine often creatively find ways that work for them. Examples of this include chewing on the ends of white straws, thus mimicking smoking a cigarette or sucking on specific mints or candies. Many persons who successfully stop using tobacco report doing so with abrupt cessation and no nicotine replacement therapy, medication, or substitute behaviors.

Nicotine, like alcohol, is a legal drug. Growing tobacco and preparing and packaging the delivery forms of cigarettes, cigars, snuff, and chewing tobacco are leading industries that provide jobs and governmental income. The health hazards of using this drug are well known and documented, yet it continues to be widely used and very legal.

OVER-THE-COUNTER MEDICATIONS (DIPHENHYDRAMINE, DEXTROMETHORPHAN, AND NASAL SPRAY)

Of the many medications available without a prescription, diphenhydramine (Benadryl) is one commonly misused (see Exhibit 17-5). It is an excellent antihistamine agent used in allergic reactions. It is the primary ingredient in over-the-counter sleeping aids and some preparations used to prevent motion sickness. It can cause sedation and euphoria in large doses or when taken intravenously.

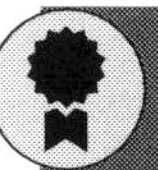

EXHIBIT 17-5: OVER-THE-COUNTER DRUGS THAT HAVE THE POTENTIAL FOR MISUSE AND ADDICTION

Diphenhydramine (Benadryl), which can cause sedation and mild euphoria

Dextromethorphan (cough syrup), which can innervate mu receptors

Pseudoephedrine (Sudafed), which can be a stimulant

Mouth rinse, cold medications, and cough syrups can be misused for alcohol content

Dextromethorphan is the reflected right rotation of the morphine molecule. It is a well known cough suppressant. Its affinity is to the kappa opiate receptor, which, when innervated, decreases the cough reflex. Misuse and dependence has been seen, although infrequently. Often, persons will misuse cough syrups for their alcohol content.

Nasal sprays with and without steroids can also be seen misused and, on occasion, in addictive disorder. As with any substance, it's the combination of the inability to stop the use in the face of negative consequences that presents as the problem.

Many substances may be misused with development of dependence and even addictive disorders, but the negative consequences if they occur are not profound (see Exhibit 17-6).

RECOVERY/RELAPSE PREVENTION

Misuse of a substance without dependence or addiction can usually be stopped by the person or by some external influence. Heavy drinkers who are not alcoholic are able to stop the minute they incur a negative consequence. Persons who regularly smoke marijuana, without addictive disorder, stop the minute they are advised to do so by their physician. Cigarette smokers, without addictive disorder, throw their pack of cigarettes out the car window when they are told they have an abnormal EKG.

Dependence and tolerance can be medically managed with attention given to medical and psychological issues. Addiction, however, is an affliction that when diagnosed, needs its own treatment.

Addictive Disorder, as a separate entity, is not the use of a mood altering substance but rather the inability to stop or refrain from the use when negative things are occurring. In many situations, persons desperately want to stop; the initial pleasure derived from the substance is far gone.

Addictive disorders have no known cure. Like many chronic ailments afflicting humans, they can be treated. With effective treatment on a day-to-day basis, the person stays healthy and can remain in remission from addiction. Like many chronic ailments, relapse is possible.

The traditional treatment for persons with addictive disorder has been the 12-step program of meeting attendance and sponsorship. For most persons who remain in remission from addiction, credit is given

EXHIBIT 17-6: CHEMICALS MISUSED AND SEEN IN ADDICTIVE DISORDERS THAT ARE NOT COVERED IN THIS CHAPTER BUT ARE WORTH NOTING

MDMA (Ecstasy) is a designer drug acting on the serotonin system; it will cause euphoria, arousal, and ultimately confusion

GHB (Gammahydroxybutyrate) is a liquid preparation that causes brief periods of euphoric and hypnotic states

PCP (Angel Dust) is the chemical phencyclidine which causes hallucinations and psychosis

Synthetic Cannabinoid (SPICE) works as an hallucinogen

MDPV or Methylenedioxypyrovalerone is the primary agent in bath salts, with variations as common as the names given to these compounds. MDPV works producing an amphetamine-like effect on the body resulting in analgesia and psychotic-like symptoms

Crystal methamphetamine (ICE), as differentiated from pharmaceutical methamphetamine (Desoxyn), is made in rudimentary laboratories by extracting pseudoephedrine from, Over the Counter (as in over the counter meds) (OTC) tablets. The many chemicals used in the preparation are extremely toxic as is the preparation itself

Metabolic Steroids

to their 12-step program. The most common reason persons give for relapsing is "I stopped going to my meetings."

The 12-step program of AA was developed by Bill Wilson, a New York stockbroker, and Dr. Robert Holbrook Smith, an Akron, Ohio, surgeon, in 1935. Noteworthy is that Sister Mary Ignatia, a Venetian Sister of Charity and originally from Ireland, assisted these two men with their new "treatment"; she developed the first hospital-based detoxification units, first at Akron's St. Thomas Hospital (known today as Ignatia Hall), then at Cleveland's St. Vincent Charity Hospital (known today as Rosary Hall). Her compassion and efforts were the very seeds of realization that addiction is not an "immoral bad habit" but a disease to be treated and managed.

Whether residential or ambulatory, whether long or short term, programs are designed to provide support and education to persons as they begin developing a personalized recovery program for themselves, a program they can practice daily. Treatment programs assist individuals as they make difficult but necessary changes in their lifestyle. Counseling, educational lectures, group therapies, occupational therapies, pastoral guidance, and spiritual development are at the core of treatment services. Medications are often a part of the treatment plan as well.

An initial "prescription" for a Recovery Program may look like this:

Daily: Attend a meeting (AA, Narcotics Anonymous)
Phone your sponsor
Practice spiritual connection (in whatever way you choose)
Follow guidance
Abstain from all mood-altering substances

Changing one's lifestyle can be very difficult; in recovery from addictions, it's essential. Traditional recovery is abstinence-based: abstinence from all forms of alcohol, recreational drugs, and mood-altering substances. Traditional recovery supports certain prescribed medications to assist one in maintaining sobriety: Antabuse, naltrexone, acamprosate, antidepressants, and mood-stabilizers and antipsychotics.

Maintenance therapies in the forms of methadone, Levo-Alpha Acetyl Methadol (LAAM), and buprenorphine are nontraditional and often rejected by traditional recovery therapies. Many persons with opiate addiction are effectively treated with maintenance therapies that allow them to function optimally and remain in remission. Harm-reduction interventions are practiced in some areas to assist persons in reducing the physical harms that are likely to happen in active addiction.

ASSISTANT MEDICATIONS

Disulfi ram (Antabuse). Disulfiram is classified as an alcohol-sensitizing agent. It has been used since the early 1970s to deter persons from using beverage alcohol.

Alcohol is metabolized by hepatic enzymes first to acetylaldehyde then to the acetyl group, which is used by the body to make acetylcholine, and the aldehyde group, which is eliminated. Disulfiram stops the hepatic enzyme that works to break up the acetylaldehyde, thus causing it to remain in the circulating blood. The specific hepatic enzyme blocked is aldehyde dehydrogenase. The circulated acetylaldehyde creates an illness that is quite unpleasant and intolerable. Disulfiram-ethanol (DER) reaction can be mild to severe.

It presents with flushing, tachycardia, palpitations, hypotension, nausea, vomiting, difficulty breathing, diaphoresis, dizziness, blurred vision, and confusion. DER is usually self-limiting; however, there have been cases where severe cardiovascular collapse or seizure occurs. In severe DER, death has occurred (Kranzler & Jaffe, 2003). Disulfiram is available in strengths of 250 mg and 500 mg. The usual dose is 250 mg daily; it can be just as effective when taken three times a week. Common side effects include drowsiness, lethargy, and fatigue.

Disulfiram is not indicated for persons with liver disease, viral hepatitis carriers, or those who are at high risk for relapse on alcohol. Persons who work in factories where fumes are inhaled should not take Antabuse. Persons should be advised against the use of mouthwash, hand sanitizer, or aftershave lotions containing alcohol. Colognes should be sprayed on clothing rather than skin. Alcohol-containing foods such as salad dressings and marinades should be avoided.

Disulfiram is only effective if a person takes it, and only if they are responsive to the knowledge that illness will occur with alcohol consumption. It is ideally used when administered by a trusted other. Receiving the drug from someone the person can visit daily and trust to oversee their taking the medication is important. The ritual of going to another person daily to receive the medication becomes a major part of a person's recovery program. It should not be prescribed to persons with minimal insight into their alcoholism, those not motivated to stop alcohol intake, those with poor judgment, and those at high risk for relapse.

Acamprosate (Campral). This drug was widely studied in Europe and the United States and found to be more effective than placebo in reducing cravings and consumption of alcohol.

The chemical calcium acetylomotaurinate is an amino acid derivative that innervates GABA and glutamate neurotransmitters (Kranzler & Jaffe, 2003).

Its major side effects are diarrhea, headache, and dizziness. There are no adverse effects if alcohol is consumed concurrently. It is available in 333 mg tablets with the recommended dosing being two tablets three times daily or one tablet three times a day if side effects occur.

Opiate antagonist (Naltrexone). This drug is approved for persons with addiction to alcohol and/or opiate drugs. The two available forms are oral tablets and depo injection (Vivitrol).

Naltrexone, as an opiate antagonist, blocks the opiate receptors. It is theorized that the reinforcing and pleasurable feelings that occur with alcohol may be due to its effects on the mu receptors in the brain; blocking them with an opiate antagonist has been shown to decrease cravings. For persons with addiction to opiates, blocking the receptors has been shown to decrease cravings and prevent effects of opiates should they be taken concurrently.

The depo form of naltrexone, marketed as Vivitrol, is a deep-muscle injection to be administered monthly. It is expensive and cumbersome to obtain, prepare, and inject. It is delivered, packaged in ice, directly from the pharmacy to the clinical site where it is to be administered. It comes with two sets of needles: one for preparation, the other for administration. The medication and its diluents must be kept refrigerated until 45 minutes before administration. It is then reconstituted into 4 ml of medication with immediate injection deep into the gluteal muscles.

Side effects include pain and induration at the injection site, insomnia, and feelings of "depersonalization." Once side effects subside, persons have reported that cravings and preoccupation are "gone"; as one young man said: "Wow, I feel normal" (29-year-old male, 2011, personal statement).

Antidepressants. Research has shown that SSRI antidepressants allow a bit more serotonin (5-HT) to linger at the neurosynaptic junction and often decrease cravings for alcohol and other drugs. Fluoxetine (Prozac), sertralin (Zoloft), and citalopram (Celexa) have all been shown to have some beneficial effect on decreasing cravings and use in persons with addiction. Indeed, the mood-altering effects of these drugs are why they are prescribed.

In summary, all of the above-mentioned medications alter physiology, either neurotransmitters or enzymes. No medication has been found to "cure" addictive disorder, but clinicians and academicians are learning much about the intricacies of the human nervous system. In reviewing the vast amount of literature on the research, it is clear that the more we learn, the more we appreciate how much we don't know.

MAINTENANCE THERAPIES

The use of aggressive community treatment and intensive case management initially developed for individuals with chronic and persistent mental illness have been modified and effectively applied to the COD population. For more information on these approaches see Chapter 10, Integrative Management of Psychotic Disorders.

Methadone Clinics. In 1965, Dole and Nyswander suggested that chronic heroin use deranges opiate receptors in the body equivalent to a metabolic disorder, thus making it difficult to remain abstinent following detoxification. They suggested that daily doses of methadone for an extended period of time corrects the disorder—thus the birth of opiate maintenance therapy (OMT) and methadone maintenance clinics (Dole, 1972).

OMT is an FDA-approved therapy for opiate dependence. The therapy and clinics are highly regulated by federal (SAMHSA) and state agencies. The clinics are located in major metropolitan areas. Candidates are evaluated and, if accepted, provided with daily doses of liquid methadone at the clinic. Some clinics are open only weekdays; others provide weekend dosing. Daily doses of methadone range from 30 mg to 120 mg per day with average doses of 40 mg to 80 mg (Pate, Zweben, & Martin, 2003).

Methadone has a half-life of 24–36 hours. In the 1970s, LAAM was introduced for OMT, administered at the OMT clinics. L-alpha-acetyl methadone is an analogue with a half-life of 72–96 hours, thus decreasing the need for daily dosing. Clients qualifying for LAAM need only report to the clinic three times weekly.

Doses of LAAM range from 20–30 mg to as high as 100 mg every 3 days. The OMT clinics all have medical, nursing, and counseling services and programs.

Methadone maintenance is the recommended standard of care for pregnant women who suffer with active opiate addiction. Miscarriage can occur due to stress on a fetus in opiate withdrawal. Methadone has not been shown to cause damage to a developing fetus, or latent effects in childhood. Following birth, a baby will need to be managed for methadone withdrawal. This is safely accomplished in a neonatal intensive care unit using morphine or tincture of opium. Pregnant women, by federal law, are cared for immediately upon referral to an OMT clinic; there is no waiting period. Most clinics have specialized programs for pregnant women.

Buprenorphine Office-Based Maintenance Therapy. Buprenorphine is a drug that itself is both an opiate agonist and antagonist. When it attaches to the mu opiate receptor, 50% of the drug innervates the receptor with the other 50% blocking it. It has some significant analgesic effects without the euphoria or "high" produced by other opiate agents. It has been used as an injectable analgesic and for brief inpatient opiate detoxification in centers that choose not to use methadone.

In 2003, sublingual buprenorphine was approved as a maintenance therapy for persons with opiate addiction, marketed as Suboxone and Subutex. Subutex is pure buprenorphine with its 50/50 effect. Suboxone is buprenorphine with added naloxone. The naloxone is added to deter misuse and prevent fatality should it be put into solution with IV injection. Sublingually, due to saliva pH, naloxone is very poorly absorbed and virtually inert. If injected, the naloxone will block the mu receptors immediately.

To prescribe sublingual buprenorphine to persons with opiate dependence, one must be a physician with a DEA number. Upon completion of a 2-day training course, the physician applies for a second DEA number known as a DEA X number. The physician can then prescribe the medication for up to 100 patients at a time. The physician may individually manage these clients with whatever guidelines they see as appropriate. As Suboxone is expensive, a person needs to determine how both the drug and the physician visits will be financed.

Typically, there is an induction phase following 24 hours of cessation of the opiate. The drug has a greater effect when the person is experiencing more severe withdrawal symptoms; if taken too close to the last dose of opiate, they may likely experience withdrawal symptoms from the antagonist property of buprenorphine.

When a dose is determined for daily maintenance, the person is required to comply with a specific agreement. Most prescribers mandate participation in an outpatient addictions treatment program and attendance at 12-step meetings. Return to clinic involves pharmacology testing to determine abstinence from mood-altering drugs and alcohol; in states that have an automatic reporting system for controlled substances, it should be routinely monitored to determine whether the person is receiving controlled drugs from other prescribers. An average daily dose of Suboxone is between 12 mg and 24 mg per day in divided doses. The drug is delivered in pill form or dissolvable strips that can be cut; both forms come in doses of 8 mg/2 mg and 2 mg/0.5 mg (buprenorphine/naloxone). The most common side effects are constipation and a bitter, unpleasant taste.

Persons should be advised to use a stool softener and laxative. Sublingual irritation and swelling are rare; it is seen more often with the strip. Persons should be advised that abrupt cessation of Suboxone will cause symptoms of opiate withdrawal.

Should opiate agents become necessary in the event of surgery or medical problems, Suboxone should be stopped 3 days before taking other opiates. Maintenance therapy is recommended for 1 to 2 years during which the person should be involved in a 12-step program of active recovery. Weaning off of Suboxone is usually done with dose reduction weekly.

Many persons have great difficulty weaning off of 2 mg/day. Once the 2 mg dose is stopped, it is recommended that the person use a small wedge of the film or portion of the tablet when the withdrawal symptoms become unbearable. Often, a person will need to be hospitalized for management with methadone detoxification. Some practitioners accept that some people will need Suboxone maintenance for their entire lives.

Candidates for Suboxone maintenance therapy should be assessed carefully. They should be responsible to safeguard their medication, keep their appointments, and take the medication as prescribed. They should advise all health care providers that they are on the medication and carry a card with name and contact information of the prescribing physician. They should be educated that any narcotic medication for analgesia will not be effective. Prior to surgery or when needing narcotic analgesic medication, they should stop taking Suboxone 36 hours before.

Suboxone is sold on the street. Persons will often keep a supply on hand to use when their supply of heroin or other opiate is unattainable; they will often sell or trade it for their preferred drug. Suboxone is the preferred preparation for office-based opiate maintenance. Subutex may be cautiously used if a person shows intolerance to or idiosyncratic reactions to Suboxone.

There is emerging evidence of safety for use during pregnancy. It is recommended that Subutex rather than Suboxone be used during pregnancy and weekly monitoring be maintained throughout. Communication between prescribing physician, obstetrician, pediatrician, and hospital staff should be maintained for the safety and well-being of the woman, the baby, and all caregivers. After delivery, the baby will need medical management of opiate withdrawal in a neonatal intensive care unit with either morphine or opium. Needless to say, this can be an emotionally tense situation for all concerned, and one in which compassion and understanding are essential.

Buprenorphine is a schedule III controlled substance. Advanced practice nurses with prescriptive authority may prescribe it for analgesia if their state board approves. Suboxone for OMT may not be prescribed by APNs. The DEA is well aware that the demand and need for Suboxone therapy far exceeds the number of physicians approved to prescribe it. Approved use by PMH-APRNs may be forthcoming.

HARM REDUCTION THERAPIES

As addictive disorder is characterized by the inability to stop the use of a substance when negative things happen, it is logical that many clinicians focus on reducing the chance of negative consequences happening, rather than a person's inability to stop. Needle exchange programs are in major cities providing sterile syringes while collecting and destroying used ones. This decreases the circulation of used syringes in communities, thus decreasing the risks that come from needle sharing.

Vaccination vans circulate in areas where drug trade occurs, encouraging persons to receive vaccinations against hepatitis A and B and be screened for other blood-borne or sexually transmitted pathogens. England offers prescription heroin in specialized clinics. Evidence-based research since 2002 has shown a drastic reduction in street use of heroin and subsequent drug-related crime. Prescribed heroin was far more effective than methadone in helping persons "stay clean," avoid crime, and have a greater quality of life (Kerr, Montaner, & Wood, 2010).

> Author's Note: Some physicians who prescribe Suboxone as maintenance therapy do not require abstinence from other drugs. Their thinking is that Suboxone is a "harm reduction" medication helping persons avoid the harmful practice of injecting opiates (G. B. Collins, october 20, 2010 personal communication, 2010).

ADJUNCTIVE TREATMENTS, ALTERNATIVE/ COMPLEMENTARY APPROACHES, AND PSYCHOTHERAPY

A human nervous system takes time to heal, adjust, and establish homeostasis in the absence of substance it has grown accustomed to. This takes time and the process is often uncomfortable, particularly with the added stress of lifestyle change. Anxiety, agitation, insomnia, and feelings of "panic" are often reported following detoxification and in early stages of recovery. This can last for several months and puts a person at risk for relapse. Medications and other forms of therapy are available to help the person as they change and develop a solid program of recovery.

WESTERN MEDICATIONS

Most persons in early recovery report increased anxiety. Often, it is latent withdrawal. More often, the fear of facing the negative consequences accrued by virtue of their addictive lifestyle is overwhelming. Anxiety, as unpleasant as it is, is a normal response in early recovery. There have been several agents that can safely be used to manage anxiety without the risk of relapse:

- Gapapentin (Neurontin) 300–600 mg every 6 hours either routinely or as needed
- Hydroxyzine (Atarax) 10–25 mg or Vistaril 25–50 mg every 6 hours as needed
- Quetiapine (Seroquel) 25–50 mg every 6 hours either routinely or as needed
- Antidepressant SSRIs that have specific "calming" effects may help; these include sertraline (Zoloft) and citalopram (Celexa)

Sleep is the last thing to return following withdrawal of a substance. The best option is to wait it out with no medication. Persons have tremendous difficulty doing this however. Safe medications to use at bedtime include gabapentin, hydroxyzine, and seroquel. Trazadone (Desyrel) is an antidepressant agent that has sedating properties; it is used often for insomnia at doses of 25–100 mg at bedtime

As a person's body and mind adjust to not having a substance, mood swings can occur. Often, a person in early recovery struggles with anger and impulsive outbursts. Medications can sometimes help minimize these symptoms.

- Valproic acid (Depakote): Begin with 125 mg twice daily to 250 mg twice daily
- Lithium (Eskalith): Begin with 150 mg twice daily to 300 mg twice daily; do not use in persons who are renally compromised or with elevations in creatinine and blood urea nitrogen (BUN)
- Topiramate (Topamax): 25 mg daily to begin then bid

When used to treat persons with bipolar disorder, these medications are prescribed in higher doses to attain a certain serum level in the blood. When used to assist persons with addictive disorder in managing mood swings, lower doses are effective.

PSYCHOTHERAPY

The energy of a group is therapeutic in helping a person in early recovery. Treatment programs are designed to teach a person to use the group process as a therapeutic tool. The group provides a place for processing feelings, reinforcing nondestructive coping, and overall exchange of energy between people. It provides education and helps one feel less isolated.

Meeting frequently with a trusted therapist, along with other modalities, can be helpful. Traditional psychotherapy is not recommended in early recovery. Addressing psychological trauma, uncovering repressed memories, and dealing with deep issues places the person at risk for relapse. A solid program of recovery including a strong support network and effective coping skills should be established before a person engages in psychodynamic therapies. However, cognitive-behavioral techniques can be especially helpful.

Eye movement desensitization and reprocessing is a unique form of therapy that assists a person to release traumatic memories that are energetically "frozen" in a person's physiological makeup. It allows the trauma to be revealed and released without the painful re-experiencing of the event. It was developed in the 1990s by Francine Shapiro. Her story is fascinating; she stumbled upon the realization that eye movement helps one cope with painful feelings (Shapiro, 1997). For persons with addictive disorder, it is best used in conjunction with a 12-Step Program.

Eriksonian hypnosis, developed by Milton Erikson, engages the unconscious mind without a person going into a deep trance. Erickson's story is also fascinating as he developed the technique through his own determination to overcome disability from polio (O'Hanlon, 2009).

Information and suggestions absorbed directly into the unconscious have a greater chance of transitioning to behavior change. This therapy has been particularly effective in helping with smoking cessation and reducing anxiety. Initial stages of recovery often find a person in a "haze"; a therapist can intervene with repeated encouragement and suggestions for recovery.

ENERGY THERAPIES

Many cultures believe that the human body, as part of our vast universe, resonates with the energy that is around us. Clearly, unseen energy is what enables us to use cell phones and wireless Internet applications (Chan, 1996). Asian cultures have taught us that the human body has specific points able to absorb and release energy: the center of the palm of the hand, the crown at the top of the head, the soles of the feet, the center of the sacral back, and the center of the clavicle (Page & Howard, 1998).

Indian culture has given us knowledge of the Chakras, the energy vortexes of the body and mind. Studying ancient Indian healing methods, one appreciates the meaning of these vortexes on disease states and the ability of the person to heal (Page & Howard, 1998). Chakras include the following:

- The Crown Chakra is located at the very center of the top of the head, which connects with energy from the cosmos.

- The Third Eye Chakra is located in the center of the forehead, which connects to the energy of archetypal wisdom.
- The Throat Chakra is located in the pharynx. It relates to the energy of communication and expression of the self.
- The Heart Chakra is at the center of the sternum, connecting with the energy of compassion for others and the world.
- The Solar Plexus Chakra is located in the center of the upper abdomen. This energy center acts as a protective radar screen for external energy fields. When we are in a situation where we need to protect ourselves, we automatically cross our arms over the Solar Plexus Chakra.
- The Pelvic Chakra is in the pelvic area between the pelvic bones; it connects with energy of creation. It generates our own creative energy in whatever form we choose to use.
- The Base Chakra is located at the coccyx. It connects with the energy of our roots. It often is firmly attached to biological family and "tribe" norms and beliefs.

There are many modes of therapy that are effective in using these energy systems of our bodies to therapeutically transform and heal disease states. The same neurotransmitters are affected as with Western Medicine technique. Noteworthy is that Western Medicine has been developed over the past 250 years. Albeit good, wholesome, and often quite effective, it's relatively new compared to some Eastern techniques that have been practiced for thousands of years.

ACUPUNCTURE: This therapy has been practiced for thousands of years by Chinese Medicine physicians. It is an established practice in Western Medicine, particularly for its effects as an analgesic. Persons with addictions have reported that acupuncture is highly effective in reducing anxiety and muscle aches that occur in latent withdrawal. Acupuncture alters neurotransmitter physiology by the careful placement of needles in points along the body's meridian system. The meridian system is parallel to the nervous system.

REIKI: This form of therapy is given to us from ancient Japanese healers. Reiki practitioners are trained and certified; they pull in energy using their own mind, transitioning it through their hands onto another. The transitioned energy works to mobilize the endogenous energy of the recipient, affecting the therapist as well. It is a safe therapy to use with persons with addictive disorder as it helps alleviate pain, anxiety, and tension.

EMOTIONAL FREEDOM TECHNIQUE (EFT): EFT is a practice of tapping on specific acupuncture meridian points while repeating affirmations; it is practiced repetitively with a specific therapeutic targeting of a symptom. It can be taught to persons for self-practice as a way to cope and deal with symptoms. It is a technique that can be used by licensed psychologists, psychiatrists, social workers, and psychiatric nurses to mobilize feelings and energies in clients suffering with the challenges of physical, emotional, and biopsychosocial problems (Lock, 2006).

The technique was developed by now-retired engineer Gary Craig. Multiple sources of training are available with EFT practitioners and in workshops (Lock, 2006).

QI GONG: Qi Gong is an ancient practice of Chinese Medicine that is actively used to this day as a mode of therapy in Chinese hospitals. Qi ("chee") and Gong are the Chinese words for energy and practice respectively; Qi Gong is "energy practice." It entails a series of various movements involving the body's points of energy exchange. The movements are designed to align the body with the universe so that energy is absorbed and released toward therapeutic balance. There are multiple movement series from simple to complex. It is most effective with daily practice and can be incorporated into the daily care plan for addiction recovery.

Qi Gong has been shown to increase energy and a sense of well-being as well as decrease anxiety and pain. It provides a gentle form of exercise (Chan, 1996).

ENERGY PSYCHOLOGY: Mind-body healing involves therapy with the body's energy fields. It utilizes a person's conscious mind along with movement techniques to mobilize feelings and energy with psychodynamic processing (Feinstein, Eden, & Craig, 2005; Myss, 1997a, 1997b; Page & Howard, 1998; Pert, Drecher, & Ruff, 2005).

MEDITATION and GUIDED IMAGERY: These are very effective ways of using the mind to influence body responses (Naperstek, 1997).

SPIRITUAL PRACTICES: Connecting with a Higher Power is a basic premise in the 12-step program. Research has shown that persons who experience a "spiritual awakening" have greater sustainable sobriety (Strobbe, 2009). While there is no defined way that a person can have a "spiritual awakening", there are practices that persons find helpful in their pursuit of sobriety. While many persons find connection with a higher power through religious practices, spiritual connectedness is not synonymous to or dependent on religion.

Obtaining a sense of spirituality involves getting out of one's self and connecting with that which is greater. Many persons in recovery connect with others in their group; many connect with nature or an object in nature. What is important is the daily practice of that which is spiritual.

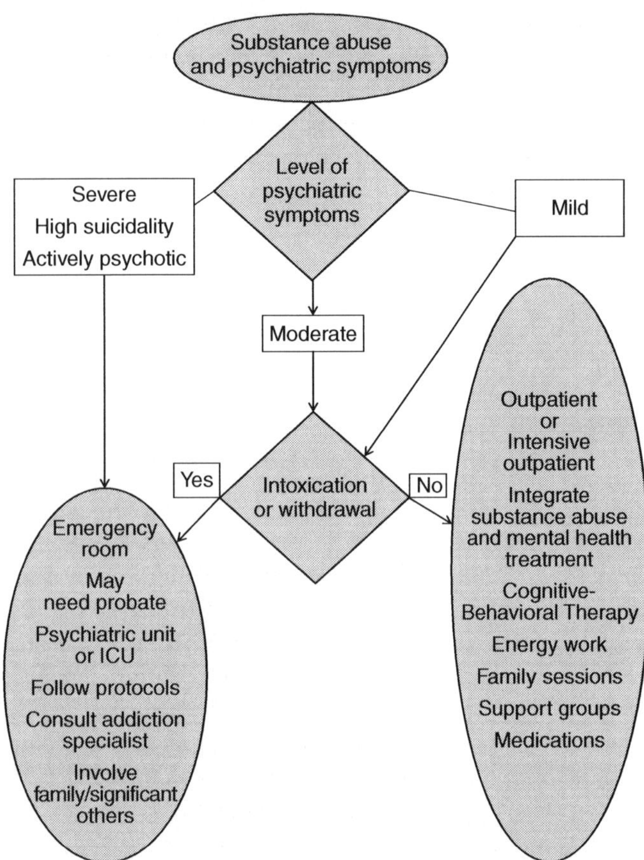

FIGURE 17-2 Decision Tree for Initiation of Treatment for Co-Occurring Substance Abuse Disorders and Psychiatric Syndromes

Veteran members of AA often advise newcomers to "get down on your knees as soon as you get out of bed in the morning, and before you get into your bed every night." Sitting on the front porch and talking to the powerful oak tree sitting in the yard is often a very effective way to develop a sense of spirituality.

Nature is a true source of renewal, energy, and spiritual connection. Popular places for retreat and vacation usually are close to mountains, forests, and water; people seek out that which is greater than themselves to renew and re-energize. Nature and the universe are true sources of energy (Chan, 1996).

Some basic guidelines to follow when working with individuals with COD (see Figure 17-2):

- Be aware of your own thoughts, feelings, and possible prejudices regarding addictive disorders and the unique situation presented to you by your client.
- Maintain a recovery perspective.
- Use a multiproblem viewpoint.
- Work with a team or colleague for support, guidance, and consultation.
- Be compassionate as you remember that a person is suffering with a chronic affliction.
- Keep a list of readily available resources.
- Address individual problems and social problems early in treatment.
- Know your practice limits and establish a relationship with area addiction specialists to contact for advice, guidance, and referral.
- Plan for cognitive and functional impairments in clients.
- Maximize support systems—formal and informal.
- Know how to access your State Board of Pharmacy's automated reporting system for controlled substances. Run a report on clients for whom you prescribe medications.

TREATMENT WITH CONSIDERATION FOR DIVERSE POPULATIONS

Substance misuse, dependence, and addiction can occur across the life span. Certain groups may seem more susceptible to its development, but no person or group is immune to it. How persons are affected by substance use and addiction may vary; and how one responds to treatment interventions certainly varies across generations and cultures.

SUMMARY

Psychiatric disorders can be the result of substance misuse, dependence, and addictions. Thoughts, feelings, and behaviors are altered with drugs and alcohol, which can cause psychosis, depression, and suicidality. Careful assessment along with a comprehensive physical and psychiatric examination is essential.

Psychiatric diagnoses in the presence of substances should always indicate the possibility that it is drug induced. Likewise, a psychiatric diagnosis should not be permanent unless made after a client is drug/alcohol free for several months or there is evidence of the psychiatric disorder before the substance use began.

Often, a person with active hallucinations will use alcohol to medicate and quiet their senses. Once stabilized with psychiatric medications, these persons use AA involvement as a way to socialize and feel a sense of belonging.

Furthermore, once the existence of an independent psychiatric disorder combined with a substance abuse disorder is established, the individual should receive seamless, concurrent treatment.

PEDIATRIC POINTERS

Children are most likely to be affected by a family member's problem with drugs and alcohol. Usually, it is their parents, but could also be siblings, grandparents, or other persons they are close to. The child exposed to repeated chemical use during fetal development may have tragic consequences.

The child abused or neglected by parents whose primary concern is obtaining and using a mood–altering chemical can suffer both physical and emotional consequences.

Children who are injured in alcohol-related car accidents or suffer burns in the kitchen when no adult is around are victims of these disorders.

Federal law mandates that health care professionals report suspicions or knowledge of child abuse or neglect to county Social Service agencies.

This law covers reporting pregnant women who are using mood-altering substances when their fetus is at a stage of development viable out of the womb.

Should a newborn test positive for opiates, alcohol, cocaine, or marijuana, reporting is mandatory. Diagnoses of addictive disorder in children before adolescence is not done.

The diagnosis is more commonly given in adolescence, but carefully. Many adolescents who use alcohol and other drugs are considered "at risk" and are provided specialized treatment to deter the development of addictive disorder.

Needless to say, alcohol, cigarette, and drug use is damaging to an adolescent body, particularly brain development. Rapid brain growth occurs in fetal development up to age 5, then slows a bit until age 13 when again it speeds up.

Adolescents are a particularly difficult group to treat in that their immaturity makes it difficult for them to grasp the reality of the problem. They are at a stage where peer relationships are both difficult and important.

Complete abstinence may be an unreasonable goal for them, whereas decreasing harmful toxic substances in quantity or frequency may be feasible.

Assessment is the first step; depending on the situation, they may be included in a special "at-risk" group for teens. Specialized treatment centers may be indicated.

Often, the focus of treatment and goal development is not abstinence, rather improved attendance at school, better grades, and better family communication.

Noteworthy is that when a teen is assessed for behavioral changes and drug use is suspected, a complete physical exam with laboratory testing should be done. A lumbar puncture may be indicated to rule out viral illness that could manifest in behavioral changes or mask as intoxication.

Young adults are another unique group to treat. The emergence into adulthood that occurs between the ages of 18 and 25 years is difficult for everyone. College, drinking, relationships, sexuality, drug experimentation, leaving home, and finding work all create a tumultuous environment. Young adults are desperate for independence yet not quite ready to function on their own. Their brains are still developing and decision making is not the best. They are at great risk for substance misuse and quite possibly have developed addictive disorder. Important to remember in planning care with young adults is to prevent your own frustration. They may be bright, motivated, and enthusiastic to "do well" yet in spite of good treatment, they may still "not get it." You need to recognize that their brains are still developing.

Patience while they are given time, education, and guidance is essential. They fear losing their girlfriend or job at the local grocery far more than fear of health or legal problems.

Education with regard to toxic effects of alcohol and drugs should be provided without expectation that it will change behavior. Many young adults report witnessing deaths among friends; often this is the motivation to ask for help.

Education with regard to addiction, along with the reassurance that continued use is "not

(*Continued*)

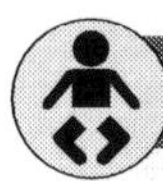

PEDIATRIC POINTERS (*Continued*)

their fault" but a real and poorly understood disorder, should be given.

Comparing addictive disorder to other chronic afflictions such as leukemia or diabetes often helps young people understand and accept their affliction. Supporting their self-esteem and giving them hope helps establish trust and more readily accept guidance. Ideally, the young person will accept residential treatment to begin maturing and developing a healthy lifestyle, which provides the best chance for sustainable recovery.

Parents will be in need of support as their young adult child begins treatment. Many parents will be traumatized at learning that their child has been injecting drugs. They are in need of education and guidance, particularly regarding their limits in "rescuing" their child from the force of addiction. Frequent communication with parents and referral to family support groups helps.

Pregnant women who are dependent on alcohol or drugs pose a unique challenge. Addictions treatment centers may be reluctant to provide detoxification services out of fear or lack of resources for prenatal care. High-risk obstetrical units may be reluctant to provide care due to inexperience or collective attitude of staff. The woman may present in early stages of pregnancy with a solid support system and a mature attitude.

The woman may present in her 8th month, and may be living on the streets, with no family support, no knowledge of the baby's paternity, and a history of sexually transmitted disease. This is one situation when the PMH-APRN needs to know community referral sources:

- Treatment centers equipped with knowledge and resources;
- Obstetrical caregivers with experience and willingness to provide care;
- Methadone maintenance treatment centers with mother-infant programs;
- Social service agencies that specialize in helping pregnant women;
- Women's residential treatment centers that will accept a pregnant woman.

In the instance of alcohol addiction, detoxification is essential to spare the fetus further toxic exposure. Detoxification is also essential with sedative addiction even though there is less toxic damage to a fetus than with alcohol.

Opiates pose less risk for toxic damage to a developing fetus. Withdrawal from opiates, however, is very stressful to a fetus. Preventing miscarriage is the goal for opiate-addicted moms. The standard of care is referral to a methadone maintenance program for continued daily dosing. Federal and state laws mandate that pregnant women be seen by the program immediately without the usual wait.

An emerging number of addiction psychiatrists are electing to manage pregnant women addicted to opiates with buprenorphine in an ambulatory, office-based setting. Subutex rather than Suboxone is used to lessen any adverse effects from naloxone. Collaboration with the obstetrician, birthing-unit staff, neonatal ICU staff, and pediatrician make the situation less stressful for all concerned.

Women managed with methadone or buprenorphine throughout their pregnancy should be advised that their infant will be born dependent on these substances and require careful monitoring throughout withdrawal and detoxification.

In some cases, if the pregnant woman is mature, responsible, and has established prenatal care and a solid family support system, she may be a candidate for detoxification. This should be done in a hospital setting with methadone. It should be done slowly to minimize risk of miscarriage. A pregnant woman should be advised of all options and resources. It is essential to document that this counseling has been done.

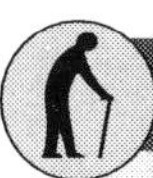

AGING ALERTS

Older adults present with their own set of beliefs and values. They may reject any diagnosis of "alcoholism" or "drug addiction." To some older adults, taking medication prescribed by a physician is not problematic, even if they take multiple controlled medications from several physicians. Often they may present with "polypharmacy" dependence, taking multiple pills for various ailments all that interact adversely with one another. Often they are dependent on "pill taking" itself, wanting a pill for everything. Challenges that may be present in caring and treating the older adult:

- They may have multiple physical, cognitive, or psychiatric disorders that indicate the use of mood-altering substances.
- They may "self-medicate" with alcohol, over-the-counter medications, and even cocaine for its energetic and sexual effects.
- They may save their medications and share them with friends/spouses.
- They will often take their spouse's medication.
- They are often faced with loss of independence, depending on others for transportation.
- The "imperfect health care system" with hurried office visits and multiple specialties tends to be rushed and "pill-focused." Benzodiazapines were the most widely prescribed drug for persons older than 65 years; and of all the benzodiazapines prescribed in the United States, the greatest percentage were to older adults.
- Symptoms of substance misuse may mimic those of other maladies common in older adults: diabetes, depression, hypertension, insomnia.
- There have been situations where older adults sell their prescribed mood-altering medications (opiates, sedatives) to supplement their income.

Treating an older adult who may suffer with misuse, dependence, or addictive disorders should start with a complete physical exam, laboratory testing, EKG, chest films, and a complete review of medications. If necessary, hospitalized medical management of withdrawal should be done. Communication and collaboration between all caregivers should be done; in this age of electronic medical records and computer communication, this should be easily accomplished.

If addiction treatment is indicated, referral to a center with a track designed for older adults is best. The older adult may have difficulty in centers with younger persons addicted to drugs unfamiliar to them. In some treatment groups designed to provide therapy to older adults, reference is not made to "alcoholism" or "drug addiction"; instead, the person is encouraged to identify themselves "as a proud member of AA" or "I became dependent on the medicine my doctor prescribed." This helps to minimize perception of societal stigma that may interfere with therapy.

Older adults may have great difficulty facing the negative consequences of alcohol or drug addiction. Rather than confrontation, it may be more beneficial to have them dialogue and reminisce about their life, while the therapist supportively reminds them of the negativity of their alcohol/drug use as appropriate.

Certain religions and cultures have fixed and long-term beliefs regarding alcohol and drug use. Many cultures encourage heavy alcohol use as a norm in their lifestyle; the term "alcoholic" is not accepted.

Muslim culture forbids the use of alcohol; admitting that one uses alcohol could bring severe punishment. A physician from a Muslim country admitted that he "never" charts alcohol abuse in cases of liver failure, even though it is the apparent cause.

The Jehovah's Witness faith supports abstinence from drugs and alcohol. They are tolerant of members of their faith who do have a problem and support their seeking help.

Cultural and religious beliefs held deeply by a person with a drug/alcohol problem can be a challenge. Feelings of shame, guilt, and remorse for going against "tribe" beliefs may be well defended, thus difficult to acknowledge

(Continued)

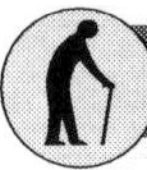

AGING ALERTS (*Continued*)

and process. The treatment provider needs to tread slowly and develop realistic goals.

Education regarding addictive disorder as a chronic affliction rather than a bad habit that is under their control may help them move forward. Referral to pastoral care or a spiritual advisor, regardless of the denomination, may be of help.

Executives—business owners, attorneys, accountants, bank presidents, pilots, and politicians—all are held in high esteem in their communities. Often, alcohol consumption is expected as part of their professional interactions. Receiving help for addiction is difficult. They fear media coverage should the secret be revealed. They fear encountering clients and people they know at AA meetings. They are reluctant to talk openly in treatment groups. Reassurance of complete confidentiality is essential to engage them in treatment. Specialized therapy groups with other executives have been tremendously helpful. The executive tends to feel safer and more anonymous in a peer-attended therapy group.

Indigent clients who are homeless or have no family support often require complete hospitalization for multiple medical concerns and referral to community resources or residential treatment centers designed for them. Free Clinics in major cities usually have ambulatory treatment programs. Persons with limited or no financial resources may be referred to free clinic chemical dependency programs. Serving these persons is another occasion when a comprehensive list of referral resources is essential. Knowledge of area hospitals and treatment centers that have "charity care" services is helpful.

Health care professionals—nurses, physicians, dentists, and pharmacists—are all subject to substance misuse, dependence, and addictive disorder. These are the professionals that people trust to care for them. They are the last that are suspected of alcohol or drug addiction. Yet they are at least as likely as anyone else to suffer with the affliction (Coombs, 1997).

Denial of a problem is profound, by both the professionals and their colleagues. Others don't want to believe that their professional colleague has a problem, even when it is openly obvious. Not knowing what to do and how to do it make it much easier to turn away from the obvious, particularly if the professional is in a supervisory position.

Alcohol dependence may be more readily detectable in these professionals. Signs may include frequent work absences and tardiness, poor work performance, disheveled appearance, complaints by patients, odor of alcohol or stale alcohol, or overt intoxication at work.

Drug addiction and, more specifically, diversion of controlled substances from the workplace may be less apparent. These professionals may be the "super workers." They may:

- Offer to work extra shifts
- Get to work early and stay late
- Come to work on their day off for "something"
- Take an assignment of difficult patients, particularly those with orders for their desired drug
- Insist that patients need certain controlled medications ordered

They take for themselves the Percocet or Vicodin refused by their sleeping patient. The pain goes away, enabling them to keep going. They tell themselves they "will never do it again," and in some instances, they never do... addiction has not set in.

For others, it happens again and again. They are unable to stop and eventually it is discovered. Many nurses, when confronted by their supervisors, are relieved: "finally I can stop." All nurses, when confronted, are thrown into a "trance-like" state. Life as they know it is about to change. They are removed from their work, their identity as a nurse, their routine, and their supply of drug.

Physicians and dentists follow a similar course, but their access may be limited.

(*Continued*)

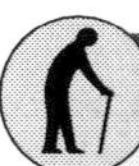

AGING ALERTS (*Continued*)

They may write prescriptions for controlled substances in another name and obtain the drug for themselves. Dentists have been known to misuse nitrous oxide typically used for patient relaxation.

Interventions and treatment of health care professionals is best done by persons specifically trained and sensitive to their issues. Denial is often profound as the underlying feelings include immense guilt and shame. Thinking is directed to "When can I go back to work?" Support and guidance are necessary to get the person to accept treatment and then the reality of the situation; this needs to extend to helping the person face their licensing board and a court of law. State laws mandate that institutions report all incidences of diversion or theft of controlled substances. State licensing boards and county prosecutors must be notified. State licensing boards in all disciplines have specific programs designed to monitor and help a professional return to practice when they attain successful recovery.

Persons suffering with chronic pain disorders are susceptible to developing dependence on prescribed narcotics, sedatives, and alcohol. Rebound pain and anxiety develop as doses of medications are increased. At some point, they may have pain and anxiety far greater than what they began with even though they are taking very large quantities of medications. Seizures may occur due to tolerance of benzodiazepines or in the case of large amounts of tramadol.

Addictive disorders can be differentiated from dependence when there is evidence of use of illegal substances, multiple prescribers, or prescription forgery. For practitioners, reviewing the automatic reporting system of their State Board of Pharmacy should be routinely done before prescribing. Open communication between client and practitioner regarding the use of controlled substances should be ongoing. Practitioners should stand firm about when and how they will prescribe controlled substances. If concerned that dependence or addiction is a problem, the goal should be having the person be assessed by an addictions professional.

RESOURCES

BOOKS

Dual Diagnosis: Counseling the Mentally Ill Substance Abuser (1990) by K. Evans and M. Sellenan

WEBSITES

Alcoholics Anonymous World Services, Inc.: www.aa.org
AA website provides online meeting and publications to purchase as well as additional resources for families and COD.

Double Trouble in Recovery: www.miepvideos.org/reachonedis.html
Website with video explaining the Double Trouble in Recovery program.

Dual Diagnosis: www.dual-diagnosis.net
Discusses COD with information on treatment and support.

Mental Health America: www.nmha.org
Mental Health America provides definitions and treatment options.

The National Institute of Mental Health: www.nimh.gov
The National Institute of Mental Health provides statistics, information on evidence-based programs, pamphlets for professionals as well as lay people, and much more.

The Substance Abuse and Mental Health Services Administration, U.S. Department of Health and Human Services: www.samhsa.gov
Provides a vast amount of information including specific guidelines for treatment (Treatment Improvement Protocols, #42 is on COD) as well as organizational structure for integrated care.

REFERENCES

American Psychiatric Association (1994). *Diagnostic and Statistical Manual of Mental Disorders, Fourth Edition.* Arlington, Va: American Psychiatric Publishing.

Borg, L., & Kreek, M. J. (2004). *Pharmacology of opiods.* In A. W. Graham, T. K. Schultz, M. F. Mayo-Smith, R. K. Ries, & B. B. Wilford (Eds.), *Principles of addiction medicine* (3rd ed., pp. 193–224). Chevy Chase, MD: American Society of Addiction Medicine.

Cadoret, R., Troughton, E., & Woodworth, G. (1994). Evidence of heterogeneity of genetic effect in Iowa adoption studies. *Annals of the New York Academy of Science, 708*, 59–71.

Center for Substance Abuse Treatment. (2002). *Substance abuse treatment for persons with co-occurring disorders: Treatment improvement protocols (TIP).* Rockville, MD: Substance Abuse and Mental Health Services Administration.

Chan, L. (1996). *101 miracles of natural healing.* London, UK: Federation of Alcoholic Residential Establishments.

Collins, G. Janesz, J., Thrope, J., & Weiss, K. (1991). A multidisciplinary approach to the treatment of drug and alcohol addiction. In N. S. Miller (Ed.), *Comprehensive handbook of drug and alcohol addiction* (pp. 981–999). New York, NY: Marcel Dekker.

Coombs, R. H. (1997). *Drug impaired professionals.* Boston, MA: Harvard University Press.

Davies-Scimeca, P. (2008). *Unbecoming a nurse: Bypassing the hidden trap of chemical dependency.* New York, NY: SeaMeca.

Dole, V. P. (1972). Narcotic addiction, physical dependence, and relapse. *New England Journal of Medicine, 286*, 998–992.

Feinstein, D., Eden, D., & Craig, G. (2005). *Principles of energy psychology.* New York, NY: Tarcher-Penguin.

Galloway, G. (2003). GHB: A new drug of abuse. In A. Graham, T. K. Schultz, M. F. Mayo-Smith, R. K. Ries, & B. B. Wilford (Eds.), *Principles of addiction medicine* (3rd ed., p. 139). Chevy Chase, MD: American Society of Addiction Medicine.

Goodwin, D. (2003). Genetic determinants of alcoholism. In J. Mendelson & N. Mello (Eds.), *Medical diagnosis and treatment of alcoholism* (pp. 201–256). New York, NY: McGraw-Hill.

Gorelick, D. & Cornish, J. (2003). Pharmacology of opioids. In A. Graham, T. K. Schultz, M. F. Mayo-Smith, R. K. Rie, & B. B. Wilford (Eds.), *Principles of addiction medicine* (3rd ed., pp. 157–177). Chevy Chase, MD: American Society of Addiction Medicine.

Greenberg, M. (2002). *Building bridges: Synopsis of the literature on co-occurring disorders.* Santa Monica, CA: Rand Health.

Kerr, T., Montaner, J. S. G., & Wood, E. (2010). Science & politics of heroin prescription. *Lancet, 375*(9729), 1849–1850.

Korsten, M., & Lieber, C. (1992). The gastrointestinal effects of alcohol. In J. Mendelson & N. Mello (Eds.), *Medical diagnosis and treatment of alcoholism* (pp. 289–340). New York, NY: McGraw-Hill.

Kranzler, H., & Jaffe, J. (2003). Pharmacological interventions for alcoholism. In A. Graham, T. K. Schultz, M. F. Mayo-Smith, R. K. Rie, & B. B. Wilford (Eds.), *Principles of addiction medicine* (3rd ed., pp. 701–718). Chevy Chase, MD: American Society of Addiction Medicine.

Leshner, A. (2003). Understanding drug addiction. In A. Graham, T. K. Schultz, M. F. Mayo-Smith, R. K. Rie, & B. B. Wilford (Eds.), *Principles of addiction medicine* (3rd ed., pp. 47–55). Chevy Chase, MD: American Society of Addiction Medicine.

Lock, C. (2006). *Emotional freedom technique: Energy therapy & the future.* Workshop conducted at the conference of the National Institute of Clinical Application of Behavioral Medicine. Hilton Head, SC.

Myss, C. (1997a). *Energy medicine and intuition.* Workshop conducted at the conference of the National Institute of Clinical Application of Behavioral Medicine. Hilton Head, SC.

Myss, C. (1997b). *Why people don't heal and how they can.* New York, NY: Harmony Books.

Naperstek, B. (1997). *Your sixth sense: Unlocking the power of your intuition.* San Francisco, CA: HarperCollins.

O'Brien, C. (2008). Prospects for a genomic approach to the treatment of alcoholism. *Archives of General Psychiatry, 65*(2), 102–116.

O'Hanlon, W. (2009). Ericksonian hypnosis. In *Master class training symposium conducted at the conference of the National Institute of Clinical Application of Behavioral Medicine*, Hilton Head, SC.

Page, C., & Howard, M. (1998). Alternative healing. In *Master class training symposium conducted at the conference of the National Institute of Clinical Application of Behavioral Medicine*, Hilton Head, SC.

Pate, J. T., Zweben, J., & Martin, J. (2003). Opioid maintenance treatment. In A. Graham, T. K. Schultz, M. F. Mayo-Smith, R. K. Rie, & B. B. Wilford (Eds.), *Principles of addiction medicine* (3rd ed., pp. 751–765). Chevy Chase, MD: American Society of Addiction Medicine.

Pert, C., Dreher, H., & Ruff, M. (2005). Foundations of mind-body medicine. In M. Schlitz, T. Amorok, & M. S. Micozzi (Eds.). *Consciousness and healing* (pp. 61–78). St. Louis, MO: Elsevier.

Rollnick, S., Miller, W., & Butler, C. (2008). Motivational interviewing in health care: Helping patients change behavior. New York: Guilford.

Rosack, J. (2004). Volkow may have unlocked the answer to the addiction riddle. *Psychiatric News, 39*(11), 32.

Saxon, A. (2003). Special issues in office-based opiod treatment. In A. Graham, T. K. Schultz, M. F. Mayo-Smith, R. K. Ries, & B. B. Wilford (Eds.), *Principles of addiction medicine* (3rd ed., pp. 767–779). Chevy Chase, MD: American Society of Addiction Medicine.

Schuckit, M. (2003). *Drug and alcohol abuse: A clinical guide to treatment* (5th ed., pp. 28–49). New York, NY: Kluwer-Plenum.

Shapiro, F. (1997). In *Keynote presentation at the conference of the National Institute of the Clinical Application of Behavioral Medicine.* Hilton Head, SC.

Stine, S., Greenwald, M., & Kosten, T. (2003). Pharmacological interventions for opiod addiction. In A. Graham, T. K. Schultz, M. F. Mayo-Smith, R. K. Rie, & B. B. Wilford (Eds.), *Principles of addiction medicine* (3rd ed., pp. 735–740). Chevy Chase, MD: American Society of Addiction Medicine.

Strobbe, S. (2009). *Alcoholics Anonymous: Personal stories, relatedness, attendance and affiliation* (Unpublished doctoral dissertation (Nursing)). University of Michigan, Ann Arbor, MI.

Victor, M. (1992). Effects of alcohol on the nervous system. In J. Mendelson & N. Mello (Eds.). *Medical diagnosis and treatment of alcoholism* (pp. 201–256). New York, NY: McGraw-Hill.

Volkow, N. D., Hitzemann, R., Wang, G. J., Fowler, J. S., Wolf, A. P., Dewey, S. L., Handlesman, L. (1992). Longterm frontal brain metabolic changes in cocaine abusers. *Synapse, 11*, 184–190.

Welch, S., & Martin, B. (2003). The pharmacology of marijuana. In A. Graham, T. K. Schultz, M. F. Mayo-Smith, R. K. Rie, & B. B. Wilford (Eds.), *Principles of addiction medicine* (3rd ed., pp. 249–269). Chevy Chase, MD: American Society of Addiction Medicine.

Woodward, J. (2003). The pharmacology of alcohol. In A. Graham, T. K. Schultz, M. F. Mayo-Smith, R. K. Rie, & B. B. Wilford (Eds.), *Principles of addiction medicine* (3rd ed., pp. 101–118). Chevy Chase, MD: American Society of Addiction Medicine.

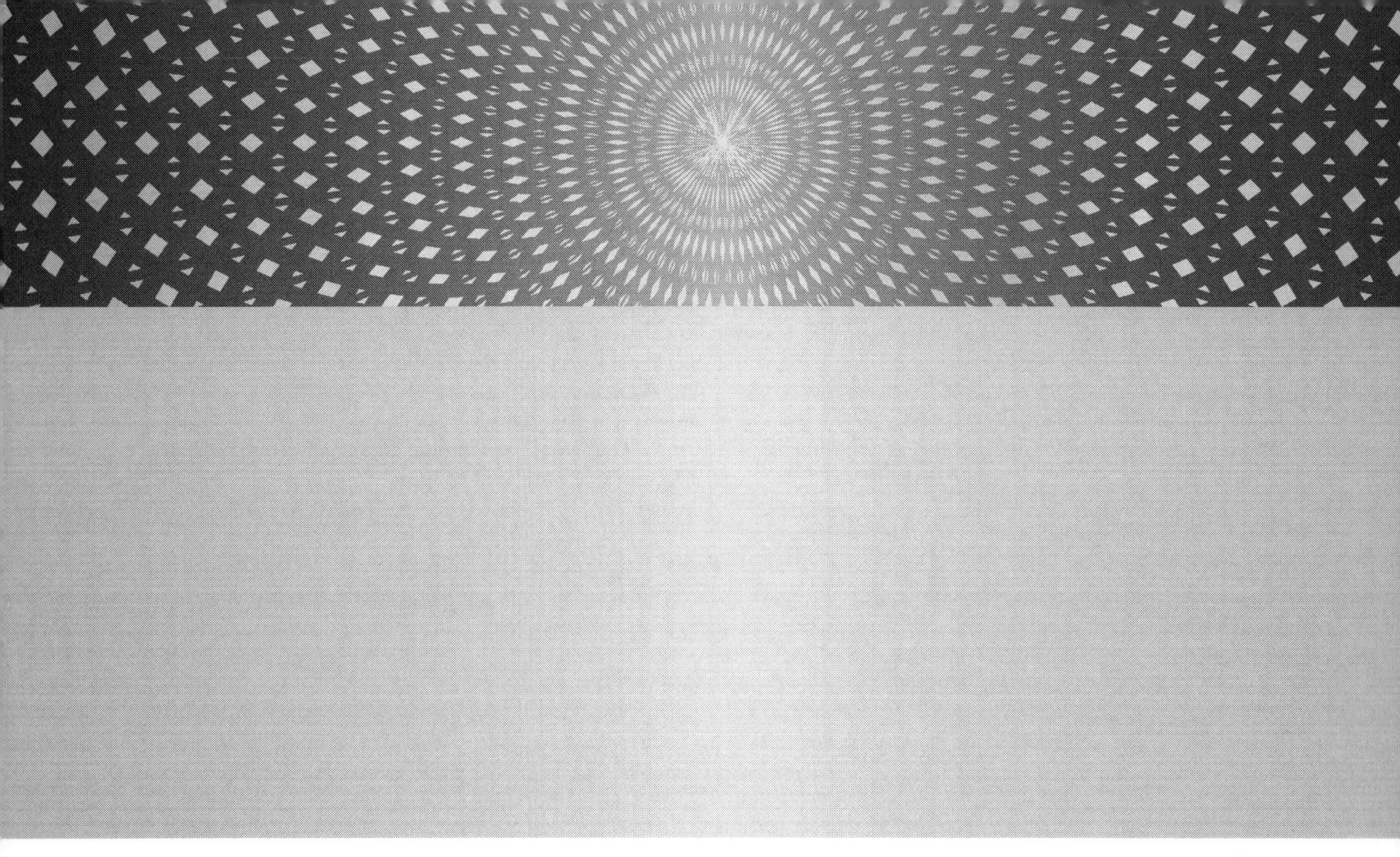

CHAPTER CONTENTS

Comorbidity refers to the occurrence of two syndromes in the same patients. The term *comorbidity* was introduced to medicine by Feinstein in 1970 to denote those cases in which a "distinct additional clinical entity" occurred during the clinical course of a patient having a diagnosis (Krishnan, & Ranga, 2005). In psychiatry, psychology, and mental health counseling comorbidity also refers to the presence of more than one diagnosis occurring in an individual at the same time. However, in psychiatric classification, comorbidity does not necessarily imply the presence of multiple diseases, but instead can reflect our current inability to supply a single diagnosis that accounts for all symptoms. For the puposes of this chapter we will focus on comorbidity as the combination of a psychiatric syndrome and one or more medical illnesses in the same patient. It is important to note that co-occurrence of mental and physical disorders in the same person happens regardless of the chronologic order in which they occurred or the causal pathway linking them. Determining whether both disorders occur in the same patient at different times or concurrently may help suggest the underlying mechanism of comorbidity.

Having a mental health disorder is a significant risk factor for developing a chronic condition and vice versa. For example, the likelihood of depression increases with the addition of chronic medical disorders. People with schizophrenia and bipolar disorder are up to three times more likely to have multiple

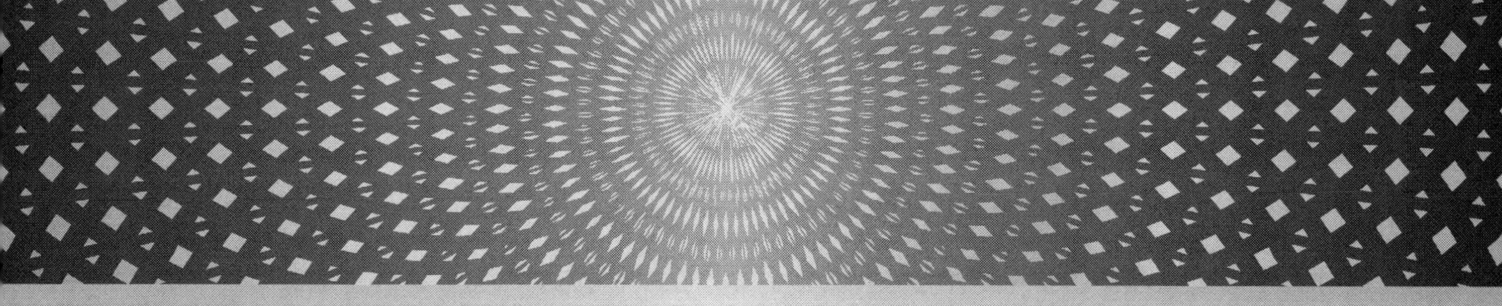

CHAPTER 18

Medical Problems and Psychiatric Syndromes

Marianne Tarraza

chronic conditions compared with those who don't. Medical conditions that are accompanied by high symptom burden such as migraine headaches or back pain can lead to depression. Major depression is a risk factor for developing medical conditions such as cardiovascular disease (CVD), that are characterized by pain or inflammation.

Sixty percent of adults with a mental disorder had at least one medical condition and 20% of those with a known medical disorder had a comorbid mental health condition. Individuals with serious mental illness (SMI) die earlier than individuals in the general population, losing on average 9 to 32 years of life (Druss, Benjamin, Walder, & Reisinger, 2011). Much of the premature mortality among persons with SMI is due to medical comorbidities such as diabetes. One of the most important drivers of the high numbers of individuals with comorbid mental and medical conditions is the prevalence of mental disorders and chronic conditions in the United States. There is evidence that having each type of disorder is a risk factor for developing the other. When assessed with the use of screening tools, there is direct inquiry regarding symptoms of a psychiatric disorder. For example, the likelihood of having major depression diagnosis via the use of a screening instrument increases with each additional reported comorbid chronic medical disorder (Druss & Walker, 2011).

IMPACT OF COMORBID PSYCHIATRIC SYNDROMES AND MEDICAL ILLNESS

The National Association of State Mental Health Program Directors conducted a multistate mortality study which revealed that the average years of life lost for people with mental illness was 25.5 and the average age at death was 56.8. Recent evidence reveals that the rate of serious morbidity in this population has accelerated. Persons with SMI are now dying 25 years earlier than the general population (Parks, Sevendsen, Singer, & Foti, 2006).

Among individuals with schizophrenia, suicide and injury account for 30% to 40% of early deaths, but 60% of early mortality is due to so-called "natural causes" including CVD, diabetes, respiratory diseases, and infectious diseases (Miller, Paschall, & Sevenden, 2008). Individuals die from CVD at more than double the rate of the general population and about triple the rate for diabetes, respiratory diseases, and infectious diseases. Approximately 22% of all adults are diagnosed with Metabolic Syndromes. This includes individuals with SMI and the general population. However, the prevalence rate for early death with individuals with SMI and Metabolic Syndrome is 30% to 60%.

Many chronic medical conditions require patients to maintain a self-care regimen in order to manage symptoms and prevent further disease progression, which may be hampered by comorbid mental conditions. Comorbid mental and medical conditions are associated with substantial individual and societal costs. Numerous studies have demonstrated higher rates of modifiable risk factors in the comorbid population. These risks factors also contribute to the acceleration of the medical conditions these patients suffer.

Higher Rates of Modifiable Risk Factors include:

1. Smoking
2. Alcohol consumption
3. Poor nutrition/obesity
4. Lack of exercise
5. "Unsafe" sexual behavior
6. IV drug use
7. Residence in group care facilities and homeless shelters (exposure to tuberculosis and other infectious diseases as well as less opportunity to modify individual nutritional practices) (Parks et al., 2006)

WHAT IS THE COST AND MORTALITY BURDEN OF COMORBIDITIES?

Melek and Norris used a national claims database to look at 10 common chronic conditions (Melek & Norris, 2008). The presence of comorbid depression or anxiety significantly increased total health care costs. Mental disorders are associated with roughly a two-fold to four-fold elevated risk of premature mortality. The bulk of these deaths are due to "natural" causes such as CVD rather than accidents or suicides. Thirty-four million American adults or 17% of the adult population had comorbid mental and medical conditions within a 12-month period. The high prevalence of this comorbidity, the complex causal connections linking medical and mental health conditions, and system fragmentation lead to problems in quality and costs related to comorbidity that are commonly even more complicated and burdensome than the problems related to the individual conditions themselves. The access to health care is also a significant burden on the patient, family, and society. Patients with comorbid disorders have a tendency not to seek preventive care, compromise the quality of their medical treatment, and often use the emergency room as their connection to the health care system (Exhibits 18-1 and 18-2).

EXHIBIT 18-1: ACCESS TO HEALTH CARE

OVERUSE:

1. Persons with severe mental illness (SMI) have high use of somatic emergency services

UNDER USE:

1. Fewer routine preventive services
2. Lower rates of cardiovascular procedures
3. Worse diabetes care

Source: Parks et al., (2006).

ASSESSMENT

DIAGNOSTIC APPROACH

The Diagnostic and Statistical Manual of Mental Disorders Text Revision (DSM-IV-TR) underscores the importance of ruling out medical disorders and substance abuse as a cause of a patient's symptoms. Common considerations in the differential diagnosis of depression include thyroid disorders and other endocrinopathies, medical side effects, malignancy, and neurological disorders (Aina & Susman, 2006). Anxiety may be caused by thyroid disorders, a variety of medication side effects including over-the-counter preparations, herbal remedies, and substance abuse.

Exhibit 18-3 summarizes the methods for determining patients with the diagnosis of mental disorders. Unlike medical disorders that can be diagnosed with a history and physical exam, and laboratory or radiographic evaluation, the diagnosis of mental disorders are made subjectively based on criteria and index of suspicion (Druss & Walker, 2011).

Mental disorders cannot be diagnosed with biological tests, unlike many medical conditions, and case definition relies on diagnostic criteria. Less than one-third of individuals meeting criteria for a mental disorder receive treatment. At any given time, 21% to 26% of patients in a primary care practice have a diagnosable mental disorder (Blexen, Perzynski, Sajatovic, & Dawson, 2011).

Half of presentations to primary care for physical problems are idiopathic or psychiatric problems. Twenty-six percent of such patients reported no improvement at follow up.

Most frequent presentations had somatic components including back pain, limb pain, headache, dyspnea, cough, abdominal problems, chest pain, dermatologic complaints, dizziness, sleep complaints, and fatigue. Of the most frequently presented medical problems the majority often had significant psychological components

EXHIBIT 18-2: PATIENT, PROVIDER, AND SYSTEM FACTORS CONTRIBUTING TO MORBIDITY AND MORTALITY IN PERSONS WITH SMI

HAVING A SMI MAY BE A RISK FACTOR BECAUSE OF:

1. Patient factors: amotivation fearfulness, social instability, unemployment, incarceration
2. Provider factors: attitude and comfort level with SMI population, coordination of care, and stigma
3. System factors: fragmentation between mental health and general health care

EXHIBIT 18-3: MEASURING MENTAL DISORDERS

- Self Report—Individuals are asked to state whether they have a diagnosis of a mental illness
- Heath Utilization Data—Diagnostic codes submitted by health care providers to insurance companies are used to determine if individuals have a mental disorder
- Screening Instruments—Interview questions—measure symptom duration and severity. These instruments are often used for screening purposes to identify potential causes of mental disorders or are included in population-based surveys
- Clinical Interviews—Interviews are based on standard diagnostic criteria designed to be administered by clinicians or lay interviewers in large epidemiological surveys

(Kroenke & Mangelsdorff, 1989). Depression is the third most frequent reason for consulting a primary care physician (Mitchell & Coyne, 2007).

More people currently receive psychological services in the primary care system rather than the specialty mental health system (Kessler, 2009).

Fifty percent of people with psychological comorbidities have higher utilization of health care. Medical patients with psychological comorbidities have higher utilization of health care resources on the order of 50% to 100% higher non–mental health medical costs. Almost any medical problem or medication capable of causing a metabolic disturbance or direct effect on the central nervous system (CNS) can present with psychiatric symptoms.

This chapter presents common comorbid conditions in individuals with psychiatric syndromes.

CONCORDANCE

Developing agreement with the client becomes more complex when comorbid conditions exist. Differentiating between medical problems and psychiatric syndromes is artificial when using a holistic approach, which most PMH-APRNs believe and practice. However, the use of specialities in practice has made this a necessity. The problems associated with this separation are obvious and amplified in individuals who have difficulty interpreting bodily sensations or lack awareness of their own sensations. Furthermore, primary care providers may feel uncomfortable in treating individuals with psychiatric problems and PMH-APRNs may not feel comfortable in providing primary health care screening to clients. This problem has been discussed a great deal with several possible solutions such as training PMH-APRNs to provide primary care or co-location of mental health treatment and primary care (Druss & Walker, 2011).

EFFECTIVE COMMUNICATION BETWEEN THE MEDICAL TEAM AND THE MENTAL HEALTH TEAM

Patients with comorbid mental and medical disorders often require multiple providers in managing their care. With the added providers, it is imperative that all of the providers maintain effective communication at all times. Providers that note significant changes or deterioration in the condition of the patient should contact others to update them on the status. Thorough and accurate documentation of interactions and changes in medical regimen need to be shared. These patients often lend best to case conference management. Patient navigators may be instituted in an effort to coordinate care.

DEPRESSIVE DISORDERS

Depressive disorders affect approximately 18.8 million American adults or about 9.5% of the U.S. population age 18 and older in a given year. This includes major depressive disorder and dysthymic disorders. Everyone will at some time in their life be affected by depression—their own or someone else's, according to government statistics. As a psychiatric syndrome, depression and numerous medical conditions have been implicated in affecting patients simultaneously or as a result of the disorder. Studies are increasingly linking more illnesses to depression, including: osteoporosis, diabetes, heart disease, some forms of cancer, eye disease, and back pain.

DEPRESSION AND HEART DISEASE

Depression is implicated in both the development and adverse outcomes of heart disease. Pathways involve the sympathetic nervous system and the hypothalamic-pituitary axis. Depressive symptoms contribute a clinically significant independent risk for the onset of coronary artery disease (CAD). Depressive symptoms were found to be a clinically significant independent risk factor for cumulative mortality following heart attack (Aina & Susman, 2006). In a recent evidence-based review of the relationship between depression and CAD, the presence of depression was determined to confer a relative risk of 1.5–2.09 for the development of CAD in healthy individuals and a relative risk of 1.5–2.5 for adverse cardiac events in patients with existing CAD. Another meta-analysis concluded that post-myocardial infarction depression is associated with a 2.0–2.5 fold increased risk for a subsequent myocardial death.

In the largest intervention trial in the treatment of patients who had depression post-myocardial infarction, the Sertraline Antidepressant Heart Attack Trial (SADHART), cardiovascular and stroke events and mortality were all positively influenced by antidepressant treatment (Glassman et al., 2006).

Among a large group of German men ages 45 to 74, obese men had significantly higher concentrations of C Reactive Protein (CRP) compared with non-obese men. CRP serves as a signal of artery inflammation and high levels of the protein may be a good predictor of future heart disease.

Depression seems to add to obese men's risk factors: CRP levels were higher in the most depressed obese men than in the less depressed obese men, according to Karl-Heinz Ludwig, PhD, of the GSF National Research Center for Environment and Health, and colleagues (Ludwig, 2003).

Depression did not affect CRP levels among non-obese men, however, suggesting that a combination of obesity and depression may be more risky for some men. The association between obesity and depression remained strong even after accounting for other factors that can affect CRP levels, including smoking, alcohol consumption, and physical activity, according to researchers.

Depression was also found to increase the risk for arrhythmias/sudden cardiac death. Metabolically it was found that depressed patients with CVD had increased platelet aggregation and alterations in lipid metabolism. These findings significantly increased their risk for sudden cardiac death. Patients with depression and CVD were less compliant in their medication adherence and less involved in alteration of lifestyle changes (i.e., smoking cessation).

In a recent prospective cohort study looking at patients with CAD, it was found that those patients with a major depressive disorder had poorer rates of adherence and completion of cardiac rehabilitation and its improved clinical outcomes (Glassman et.al., 2006).

DEPRESSION AND DIABETES MELLITUS

Ten percent to 20% of individuals with diabetes suffer from depression. Japanese men and those with depressive symptoms were at a higher risk of having type 2 diabetes mellitus and developing insulin resistance. Depression and diabetes are intimately linked. Patients with diabetes are twice as likely to experience depression as those without diabetes. The odds of depression are similar in type 1 and type 2 diabetes and are significantly higher in women than in men (Hirshfield et al., 2003).

The course of depression in diabetes tends to be severe, with recurrences being the norm and not the exception. Following successful treatment, fewer than 10% of patients remained depression-free over the ensuing 5 years.

Just why diabetes sufferers are so prone to depression is unknown. It probably involves a complex interaction of psychological and genetic factors as well as the strain of coping with a very difficult disease. However, there is a growing body of evidence showing that depression may, in fact, cause the illness.

A number of recent studies have shown increased insulin resistance in depressed patients without diabetes and recent studies that controlled for conventional risk factors (e.g., age, obesity, body mass index [BMI]) found that depression was associated with a two-fold increased risk of type 2 diabetes.

One of the main problems has been that despite all the evidence linking diabetes and depression, providers have ignored the mood disorder in treating the disease. This situation has been blamed on a variety of factors, including the presumption by clinicians that depression is merely a secondary reaction to the medical illness, and the view (often shared by patients and family members) that the diagnosis conveys an additional burden.

Primary care physicians may also lack sufficient training and face financial disincentives to perform psycho diagnostic testing. The average provider-patient interaction in the United States is currently about 15 minutes which does not allow for adequate screening (Goodell, Druss, Reisinger, & Walker, 2011).

DEPRESSION AND HIV INFECTION/AIDS

Rates of depression in people with HIV are as high as 60%. HIV/AIDS does not directly cause depression. High prevalence of depression in persons with HIV/AIDS is well documented. Persons with HIV/AIDS are prone to depression as a result of the neurotropic effects of the HIV on the subcortical brain structures. Some HIV symptoms and side effects of HIV drugs are the same as those of depression. These include fatigue, low sex drive, little appetite, confusion, nightmares, nervousness, and weight loss. Several of the drugs used to treat AIDS may cause depressive symptoms. The most common one associated with depression is Sustiva. In advanced symptomatic HIV disease, a number of opportunistic infections, as well as HIV itself, can produce symptoms of depression. But a true loss of interest in activities that someone used to enjoy is a sign that a person is depressed.

HIV-infected patients do not become depressed simply because their disease progresses; however, it is particularly important to screen for depression during the crisis points. Depression can lead people to miss doses of their medication. It can increase high-risk behaviors that transmit HIV infection to others. Depression might cause some latent viral infections to become active. Depression can make HIV disease progress faster (National Institute for Mental Health, 2002).

DEPRESSION AND ASTHMA

Asthma, a chronic disease of the airways, affects more than 22 million people in the United States. Asthma is a chronic inflammatory disease. When the presence of inflammation in the body is communicated to the brain, neural changes take place. The neural changes can modify behaviors that resemble those seen in depression. Symptoms may include depressed mood, lethargy, decreased appetite, and decreased interest in social interaction. People reporting a diagnosis of asthma were 2.3 times more likely to screen positive for current depression compared to people without asthma.

Rosenkranz, published in the journal *Neuroimage*, analyzed clues that may link depression and asthma. Her findings show that as depressive symptoms improve, so does the asthma. In fact, a reduction in depressive symptoms is linked to a decreased use of asthma medications (Rosenkranz & Davidson, 2009).

Poorly managed asthma keeps people from being active. When inactivity combines with difficulty breathing, it triggers a downward spiral that includes:

- Social isolation
- Increased feelings of depression
- Poor asthma management
- Worsening of asthma symptoms

Depression with asthma is also a side effect of steroid use. This includes anti-inflammatory inhalers and oral steroids commonly used to treat asthma.

Findings show that other nonsteroid asthma drugs may cause irritability, depression, and even suicidal ideation or completion.

ANXIETY DISORDERS

People with anxiety disorders are more likely to see a family doctor before a mental health specialist, since their symptoms are often physical. Symptoms can include muscle tension, trembling, twitching, aching, soreness, cold and clammy hands, dry mouth, sweating, nausea or diarrhea, or urinary frequency. Anxiety attacks can mimic or accompany nearly every acute disorder of the heart or lungs, including heart attacks and angina (chest pain). In fact, nearly all individuals with panic disorders are convinced that their symptoms are physical and possibly life-threatening. It is also important to consider endocrine (thyroid disorders, pheochromocytoma, or disturbances in sugar metabolism), cardiovascular (dysrhythmias, congestive heart failure [CHF]), and neurologic disorders. The presentation of anxiety may be confused by the presence of comorbid psychiatric disorders as well, such as depression or substance abuse. In particular, depression and anxiety are noted to often be comorbid and may need to be addressed separately.

Patients with chronic medical illness and comorbid anxiety compared to those with chronic medical illness alone reported significantly higher numbers of medical symptoms when controlling for severity of medical disorder. Across the four categories of common medical disorders examined (diabetes, pulmonary disease, heart disease, arthritis), somatic symptoms were at least as strongly associated with anxiety as were objective physiologic measures. Two treatment studies also showed that improvement in anxiety outcome was associated with decreased somatic symptoms without improvement in physiologic measurements (Merikangas & Swanson, 2010).

After controlling for gender, comorbid substance abuse/dependence and/or depression, patients with a lifetime anxiety disorder have higher rates of: cardiac disorders, hypertension, gastrointestinal problems, genitourinary disorders, and migraines. Individuals presenting with anxiety disorders or medical illness need, therefore, to be evaluated carefully for comorbidity. In a review of symptoms of 1,000 patients presenting with somatic symptoms that eventually were diagnosed as having a comorbid medical condition and anxiety disorders, Kroenke found 33% had cardiovascular disorders, 32% insomnia, and 30% irritable bowel syndrome (Kroenke & Manglesdroff, 1989).

ANXIETY DISORDER AND DIABETES

Anxiety disorders are twice as prevalent among people with diabetes as those without diabetes. Patients with major anxiety disorders have 3 to 5 times higher incidence of diabetes than the general population. Anxiety in diabetics has been associated with increased diabetic complications, lower adherence to diet and medications, and poor glycemic control when compared to diabetics without anxiety. The total health expenditures for persons with diabetes and anxiety are 4.5 times higher than for people with diabetes without anxiety (Merikangas & Swanson, 2010).

ANXIETY AND ASTHMA

Several studies have examined the association between anxiety disorders and asthma as well as other respiratory illnesses in adults. Researchers' interest in this association stems from overlapping symptoms these illnesses share such as sensations of being smothered, choking, hyperventilation-induced dyspnea, and increased anxiety. The prevalence of panic disorder in adults has been estimated as 1% to 3% in community populations and 4% to 8% in primary care populations. Twelve cross-sectional studies in adult populations have suggested that the prevalence of panic disorder among patients with asthma ranges from 6.5% to 24%. Most of the adult and child studies of patients with asthma have shown an increased rate of comorbid anxiety disorders. However, there are important limitations in many of the studies. Only six of the studies examined more than 150 subjects. In the six larger studies, only two had physician verification of asthma. Only one of the larger studies (the German community study) controlled for asthma severity. This community study found a significantly higher likelihood of having one or more anxiety disorders in patients with severe compared with non-severe asthma.

Most studies did not attempt to control for all possible socioeconomic and clinical confounders such as the severity of asthma (Merikangas & Swanson, 2010).

BIPOLAR DISORDER

There is a strong association between bipolar disorder and substance abuse. Medical disorders also accompany bipolar disorder at rates greater than predicted by chance. It is often unclear whether a medical disorder is truly comorbid, a consequence of treatment, or a combination of both. The clinician must evaluate and monitor patients with bipolar disorder for the presence and the development of comorbid psychiatric and medical conditions. Rates of chronic fatigue syndrome, migraine, asthma, chronic bronchitis, multiple chemical sensitivities, hypertension, and gastric ulcer were significantly higher in the bipolar disorder groups (Krishnan & Ranga, 2005) (see Table 18-1). Comorbid medical disorders in bipolar disorder are associated with several indices of harmful dysfunction decrements in functional outcomes and increased utilization of medical services. Patients with affective disorders are an at-risk group for myriad medical disorders, which are often undiagnosed and subsequently left untreated.

Medical disorders that coexist with bipolar disorder at rates greater than predicted by chance include those comorbid with symptomatic mania and bipolar disorder and those related to the treatment of bipolar disorder. Strokes, tumors, head trauma, CNS infections, and degenerative disorders define these as "mood disorders" due to a general medical condition with manic features.

BIPOLAR DISORDER AND MIGRAINE

Between 25 and 40% of people who have bipolar disorder also have migraines. In a study looking at the relationship between the two entities, the adjusted lifetime prevalence of migraine headaches was 15.2% among the 3.7% of the sample that screened positive for bipolar disorder, compared with 7.09% for those who screened negative. Bipolar disorder and migraine are linked in a unique way: They share common triggers, such as stress, anxiety, and sleep disruption (Hirshfield et al., 2003).

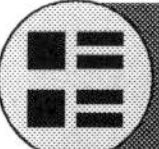

TABLE 18-1: PREVALENCE (WEIGHTED PERCENTAGES) OF CHRONIC MEDICAL DISORDERS AMONG 36,984 CANADIANS AGED 15 YEARS AND OLDER WITH PRESENCE OF A MANIC EPISODE OVER THE LIFETIME

CHRONIC CONDITIONS	EPISODE N = 938	MANIC EPISODE N = 35,848
At lease one chronic condition	64.3	48.5
Migraine	24.8	10.3
Arthritis	20.6	17.4
Asthma	15.9	8.3
Gastric ulcer	10.8	3.9
Hypertension	10.4	14.9
Chronic bronchitis	7.9	3.1
Thyroid disease	7.4	5.6
Multiple chemical sensitivities	4.6	2.3
Heart disease	4.4	5.4
Diabetes	4.3	4.8
Crohn's Disease	4.0	2.7
Chronic fatigue syndrome	3.8	1.1
Fibromyalgia	2.8	1.4
Cataract	1.8	4.7
Cancer	1.3	2.0

Source: Druss & Walker (2011).

BIPOLAR DISORDER AND VELOCARDIO-FACIAL SYNDROME

Velocardio-facial syndrome (VCFS) is a genetic syndrome that involves over 40 somatic anomalies, learning disabilities, and behavioral disorders and is associated with a micro deletion on chromosome 22q11. Psychiatric disorders in excess of population norms in VCFS patients include schizophrenia, bipolar disorder, and attention deficit hyperactivity disorder (ADHD). In one study, 64% (N = 16 of 25) of an unselected series of patients with VCFS met *DSM-III-R* criteria for a spectrum of bipolar disorders with full syndrome onset in late childhood or early adolescence (mean age at onset = 12 years, SD = 3) (Papolos, 1996).

BIPOLAR DISORDER AND MULTIPLE SCLEROSIS

Multiple Sclerosis is the neurological disorder most consistently identified as comorbid with bipolar disorder. Bipolar disorder is seen in more than 10% of Multiple Sclerosis patients. The comorbidity of bipolar disorder is related to the location of the genetic defects. It has been postulated that genes very close to the human leukocyte antigen (HLA) region on chromosome 6 may constitute one of the elements in the multifactorial etiology of bipolar disorder and multiple sclerosis (O'Donovan, Kusumaker, Graves, & Bird, 2002).

BIPOLAR DISORDER AND ASTHMA

In a study to determine the association between asthma and mental disorders, Goodwin et al. found a two-fold increase in the incidence of bipolar disorder among asthmatics compared to the general population. Lifetime severe asthma was also found to be associated with a five-fold increase in the probability of bipolar disorder (Goodwin, Jacobi, & Thefield, 2003).

BIPOLAR DISORDER AND DIABETES MELLITUS

The prevalence of diabetes mellitus was significantly higher in 345 hospitalized bipolar patients with manic or mixed subtype than in the overall general population. Diabetes is found in people with bipolar disorder nearly three times more often than in the general population. This has prompted much research into the link between diabetes and bipolar disorder. Studies have found that people with bipolar disorder tend to be overweight or obese, a key risk factor in developing diabetes (Cassidy, Ahern, & Carroll, 1996).

BIPOLAR DISORDER AND POLYCYSTIC OVARIAN SYNDROME

Women with bipolar disorder are prone to have high rates of gynecologic disturbances including menstrual abnormalities, hyperandrogenism, and polycystic ovarian syndrome (PCOS). PCOS in bipolar disorder (along with other mental disorders) has also been linked pharmacologically to the use of valproate (Keck & McElroy,2003).

BIPOLAR AND OBESITY

Bipolar patients tend to be overweight and treatment of bipolar disorder may worsen obesity and increase the risk of comorbid medical disease. Forty percent of patients in the Bipolar Treatment Outcomes Network were overweight, 21% were obese, and 5% were extremely obese. Twenty-eight percent gained at least 5% of their baseline BMI during maintenance treatment and 13 subjects gained more than 5% of their BMI. Higher scores on the Hamilton Rating Scale for Depression and negative scores on the Bech-Rafaelsen Mania Scale predicted an increase of BMI during acute treatment (McElroy et al., 2005). Lithium has been associated with weight gain. Valproate may also increase risk of weight gain (Keck & McElroy, 2003).

SCHIZOPHRENIA

More than 50% of patients with schizophrenia have one or more comorbid psychiatric or general medical conditions. In a study looking at hospital discharge records with a primary diagnosis of schizophrenia, patients consistently showed higher proportions of all comorbid psychiatric conditions examined and of some general medical conditions, including acquired hypothyroidism, contact dermatitis and other eczema, obesity, epilepsy, viral hepatitis, diabetes type II, essential hypertension, and various chronic obstructive pulmonary diseases. Knowledge of the risks of comorbid psychiatric and general medical conditions is critical both for clinicians and for patients with schizophrenia. Closer attention to prevention, early diagnosis, and treatment of comorbid conditions may decrease associated morbidity and mortality and improve prognosis among patients with schizophrenia.

Schizophrenia symptoms include memory and attention problems, hallucinations, disorganized thinking and behavior, and delusions. Psychotic symptoms typically start in late adolescence and early adulthood. But researchers believe that developmental abnormalities they don't yet know about also increase diabetes risk.

One recent study—based on data from the Clinical Antipsychotic Trials of Intervention Effectiveness Schizophrenia Trial—showed the prevalence rate of metabolic syndrome, a group of risk factors that include abdominal obesity, high lipid and cholesterol blood levels, and insulin resistance, is more than 50% in women and about 37% in men with schizophrenia. Sixty percent of premature deaths in persons with schizophrenia are due to medical conditions such as cardiovascular and pulmonary conditions or infectious diseases (NIMH, 2006).

SCHIZOPHRENIA AND CVD

Heart disease is the leading cause of death in the United States, and it's about twice as deadly for people with schizophrenia. Relative risk of cardiovascular death was 4 to 6 times higher for the schizophrenic population compared to the Massachusetts age-matched population (Duckworth, 2009). People with schizophrenia are more likely than others to have one or more of the major risk factors for heart disease. They are also less likely to receive good preventive care, in large part because they are more likely to see a psychiatrist than a primary care physician or cardiologist. Research indicates that at least half of people with schizophrenia will stop taking their antipsychotic medication at some point, so clinicians may assume that compliance with other medications will also be poor. Basic monitoring and treatment of CVD risk factors in severely mentally ill patients falls far short of that in the general population in most respects, according to results of a U.S. study.

SCHIZOPHRENIA AND DIABETES

Researchers have long suspected that schizophrenia leads to an increased risk of diabetes. Diabetes, hyperlipidemia, and hypertension are highly prevalent in populations with schizophrenia, with rates in excess of 50% reported in some studies. In a study of 50 people newly-diagnosed with schizophrenia or a related psychotic disorder with no other known risk factors, 16% had either diabetes or an abnormal rate of glucose metabolism.

In the last few years, there has been heightened awareness of the potential interactions between diabetes, schizophrenia, and antipsychotic medications. A recent review concluded that metabolic syndrome at the onset of schizophrenia (i.e., prior to treatment) as well as poor diet, lack of exercise, and high rates of smoking may account for this trend (Duckworth, 2009).

Newer atypical anti-psychotic agents (for example: clozapine/Clozaril, olanzapine/Zyprexa, resperidone/Resperdal, quetiapine/Seroquel, and ziprasidone/Geodon) have been given a "black box" warning by the Food and Drug Administration (FDA) because of an association with diabetes in people taking these compounds (Duckworth, 2009).

PARKINSON'S DISEASE

Although Parkinson's disease (PD) is primarily considered a neurodegenerative disorder, the high prevalence of psychiatric complications suggests that it is more accurately conceptualized as a neuropsychiatric disease (Weintraub & Stern, 2008). The major neuropsychiatric comorbidities are depression, anxiety, and psychotic symptoms. Affective disorders (depression and anxiety), cognitive impairment or dementia, and psychosis are common in patients affected by PD. Other common but less well-studied psychiatric disorders include apathy, impulse control disorders, disorders of sleep and wakefulness, and pseudo bulbar affect. Nonmajor depression (minor or subsyndromal depression) is more common than major depression in patients with PD. Experts state that atypical depressive disorders such as recurrent brief depressive disorder better capture the symptom variability that many patients with PD experience. Depressive symptoms can also be specifically related to motor symptoms, as in patients who experience temporary dysphoria during "off" periods. Most patients with PD and depression also meet criteria for an anxiety disorder, and those with PD and anxiety disorder also meet the criteria for depression. Although apathy is a distinct psychiatric syndrome, there is extensive overlap between depression and apathy in PD. Executive impairment, which in particular has been associated with depression in patients with PD, may be related to the additive effects of PD and depression.

Depression is present in both early and late stages and is seen in approximately 30% of patients, although some estimates are as high as 75%. Diagnosis is made difficult by the confounding and overlapping nature of the typical symptoms, which include loss of motility, facial mimesis, and apathy. Reactive states are more common in the early stages when patients begin to be aware of the disease's impact on their lives, and biological depression is more common in later stages, perhaps as a direct effect of the ongoing neurodegenerative processes. Anxiety is also common in patients with PD, and psychosis may occur in as many as 50% of patients.

Treatment of these comorbid conditions, whether they are reactive or inherent in the disease, is complicated by the fact that most of the current medications interact poorly with the underlying pathology of PD. More studies need to be carried out to develop psychiatric medications that aide patients with PD.

Exhibit 18-4 outlines the common medical conditions that can be associated with depression, mania, anxiety, cognitive impairment and/or psychosis. It is important to realize that there is a significant crossover in the diagnosis of these conditions with psychiatric syndromes (Druss & Walker, 2011).

MEDICAL AND PSYCHIATRIC COMORBIDITES RELATED TO PHARMACOLOGY

THE IMPACT OF COMMON MEDICATIONS CAUSING PSYCHIATRIC SYNDROMES

Many of the most common treatments for diseases may actually worsen the cormorbid psychiatric or medical problems. Exhibit 18-5 lists commonly used drugs that are capable of causing psychiatric symptoms such as depression, mania, anxiety, cognitive impairment, or psychosis. Patients, families, and providers need to be on a constant vigil for these potential side effects (Druss & Walker, 2011).

THE IMPACT OF COMMON PSYCHIATRIC MEDICATIONS CAUSING MEDICAL COMORBIDITY

Psychiatric medications have also been implicated in causing medical problems that can lead to comorbid situations.

Antidepressants

The most popular types of antidepressants are called selective serotonin reuptake inhibitors (SSRIs). These include: fluoxetine (Prozac), citalopram (Celexa),

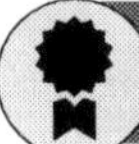

EXHIBIT 18-4: MEDICAL CONDITIONS THAT CAN BE ASSOCIATED WITH DEPRESSION, MANIA, ANXIETY, COGNITIVE IMPAIRMENT, AND/OR PSYCHOSIS

1. Neurodegenerative: Alzheimer's disease, frontotemporal, Lewy body (D, A, C, P); Parkinson's Disease, Huntington's Disease (D, M, A, C, P)
2. Metabolic: electrolyte abnormality, hepatic or renal failure, anemia, porphyria (D, A, C, P); hypoxia, hypercarbia (D, A, C)
3. Endocrine: hypothyroidism (D, C, P); hyperthyroidism (D, M, A, C, P); hyperparathyroidism, Cushing's syndrome, Addison's Disease (D, A, C, P); hypoglycemia (A, C), diabetes (D, A, C)
4. Cardiac: congestive heart failure (D, A, C), mitral valve prolapse, angina (A)
5. Normal pressure hydocenphalus (C, P)
6. Nutritional deficiencies: B12, folate, niacin, thiamine (D, M, A, C, P)
7. CAN trauma (D, A, C, P)
8. Cancer (D, M, A, C, P)
9. Infection: CAN, sepsis, pneumonia, urinary tract (D, M, A, C, P)
10. Stroke (D, M, A, C, P)
11. Pulmonary embolus (A)
12. Seizures (D, A, C, P)
13 Immunological: lupus, sarcoidosis, CNS vasculitis (D, A, C, P)
14. Sleep apnea (D, C)
15 Toxicity: e.g., heavy metals (A, C, P) drugs
16. Chronic pain (D, A)

D = depression; M = manic; A = anxiety; C = cognitive impairment; P = psychosis.

sertraline (Zoloft), paroxetine (Paxil), and escitalopram (Lexapro).

Other types of antidepressants are serotonin and norepinephrine reuptake inhibitors (SNRIs). SNRIs are similar to SSRIs and include venlafaxine (Effexor) and duloxetine (Cymbalta). Another antidepressant that is commonly used is bupropion (Wellbutrin). Bupropion, which works on the neurotransmitter dopamine, is unique in that it does not fit into any specific drug type.

SSRIs and SNRIs are popular because they do not cause as many side effects as older classes of antidepressants. The most common side effects associated with SSRIs and SNRIs include: Headache, which usually goes away within a few days, nausea which usually goes away within a few days, sleeplessness or drowsiness, which may happen during the first few weeks but then goes away, agitation, and sexual disfunction, which can affect both males and females.

Antipsychotics

Antipsychotic medications are used to treat schizophrenia and schizophrenia-related disorders. In the 1990s, atypical antipsychotics were developed. One of these medications was clozapine (Clozaril). It is a very effective medication that treats psychotic symptoms. But clozapine can sometimes cause a serious problem called agranulocytosis. Following the introduction of clozapine, other atypical antipsychotics were approved for use in the United States. All of them are effective in managing the symptoms of schizophrenia. These include risperidone (Risperdal), olanzapine (Zyprexa), quetiapine (Seroquel), ziprasidone (Geodon), aripiprazole (Abilify), and paliperidone (Invega).

Side effects of many antipsychotics include: drowsiness, dizziness when changing positions, blurred vision, rapid heartbeat, sensitivity to the sun, skin rashes, and menstrual disorders. Most psychotropic medications, particularly antipsychotic medications, can cause weight gain, obesity, and type 2 diabetes.

A recent ranking of atypical antipsychotic medications based on currently available literature rated the relative risk highest for clozapine and olanzapine, moderately high for quetiapine, and rather low for risperidone and ziprasidone.

EXHIBIT 18-5: DRUGS CAPABLE OF CAUSING PSYCHIATRIC SYMPTOMS; DEPRESSION, MANIA, ANXIETY, COGNITIVE IMPAIRMENT, AND/OR PSYCHOSIS

1. Alcohol intoxication/withdrawal (D, A, C, P)
2. Analgenics, anti-inflammatory agents: neurotics, Non steroidal anti-inflammatory drugs (NSAIDs) (D, A, C, P)
3. Antiarrthythmics (D, A, C, P)
4. Antibiotics: for example, gatifloxacin (D, A, C, P)
5. Anticholinergics (A, C, P)
6. Anticonvulsants (D, A, C, P)
7. Antidiarrheals (A, C, P)
8. Antihistamines (A, C, P)
9. Antipertensives (D, A, C, P)
10. Antineoplastics: for example, cisplatin (C, P)
11. Antitussives: for example, dextromethorphan (M, C)
12. Antivirals: for example, Interferon (D, A, C, P)
13. Antidepressants: selective serotonin reuptake inhibitors (M, A), tricyclics (M, A, C, P)
14. Antipsychotic: atypical (D, M, A, C, P), typical (D, A, C, P)
15. Anti-Parkinsonians: dopaminergic (D, M, A, C, P)
16. Beta blockers (C, P)
17. Bronchodilators: theophylline, isoproterenol (A)
18. Cardiac drugs: calcium channel blockers, digoxin (D, A, C, P)
19. Cholinesterase inhibitors (D, A, C, P)
20. Decongestants: for example, pseudo ephedrine (A)
21. Diuretics: for example, thiazides (D)
22 H2 blockers: for example, cimetidine (D, M, C, P), ranitdine (C, P)
23. Hormones: steroids, thyroxine (D, M, A, C, P)
24. Lithium (A, C)
25. Organophosphates (A, C)
26. Sedatives, hypnotics, tranquillizers (D, A, C, P)
27. Stimulants, caffeine (A)

D = depression; M = manic; A = anxiety; C = cognitive impairment; P = psychosis.

Medications Used for Bipolar Disorders

The first line of treatment in bipolar disorders are mood stabilizers. Lithium is a very effective mood stabilizer. It was the first mood stabilizer approved by the FDA in the 1970s for treating both manic and depressive episodes.

Anticonvulsant medications also are used as mood stabilizers. They were originally developed to treat seizures, but work well to control moods. An anticonvulsant commonly used as a mood stabilizer is valproic acid, also called divalproex sodium (Depakote). Other anticonvulsants used as mood stabilizers include carbamazepine (Tegretol), lamotrigine (Lamictal), and oxcarbazepine (Trileptal).

Lithium can cause modest side effects. They include loss of coordination, excessive thirst, slurred speech, irregular heart rhythm, seizures, visual disturbances, and swelling of the extremities. Patients on lithium should have their lithium levels, renal function, and thyroid levels checked periodically. Valproic acid may cause damage to the liver or pancreas. Valproic acid may increase testosterone levels in teenage girls and lead to the development of PCOS.

Atypical antipsychotic medications are sometimes used to treat symptoms of bipolar disorder. Often, antipsychotics are used along with other medications.

Antipsychotics include aripiprazole (Abilify), risperidone (Risperdal), ziprasidone (Geodon), olanzapine (Zyprexa), clozapine (Clorazil).

Antidepressants are sometimes used to treat symptoms of depression in bipolar disorder. These include fluoxetine (Prozac), paroxetine (Paxil), or sertraline (Zoloft). Patients with bipolar disorder should not bet treated with antidepressants as a solo agent because of the risk of inducing mania and also increasing the rate of cycling between episodes.

Anti-anxiety Medications

Antidepressants were originally developed to treat depression, but they can be used to treat patients with anxiety disorders. SSRIs such as fluoxetine (Prozac), sertraline (Zoloft), escitalopram (Lexapro), paroxetine (Paxil), and citalopram (Celexa) are commonly prescribed for panic disorder, obsessive compulsive disorder (OCD), post-traumatic stress disorder (PTSD), and social phobia. The SNRI venlafaxine (Effexor) is commonly used to treat Generalized Anxiety Disorders (GAD). The antidepressant bupropion (Wellbutrin) can be used in this setting. Some tricyclic antidepressants work well for anxiety. Imipramine (Tofranil) is prescribed for panic disorder and GAD. Clomipramine (Anafranil) is used to treat OCD. Monoamine oxidase inhibitors (MAOIs) are also used for anxiety disorders.

The benzodiazepines have a therapeutic benefit faster than the antidepressants. These include lorazepam (Ativan), alprazolam (Xanax), and clonazepam (Klonopin). Buspirone (Buspar) is an anti-anxiety medication used to treat GAD. Unlike benzodiazepines, its effects can take up to 2 weeks.

Beta-blockers such as propanolol (Inderal) control some of the physical symptoms of anxiety, such as trembling and sweating. Common side effects from beta-blockers include fatigue, cold hands, dizziness, and weakness. Beta-blockers are not recommended for people with asthma or diabetes.

OVERVIEW OF TREATMENT

The management of patients with psychiatric syndromes and medical comorbidity is complex and requires significant coordination of care. A "collaborative care" approach that uses a multidisciplinary team to provide care for both medical and mental conditions is paramount. The multidisciplinary team needs to adopt the following six parameters to effectively manage patients with comorbid illness.

1. Use of appropriate medical and mental health screening tools at first encounters
2. Evaluate for underlying medical conditions that may be causing psychiatric syndromes and mental health conditions that may be causing medical problems
3. Use of medication reconciliation at all encounters
4. Effective communication between the medical team and the mental health team
5. Appropriate and timely referrals between caregivers
6. Holistic approach to the patient

USE OF APPROPRIATE MEDICAL AND MENTAL HEALTH SCREENING TOOLS AT FIRST ENCOUNTERS

Patients with psychiatric syndromes will commonly present to primary care providers. Psychiatric patients often will manifest medical issues to their mental health providers. In an effort to adequately assess these patients, all providers (regardless of discipline) need to conduct both medical and mental health screening assessments. Screening assessment tools can be used in determining what conditions and possible comorbidities the patient has. Communities need to determine which screening tool will serve best their community and incorporate them as part of best practice.

EVALUATE FOR UNDERLYING MEDICAL CONDITIONS THAT MAY BE CAUSING PSYCHIATRIC SYNDROMES AND MENTAL HEALTH CONDITIONS THAT MAY BE CAUSING MEDICAL PROBLEMS

Patients presenting to a provider need careful attention to evaluate their symptoms as possibly a psychiatric syndrome, a medical condition or even both. Chest tightness may be CAD, anxiety, or both. Sadness may be depression, hypothyroid, or both. A clear understanding of the symptoms with correlation of the physical findings, and other medical tests can help delineate the pathophysiology and help determine if it is medical, mental, or both.

USE OF MEDICATION RECONCILIATION AT ALL ENCOUNTERS

Medications play an important role in the management of both psychiatric and medical conditions. Providers need to assess the exact medications the patient is currently on, the doses and adherence at every encounter. A medication reconciliation allows for accuracy, patient safety, and assessment of intervention. All providers need to reconcile at every encounter and intervene if there is an error or adherence has become an issue.

APPROPRIATE AND TIMELY REFERRALS BETWEEN CAREGIVERS

Patients with comorbid conditions often have complex issues requiring appropriate and timely referrals. Morbidity and even mortality can be diminished if these patients are appropriately and expeditiously referred.

HOLISTIC APPROACH

Managing patients with psychiatric syndrome in the setting of medical problems or caring for a complicated medical issue in a patient who has a mental disorder can be difficult. Often the focus becomes symptom management with no attention played to the "big picture." The mental health provider can focus on the psychiatric issues and not take into account the medical comorbidity and its impact on the patient. The primary care provider can focus on the laboratory or radiographic abnormalities and not fully understand or attend to the severe anxiety or other psychiatric disorder of the patient. Both providers can totally miss the main issues if they do not approach it holistically. It is only then that providers and the health care system can have a major impact on decreasing the morbidity and mortality of these complex patients.

DECISION TREE

The decision tree for patients with Comorbid Psychiatric and Medical disorders can be divided into two important steps. Step 1 outlines the initial step in managing patients. Commonly, patients present with symptoms to the provider. Symptoms can be classified as somatic symptoms (abdominal pain, headache, nausea, vomiting, etc.) or psychiatric symptoms (anxiety, depression, psychosis, etc.). Patients require a physical exam and/or mental health exam respectively. By following the Decision Tree—Step 1 (Figure 18-1), providers can determine if the patient has a medical diagnosis, a psychiatric diagnosis, or both in a comorbid fashion. Patients then can have a treatment plan proposed to address the problems. Decision Tree—Step 2 (Figure 18-2) focuses on how once a treatment plan is developed for the medical and psychiatric disorders, providers need to coalesce them and evaluate the impact that each of the treatment plans has on the other conditions. What effect does the psychiatric medication have on the medical condition? What can happen to the psychiatric situation when a proposed medical treatment is implemented? Issues such as efficacy, compliance, side effects, and interaction are essential to monitor both initially as well as ongoing.

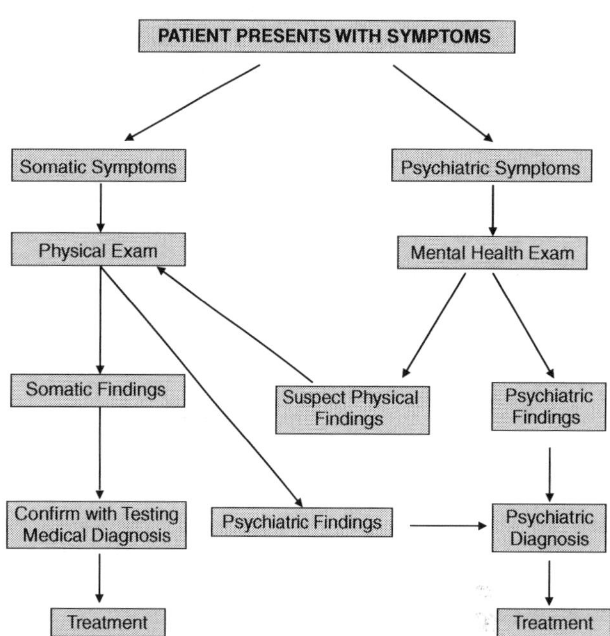

Figure 18-1 Decision Tree Step 1

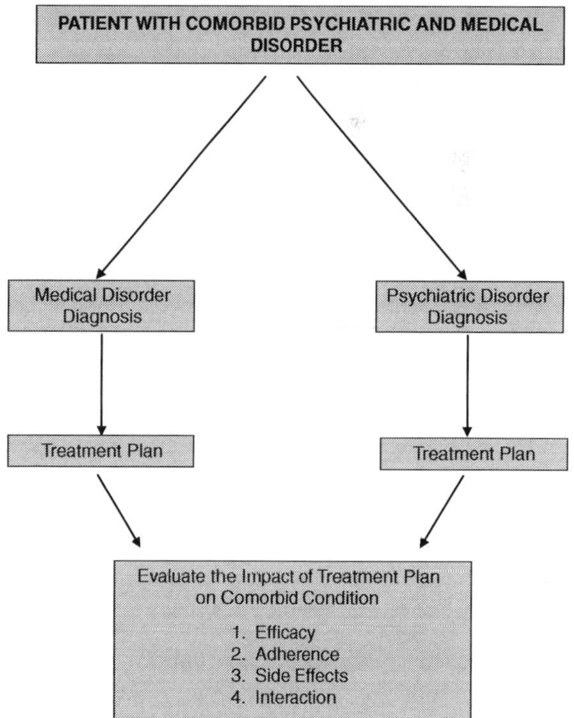

Figure 18-2 Decision Tree Step 2

A final area of importance is the situation where a patient presents with symptoms and the medical and psychiatric evaluation is not clear and does not lead to a definitive diagnosis in either area. These patients historically have been ignored because of the practitioner's inability to categorize their symptoms into a defined diagnosis. These patients would benefit from a psycho education evaluation and management of the mind-body connection in an effort to understand and manage their symptoms. This approach allows the provider to work with the patient in a comprehensive manner when caring for his or her needs.

SUMMARY POINTS: PSYCHIATRIC COMORBIDITIES

Summary: Essential Points

1. Individuals with serious mental illness face an increased risk of chronic medical conditions.
2. Individuals with serious mental illness die 25 years earlier than other Americans largely to treatable disorders (NAMI).
3. A multidisciplinary approach is critical in the management of patients with comorbid disorders.
4. It is important to use both mental health and medical screening tools at first encounters.
5. It is important to evaluate medical conditions that may cause psychiatric syndromes and mental health conditions that may be causing medical problems.
6. Medical comorbidities are prevalent across the life span but are particularly common in the aging population.
7. Medications can play an important role in management of comorbidities and can also be a cause of comorbidities.
8. Given the advances in biological psychiatry, treatments of mental health, and medical disorders, a holistic approach that includes a biopsychosocial perspective should be an intricate component of treatment.
9. Managing patients with comorbid conditions is associated with complex issues that impact treatment from either perspective.
10. The management of children with comorbid medical and psychiatric disorders should be treated from the perspective of lifelong impact of disease management.

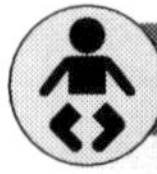

PEDIATRIC POINTERS

As with the adult population, childhood mental health disorders often are closely correlated with complex medical disorders. The impact of medical and psychiatric disorders occurring simultaneously is multifaceted since the growth and development of the child can be altered and have lifelong implications.

In the last several years there has been an increase use of psychotropic medications with children. This has been in response to a refined diagnostic application of adult disorders to children and a focus on prevention. Subsequently, prevention and recognition of prodronal symptoms has improved outcomes psychiatrically but has also contributed to metabolic and other concerns when initiating medications at early ages. The endocrine system in particular has been impacted by the use of these medications.

Childhood obesity and type 2 diabetes rates have increased over the past few years (Szydio, Van Wattum, & Woodston, 2003). The rate of type 1 and type 2 diabetes is associated with childhood obesity, family history, and the use of psychotropic medications (Szydio et al., 2003). The stressors related to the care of children with diabetes are complex in relationship to dietary, environment, peers, and family impact. This too is similar in reverse, whereas the child who is diagnosed with type 1 diabetes often exhibits depression, anxiety, and eating disorders causing lifelong impact (Fristch, Overton, & Robbins, 2010).

Childhood psychiatric disorders are common. As discussed in Chapter 15, the prevalence has been estimated that 5% to 15% of children will experience a psychiatric disturbance that is sufficiently severe to require treatment or to impair their functioning during the course of a year (Andreasen & Black, 2006). The incidence of childhood onset of psychiatric disorders, lends itself to an

(Continued)

PEDIATRIC POINTERS (*Continued*)

increased risk of illness burden and medical comorbidity since childhood onset impacts the degree of both indicators. For example, in the treatment of bipolar disorder, the NIMH-Funded Systematic Treatment Enhancement Program for Bipolar Disorder (Step-BD) algorithm identified an increase incidence of medical burden in patients who had a childhood onset of bipolar disorder (Magalhaes et al., 2011). As discussed in Chapter 15, children with autistic spectrum disorder are more prone to more physician visits, food allergies, and skin allergies than children of their same age (Gurney, Mc Pheeters, & Davis, 2006).

Less commonly thought of disorders such as strabismus, are associated with the development of mental health disorders (Mohoney, McKenzie, Capa, Nusz, Mirazek & Diehl, 2008). Extropia is particularly concerning. These patients have a higher risk of emergency room visits, psychiatric hospitalizations, and suicide attempts (Mohoney, et al., 2008). The relationship is considered temporal and there is currently no causal relationship established.

Essentially, any chronic medical disorder can impact the mental health of a child and should be considered in all psychiatric diagnoses. In the reverse, a child that is diagnosed with a psychiatric disorder should be screened for medical illnesses that are part of the differential diagnosis.

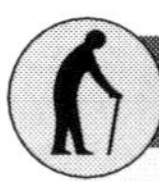

AGING ALERTS

As discussed in Chapter 11, the prevalence of mental health disorders in elderly individuals can be up to 25% of the population (Sadock & Sadock, 2008). When combined with the prevalence of medically diagnosed conditions that are impacted by or coincide with psychiatric disorders, this number increases. Psychopharmacologic interventions in this population requires that the clinician is aware of all medical comorbidities and ongoing consistent medication reconciliation to minimize drug interactions and side effects which can be lethal in this population.

The onset of severe and persistent psychiatric disorders such as schizophrenia is rare in this age group. However, it is not unusual to exhibit a first diagnosed episode of depression or anxiety that may be triggered by stage of life and or medical disorders such as PD. Psychotic symptoms that were previously non-exhibited may be related to emerging Alzheimer's, Dementia, or simple cognitive decline. One of the more common presenting symptoms that must be considered in a differential is the presence of delirium which can be caused by the onset of a psychiatric disorder, a medical problem or simply as a result of a medication including over-the-counter meds.

Delirium in itself is not a disorder but rather is a syndrome. It is a constellation of neurological symptoms that are considered a medical emergency and must be treated in the same manner. It has a classic waxing and waning presentation and is often mistaken for dementia. It is an acute onset, often noting a mental status change within hours. It is estimated that up to 42% of patients referred for depression while hospitalized for a medical disorder may experience delirium (Farrel & Ganzani, 1995).

Depression in late life can be associated with several medical disorders such as PD, cerebral vascular deficiencies, diabetes, obesity, or in some instances hypertension. Certain medications such as beta-blockers have been historically considered "depressongenic" with some association of inducing

(*Continued*)

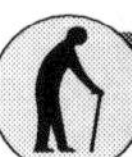

AGING ALERTS (*Continued*)

depression, although more recently studies have not supported this hypothesis (Leard-Hansson, 2011).

Insomnia and sleep disorders, although not unique to the elderly persons, can cause significant distress in an elderly person. A thorough assessment of sleep patterns is a necessary component of all psychiatric evaluations and particularly important in the elderly population. Sleep can be considered the blood pressure of mental health, meaning that changes in sleep often are indicative of clinical status. Quality, quantity, and degree of restorative sleep are subsets of a thorough sleep assessment that can be implicated in a disorder that is related to either psychiatric health or physical health.

Clinical concerns that should remain on the forefront for the clinician are the consideration of drug to drug interactions, ability to remain compliant to treatment plans, risk of suicide (higher incidence in men over 65), and collaboration with the medical provider to facilitate integrated treatment. As a general rule, elderly individuals require a slower titration schedule when beginning mediations and are often stabilized at a lower dose. Side effects that are inherently part of the aging process, like constipation and insomnia, are often more problematic for an elderly person. Careful history and evaluation at every session will help to manage the delicacies of medication treatment in this population.

Psychiatric comorbidities are inherent in everyday practice and require skill and expertise to differentiate possible related diagnosis so that integrated treatment can be initiated. The role of the advanced practice nurse is to distinguish the existence of the differential diagnosis and initiate treatment modalities that address both ends of the sphere. This emphasizes the holistic approach that is at the core of the advanced practice role of the nurse.

REFERENCES

Aina, Y., & Susman, J. (2006). Understanding comorbidity with depression and anxiety disorders. *Journal of the American Osteopathic Association, 106*(5), (Suppl. 2), 9–14.

Andreason N., & Black D. (2006). *Introductory textbook of psychiatry* (4th ed.). Washington, DC: American Psychiatric Publishing.

Blexen, C., Perzynski, A., Sajatovic, M., & Dawson, N. (2009). Treating severe mental illness and co morbid medical conditions in the primary care setting: An idea whose time has come. *Cutting Edge Psychiatry in Practice, 3*(3), 109–119.

Cassidy, F., Ahern, E., & Carroll, B. J. (1999). Co morbidities of Bipolar disorder. *American Journal of Psychiatry, 2156*, 1417–1420.

Chwastiak, L., Rosenheck, R. J., McEvoy, J., Keefe, R., Swartz, M., & Lieberman, J. (2006). Interrelationships of psychiatric symptom severity, medical comorbidity and functioning schizophrenia. *Psychiatric Services, 57*(8), 1102–1109.

Druss, B. G., & Walker, E. R. (2011). *The synthesis project research synthesis* (Report No. 21). Princeton, NJ: Robert Wood Johnson Foundation.

Druss B., Walder, E. (2011, February). *The Synthesis Project Research Synthesis* (Report no. 21).

Duckworth, K. (2009). *Medical comorbidities and schizophrenia—A guide for medical professionals and trainees* (pp.105–138). New York, NY: Blackwell.

Farrell K. R, & Ganzini, L. (1995). Misdiagnosing delirium as depression in medically ill elderly patients. *Archives of Internal Medicine, 155*(22), 2459–2464.

Fritsch, S. L., Overton, M. W., & Robbins, D. R. (2010). The interface of child mental health and juvenile diabetes. *Child Adolescent Psychiatric Clinics of America, 19*(2), 335–352.

Glassman, A., O'Connor, C., Califf, R., Swedberg, K., Schwartz, P., & Bigger, J. T. (2002). Understanding comorbidity with depression and anxiety disorders. *The Journal of American Medical Association, 288*, 701–709.

Goodell, S., Druss, B., Reisinger, E., & Walker, E. (2011). *Mental disorders and medical comorbidity (Synthesis Project Policy Brief No. 21)*. Priceton, NJ: Robert Wood Johnson Foundation.

Goodwin, R. D., Jacobi, F., & Thefield, W. (2003). Mental disorders and asthma in the community. *Archives of General Psychiatry, 60*, 1125–1130.

Gurney G. J., McPheeters L. M., Davis M. M. (2006). Parental report of health Conditions and Health Care Use Among Children With and Without Autism: National Survey of Children's Health Copyright 2006 American Medical Association. *Archives of Pediatrics & Adolescent Medicine, 160*(8), 825–830.

Hirschfeld R. M., Calabrese, J. R., Weissman, M. M., Reed, M., Davies, M. A., Frye, M. A.,...Wagner, K. D. J. (2003). Comorbidities of bipolar disorders. *Journal of Clinical Psychiatry, 64*, 53–59.

Keck, P. E., & McElroy, S. I. (2003). Psychiatric comorbidities. *Journal of Clinical Psychiatry, 64*, 1426–1435.

Kessler, R. (2009). Identifying and screening for psychological and comorbidity medical and psychological disorders in medical settings. *Journal of Clinical Psychology, 65*(3), 253–267.

Krishnan, K., Ranga R. (2005). Psychiatric and medical comorbidities of bipolar disorders. *Psychosomatic Medicine, 67*, 1426–1435.

Kroenke, K., & Mangelsdorff, A., (1989). Common symptoms in ambulatory care. *American Journal of Medicine, 86*, 262–266

Leard-Hansson, J. (2011). Do beta-blockers cause depression? *Clinical Psychaitry News*, Retrieved from http://www.FindArticles.com

Magalhaes, P. V., Kapczinski, F., Nierenberg, A. A., Deckersbach, T., Weisinger, D., Dodd, S., & Beck, M. (2011). Illness burden and medical comorbidity in the systemic treatment enhancement program for bipolar disorder. *Acta Psychiatrica Scandinavica, 125*(4), 303–308.

McElroy, F., Suppes, T., Dhavale, D., Keck, P. E., Leverich, G., Altshuler, L.,...Post, R. (2005). Comorbidities of bipolar disorder. *Psychosomatic Medicine, 67*, 1–8.

Melek, S., & Norris, D. (2008). *Chronic conditions and comorbid psychological disorders.* Milliman research reports. Seattle, WA: Milliman.

Merikangas K. R., & Swanson S. A. (2010). Comorbidity in anxiety disorders. *Current Topics in Behavioral Neurosciences, 2*, 37–59.

Miller, B. J., Paschall, C. B., & Sevenden, D. P. (2008). Mortality and medical comorbidity among patients with serious mental illness. *American Psychiatric Association Focus, 6*, 239–243.

Mitchell A., & Coyne J. (2009). *Screening for depression in clinical practice: An evidence-based guide.* Oxford, UK: Oxford University press.

Mohoney, B. G., McKenzie, J. A., Capo, J. A., Nusz, K. J., Mirazek, D., & Diehl, N. N. (2008). Mental illness in young adults who had strabismus as children. *Pediatrics, 122*(5), 1033–1038.

National Institutes for Mental Health Depression and HIV. (2002). Retrieved from http://www.dhs.wisconsin.gov/aids-hiv/PDFdocuments/CMResManual0309/Section%203-%20Mental%20Health/Depression.pdf

NIMH Clinical Antipsychotic Trials of Intervention Effectiveness (CATIE). (2006). Retrieved from http://mentalhealth.gov/trials/practical/catie/index.shtml

O'Donovan, C., Kusumaker, V. G., & Bird, D. C. (2002). Medical and psychiatric comorbidities. *Journal of Clinical Psychiatry, 63*, 322–330.

Parks, J., Sevendsen, D., Singer, P., & Foti, M. E. (2006). *Morbidity and mortality in people with serious mental illness.* Alexandria, VA: Association of State Mental Health Program Directors (NASMHPD) Medical Directors Council.

Rosenkranz, M. A., & Davidson, R. J. (2009). Affective neural circuitry and body influences in asthma. *NeuroImage, 47*, 972–980.

Sadock, B. J., & Sadock, V. A. (2008). *Kaplan and Sadock's concise textbook of clinical psychiatry* (3rd ed.). Philadelphia, PA: Lippincott Williams and Wilkins.

Szydio, D., Van Wattum, P. J., & Woodston, J. (2003). Psychological aspects of diabetes mellitus. *Childhood Adolescent Clinics of North America, 12*(3), 439–458.

Weintraub D., & Stern M. (2008) *Recognizing psychiatric and cognitive complications in Parkinson's disease.* Retrieved from http://www.medscape.org/viewarticle/590850

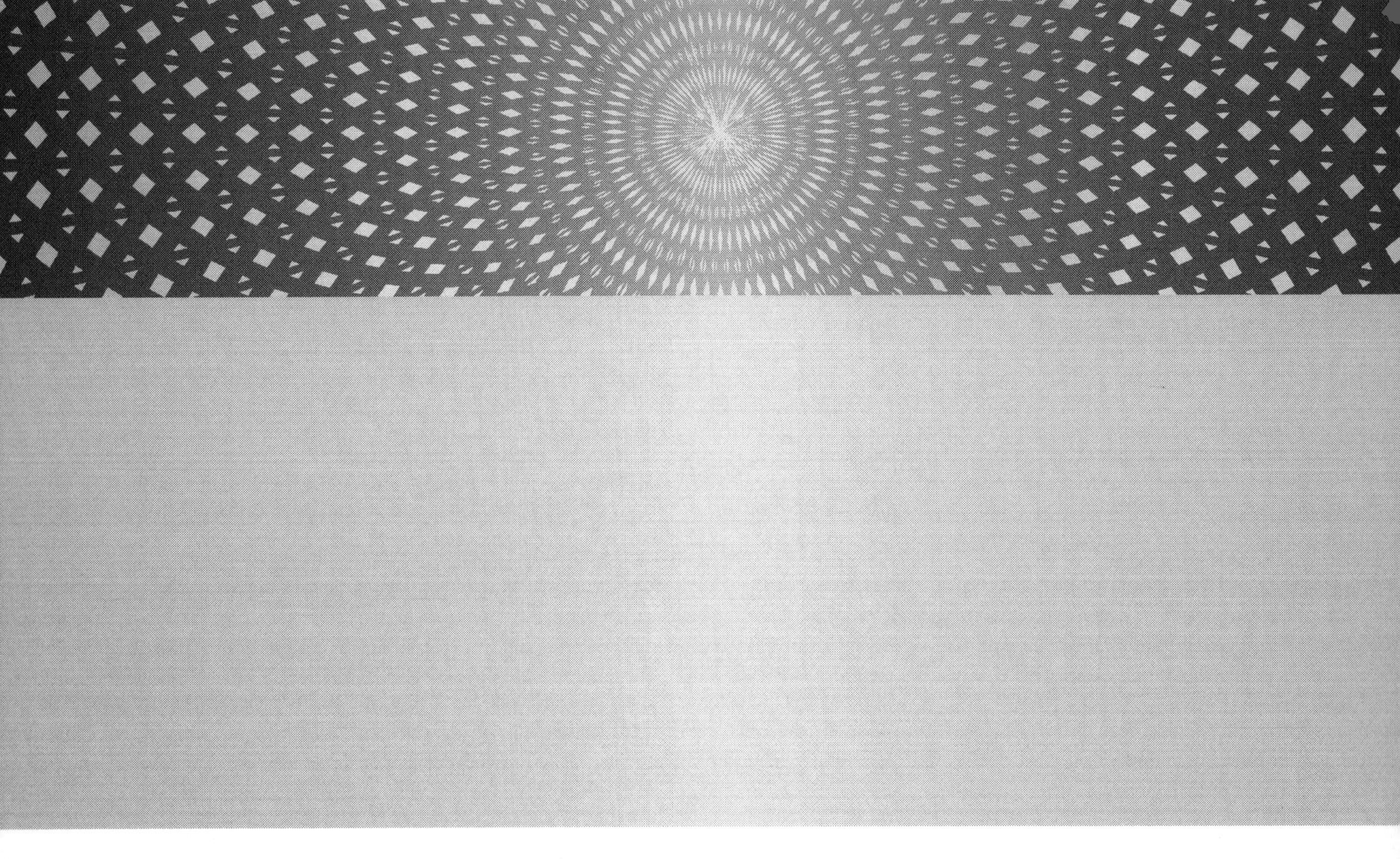

CHAPTER CONTENTS

The purpose of this chapter is to discuss various psychiatric disorders in the context of pregnancy. Complications such as hyperemesis gravidarum, intimate partner violence (IPV), miscarriage, stillbirth, and pregnancy after loss will also be addressed. Assessment, etiology, treatment options, expected outcomes for the patient and for the baby, and consequences for the partner will be reviewed. Research investigating various pharmacologic and nonpharmacologic interventions and select case reports will be discussed to arm the clinician in providing evidence-based treatment.

Pregnancy is divided into 3 trimesters. The first trimester involves bodily changes resulting in nausea, fatigue, breast tenderness, and mood lability. Next trimester most women begin feeling better and begin to look pregnant. The final trimester there is usually physical discomfort such as dyspnea, weight gain influencing balance and appearance, exertional dyspnea, and often heartburn. Psychological changes are also present in the mother as well as the father.

Reactions to the pregnancy are determined by many factors. Some include cultural expectations and beliefs about reproduction, relationships with the father and extended family members, whether the pregnancy was planned, age of the mother, and sense of one's own identity. Some women may see pregnancy as self-fulfilling and a creative act while others may view it as unwanted and a punishment.

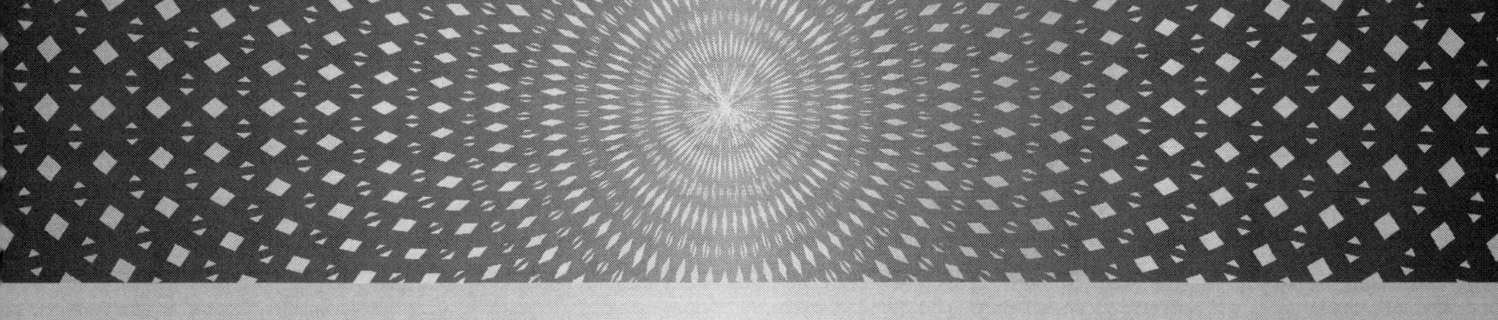

CHAPTER 19
Pregnancy During Psychiatric Syndromes

Carrie Cichocki

Even before birth, the fetus is viewed as having a personality and parents project hopes and dreams upon their unborn child. Fathers may view the child as evidence of their potency and generativity or fear of the added responsibility.

Psychiatric Mental Health Advanced Practice Nurses (PMH-APRNs) are in a position to promote stability, help maximize the quality of life, and minimize the chance of poor outcomes with patients. Treating patients with mental health issues can be challenging. Adding the variable of pregnancy makes the challenge ever more so. Interventions for the mother generate returns for the patient, her baby, and her family.

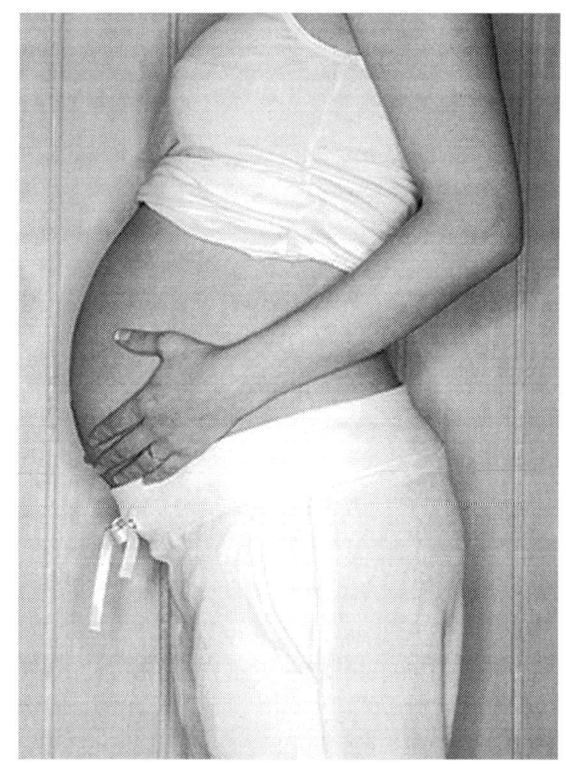

Source: http://www.flickr.com/photos/newlifehotels/3492728122/. "Swangerschaft."

CONCORDANCE

Ideally, patients would involve PMH-APRNs in their pregnancy planning, allowing for education and adjustments in the treatment plans prior to conception. Such planning time would permit psychiatric and obstetrical clinicians to coordinate care, collaborate in educating the patient, and send a consistent and cohesive message to the patient.

This time would allow for the psychiatric team to explore and assist the patient in planning for the pregnancy and the baby. Patients may not have considered the emotional and nurturing needs of the baby nor the physiological needs including feeding and sleeping schedules. Another need which may require exploration is the financial needs of the baby including bottles, diapers, clothing, and child care. The demands of a baby may be extremely underestimated and the mother may be ill prepared to care for a new life. An investment of time in planning would also allow the patient to approach key people to enlist assistance such as the father of the baby, family members, and friends.

Another advantage of pregnancy planning is to help minimize multiple medication exposures to the baby. Pregnancy planning discussions provide the opportunity for a "trial run" of a new agent or regimen with which the patient and PMH-APRN would be mutually accepting of use during a pregnancy. Should the newer regimen not achieve the desired remission of symptoms or patient stability, further adjustments and trials could be attempted at no risk to a baby. The luxury of time would also offer additional opportunities for patient and provider discussions.

Alternative family planning could be discussed. Patients with a history of severe mood or psychotic episodes who also have sufficient resources may consider using a surrogate rather than carrying a pregnancy. Surrogate use may minimize the risk of patient decompensation and may also avoid negative fetal outcomes. Despite the numerous benefits of planning a pregnancy, patients often do not involve their clinicians in family planning. Also, it is not unusual for patients to become pregnant without planning. According to the Centers for Disease Control (CDC), nearly half of all pregnancies in the United States in 2001 were unplanned such that the CDC had the goal of reducing unplanned pregnancies to 30% by 2010 (www.CDC.gov/ReproductiveHealth/Unintended Pregnancy/ extracted on August 6, 2011). Given that many pregnancies are unplanned, it may behoove the clinician to discuss the medication Category and discuss the potential risks and benefits (see Table 19-1) to both the patient and a fetus in routine visits irrespective of the patient's pregnancy status.

It may be the impulse of the patient to immediately discontinue the use of psychiatric medication upon discovering she is pregnant without involving the PMH-APRN. If this does occur, the patient may be unaware of the risks for the emergence of symptoms, decompensation, and risks to the fetus in choosing to discontinue medications. These changes in treatment can contribute to relapse for the patient, increase the chance for multiple medication exposures and medication withdrawal for the fetus. These variables can translate into poor outcomes for the fetus.

The risks of no treatment as well as treatment risks must be explored with the patient. Many pregnant women want to be medication free; however, being medication free and psychiatrically stable is not realistic for all patients. Considerations such as fetal toxicity, fetal malformations, and neurobehavioral consequences must also be considered and discussed with the patient and her partner if one is involved. It is only through informed mutual decision making that concordance can be reached.

Clinicians should be mindful that physiological changes within the patient during pregnancy may require increased doses for therapeutic effect. Shifts in hormones, hemodilution, increased liver metabolism, changes in renal functioning, and changes in gastrointestinal motility can all require such adjustments. For medications which require monitoring of therapeutic levels, it may be fruitful to obtain baseline levels at the beginning of pregnancy. Given the above changes that occur during pregnancy, such a baseline and drawing levels during pregnancy may be of benefit. There are many issues to be explored and discussed when an individual with psychiatric problems becomes pregnant.

In addition to the discussions in previous chapters about relationship building and reaching concordance, there are additional issues specific to working with the woman who is pregnant and experiencing psychiatric symptoms. First, it is imperative to assess the mother's attitude toward the pregnancy. It cannot be assumed that this is all positive and the PMH-APRN needs to be aware of their own biases about pregnancy. The direct approach involves simply asking what her thoughts are about the pregnancy and then continuing with the exploration of her thoughts and feelings. Sometimes, women are not quick to share reservations and concerns and a more indirect approach may involve questions about the father's reaction as well as others who are important in her support system. Also, an exploration of sleep patterns and dreams may reveal other concerns. Freud has written about dreams as the royal road to the unconscious, and more recently Hall and Van de Castle have described the emotional content of dreams as a revealing processing of daytime issues. See http://psych.ucsc.edu/dreams/DreamsSAT/index.html for a complete description of their work. Depending upon the PMH-APRN's familiarity with dream work, this may be one indirect approach to determine and assist a woman with her reactions to a pregnancy.

Another aspect unique to pregnancy is the awareness of any intervention influencing the fetus as well as

TABLE 19-1: COMMON PSYCHOTROPIC MEDICATIONS AND ADVERSE EFFECTS DURING PREGNANCY

MEDICATION	TYPICAL DOSAGE	CLASSIFICATION	PREGNANCY CATEGORY	MATERNAL ADVERSE EFFECTS	FETAL ADVERSE EFFECTS	BREASTFEEDING PER AAP
Alprazolam (Xanax)	0.5–6 mg/day	Benzodiazepine	D	Drowsiness, depression, memory impairment, appetite changes; risk for dependence	Increased risk for congenital malformation; neonatal withdrawal	Drug for which the effect on nursing infants is unknown but may be of concern
Amitriptyline (Elavil)	50–300 mg/day	Tricyclic antidepressant	C	Orthostatic hypotension, sedation, EKG changes, urinary retention; risk for toxicity; risk for bone marrow suppression	Central nervous system effects, limb deformities, development delays per case reports	Drug for which the effect on nursing infants is unknown but may be of concern
Buproprion (Wellbutrin)	sustained release (SR) 150–400 mg/day Extended release (XL) 150–450 mg/day	Dopamine reuptake inhibitor	C	Tachycardia, headache, insomnia, dizziness, xerostomia, weight loss, pharyngitis; risk for seizure; risk for treatment emergent hypertension	Possible increase for spontaneous abortion, possible neonatal withdrawal	Drug for which the effect on nursing infants is unknown but may be of concern
Chlorpromazine (Thorazine)	30–800 mg/day	Typical antipsychotic	C	EPS, prolonged QT, akathisia, altered temperature regulation, sedation; risk for NMS; risk for tardive dyskinesia	Third trimester use increases risk of neonatal EPS; risk of neonatal withdrawal: agitation, altered feeding, respiratory distress, lethargy	Drug for which the effect on nursing infants is unknown but may be of concern
Citalopram (Celexa)	20-40 mg/day	SSRI antidepressant	C	Somnolence, insomnia, nausea, xerostomia, diaphoresis, anorexia	Third Trimester Exposure: respiratory distress, cyanosis, apnea, seizures, unstable temperature, feeding difficulties, hyper or hyptononia, irritability, tremor, increased risk for lower Apgar and lower birth weight; persistent pulmonary hypertension (PPHN) risk use after week 20	Not included
Clonazepam (Klonopin)	0.25–4 mg/day	Benzodiazepine	D	Drowsiness, depression, memory impairment, appetite changes; risk for dependence	Increased risk for congenital malformation; neonatal withdrawal	Not included

(*Continued*)

TABLE 19-1: COMMON PSYCHOTROPIC MEDICATIONS AND ADVERSE EFFECTS DURING PREGNANCY (*Continued*)

MEDICATION	TYPICAL DOSAGE	CLASSIFICATION	PREGNANCY CATEGORY	MATERNAL ADVERSE EFFECTS	FETAL ADVERSE EFFECTS	BREASTFEEDING PER AAP
Clozapine (Clozaril)	12.5–900 mg/day	Atypical antipsychotic	B	Tachycardia, sedation, dizziness, constipation, weight gain, sialorrhea; EPS; risk for NMS, risk for tardive dyskinesia; risk for seizure, risk for agranulocytosis	Third trimester use increases risk of neonatal EPS; risk of neonatal withdrawal: agitation, altered feeding, respiratory distress, lethargy	Drug for which the effect on nursing infants is unknown but may be of concern
Escitalopram (Lexapro)	10–20 mg/day	SSRI antidepressant	C	Headache, somnolence, insomnia, nausea, anorexia	Third Trimester Exposure: respiratory distress, cyanosis, apnea, seizures, unstable temperature, feeding difficulties, hyper or hypotonia, irritability, tremor, lower Apgar and lower birth weight; PPHN risk use after week 20	Not included
Fluoxetine (Prozac, Sarafam)	20–80 mg/day	SSRI antidepressant	C	Insomnia, headache, somnolence, anxiety, nausea, diarrhea, anorexia, weakness	Third Trimester Exposure: respiratory distress, cyanosis, apnea, seizures, unstable temperature, feeding difficulties, hyper or hypotonia, irritability, tremor, lower Apgar and lower birth weight; PPHN risk use after week 20	Drug for which the effect on nursing infants is unknown but may be of concern
Fluvoxamine (Luvox)	50–300 mg/day	SSRI antidepressant	C	Headache, insomnia, somnolence, dizziness, anxiety, nausea, diarrhea, anorexia, weakness	Third Trimester Exposure: respiratory distress, cyanosis, apnea, seizures, unstable temperature, feeding difficulties, hyper or hypotonia, irritability, tremor, lower Apgar and lower birth weight; PPHN risk use after week 20	Drug for which the effect on nursing infants is unknown but may be of concern
Haloperidol (Haldol)	0.5–30 mg/day	Typical antipsychotic	C	extrapyrimidal symptoms (EPS), prolonged QT, akathisia, altered temperature regulation, sedation; risk for neuroleptic malignant syndrome (NMS); risk for tardive dyskinesia	Third trimester use increases risk of neonatal EPS; risk of neonatal withdrawal: agitation, altered feeding, respiratory distress, lethargy	Drug for which the effect on nursing infants is unknown but may be of concern

Lamotrigine (Lamictal)	25–200 mg/day	Anticonvulsant mood stabilizer	C	Nausea; risk for Stevens-Johnson Syndrome	Increased risk for cleft palate in first trimester use	Drug for which the effect on nursing infants is unknown but may be of concern
Lithium (Escalith, Lithobid, Lithostat)	600–2400 mg/day	Antimanic agent	D	Arrhythmia, hypotension, dizziness, sedation, headache; risk for toxicity	Cardiac malformations in first trimester use; shallow respiration, lethargy, hypotonia, thyroid depression in the neonate; risk for toxicity	Drugs that have been associated with significant effects on some nursing infants and should be given to nursing mothers with caution
Lorazepam (Ativan)	1–6 mg/day	Benzodiazepine	D	Drowsiness, depression, memory impairment, appetite changes; risk for dependence	Increased risk for congenital malformation; respiratory depression, neonatal withdrawal, hypotonia with use later in pregnancy	Drug for which the effect on nursing infants is unknown but may be of concern
Mirtazapine (Remeron)	15–45 mg/day	Alpha 2 antagonist	C	Somnolence, increased cholesterol, constipation, xerostomia, weight gain; risk of neutropenia	Increase in fetal loss, decrease birth weight	Not included
Olanzapine (Zyprexa)	5–20 mg/day	Atypical antipsychotic	C	Sedation, dizziness, constipation, weight gain; EPS; risk for NMS, risk for tardive dyskinesia	Third trimester use increases risk of neonatal EPS; risk of neonatal withdrawal: agitation, altered feeding, respiratory distress, lethargy	Not included
Paroxetine (Paxil)	20–60 mg/day	SSRI antidepressant	D	Somnolence, insomnia, headache, dizziness, nausea, diarrhea, weakness, tremor, anorexia	Increased risk for congenital and cardiovascular malformations; Third Trimester Exposure: respiratory distress, cyanosis, apnea, seizures, unstable temperature, feeding difficulties, hyper or hypotonia, irritability, tremor, lower Apgar and lower birth weight; PPHN risk use after week 20	Drug for which the effect on nursing infants is unknown but may be of concern

(Continued)

TABLE 19-1: COMMON PSYCHOTROPIC MEDICATIONS AND ADVERSE EFFECTS DURING PREGNANCY (*Continued*)

MEDICATION	TYPICAL DOSAGE	CLASSIFICATION	PREGNANCY CATEGORY	MATERNAL ADVERSE EFFECTS	FETAL ADVERSE EFFECTS	BREASTFEEDING PER AAP
Quetiapine (Seroquel)	50–600 mg/day	Atypical antipsychotic	C	Sedation, headache, dizziness, increased cholesterol, weight gain; EPS; risk for NMS, risk for tardive dyskinesia	Third trimester use increases risk of neonatal EPS; risk of neonatal withdrawal: agitation, altered feeding, respiratory distress, lethargy	Not included
Risperidone (Risperdol)	1–6 mg/day	Atypical antipsychotic	C	Sedation, dizziness, weight gain; EPS; risk for NMS, risk for tardive dyskinesia	Third trimester use increases risk of neonatal EPS; risk of neonatal withdrawal: agitation, altered feeding, respiratory distress, lethargy	Not included
Sertraline (Zoloft)	25–200 mg/day	SSRI antidepressant	C	Dizziness, fatigue, headache, insomnia, somnolence, anorexia, diarrhea, nausea, tremors	Third Trimester Exposure: respiratory distress, cyanosis, apnea, seizures, unstable temperature, feeding difficulties, hyper or hypotonia, irritability, tremor, lower Apgar and lower birth weight; PPHN risk use after week 20	Drug for which the effect on nursing infants is unknown but may be of concern
Trazodone (Desyrl)	150–600 mg/day	Serotonin reuptake inhibitor antagonist	C	Dizziness, sedation, headache, nausea, xerostomia, blurred vision	Possible neonatal withdrawal	Drug for which the effect on nursing infants is unknown but may be of concern
Valproic acid (Depakote)	750 mg/day to 60mg/kg/day	Antimanic agent	D	Headache, somnolence, dizziness, nausea, emesis, diarrhea, thrombocytopenia, weakness; risk for toxicity	Neural tube defects, facial defects, cardiac defects, skeletal defects have been reported. Afibrinogenemia resulting in fetal hemorrhage and hepatotoxicity have been reported	Drugs that have been associated with significant effects on some nursing infants and should be given to nursing mothers with caution

Note: Definitions of Pregnancy Categories can be found in Exhibit 19-1 on page 503.

the father. Therefore, when making treatment decisions it is wise to involve the father if available and also the mother's gynecologist.

The screening, etiology, and treatment of anxiety, depression, psychotic disorders, and chemical dependency during pregnancy are discussed.

ANXIETY DISORDERS

SCREENING AND ETIOLOGY

While completing the psychiatric evaluation on the patient planning a pregnancy or the already pregnant patient, the PMH-APRN will inquire about panic attacks, generalized anxiety, obsessions, and compulsions in both the patient's history and family psychiatric history. Further, it can be helpful to discern if these symptoms existed prior to pregnancy or emerged during pregnancy. Current abuse or a past history of abuse and trauma also needs to be identified. Patients rarely spontaneously report past miscarriages or difficulties during past pregnancies or delivery, so clinicians should inquire about this directly during interviews with pregnant patients. Details and patterns from the history of present illness that parallels events from the patient's social history may be uncovered with the patient lacking awareness of these connections. This clinical data provides another opportunity for the PMH-APRN to address past and current issues in the treatment plan and therapeutic process.

During pregnancy, patients may develop anxiety disorders. Also, patients with preexisting anxiety disorders may experience an exacerbation of their symptoms given the changes associated with pregnancy. During pregnancy, bodies and lifestyles change. For some patients, the necessary changes in diet may cause or exacerbate symptoms of anxiety. Increasing weight and adjustments in weight distribution, and shopping for and purchasing properly fitting clothing may be distressing to some patients. Increased need for sleep and decreased energy during pregnancy may interfere with the patient's work in and outside the home, which can also be a source of distress. Family, friends, colleagues, and strangers may overstep the patient's boundaries in attempts to make a physical connection with the baby by touching the patient's abdomen. This simple touch may be perceived as an invasion of boundaries and ultimately provoke anxiety. Finally, contemplating the demands of a newborn baby and the associated changes in not only day-to-day life but also changes within the family dynamic may heighten distress for the patient with newly developed anxiety or preexisting anxiety.

Another source of anxiety may be the screening and tests required during pregnancy. Kowalcek et al. (2003) investigated anxiety in the context of prenatal testing. They reported anxiety in 11.1% of patients who received prenatal testing. Advanced maternal age, positive family history, or exclusion of malformation are indications for prenatal testing. Patients in this study reported anxieties about pain, the exam itself, preterm delivery, having a miscarriage, detection of malformation, and missed malformation detection. During the psychiatric assessment of the pregnant patient, inquiries about the patient's concerns and attitude toward prenatal testing should be included. The PMH-APRN is in a position to assist the patient in processing and facilitating acceptance of the results of the prenatal testing.

Another important element is the presence of current or past verbal, physical, or sexual abuse or trauma. A past history of sexual abuse can also reawaken issues for the patient as her body undergoes changes during pregnancy. Different sensations in her anatomy from the pregnancy and during delivery can bring back memories of past trauma, possibly pulling the patient back to regressed behaviors and past patterns of maladaptive coping. Sensations during vaginal birth and interventions such as checking dilation may be intolerable for patients with a past history of sexual abuse. Rather than generate another negative and traumatic experience for these patients, in these cases it may behoove the patient to discuss the possibility of a caesarian section with her midwife or obstetrician. This is another opportunity for the PMH- APRN to collaborate with the obstetrical clinician to help the patient be physically and emotionally stable during her delivery experience and prenatal checks leading up to the delivery. The PMH-APRN can assist the patient in preparing for and processing prenatal checks and the delivery itself.

Also at risk for anxiety symptoms and disorders are patients with a history of stillbirth or miscarriage. The anxieties of losing another pregnancy can negatively impact the patient and consequently the fetus. Screening for prior fetal loss during the psychiatric appointments in a patient who is planning or is already pregnant gives the clinician and patient an opportunity to address and process this loss. This work sets the stage for a more comfortable and stable outlook for the pregnancy and delivery.

In addition to concerns for the mother's welfare, the hormone shifts of anxiety may be dangerous to the fetus. Increases in corticotrophin-releasing factor in the context of anxiety and stress are a concern. Specifically, increases in maternal corticotrophin-releasing factor have been found to negatively impact the fetus. Dayan et al.

(2002) investigated the impact of anxiety and depression on spontaneous preterm labor. They found women with high depression scores were twice as likely as unaffected women to have spontaneous preterm labor. Depression was correlated with low prepregnancy body mass index (BMI). In pregnant women with stated anxiety, they found a not statistically significant increase in the incidence of vaginal bleeding. The investigators hypothesized that depression and anxiety impact placental secretion of corticotropin-releasing factor, which may act as a stimulant. They also proposed that a low BMI could further deepen depression by increasing the release of corticotropin-releasing factor and increasing serum cortisol levels.

Not surprisingly, the act of delivery can also be a source of anxiety. The most carefully constructed birthing plan may be replaced by alternative interventions when necessity demands. Complications can occur and less than desirable outcomes can result. Women on the day of caesarian delivery were found to have anxiety 10 points higher as compared with women of reproductive age, suggesting women's anxiety increases prior to delivery (Uppal, Rooney, & Young, 2009).

Acute and post-traumatic stress disorders after first trimester spontaneous abortion were explored in a small study (Bowles et al., 2006). Twenty-eight percent of patients met criteria for acute stress disorder and 39% met criteria for Post-Traumatic Stress Disorder (PTSD) one month after spontaneous abortion. History of emotional, physical, or sexual abuse was one of the predictors for developing these disorders. Other risk factors identified for the development of stress disorders following spontaneous abortion included the perception of feeling responsible for the spontaneous abortion, lacking a sense of control in one's life, and feeling bonded with the fetus. These findings suggest the importance of screening for PTSD at the one month follow up appointment. Identifying PTSD in a new mother holds the potential for referral and psychiatric treatment leading to a more secure bonding between mother and child and an overall higher level of wellness for the family.

In addition to generalized anxiety and PTSD, pregnancy can be a time of increased compulsions and obsessive symptoms within an Obsessive Compulsive Disorder (OCD). Changes during pregnancy and anticipating the demands of a newborn can further heighten OCD symptoms or cause OCD symptoms to emerge. Compulsive behaviors and obsessions can be distracting and disruptive to the patient during the time of pregnancy. These symptoms can interfere with the patient's functioning and interfere with her achieving or maintaining her maximal level of functioning.

A strong association between OCD and pregnancy has been identified. For those with preexisting OCD, obsessive and compulsive symptoms can worsen during pregnancy. Worsening in OCD symptoms dependent upon timing of menstruation may be an indicator of risk for increase of OCD symptoms during pregnancy. For others, OCD can emerge during pregnancy or during postpartum. Often, obsessions and compulsions during or after pregnancy revolve around contamination.

Buttolph and Holland (1990) reported that 52% of women with OCD had onset during pregnancy. A case report of pregnancy-induced obsessive disorder described a primigravid patient who was consumed by obsessions of fetal contamination and cleaning compulsions starting the fourth month of gestation and resolving two weeks postpartum (Kalra, Tandon, Trivedi, & Janca, 2005). Flouoxetine 20 mg/day one month after initial assessment was ordered and titrated to 60 mg/day. At eight months gestation, the patient discontinued flouxetine at the advice of family and experienced a reemergence of OCD symptoms. Two weeks postpartum the patient reported resolution of OCD symptoms and through one month follow up showed no reemergence of OCD symptoms. The investigators hypothesized involvement of caudate nucleus pathology contributed to the development and eventual resolution of OCD in this case. So, it is wise to consider the possibility of an anxiety disorder during any stage of pregnancy.

TREATMENT

The decision to not treat or the consequences of undertreating anxiety during pregnancy can have long-lasting consequences for the newborn. See Figure 19-1 for the process to assist with decision making when considering psychiatric treatment during pregnancy. A correlation between third trimester anxiety and behavioral problems in offspring at four years has been identified. (O'Connor, Heron, Golding, Beveridge, & Glover, 2002). Furthermore, late gestational anxiety was correlated with hyperactivity and inattention in boys and with total behavioral and emotional problems in both boys and girls, even after controlling for antenatal and obstetrical risks such as gestational age and birth weight. Therefore, treatment of anxiety during pregnancy is quite important for current as well as future functioning of the mother and child.

In addition to medications, many complimentary treatments are available for anxiety during pregnancy. These interventions are appealing and effective. Both individually and in concert, massage and aromatherapy have long been used to aid in relaxation. Many labor and delivery nurses are trained in massage and aromatherapy. Hospitals often have programs to support use of massage or aromatherapy in obstetrical or labor and delivery units. These nonpharmacologic interventions can be easily implemented during pregnancy. The patient's partner can perform the massage and assist in the aromatherapy. One could surmise that these interactions can increase the couples bond and include the partner in bonding with the baby. Burns, Blamey, Ersser, Lloyd, and Barnetson (2000) found patients who used aromatherapy during delivery reported it beneficial. Specifically, 50% reported it reduced their levels of fear and anxiety, and almost 60% reported reduction in pain. The oils most frequently used were lavender and frankincense. Other oils available included eucalyptus, mandarin, lemon, chamomile, clary sage, and peppermint administered via skin absorption or inhalation. Within this study, only 1% of patients reported adverse reactions, such as mild skin irritation or nausea. Patients included those with low-risk births, patients who were induced, and patients awaiting caesarean section. Of course, preference of scent for each individual is a consideration.

Another option is ongoing massage therapy used to complement treatment for anxiety during pregnancy as well as pain during labor (Chang, Wang, & Chen, 2002). Massage is thought to block pain impulses and is also thought to increase the release of endorphins, and its benefits include decreased sensation of pain, increased relaxation, and decreased anxiety. These interventions

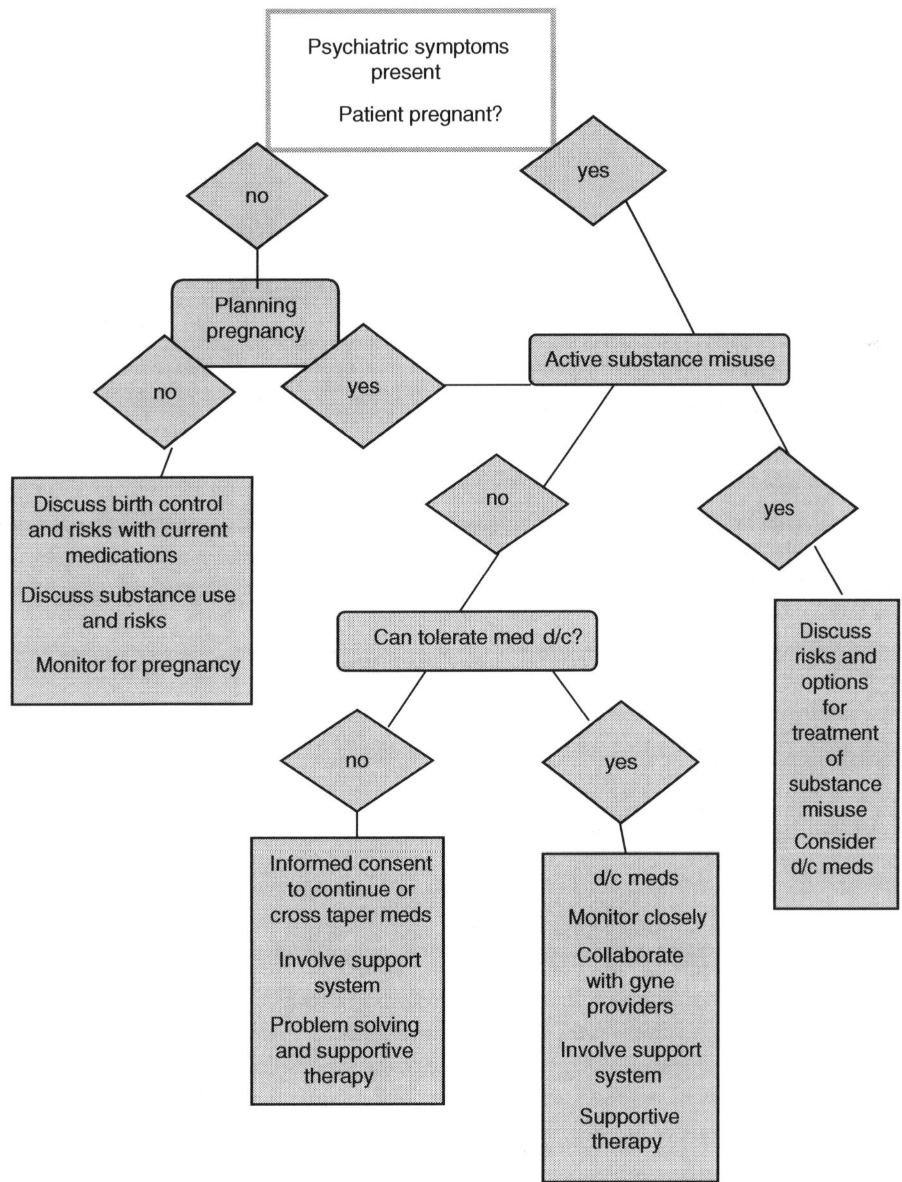

FIGURE 19-1 Decision Tree on Initiation of Treatment of Psychiatric Symptoms in Pregnant Women

contributed to a positive birthing experience and may prevent PTSD symptoms.

For patients with anxiety, many find education and anticipatory guidance also helpful. Education from the obstetrician, midwife, and anesthetist about the events during labor and delivery can provide anticipatory guidance for the patient and decrease anxiety. Learning beyond indication, risk, benefit, and alternatives about various interventions and outcomes can further help quell anxiety. Having the partner be a part of this process can further provide support to the patient.

However, increased education and dialogue above the standard discussion of labor pain management may not necessarily make a positive impact. Uppal et al. (2009) reported no significant reduction in anxiety at the time of caesarean delivery nor improved sleep in preoperative nights in patients who received the intervention of intensive antenatal counseling by the anesthesia provider prior to delivery, as compared with standard pain management education. Of course, one must consider the content and the relationship issues of this educational process and further studies are needed to identify factors contributing to positive impact.

Another nonpharmacological intervention that is beneficial to the mother, parent dyad, or family unit is engagement with a doula. Doulas are professionals trained to provide support to patients during and following labor. Doulas remain present throughout labor and provide emotional support and attend to the patient's physical comfort. Doulas present during labor can guide the patient through delivery and help preserve positive memories of the experience. Some doulas are certified in providing postpartum support to the parents. Postpartum doulas provide the parents and other family members with education, emotional support, and assistance in developing the relationship with the newborn and shifting the other relationships within the family. They are usually trained to screen for postpartum depression and anxiety and to make appropriate referrals. Some postpartum doulas provide hands-on assistance in the care of the newborn and are present with the family during the day and night.

The use of benzodiazepines can be helpful in treating anxiety disorders. As with any other class of medications, the use of benzodiazepines does not come without risk. During pregnancy, the patient and clinician discussion of indication, risk, benefit, and alternatives in benzodiazepine use becomes more complicated. Dependent upon the timing of fetal exposure, certain fetal malformations and syndromes can occur in benzodiazepine use.

In their review of the literature, Altshuler et al. (1996) reported an increased risk of oral cleft in first trimester benzodiazepine exposure. While not fatal, children with such defects can have difficulty breastfeeding, require special formula, and can have lifelong ear, nose, and throat issues. The palate can be corrected surgically, but a series of such surgeries is an additional burden on the newborn, and her family. The physical appearance in the newborn in the interim may impact bonding with the newborn and parents. Some parents may limit contact between the child and the community if they are ashamed of the newborn's appearance.

Furthermore, complications can arise at delivery in newborns exposed to benzodiazepines including "floppy infant syndrome." Floppy infant syndrome symptoms can include fetal hypothermia, lethargy, poor respiratory effort, and feeding impairments. Other complications reported after third trimester or parturition benzodiazepine exposure include low Apgar scores, poor feeding, apnea, temperature dysregulation, and muscular hypotonicity (Altshuler et al., 1996).

In addition, just as patients can become physiologically dependent upon benzodiazepines, so does the newborn. The symptoms of neonatal benzodiazepine withdrawal can include restlessness, hyperreflexia, tremors, apnea, diarrhea, emesis, hypertonia. Treatment for withdrawal can require increased newborn monitoring and prolong the length of stay in the hospital nursery. Such delays in discharge to home can interfere with parental bonding and contribute to stress within the family.

The indications, risks, benefits, and fetal outcomes in use of selective serotonin reuptake inhibitors during pregnancy will be reviewed in the depression portion of this chapter. See Chapter 9 in this text for a more detailed description of psychotherapy for anxiety as well as pharmacological treatment.

DEPRESSION

SCREENING AND ETIOLOGY

Depression is not uncommon during pregnancy and postpartum. Studies have reported various rates of depression in these categories. Roughly 10% to 16% of pregnant patients meet criteria for depression, and up to 70% of pregnant patients display depressive symptoms during pregnancy. Furthermore, approximately 12% of women during postpartum meet criteria for depression (1984), with an emergence of depressive symptoms one week following delivery (Gotlib, Whiffen, Mount, Milne,

& Cordy, 1989; O'Hara, Neunaber, & Zekoski, 1984) Risk factors for developing depression during pregnancy were younger age at delivery, history of depression, less education, greater number of children in the household, and stay-at-home mothers. However, the status of stay-at-home mothers was the only risk factor correlated with postpartum depression.

Hostetter, Stowe, Strader, McLaughlin, and Llewellyn (2000) found that of patients taking antidepressants for depression at conception, 57% required an antidepressant increase during pregnancy. Patients with and without prior depressive episodes comprised the study; of this total, 65% required increases in antidepressants during their pregnancies. PMH-APRNs should be mindful of these risk factors while completing their psychiatric assessments on patients. Patients who possess these risk factors require heightened vigilance during pregnancy including more frequent follow-up appointments, continual collaboration with other members of the psychiatric care team, continual collaboration with obstetrical providers, and involvement with the patient's partner or other support person.

During each follow-up appointment, it is imperative for the clinician to inquire if the patient has continued with medications as they have been prescribed. This is important for several reasons. First, patients who discontinued antidepressant use at time of discovery of pregnancy and patients who required initiation of antidepressant during pregnancy had a significant increase risk of requiring higher doses of antidepressant. Second, depression during pregnancy has negative consequences for the mother as well as the baby. Depression during pregnancy has been correlated with preterm delivery, low birth weight, decreased head circumference, lower Apgar scores, higher neonatal cortisol levels, bleeding during gestation, and spontaneous abortion (Bonari et al., 2004; Nonacs & Cohen, 2003). Disruptions of the hypothalamic pituitary adrenal axis and increased levels of cortisol and catecholamine are found in depressed patients; it has been postulated that these changes negatively affect uterine blood flow and fetal development. For those clinicians who suspect that antidepressant medications themselves impact infant hypothalamic pituitary adrenal reactivity, Oberlander et al. (2008) support an alternative. They suggest maternal mood at third trimester rather than antidepressant exposure is correlated with increased infant hypothalamic-pituitary-adrenal axis (HPA) reactivity. The HPA contributes to one's response to stressors. Although the etiology remains unclear, it is generally accepted that maternal depression during pregnancy has negative outcomes for the baby.

Mother's behavior associated with depression during pregnancy includes lower use of prenatal care, poor nutrition, and substance abuse. After presenting these complications, the dilemma of screening and treating depression during pregnancy becomes apparent. Depressive symptoms ranging from isolation, withdrawal, sleep impairment, impaired appetite, to self-neglect and suicidal ideation must be addressed. The severity of prior depressive episodes and previous episodes of depression during pregnancy can help guide the clinician to judicious use of antidepressants, psychotherapy, or interventions such as psychiatric hospitalizations or electroconvulsive therapy. For some patients, antidepressants are a necessity in targeting mood symptoms during pregnancy.

TREATMENT

A variety of treatments for depression are available for use during pregnancy. The patient's current presentation, current treatment linkage, current support system, and past psychiatric history will help provide context and guide the clinician in making appropriate recommendations for care. Some patients may benefit from therapy alone, some may require antidepressants, and some may require inpatient psychiatric hospitalization and or Electroconvulsive therapy (ECT). See Chapter 8 for an in-depth discussion of levels of depression and treatment options.

Individual therapy has been found to be helpful in the treatment of mood disorders. The therapeutic process helps the patient acknowledge and address cognitive distortions. As cognitive distortions are addressed, symptoms are reduced and quality of life is enhanced. This reduction of symptoms is believed to be of benefit to the fetus. Participating in weekly individual therapy sessions is also a source of support for the patient. The therapeutic interaction of sessions can set the stage for a more confident and secure birthing and parenting experience for the patient. This will be of benefit for the patient, her partner, newborn, and other members of the patient's support system. As the patient engages in more healthful and positive interpersonal interactions, positive and healthful exchanges will be readily mirrored by others toward the patient.

Spinelli and Endicott (2003) investigated interpersonal psychotherapy versus parenting education in a bilingual controlled clinical trial of depressed pregnant women. Women receiving interpersonal psychotherapy experienced a significant improvement in mood as compared with the education controls. Women receiving interpersonal psychotherapy also had a significant difference in recovery as compared with the controls. Of note, depression scores improved by week 7 of the 16-week program, supporting the typical model of 12 weekly sessions of therapy.

There are times when antidepressant medications are a necessary treatment modality in helping the patient restore psychiatric balance. A variety of antidepressants are available to the clinician to prescribe during pregnancy. Each antidepressant comes with possible risks for patient and fetus. Some possible risks are more concerning than others. The decision to not treat with antidepressants can also generate negative outcomes for patient and fetus. A patient may desire to receive suboptimal treatment for symptoms in the hopes of minimizing risk to the fetus. However, inadequately treating disease exposes the mother and fetus to risks without receiving the full benefit of the treatment.

Not all patients may require antidepressant initiation or continue with antidepressant therapy during pregnancy. For the patient stabilized on an antidepressant who then learns she is pregnant and elects to pursue a discontinuation of antidepressant treatment, a gradual antidepressant reduction may be feasible. Such patients should be closely monitored for reemergence of mood symptoms. Collateral information from support persons can help the clinician monitor the patient's response to such changes.

For those who require antidepressant use during pregnancy but wish to reduce the dose closer to delivery to minimize adverse effects to the neonate, Miller, Bishop, Fischer, Geller, and Macmillan (2008) advise consideration of a reduction of 25% in the initial 2 weeks of a taper starting at around 35 weeks, followed by a total reduction of 50% until delivery, after which time the full antidepressant dose can be restarted. They describe a candidate for such a taper as a woman with stable mood symptoms, past history of treatment responsiveness, possessing good insight, and receiving ample social support from individuals who can assist in reporting emergence of symptoms should they occur. However, some patients with a history of depression will not tolerate discontinuation or a reduction in antidepressant medication. Some patients who develop depression after becoming pregnant may not do sufficiently well with non-pharmacologic interventions alone to target mood symptoms.

According to the most recent guidelines jointly published by the American Psychiatric Association and the American College of Obstetricians and Gynecologists (2009), prescribing practice during pregnancy should reflect prescribing outside of pregnancy, that is, preferentially using selective serotonin reuptake inhibitors and infrequently utilizing tricyclic antidepressants or monoamine oxidase inhibitors.

According to this joint report, decreased birth weight and small for gestational age have been associated with selective serotonin reuptake inhibitator (SSRI) use during pregnancy. There may be an increased risk for preterm delivery in SSRI use. First trimester exposure to paroxetine carries a higher risk for cardiac malformations. Other SSRI use during pregnancy is not known to carry this same risk. "Poor neonatal adaptation" has been identified wherein the neonate experiences symptoms including tachypnea, unstable temperature, low blood glucose, seizures, and irritability. Persistent pulmonary hypertension can also occur in the context of SSRI use after week 20 of pregnancy wherein the neonate can experience symptoms including neonatal hypoxia and in some instances, neonatal right heart failure. Some research has not demonstrated an association between SSRI gestational exposure and adverse cognitive effects; the American Psychological Association (APA) and American Congress of Obstetricians and Gynecologists (ACOG) advise close monitoring of the neonates development.

The aggregate of studies investigating use of tricyclic antidepressant (TCA) in the context of pregnancy has not yielded an association between TCA use and structural malformations. There may be an increased risk for preterm delivery in TCA use. TCA use has been associated with neonatal complications after birth including irritability, jitters, and, rarely, convulsions. Long-term behavioral effects in offspring exposed to TCA is unclear; therefore, the APA and ACOG advise careful monitoring of the development of exposed infants be tracked.

The APA and ACOG report that research on use of agents including bupropion, venlafaxine, duloxetine, nefazodone, and mirtazepine is sparse. They do report that existing research has shown an increase in preterm delivery and neonatal convulsions, low blood glucose, and respiratory difficulties. According to APA and ACOG, no increased risk for congenital malformations and use of newer antidepressant agents has been identified.

For a select set of patients, the severity of depression is such that immediate results are required. For these patients, electroconvulsive therapy can be a treatment option (Rabheru, 2001).

Potential risks with ECT during pregnancy include placental abruption, preterm labor, and spontaneous abortion. Special considerations include using a wedge beneath the patient's right hip at 20 weeks or more gestation during ECT. Additionally, fetal cardiac monitoring may be of benefit (Solari, Dickson, & Miller, 2009).

In a case report of a 30-year-old at 8 weeks gestation admitted for manic and psychotic symptoms, and who had discontinued maintenance carbamazepine (200 mg/day) upon discovering she was pregnant, Ghanizadeh, Ghanizadeh, Moini, and Ekramzadeh (2009) reported vaginal bleeding in the course of ECT. The patient experienced approximately 12 hours of vaginal bleeding after treatments number 3 through 6. However, her psychiatric symptoms improved such that she was discharged medication free. She was readmitted for mania 20 days postdischarge and again underwent ECT; ECT was discontinued as vaginal bleeding reoccurred. An obstetrical consultation found no placenta previa, abnormalities in amniotic fluid, miscarriage, premature labor, or other pathological findings.

SUICIDE

SCREENING AND ETIOLOGY

Few psychiatric emergencies are more urgent than the instance of a patient who is suicidal. The issue is even more of a crisis when the patient is also pregnant. Bonari et al. (2004) report that of women who are not treated for depression during pregnancy, 15% attempt suicide.

Furthermore, Newport, Levey, Pennell, Ragan, and Stowe (2007) found that 16.7%–27.8% of pregnant women referred to a tertiary clinic for neuropsychiatric evaluation reported suicidal ideation. Suicidal ideation was found to be more likely among patients with the following characteristics: unmarried, less than college education, unwanted pregnancy, and unplanned pregnancy. Within this pregnancy sample, suicidal ideation was more likely to occur in patients with a history of mood disorder, anxiety disorder, or substance abuse disorder. For a detailed presentation of assessment and treatment of suicidal individuals, see Chapter 15, Integrative Management of Self-Directed Violence.

TREATMENT

Maintaining safety and swiftly adjusting the treatment plan of the suicidal pregnant patient is paramount. If the patient is medically stable, the clinician should pursue an inpatient psychiatric hospitalization for the patient. Obstetrical services should be used on a consultative basis, contribute to the treatment plan, and dialogue with the treatment team. In such instances, it is beneficial for the psychiatric nursing staff to receive in-service education from the obstetrical team. This in-service helps the psychiatric nursing staff be better prepared to address the obstetrical needs and deliver care to the pregnant patient.

Due to the myriad of medical complications that can arise during pregnancy, it is not always feasible to admit a suicidal pregnant patient to a psychiatric unit. During such instances, the suicidal pregnant patient requires medical stabilization on a high-risk obstetrical unit, intensive care unit, medical surgical unit, or other non-psychiatric unit. On such units, neither the physical environment of the unit nor the staff supporting it is an equal substitute for an inpatient psychiatric unit. However, efforts can be made to make the physical surroundings as safe as possible and prepare the staff to better therapeutically interact with the patient. Interventions such as removing unnecessary tubes and cords, removing sharp instruments, providing the patient with a safety meal tray including finger foods and eliminating cans, and using one-to-one supervision can all enhance the safety of the suicidal patient on a non-psychiatric unit. As the nurses and support staff are not necessarily familiar with psychiatric issues and therapeutic ways in which to contribute to psychiatric care of the patient, in-services with staff to provide such education can be helpful. During such occasions, it is especially important for the psychiatric team to dialogue with the obstetrical staff, attending provider, and affiliated nursing and ancillary staff. For patients who require longer-term stabilization on such units, weekly meetings to permit the staff to ventilate their frustrations and have their concerns addressed can be of benefit.

MANIA, HYPOMANIA, AND MIXED STATES

Mania, hypomania, and mixed states can involve sleep deprivation, impulsivity, increased goal-directed activity, decreased self-care, grandiosity, agitation, and risk-taking behavior. Such symptoms can contribute to partial compliance or treatment noncompliance for mental health, medical, and prenatal care needs. Such symptoms can lead to alcohol and illicit substance use. Manic, hypomanic, and mixed symptoms can jeopardize relationships with partners, family, colleagues, employers, and other social supports. The above symptoms and consequences can very quickly cause negative consequences to the mother, her fetus, and her family.

Although select fetal defects and complications are known to be associated with the treatments for mania, such states themselves have been found to be associated with obstetrical complications. Jablensky, Morgan, Zubrick, Bower, and Yellachich (2005) investigated reproductive pathology in pregnant patients with histories of schizophrenia or major affective disorders in a sample resulting in more than 3,000 births. A significantly increased incidence of placenta previa and antepartum hemorrhage was detected within patients with bipolar disorder.

ASSESSMENT AND SCREENING

Hormonal changes during pregnancy can contribute to fluctuations in mood and mood stability. Mood episodes in the context of pregnancy are more likely to be depressive and the postpartum psychosis in patients with bipolar disorder can occur in as many as 46% of pregnancies (ACOG, 2008). Given the limited insight patients can have when they are in such states, it is imperative that PMH-APRNs collect collateral information and involve the partner in assessing for symptoms of manic, hypomanic, mixed states, and psychotic features. Both the patient and the PMH-APRN can find it helpful to increase the frequency of outpatient appointments to monitor for such symptoms and provide more opportunities to discuss the patient's transitioning within the pregnancy.

Findings by Grof et al. (2000) can help guide the PMH-APRN in honing in on mood symptoms during specific at-risk times during the pregnancy. Grof et al. (2000) reported pregnant Bipolar I patients experienced fewer and shorter mood episodes during pregnancy as compared with the ante and postpartum. Mood episodes that did emerge during pregnancy did so within the last five weeks of pregnancy. Twenty five percent experienced postpartum episodes. The investigators posit that corticotropin releasing hormone (CRH) produced by the hypothalamus and placenta both may offer protective effects toward maternal mood. Given that this hormone declines after delivery, mood is negatively impacted. Further, they posit there may be instances where CRH declines prior to delivery, which may explain episodes toward the last few weeks of pregnancy.

PMH-APRNs should be aware of specific risk factors associated with relapse during pregnancy. PMH-APRNs should also be mindful of the rates of relapse given certain variables.

Patients who discontinue mood stabilizing medications upon discovery of pregnancy are at increased risk for relapse of depression or mania. Viguera et al. (2007) followed bipolar patients through the end of their pregnancies and one year postpartum. The overall risk of recurrence of mood instability during pregnancy was 71%. In pregnant patients who discontinued mood stabilizer medications, the risk of recurrence was doubled. Further, the time to recurrence of symptoms was four times shorter and the period of mood instability was five times longer in these patients who discontinued mood stabilizers during pregnancy. Those patients who continued mood stabilizers throughout pregnancy spent almost 9% of pregnancy in an illness episode. The first recurrences were found to be depressed (41.3%), mixed (38.1%), hypomanic (11.1%), and manic (9.5%); less than half occurred during trimester one. Younger age of onset, longer duration of illness, more frequent recurrences, rapid cycling history, suicide attempt history, antidepressant use, and comorbid disorders were predictors of illness recurrence during pregnancy. Screening patients for these risk factors and candid discussions about mood relapse during pregnancy are necessary. Further, PMH-APRNs must discuss with the patient the risks associated with treatment noncompliance.

PMH-APRNs may be shocked to learn the frequency with which pregnant patients with histories of manic, hypomanic, or mixed states are noncompliant with their mental health medication treatments. Peindl, Masand, Mannelli, Narasimhan, and Patkar (2007) conducted a descriptive study of 115 pregnant patients with bipolar or schizoaffective disorders who were followed for two years. The investigators reported most concerning findings on treatment compliance during pregnancy. On average, pregnant patients took a mood stabilizer or antidepressant for less than 3 months. Only half of the patients were taking medications for their psychiatric illnesses during their pregnancies.

TREATMENT

In their joint practice guideline, the APA and ACOG (2009) advise avoidance of antiepileptic and newer atypical antipsychotic agents in the first trimester when possible as antiepileptics can become teratogens and as there is a limited amount of safety information on the use of atypical antipsychotics during pregnancy. In general, the APA and ACOG advise prescribers to be mindful of the medication safety profile, patient's current symptoms, patient's past history of mental health issues and treatment, and the patient's treatment preferences.

Lithium

There are a variety of medications available to use to stabilize mood. Mood stabilizers can come with specific risks in the pregnant patient. The patient's past history of manic, hypomanic, and mixed states; severity of such episodes; and past treatment responses can help guide the PMH-APRN in selecting with the patient the most appropriate treatment. An open discussion of the indications, benefits, alternatives, and risks to the patient and risks to the fetus must take place. Specifically, risks for fetal defects and complications found to be associated with the treatments for mania, hypomania, and mixed states must also be discussed for concordance to be achieved.

Although often the drug of choice to promote mood stability, lithium is not a first-line agent for patients with a history of manic, hypomanic, or mixed states during pregnancy. Additional factors must be considered in the use of lithium in the context of pregnancy. Specific malformations and toxicity can occur in the fetus exposed to lithium.

Prenatal lithium exposure has been correlated with an increase in the cardiovascular malformation Ebstein's anomaly. Ebstein's anomaly is a cardiac defect wherein the tricuspid valve is misplaced and ventricular hypoplasia is present. Cohen, Friedman, Jefferson, Johnson, and Weiner (1994) reported an increased risk of Ebstein's anomaly to be 4% to 12% in the context of first trimester lithium gestational exposure as compared with 2% to 4% for untreated comparitors (Cohen et al., 1994).

Despite the above delineated risks, for those patients who have responded poorly to other agents and well to lithium prepregnancy, lithium can be a viable option. Some patients decline a cross tapering or medication switch to other mood stabilizing agents. Some patients have previously poorly responded to other mood stabilizing agents.

The American College of Obstetricians and Gynecologists (2008) have specific guildelines for patients who wish to conceive. ACOG recommend gradually discontinuing lithium prior to conception in bipolar patients with mild and rare episodes of mood instability. For patients with a history of severe episodes but are at moderate risk for relapse, lithium should be gradually tapered prior to conception and restarted following organogenesis. Finally, for patients with a history of both severe and frequent episodes, lithium should be continued throughout pregnancy and the patient receive counseling in risks to the fetus related to lithium use.

In patients who have used lithium during the first trimester, the ACOG encourages the clinician to consider fetal echocardiography. The ACOG does not recommend any specific frequency with which to monitor lithium levels or taper lithium prior to delivery.

In such patients, lithium serum levels must continue to be carefully monitored.

Galbally, Snellen, Walker, and Permezel (2010) advise checking lithium levels monthly during pregnancy until 36 weeks after which time weekly lithium level checks are advised. They advise obtaining a lithium level check immediately prior to delivery and withholding lithium at delivery or 24 to 48 hours prior to delivery if possible.

Cohen et al. (1994) advise a preconception gradual tapering of lithium in patients with mild or infrequent episodes of illness and a reintroduction of lithium once organ generation is completed. In instances of patients with a history of more severe episodes, they advise continued lithium treatment. Newport et al. (2005) advise withholding lithium 24 to 48 hours before scheduled delivery or at the onset of labor and restarting prepregnancy lithium dosing upon medical stabilization following delivery.

A case report from years past serves as a good reminder to carefully consider stopping or reducing lithium prior to delivery. Woody, London, and Wilbanks (1971) reported poor suck reflex, lethargy, and flaccidity in a neonate who had gestational exposure to lithium including immediately prior to delivery. On the second day of the neonate's life, its lithium level was 2.4. Symptoms continued for ten days as the lithium level trended down. Following delivery, the mother's lithium level spiked to 4.4. Both mother and patient survived and the child was found to be healthy at one year of age.

Lithium toxicity in the fetus and newborn can include hypotonia, cyanosis, bradycardia, thyroid abnormalities, cardiomegaly, diabetes insipidus, seizures, and polyhydramnios (Ward & Wisner, 2007).

Hypothermia, electrocardiogram (EKG) changes, and lethargy have been observed in breastfed newborns of mothers on lithium (Woody et al., 1971). No statistically significant neurobehavioral differences were detected at 5 years follow up in a lithium gestational exposure study of 60 children (Schou, 1976).

Antiepileptics

It is important to acknowledge that much of the information available on use of antiepileptics during pregnancy is for the seizure disorder indication rather than bipolar disorder. As each of these diseases are unique, it is therefore important to consider that use of antiepileptics in pregnancy in these differing illnesses may not necessarily share the same outcomes. However, this valuable information about gestational exposure to antiepileptics should be carefully discussed with the patient.

Gentile (2006) reports a fivefold increased risk of major malformations in valproate use for mood stability during pregnancy. Risks related to valproate gestational exposure can include spina bifida, skeletal malformations, cardiovascular abnormalities, coagulapothies, hepatotoxicity, and hypoglycemia. Wyszyniski and colleagues report the risk for neural tube defect with valproate gestational exposure to range from 2% to 5% and the risk for other major malformations is significantly higher (Wyszynski, Nambisan, Surve, Alsdorf, Smith, & Holmes, 2005).

Specific facial features have been noted in those exposed to valproate during gestation. In investigating children with gestational exposure to valproate for their mother's seizure disorders, Moore et al. (2000) describe fetal valproate syndrome. Fetal valproate syndrome includes a stigmata of epicanthic folds, infraorbital groove, flattened nasal bridge, shortened nose, shallowed or smoothed philtrum, small mouth with thinned and elongated upper lip and thickened lower lip. Although the indication in this study was for seizure disorder rather than bipolar disorder, this information should still be shared with the pregnant patient in discussing the risks of use.

Given the teratogenic risks associated with valproate use during pregnancy, the ACOG (2008) advocates for the avoidance of its use during pregnancy and especially during the first trimester when possible. ACOG advises 4 mg/day of folate supplementation prior to conception and during the first trimester despite lack of evidence supporting its benefit in the context of antiepileptic use. Testing advised by ACOG includes maternal serum alpha fetoprotein, fetal echocardiography, and/or a fetal ultrasound. Cohen et al. (2010) advise fetal ultrasound at 18 to 22 weeks. Galbally et al. (2010) advise checking valproate levels at least each trimester.

The frequency with which to check levels or whether to gradually decrease immediately prior to delivery is not addressed by the ACOG in their 2008 clinical management guideline bulletin.

Fetal valproate withdrawal can include jitteriness, irritability, feeding problems, seizures, and abnormality of tone (Thisted & Ebbesen, 1993). To minimize the risk of this withdrawal syndrome, the authors advise using the lowest therapeutic dose of valproate. Although this is a study of patients with seizure disorders, patients on valproate for mood stability should be made aware of the possibility of withdrawal for the neonate exposed to this medication.

Longer lasting consequences have found to be possible as well. Valproate gestational exposure has been linked with lower IQ (Adab, Jacoby, Smith, & Chadwick, 2001). Adab et al. (2001) found behavioral issues such that there was a greater need for additional educational resources in children with gestational valproate exposure. Thirty percent of the children who had been exposed to valproate during gestation required additional educational needs, as compared with 3.2% of the carbamazepine exposed group, and the 6.5% of the other monotherapy groups. Gaily et al. (2004) reported significantly reduced IQ scores in children with valproate gestational exposure; further, a negative relationship was found between maternal valproate dose and the resulting child's verbal IQ.

Congenital malformations are also known to occur in the context of carbamazepine gestational exposure. Gentile (2006) reports the overall incidence of carbamazepine-related fetal malformations for use in bipolar disorder is 5.7%. Such malformations can include microcephaly, growth retardation, cardiac defects, spina bifida, and skeletal defects (Gentile, 2006). Matalon, Schechtman, Goldzweig, and Ornoy (2002) found no statistical difference in the rate of abnormalities in the neonate in untreated epileptic and control pregnancies. Matalon et al. (2002) found in neonates with gestational carbamazepine exposure for seizure indication, there was greater than twice but less than thrice increased risk of major malformations including congenital heart defects, anomalies of the urinary tract, cleft palate, and mental retardation.

Carbamazapine was not found to be linked with lower IQ (Gaily et al., 2004). However, 3.2% of children with gestational exposure to carbamazapine had additional educational needs (Adab et al., 2001).

Given the risks associated with gestational exposure to carbamazapine, ACOG (2008) advises avoidance of its use during pregnancy, especially during the first trimester. As in the use of valproate, ACOG also advises supplementation of folate 4 mg/day prior to conception and during the first trimester. Testing advised by ACOG includes maternal serum alpha fetoprotein, fetal echocardiography, and/or a fetal ultrasound. ACOG reports that it is unclear if carbamazapine increases risk for hemorrhage in the neonate or if Vitamin K supplementation is of help. The frequency with which to check levels or whether to gradually decrease immediately prior to delivery is not addressed by the ACOG in their 2008 clinical management guideline bulletin. Galbally et al.

(2010) advise checking carbamazepine levels at least each trimester.

Moore et al. (2000), in a study of outcomes of gestational antiepileptic exposure including valproate and carbamazepine monotherapy in seizure disorder patients reported speech delay, impaired motor skills, and hyperactivity in offspring. Seventy-five percent of the children had developmental delay, 74% of school-age children required educational assistance, 39% had hyperactivity or inattention, and 16% were formally diagnosed with a behavioral disorder.

First trimester lamotrigine gestational exposure without specification of indication has been found to increase the risk of cleft palate (Holmes et al., 2006).

Given the risks associated with lamotrigine and pregnancy at the time, ACOG in its 2008 Clinical Management Guideline stated it is a potential maintenance therapy option for pregnant bipolar patients. Galbally et al. (2010) advise lamotrigine levels be checked at least monthly during the course of pregnancy as fluctuating levels of the medication can occur during pregnancy.

The following case study by Gentile and Vozzi (2007) illustrates the incremental fluctuation of treatment of a mood disorder during the course of pregnancy. A 30-year-old with cyclothymic disorder was on 100 mg/day of lamotrigine when it was discovered that she was three weeks pregnant. Lamotrigine was discontinued at that time but was restarted at 20 weeks due to relapse. Lamotrigine was again stopped at 24 weeks due to poor response and citalopram introduced at that time. Citalopram was reduced and discontinued in the last month of pregnancy. The baby was born vaginally and without complications. Citalopram was restarted postpartum day 5 and the baby was breastfed until age 6 months. Per the pediatrician, the baby showed no perinatal or neuropsychological issues at age 18 months (Gentile & Vozzi, 2007). Such a case highlights the need of the patient and APRNs to be willing to shift treatment to better address the moving target of symptoms while simultaneously attempting to limit the number of agents to which the fetus is exposed.

Antipsychotics

Pregnancy classes (see Exhibit 19-1) give the APRN some initial and rudimentary guidance in selecting mood stabilizing antipsychotics. The use of haloperidol during

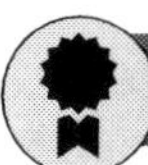

EXHIBIT 19-1: FOOD AND DRUG ADMINISTRATION (FDA) ASSIGNED PREGNANCY CATEGORIES

Category A

Adequate and well-controlled studies have failed to demonstrate a risk to the fetus in the first trimester of pregnancy (and there is no evidence of risk in later trimesters).

Category B

Animal reproduction studies have failed to demonstrate a risk to the fetus and there are no adequate and well-controlled studies in pregnant women.

Category C

Animal reproduction studies have shown an adverse effect on the fetus and there are no adequate and well-controlled studies in humans, but potential benefits may warrant use of the drug in pregnant women despite potential risks.

Category D

There is positive evidence of human fetal risk based on adverse reaction data from investigational or marketing experience or studies in humans, but potential benefits may warrant use of the drug in pregnant women despite potential risks.

Category X

Studies in animals or humans have demonstrated fetal abnormalities and/or there is positive evidence of human fetal risk based on adverse reaction data from investigational or marketing experience, and the risks involved in use of the drug in pregnant women clearly outweigh potential benefits.

Retrieved on 3/16/12 from: http://depts.washington.edu/druginfo/Formulary/Pregnancy.pdf

pregnancy has been well studied. Unfortunately there is only limited information on the use of other antipsychotic medications to target pregnancy mood instability. Given this limited information, treatment guidelines from national bodies and information from case reports can provide the clinician with guidance of risks, benefits, and alternative choices in the treatment of the pregnant patient who is considering the use of such agents.

In its most recent Clinical Management Guideline, the ACOG does not address the use of antipsychotics in the context of bipolar disorder and pregnancy. Galbally et al. (2010) advise obtaining a glucose tolerance test at 14 to 16 weeks and again at 28 weeks given the potential diabetogenic effects of that class of medications.

Although the education for APRNs and various national bodies direct the clinician to use the least amount of medications possible, monotherapy is not always possible. Cabuk, Sayin, Derinoz, and Biri (2007) published a case report in which a 30-year-old patient at 21 weeks gestation was hospitalized for mania. The patient was started on quetiapine 400 mg/day that was gradually titrated to her discharge dose of quetiapine 1200 mg/day in conjunction with haloperidol 15 mg/day. One week postdischarge she was maintained on quetiapine 1200 mg/day alone with a gradual reduction over 9 weeks; quetiapine was discontinued immediately prior to delivery. A male infant was born at 39 weeks without defect and with a normal neurological examination at birth. At follow-up at day 80, the baby was found to have a normal neurological examination and normal psychomotor development at repeat assessment.

Burt, Bernstein, Rosenstein, and Altshuler (2010) did a case report on a 29-year-old bipolar patient who had a past history of numerous medication trials and ECT and who had been maintained on a combination of clozapine 400 mg/day, lithium 900 mg/day, and lamotrigine 75 mg/day. The patient presented prior to pregnancy seeking assistance in maintaining stability and planning for the pregnancy. A prepregnancy crosstaper of olanzapine and clozapine were attempted; however, the patient decompensated and required an inpatient admission and an increase of lithium. Upon restabiliztion and discharge to the community, the patient became pregnant but miscarried at 6 weeks while maintained on olanzapine, fluoxetine, lithium, and lamotrigine. Testing of fetal tissue found a chromosomal abnormality that was determined to be unrelated to the use of psychiatric medications. The patient again became pregnant 4 months after miscarriage; at 30 weeks gestation, signs of placental degradation and fetal decelerations were detected. The patient was admitted to an obstetrical unit for monitoring at which time olanzapine was reduced to 10 mg/day, fluoxetine reduced to 40 mg/day, lithium continued at 1350 mg/day, and lamotrigine was discontinued as fetal demise appeared imminent. The patient became depressed and developed thoughts of self-harm, which improved when olanzapine was increased. At 36½ weeks, rupture of membranes occurred. An infant girl was born via caesarian section. At delivery, the infant had transient tachypnea and received Neonatal intensive care unit (NICU) monitoring for 12 hours. Occasional jerking movements were observed during the infant's first week but resolved. During her first year, the girl had hypotonic muscle tone, was unable to walk at 18 months; however, there was a maternal and paternal family history of motor delay. At the 29-month follow-up, the girl was found to be cognitively bright and emotionally stable. Following this experience, the patient told her clinicians she would use a surrogate for future pregnancies.

PSYCHOTIC DISORDERS

The peak age for onset of schizophrenia for women is 25 to 35 years of age, which are also fertile years (Einarson & Boskovic, 2009). Howard, Kumar, and Thornicroft (2001) reported that slightly more than 60% (63%) of women with psychotic disorders become mothers, with the majority having at least two children. Of these, 10% had a history of social services involvement for the benefit of the child. By screening for pregnancy, monitoring mental health symptoms, communicating with collaborating providers, and engaging the patient in services and resources, the APRN has the unique opportunity to effect healthful change in a patient's life and in the lives of her children.

Given the turmoil and dysfunction that psychotic disorders can create, one could infer that a portion of pregnancies of women with psychotic disorders are unplanned or unwanted. Logic follows that an unplanned or unwanted pregnancy is less likely to receive proper prenatal care or preparation for new life entering the family.

Women with schizophrenia are more likely to engage in high-risk behaviors and be the victims of circumstances that are harmful to both the patient and her fetus. Women with schizophrenia have a significantly higher number of lifetime sexual partners, significantly higher rate history of rape, significantly higher history of trading sex for money or other currency, significantly less likely to be checked for HIV, significantly less likely to have planned or wanted their pregnancies, significantly less likely to use prenatal care, significantly more likely to have been a victim of IPV during pregnancy, and significantly more likely to have an abortion (Miller & Finnerty, 1996).

In addition to lacking in family planning, suboptimal outcomes are well known to occur in the pregnancies of women with psychotic disorders. One could surmise that the decreased nutrition, decreased use of health care, and increased use of illicit substances, alcohol, and nicotine one often observes in patients with psychotic disorders is no different when said patients are pregnant. Patients with a history of psychosis reported significantly more anxiety, more interpersonal problems, and lack of confidence in parenting ability during their pregnancies as compared with pregnant controls (McNeil, Kaij, & Malmquist-Larsson, 1983). Thirty-three percent of the pregnancies were unplanned and 6% of the patients had denial of pregnancy.

Nilsson, Lichtenstein, Cnattingius, Murray, and Hultman (2002) found rate of stillbirth, infant death, preterm delivery, low birth weight, and small for gestational age to be significantly higher in patients with schizophrenia as compared with non-schizophrenic women. They also reported that women admitted to inpatient psychiatric settings during pregnancy carried the highest risks for adverse outcomes in the pregnancy.

Specific malformations and obstetrical risks have been associated with the illness of schizophrenia. Risks have been found to be associated with the onset of the disease. Jablensky et al. (2005) have reported an association between schizophrenia and cardiac anomalies. In their study investigating pregnant patients with histories of schizophrenia or major affective disorders in a sample resulting in 3,174 births, women with schizophrenia were found to have a significantly increased risk of placental abruption, to have given birth to infants with cardiovascular abnormalities, and to have given birth to infants in the lowest weight and/or growth decile. Also, 46.3% of women with schizophrenia had two or more obstetrical complications and 7.3% of women with schizophrenia had five or more obstetrical complications, as compared with the 40.5% and 4.8% unaffected controls. A 2.50 odds ratio after adjustment for cardiovascular defects including ventricular septal defects, atrial septal defects, patent ductus arteriosis, and aortic abnormalities was found in mothers with schizophrenia. Mothers who had schizophrenia prior to pregnancy were found to be significantly more likely to have serious obstetric complications; mothers with onset of schizophrenia at pregnancy had the same rate of risk as the controls. Specific complications of placental abruption, low birth weight for gestational age, and cardiovascular defects were equally occurring in the premorbid and schizophrenia at onset of pregnancy groups. Specifically, the risk of patent ductus arteriosis was found to have a tenfold increase in frequency as compared with controls, ventricular septal defect to have a threefold increase in frequency as compared with controls, and atrial septal defects to have a twofold increase in frequency as compared with controls. Fetal distress during labor was significantly increased in the patients with schizophrenia. Bennedsen, Mortensen, Olesen, and Henriksen (2001) found a significantly increased risk of sudden infant death syndrome (SIDS) in children of women with schizophrenia.

ASSESSMENT AND SCREENING

At the detection of pregnancy, it is imperative that the APRN assess for delusions specific to the pregnancy. Delusions specific to the pregnancy can encompass concerning content including but certainly not limited to the fetus being a non-human life, being connected to a religious deity, or being linked with the demise of mankind. It is not difficult to imagine how such content can lead to tragic outcomes.

An especially high-risk delusion is psychotic denial of pregnancy. Psychotic denial of pregnancy is when the patient does not believe or accept that she is pregnant. Since they do not believe they are pregnant, these patients do not seek prenatal care, do not properly interpret labor, do not seek assistance in delivery, and do not bond with the infant. Psychotic denial of pregnancy is a high-risk situation in which the APRN must carefully proceed and collaborate with other providers. One of the treatment goals is to reduce delusions based upon misinterpretation of the reality of the changes in the body during pregnancy.

TREATMENT

Although atypical antipsychotics better target negative symptoms and are frequently better tolerated than typical antipsychotics, the risk of teratogenesis and long-term neurobehavioral consequences has not been well studied. Converesely, typical antipsychotics have been better researched and have been used for decades. Given this, the American College of Obstetricians, per their 2008 Clinical Management Guideline, supports the use of typical antipsychotics for psychotic disorders. Specifically, they advise the use of the smallest therapeutic doses possible during pregnancy. In instances where a patient conceives while on an atypical antipsychotic, the ACOG advises the clinician to have a thorough discussion of the risk and benefit of continuing on the atypical versus switching to a typical antipsychotic and exposing the fetus to multiple medications.

Further contributing to the concern of use of atypicals during pregnancy includes a recent labeling change in atypical antipsychotics. In February of 2011, the Food and Drug Administration updated the labeling on antipsychotic medications to show risk of side effects in use during the third trimester. Possible symptoms include sleepiness, respiratory difficulty, feeding difficulty, and tremor.

Diav-Citrin et al. (2005) investigated the use of haloperidol and penfluridol in a sample of 215 pregnancies. Rate of congenital malformations did not differ between the two medication groups and the control group. However, decreased birth weight and a double risk of preterm birth were found in the two medication groups as compared with the control group.

Typical antipsychotic toxicity has been reported in fetuses and neonates. Exposure to typical antipsychotics can result in respiratory depression, hypertonicity, jaundice, and neuroleptic malignant syndrome (ACOG, 2008).

In the instances where a patient has been on an atypical antipsychotic and conceives, the following case studies and research findings can provide some pertinent information for the APRN to discuss with the patient. As more use and more research is conducted on the use of atypical antipsychotics in pregnancy, APRNs will be better informed and more able to discuss the risks and benefits of their use during pregnancy.

McKenna et al. (2005) found no association in risk for major malformations and use of atypical antipsychotics in a sample using olanzapine, risperidone, quetiapine, or clozapine during pregnancy. A significantly increased maternal BMI in quetiapine use was detected.

Grover and Avasthi (2004) report a case of risperidone gestational exposure for psychotic disorder and oligohydraminos at 39 weeks such that labor was induced. No congenital malformations were detected.

Mendhekar and Lohia (2008) report a patient with undifferentiated schizophrenia who used risperidone through two pregnancies had uneventful deliveries. Both infants were healthy and found to be without behavioral or neurodevelopmental issues.

Dabbert and Heinze (2006) offer a case report of a 30-year-old pregnant patient with paranoid schizophrenia who received risperidone microspheres 25 mg every 2 weeks between weeks 4 and 20 gestation; medication was discontinued upon discovery she was pregnant but was reinstituted when the patient became malnourished, decompensated, and required inpatient admission at week 38 gestation. At birth, the newborn was small for date, but without malformations. The newborn was adopted outside of the biological family and at follow-up at 2½ years, was neurobehaviorally healthy.

Yeshayahu (2007) reports a case study of a 25-year-old patient with schizophrenia stabilized on olanzapine 10 mg/day who delivered an infant with atrioventricular canal defect and unilateral clubfoot. Mendhekar, War, Sharma, and Jiloha (2002) report a case wherein a psychotic woman at 24 weeks required psychiatric admission and was started on olanzapine. Olanzapine was continued for one month and then gradually tapered and eventually discontinued 10 days prior to delivery. At three months follow-up, the baby was free from abnormalities and had achieved his developmental milestones. Littrell, Johnson, Peabody, and Hilligoss (2000) share a report of a patient with an extensive history of psychiatric hospitalizations, suicide attempts, and diagnosis of schizophrenia who was maintained on olanzapine throughout pregnancy and delivered a viable infant at 30 weeks.

Mervak, Collins, and Valenstein (2008) report aripiprazole use in a 24-year-old patient with schizoaffective disorder who discontinued aripiprazole upon learning she was pregnant. The patient remained off medication until emergence of depressive, suicidal, and psychotic symptoms at 8 weeks, at which time she was tapered back to her prior 20 mg/day dose. The patient was started on bed rest at 39 weeks gestation for elevated blood pressure. The patient delivered a healthy infant at 40 weeks gestation. The infant was formula fed and found to be in good health at follow-up at 6 weeks, 6 months, and 12 months.

Mendhekar, Sharma, and Srilakshmi (2006) offer a case report of third trimester use of aripiprazole from weeks 29 gestation at 10 mg/day, to 15 mg/day at 31 weeks gestation, through six days before delivery, in a 22-year-old with paranoid schizophrenia. No adverse antenatal or events following birth were detected; the infant boy was found to be healthy at 6 months follow-up.

Mendhekar (2007) shares a case study of a 30-year-old patient with schizophrenia maintained on clozapine throughout her entire pregnancy and during one year of breastfeeding. The baby was born to term and without perinatal complication. Speech was delayed; other developmental milestones achieved on time; at 5-year follow-up, the child had attained normal speech.

Nonpharmacological interventions can also be of great benefit for pregnant patients with psychosis. Nishizawa, Sakumoto, Hiramatsu, and Kondo (2007) report reduction in Positive and Negative Syndrome Scale when nonpharmacological-related supports were used in women with schizophrenia during pregnancy. These nonpharacological supports included: child care support, public health nurse consultation, regular meetings between psychiatric obstetric clinicians, midwife, psychiatrist, and public health nurse group conferences, psychiatric hospitalization, mother-baby skill training and education, visiting child care support from regional resources, child welfare center consultation, nursery use, and follow-up consultation with obstetrician and psychiatrist. The investigators also found a high frequency of obstetric complications for both neonates and mothers, including a need for caesarian section in 25%, and 15% requiring induction of labor. It is easy to see how many of the above nonpharmacological interventions may be of benefit to patients with disorders other than schizophrenia.

In patients with psychotic disorders, it can be especially helpful to highlight psychoeducation in addition to the standard psychiatric interview and assessment. Solari et al. (2009) advise the clinician to assess the patient's understanding of pregnancy-related changes. They also advise the clinician to assess the patient's understanding of labor and its signs of onset. They remind the clinician to specifically search for psychotic symptoms pertaining to the fetus and the pregnancy. They recommend having the patient draw self-portraits and portraits of the baby during pregnancy to help unveil delusional content. Developing the birthing plan, identifying who will be the support person present at birth, and touring a birthing center can also be interventions that will help enhance the patient's treatment plan.

CHEMICAL DEPENDENCY

Tobacco, alcohol, illicit substance use, and controlled substance prescription medication abuse are all chemical dependency disorders that PMH-APRNs treat and help patients address. It is well known that use of these substances is harmful to the mother and fetus both. The abuse and dependence of such substances can contribute to negative effects toward the family. Assisting a patient in abstaining from use or minimizing use can help minimize the damage to the fetus. Being mindful of the management of fetal toxicity or withdrawal from such substances and discussing this with the patient also falls within the purview of the PMH-APRN.

According to the Substance Abuse and Mental Health Services Administration's (2006) national survey on drug use, 11.8% of pregnant women aged 15 to 44 years reported alcohol use in the prior month and 0.7% reported heavy alcohol use. In that same survey, 4% of pregnant women reported illicit substance use. Among pregnant 15 to 17 year olds, illicit substance use was reported at 15.5%.

The U.S. Preventive Services Task Force (USPSTF) (2009) recommends that all clinicians assess pregnant patients for tobacco use and provide counseling for tobacco users. Per USPSTF, smoking during pregnancy is not only associated with higher risk for premature birth and intrauterine growth retardation, but also results in the death of 1,000 infants each year. The USPSTF did not find adequate evidence to evaluate the efficacy or safety of smoking cessation pharmacotherapy during pregnancy, but did find evidence that smoking cessation counseling and self-help materials increase abstinence rates of smoking during pregnancy.

In their 2008 Committee Opinion, the American College of Obstetricians and Gynecologists advise clinicians to screen for alcohol misuse with the four-item questionnaire, T-ACE (see Table 19-2) which can be downloaded at www.beststart.org/resources/alc_reduction/pdf/bs_bookmark_lr.pdf.

Or TWEAK, a five-item questionnaire reported to be more accurate than T-ACE and can be downloaded at http://www.alcoholism.about.com/od/tests/a/tweak.htm.

The BNI-ART Institute Intervention Algorithm can be helpful w all patients in screening and intervening w substance abuse and referring to treatment. The questionnaires are less than 10 questions each and are

TABLE 19-2: SCREENING TOOLS SPECIFIC TO PREGNANCY

NAME	FOCUS
T-ACE (tolerance, annoyance, cut-down, eye opener)	Alcohol screen
TWEAK (tolerance, worried, eye opener, amnesia, cut down)	Risk drinking during pregnancy
Abuse Assessment Screen	Domestic violence and pregnancy
Danger Assessment Tool	Domestic violence
Edinburgh Postnatal Depression Scale	Depression
Postpartum Depression Screening Scale	Depression

easily scored. The BNI-ART is an algorithm that guides the interview and assessment of substance abuse and can be downloaded at http://www.ed.bmc.org/sbirt/docs/aligo_adult.pdf

Education is an essential intervention that the APRN uses on a daily basis. O'Connor and Whaley (2007) found that pregnant women who received a workbook-driven brief intervention were five times more likely to report abstinence from alcohol as compared with pregnant women in an assessment-only comparative group. Mothers who had received the brief intervention had infants with higher birth weights, higher birth lengths, and a 0.9% fetal mortality rate as compared with the fetal mortality rate of 2.9% in the assessment-only group. Women were assessed every month at prenatal visits and provided with brief intervention if they endorsed continued alcohol use.

The CDC advise health care providers to routinely screen childbearing-age women for alcohol use and educate them on risks associated with alcohol use during pregnancy. The CDC reports that prenatal drinking patterns are highly predictive of pregnancy drinking patterns. Unmarried and older pregnant women tend to have higher rates of alcohol use (CDC, 2002).

Grant et al. (2009) followed 12,526 pregnant women over the course of years 1989–2004 and found that both women less than 25 years of age and unmarried women had higher rates of binge drinking than other women in the month before pregnancy. Also in this study, smokers were found to have higher rates of alcohol and binge alcohol drinking during pregnancy. Finally, women were more likely to report alcohol use than to report illicit substance use.

Of their sample in their 2007 study, O'Connor and Whaley found that 54% of women reported consuming a maximum of one drink per occasion, 21% reported consuming a maximum of two drinks; and 25% reported consuming three or more drinks per occasion. Furthermore, 61% of their sample scored on the TWEAK such that the fetal alcohol exposure put the fetus at risk. Women in the brief intervention group were five times more likely to report alcohol abstinence by the third trimester as compared with the assessment only group. Participants in the same study also reported drinking before pregnancy recognition at a rate of 62%, with pregnancy recognition occurring at about week seven. Delayed enrollment was associated with lower abstinence rates.

Even minimal or moderate consumption of alcohol during pregnancy has been found to have negative consequences for the fetus. Consuming more than one drink per day is risky drinking behavior during pregnancy. Patterns of drinking as low as one alcoholic beverage per week during pregnancy were found to be associated with aggressive and delinquent behavior in children at 6 to 7 years follow-up. (Sokol, Delaney-Black, & Nordstrom, 2003).

Fetal alcohol syndrome (FAS) is characterized by distinctive facial features including head circumference below the 10th percentile, intrauterine and postnatal growth deficiency, smooth philtrum, smaller palpebral fissures, thinned vermillion border, and absent or small corpus callosum. FAS also includes behavioral abnormalities in infancy including sleep impairment, poor sucking, poor feeding, diminished muscle tone, texture aversions, (Boyce, 2010; Sokol et al., 2003). The prevalence of FAS is 0.2. to 1.5 per 1,000 live births (Boyce, 2010). Bailey et al. (2004) reported IQ scores 1.7 times more likely to be in the mental retardation range and 2.5 times more likely to engage in delinquent behavior in children 7 years of age at follow-up, who had gestational exposure to alcohol in mothers with binge drinking patterns.

Given the above-stated research, risk factors of binge patterns of alcohol use, unmarried status, and older age should be an alert. Past patterns of alcohol use should also help anticipate the patient's pattern of alcohol use during pregnancy. The PMH-APRN must acknowledge these risks with the patient and properly address these risks and behaviors.

For the patient who considers marijuana to be a benign street drug or refers to it as an "herbal supplement," the PMH-APRN should make the patient aware of risks involved during pregnancy. Use of marijuana during pregnancy has been associated with meconium staining, abruptio plaentae, and troubled sleep in the neonate (Behnke & Eyler, 1993).

Kennare, Heard, and Chan (2005) reported of 89,080 obstetrical cases, 0.8% reported drug misuse during pregnancy. Of these, 23.6% reported tobacco use, 39.9% reported marijuana use, 29.9% methadone, 14.6% methamphetamine, 12.5% heroin, and 18.8% reported polysubstance abuse. Further, they reported increased risks of placental abruption, stillbirth, neonatal death, prematurity, small for gestational age, and need to remain in nursery more than one week in patients who abused these substances.

Salisbury, Ponder, Padbury, and Lester (2009) state that cocaine is associated with vasoconstriction, which decreased placental blood flow and consequently reduces oxygenation and nutrition delivery to the developing fetus. Cocaine gestational exposure is associated with decreased fetal growth, decreased birthweight, and increased risk of abruptio placentae and preterm delivery (Behnke & Eyler, 1993; Feldman, Minkoff, McCalla, & Salwen, 1992).

Fulroth, Philips, and Durant (1989) investigated outcomes in infants with heroin and/or cocaine exposure in a sample of 86 infants. Of those exposed to cocaine, 14% were born prematurely and 34% had meconium staining. The investigators opine that cocaine causes placental vasoconstriction thereby decreasing fetal blood flow and diminishing fetal oxygenation. Microcephaly and growth retardation were associated with cocaine use. Six percent of the cocaine exposed group required treatment for withdrawal and 14% exposed to heroin required treatment for withdrawal. Those infants withdrawing were treated with phoneobarbital sodium. The investigators note that method of cocaine use is of consequence, as freebasing (smoking crack cocaine) appears to cause more vasoconstriction than insufflating cocaine does.

Irregular menstruation often occurs during opiate use; this can very easily contribute to a delay in the patient's awareness of pregnancy and consequently delay presentation for prenatal care. Also deleterious to the fetus is malnourishment, which is not unusual in patients who use opiates. Another risk with negative fetal outcomes includes exposure to infection in opiate use given the prostitution and needle-sharing behaviors that often occur. Patients under the influence of their opiate addiction may also be less likely to participate in prenatal care and their prenatal treatment plan. It is important for patients abusing opiates to understand the risks conferred to their developing fetus. At the very least, need for neonatal abstinence syndrome may be required, which can involve use of medications such as opium solutions, phenobarbitol, and paregoric.

Hulse, Milne, English, and Holman (1997) reported decreased birthweight in infants with opiate gestational exposure. Specifically, they reported a reduction of 489 g or more in infants with heroin gestational exposure and reduction of 557 g or more in infants with mixed heroin and methadone gestational exposure.

Liu, Sithamparanathan, and Jones (2010) identified an intrauterine growth restriction association with maternal BMI rather than nicotine use or opiate dosing in methadone-maintained, opiate-dependent pregnant patients. Nineteen percent of the opiate-dependent mothers had babies with intrauterine growth retardation. An association with decreased head circumference and length was also significantly lower in the opiate-exposed infants. Mean BMI in opiate-dependent pregnant patients was significantly lower than the BMI of the controls.

Fulroth et al. (1989) reported meconium staining occurring in 36% of the infants with gestational opiate exposure, the mechanism thought to be fetal hypoxia. Thirty-four percent of the infants with gestational cocaine exposure had meconium staining.

McGlone et al. (2008) reported lower birth weights, smaller occipito-frontal circumferences, and earlier gestation in methadone-exposed neonates. Also, Dashe et al. (2002) report that maintenance doses of methadone less than 20mg/day decrease the risk of neonatal abstinence syndrome. Such symptoms can include hyperactivity, hyperreflexia, abnormal cry, irritability, loose stools, emesis, tachypnea, and can progress to seizures and coma if untreated. Various treatment protocols can include use of phenobarbital, paregoric, or opium solution.

Perhaps counter intuitively, patients maintained on higher methadone doses were found to be significantly more likely to also be concurrently using heroin. Higher maternal methadone use was significantly associated with neonatal abstinence syndrome in this study. Interestingly, the clinicians of this group offer opiate detoxification for select pregnant patients after 24 weeks, utilizing inpatient observation and use of medications including methadone and clonidine according to a specific protocol.

Jones et al. (2010) compared gestational exposure in buprenorphine or methadone in pregnant opiate dependent patients in this double-blind, randomized, controlled study. They found 33% of the buprenorphone group discontinued treatment as compared with 18% of the methadone group. The neonates of the buprenorphine group required less morphine and had a shorter length of treatment for neonatal abstinence syndrome which can include symptoms of diarrhea, feeding problems, weight loss, seizures, and possible death. No significant differences in neonatal abstinence syndrome scores were detected between the two groups. However, the buprenorhine-exposed neonates required 89% less morphine as compared with the methadone neonates and required 43% less hospitalization time.

Fetal opiate abstinence syndrome is a concern. Studies have provided helpful information to consider while treating the pregnant patient for opiate dependence. Many have discouraged attempts to detoxify pregnant patients from opiates. Given fluid adjustments that occur during pregnancy, it may be necessary to increase methadone doses to properly treat the patient as pregnancy progresses. It is not advised to attempt opiate withdrawal after 32 weeks (Bell & Harvey-Dodds, 2008).

Seligman et al. (2010) found no correlation between methadone dose and rate of neonatal abstinence syndrome. Higher methadone dose was found to be associated with decreased illicit opiate use in this study of 330 pregnant women treated for opiate dependence for whom the average methadone dose at delivery was 117 mg/day. Women taking methadone at conception were found to require higher mean methadone doses at the time of delivery. Within this sample, 77 women were also prescribed psychiatric medications; 35% used illicit substances at delivery as compared with the 20% rate of those on methadone alone; 27% of births were preterm. No significant differences in gestational age at delivery, head circumference, or preterm birth rate were detected between the various methadone dosage groups (less than or equal to 80, 81–120, 121–160, 161 or more mg/d). Of this sample, 62% of neonates required treatment for neonatal abstinence syndrome (NAS) but no correlation was found between maternal methadone dose and NAS. NAS was found to be more likely in neonates with maternal tobacco use, illicit opiate use, cocaine use at delivery, and preterm birth.

Methamphetamine use can contribute to malnourishment as this substance decreases the appetite. Consequently, methamphetamine use during pregnancy can negatively impact fetal nutrition. Salisbury et al. (2009) report that among other effects, methamphetamine causes vasoconstriction, increases fetal blood pressure, reduces fetal oxyhemoglobin saturation, and can lead to chronic fetal hypercortisolism.

Chang, Carroll, Behr, and Kosten (1992) found that pregnant opiate-dependent women participating in an enhanced outpatient chemical dependency program showing less illicit substance use received more prenatal care, and delivered healthier neonates as compared with controls who simply received methadone maintenance, group counseling, and random urine toxicology testing. The intervention consisted of a group that met weekly, weekly prenatal care, urine toxicology checks occurring three times per week, child care during group, and positive contingency for abstinence from substances.

Although findings may not be as generalizable to patients in the United States as the study was conducted in Hong Kong, certain details bear careful consideration. Lam, To, Duthie, and Ma (1992) findings reported that pregnant patients dependent upon narcotics first presented for prenatal care at an average of 9 weeks later than controls, at an average of 28 weeks. Within the study, 29% of patients with narcotic dependence were first assessed for their pregnancy upon the onset of labor. Almost half the subjects reported irregular periods.

TREATMENT

Patients who are dependent upon alcohol, benzodiazepines, or opiates and are agreeable to treatment will be best served with admission to a chemical dependency inpatient rehabilitation unit to manage withdrawal or start methadone or alternate agent maintenance. The PMH-APRN can help coordinate this transfer.

In the instance where abuse rather than dependency is occurring, education and promotion of abstinence from the substances should be encouraged. Patients who are agreeable to a recommendation of an intensive outpatient or partial hospital program should be assisted in enrollment. Many community mental health agencies even have day programs for chemical dependency in mothers wherein free childcare is provided during groups. Patients who use tobacco should be provided with education on the risks of smoking and be encouraged to abstain from tobacco use.

When possible, it is helpful to involve the patient's support system such as spouse, partner, or family. The PMH-APRN should refer these support members to Al-Anon and provide education to these support members.

SPECIAL CONSIDERATIONS

HYPEREMESIS GRAVIDARUM

Fifty to 80% of pregnant patients experience nausea and vomiting during pregnancy, which typically starts at the fourth week and concludes by the 12th week. However, 1% to 3% of pregnant patients have hyperemesis gravidarum, a more severe expression of these symptoms that can continue throughout pregnancy; 55% of women with nausea and vomiting in pregnancy endorse depression and almost half claim it interferes with their relationship with their partners (Miller, 2002). Hyperemesis gravidarum has been associated with risk of fetal loss, lower birth weight, central nervous malformations, and prematurity (Mazzota, Magee, & Koren, 1997).

The troublesome nausea and vomiting that frequently occurs during weeks 4 through 12, or in some instances beyond, can evolve into a more severe form. Hyperemesis gravidarum involves loss of more than 5% prepregnancy weight and dehydration due to intractable vomiting and nausea. Hyperemesis gravidarum not only interferes with the quality of life and day-to-day functioning of a patient, but can require hospitalization for electrolyte derangements and can contribute to negative outcomes for the fetus. Hyperemesis gravidarum can also contribute to maternal depression and anxiety. In some instances, the severity of symptoms can prompt the patient to seek termination of the pregnancy.

In the past, hyperemesis gravidarum was thought to be an expression of rejection of pregnancy, rejection of the patient's mother targeted through the fetus, or dissatisfaction with the marital relationship. Buckwalter and Simpson (2002) reviewed the literature and reported flaws in the methods of empirical studies investigating these hypotheses. One can infer that clinicians who ascribe to these hypotheses may not be fully invested in exhausting the treatment options for patients with hyperemesis gravidarum.

Rohde, Dembinski, and Dorn (2003) present a case study of a patient with treatment-resistant hyperemesis gravidarum during her 15th week of gestation with 13 kg of weight loss. Her symptoms were such she requested termination of the pregnancy and endorsed suicidal ideation. While on an inpatient psychiatric unit, the patient was started on mirtazapine. Nausea and vomiting resolved, as did suicidal ideation and the desire to terminate the pregnancy. The patient delivered at 36 weeks via caesarian section. At the 6-month checkup, no abnormalities were noted in either of the twins. At 6-month follow-up, mood was stable and somatic symptoms had not reemerged for the patient.

TREATMENT

Current treatment for hyperemesis gravidarum typically starts with nonpharmacological interventions such as avoiding of spicy foods, eating small and frequent meals, drinking small and frequent amounts of fluids, and wearing accupressure wristbands. Should these nonpharmacological interventions fail, antihistamines and or vitamin B6 are typically the next step. Should these fail, dopamine antagonists such as promethazine are often used. Should these fail, chlorpromazine has been used. Some instances require intravenous rehydration, hospitalization, or parenteral nutrition. Should depression emerge in the presence of hyperemesis gravidarum, the PMH-APRN should offer appropriate interventions including therapy and pharmacomanagement as described above.

INTIMATE PARTNER VIOLENCE

The American College of Obstetricians and Gynecologists recommends domestic violence screening during each trimester and postpartum. The frequency of visits to the obstetrical provider during pregnancy represents numerous opportunities for the clinician to assess for Intimate Partner Violence (IPV). PMH-APRNs remaining connected to and collaborating with the obstetrical providers can further assess if the patient is in an unsafe relationship and willing to leave.

Some women may believe that having a baby can strengthen or secure her relationship with the partner, thereby ending abuse. Some women may believe that being in a vulnerable state such as pregnancy may deter the father of the baby from continuing to physically abuse her. Despite these possible motivations for pregnancy, cessation of abuse is not always the outcome.

SCREENING AND ASSESSMENT

Screening for a history of sexual, physical, verbal, and exposure to trauma is a component of a standard psychiatric examination. Patients who are abused by their partners are at risk for continued abuse during pregnancy. Physical abuse can harm the patient and the developing fetus. Blows to the abdomen can cause fractures to the fetus, uterine rupture, antepartum hemorrhage, preterm delivery, or fetal loss (Sagrestano, Carroll, Rodriguez, & Nuwayhid, 2004). Given these risks, the PMH-APRN should continue to screen for abuse throughout the patient's pregnancy in follow-up visits and provide education, supportive therapy, and information on resources available should the patient be prepared to leave the relationship.

In patients who do not disclose abuse but which the PMH-APRN suspects abuse may be occurring, patients can still benefit from education, supportive therapy, and information on referrals. Substance use, younger age, unmarried status, unemployed status, unwanted pregnancy, consideration for termination of pregnancy can all be risk factors for IPV. A past history of IPV or exposure to IPV in childhood is not unusual in patients who are being abused. A past history of perpetrating IPV on the partner's behalf can also increase the risk for IPV in the current relationship.

Wiemann, Agurcia, Berenson, Volk, and Rickert (2000) reported 11.9% of adolescents reported physical assault by the father of their babies; assaulted adolescents were significantly more likely to have been exposed to other forms of violence within the past year and carried a weapon for protection. Such adolescents were also more likely to engage in noncomforming behavior and use substances.

Lutgendorf et al. (2009) investigated IPV in 1,162 pregnant patients presenting for prenatal care at a Naval hospital. Of these, 14.5% reported a history of IPV and

1.5% reported current IPV during pregnancy. Marriage was found to decrease the odds of IPV. Family history of IPV was found to increase the risk of IPV in the past year.

Li et al. (2010) investigated IPV in a sample of 2887 pregnant women. They found 7.4% of these women reported IPV within the past year. The investigators found an association with IPV and the variables of unmarried status, welfare use, older maternal age, alcohol use, and women performing the majority of the housework. Protective factors included a greater sense of mastery and later age of first vaginal intercourse.

Gazmararian et al. (1995) reported higher rates of physical violence in pregnant women who had the following risk factors: less than a 12th-grade education, receiving Women Infant Children (WIC) assistance, living in crowded quarters, receiving no or delayed prenatal care, race other than white, younger than twenty years of age, and unmarried status. The patients reporting unplanned or mistimed pregnancy comprised more than 70% of the pregnant patients reporting physical violence from their partners. Nearly 43% of the more than 12,000 patients of the study reported unintended pregnancy.

Rodrigues, Rocha, and Barros (2008) investigated IPV in 2,660 pregnant patients. They found an association between IPV and preterm birth. Of the preterm birth mothers, 24% reported physical abuse during pregnancy. Of the sample, 9.7% reported physical abuse during pregnancy. In this study, women reporting physical abuse were found to be younger than 20 years, domiciled apart from the partner, unemployed, less educated, higher parity, unplanned pregnancy, no or late initiate antenatal care, smoke cigarettes, and use alcohol and/or illicit substances. These abused women were found to have an increased risk for small for gestational age newborns.

Silverman, Decker, Reed, and Raj (2006) investigated IPV prior to and during pregnancy in 118,579 women in 26 of the United States. They found women reporting IPV in the year prior to pregnancy had an increased risk for elevated blood pressure, edema, vaginal bleeding, severe nausea, vomiting or dehydration, urinary tract infections, preterm delivery, decreased birthweight, and/or NICU admission. Of this sample, 5.8% reported physical abuse in the year prior to pregnancy or during pregnancy. Women reporting IPV in the year prior to pregnancy or during pregnancy were found to be less likely to receive first trimester prenatal care and more likely to report third trimester smoking. Third trimester alcohol use was found to be more common in those who had IPV in the year prior to pregnancy but not during pregnancy.

Koenig et al. (2006) investigated IPV during and after pregnancy; they found 8.9% of the sample reported IPV during pregnancy and 4.9% IPV after delivery in their sample of more than 600 pregnant women. Factors associated with IPV were found to include lower income, frequent residential moves, and not financially assisted by their partners or family. The odds of experiencing IPV were 3 to 4 times higher in pregnant women who had recently used marijuana or cocaine and 6 times higher in those who recently injected drugs. Odds of experiencing IPV were twice as high during pregnancy as compared with after delivery.

Some insight into perpetrators of IPV can better help the APRN appreciate the frequency of IPV during pregnancy. Burch and Gallup (2004) surveyed 258 men convicted of domestic violence. Nearly one-third of the participants admitted to perpetrating violence toward their current partners during pregnancy and 4.2% admitted to violence toward prior partners during pregnancies. Amplifying the import of these rates is the fact that several participants refused to answer these questions.

Elective termination of pregnancy also carries a specific set of risks for IPV. Saftlas et al. (2010) investigated IPV in 986 patients electing abortions. Of these patients, 11.5% reported abuse within the past year, of which 8.4% reported abuse occurring in the current relationship.

Silverman et al. (2010) investigated IPV in male partners of patients who elected to abort; 31.9% reported having perpetrated physical or sexual violence against a partner. Having been involved in three prior abortions was greater in abusive men.

Koenig et al. (2006) followed patients from pregnancy to the postpartum in four different states in the United States. The investigators found 8.9% of patients reported IPV during pregnancy and 4.9% reported IPV after delivery. Predictors of IPV included bartering sex, use of illicit substances, frequent moves in residency, and HIV diagnoses.

TREATMENT

PMH-APRNs treating patients who are being abused by their partners should educate patients and provide referrals. These interventions should be employed even if the patient is in the precontemplative stage of change. Referral information and contact numbers for shelters, legal aid, and police assistance should be provided to the patient. Such information can be reduced via photocopier such that the information can be stored in a concealed area such as under the innersole of a shoe, away from the eyes of the abuser.

In the instances where pregnancy has resulted from rape, some treatment centers specialize in rape crisis and may be especially helpful to the patient. If the sexual assault has been recent enough, Sexual Assault Nurse Examiners (SANE) nurses who often work in Emergency Room settings can collect evidence that can be used against the perpetrator should the case go to trial. SANE clinicians conduct medicolegal assessments, serve as expert witnesses, and operate under the position statements and standards of practice as deemed by the International Association of Forensic Nurses and the Emergency Nurses Associations. SANE clinicians are moving beyond providing care to patients who have been sexually assaulted and are incorporating medicolegal assessments to victims of domestic violence as well.

As pregnancies resulting from abuse can be unwanted by the patient, patients should be made aware of safe surrender options in case the patient changes her mind in the future. Safe Surrender programs are available in many states in the United States. Some states require that the surrendered infant be younger than 72 hours, some accept infants younger than one month. In some states, only hospitals are approved surrender sites. In others, churches, police stations, and fire stations are approved surrender sites. The level of anonymity varies from state to state as well. One can review http://www.childwelfare.gov/systemwide/laws_policies/statutes/safehaven.cfm to check individual state statutes. For patients who decide to put the baby up for adoption, helpful resources can be located at http:www.childwelfare.gov/adoption/birth/for which contains links about different facets of adoptiong including types of adoption arrangements and legal considerations.

Within the legal system, some communities have victim's advocates available who can assist the patient through the legal system and provide support during the hearing process. The National Organization for Victim Assistance (NOVA) promotes the support and advocacy for victims of crime. Their hotline, 1–800-TRY-NOVA, is available to help victims access assistance within their communities. In addition to NOVA, victim advocates can be located through local law enforcement agencies or a prosecutor's office. For victims of federal crimes, federal victim witness coordinators can provide assistance.

Patients should be encouraged by the APRN to document their bruises and wounds via photograph and calendar in addition to making the patient aware she can report the incident to the police. PMH-APRNs should also make note in the physical appearance portion of a psychiatric evaluation or within the body of the follow-up note stating the presence of bruises, documenting the patient's response when asked how the bruises came to be, documenting the education and interventions the PMH-APRN made available to the patient, and the patient's interest in or declining of the intervention. In certain settings, photography may be available to document bruises and marks with the patient's signed permission.

Irrespective of the patient's decision to stay or leave the abusive relationship, the APRN should maintain a nonjudgmental attitude. The PMH-APRN should continue to offer the various interventions to the patient in future follow-up appointments. As in the case of all patients, the strengths of the patient should be reviewed and discussed between the PMH-APRN and patient. The PMH-APRN can highlight health-seeking and positive behaviors with which the patient engages and encourage the patient to use these skills to cope with her situation.

Kiely, El-Mohandes, El-Khorazaty, and Gantz (2010) investigated cognitive-behavioral integrated intervention versus regular prenatal care in a multisite, randomized controlled trial. The intervention was multifaceted and included education on types of abuse, education on the cycle of abuse, education on preventative options available, construction of a safety plan, education on resources available, a cognitive behaviorally based intervention for smoking cessation, and a cognitive and behaviorally based intervention to address depression over the course of at least four sessions. Women in the intervention group were less likely to be abused by their partners at the first or second follow-up session (occurring during the second or third trimester). The investigators also identified a significant association between IPV and illicit substance use and cigarette smoking. Among the subjects endorsing IPV at baseline, 62% reported depression and 32% reported alcohol use during pregnancy. Women in the intervention group gave birth to significantly fewer very preterm neonates and also had an increased mean gestational age.

FETAL DEMISE

The sadness and despair experienced in the loss of a pregnancy can plunge to indefinable depths for both the patient and her partner. The aspirations, dreams, and intentions for starting a family or adding to a family can swiftly come to an abrupt end or diminish with minimal warning of fetal loss. Time allowing for preparation of loss may or may not be of benefit. The impact of such a loss can extend into future pregnancies, referred to as Pregnancy After Loss (PAL) in the literature.

The nomenclature of loss is defined by the duration of gestation. Miscarriage is defined as loss during first 19 weeks. Stillbirth is defined as loss at week 20 or later (American Family Physician, [AFP] 2007). One in five pregnancies ends within 24 weeks. Second trimester loss occurs in one to five pregnancies out of every 100. Less than one in one hundred pregnancies end in stillbirth (AFP, 2007).

Swanson, Connor, Jolley, Pettinato, and Wang (2007) investigated 85 participants' feelings about miscarriage at 20 weeks or less at specific intervals in the year following miscarriage (weeks 1, 6, 16, 52 post loss). Significant differences between responses were found at weeks 1 and 6 in those who were overwhelmed or grieving, suggesting miscarriage-related crisis lasts about 6 weeks. How women reported feeling at 6 weeks was an indicator of how they would feel at 52 weeks; responses at 6 weeks were not significantly different at 52 weeks.

Cumming et al. (2007) investigated anxiety and depression in women and their partners during the 13 months following miscarriage; women reported higher scores for anxiety and depression than men. Thus, 28.3% of women were found to have anxiety and 10% depression at baseline as compared with 12.4% anxiety and 4.0% depression for men at baseline. In men, no significant differences between baseline and 13 months in either anxiety or depression was noted as compared with the women's group wherein anxiety and depression were significantly higher at baseline as compared with 13 months after miscarriage.

Kong, Chung, Lai, and Lok (2010) investigated the psychological reactions of miscarrying couples at baseline and specific intervals post loss. Tools used included the General Health Questionnaire-12 (GHQ), a tool that measures general psychological distress and the Beck Depression Inventory, a tool that measures the severity of depression. Results showed that 51.8% of women rated high on GHQ immediately after miscarriage, 21.1% rated high 3 months after miscarriage, and 7.7% rated high 12 months after miscarriage. Also, 43.4% of men rated high on GHQ immediately after miscarriage, 7% rated high 3 months after miscarriage, and 5% at 12 months after miscarriage. Scores decreased sharply within the first 3 months then plateaued in men as compared with a gradual reduction over 12 months in women. For men, planned pregnancy was a risk factor associated with depression. For women, marital discord and seeing the fetus on ultrasound were risk factors for depression.

Cote-Arsenault and Donato (2007) investigated women's PAL experiences via thematic data analysis from weeks 25 gestation and beyond. From week 25 on, women changed from worrying that it would end to guardedly anticipating that the baby would survive. Patients reported feeling affirmed in the fetus's safety by its movement. Women had a higher frequency of prenatal visits as compared with routine visits for low-risk pregnancies; the investigators inferred these visits provided the patient with increased information and security.

Woods-Giscombe, Lobel, and Crandell (2010) investigated pregnancy after loss in 363 participants at three interview points during each trimester of pregnancy. No statistically significant difference was found between women with pregnancy after loss and controls at first trimester. Women with pregnancy after loss had higher stated anxiety in second trimester and third trimester as compared with pregnant women without a history of miscarriage. No statistically significant difference was found between the two groups at first trimester. Younger age and unemployment were risk factors significantly associated with anxiety throughout the trimesters.

Cumming et al. (2007) investigated the emotional responses to miscarriage one year following loss—28.3% of women and 12.4% of men were found to have anxiety immediately following miscarriage. Thus, 10% of women and 4.0% of men were found to have depression immediately following miscarriage. Women had a significantly higher level of anxiety and depression immediately after miscarriage as compared with 13 months following loss; no significant difference in depression or anxiety was detected in men in the same time period.

TREATMENT

PMH-APRNs should monitor for mood and anxiety symptoms in patients who experience fetal loss. Education and support to the patient during the bereavement process are needed. PMH-APRNs can provide individual therapy to patients and provide referrals to therapists who specialize in loss. Pharmacological interventions should be offered in instances where depressive, anxiety, or PTSD symptoms are present. Patients may find it helpful to join a support group for women who have experienced loss. Referrals for other family members including the partner and children should also be provided.

Nonpharmacological Therapies

Spinelli (1997) reported interpersonal therapy significantly reduced depression ratings in pregnant patients participating in 16 weeks of this intervention. At the conclusion of interpersonal psychotherapy, all the subjects recovered from depression. Of the patients available at three months follow-up, none reported depressive symptoms.

Therapies for use during pregnancy include:

- Behavioral Therapy
- Cognitive Therapy
- Psychoeducation

- Parenting Education
- Pharmacotherapy
- Meditation
- Yoga
- Massage
- Aromatherapy
- Exercise

Complementary therapies may be of benefit to the pregnant patient. Further, patients may be more inclined to use such interventions, with or without a prior discussion with the psychiatric clinician. Some complementary treatments have more scientific support of positive outcomes than others. Irrespective of the efficacy, a clinician is typically not going to know about patient implementation of such interventions unless the clinician asks.

Acupuncture

Guerreiro da Silva (2007) found acupuncture to be an effective intervention in decreasing symptoms including mood and sleep disturbance in pregnant women with emotional complaints. Acupuncture and electroacupuncture have been found to release serotonin and norepinephrine (Han, 1986). Luo, Meng, Jia, and Zhao (1998) reported an antidepressant effect better than amitriptyline in electroacupuncture. Better effect in anxious somatization in electroacupuncture use as compared with amitriptyline was also reported. Guerreiro da Silva reported an eight-week treatment study sample of 51 pregnant patients reporting mild or moderate emotional complaints with 28 receiving acupuncture and 23 controls receiving standard care. No significant adverse effects were reported by the acupuncture group. Reported symptom intensity decreased in 60% of the sample group as compared with 26% of the control group. Seven control patients as compared with one study group patient received *Passiflora edulis* or *Hypericum perforatum* as supplemental treatment. Sleep was also found to show improvement with the study group as compared with the control. Although there is the concern that some points may trigger uterine contractions, no such effects were observed in this study.

Lavender and rosemary are scents frequently used in aromatherapy to promote a sense of calm and well being. (Bastard & Tiran, 2006).

Chang et al. (2002) investigated massage and anxiety and pain during labor in a randomized controlled trial as massage is thought to decrease pain intensity, distract from pain, increase physical activity, promote relaxation, decrease anxiety, and in some instances strengthen relationships. Massage is thought to increase endorphin levels and reduce cortisol levels. The investigators point out that massage is an opportunity for a partner to actively participate in supporting the laboring mother. The experimental subjects received 30-minute massages during phase one of labor from researcher and repeat 30-minute massages during phases 2 and 3 of labor from their partners who were newly trained in massage. Thirty minutes after delivery, the subjects and their partners were interviewed. Although not statistically significant, experimental subjects more frequently reported a sense of satisfaction from massage as compared with the controls; 87% reported more than moderate benefit from massage during labor. They posited that appropriate physical touch "may help the woman to feel in control of her body and maintain a sense of body boundary integrity."

Beddoe, Yang, Kennedy, Weiss, and Lee (2009) investigated the experiences of 16 pregnant patients with Iyengar yoga and mindfulness-based stress reduction; they found women in their third trimester reported decreases in perceived stress and trait anxiety. Study subjects participated in a 7-week mindfulness-based yoga intervention. Almost one-third of the sample reported a past history of anxiety or depression, and none reported mental health issues during the pregnancy. Additionally, no significant postintervention differences in second and third trimester cortisol levels were detected which suggest stronger circadian rhythmicity as a result of the intervention.

The Motherisk Program investigated the use of St. John's Wort (*Hypericum perforatum L.*) in pregnancy (Moretti, Maxson, Hanna, & Koren, 2009). The average daily dose of St. John's Wort (SJW) used was 615 mg in tablet form in the 54 depressed subjects. SJW gestational exposures were compared with a total of 108 matched pregnancies, including a depressed group treated with conventional pharmacoligics and a non-depressed group. Of the SJW group, 49 were exposed during first trimester only, 7 during first and second or first through third trimester, and 5 began use in second or third trimester. The SJW exposed and conventional pharmacological intervention groups both had higher rates of spontaneous abortion as compared with the nondepressed group. The SJW group was found to have depression scores between that of the conventional treatment group and the healthy group. Other studies have shown a correlation between spontaneous abortion and SJW (Hemels, Einarson, Koren, Lanctot, & Einarson, 2005) and (Way, 2007).

POSTPARTUM

Postpartum blues can include crying, irritability, and disturbance of mood lasting up to the 10th day postpartum.

Postpartum blues are not considered pathological and do not require treatment. Should these symptoms persist longer than two weeks, other factors are at play and warrant further assessment and possibly intervention.

Gotlib et al. (1989) investigated antepartum and postpartum depression in a sample of 295 pregnant women. Of the sample, 3.4% developed postpartum depression in the absence of depressive symptoms during pregnancy. One-third of the sample experiencing postpartum depression were also depressed during pregnancy. Within the depressed patients, risk factors were found to include younger, less educated, more children, and described themselves as housewives. Within the postpartum depression patients, housewife status was the sole demographic risk factor identified. The clinician should assess patients with these select risk factors more frequently.

Freeman et al. (2002) report 67% of patients experience a relapse in mood symptoms within one month postpartum. In their study of 50 patients, depression was the most common bipolar relapse after delivery. Of the patients who experienced a postpartum mood episode after the first pregnancy, all experienced mood episodes in subsequent pregnancies. Of those who did not have a relapse following their first delivery, 46% did after a subsequent delivery. Worsening mood symptoms during pregnancy significantly correlated with postpartum relapse.

Kendell, Chalmers, and Platz (1987) reported an increased rate of psychiatric admissions remained significantly elevated for 2 years after delivery and the relative risk of admission to a psychiatric hospital with psychosis was extremely high during the first month after delivery.

Postpartum psychosis is estimated to occur at a rate of 1.1 through 4 per thousand births, with onset typically within the two weeks after birth (Weissman & Olfson, 1995).

Marks and colleagues reported the risk of postpartum psychosis approaching 46% in bipolar patients (Marks, Wieck, Checkley, & Kumar, 1992). Serious consequences to both the patient and fetus can occur when the patient is not operating within reality and is influenced by psychotic symptoms. They also reported a history of schizophrenia, mania, hypomania, recent psychiatric hospitalization, and marital discord to be predictors of postpartum psychosis.

Howard, Goss, Leese, Appleby, and Thornicroft (2004) found that 55% of patients with schizophrenia experienced a psychotic episode within one year after delivery, with the episode most frequently occurring during the first three postpartum months. Per Howard, these patients are also likely to be more depressed as compared with controls.

Trixler, Gati, and Tenyi (1995) reported decompensation in 11.9% of schizophrenic postpartum patients within six months of delivery, as compared with 0.32% decompensating during pregnancy.

TREATMENT

Treatment for the postpartum variants of the anxiety, mood, and psychotic disorders is less restrictive as compared with during pregnancy treatment. For patients who have not had severe episodes of their illnesses and who have moderate symptoms, individual and/or group therapies can be an option. For those who require medication, such therapies are appropriate components of the treatment plan. Some community mental health centers and teaching hospitals have intensive outpatient or partial hospital programs wherein patients not only receive therapies, but transportation, light meals, and childcare is provided.

Should the patient want to breastfeed, the PMH-APRN should make medication choices to reflect that option if possible. As always, it is imperative to discuss the indication, risks, benefits, and alternatives of the treatment with the patient. It is also important to be mindful of the patient's past history of symptoms, past history of treatment response, and current presentation when selecting the most appropriate treatment for the postpartum patient.

PMH-APRNs should involve the partner and support members for the patient. Such key support people can help bottle feed the infant during the night, permitting the patient to get adequate rest, and provide assistance in the other basic needs of the infant, while being aware and ready to call for an earlier follow-up appointment should concerning symptoms emerge.

INFANTICIDE AND FILICIDE

The killing of a child by a parent naturally makes one question what exactly transpired and contemplate how such a tragedy could occur. Perhaps the more fruitful train of thought for the majority of clinicians is to be aware of the risk factors for such events, how to effectively screen for these risks, and how to treat the patients and their remaining family members following such events.

Neonaticide is the killing of a human younger than 1 day old irrespective of the perpetrator. Infanticide is the killing of an infant irrespective of the perpetrator. Filicide is the murder of a child by a parent older than the age of 1 day. All can be perceived as morally repellent and subjects from which people recoil. They can also be perceived as instances wherein there are multiple victims; one may contemplate that the tragedy could have been avoided. In the United States, those who kill their children and are not sentenced to death are often required to receive psychiatric treatment as part of their sentencing.

In some instances, the killing of the children is motivated by selfish, vindictive, or sadistic motivators. In other instances, the motivation to kill is rooted in psychosis, is an attempt to mitigate danger to the child and/or mother, and is an ego-dystonic act.

Resnick (1969) reviewed more than 100 cases of child murder, provides comment on the psychodynamics of filicide, and discusses strategies for prevention. Resnick reports the time of highest risk for filicide is the first 6 months of the infant's life. The younger the child is, the more likely the mother perceives the child to be inseparable from the mother, which increases the risk for filicide. Resnick found that 40% of the perpetrators of filicide had been assessed by a health care provider shortly before the filicide.

Button and Reivich (1972) reviewed more than 40 cases of patients with obsessions of infanticide. Of those patients, 86% had traumatic events during their childhoods, often including physical abuse, 14% of the sample were men. In the nonpsychotic patients, the infanticide obsessions had a quality of fear that the impulse might come to fruition. From this, the child became a phobic object for the patient. This leads to feelings of increased guilt, self-deprication, and contributed to feelings of decreased control. Patients received treatments available during that time period, with 80% returned to the community and functioning.

Kaye, Borenstein, and Donnelly (1990) investigated neonaticide. They report that 90% of mothers who commit neonaticide are younger than 25 years, less than 20% are married, and less than 30% are perceived as psychotic or depressed. The majority of mothers who commit neonaticide hide their pregnancies, give birth in secret, and swiftly dispose of the body.

Kunst (2002) delineates two types of personality structures involved in maternal filicide: the disorganized type and the organized type. The disorganized type does not experience bonding, as the patient's mother was either toxic or not present. The disorganized type does not perceive the infant as a human, but rather "a lifeless part-object into which she can project split-off and unwanted parts of her own fragmented ego." Disorganized patients poorly respond to treatment given the severity of their illnesses and nonexistent or sparse ability to process the filicide, whereas the organized type are better able to process the filicide and move forward from the filicide.

The organized type often also has poor attachments to their parents, including mothers who although present during the patient's childhood were also mentally ill, abusive, or unable to properly care for the patient as a child. As adults, these women seek partners to fulfill their needs unmet during childhood; they ultimately seek their needs to be met through their own children, looking to their children to serve the role of their own mother during their childhood. Such patients may expect their children to run the household while they are withdrawn and not properly functioning. The organized type mother perceives the child as a transformational object and not as a separate being. Such a mother becomes enmeshed with the child and sees the mother role in her child. According to Kunst, such women do benefit from psychotherapy, are well served with filicide group therapy, and with time can process the filicide.

Spinelli (2004) provides the psychiatric clinician with some direction in screening for patients who are at risk for filicide. She highlights the import of the clinician being aware of mood lability, the waxing and waning of disorganization, and the waxing and waning of perceptual disturbances to be a presentation consistent with a mother who completes filicide. A sense of denial or stigma can also be a risk factor for filicide. The need to screen for past history of mental illness, past history of mental illness in the context of pregnancy and postpartum, family psychiatric history, and the role of providing education, appropriate use of medication, and involvement of the family is advised.

TREATMENT

Stanton and Simpson (2006) conducted a qualitative study of six women who committed filicide, of which one had major depression, two schizoaffective disorder, three with schizophrenia, and one had a comorbidity of alcohol abuse. The women reported having an awareness of the filicide but reported incomplete memories of the filicide. All of the women used statements such as "the day my son died" and none used statements such as "the day I killed my son." Some were ambivalent about having more children, some articulated concern for the high risk in having more children, and some denied any concern in having more children. One did have a child after the filicide, and reported surprise at the reemergence of past memories and the weight of the need to make sure the baby remained alive and unharmed. Most of the women reported receiving support from friends and family as extremely helpful in moving forward and recovering. They advise a clear delineation of the arc of treatment including building a therapeutic alliance, education and discussion of the illness, mutual decision making of the treatment goals, and initially discussing the filicide using language such as "when your son died" when that stage of treatment arrives. This process will assist the patient in accepting their role in the death of their child in the context of their illness, and on proper cognitive processing, impulse control, and self-forgiveness.

According to Kunst (2002), organized type female filicide completers benefit from psychotherapy, are well served with filicide group therapy, and with time can process the filicide. PMH-APRNs treating patients who have killed their children should use supervision in such cases lest their countertransferance interfere with treatment.

BREASTFEEDING

Extra consideration should be made in instances of premature and young neonates in breastfeeding as their liver and renal functioning can be limited. In general, mothers should be advised to monitor their breastfed infants for feeding difficulties, irritability, and sleep disturbances. Should such issues emerge, the mother should consider formula feeding.

Medication exposure can be minimized by dosing immediately after breastfeeding or shortly before the baby is due for a sleep. Pumping prior to dosing and bottle feeding can also be a strategy to minimize medication exposure to the infant. Certain medications such as lithium carry risks to the infant such that breastfeeding is not recommended.

Kendall-Tackett and Hale (2010) report that of the SSRIs, fluoxetine has the highest proportion of detectable infant levels. Citalopram as compared with ecitalopram may lead to higher infant levels. Paroxetine, sertraline, and nortriptyline were reported to be unlikely to yield elevated infant levels.

Viguera et al. (2007) evaluated breastfeeding and lithium. Lithium levels in the breastfed newborns were roughly one-quarter of the maternal serum levels. Guidelines include monitoring infant lithium level, thyroid stimulating hormone, blood urea nitrogen, and creatinine immediately after birth and up to 6 weeks of life. In addition to the before-mentioned risks in use with lithium, the mother must also be informed of the risks of infant hypothyroidism for concordance to be achieved. As lithium is hydrophilic, concentrations of lithium in breastmilk are relatively constant as compared with hydrophilic medications that have higher concentrations in hindmilk.

Burt et al. (2001) from their literature review encourage mothers to consider formula supplementation to decrease infant exposure. They also encourage mothers on SSRIs to avoid caffeine use as metabolism is inhibited. They encourage patients maintained on clozapine not breastfeed given the known risk of agranulocytosis for adults and lack of data on breastfed infants.

Lester, Cucca, Andreozzi, Flanagan, and Oh (1993) report a case study in which the investigators discover an incidental finding in a mother enrolled in a study and taking fluoxetine. The mother had started fluoxetine three days postpartum and noticed inconsolable crying, poor sleep, watery stools, and vomiting in her infant. Per the study protocol, the mother switched feeding to a formula for three weeks during which time she noticed resolution of the colicky symptoms. The patient then reverted to breastfeeding shortly after which time the colicky symptoms returned such that she decided to resume formula feeding her infant. Such an exercise of documenting the nursing infant's response following breastfeeding can help guide the PMH-APRN to encouraging the mother on pharmacotherapy to cease breastfeeding when adverse reactions are resulting.

The American Academy of Pediatrics Committee on Drugs report (2001) provide these general guidelines in prescribing to lactating women: use medications only when necessary, use the safest medication possible, consider the measurement of blood concentrations in the nursing infant of medications, and attempt to minimize the infant's exposure to medication by the mother taking the medication just after breastfeeding or just before the infant will have a lengthy sleep.

The anxiolytics alprazolam, diazepam, lorazepam, and temazepam; the antidepressants amitriptyline, amoxapine, bupropion, clomipramine, desipramine, dothiepin, doxepin, fluoxetine, fluvoxamine, imipramine, nortriptyline, paroxetine, sertraline, and trazodone; the antipsychotics chlorpromazine, chlorprothixene, clozapine, haloperidol, mesoridazine, trifluoperazine, and lamotrigine are considered "drugs for which the effect on nursing infants is unknown but may be of concern." The American Association of Pediatricians (AAP) comments for this category that after ingestion of these medications, the concentration of them in milk is low; however, the half lives of these agents can be long enough that infants may have amounts in their plasma which can pass into the brain. The ACOG (2008) reports infant sedation occurs in benzodiazepine use and no considerations in lactation in antidepressants and antipsychotics. The ACOG advises monitoring of the infant Complete Blood Count (CBC), Liver Functioning Tests (LFTs), and drug level (which they also advise in other antiepileptic medications).

Under the category of "drugs that have been associated with significant effects on some nursing infants and should be given to nursing mothers with caution" include lithium, valproic acid, and zolpidem. The ACOG (2008) encourages monitoring of the infant's complete blood count, thyroid stimulating hormone (TSH), and lithium levels. The ACOG (2008) advises immediate discontinuation of breastfeeding wherein an infant develops abnormal symptoms likely attributable to medication use.

The American Academy of Pediatrics Committee on Drugs report (2001) states that smoking cessation should be encouraged by the provider, and that smoking during breastfeeding has been linked with increased respiratory illnesses in the infant. Given the lack of information on outcomes on the infant in the context of smoking cessation aides, these are not recommended by the AAP. The AAP encourages nursing mothers to abstain from use of amphetamines, cocaine, heroin, marijuana, and phencyclidine as they are hazardous to infant safety and compromise the mother's health. Specifically, they state amphetamines cause irritability and poor sleep; cocaine causes irritability, emesis, diarrhea, tremors, and seizures; heroin causes tremors, restlessness, poor feeding and emesis; marijuana has a long half-life; and phencyclidine is a hallucinogen. The AAP advises that caffeine, alcohol, and methadone use in nursing mothers is associated with significant effects on the infant and should be used with caution. Risks with caffeine use include poor sleep and irritability. Risks with alcohol use include drowsiness, weakness, decreased linear growth, deep sleep, and abnormal weight gain. AAP does not specify symptoms to the infant with methadone-using nursing mothers.

CONCLUSION

It is imperative for the APRN to be aware of unintended consequences to the patient and fetus during pregnancy and consequences to both following delivery. The discussion of indications, risks, benefits, and alternatives enter a whole new level of import when a developing fetus is involved in this patient-clinician-shared decision-making process. The decision to treat or not treat has consequences to both patient and fetus. APRNs have the opportunity to treat the patient along the childbearing continuum from pregnancy planning to postpartum. Given the limited research on treatments in the context of pregnancy, clinicians also have an opportunity to contribute to the literature and help patients in future pregnancies.

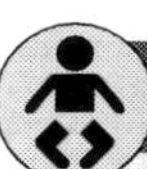

PEDIATRIC POINTERS

Adolescents carries a high risk of exposure to traumatic situations including sexual abuse and dating violence (Pelcovitz et al., 2000). When an adolescent becomes pregnant it is important to screen for abuse. Furthermore, the development of post-traumatic stress disorder following delivery may become a problem. Adolescents who go through delivery may have these painful experiences superimposed upon prior traumas and untreated chronic post-traumatic stress symptoms.

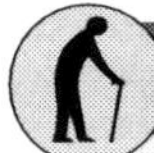

AGING ALERTS

Women over 35 years of age are at increased risk for their child to have a chromosome abnormality and usually require an aminocentesis. Approximately one in 300 women will miscarry after the procedure. Therefore, women over 35 who are pregnant often require additional support and screening for anxiety or depression. These women may require assistance in making a decision about terminating a pregnancy with a known defect in the fetus.

PROVIDER RESOURCES

Bereavement Support Work Team of the National SIDS and Infant Death Program Support Center: "The Guidelines for Medical Professionals Providing Care to the Family Experiencing Perinatal Loss, Neonatal, Death, SIDS, or Other Infant Death": www.sidscenter.org/TopicalBib/BereavementForProfessionals.html

BNI-ART Institute Intervention Algorithm: www.ed.bmc.org/sbirt/docs/aligo_adult.pdf

National Institute on Alcohol Abuse and Alcoholism: http://pubs.niaa.nih.gov/publications/arh28–2/78–79.htm

Nursing Network on Violence Against Women, International: www.nnvawi.org

Reprotox: (Reproductive Toxicology Center): www.reprotox.org

Safe Surrender: www.childwelfare.gov/systemwide/laws_policies/statutes/safehaven.cfm

Substance Abuse During Pregnancy (guidelines for screening): http://here.doh.wa.gov/materials/guidelines-substance-abuse-pregnancy/15-PregSubs-E10H.pdf

TERIS (Teratogen Information System): http://depts.washington.edu/terisweb

PATIENT RESOURCES

Centre for Addiction and Mental Health: www.camh.net

National Institute of Mental Health: www.nimh.nih.gov

National Organization on FAS: www.nofas.org

Online support for postpartum: www.marcesociety.com; www.postpartum.net

Online support after death of a baby: www.babyloss.com; www.hygeia.org; www.miscarriagesupport.org 1-800-TRY-NOVA (1-800-879-6682)

REFERENCES

Adab, N., Jacoby, A., Smith, D., & Chadwick, D. (2001). Additional educational needs in children born to mothers with epilepsy. *Journal of Neurology, Neurosurgery, and Psychiatry, 70,* 15–21.

Altshuler, L., Cohen, L., Szuba, M., Burt, V., Gitlin, M., & Mintz, J. (1996). Pharmacologic management of psychiatric illness during pregnancy: Dilemmas and guidelines. *American Journal of Psychiatry, 153,* 592–606.

American Academy of Pediatrics (2001). Committee on drugs: The transfer of drugs and other chemicals into human milk. *Pediatrics, 108,* 776–789.

American College of Obstetricians and Gynecologists Committee Opinion (2008). At-risk drinking and illicit drug use: Ethical issues in obstetric and gynecologic practice. *Obstetrics and Gynecology, 112*(6), 1449–1460.

American College of Obstetricians and Gynecologists Practice Bulletin Number 92 (2008). Use of psychiatric medications during pregnancy and lactation. *Obstetrics & Gynecology, 111*(4), 1001–1020.

American Family Physician (2007). Pregnancy loss: What you should know. *76*(9), 1347–1348.

Bailey, B., Delaney-Black, V., Covington, C., Ager, J., Janisse, J., Hannigan, J., & Sokol, R. (2004). Prenatal exposure to binge drinking and cognitive and behavioral outcomes at age 7 years. *American Journal of Obstetrics and Gynecology, 191,* 1037–1043.

Bastard, J., & Tiran, D. (2006). Aromatherapy and massage for antenatal anxiety: Its effect on the fetus. *Complementary Therapies in Clinical Practice, 12,* 48–54.

Beddoe, A., Yang, C., Kennedy, H., Weiss, S., & Lee, K. (2009). The effects of mindfulness-based yoga during pregnancy on maternal psychological and physical distress. *Journal of Obstetric, Gynecologic, and Neonatal Nursing, 38,* 310–319.

Behnke, M., & Eyler, F. D. (1993). The consequences of prenatal substance use for the developing fetus, newborn, and young child. *International Journal of Addiction, 28*(13), 1341–1391.

Bell, J., & Harvey-Dodds, L. (2008). Pregnancy and injecting drug use. *British Medical Journal, 336,* 1303–1305.

Bennedsen, B., Mortensen, P., Olesen, A., & Henriksen, T. (2001). Congenital malformations, stillbirths, and infant deaths among children of women with schizophrenia. *Archives of General Psychiatry, 58,* 674–679.

Bonari, L., Pinto, N., Ahn, E., Einarson A., Steiner, M., & Koren, G. (2004). Perinatal risks of untreated depression during pregnancy. *Canadian Journal of Psychiatry, 49*(11), 726–735.

Bowles, S. V., Bernard, R. S., Epperly T., Woodward, S., Ginzburg, K., Folen, R.,...Koopman, C. (2006). Traumatic stress disorders following first-trimester spontaneous abortion. *Journal of Family Practice, 55*(11), 969–973.

Boyce, M. (2010). A better future for baby: Stemming the tide of fetal alcohol syndrome. *Journal of Family Practice, 59*(6), 337–344.

Buckwalter, J., & Simpson, S. (2002). Psychological factors in the etiology and treatment of severe nausea and vomiting in pregnancy. *American Journal of Obstetric Gynecology, 186,* S210–S214.

Burch, R., & Gallup, G. (2004). Pregnancy as a stimulus for domestic violence. *Journal of Family Violence, 19*(4), 243–247.

Burns, E., Blamey, C., Ersser, J., Lloyd, A., & Barnetson, L. (2000). The use of aromatherapy in intrapartum midwifery practice an observational study. *Complementary Therapies in Nursing and Midwifery, 6,* 33–34.

Burt, V., Bernstein, C., Rosenstein, W., & Altshuler, L. (2010). Bipolar disorder and pregnancy: Maintaining psychiatric stability in the real world of obstetric and psychiatric complication. *American Journal of Psychiatry, 167*(8), 892–897.

Burt, V., Suri, R., Altshuler, L., Stowe, Z., Hendrick, V., & Muntean, E. (2001). The use of psychotropic medications during breast-feeding. *American Journal of Psychiatry, 158,* 1001–1009.

Buttolph, M., & Holland, A. (1990). Obsessive compulsive disorders in pregnancy and childbirth. In M. Jenike, I. Baer, & W. Minichiello (Eds.), *Obsessive Compulsive Disorders. Theory and Management* (pp. 89–97). Chicago, IL: Yearbook Medical Publishers.

Button, J., & Reivich, R. (1972). Obsessions of infanticide. *Archives of General Psychiatry, 27,* 235–240.

Cabuk, D., Sayin, A., Derinoz, O., & Biri, A. (2007). Quetiapine use for the treatment of manic episode during pregnancy. *Archives of Women's Mental Health, 10,* 235–236.

Centers for Disease Control and Prevention. (2002). Alcohol use among women of childbearing age-United States, 1991–1999. MMWR Morb Mortal Wkly Rep. April 5, 2002; 51(13): 273–276.

Chang, G., Carroll, K., Behr, H., & Kosten, T. (1992). Improving treatment outcome in pregnant opiate-dependent women. *Journal of Substance Abuse Treatment, 9,* 327–330.

Chang, M., Wang, S., & Chen, C. (2002). Effects of massage on pain and anxiety during labour: A randomized controlled trial in Taiwan. *Journal of Advanced Nursing, 38*(1), 68–73.

Cohen, L., Friedman, J., Jefferson, J., Johnson, E., & Weiner, M. (1994). A reevaluation of risk of in utero exposure to lithium. *Journal of the American Medical Association, 271*(2), 146–150.

Cole, J., Modell, J., Haight, B., Cosmatos, I., Stoler, J., & Walker, A. (2007). Bupropion in pregnancy and the prevalence of congenital malformations. *Pharmacoepidemiology and Drug Safety, 16*(5), 474–484.

Cote-Arsenault, D., & Donato, K. (2007). Restrained expectations in late pregnancy following loss. *Journal of Obstetric, Gynecologic, & Neonatal Nursing, 36*(6), 550–557.

Cumming, G., Klein, S., Bolsover, D., Lee, A., Alexander, D., Maclean, M., & Jurgens, J. (2007). The emotional burden of miscarriage for women and their partners: Trajectories of anxiety and depression over 13 months. *British Journal of Obstetrics and Gynecology, 114,* 1138–1145.

Dabbert, D., & Heinze, M. (2006). Follow-up of a pregnancy with risperidone microspheres: Letter to the editor. *Pharmacopsychiatry, 39,* 235.

Dashe, J., Sheffield, J., Olscher, D., Todd, S., Jackson, G., & Wendel, G. (2002). Relationship between maternal methadone dosage and neonatal withdrawal. *Obstetrics and Gynecology, 100*(6), 1244–1249.

Dayan, J., Creveuil, C., Herlicoviez, M., Herbel, C., Baranger, E., Savoye, C., & Thouin, A. (2002). Role of anxiety and depression in the onset of spontaneous preterm labor. *American Journal of Epidemiology, 155*(4), 293–301.

Diav-Citrin, O., Shechtman, S., Ornoy, S., Arnon, J., Schaefer, C., Garbis, H.,... Ornoy, A. (2005). Safety of haloperidol and penfluridol in pregnancy: A multicenter, prospective, controlled study. *Journal of Clinical Psychiatry, 66,* 317–322.

Einarson, A., & Boskovic, R. (2009). Use and safety of antispychotic drugs during pregnancy. *Journal of Psychiatric Practice, 15*(3), 183–192.

Feldman, J., Minkoff, H., McCalla, S., & Salwen, M. (1992). A cohort study of the impact of perinatal drug use on prematurity in an inner-city population. *American Journal of Public Health, 82*(5), 726–728.

Freeman, M., Wosnitzer Smith, K., Freeman, S., McElroy, S., Kmetz, G., Wright, R., & Keck, P. (2002). The impact of reproductive events on the course of bipolar disorder in women. *Journal of Clinical Psychiatry, 63*(4), 284–287.

Fulroth, R., Philips, B., & Durant, D. (1989). Perinatal outcome of infants exposed to cocaine and/or heroin in utero. *American Journal of Diseases of Children, 143,* 905–910.

Gaily, E., Kantola-Sorsa, E., Hiilesmaa, V., Isoaho, M., Matila, R., Kotila, M.,... Granstrom, M. (2004). Normal intelligence in children with prenatal exposure to carbamazepine. *Neurology, 62,* 28–32.

Galbally, M., Snellen, M., Walker, S., & Permezel, M. (2010). Management of antipsychotic and mood stabilizer medication in pregnancy: Recommendations for antenatal care. *Australian and New Zealand Journal of Psychiatry, 44,* 99–108.

Gazmararian, J., Adams, M., Saltzman, L., Johnson, C., Bruce, C., Marks, J.,... the PRAMS Working Group (1995). The relationship between pregnancy intendedness and physical violence in mothers of newborns. *Obstetrics & Gynecology, 85*(6), 1031–1008.

Gentile, S. (2006). Prophylactic treatment of bipolar disorder in pregnancy and breastfeeding: Focus on emerging mood stabilizers. *Bipolar Disorders, 8,* 207–220.

Gentile, S., & Vozzi, F. (2007). Consecutive exposure to lamotrigine and citalopram during pregnancy. *Archives of Women's Mental Health, 10,* 299–300.

Ghanizadeh, A., Ghanizadeh, M., Moini, R., & Ekramzadeh, S. (2009). Association of vaginal bleeding and electroconvulsive therapy use in pregnancy. *Journal of Obstetrics and Gynaecology Research, 35*(3), 569–571.

Gotlib, I., Whiffen, V., Mount, J., Milne, K., & Cordy, N. (1989). Prevalence rates and demographic characteristics associated with depression in pregnancy and the postpartum. *Journal of Consulting Clinical Psychology, 57*(2), 269–274.

Grant, T., Huggins, J., Sampson, P., Ernst, C., Barr, H., & Streissguth, A. (2009). Alcohol use before and during pregnancy in western Washington 1989–2004: Implications for the prevention of fetal alcohol spectrum disorders. *American Journal of Obstetrics & Gynecology, 200,* 278.e1–278.e8.

Grof, P., Robbins, W., Alda, M., Berghoefer, A., Vojtechovsky, M., Nilsson, A., & Robertson, C. (2000). Protective effect of pregnancy in women with lithium-responsive bipolar disorder. *Journal of Affective Disorders, 61,* 31–39.

Grover, S., & Avasthi, A. (2004). Risperidone in pregnancy: A case of oligohydramnios. *German Journal of Psychiatry, 7,* 56–57.

Guerreiro da Silva, J. (2007). Acupuncture for mild to moderate emotional complaints in pregnancy—A prospective, quasi-randomised, controlled study. *Acupuncture in Medicine, 25*(3), 65–71.

Han, J. (1986). Electroacupuncture: An alternative to antidepressants for treating affective diseases? *International Journal of Neuroscience, 29,* 79–92.

Hemels, M., Einarson, A., Koren, G., Lanctot, K., & Einarson, T. (2005). Antidepressant use during pregnancy and the rates of spontaneous abortions: A meta-analysis. *Annals of Pharmacotherapy, 39,* 803–809.

Holmes, L., Wyszynski, D., Baldwin, E., Habecker, E., Glassman, L., & Smith, C. (2006). Increased risk for non-syndromal cleft palate among infants exposed to lamotrigine during pregnancy [abstract]. *Birth Defects Research Part A: Clinical Molecular Teratology, 76,* 318.

Hostetter, A., Stowe, Z., Strader, J., McLaughlin, E., & Llewellyn, A. (2000). Dose of selective serotonin uptake inhibitors across pregnancy: Clinical implications. *Depresion and Anxiety, 11,* 51–57.

Howard, L., Goss, C., Leese, M., Appleby, L., & Thornicroft, G. (2004). The psychosocial outcomes of pregnancy in women with psychotic disorders. *Schizophrenia Research, 71,* 49–60.

Howard, L., Kumar, R., & Thornicroft, G. (2001). Psychosocial characteristics and needs of mothers with psychotic disorders. *British Journal of Psychiatry, 178,* 427–432.

Hulse, G., Milne, E., English, D., & Holman, C. (1997). The relationship between maternal use of heroin and methadone and infant birth weight. *Addiction, 92*(11), 1571–1579.

Jablensky, A., Morgan, V., Zubrick, S., Bower, C., & Yellachich, L. (2005). Pregnancy, delivery, and neonatal complications in a population cohort of women with schizophrenia and major affective disorders. *American Journal of Psychiatry, 162*(1), 79–91.

Jones, H., Kaltenbach, K., Heil, S., Stine, S., Coyle, M., Arria, A.,... Fischer, G. (2010). Neonatal abstinence syndrome after methadone or buprenorphine exposure. *New England Journal of Medicine, 363*(24), 2320–2331.

Kalra, H., Tandon, R., Trivedi, J., & Janca, A. (2005). Pregnancy-induced obsessive compulsive disorder: A case report. *Annals of General Psychiatry, 4,* 12.

Kaye, N., Borenstein, N., & Donnelly, S. (1990). Families, murder, and insanity: A psychiatric review of paternal neonaticide. *Journal of Forensic Sciences, 35*(1) 133–139.

Kendall-Tackett, K., & Hale, T. (2010). The use of antidepressants in pregnant and breastfeeding women: A review of recent studies. *Journal of Human Lactation, 26*(2), 187–195.

Kendell, R., Chalmers, J., & Platz, C. (1987). Epidemiology of puerperal psychoses. *British Journal of Psychiatry, 150,* 662–673.

Kennare, R., Heard, A., & Chan, A. (2005). Substance use during pregnancy: Risk factors and obstetric and perinatal outcomes in South Australia. *Austrialian and New Zealand Journal of Obstetrics and Gynaecology, 45,* 220–225.

Kiely, M., El-Mohandes, A., El-Khorazaty, M., & Gantz, M. (2010). An integrated intervention to reduce intimate partner violence in pregnancy: A randomized trial. *Obstetrical Gynecology, 115,* 273–283.

Koenig, L., Whitaker, D., Royce, R., Wilson, T., Ethier, K., & Fernandez, M. (2006). Physical and sexual violence during pregnancy and after delivery: A prospective multistate study of women with or at risk for HIV infection. *American Journal of Public Health, 96*(6), 1052–1059.

Kong, G., Chung, T., Lai, B., & Lok, I. (2010). Gender comparison of psychological reaction after miscarriage—A 1-year longitudinal study. *British Journal of Obstetrics & Gynecology, 117,* 1211–1219.

Kowalcek, I., Huber, G., Lammers, C., Brunk, J., Bieniakiewicz, I., & Gembruch, U. (2003). Anxiety scores before and after prenatal testing for congenital abnormalities. *Archives of Gynecology and Obstetrics, 267,* 126–129.

Kunst, J. (2002). Fraught with the utmost danger: The object relations of mothers who kill their children. *Bulletin of the Menninger Clinic, 66*(1), 19–38.

Lam, S., To, W., Duthie, S., & Ma, H. (1992). Narcotic addiction in pregnancy with adverse maternal and perinatal outcome. *Australian and New Zealand Journal of Obstetrics and Gynaecology, 32*(3), 216–221.

Lester, B., Cucca, J., Andreozzi, L. Flanagan, P., & Oh, W. (1993). Possible association between fluoxetine hydrochloride and colic in an infant. *Journal of the American Academy of Child & Adolescent Psychiatry, 32*(6), 1253–1255.

Li, Q., Kirby, R., Sigler, R., Hwang, S., LaGory, M., & Goldenberg, R. (2010). A Multilevel analysis of individual, household, and neighborhood correlates of intimate partner violence among low-income pregnant women in Jeffersson County, Alabama. *American Journal of Public Health, 100*(3), 531–539.

Littrell, K., Johnson, C., Peabody, C., & Hilligoss, N. (2000). Antipsychotics during pregnancy. *American Journal of Psychiatry, 157*(8), 1342.

Liu, A., Sithamparanathan, S., Jones, M., Cook, C., & Nanan, R. (2010). Growth restriction in pregnancies of opioid-dependent mothers. *Archives of Disease in Childhood Fetal and Neonatal Edition, 95,* F258–F262.

Luo, H., Meng, F., Jia, Y., & Zhao, X. (1998). Clinical research on the therapeutic effect of the electro-acupuncture treatment in patients with depression. *Psychiatry and Clinical Neurosciences, 52*(Suppl.), S338–S340.

Lutgendorf, M.A., Busch, J.M., Doherty, D.A., Conza, L.A., Moone, S.O., & Magann, E.F. (2009). Prevalence of domestic violence in a pregnant military population. *Obstetrics & Gynecology, 113*(4), 866–872.

Marks, M., Wieck, A., Checkley, S., & Kumar, R. (1992). Contribution of psychological and social factors to psychotic and nonpsychotic relapse after childbirth in women with previous histories of affective disorder. *Journal of Affective Disorders, 29,* 253–264.

Matalon, S., Schechtman, S., Goldzweig, G., & Ornoy, A. (2002). The teratogenic effect of carbmazepine: A meta-analysis of 1255 exposures. *Reproductive Toxicology, 16,* 9–17.

Mazzota, P., Magee, L., & Koren, G. (1997). Motherrisk update: Therapeutic abortions due to severe morning sickness: Unacceptable combination. *Canadian Family Physician,* 43, 1055–1057.

McGlone, L., Mactier, H., Hamilton, R., Bradnam, M., Boulton, R., Borland, W.,...McCulloch, D. (2008). Visual evoked potentials in infants exposed to methadone in utero. *Archives of Disease in Childhood, 93,* 784–786.

McKenna, K., Koren, G., Tetelbaum, M., Wilton, L., Shakir, S., Diav-Citrin, O.,...Einarson, A. (2005). Pregnancy outcome of women using atypical antipsychotic drugs: A prospective comparative study. *Journal of Clinical Psychiatry, 66,* 444–449.

McNeil, T., Kaij, L., & Malmquist-Larsson, A. (1983). Pregnant women with nonorganic psychosis: Life situation and experience of pregnancy. *Acta Psychiatrica Scandinavica, 68,* 445–457.

Mendhekar, D. (2007). Possible delayed speech acquisition with clozapine therapy during pregnancy and lactation. *Journal of Neuropsychiatry & Clinical Neurosciences, 19*(2), 196–197.

Mendhekar, D., & Lohia, D. (2008). Risperidone therapy in two successive pregnancies. *Journal of Neuropsychiatry & Clinical Neurosciences, 20*(4), 485–486.

Mendhekar, D., Sharma, J., & Srilakshmi, P. (2006). Use of aripiprazole during late pregnancy in a woman with psychotic illness. Letter to the editor. *Annals of Pharmacotherapy, 40,* 575.

Mendhekar, D., War, L., Sharma, J., & Jiloha, R. (2002). Olanzapine and pregnancy. *Pharmacopsychiatry, 35,* 122–123.

Mervak, B., Collins, J., & Valenstein, M. (2008). Case report of aripiprazole usage during pregnancy. *Archives of Women's Mental Health, 11,* 249–250.

Miller, F. (2002). Nausea and vomiting in pregnancy: The problem of perception—Is it really a disease? *American Journal of Obstetrics and Gynecology, 186,* S182–S183.

Miller, L., Bishop, J., Fisher, J., Geller, S., & Macmillan, C. (2008). Balancing risks: Dosing strategies for antidepressants near the end of pregnancy. *American Society of Clinical Psychopharmacology, 69*(2), 323–324.

Miller, L., & Finnerty, M. (1996). Sexuality, pregnancy, and childrearing among women with schizophrenia-spectrum disorders. *Psychiatric Services, 47*(5), 502–506.

Moore, S., Turnpenny, P., Quinn, A., Glover, S., Lloyd, D., Montgomery, T., & Dean, J. (2000). A clinical study of 57 children with fetal anticonvulsant syndromes. *Journal of Medical Genetics, 37,* 489–497.

Moretti, M., Maxson, A., Hanna, F., & Koren, G. (2009). Evaluating the safety of St. John's Wort in human pregnancy. *Reproductive Toxicology, 28,* 96–99.

Newport, D., Levey, L., Pennell, P., Ragan, K., & Stowe, Z. (2007). Suicidal ideation in pregnancy: Assessment and clinical implications. *Archives of Women's Mental Health, 10,* 181–187.

Newport, D., Viguera, A., Beach, A., Ritchie, J., Cohen, L., & Stowe, Z. (2005). Lithium placental passage and obstetrical outcome: Implications for clinical management during late pregnancy. *American Journal of Psychiatry, 162,* 2162–2170.

Nilsson, E., Lichtenstein, P., Cnattingius, S., Murray, R., & Hultman, C. (2002). Women with schizophrenia: Pregnancy outcome and infant death among their offspring. *Schizophrenia Research, 58,* 221–229.

Nishizawa, O., Sakumoto, K., Hiramatsu, K., & Kondo, T. (2007). Effectiveness of comprehensive supports for schizophrenic women during pregnancy and puerperium: Preliminary study. *Psychiatry and Clinical Neuroscience, 61,* 665–671.

Nonacs, R., & Cohen, L. (2003). Assessment and treatment of depression during pregnancy: An update. *Psychiatric Clinics of North America, 26,* 547–562.

Oberlander, T., Weinberg, J., Papsdorf, M., Grunau, R., Misri, S., & Devlin, A. (2008). Prenatal exposure to maternal depression, neonatal methylation of human glucocorticoid receptor gene (NR3C1) and infant cortisol stress responses. *Epiegenetics, 3*(2), 97–106.

O'Connor, M., & Whaley, S. (2007). Brief intervention for alcohol use by pregnant women. *American Journal of Public Health, 97*(2), 252–258.

O'Connor, T., Heron, J., Golding, J., Beveridge, M., & Glover, V. (2002). Maternal antenatal anxiety and children's behavioural/emotional problems at 4 years: Report from the Avon longitudinal study of parents and children. *British Journal of Psychiatry, 180,* 502–508.

O'Hara, M., Neunaber, D., & Zekoski, E. (1984). Prospective study of postpartum depression: Prevalence, course, and predictive factors. *Journal of Abnormal Psychology, 93*(2), 158–171.

Peindl, K., Masand, P., Mannelli, P., Narasimhan, M., & Patkar, A. (2007). Polypharmacy in pregnant women with major psychiatric illness: A pilot study. *Journal of Psychiatric Practice, 13*(6), 385–392.

Rabheru, K. (2001). The use of electroconvulsive therapy in special patient populations. *Canadian Journal of Psychiatry, 46,* 710–719.

Resnick, P. (1969). Child murder by parents: A psychiatric review of filicide. *American Journal of Psychiatry, 126*(3), 325–334.

Rodrigues, T., Rocha L., & Barros, H. (2008). Physical abuse during pregnancy and preterm delivery. *American Journal of Obstetrics and Gynecology, 198,* 171.e1–171.e6.

Rohde, A., Dembinski, J., & Dorn, C. (2003). Mirtazapine for treatment resistant hyperemesis gravidum: Rescue of a twin pregnancy. *Archives of Gynecology & Obstetrics, 268,* 219–221.

Saftlas, A., Wallis, A., Shochet, T., Harland, K., Dickey, P., & Peek-Asa, C. (2010). Prevalence of intimate partner violence among an abortion clinic population. *American Journal of Public Health, 100*(8), 1412–1415.

Sagrestano, L., Carroll, D., Rodriguez, A., & Nuwayhid, B. (2004). Demographic, psychological, and relationship factors in domestic violence during pregnancy in a sample of low-income women of color. *Psychology of Women Quarterly, 28,* 309–322.

Salisbury, A., Ponder, K., Padbury, J., & Lester, B. (2009). Fetal effects of psychoactive drugs. *Clinical Perintology, 36*(3), 595–619.

Schou, M. (1976). What happened to the lithium babies? A follow-up study of children born without malformations. *Acta Psychiatrica Scandinavica, 54,* 193–197.

Seligman, N., Almario, C., Hayes, E., Dysart, K., Berghella, V., & Baxter, J. (2010). Relationship between maternal methadone dose at delivery and neonatal abstinence syndrome. *Journal of Pediatrics, 157,* 428–433.

Silverman, J., Decker, M., McCauley, H., Gupta, J., Miller, E., Raj, A., & Goldberg, A. (2010). Male perpetration of intimate partner violence and involvement in abortions and abortion-related conflict. *American Journal of Public Health, 100*(8), 1415–1417.

Silverman, J., Decker, M., Reed, E., & Raj, A. (2006). Intimate partner violence victimization prior to and during pregnancy among women residing in 26 U.S. states: Associations with maternal and neonatal health. *American Journal of Obstetrics and Gynecology, 195,* 140–148.

Sokol, R., Delaney-Black, V., & Nordstrom, B. (2003). Fetal alcohol spectrum disorder. *JAMA, 290*(22), 2996–2999.

Solari, H., Dickson, K., & Miller, L. (2009). Understanding and treating women with schizophrenia during pregnancy and postpartum. *Canadian Journal of Clinical Pharmacology, 16*(1), e23–e32.

Spinelli, M. (1997). Interpersonal psychotherapy for depressed antepartum women: A pilot study. *American Journal of Psychiatry, 154*(7), 1028–1030.

Spinelli, M. (2004). Maternal infanticide associated with mental illness: Prevention and the promise of saved lives. *American Journal of Psychiatry, 161,* 1548–1557.

Spinelli, M., & Endicott, J. (2003). Controlled clinical trial of interpersonal psychotherapy versus parenting education program for depressed pregnant women. *American Journal of Psychiatry, 160,* 555–562.

Stanton, J., & Simpson, A. (2006). The aftermath: Aspects of recovery described by perpetrators of maternal filicide committed in the context of severe mental illness. *Behavioral Sciences and the Law, 24,* 103–112.

Substance Abuse and Mental Health Services Administration. (2007). *Results from the 2006 National survey on drug use and health: National findings* (Office of Applied Studies, NSDUH Series H-32, DHHS Publication No SMA 07–4293). Rockville, MD: SAMSHA. Retrieved from http://www.oas.samsha.gov/nsduh/2k6nsduh/2k6Results.pdf

Swanson, K., Connor, S., Jolley, S., Pettinato, M., & Wang, T. (2007). Contexts and evolution of women's responses to miscarriage during the first year after loss. *Resarch in Nursing & Health, 30,* 2–16.

Thisted, E., & Ebbesen, F. (1993). Malformations, withdrawal manifestations, and hypoglycaemia after exposure to valproate in utero. *Archives of Disease in Childhood, 95,* 159–162.

Trixler, M., Gati, A., & Tenyi, T. (1995). Risks associated with childbearing in schizophrenia. *Acta Psychiatrica Serv, 47,* 159–162.

U.S. Preventive Services Task Force (2009). Counseling and interventions to prevent tobacco use and tobacco-caused disease in adults and pregnant women: U.S. preventive Services Task Force reaffirmation recommendation statement. *Annals of Internal Medicine, 150*(8), 551–556.

Uppal, V., Rooney, K. D., & Young, S. J. (2009). Better antenatal education is a good idea, but does not reduce maternal anxiety regarding anaesthesia for emergency caesarean delivery. *International Journal of Obstetric Anesthesia, 18*(1), 97–98.

Viguera, A., Newport, D., Ritchie, J., Stowe, Z., Whitfield, T., Mogielnicki, J.,...Cohen, L. (2007). Lithium in breast milk and nursing infants: Clinical implications. *American Journal of Psychiatry, 164,* 342–345.

Viguera, A., Whitfield, T., Baldessarini, R., Newport, D., Stowe, Z., Reminick, A.,...Cohen, L. (2007). Risk of recurrence in women with bipolar disorder during pregnancy: Prospective study of mood stabilizer discontinuation. *American Journal of Psychiatry, 164*(12), 1817–1824.

Ward, S., & Wisner, K. (2007). Collaborative management of women with bipolar disorder during pregnancy and postpartum: Pharmacologic considerations. *Journal of Midwifery and Women's Health, 52*(1), 3–13.

Way, C. (2007). Safety of newer antidepressants in pregnancy. *Pharmcotherapy, 27*(4), 546–552.

Weissman, M., & Olfson, M. (1995). Depresison in women: Implications for health care research. *Science, 269,* 799–801.

Wiemann, C., Agurcia, C., Berenson, A., Volk, R., & Rickert, V. (2000). Pregnant adolescents: Experiences and behavior associated with physical assault by an intimate partner. *Maternal and Child Health Journal, 4*(2), 93–101.

Woods-Giscombe, C., Lobel, M., & Crandell, J. (2010). The impact of miscarriage and parity on patterns of maternal distress in pregnancy. *Research in Nursing and Health, 33,* 316–328.

Woody, J., London, W., & Wilbanks, G. (1971). Lithium toxicity in a newborn. *Pediatrics, 47,* 94–96.

Wyszynski, D., Nambisan, M., Surve, T., Alsdorf, R., Smith, C., & Holmes, L. (2005). Increased rate of major malformations in offspring exposed to valproate during pregnancy. *Neurology, 64,* 961–965.

Yeshayahu, Y. (2007). The use of olanzapine in pregnancy and congenital cardiac and musculoskeletal abnormalities. *American Journal of Psychiatry, 164*(11), 1759–1760.

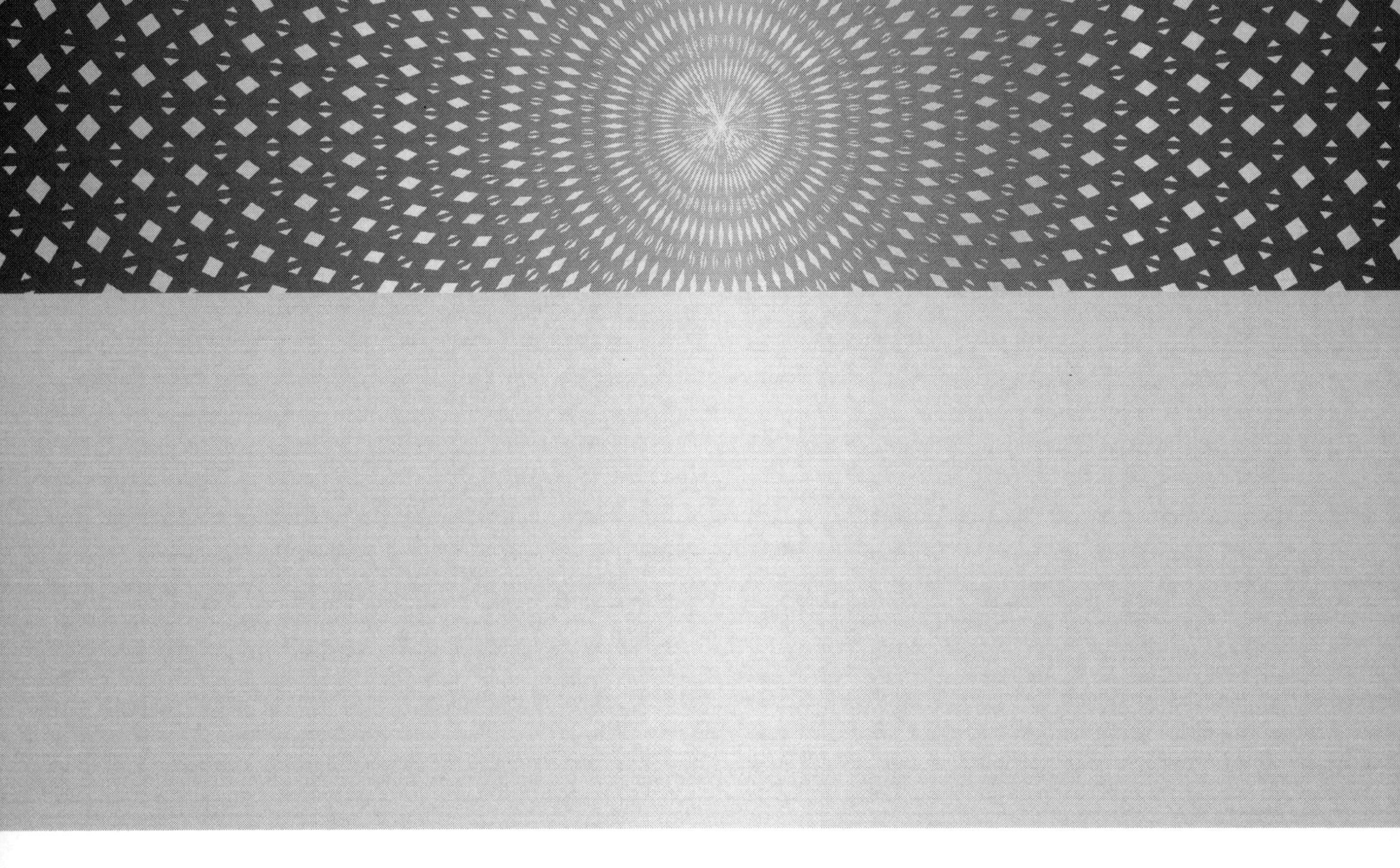

CHAPTER CONTENTS

OVERVIEW

Over the past decade the role of the Psychiatric Mental Health Advanced Practice Registered Nurse (PMH-APRN) has become a more visible presence in the specialty of forensics. The term *forensic* means "relating to or dealing with the application of scientific knowledge to legal problems" (Merriam-Webster, 2011). While corrections are the predominant area of PMH-APRN presence in the forensic specialty, the term *forensics* can actually encompass several areas beyond this. This would include Legal Nurse Consulting (LNC) and programs such as the Sexual Assault Nurse Examiner (S.A.N.E).

LNC is one such specialty area. A PMH-APRN choosing to specialize as an LNC would find him or herself working with attorneys and law firms either for the defense or plaintiff. The work could encompass reviewing of psychiatric malpractice cases for merit, development of interrogatories, case analysis and development of written timelines, and serving as an expert witness. The training and education to become an LNC does vary from state to state and program to program. Most of the reputable/recognized programs are postgraduate and are American Bar Association (ABA) approved.

S.A.N.E. programs have been around for several decades and also vary in training and certification requirements from state to state and program to program. While some psychiatric APRNs do function in this capacity, at the present, PMH-APRN credentialing is not a requirement.

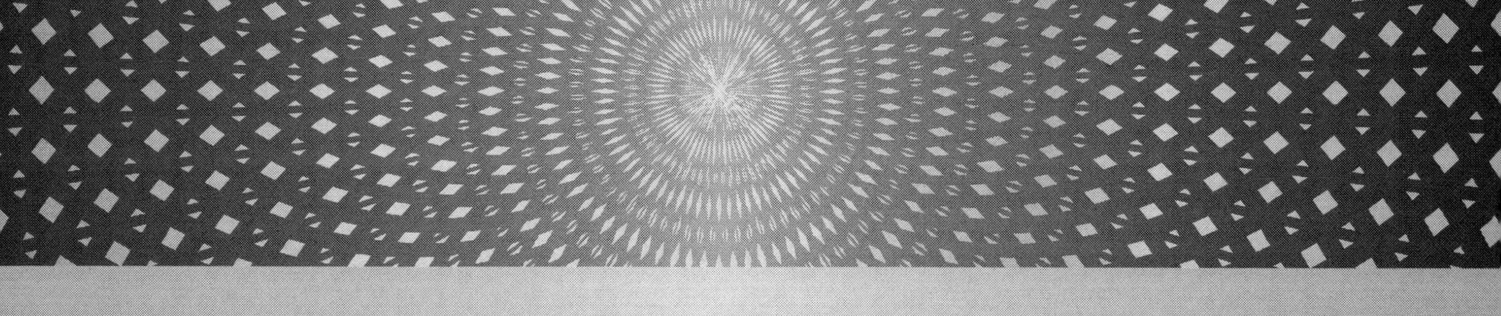

CHAPTER 20

Forensic Issues and Psychiatric Syndromes

Jeffrey S. Jones

Some of the functions of the S.A.N.E. nurse may include performing a physical examination on a victim of sexual assault, collecting evidence, providing expert testimony regarding the forensic evidence collected, and working collaboratively with law enforcement and the prosecutors.

CORRECTIONS

The largest area of forensic practice for PMH-APRNs is in corrections. Corrections mean that they are housed in jails or prisons. The increased needs for an organized delivery of mental health care in the correctional system is in response to a higher number of inmates being diagnosed with a mental illness. The higher numbers are partially the result of **deinstitutionalization** and **transinstitutionalization.** Deinstitutionalization of state mental hospitals in 1955 led to approximately 560,000 patients being released into the community. With many severely mentally ill patients no longer being housed in long-term state-run hospitals, by the 1990s community mental health centers with floundering budgets were unable to provide the comprehensive care that was once envisioned. Some of the Severely Mentally Disabled (SMD) population began falling through the cracks in service, became homeless, and ended up in the legal system for a variety of reasons (vagrancy, trespassing, etc.). Transinstitutionalization refers to the transfer of psychiatric care to jails and prisons (Lint, 2012). Estimates indicate that between 10% and 16% of people in state prisons can be considered to have a true severe mental illness (Metraux, 2008). The increase in mental health services in corrections is also due to subsequent state mandates that require inmates be treated humanely and comprehensively with regard to their total health care needs. When incarcerated, the SMD population is very vulnerable and easily exploited by other inmates. Properly diagnosing them, treating them, and assuring that they are being cared for humanely by staff and are safe from harm by other inmates falls squarely within the realm of the advocacy role of the nurse and PMH-APRN.

The opportunity to provide much-needed, compassionate care to the incarcerated mentally ill can be very rewarding. However, the forensic environment of corrections is comprised of multiple dynamics that make the work of treating the truly mentally ill very challenging. There is a fine line between providing care, while maintaining security and promoting advocacy (Peternelj-Taylor & Johnson, 1995). Determining which inmate is truly mentally ill is not as straightforward as say assessing patients in the hospital or clinic setting. Before a discussion of common treatment protocols for the mentally ill in corrections can take place several important areas must be addressed.

INTERPERSONAL PROCESS

The practice of nursing in general can be said to be an interpersonal process in that the relationship dynamic between two people plays as significant part in the practice (Peplau, 1991). Psychiatric-mental health nursing can then be said to focus this concept even further as to be the total foundation for practice. The navigation of the interpersonal process and the attempts at development of the therapeutic relationship in corrections has many challenges.

CONCEPT OF NURSING CARE AND THE CRIMINAL

The first and foremost important personal and professional reconciliation the PMH-APRN must come to terms with is the concept of criminal behavior and their own value/belief system. Much has been written about working with criminals and much has been written about nurses' behavior and what is at risk in forensic situations. Nurses and other forensic workforce are at risk for slowly being pulled into inappropriate relationships with inmates (Hackett, 2011). Nursing is a profession that inherently wants to "care for" others. Thus, the PMH-APRN may find they are struggling with how to function in a correctional environment and deliver caring nursing services to clients that could be considered evil. This concept can be processed at a deeper level in terms of the significance to nursing practice. Many nurse theorists identify the nurse's ability to experience empathy as a key component to the actual practice of nursing (Travelbee, 1971). We can define empathy as being characterized by the ability to share in the other person's experience as it is "an intellectual process and, to a lesser extent, emotional comprehension of another" (Travelbee, 1964). Nurses functioning in many settings, such as the emergency department (ED), oncology unit, pediatric unit, etc., can dialogue about their experience of empathy as driving nursing actions designed to deliver care. How then can the practice of nursing be delivered in a prison setting with individuals who have raped, murdered, assaulted, and robbed others in a manner that can be argued exhibited a lack of empathy? Does someone who has little to no capacity to experience empathy (inmates) deserve our (nurses) empathy?

The PMH-APRN must remember at all times that for the most part these individuals are characterologically disturbed. Axis II diagnosis is prevalent in corrections with predominance of Antisocial Personality Disorder, which will be discussed more elsewhere. Other common personality disorders range from Borderline Personality Disorder to Narcissistic Personality Disorder. The main impedance then with the development of the therapeutic relationship is that the individual is so characterologically damaged, and your time with them is so fragmented, that the long-term healing benefits of stewarding the therapeutic relationship is actually potentially more dangerous than helpful. This is not to say that each inmate shouldn't be treated initially with respect and offered general courtesy. This does mean that by and large once you have been perceived as "being nice" the criminal will likely try to exploit you to get needs met. This may present as staff splitting and pitting you against another staff on the compound to get something they want. They may flatter you regarding how you have been treating them in an attempt at manipulation. They may see you as being able to help them in some manner, that is,....want you to advocate for an early parole, want you to become involved in a request for a cell change, and so on. In short, the common mental health field practice of unconditional acceptance, therapeutic use of self, and nurturance of the interpersonal process, becomes a veritable field of landmines as any one of these approaches could backfire and be exploited by the inmate due to their pathology. So, if an interpersonal model of practice is not ideal for the corrections environment, what practice model is? Perhaps adapting a medical model mindset for this population is more effective and certainly with merit. Recent studies into the neurobiology of the criminal mind have revealed key findings into areas of the brain responsible for emotions such as empathy. There are several key areas in the prefrontal cortex that appear to be responsible for this but in particular the amygdala seems to play a "key role in the ability to experience empathy" (Baron-Cohen, 2011, pg 39). In the same way that ED nurses speak of "detaching" in the face of gruesome scenarios to be able to function and get through what needs to be done, corrections nurses need to not become emotionally driven in their work but rather see the inmate from a purely biological perspective. Practicing from this paradigm may be protective in terms of helping reconcile the ability to offer care in corrections, but is not without its drawbacks. Over the long haul, this may begin to feel counter to what nursing is supposed to be in the first place, and just as important as not becoming overinvolved, the nurse must guard against becoming underinvolved due to this self-imposed detachment. There are no easy answers to this dilemma and it certainly speaks to the multiple issues and difficulties of working in corrections. This aspect of managing yourself and the care you provide invites a reflection on boundary navigation because underinvolvement can be viewed as much of a boundary violation as overinvolvement, (Jones, Fitzpatrick, & Drake, 2008).

BOUNDARIES

Because of the challenging issues that present with regard to attempts at establishment and maintenance of a therapeutic relationship with the criminal population it is imperative that the clinician have a mastery of boundary navigation (see Exhibit 20-1). Far too often nurses find themselves the focus of a disciplinary process for a boundary violation with a client and they seemingly have no clue as to how they ended up there. Nurses have been walked out of prisons

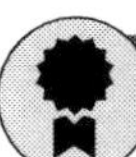

EXHIBIT 20-1: RED FLAGS OF A PENDING BOUNDARY VIOLATION IN CORRECTIONS

- You find yourself looking forward to the appointment with the inmate (disproportionately so when compared to other inmates).
- You schedule more frequent appointments than may be needed with a particular inmate.
- You find yourself deviating from standard treatment protocols for this inmate.
- You find that you want to become involved in other aspects of the inmate's treatment (housing, release, work assignment, disciplinary actions, etc.).
- You self-disclose personal information too liberally and without forethought.
- You tend to become protective of this inmate and see him/her as "the victim."
- You begin to feel as though you are the only one who understands the inmate and subsequently are the only one who can help them.

by security staff for having personal relations with inmates. Not only have they now lost their job, but they then have to answer to their state's board of nursing and may find their licensure in jeopardy. Most of these situations occur because the clinician failed at monitoring transference/countertransferance. Nurses can find themselves slowly being seduced into becoming involved in any number of inappropriate matters that really have nothing to do with the plan of care. Access to clinical supervision can greatly help in this regard. The ability to process the multitude of feelings generated from working with the incarcerated population is very helpful in catching a boundary violation before it happens. There are some red flags that may alert you that you may be in trouble. See Exhibit 20-1.

THERAPY

At the advanced practice level it is expected that the PMH-APRN has mastered the interpersonal skill set and also incorporated therapeutic modalities such as motivational interviewing, cognitive behavioral therapy, or psychodynamic-insight-oriented strategies into their repertoire. Attempting to use these approaches with the incarcerated population presents several challenges. First, many inmates have not graduated high school, have limited reading and writing ability, and may be low functioning on the IQ spectrum. These cognitive limitations may limit the ability for insight-oriented strategies or cognitive behavioral changes. Yet, some success has been reported with regard to forms of therapy aimed at personality disordered individuals such as Dialectical Behavioral Therapy (Shelton, Kesten, Zhang, & Trestman, 2011). In this study a modified version of this therapy was utilized with adolescent incarcerated males. Some degree of success was reported in changes in physical aggression and number of rule violations.

ANTISOCIAL PERSONALITY DISORDER

A vast majority of inmates will have an axis II diagnosis and of these Antisocial Personality Disorder is the most prominent. Many inmates will meet the criteria by virtue of the nature of their crime (murder, rape, arson, assault, etc). A review of the diagnostic criteria, though, will help you come to a better understanding if the inmate you are working with has this diagnosis. There will be a defined pattern since midadolescence for the flagrant disregard of the rights of others as well as a pattern of violations of societal norms. In addition to these patterns, there will have been evidence of the following behaviors:

A. Breaking the law.
B. Conning, repeated lying, or the use of others.
C. Failure to plan ahead and being impulsive.
D. Assaults on others.
E. Recklessness when it comes to safety.
F. Poor work history and irresponsible financial management.
G. Exhibits no empathy regarding pain they inflict on others.

It's also worth exploring if there is a history of cruelty to animals. The torture and killing of cats and dogs and other small animals is not unusual for individuals with antisocial personality disorder. Sometimes this behavior is disguised as "hunting." Careful eliciting of these "hunting excursions" though will reveal that they may have used a bow and arrow or some other weapon and shot the animal in an area with intent to wound rather than kill so as to witness the suffering. They may also have held a job at a slaughterhouse and are able to talk about how they "enjoyed the work." These individuals frequently seek mental health services as a means of escaping punishment. Their goal is to either have their sentence reduced or changed because of the claim of mental illness.

MALINGERING

Probably nowhere else in the arena of mental health care does the clinician have to be adeptly skilled at diagnosing because of the pervasiveness of malingering. Malingering, the intentional feigning of symptoms for ulterior gain is particularly problematic in corrections as some inmates believe that having a mental illness will help their case. Most clinicians detect only approximately 50% of lies in interviews, which is no better than that which would be discovered by chance. The assessment of malingering presents a significant challenge for mental health clinicians. The traditional clinician-patient relationship is based on the assumption that a patient is in genuine need of treatment, so clinicians may feel uneasy about initiating malingering assessment. This uneasiness is understandable given the potential for escalation of an individual's behavior when confronted with the clinician's suspicions of malingering, not to mention the rare potential for lawsuits alleging malpractice following a diagnosis of malingering.

Inmates have become very savvy regarding how to feign symptoms and will share with each other what words to use and what symptoms to claim. There are underground manuals and websites devoted to helping individuals learn how to "feign" mental illness to obtain disability, and so on. These are well known among the criminal population. There are diagnostic aids that will be discussed later that may help rule out malingering.

THE DIAGNOSTIC INTERVIEW

While malingerers may be referred for evaluation by other custodial staff because of their "bizarre behavior," most malingerers will initiate services themselves. They frequently present with claims of "seeing things" or "hearing things." It is first and foremost important to understand that most individuals suffering from a true mental illness of a psychotic nature rarely are comfortable discussing it at length. The malingerer will usually have no problem describing their alleged hallucination or delusion in detail (Resnick & Knoll, 2005). The importance of assessing for positive as well as negative symptoms is key. Frequently, malingerers will discuss at length and in detail their hallucinations while smiling and exhibiting a full range of affect. The other important point to remember is that you may be seeing them for a full hour. If they have been able to hold an articulate and focused conversation that illustrated their ability to track your lead in the flow of content, then this is counterintuitive to someone who claims to be plagued by voices or visions to the extent that they can't function and need medication or to be excused from work. Please see Exhibit 20-2 for common motivating factors for malingering.

EXHIBIT 20-2: COMMON REASONS FOR MALINGERING

- To avoid punishment or reduce sentence
- To seek financial gain (SSI disability, workers compensation, etc.)
- To avoid working
- Seeking drugs (pain meds, benzodiazepines)

Source: Resnick & Knoll (2005).

FOLLOW-UP WORK

When malingering is suspected it is always helpful to utilize some screening or diagnostic tools to aid in your r/o diagnosis Exhibit. One of the quickest and most reliable tools available is the Miller Forensic Assessment of Symptoms Test™ (M-FAST™). It is a reliable, psychometrically sound screening tool and takes only 10–15 min to administer. After scoring, the clinician has a fairly good idea whether the subject is faking or not. Another useful tool is the Structured Interview of Reported Symptoms™ (SIRS™). This test is longer (30–45 minutes) to take and takes approx 10 to 15 minutes to score, but also has a high validity and reliability rate. If these tools still prove inconclusive, you may need to order a Minnesota Multiphasic Personality Inventory, Revised™ (MMPI-2™). The F-scale and F-K Index are the most frequently used tests for evaluating suspected malingering.

If these screening tools produce the results that you suspected, then you should meet with the treatment team to discuss your findings and explore strategies on confronting the inmate. Probably the most preferable would be to do so in a group treatment team setting with a security officer present. How you reveal your findings can range from "Mr. Smith, I am pleased to tell you that based on the results of our testing we find that while you may be experiencing something that is causing you discomfort, it doesn't appear as though it is due to any serious mental illness" to "Mr. Smith, your symptoms are not consistent with anything that we can help you with as we believe you are fabricating your illness for other reasons." How you disclose your findings will be based on the individual situation and it is important to have documented all the steps you took leading up to your final conclusion in case the inmate files a grievance or initiates litigation (Resnick & Knoll, 2005).

The PMH-APRN desiring to practice in forensics would be well advised to engage in additional diagnostic coursework on ruling out malingering with this regard.

ASSESSMENTS

Most mental health departments in corrections will have a standard mental health assessment and a classification form as authorized by that state's Department of Corrections. Most of these assessments will cover reason for referral, presenting problem, psychiatric history, medical history, family history of mental illness, personal history, social history, and legal history. There may also be a section for past psychological testing. Some institutions utilize the Beck Depression Inventory™, particularly if an inmate is being seen for depression related to Interferon treatment for hepatitis. Inmates are classified in the correctional system by severity of their mental illness. You will have to complete this paperwork based on their diagnosis.

If an inmate has been placed in segregation on suicide watch, you will have to complete a departmental self-harm risk assessment form if you are the one performing the evaluation for continuance or release. Other standardized assessment would be a routine Abnormal and Involuntary Movement Scale (AIMS) on inmates being treated with antipsychotics and possibly a Mini Mental Status Exam (MMSE) if dementia is suspected.

ETIOLOGY

Most of the etiologies of specific disorders will have been discussed elsewhere in this text. For the purpose of this chapter we will focus on what is currently known regarding represented percentages of diagnosis discussed in the incarcerated population.

TRUE SEVERE AND PERSISTENT MENTAL ILLNESS

The inmate who presents with symptoms of bipolar disorder and any one of the thought disorders (schizophrenia, schizoaffective, etc.) has been estimated to be legitimately between 10% and 16% of the general incarcerated population (Metraux, 2008). McNiel, Binder, and Robinson (2005) had previously suggested the numbers to be between 16% & 18% of the general incarcerated population.

MALINGERING

Although sometimes difficult, but imperative to determine, one recent study indicated that the numbers are quite high (66%) of inmates that are feigning a mental illness (McDermott & Sokolov, 2009).

ANTISOCIAL PERSONALITY DISORDER

The prevalence of antisocial personality disorder has been studied extensively in incarcerated populations. One recent study indicates at least a 35% rate of prevalence among inmates (Black, Gunter, Loveless, Allen, & Sieleni, 2010).

CONCORDANCE (SHARED DECISION MAKING, PLANNING WITH CLIENT)

Concordance can be initially difficult with a mentally ill inmate. He or she may have had treatment experience on the street that they felt worked, that is, a combination of Seroquel XR and lamictal ODT for treatment of bipolar disorder. In corrections your choice of what you can and can't prescribe is severely limited to a state-developed formulary. It is very likely that a name brand expensive drug such as Seroquel (in any form) will not be allowed and only the generic regular form of lamictal is available. You will have to work with the inmate to arrive at an alternative regimen that will manage their symptoms as best as possible within the limitations of what you are allowed to prescribe. This will call for you to utilize previously mentioned skills on boundaries, monitoring of the interpersonal process, and possibly thinking about the case from a purely medical model viewpoint.

EXPECTED OUTCOMES

In corrections, the goal for expected outcomes can be fairly straightforward.

Inmates:

1. will not have to go to segregation due to behavioral problems.
2. will not need to be transferred to a residential treatment unit (RTU, a psychiatric hospital within a correctional facility).
3. will take their medicine as prescribed.
4. will show up for all psych appointments.
5. will be able to work as assigned on the compound.
6. will report a decrease of problematic symptoms.

TREATMENT INITIATION

In corrections, inmates can either self-refer to mental health service or be referred by correctional staff. As a PMH-APRN you can establish a diagnosis, determine level of severity and classification, schedule frequency of appointments, initiate medication, and order any testing (psychological or lab) as seen fit. You can also refer the inmate to any programming offered by the facility/department, for example, stress management, anger management, and so on. If a co-occurring substance abuse problem is diagnosed, a referral to the substance abuse treatment program is indicated.

TREATMENT OF SEVERE AND PERSISTENT CHRONIC MENTAL ILLNESS

If diagnoses of a true severe mental illness is arrived at, the initiation or continuation of a treatment regimen appropriate for the diagnosis is implemented. All med-somatic providers working in corrections must follow the state's authorized formulary and protocol for the arrived at diagnosis. Some may find this very limiting, that is, most of these formularies allow only generic versions of medications and severely restrict attempts at polypharmacy.

TREATMENT OF MALINGERING

Malingering as a rule should always be ruled out in the criminal population. If after careful assessment and screening you have arrived at this conclusion, then the most prudent approach is to not treat. This may become a true ethical dilemma for the PMH-APRN who may feel that they must treat all clients who present with complaints. As a prescriber, you may also feel pressure to "do something" for a persistent inmate who keeps complaining of symptoms. Educating your peers about malingering with emphasis on the subsequent wasting of provider resources may help. If pressure from the institution to treat persists, then ask that a second opinion by a colleague or collaborating psychiatrist be rendered. If this second opinion reaches a different diagnosis then they can take over and treat the case in question.

TREATMENT OF ANTISOCIAL PERSONALITY DISORDER

This may be one of the most difficult struggles you will have as a provider. The inmate with antisocial personality disorder may present with a variety of symptoms ranging from irritability, anger, threats of violence, to moodiness. All of this is truly often just part of the antisocial profile. Some modest benefit can occasionally be achieved with use of medications such as mood stabilizers (e.g., lamotrigine), to reduce explosiveness if this symptom presents as a major concern. Overall though, aggressive treatment for someone whose primary diagnosis is antisocial personality disorder is futile. Some have even discovered that engagement in psychotherapy actually backfires as the antisocial inmate uses the skills learned in therapy to further hone antisocial traits. The area becomes very grey when there is a true affective disorder superimposed on the antisocial personality disorder. In such cases it is reasonable to treat the mood disorder, always being mindful of the psychopathology underneath.

ADJUSTMENT DISORDERS

It has been said that most inmates will have some variety of an adjustment disorder by virtue of the incarceration

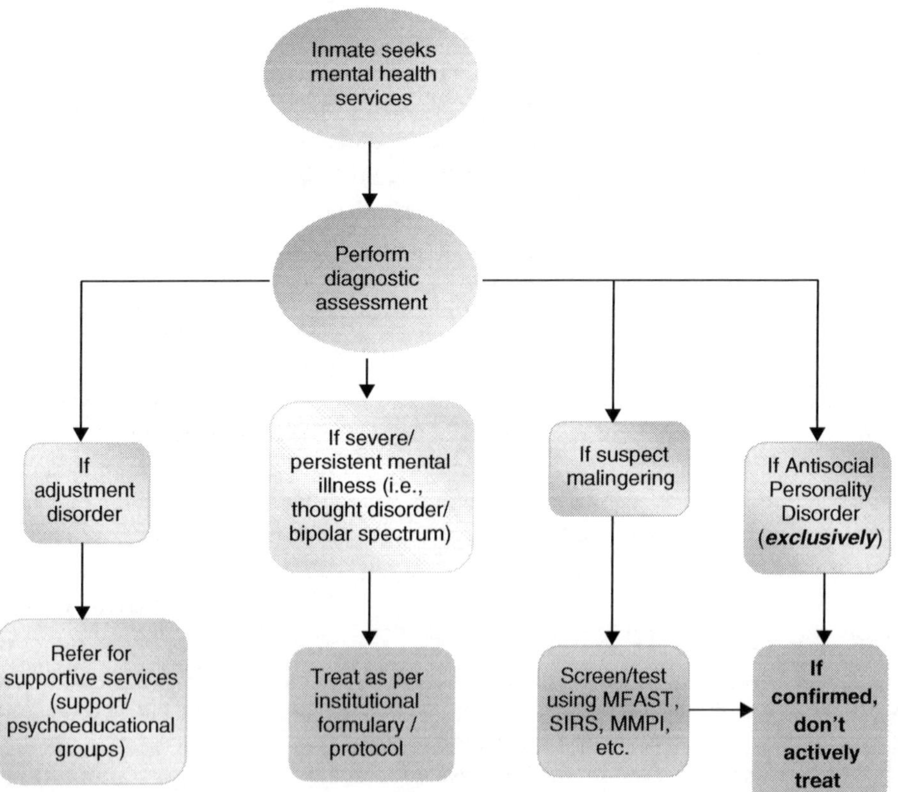

Figure 20-1 Decision Tree

Source: Forensic APRN Practice Conceptual Model (Jones, 2012).

experience. Sleep becomes altered, appetite may change, mood may fluctuate, and episodes of transient anxiety may manifest. Taken within the context of the correctional setting, this is normal and expected. Yet, conservative treatment may be offered in the form of support groups or psychoeducational groups aimed at sleep hygiene or stress management. It is not prudent to treat a suspected adjustment disorder aggressively with psychotherapy and medication as this becomes counterproductive to the intent of being incarcerated. Please refer to Figure 20-1 for a quick general decision tree to providing care to the incarcerated.

SPECIAL CONSIDERATIONS

All psychotropic medication, whether habit forming or not, can become a monetary commodity in prison. For example, if you are prescribing substances that require blood monitoring (e.g., anticonvulsants), and the results keep coming back subtherapeutic regardless of your adjustments, strongly suspect that the inmate in question has been selling his/her medication for money. Requests for increasingly higher doses of sedating medications should also be suspect.

SUMMARY

The desire to work in corrections can be a very noble calling, for the opportunity to provide mental health care to the incarcerated mentally ill can be rewarding. Working in the correctional area of forensics though is not without its difficulties. Severely character-disturbed patient populations challenge the use of interpersonal approaches and compel the practitioner to adapt a medical model approach to be able to deliver competent care. But for the truly severelymentally ill (SMI) population who deserve compassionate care in a very vulnerable setting, some may find these challenges worthwhile.

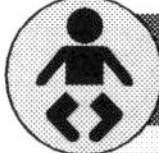

PEDIATRIC POINTERS

There is a lack of extensive data on the actual prevalence of mental illness among incarcerated youth. Some recent data suggest percentages fluctuating between 17% to 27%, (Erickson, 2011).

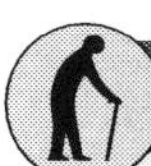

AGING ALERTS

There may be elderly inmates on your caseload. Normal adherence to the well-established cautions in use of psychotropics as related to this population is advised.

REFERENCES

Baron-Cohen, S. (2011). *The science of evil.* New York, NY: Basic Books.

Black, D. W., Gunter, T., Loveless, P., Allen, J., & Sieleni, B. (2010). Antisocial personality disorder in incarcerated offenders: Psychiatric comorbidity and quality of life. *Annals of Clinical Psychiatry, 22*(2), 113–120.

Erickson, C. D. (2012). Using systems of care to reduce incarceration of youth with serious mental illness. *American Journal of Community Psychology, 49*(3–4): 404–416.

Hackett, M. (2011). Commentary: Female forensic worker sexual misconduct—Who is the captive? *The Journal of the American Academy of Psychiatry and the Law, 39*, 166–169.

Jones, J., Fitzpatrick, J. J., & Drake, V. (2008). Frequency of post-licensure registered nurse boundary violations with patients in the state of Ohio: A comparison based on type of pre-licensure registered nurse education. *Archives of Psychiatric Nursing, 22*(6), 356–363.

Lint, M. (2012). Vulnerable populations and the role of the forensic nurse. In J. Jones, J. Fitzpatrick, and V. L. Rogers (Eds.), *Psychiatric mental health nursing, an interpersonal approach.* New York, NY, Springer.

McDermott, B. E., & Sokolov, G. (2009). Malingering in a correctional setting: The use of the structured interview of reported symptoms in a jail sample. *Behavioral Sciences & the Law Special Issue: Correctional Mental Health Care, 27*(5), 753–765.

McNiel, D. E., Binder, R.L., & Robinson, J.C. (2005). Incarceration associated with homelessness, mental disorder, and co-occurring substance abuse. *Psychiatric Services, 56*(7), 840–846.

Merriam-Webster. (2011) Retrieved from http://www.merriam-webster.com/dictionary/forensic

Metraux, S. (2008). Examining relationships between receiving mental health services in the Pennsylvania prison system and time served. *Psychiatric Services, 59*(7), 800–802.

Peplau, H. (1991). *Interpersonal relations in nursing.* New York, NY: Putnam.

Peternelj-Taylor, C. A., & Johnson, R. L. (1995). Serving time: Psychiatric mental health nursing in corrections. *Journal of Psychosocial Nursing and Mental Health Services, 33*(8), 12–9.

Renick, P. J., & Knoll, J. (2005). Faking it, how to detect malingered psychosis. *Current Psychiatry, 4*(11), 13–25.

Shelton, D., Kesten, K., Zhang, W., & Trestman, R. (2011). Impact of a dialectic behavior therapy-corrections modified (DBT-CM) upon behaviorally challenged incarcerated male-adolescents. *Journal of Child and Adolescent Psychiatric Nursing, 24*(2), 105–113.

Travelbee, J. (1964). What's wrong with sympathy? *American Journal of Nursing, 64*(1), 68–71.

Travelbee, J. (1971). *Interpersonal aspects of nursing* (2nd ed.). Philadelphia, PA: F. A. Davis.

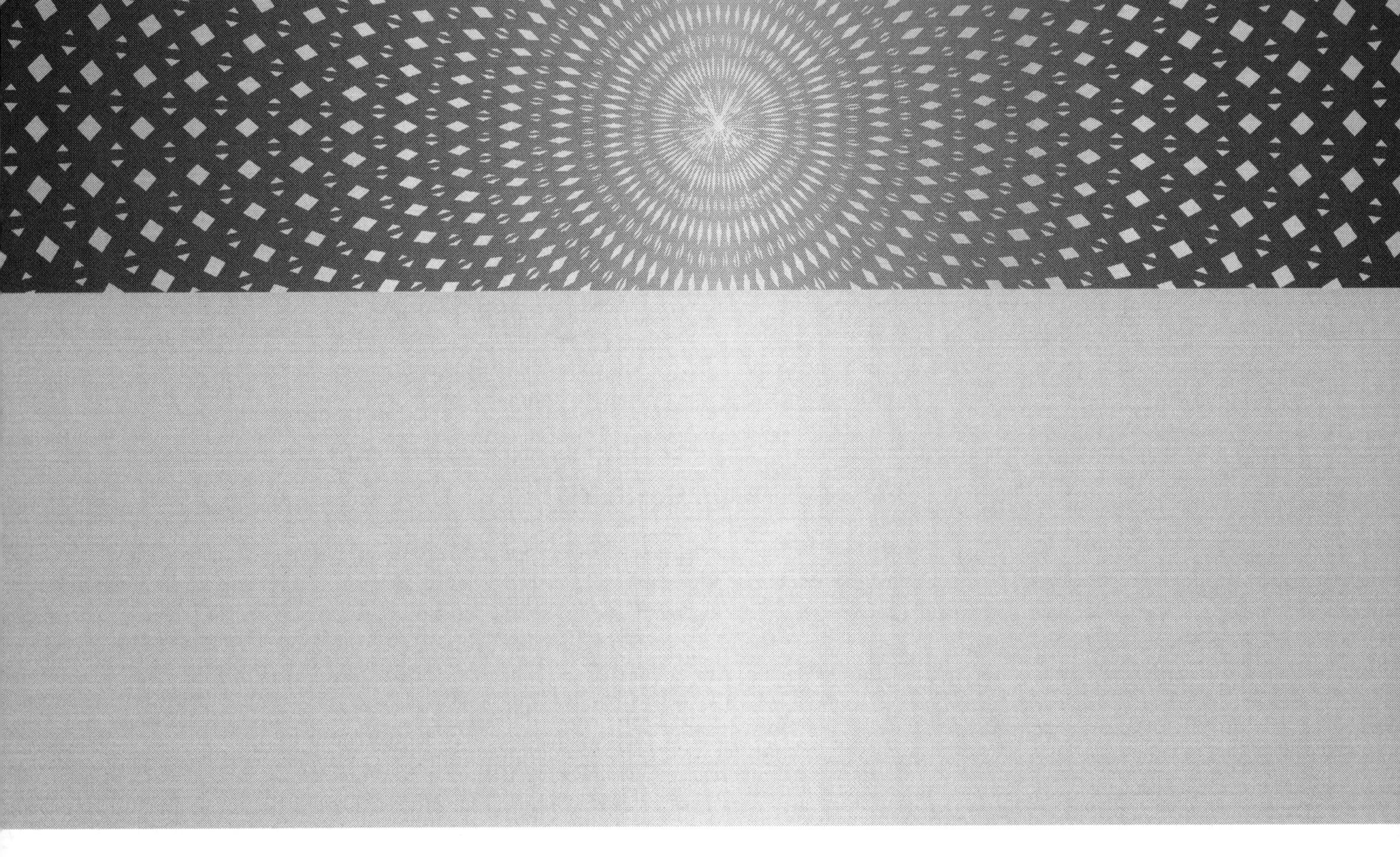

CHAPTER CONTENTS

The 21st century in nursing has been characterized by a renewed commitment to the goal of "health for all" globally. While there are many health care challenges, the burden of mental illness compels us to address the needs of individuals, families, and communities that are at risk for, or experiencing, mental health problems. Advanced practice psychiatric mental health nurses (PMH-APRNs) can be at the forefront of programmatic efforts to address these issues.

GLOBAL INITIATIVES IN PSYCHIATRIC NURSING

Although the advanced practice movement in nursing began in the United States in the 1960s, there are now many countries in which nurses practice at the advanced practice level. Presently there are no efforts to develop a common educational or credentialing model for advanced nursing practice. But this may be possible in the future.

The International Council of Nurses (ICN, 2011) is the official professional organization for nurses globally. The ICN, founded in 1899, is a federation of 130 national professional organizations representing more than 13 million nurses worldwide. The American Nurses Association (ANA) represents the United States in the ICN. The ICN mission is to represent nurses worldwide, advancing the profession and influencing health policy. Within the past decade ICN launched a Nurse

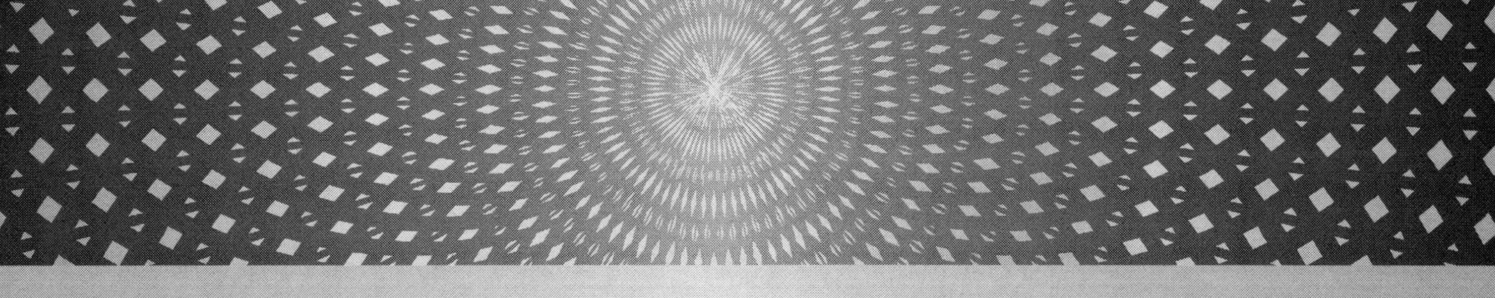

CHAPTER 21

Global Perspectives and the Future of Advanced Practice Psychiatric Mental Health Nursing

Joyce J. Fitzpatrick

Practitioner/Advanced Practice Nurse (APRN) Network which serves as a global resource for APRNs across specialty areas. This Network sponsors a web-based Forum which APRNs can use for connections with colleagues in other countries.

In addition to the work of ICN, there are professional organizations that are specifically targeted to psychiatric mental health nurses. These include organizations at the global, regional, and national levels.

The International Society of Psychiatric Mental Health Nurses (ISPN) has as its mission to unite and strengthen the presence and the voice of specialty psychiatric mental health nursing while influencing health care policy to promote equitable, evidence-based, and effective treatment and care for individuals, families, and communities (ISPN, 2011). ISPN has developed a comprehensive Strategic Plan to address the mission and goals and is active in conference sponsorship and development of policy papers to influence psychiatric mental health care provision and delivery. Membership is open to all psychiatric mental health nurses yet there is also a direct focus on advancing the specialty at the advanced practice level.

The European Psychiatric Nursing organization is known as Horatio. The aims of this organization are: to advocate for the interests of the members by providing input on decision-making processes on issues relevant to psychiatric and mental health nursing in Europe and to promote the development of psychiatric and mental health nursing practice, education, management, and research (Horatio, 2011). This organization accomplishes its goals through its conferences, newsletters, and website postings.

The American Psychiatric Nurses Association (APNA) is the organization in the United States that serves all PMH nurses, from those prepared at the basic professional practice level to those with doctorates. APNA was founded in 1987 and is now the largest PMH nursing specialty organization. APNA is focused on PMH nursing and their role in wellness promotion, prevention of mental health problems, and the care and treatment of persons with psychiatric disorders (APNA, 2011). The strategic plan for APNA calls for collaboration with consumer groups that can help guide advancements in recovery-focused assessment, diagnosis, treatment, and evaluation of persons with mental conditions and substance abuse disorders (APNA). The goals of APNA are accomplished through a state-based chapter model, and through conferences, newsletters, and web-based programming.

Like APNA in the United States, other countries have specialty organizations for psychiatric mental health nurses. Examples are the Canadian Federation of Mental Health Nurses, the Psychiatric Nurses Association of Ireland, the New Zealand College of Mental Health Nurses, and the Australian College of Mental Health

Nurses. Through these national, regional, and international organizations there are many opportunities for advanced practice psychiatric mental health nurses to network and collaborate in educational, practice, and research arenas.

EXEMPLARY PSYCHIATRIC MENTAL HEALTH NURSE: A GLOBAL ROLE MODEL

In 2001, Dr. Susie Kim, the first nurse from South Korea to receive a doctorate in nursing, was recognized by ICN with the Florence Nightingale Foundation International Achievement Award. Dr. Kim is a psychiatric mental health nurse who was the first nurse ever to receive funding from the United Nations Development Program (UNDP). Her UN-funded project was focused on deinstitutionalizing the chronically mentally ill in South Korea, and, with 20 other advanced practice psychiatric nurses, on developing and providing mental health services that were community based. Through Dr. Kim's leadership, these nurses opened 15 community-based centers for the chronically mentally ill. As a result of the positive outcomes in quality and cost of the services provided, the government of South Korea made policy changes for care of the mentally ill, and 44 additional localities adopted the community-based model of care. Also, her project led to the formation of a Mental Health Interdisciplinary Association which serves as a policy advisory group to the South Korean government. She was instrumental in introducing advanced practice psychiatric nursing to her country, and continues to provide inspiration to the many nurses globally who aspire to achieve positive changes in care delivery, particularly to those who are marginalized by societies.

STRATEGIES FOR GLOBAL CONNECTIONS

There are many opportunities for global connections based on one's area of expertise and the model for partnership development that is desired. Individuals can connect with other individuals found through publications or presentations at international scientific forums. With the easy access to information through the Internet, each of us is only a few keystrokes away from connecting with colleagues who are engaged in similar research, theory development, education, or professional practice. Professional colleagues across the globe are enthused about these professional connections and eager to decide how to collaborate.

Several professional organizations offer opportunities for networking. The interested psychiatric nurse can reach out to colleagues who are participants and/or presenters at conferences, and develop partnerships for future collaboration. Further, there are many avenues for serving within professional organizations and assuming a leadership role in shaping the professional and public response to mental illness. Professional organizations in nursing rely on the volunteers at both the elected and appointed levels to make certain that the organizational goals and activities are successfully accomplished.

PROFESSIONAL SELF-DEVELOPMENT

There are many ways that individual nurses can advance their own professional development in addition to the avenues discussed above. One of the key strategies is to find a mentor, someone who is willing to shepherd you through the professional development process, to guide you in choices to make to advance your career, and to listen as you shape your journey and advance your own goals and those of the individuals you serve. You can reach out to a mentor through electronic communications, through professional association memberships, or thorough networking. Most professional nurses, particularly those who are in leadership positions, are interested in preparing future generations of nurse leaders, and will often accept the invitation to mentor others.

One of the most important responsibilities that advanced practice nurses share is that of improving future generations of clinicians through education and dissemination of scholarship. As a leader within the discipline, the professional responsibilities to disseminate scholarship (including clinical knowledge) cannot be overstated. The ripple effect that this will have on others in clinical practice is important to recognize. All new clinical insights, and all pilot work, including both research and evidence-based practice initiatives, are important to share.

INTERDISCIPLINARY PARTNERSHIPS

In addition to the disciplinary partnerships within nursing, there are multiple opportunities for interdisciplinary partnerships. Some of the same strategies for connecting to colleagues that were discussed above would work for connecting to colleagues from other disciplines. The important common denominator is the content area of interest, and this should serve as the core of introduction and connection.

FUTURE DIRECTIONS FOR PRACTICE AND RESEARCH IN PSYCHIATRIC MENTAL HEALTH NURSING

There are many opportunities for the APRN within PMH nursing. These opportunities abound in clinical practice, education, and research. Also, APRNs can assume leadership positions and influence policy development on local, national, and global levels. PMH-APRNs can lead research projects that address the various dimensions of clinical research. There are funding resources available through the National Institute of Mental Health (NIMH) of the National Institutes of Health (NIH).

How large are the opportunities? Consider the extent of the mental health issues globally and the effects on family members and communities.

According to the first U.S. Surgeon General's Report on Mental Health, few families in the United States are untouched by mental illness and at least one in five people has a diagnosable mental disorder during the course of a year (i.e., 1-year prevalence) (Satcher, 1999). And, according to the World Health Organization (WHO) statistics, as many as 450 million people suffer from a mental or behavioral disorder, nearly 1 million people commit suicide each year, and one in four families has at least one member with a mental illness (WHO, 2003). The extent of the burden of mental illness is great, on individuals, families, and societies. In addition to the illness itself, those affected by mental illness often suffer human rights abuses, stigma, and discrimination (WHO, 2003). Overall the societal costs of mental illness are great, and efforts directed toward prevention of illness and promotion of mental health are needed.

The WHO presented a Mental Health Atlas in 2011 detailing the extent of the mental health problems globally (WHO, 2011). The important messages from this comprehensive report on the global situation in relation to mental health and illness are as follows:

- Resources to treat and prevent mental disorders remain insufficient.
- Resources for mental health are inequitably distributed.
- Resources for mental health are inefficiently utilized.
- Institutional care for mental disorders may be slowly decreasing worldwide.

Further, only 60% of the countries reported having a dedicated mental health policy, with high-income countries more often reporting the existence of a mental health policy. A significant percentage (77%) of individuals who are institutionalized remain there for more than a year, and only 32% of the countries provide any follow-up care after discharge. An important finding in relation to nursing was that globally, nurses represent the most prevalent professional group working in the mental health sector. The median rate of nurses per population was found to be 5.8 per 100,000 population; this is compared to the rate of psychiatrists at 0.05 per 100,000 population. The needs for care delivery worldwide are significant, yet so also are there concomitant needs for new knowledge generation through research and for the preparation of future generations of professional nurses through education.

While the challenges are great in the mental health fields, the opportunities for nurses to demonstrate comprehensive, effective care are many. In 2007, WHO and ICN published summary information on the numbers, training, roles, and responsibilities of nurses in the mental health field. The most consistent finding in the study was the severe shortage of nurses providing mental health care in most low- and middle-income countries. This information has been collected from 172 countries from all regions of the world (WHO, 2007).

Research opportunities exist at both the disciplinary and multidisciplinary levels. While there is an emphasis on outcome research, including clinical, functional, satisfaction, and financial outcomes, there also is a need for research on the structures for delivering mental health services and the processes of therapeutic interventions that lead to positive outcomes. Advanced practice psychiatric mental health nurses have a responsibility to participate in the development and dissemination of scholarship through their professional work.

In summary, PMH-APRNs have many professional opportunities. The potential is great to make a difference in the lives of patients and families in need of mental health services. One way to insure the success is to pass along the knowledge and connections with colleagues, and continue to strengthen future generations of PMH-APRNs.

REFERENCES

American Psychiatric Nurses Association. (2011). *About the American Psychiatric Nurses Association.* Retrieved October 1, 2011, from http://www.apna.org/i4a/pages/index.cfm?pageid=3277

Horatio. (2011). *Horatio European psychiatric nurses*. Retrieved October 31, 2011, from http://www.horatio-web.eu

International Council of Nurses. (2011). *International Council of Nurses*. Retrieved October 2, 2011, from http://www.icn.ch

International Society of Psychiatric Nurses. (2011). *International Society of Psychiatric-Mental Health Nurses.* Retrieved October 1, 2011, from http://www.ispn-psych.org

Satcher, D. (1999). *Mental health: A report of the Surgeon General.* Retrieved October 1, 2011, from http://www.surgeongeneral.gov/library/mentalhealth/home.html

World Health Organization. (2003). *Investing in mental health.* Retrieved October 20, 2011, from http://www.who.int/mental_health/en/investing_in_mnh_final.pdf

World Health Organization. (2007). *Atlas: Nurses in mental health 2007.* Retrieved November 1, 2011, from http://www.who.int/mental_health/evidence/nursing_atlas_2007.pdf

World Health Organization. (2011). *Mental health Atlas 2011.* Geneva, Switzerland: Author.

INDEX

Made in the USA
Lexington, KY
30 August 2016